Reid's

CONTROVERSY IN OBSTETRICS AND GYNECOLOGY—III

FREDERICK P. ZUSPAN, M.D.

*Professor and Chairman, Department of Obstetrics
and Gynecology, The Ohio State University College of Medicine*

C. D. CHRISTIAN, M.D., Ph.D.

*Professor and Head, Department of Obstetrics
and Gynecology, University of Arizona College of Medicine*

1983

W. B. SAUNDERS COMPANY

Philadelphia / London / Toronto / Mexico City / Rio de Janeiro / Sydney / Tokyo

W. B. Saunders Company: West Washington Square
Philadelphia, PA   19105

1 St. Anne's Road
Eastbourne, East Sussex BN21 3UN, England

1 Goldthorne Avenue
Toronto, Ontario M8Z 5T9, Canada

Apartado 26370—Cedro 512
Mexico 4, D.F., Mexico

Rua Coronel Cabrita, 8
Sao Cristovao Caixa Postal 21176
Rio de Janeiro, Brazil

9 Waltham Street
Artarmon, N.S.W. 2064, Australia

Ichibancho, Central Bldg., 22-1 Ichibancho
Chiyoda-Ku, Tokyo 102, Japan

**Library of Congress Cataloging in Publication Data
(Revised)**

Main entry under title:

Controversy in obstetrics and gynecology.

Vol. 2 by D. E. Reid and C. D. Christian; vol. 3 edited by
Frederick P. Zuspan, C. D. Christian has title: Reid's controversy in obstetrics and gynecology.

Includes bibliographies.

1. Obstetrics—Addresses, essays, lectures.   2. Gynecology—
   Addresses, essays, lectures.   I. Barton, Theodore C., 1929–
        II. Reid, Duncan E.   III. Christian, Charles Don-
   ald, 1930–   IV. Title: Reid's controversy in obstetrics
   and gynecology.

RG123.R42   618   68–10408

Reid's Controversy in Obstetrics and Gynecology—III   ISBN 0-7216-2565-7

Last digit is the print number: 9   8   7   6   5   4   3   2   1

Dedication

DUNCAN EARL REID, M.D. (1905–1973)

Duncan Reid was a special person to everyone who was fortunate enough to have known him. His efforts are the reason that *Controversy in Obstetrics and Gynecology* exists, and it is a privilege for us to carry on this splendid tradition.

Duncan Reid was born in the small community of Burr Oak, Iowa, and did his premedical studies at Ripon College, where he worked his way through school, as well as participating in football, basketball and track. He continued to support himself while attending Northwestern University Medical School, where he received the M.D. degree in 1931. He received gynecologic and surgical training at St. Luke's Hospital in Chicago, then went to Boston Lying-In Hospital as a resident in obstetrics, and was the first non-Harvard trained individual to assume this role. His faculty appointment at Harvard began in 1935 and continued until 1971, when he retired as Chairman of Obstetrics and Gynecology.

Dr. Reid published his important *Textbook of Obstetrics* in 1962, later revising it with others under a new title, *Principles and Management of Human Reproduction*. Dr. Reid was a consistent contributor to the scientific media and wrote over 140 original papers.

What made him special was his perception and his absolute honesty to himself and to each of his patients. He took courageous stands when issues seemed more emotional than scientific, and his courage was always on behalf of the female patient. He was the president of a number of national societies, and while his importance in the arena of obstetrics in the United States became ever stronger, he remained an unpretentious, human and personable individual. It is to the memory of this man that we dedicate this book.

FREDERICK P. ZUSPAN

C. D. CHRISTIAN

Contributors

KARLIS ADAMSONS, M.D., Ph.D.
Professor and Chairman, Department of Obstetrics and Gynecology, University of Puerto Rico School of Medicine. Director, Department of Obstetrics and Gynecology, University Hospital, San Juan, Puerto Rico.

MARVIN S. AMSTEY, M.D., F.A.C.O.G.
Professor of Obstetrics and Gynecology, University of Rochester School of Medicine and Dentistry. Chairman, Department of Obstetrics and Gynecology, Highland Hospital; Consultant, Department of Obstetrics and Gynecology, Genesee Hospital; Attending Obstetrician-Gynecologist, Strong Memorial Hospital, Rochester, New York.

FERNANDO ARIAS, M.D., Ph.D.
Professor of Obstetrics and Gynecology and Director, Division of Maternal-Fetal Medicine, Washington University School of Medicine. Attending Obstetrician, Barnes Hospital, Jewish Hospital, and County Hospital; Consultant, St. Louis Children's Hospital, St. Louis, Missouri.

SUSAN A. ARNOLD, M.D.
Research Fellow in Maternal and Fetal Medicine, University of Puerto Rico, San Juan, Puerto Rico.

DAVID A. BAKER, M.D.
Assistant Professor, Department of Obstetrics and Gynecology; Director of Maternal-Fetal Medicine, State University of New York at Stony Brook.

TOM P. BARDEN, M.D.
Professor and Chairman, Department of Obstetrics and Gynecology, University of Cincinnati College of Medicine. Chief of Obstetrics and Gynecology, University of Cincinnati Hospitals; Chief of Gynecology, Cincinnati Children's Hospital, Cincinnati, Ohio.

ROSS S. BERKOWITZ, M.D.
Assistant Professor of Obstetrics and Gynecology, Harvard Medical School. Associate Director, New England Trophoblastic Disease Center; Gynecologic Oncologist, Brigham and Women's Hospital; American Cancer Society Junior Faculty Clinical Fellow, Boston, Massachusetts.

JOSEPH BIENIARZ, M.D.
Professor Emeritus, Department of Obstetrics and Gynecology, University of Chicago Pritzker School of Medicine. Director, Laboratory of Uterine Physiology, Michael Reese Hospital, Chicago, Illinois.

BENGT BJERRE, M.D.
Associate Professor, Department of Obstetrics and Gynecology, University of Lund. Allmänna Sjukhuset, Malmö, Sweden.

EDWARD H. BISHOP, M.D.
Professor of Obstetrics and Gynecology, University of North Carolina School of Medicine. Attending Physician, North Carolina Memorial Hospital, Chapel Hill, North Carolina.

WATSON A. BOWES, Jr., M.D.
Professor of Obstetrics and Gynecology, University of Colorado School of Medicine. Staff Physician, University Hospital, University of Colorado Health Sciences Center, Denver, Colorado.

WILLIAM E. BRENNER, M.D.
Staff Physician, Durham County Hospital, Chapel Hill, North Carolina.

I. BROSENS, M.D., Ph.D.
Professor of Obstetrics and Gynecology; Head of the Clinic for Gynecological Endocrinology and Infertility, Unit for the Study of Human Reproduction, University of Leuven, Belgium.

LAURENCE BURD, M.D.
Associate Professor of Obstetrics and Gynecology, University of Chicago Pritzker School of Medicine. Director, Division of Obstetrics; Director, Division of Fetal and Maternal Medicine, Michael Reese Hospital, Chicago, Illinois.

STEVE N. CARITIS, M.D.
Associate Professor of Obstetrics and Gynecology and Pediatrics, University of Pittsburgh School of Medicine. Attending Obstetrician-Gynecologist, Magee-Womens Hospital, Pittsburgh, Pennsylvania.

WILLIAM J. CASHORE, M.D.
Associate Professor of Pediatrics, Brown University Program in Medicine. Neonatologist, Women and Infants Hospital of Rhode Island, Providence, Rhode Island.

PATRICK M. CATALANO, M.D.
Instructor of Obstetrics and Gynecology, University of Vermont College of Medicine. Attending Obstetrician and Gynecologist, Medical Center Hospital of Vermont, Burlington, Vermont.

R. JEFFREY CHANG, M.D.
Assistant Professor, Department of Obstetrics and Gynecology, Division of Reproductive Endocrinology, University of California, Los Angeles, California.

ARTHUR C. CHRISTAKOS, M.D., F.A.C.O.G.
Professor, Obstetrics and Gynecology, Duke University School of Medicine. Attending Staff, Duke Hospital; Consultant, Durham County General Hospital, Cape Fear Valley Hospital, Cabarras County Memorial Hospital, Durham, North Carolina.

LUIS A. CIBILS, M.D.
Mary Campau Ryerson Professor of Obstetrics and Gynecology, University of Chicago Pritzker School of Medicine. Consultant, Chicago Lying-in Hospital, Chicago, Illinois.

JOSEPH V. COLLEA, M.D.
Associate Professor of Obstetrics and Gynecology, Georgetown University School of Medicine. Attending Perinatologist, Georgetown University Hospital, Columbia Hospital for Women, Sibley Memorial Hospital, Washington, D.C.

LEANDRO CORDERO, M.D.
Professor of Pediatrics and Obstetrics and Gynecology, Ohio State University College of Medicine.

Director, Newborn Services, Ohio State University Hospitals, Columbus, Ohio.

JAMES J. CORRIGAN, M.D.
Professor of Pediatrics; Lecturer in Internal Medicine; Chief, Section of Pediatric Hematology/Oncology, University of Arizona Health Sciences Center, Tucson, Arizona.

WILLIAM T. CREASMAN, M.D.
Professor of Obstetrics and Gynecology, Department of Obstetrics and Gynecology, Duke University Medical Center, Durham, North Carolina.

CARLYLE CRENSHAW, M.D.
Professor and Chairman, Department of Obstetrics and Gynecology, University of Maryland School of Medicine; Chief, Obstetric and Gynecologic Service, University of Maryland Hospital. Attending Physician, Maryland General Hospital, Mercy Hospital, Baltimore, Maryland.

WILLIAM R. CROMBLEHOLME, M.D.
Assistant Professor of Obstetrics and Gynecology, SUNY-Downstate Medical Center. Director, Obstetrical Service, State University Hospital, Brooklyn, New York.

JOHN R. DAVIS, M.D.
Professor of Pathology, University of Arizona College of Medicine, Tucson, Arizona; Chief, Anatomical Pathology, University of Arizona Health Sciences Center.

GUNTER DEPPE, M.D.
Associate Professor, Obstetrics and Gynecology, Rush Medical School. Director of Gynecology and Gynecological Oncology, Mt. Sinai Hospital, Chicago, Illinois.

W. PAUL DMOWSKI, M.D., PH.D.
Professor and Director of Section of Reproductive Endocrinology and Infertility, Department of Obstetrics and Gynecology, Rush Medical College. Senior Attending Physician, Rush-Presbyterian-St. Luke's Medical Center, Chicago, Illinois.

WILLIAM DROEGEMUELLER, M.D.
Professor and Chairman, Department of Obstetrics and Gynecology, University of North Carolina School of Medicine. North Carolina Memorial Hospital, Chapel Hill, North Carolina.

JOHANN H. DUENHOELTER, M.D.
331 South Mendian, Puyallup, Washington.

D.V.I. FAIRWEATHER, M.D., F.R.C.O.G.
Professor and Director, Department of Obstetrics
and Gynecology, School of Medicine, University
College. Honorary Consultant Obstetrician and Gy-
naecologist, University College Hospital, London,
England.

ROGER K. FREEMAN, M.D.
Professor of Obstetrics and Gynecology, University
of California, Irvine. Medical Director, Women's
Hospital, Memorial Medical Center of Long Beach,
California.

RUDOLPH P. GALASK, M.D.
Professor of Obstetrics and Gynecology and Profes-
sor of Microbiology, University of Iowa College of
Medicine. Department of Obstetrics and Gynecol-
ogy, University of Iowa Hospitals and Clinics, Iowa
City, Iowa.

NORMAN F. GANT, M.D.
Professor and Chairman, Department of Obstetrics
and Gynecology, University of Texas Southwestern
Medical School. Chief of Service, Obstetrics and
Gynecology, Parkland Memorial Hospital, Dallas,
Texas.

HERMAN L. GARDNER, M.D.
Clinical Professor of Obstetrics and Gynecology,
Baylor College of Medicine, Houston, Texas.

THOMAS J. GARITE, M.D.
Assistant Professor, Department of Obstetrics and
Gynecology, University of California, Irvine. As-
sociate Medical Director for Perinatology, Women's
Hospital, Memorial Medical Center of Long Beach,
California.

HARLAN R. GILES, M.D.
Department of Obstetrics and Gynecology, University of Arizona, Tucson, Arizona

DONALD P. GOLDSTEIN, M.D.
Assistant Clinical Professor of Obstetrics and Gynecology, Harvard Medical School. Chief, Division
of Gynecology, Children's Hospital Medical Center; Attending Obstetrician-Gynecologist, Brigham
and Women's Hospital, Boston, Massachusetts.

RAPHAEL S. GOOD, M.D.
Vice-Chairman, Department of Psychiatry and Behavioral Sciences; Associate Professor of Psychiatry
and Obstetrics-Gynecology, University of Texas
Medical Branch, Galveston, Texas.

JUAN L. GRANADOS, M.D.
Associate Professor of Obstetrics and Gynecology;
Director, Maternal and Fetal Medicine, University
of West Virginia School of Medicine, Morgantown,
West Virginia.

DAVID A. GRIMES, M.D.
Chief, Abortion Surveillance Branch, Family Plan-
ning Evaluation Division, Centers for Disease Con-
trol. Clinical Assistant Professor, Department of
Gynecology and Obstetrics, Emory University
School of Medicine, Atlanta, Georgia.

S. B. GUSBERG, M.D., D.Sc.
Professor and Chairman Emeritus, Department of
Obstetrics and Gynecology, Mt. Sinai School of
Medicine. Consultant, Director Emeritus, Mt.
Sinai Hospital, New York, New York.

CHARLES B. HAMMOND, M.D.
E. C. Hamblen Professor and Chairman, Department of Obstetrics and Gynecology, Duke University Medical Center, Durham, North Carolina.

GUY M. HARBERT, Jr., M.D.
Mamie A. Jessup Professor, University of Virginia
School of Medicine. Director, Division of Maternal-
Fetal Medicine, University of Virginia School of
Medicine, Charlottesville, Virginia.

DOROTHY J. HICKS, M.D.
Professor, Department of Obstetrics and Gynecol-
ogy, University of Miami School of Medicine. Di-
rector, Rape Treatment Center; Director, Pediatric
Gynecology Clinic; Medical Director, Ob-Gyn
Emergency Room; Medical Director (Interim),
Emergency Room, Jackson Memorial Hospital,
Miami, Florida.

FREDERICK J. HOFMEISTER, M.D.
Clinical Professor of Gynecology and Obstetrics,
Medical College of Wisconsin. Attending Staff,
Good Samaritan Hospital, Lutheran Campus; Elm-
brook Hospital; Milwaukee County Hospital;
Froedtert Memorial Lutheran Hospital, Milwau-
kee, Wisconsin.

FRANKLIN C. HUGENBERGER, M.D.
Associate Clinical Professor Emeritus, Ohio State
University College of Medicine. Attending Staff,
Grant Hospital, Columbus, Ohio.

JOHN H. ISAACS, M.D.
Professor, Department of Obstetrics and Gynecology, Stritch School of Medicine, Loyola University
of Chicago. Director of Gynecologic Oncology,

Loyola University Medical Center; Chairman, Department of Obstetrics and Gynecology, Saint Francis Hospital, Evanston, Illinois.

SUSAN R. JOHNSON, M.D.
Assistant Professor, Department of Obstetrics and Gynecology, University of Iowa College of Medicine. University of Iowa Hospitals and Clinics, Iowa City, Iowa.

HOWARD L. JUDD, M.D.
Professor, Department of Obstetrics and Gynecology, Division of Reproductive Endocrinology, University of California, Los Angeles, California.

RAYMOND H. KAUFMAN, M.D.
Professor and Ernst Bertnec Chairman, Department of Obstetrics-Gynecology; Professor of Pathology, Baylor College of Medicine, Houston, Texas.

KIRK A. KEEGAN, JR., M.D.
Assistant Professor of Obstetrics and Gynecology, University of California, Irvine Medical Center. Director of Medical Education, Department of Obstetrics and Gynecology, University of California, Irvine Medical Center, Orange, California.

DAVID W. KELLER, M.D.
Associate Professor of Obstetrics and Gynecology, Washington University School of Medicine. Associate Obstetrician-Gynecologist, Washington University School of Medicine, Barnes and Jewish Hospitals, St. Louis, Missouri.

ALLEN P. KILLAM, M.D.
Professor, Department of Obstetrics and Gynecology, Duke University Medical Center, Durham, North Carolina.

MOON H. KIM, M.D.
Professor and Vice-Chairman, Director, Division of Reproductive Endocrinology, Department of Obstetrics and Gynecology, Ohio State Univesity College of Medicine. Attending Staff, University Hospital, Columbus, Ohio.

ALFRED B. KNIGHT, M.D.
Assistant Professor, Department of Obstetrics and Gynecology, Washington University School of Medicine. Attending Staff, Barnes and Jewish Hospitals, County Hospital of St. Louis, St. Louis, Missouri.

ROBERT A. KNUPPEL, M.D., M.P.H.
Associate Professor of Obstetrics and Gynecology,

Director, Division of Maternal-Fetal Medicine, University of South Florida College of Medicine. Consultant, Bayfront Medical Center, St. Petersburg; Attending Obstetrician, St. Joseph's Hospital and Women's Hospital, Tampa, Florida.

JOSEPH JOHN KRYC, M.D.
Assistant Professor, Department of Anesthesiology and Department of Obstetrics and Gynecology, Ohio State University School of Medicine, Columbus, Ohio.

ROBERT LANDESMAN, M.D.
Professor of Clinical Obstetrics and Gynecology; Attending Obstetrician and Gynecologist, New York Hospital, New York; Consultant Obstetrician and Gynecologist, Vassar Brothers Hospital, Poughkeepsie, New York.

RONALD S. LEUCHTER, M.D., F.A.C.O.G.
Assistant Professor of Obstetrics and Gynecology, UCLA Medical Center. Assistant Professor in Residence, Department of Obstetrics and Gynecology, Cedars-Sinai Medical Center, Los Angeles, California.

JAMES A. LOW, M.D.
Professor and Chairman of Obstetrics and Gynecology, Queens University. Attending Staff, Kingston General Hospital, Kingston, Ontario, Canada.

DAVID A. LUTHY, M.D.
Clinical Associate Professor, Department of Obstetrics and Gynecology, University of Washington. Associate Director, Department of Obstetrics and Gynecology, Swedish Hospital Medical Center, Seattle, Washington.

HUGH M. MacDONALD, M.D.
Attending Neonatologist, Medical Center of Tarzana, Tarzana, California.

LEON I. MANN, M.D.
Professor and Chairman, Department of Obstetrics and Gynecology; Associate Dean, University of Vermont College of Medicine. Chief of Obstetrics and Gynecology Service, Medical Center Hospital of Vermont, Burlington, Vermont.

HEIDI McNANEY, M.D.
University of South Florida College of Medicine, Tampa, Florida.

PHILIP B. MEAD, M.D.
Professor of Obstetrics and Gynecology, University of Vermont College of Medicine. Attending Obste-

trician and Gynecologist, Medical Center Hospital of Vermont, Burlington, Vermont.

ROBERT H. MESSER, M.D.
Professor and Chairman, Department of Obstetrics-Gynecology, University of New Mexico School of Medicine, Albuquerque, New Mexico.

JOSEPH M. MILLER, Jr., M.D.
Assistant Professor of Obstetrics and Gynecology, Medical University of South Carolina, Charleston, South Carolina.

DANIEL R. MISHELL, Jr., M.D.
Professor and Chairman, Department of Obstetrics and Gynecology, University of Southern California School of Medicine. Chief of Professional Services, Women's Hospital, Los Angeles County-USC Medical Center, Los Angeles, California.

SANGITHAN MOODLEY, M.B., Ch.B., M.D.
Assistant Professor of Obstetrics-Gynecology, University of Rochester School of Medicine and Dentistry. Assistant Attending Obstetrician-Gynecologist, Strong Memorial Hospital, Division of Maternal-Fetal Medicine, Rochester, New York.

PATRICK W. MORELL, M.D.
Chief Resident, Obstetrics and Gynecology, University of Arizona, Tucson, Arizona.

JOHN C. MORRISON, M.D.
Professor and Director, Division of Maternal-Fetal Medicine, Department of Obstetrics and Gynecology, University of Mississippi, Jackson, Mississippi.

EBERHARD MUELLER-HEUBACH, M.D.
Associate Professor of Obstetrics and Gynecology and Pediatrics, University of Pittsburgh School of Medicine. Attending Obstetrician-Gynecologist, Magee-Womens Hospital, Pittsburgh, Pennsylvania.

WILLIAM OH, M.D.
Professor of Pediatrics and Obstetrics, Brown University Program in Medicine. Pediatrician in Chief, Women and Infants Hospital of Rhode Island, Providence, Rhode Island.

MARILYN OHM-SMITH, M.S., M.T. (A.S.C.P.)
Senior Clinical Laboratory Technologist Specialist, Department of Obstetrics and Gynecology, San Francisco General Hospital, San Francisco, California.

JAMES A. O'LEARY, M.D.
Professor of Gynecology and Obstetrics, University of Buffalo School of Medicine. Attending Physician, Erie County Medical Center, Buffalo, New York.

WILLIAM W. PASLEY, M.D.
Attending Physician, University of South Alabama Medical Center, Mobile, Alabama.

LILLIE-MAE PADILLA, M.D.
Assistant Professor of Obstetrics and Gynecology, Indiana University School of Medicine. Attending Obstetrician/Gynecologist, Indiana University Hospitals (University Hospital and Wishard Memorial Hospital), Indianapolis, Indiana.

RICHARD H. PAUL, M.D.
Professor of Obstetrics and Gynecology, University of Southern California. Director, Division of Maternal-Fetal Medicine, Women's Hospital, Los Angeles County/University of Southern California Medical Center, Los Angeles, California.

JACK W. PEARSON, M.D.
Professor of Obstetrics and Gynecology, Indiana University School of Medicine. Chief, Obstetrics and Gynecology, Wishard Memorial Hospital; Attending Obstetrician/Gynecologist, Indiana University Hospitals, Indianapolis, Indiana.

L. L. PENNEY, M.D.
Chief, Department of Clinical Investigation, William Beaumont Army Medical Center. Attending Physician, Reproductive Endocrinology and Infertility, William Beaumont Army Medical Center and Texas Tech University Regional Academic Health Center, El Paso, Texas.

DAVID PENT, M.D.
Clinical Associate, Obstetrics and Gynecology, University of Arizona College of Medicine, Tucson, Arizona. Director, Urodynamics Unit, St. Joseph's Hospital, Phoenix, Arizona.

EDWARD J. QUILLIGAN, M.D.
Professor and Head, Division of Maternal-Fetal Medicine, University of California, Irvine, California College of Medicine, Irvine; University of California, Irvine, Medical Center, Orange, California.

BROOKS RANNEY, M.D., M.S.
Professor of Obstetrics and Gynecology, University of South Dakota School of Medicine. Chairman, Department of Obstetrics and Gynecology, Sacred Heart Hospital; Consulting Gynecologist, Human Services Center, Yankton, South Dakota.

JACK R. ROBERTSON, M.D.
Clinical Professor, Department of Obstetrics and Gynecology, University of California, Irvine, California

SUBIR ROY, M.D.
Associate Professor, Department of Obstetrics and Gynecology, University of Southern California School of Medicine. Physician Specialist, Women's Hospital, Los Angeles County-USC Medical Center, Los Angeles, California.

IVOR L. SAFRO, M.D.
Clinical Associate Professor of Obstetrics and Gynecology, Baylor College of Medicine, Houston, Texas.

BARRY S. SCHIFRIN, M.D.
Professor, Obstetrics and Gynecology, University of Southern California School of Medicine. Attending Staff, Los Angeles County-USC Medical Center, Los Angeles, California.

HERBERT J. SCHMIDT, M.D.
Associate Professor, Obstetrics-Gynecology, Arizona Health Sciences Center, College of Medicine, University of Arizona-Tucson. Assistant Director, St. Johns Regional Oncology Center, Joplin, Missouri.

JACK M. SCHNEIDER, M.D.
Director, The Perinatal Center, Sutter Memorial Hospital, Sacramento, California.

RICHARD H. SCHWARZ, M.D.
Professor of Obstetrics and Gynecology, SUNY-Downstate Medical Center. Chairman, Department of Obstetrics and Gynecology, State University Hospital and Kings County Hospital, Brooklyn, New York.

ANTONIO SCOMMEGNA, M.D.
Professor, Department of Obstetrics and Gynecology, University of Chicago Pritzker School of Medicine. Chairman, Department of Obstetrics and Gynecology, Michael Reese Hospital, Chicago, Illinois.

D. E. SCOTT, M.D.
Professor, Department of Obstetrics and Gynecology, University of Texas Health Science Center at Dallas. Chairman and Chief, Department of Obstetrics and Gynecology, Presbyterian Hospital of Dallas. Senior Attending Physician, Parkland Memorial Hospital; Senior Consultant, Baylor University Hospital and St. Paul Hospital, Houston, Texas.

WILLIAM C. SCOTT, M.D.
Associate Professor, Obstetrics and Gynecology, Arizona Health Sciences Center, College of Medicine, University of Arizona-Tucson. Attending Gynecologist, Chief of Staff, University Hospital, Arizona Health Sciences Center, Tucson, Arizona.

A. E. SEEDS, M.D.*
Professor and Chairman, Department of Obstetrics and Gynecology, University of Cincinnati School of Medicine, Cincinnati, Ohio.

STEFAN SEMCHYSHYN, M.D.
Director, Maternal-Fetal Medicine, Department of Obstetrics and Gynecology, St. Barnabas Medical Center, Livingston, New Jersey.

JOE LEIGH SIMPSON, M.D.
Head, Section of Human Genetics, Professor, Department of Obstetrics and Gynecology, Northwestern University Medical School, Chicago, Illinois.

NILS-OTTO SJÖBERG, M.D.
Professor in Obstetrics and Gynecology, Department of Obstetrics and Gynecology, University Hospital, Lund, Sweden.

KENNETH R. SPISSO, M.D.
Associate Professor, Rutgers University. Director, Obstetrics and Gynecology, Dhahran Health Center, Saudi Arabia.

C. ROBERT STANHOPE, M.D.
Gynecologic Surgeon, Mayo Clinic, Rochester, Minnesota.

MORTON A. STENCHEVER, M.D.
Professor and Chairman, Department of Obstetrics and Gynecology, University of Washington School of Medicine. Attending Physician, University Hospital, Harborview Hospital, and Swedish Hospital, Seattle, Washington.

ANN L. STEWART, M.B., Ch.B., D.C.H.
Senior Lecturer in Perinatal Medicine, Department of Obstetrics and Paediatrics, School of Medicine, University College, London. Consultant in Perinatal Medicine, University College Hospital, London, England.

THOMAS N. SUCIU, M.D.
Assistant Professor, Department of Obstetrics and

---

*Dr. Seeds died on May 12, 1980.

Gynecology, Division of Gynecologic Oncology, University of Arizona Health Sciences Center, Tuscon, Arizona.

JAMES E. THOMASSON, M.D.
Clinical Associate, Department of Obstetrics and Gynecology, University of Arizona, Tucson, Arizona.

CARL W. TYLER, Jr., M.D.
Assistant Director, Science Center for Health Promotion and Education, Centers for Disease Control. Clinical Associate Professor, Department of Gynecology and Obstetrics, Emory University School of Medicine, Atlanta, Georgia.

UMBERTO VILLASANTA, M.D.
Professor of Obstetrics and Gynecology; Director, Gynecologic Oncology, University of Maryland School of Medicine, Baltimore, Maryland.

HELMUTH VORHERR, M.D.
Professor of Obstetrics-Gynecology and of Pharmacology, The University of New Mexico School of Medicine, Albuquerque, New Mexico.

JAMES C. WARREN, M.D., Ph.D.
Professor and Chairman, Department of Obstetrics and Gynecology, Washington University School of Medicine. Obstetrician-Gynecologist-in-Chief, Barnes and Allied Hospitals, St. Louis, Missouri.

JOHN C. WEED, Jr., M.D.
Department of Obstetrics and Gynecology, University of South Alabama College of Medicine, Mobile, Alabama.

LOUIS WEINSTEIN, M.D.
Associate Professor, Department of Obstetrics and

Gynecology, University of Arizona Health Sciences Center. Department of Obstetrics and Gynecology, Arizona Health Sciences Center, Tucson, Arizona.

STUART A. WEPRIN, M.D.
Assistant Clinical Professor, Wright State University School of Medicine. Active Staff, Good Samaritan Hospital and Miami Valley Hospital; Courtesy Staff, St. Elizabeth Medical Center, Kettering Medical Center, Sycamore Medical Center, Dayton, Ohio.

JOHN A. WIDNESS, M.D.
Assistant Professor of Pediatrics, Brown University Program in Medicine. Neonatologist, Women and Infants Hospital of Rhode Island, Providence, Rhode Island.

KATHLEEN H. WILSON, B.S.
Technical Assistant, Physiologist, New York, New York.

DENNIS WORTHINGTON, M.D.
Associate Professor, Department of Gynecology and Obstetrics, Medical College of Wisconsin, Milwaukee, Wisconsin.

MARVIN A. YUSSMAN, M.D.
Professor of Obstetrics and Gynecology; Director, Division of Reproductive Endocrinology, University of Louisville School of Medicine, Louisville, Kentucky.

FREDERICK P. ZUSPAN, M.D.
Professor and Chairman, Department of Obstetrics and Gynecology, Ohio State University College of Medicine. Obstetrician-Gynecologist-in-Chief, University Hospital, Columbus, Ohio.

Preface

The contributors to the third edition of *Controversy in Obstetrics and Gynecology* were selected because each has made basic and worthwhile contributions to the area about which he or she writes and each is an accomplished clinician. The fact that they have different points of view and differ in methods of management is expected and appropriate in a discipline that has the breadth and depth that Reproductive Medicine has come to encompass.

The topics selected are not intended to cover the entire gamut of the specialty but do represent areas of everyday concern to the practitioner and the house officer in training. It has been noted that the two previous editions have been used extensively by physicians in training programs and busy clinicians who can find two or three points of view capsulized and directed toward management with appropriate reference being made to the rationale for such management. We have also noted that physicians who are called upon to teach find this format helpful because of the varying points of view that are available in a single source. It is our hope that this third edition will likewise be of benefit to the readers.

Our editor, Mr. Albert Meier, has been most helpful during the gestation of this edition and we offer him our special thanks.

FREDERICK P. ZUSPAN

C. D. CHRISTIAN

Contents

6

The Management of Breech Presentations 226

7

Identification and Management of Intrauterine Growth Retardation and the Post-Term Pregnancy 242

1
Antepartum Fetal Monitoring

Alternative Points of View

by Richard H. Paul and Kirk A. Keegan, Jr.

by Ronald S. Leuchter and Barry S. Schifrin

by Roger K. Freeman and Thomas J. Garite

Editorial Comment

Antepartum Fetal Monitoring: The Optimal Method and Role

Richard H. Paul, M.D.

Kirk A. Keegan, Jr., M.D.

University of Southern California

Evaluation of the antepartum fetus has long frustrated the obstetrician. The past decade has seen some advances in biophysical and biochemical monitoring, which have helped to elucidate fetal status. Antepartum fetal heart rate testing (AFHRT) is playing an ever-increasing role in prenatal fetal evaluation, and is today a mainstay in the management of most high-risk obstetric patients. Despite popular acceptance, controversy still exists on which is the best type of testing approach, on technique and interpretation, and on the course of action to be followed when an abnormal test is encountered.

The major experience in AFHRT in the United States has been with the contraction stress test (CST). Suggested approaches to testing using other stress factors such as exercise and hypoxia have failed to achieve clinical acceptance.[1] The CST, or oxytocin challenge test (OCT), in which oxytocin is used to provoke uterine contractions, evolved from intrapartum observations by Hon, Quilligan,[2] and others,[3] who defined the association of late deceleration of fetal heart rate and fetal hypoxia in labor. Thus, the occurrence of late decelerations in an antepartum CST, a positive result, was associated with an increased incidence of low Apgar scores and fetal and neonatal deaths.[4] However, "false-positive CSTs" in which the fetus subsequently tolerated labor without late deceleration occurred in as many as 20 to 50 per cent of reported cases.[5, 6] A negative or "normal" CST more reliably identifies the fetus that is not at risk. Fetal death within a week of a negative CST, while reported, is a rare event, occurring at a rate of less than 0.4 to 1 per cent.[7]

Although the use of a CST provides useful clinical direction, it has serious drawbacks as a method of antepartum testing. The test is time-consuming, requiring 50 to 90 minutes to complete, a disadvantage for both patient and medical personnel. An intravenous infusion of oxytocin and operation of its delivery system requires specially trained personnel and close proximity to a labor and delivery facility for management of potential complications. Contraindications to oxytocin in the antepartum period, such as third trimester bleeding, premature labor, uterine scar, incompetent cervix and multiple gestation, all are relative contraindications to the performance of the CST. In addition, quantifying the stress imposed by the uterine contractions is difficult. Interpretation of the end result, especially the suspicious, equivocal or even positive test, can be confusing. Finally, 2 to 14 per cent of tests are interpreted as unsatisfactory for one reason or another.[8, 9]

An effective antepartum test should be convenient, noninvasive and technically simple, with easily recognizable end points for evaluation. For these reasons, the CST is not applicable for rapid screening of large numbers of high-risk obstetric patients, especially in the office or clinical setting.

The limitations of contraction stress testing have generated renewed interest in the characteristics of the fetal heart rate under "nonstressed" conditions, as observed by Hammacher in the 1960s.[10] Characteristics of heart rate in the healthy fetus are the presence of fluctuations and accelerations associated with fetal movement. These accelerations are presumably reflex mediated, and when present, indicate intact, responsive mechanisms that control fetal heart rate. Depression of normal fluctuations and accelerations associated with fetal movement are seen in fetal sleep-like states, hypoxia, acidosis and use of certain narcotic-sedative drugs. Hammacher categorized antepartum nonstress fetal heart rate patterns by their amount of fluctuation or oscillation and noted an increased incidence of low Apgar scores when these characteristics were diminished or absent. He also advocated stimulation of the fetus with decreased oscillations to rule out sleep-like states as a possible etiology. Kubli,[11] using a multiassessment approach to antepartum evaluation consisting of electronic monitoring, estriol, ultrasound and amniotic fluid analysis, confirmed Hammacher's observations regarding fetal heart rate

fluctuation. He believed that oxytocin administration for antepartum testing was rarely necessary.

The presence of fluctuations or movement-associated fetal heart rate accelerations, either preceding or during the CST, has been analyzed with respect to CST result and subsequent perinatal outcome. Schifrin[12] reviewed 189 CSTs and noted that if accelerations associated with fetal movement were present during the test, no subsequent late decelerations were noted.

Trierweiler[13] reported on a retrospective review of 255 OCTs in which the baseline fetal heart rate was examined for accelerations prior to the stress testing. The accelerations noted had to exceed 20 beats per minute (bpm) associated with spikes on the tocodynamometer, presumed to be fetal movement. Accelerations, although not quantified as to duration or number, were present in 75 of 255 tests. In none of these 75 cases of accelerations was positive CST subsequently noted. Lack of acceleration was noted in 180 tests and a positive CST result was noted in 25 tests. Farahani[14] performed a similar study in which accelerations were evaluated both prior to and during the CST. Accelerations were classified as minimum (less than 10 bpm), average (10 to 20 bpm) and marked (20 to 50 bpm). Duration or frequency of accelerations was not noted. A negative CST result was obtained in 1478 tests on 492 fetuses. Heart rate accelerations were averaged or marked in all but 18 fetuses (96 per cent). The CST was positive on 40 occasions in 38 fetuses. In 27 of these 38, minimal or no accelerations were seen, and thick meconium, low Apgar scores or fetal dysmaturity was subsequently noted at delivery. Of interest is that 8 of the 38 patients with positive CSTs had normal outcome. In 6 of these 8, the CST showed average to marked accelerations.

Fox[8] evaluated accelerations in 215 patients having contraction stress testing. He noted a good outcome without increased perinatal morbidity in 133 of 148 patients (90 per cent) who demonstrated accelerations during stress testing. Increased morbidity was defined as the presence of intrapartum fetal distress, falling estriol levels, low Apgar score, or neonatal morbidity. Conversely, a good outcome was noted in only 36 of 67 patients (54 per cent) who demonstrated no accelerations during stress testing.

Lee,[15] after noting accelerations in 63 of 81

negative CSTs and the absence of accelerations in 6 positive CSTs, performed nonstress testing (fetal activity acceleration determination [FAD]) prior to CST in 298 fetuses. Tests that revealed 3 to 4 accelerations in the nonstress period were followed by negative CSTs in 296 of 324 tests (91 per cent). In four instances accelerations were not shown, and in all four positive CSTs were subsequently recorded. The combination of fetal accelerations and negative CSTs resulted in good fetal outcome with the exception of one fetal death secondary to abruptio placenta. Fetuses that did not demonstrate accelerations and had a positive CST were delivered by cesarean section, again with good outcome.

These studies support the convention that the presence of acceleration preceding or during the CST connotes fetal well-being and corrolates not only with the outcome of the CST but with perinatal outcome. This information seems to corroborate reports from Europe where the nonstress method has been used, in some instances, as the sole method of AFHRT. Rochard[16] reported a series of 125 patients, of whom 40 per cent were Rh isoimmunized, who underwent 641 tests using only the nonstress approach. The fetal heart rate pattern was classified as reactive if the rate was between 120 to 160 bpm, variability was greater than 6 bpm, and accelerations accompanied fetal movement. A test was considered nonreactive if any of these criteria were not met. Fifty-one patients had consistently reactive tests. Forty-one of 51 (80 per cent) showed no evidence of intrapartum fetal distress and had normal neonatal outcomes. In 6 of 41 patients (12 per cent) fetal distress developed in labor and 4 (8 per cent) of 51 had perinatal morbidity. All 51 with a reactive test survived. Nineteen had persistently nonreactive tests. Three of 19 patients had mild fetal distress but recovered in labor, 11 of 19 required prolonged neonatal care, and 5 of 19 died in utero. Seventy-six of the 125 patients had a reactive pattern equal to or more than 50 per cent of the time. In this group, only 8 (10.5 per cent) required prolonged hospitalization. Forty-nine of 125 patients (39 per cent) had a nonreactive pattern equal to or more than 50 per cent of the time. Twenty-three (47 per cent) required prolonged neonatal care and 21 (41 per cent) died either in utero or in the neonatal period.

Tushuizen[17] studied 386 patients using a nonstressed approach. He defined a normal test result as a heart rate of 120 to 160 bpm, with no decelerations of longer than 30 seconds' duration or greater than 30 bpm, with normal beat-to-beat variation and the presence of accelerations with fetal movement. An abnormal result was the absence of any of these characteristics. A significant difference was noted in perinatal mortality when the fetal heart rate was normal as opposed to when it was abnormal or recurrently abnormal. There was 1 fetal death and 4 neonatal deaths in 325 patients with a normal heart rate pattern (PNM 15.4/1000). In the abnormal heart rate group, there were 3 neonatal deaths in 37 patients (PNM 81.4/1000) and in the recurrently abnormal group, there were 5 fetal deaths and 4 neonatal deaths in 24 patients (PNM 375/1000). Tushuizen also noted lower Apgar scores and a higher incidence of asphyxia as measured by pH and standard bicarbonate in fetuses with abnormal nonstress cardiotocograms.

Viser[18] employed nonstressed cardiotocography in 454 patients. In a normal nonstress test, baseline irregularity of more than 10 bpm was noted and accelerations were noted with fetal movement. Abnormal test results were defined as: (1) suboptimal, when there was decreased accelerations and irregularity, and (2) decelerative, showing a decrease in irregularity and accelerations with absence of repetitive late decelerations provoked with spontaneous contractions. He also described (3) terminal pattern, which showed almost a complete lack of irregularity and accelerations, with late decelerations occurring in response to spontaneous uterine contractions. In the terminal group, there were 9 fetal and 3 neonatal deaths in 26 patients (PNM 460/1000). No perinatal deaths were noted in the groups with suboptimal, decelerative, or normal patterns. An increased incidence of cesarean section for fetal distress, as well as a higher incidence of small for gestational age (SGA) infants, was noted in those who had decelerative and suboptimal patterns.

Flynn[19] reported on 800 cases in 301 fetuses, using nonstress testing. For the first time, a clear, concise, composite description of both accelerations and timing of the test was given in this report. A reactive pattern or test was defined as the presence of 4 accelerations of more than 15 bpm associated with fetal movement in one of two 20-minute periods. The "last test" was reactive in 245 and nonreactive in 56 fetuses. Four stillbirths and one neonatal death occurred in the nonreactive group (PNM 89 to 1000). No perinatal deaths occurred in the reactive group. Those with nonreactive patterns revealed a higher incidence of "pathological fetal heart rate patterns in labor" (45 per cent) than did the reactive pattern group (1.0 per cent). Cesarean delivery or fetal distress occurred in 14 per cent with nonreactive patterns and 0.4 per cent with reactive patterns. Five-minute Apgar scores equal to or less than 6 occurred in 3.6 per cent of the reactive group and in 23 per cent of those with a nonreactive pattern.

These studies support the hypothesis that the presence of fetal heart rate accelerations, either in conjunction with a CST or during nonstress testing, identifies the fetus that is at low risk. In addition, most mortality and morbidity occurs in fetuses that do not demonstrate heart rate accelerations. However, in spite of an abnormal result on AFHRT, the majority of these newborns do well as measured by Apgar score, normal heart rate patterns in labor and perinatal mortality. Therefore, were the nonstress test to be used as the sole method of AFHRT, an unacceptably high incidence of false-positive results would occur. Although the false-positive rate for the CST is high, one would anticipate only 3 to 10 per cent positive CSTs, whereas as many as one third have nonreactive (abnormal) nonstress tests. Aggressive intervention for the patient with a nonreactive pattern would seem to be unwarranted in view of the high false-positive rate, and further evaluation of the significance of such a test is mandatory.

The role of the AFHRT in prenatal evaluation is thus hampered by the many disadvantages of the CST and the high false-positive rate of the NST. A logical approach to this dilemma has been suggested by Martin and Schifrin,[20] Evertson,[21] and Nochimson.[22] The NST approach, which is quicker, safer, easier and allows more patients to be tested, was utilized as a screening test. In Nochimson's series, a reactive test required 4 accelerations with fetal movement in one of two 20-minute periods. Reactive tests were repeated in 1 week or as dictated clinically. Nonreactive tests were followed by CSTs. A total of 786 NSTs were performed on 421 fetuses, of which 594 (75.5 per cent) were reactive, 187 (23.8 per cent) nonreactive and 5 (0.63 per cent) unsatisfactory. Of the 187 CSTs, 42 were abnormal (23 per cent 13 positive and 29 suspicious) following nonreactive patterns. Re-

peat testing in 27 of 29 fetuses with suspicious results produced a negative CST or a reactive NST. The outcome in the 13 instances of nonreactive NST with positive CST was not discussed. A total of 401 patients entered labor with either a reactive NST or negative CST. Apgar scores were equal to or more than 5 minutes in all but 8 instances; each of these newborns had a specific intrapartum etiology for the low Apgar score. The nonreactive test seemed to screen adequately for the fetus that would demonstrate a positive CST and the reactive test predicted perinatal outcome equivalent to the negative CST.

Evertson, using a similar management protocol at Los Angeles County–University of Southern California Medical Center, Women's Hospital, studied 2422 NSTs in 1169 fetuses. Reactive tests required 5 accelerations with fetal movement in one of two 20-minute periods. A reactive pattern was noted in 1547 tests (64 per cent) and a nonreactive pattern in 829 tests (35 per cent). CSTs were performed 939 times with 851 (91 per cent) negative, 13 (1.4 per cent) equivocal, 29 (3 per cent) positive and 46 (5.0 per cent) unsatisfactory. There were 5 perinatal deaths in 493 patients within one week of a reactive test— PNM rate 10/1000; 10 deaths in 302 patients with nonreactive test—PNM 33/1000. There was a statistical difference in PNM in patients with reactive and nonreactive tests (p = 0.05). The perinatal mortality rate for a nonreactive test coupled with a negative CST was 27/1000, with a positive CST, 87/1000. No statistical difference existed in patient groups with a "normal" test—reactive NST or negative CST. A reactive NST was as predictive of perinatal outcome as a negative CST. Evertson also noted that if a minimum of 2 accelerations in 20 minutes was present during the NST, no abnormal CSTs followed. In addition, fetuses that had accelerations with movement or a reactive pattern during oxytocin infusion for stress uniformly had normal CSTs.

Testing Method

Based on Evertson's observations, the following working protocol was implemented on July 1, 1977, for AFHRT at Los Angeles County–University of Southern California Medical Center, Women's Hospital. The protocol is readily adaptable to both inpatient and

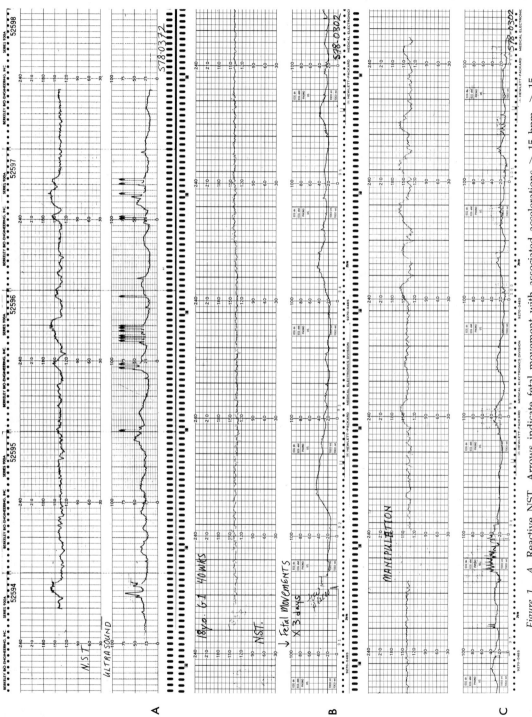

Figure 1. A, Reactive NST. Arrows indicate fetal movement with associated accelerations > 15 bpm, > 15 seconds. *B* and *C,* Nonreactive NST with absence of fetal movement (FM) and fetal heart rate acceleration. Manipulation (C) followed by FM and acceleration.

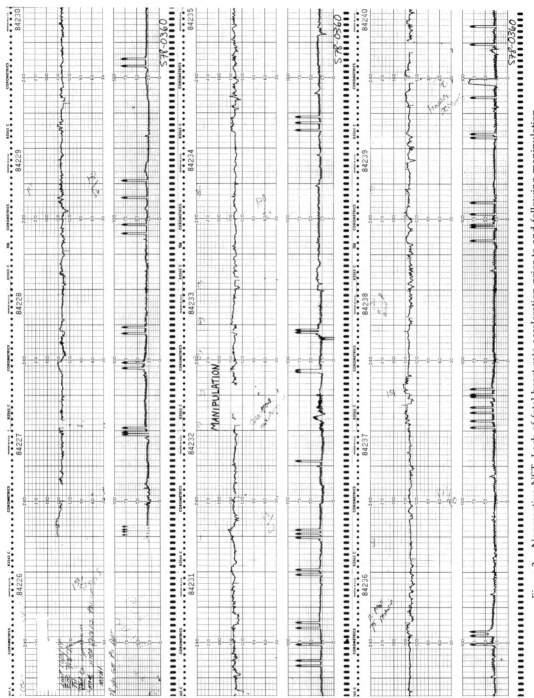

Figure 2. Nonreactive NST. Lack of fetal heart rate acceleration prior to and following manipulation.

outpatient facilities. Patients are placed in the semi-Fowler's position and blood pressures are taken at 10-minute intervals to identify and correct supine hypotension. External techniques are employed, using standard monitors, and abdominal wall FECG, modified phonocardiogram or ultrasound for deviation of FHR data. If contractions are present, the frequency and duration are detected by using a tocodynamometer. Fetal movement is detected by the woman or the nurse observer or both and recorded on the strip chart. A pattern is considered reactive when 2 or more accelerations of more than 15 bpm and longer than 15 seconds' duration are present in one of two 20-minute observation periods. Minimal observation time for a reactive test is 10 minutes (Fig. 1A).

The absence of 2 accelerations in the two observation periods is considered a nonreactive (NR) pattern. If a nonreactive pattern is found in the initial 20-minute period, the fetus is stimulated by grasping of both fetal poles and manipulation for 60 seconds. This is done in an attempt to alter the presumed sleep-like state in the fetus. The 5 minutes of recording during and following stimulation are eliminated to preclude accelerations evoked solely from the direct stimulus. The subsequent 20 minutes are then evaluated. Fetuses demonstrating reactive patterns are presumed "normal" and retested in 1 week (Fig. 1B,C). If a nonreactive pattern persists, a CST is performed (Fig. 2). If 2 accelerations of more than 15 bpm, longer than 15 seconds are noted during the performance of CST, the result is considered reactive, the test is terminated, and the fetus retested in 1 week. A test that remains nonreactive during the CST is completed as defined by Martin and Schifrin (3 contractions in 10 minutes).[20] A nonreactive NST with negative CST is repeated in 1 week. A nonreactive NST with an equivocal CST is repeated within 24 hours. A positive CST is managed according to the clinical situation. Following completion of NST or CST, suprapubic and fundal pressure is applied to the fetus for 1 minute to ascertain the possibility of a vulnerable cord as evidenced by variable deceleration or prolonged bradycardia of the fetal heart rate.

Preliminary Results

Preliminary data obtained from July through December 1977 using the protocol just de-

TABLE 1. Nonstress Testing During 1975–1977*

	May 1975–April 1977	July 1977–December 1977
Patients	1169	411
NSTs	2422	787
Reactive	1547 (64%)	726 (92%)
Nonreactive	829 (34%)	61 (7.7%)
Unsatisfactory	43	2

*Data in Tables 1–4 from Los Angeles County–University of Southern California Medical Center, Women's Hospital.

scribed are presented in Tables 1 through 4. Of interest is the significantly increased incidence of reactive tests, 95 per cent as opposed to 64 per cent, when the new criterion of two accelerations is required for a reactive pattern. A CST was performed in only 8 per cent of cases, and in 52 per cent of these CSTs, the pattern became reactive and the CST was terminated (Table 2).

CSTs performed after a nonreactive pattern requiring 5 accelerations (1975 to 1977) revealed 91 per cent normal and 4 per cent abnormal results (positive or equivocal CSTs) (Table 2). This indicated that most of these fetuses were, in retrospect, normal and that 5 accelerations was possibly too stringent a screening requirement. In contrast, the tests in which two accelerations were not achieved seemed to predict a group at greater risk for an abnormal CST. Using the current protocol for screening, an abnormal CST was noted in 31 per cent of cases in contrast to the previous occurrence of 4 per cent.

Table 3 indicates test results on 290 patients who had a test within 7 days of delivery. A reactive pattern was seen in 257 (88.6 per cent) and a nonreactive pattern in 33 (11.4 per cent). In the reactive group, 160 fetuses were

TABLE 2. Contraction Stress Testing During 1975–1977

	May 1975–April 1977	July 1977–December 1977
CST attempted	939	61
CST reactive (52%)		32
CST completed (48%)	893 (5% unsat.)	29
Negative CST	851 (91%)	20 (69%)
Positive CST	29 (3%)	6 (21%)
Equivocal CST	13 (1%)	3 (10%)

TABLE 3. RESULTS OF NST-CST WITHIN 7 DAYS OF DELIVERY

	No. PATIENTS
Reactive	205
Reactive (stim.)	47
Reactive (CST)	5
TOTAL	257 (88.6%)
NR negative CST	17
NR equivocal CST	3
NR positive CST	5
NR prolonged bradycardia	1
TOTAL	33 (11.4%)

monitored during labor (Table 4). Late decelerations requiring cesarean section for fetal distress occurred in only one instance in this group. In the nonreactive group, 22 fetuses were monitored and late decelerations requiring cesarean section occurred in four patients. One fetal death occurred in the reactive group. At delivery, the umbilical cord was wrapped tightly around the leg, possibly indicating a cord accident as an etiologic factor. No fetal deaths occurred in the nonreactive group. However, in 9 of 33 patients (27 per cent) intervention was performed for presumed fetal indications on the day of the abnormal test. There were no neonatal deaths in either group.

Summary

In summary, a combination of the contraction stress test and the nonstress test seems best suited for fetal evaluation. A reactive nonstress test predicts outcome as well as does a negative CST. Furthermore, this approach provides the advantages of time savings, simple technique and clear interpretation. A nonreactive nonstress test requires further clarification of fetal status, which is currently accomplished by performing a CST. Future approaches will likely explore more frequent testing intervals and observations regarding other signs of fetal well-being, such as fetal breathing movements.

The appeal of a simple, reliable and inexpensive test of fetal well-being is apparent. The NST appears to hold this potential and may be conveniently used in an outpatient setting. The role of such an approach as a screening method, in an attempt to reduce the occurrence of fetal deaths, would appear to be a valid area for further clinical study.

REFERENCES

1. Hon, E. H., and Wohlgemuth, R.: The electronic evaluation of fetal heart rate: IV. The effect of maternal exercise. Am. J. Obstet. Gynecol. 81:361, 1961.
2. Hon, E. H. and Quilligan, E. J.: Classification of fetal heart rate: II. A revised working classification. Connecticut Med. 31:779, 1967.
3. Caldeyro-Barcia, R. et al.: Control of Human Fetal Heart Rate During Labor. *In* Cassels, D. E. (ed.): The Heart and Circulation of the Newborn Infant. New York, Grune and Stratton, Inc., 1966, p. 7.
4. Ray, M. J. et al.: Clinical experience with the oxytocin challenge test. Am. J. Obstet. Gynecol. 114:1, 1972.
5. Braly, P. and Freeman, R. K.: The significance of fetal heart rate reactivity with a positive oxytocin challenge test. Obstet. Gynecol. 50:689, 1977.
6. Weingold, A. B., DeJesus, T. P. and O'Keiffe, J.: Oxytocin challenge test. Am. J. Obstet. Gynecol. 123:466, 1975.
7. Evertson, L. R., Gauthier, R. J. and Collea, J. V.: Fetal demise following negative contraction stress tests. Obstet. Gynecol. 51:671, 1978.
8. Fox, H. E., Steinbrecher, M. and Ripton, B.: Antepartum fetal heart rate and uterine activity studies. I. Preliminary report of accelerations and the oxytocin challenge test. Am. J. Obstet. Gynecol. 126:61, 1977.
9. Garite, T. J., Freeman, R. K., Hochleutner, I. and Linzey, E. M.: Oxytocin challenge test: achieving the desired goals. Obstet. Gynecol. 51:614, 1978.
10. Hammacher, K.: The Clinical Significance of Cardiography. *In* Huntingford, P. S. et al. (eds.): Perinatal Medicine. New York, Academic Press, Inc., 1969, pp. 80–93.
11. Kubli, F. W., Kaeser, O. and Kinselman, M.: Diag-

TABLE 4. PREGNANCY OUTCOME IN REACTIVE AND NONREACTIVE GROUP TESTED WITHIN 7 DAYS OF DELIVERY

	No. PATIENTS	LABOR MONITORED	C/S FOR LATE DECELERATIONS	PND*	PNDR
Reactive	257	160	1 (0.6%)	1	3.9/1000
Nonreactive	33	22	4 (18%)†	0‡	0

*PND = prenatal death; PNDR = prenatal death rate.
†P < 0.001
‡9/33 delivery induced on day of test.

nostic Management of Chronic Placental Insufficiency. *In* Pecile, A. and Finzi, C. (eds.): The Foeto-Placental Unit. Amsterdam, Excerpta Medica Foundation, 1969, pp. 323–339.

12. Schifrin, B. S., Lapidus, M., Doctor, G. S. and Leviton, A.: Contraction stress test for antepartum fetal evaluation. Obstet. Gynecol. 45:43, 1975.

13. Trierweiler, M. W., Freeman, R. K. and James, J.: Baseline fetal acceleration heart rate characteristics as an indicator of fetal status during the antepartum period. Am. J. Obstet. Gynecol. 125:618, 1976.

14. Farahani, G. and Fenton, A. N.: Fetal heart rate acceleration in relation to the oxytocin challenge test. Obstet. Gynecol. 49:163, 1977.

15. Lee, C. Y., Di Loreto, P. C. and Logrand, B.: Fetal activity acceleration determination for the evaluation of fetal reserve. Obstet. Gynecol. 48:19, 1976.

16. Rochard, F., Schifrin, B. S., Goupil, F., LeGrad, H., Blottiere, J. and Sureau, C.: Non-stressed fetal heart rate monitoring in the antepartum period. Am. J. Obstet. Gynecol. 126:699, 1976.

17. Tushuizen, P., Stoot, J. and Ubachs, J.: Clinical experience in nonstressed antepartum cardiotocography. Am. J. Obstet. Gynecol. 128:507, 1977.

18. Viser, G. H. A. and Huisies, H. J.: Diagnostic value of the unstressed antepartum cardiotocogram. Br. J. Obstet. Gynaecol. 54:321, 1977.

19. Flynn, A. M. and Kelly, J.: Evaluation of fetal well being by antepartum fetal heart monitoring. Br. Med. J. 1:936, 1977.

20. Martin, C. B., Jr. and Schifrin, B. S.: Prenatal Fetal Monitoring. *In* Aladjem, S. and Brown, A. K. (eds.): Perinatal Intensive Care. St. Louis, C. V. Mosby Co., 1977, pp. 155–173.

21. Nochimson, D. J., Turbeville, J. S., Terry, J. E., Petrie, R. H. and Lundy, L. E.: The nonstress test. Obstet. Gynecol. 51:419, 1978.

22. Evertson, L. R., Gauthier, R. J., Schifrin, B. S. and Paul, R. H.: Antepartum fetal heart rate testing: I. Evolution of the nonstress test. Am. J. Obstet. Gynecol. 133:29–33, 1979.

Antepartum Assessment of the Fetus

Ronald S. Leuchter, M.D.

Barry S. Schifrin, M.D.

Cedars–Sinai Medical Center, Los Angeles

There has been a continuing search for means of identifying those pregnant patients who are at increased risk of poor outcome. The search has brought about significant advances but proved frustrating as well. Initially, only those patients with obvious medical clinical risk factors or history of problem pregnancy were selected for specialized care. Information regarding the well-being of the individual fetus was minimal; treatment of the fetus directly was nonexistent and the timing of delivery empirical. Improvement in this situation awaited the development of methodologies to define the condition of the individual fetus. This goal has been achieved over the last 20 years with the widespread availability of reliable fetal information. Estrogen excretion measurement, fetal heart rate monitoring, blood sampling, ultrasound, and amniocentesis have removed considerable guesswork about the condition of the fetus and permitted more appropriate timing of delivery. In this article we will discuss several biochemical and biophysical tests currently available for the antenatal assessment of fetal well-being.

Biochemical Tests

ESTRIOL

Estriol is the major estrogen secreted in pregnancy. Its excretion represents a complex interaction between fetus, placenta and mother (Fig. 1). Virtually all of the estriol produced in pregnancy originates within the fetal/placental compartment from precursors supplied by the mother. The fetal adrenal gland forms dehydroepiandrosterone sulfate (DHEA-S), a weak androgen. This compound, in turn, is hydroxylated at the 16 position in the fetal liver (the placenta lacks the capacity for 16 hydroxylation) and then transported to the placenta. In the placenta, sulfatase enzyme converts the 16 hydroxylated androgen to estriol. Estriol in its unconjugated, or "free," form is then transferred to the mother, in whose liver and kidney it is reconjugated with sulphate or glucuronide or both. About half of the estriol conjugates are excreted into the bile and take part in the enterohepatic circulation. In the intestine, estriol conjugates are again cleaved and reabsorbed by the gut,

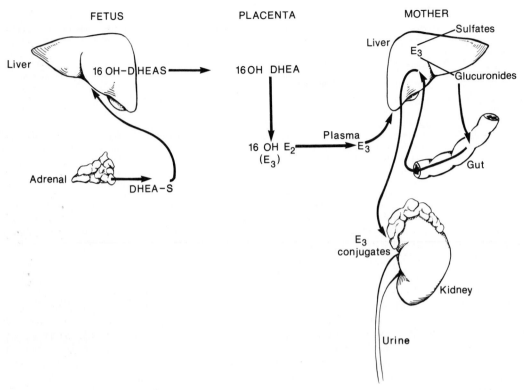

Figure 1. Estriol synthesis.

which yields yet other such conjugates. Estriol excreted by the kidneys circulates in the plasma in various forms; about 10 per cent represents the free or unconjugated form, while 90 per cent represents a rich variety of various conjugates. It is obvious that there are many steps involved in the production and disposition of estriol, and the various forms in which it exists pose potential pitfalls in laboratory determination and clinical interpretation.

As pregnancy advances, plasma levels and urinary excretion of estriol increase. In normal pregnancies excretion of urinary estriol at term is about 28 mg/24 hr and the total estrogen output is 53 mg/24 hr.[1] Not only does interpretation of estriol values depend upon gestational age, but, as shown by Beischer et al., daily estriol excretion varies considerably, particularly in the third trimester.[2] The coefficient of variation for urinary estriol over a 24-hour period is 20 per cent, while the coefficient of variation for plasma estriol is about 15 per cent. These statistics presumably prevail in the absence of either collection or laboratory error. Owing to the cooperative efforts required on the part of fetus, placenta and mother for the production of estriol, any con-

dition that affects any one of these contributors can result in misleading values, which make the assessment of the fetal condition difficult. Similarly, difficulties in collection and determination of estriol may further confound accurate interpretation.

In the fetal compartment, enzyme deficiencies associated with congenital adrenal hyperplasia can result in an excess of androgenic precursors and elevated estriol values. Likewise, anencephalic fetuses with hypoplastic adrenal glands lack available precursors for estriol synthesis, causing values to be low.

Conditions that increase placental mass, such as maternal diabetes mellitus and Rh isoimmunization, can result in normal or elevated estriol levels at a time when the fetus may be severely compromised. On the other hand, the rare patient with placental sulfatase deficiency will be unable to convert androgenic precursors to estrogens. Estriol values will be markedly low, yet the fetal condition will likely be normal. Similarly, any condition that diminishes the mother's ability to conjugate and excrete estrogens will affect the interpretation of estriol values. With maternal liver disease, the ability to conjugate estriol is diminished and the amount of conjugated deriv-

TABLE 1. INTERPRETATION OF ESTRIOL VALUES

	FETUS	PLACENTA	MOTHER	MISCELLANEOUS
Elevation	CAH	Diabetes mellitus Rh hemolytic disease		
Depression	Anencephaly, maternal use of steroids	Sulfatase deficiency	Liver disease, renal disease, glucosuria, use of ampicillin	Collection error, laboratory error

ative in urine will be decreased while the amount of free unconjugated estriol in the serum will be increased. Antibiotics such as ampicillin can reduce intestinal flora and interfere with the enterohepatic circulation of estriol. In this situation, the amount secreted in the urine will likewise be diminished. Any compound that inhibits renal tubular secretion of estriol will diminish its excretion: Glucosuria acts in this fashion to inhibit estriol excretion. Similarly, renal disease in the mother will tend to diminish urinary estriol and at the same time elevate plasma estriol.

Excretion of estriol is highly variable; this is shown especially if tests are performed on random urine samples. To minimize some of this variability, a 24-hour collection is necessary. Even with this standard, estriol determinations are plagued with both collection and laboratory error. In many institutions, creatinine collections are performed along with the urine estriol test and corrections are made if the creatinine excretion is decreased. In the presence of an adequate collection, there is little value to the estriol/creatinine ratio. In addition, normal values of estriol must be determined because techniques of measurement vary among laboratories.

The frequency of collections may also have a bearing on outcome. Freeman and others have shown that about 65 per cent of clinically significant decreases in urinary estriol values in diabetics will be missed with collections taken every other day.[3] Because of numerous factors prevailing in the diabetic, there is an extremely narrow margin of safety between normal and abnormal estriol results.[3, 4] For this reason, Goebelsmann et al. considered daily collections of urinary estriol necessary if one is to provide optimal care for the diabetic. They consider fetal jeopardy as existing if the levels fall 35 per cent or more from the mean of the previous 3 days' excretion. With an accurate collection and laboratory evaluation,

estriol excretion levels indicate the condition of the fetus during the previous 24 hours but cannot give information regarding its present condition. This time lapse may prove critical in some instances.

In most high-risk situations, rising estriol values provide reassurance of fetal well-being. Critical values have not been defined in the presence of Rh disease, twin gestation, and maternal diabetes, and should be used with extreme caution in these circumstances. These conditions are associated with large placentas, which apparently elaborate increased levels of estriols, compared to normals. Estriol excretion testing is best applied in those high-risk conditions associated with slowly deteriorating placental function, such as the post-term pregnancy and maternal hypertension.

Because of numerous pitfalls involved in estriol determination, falsely low (false-positive) values are common. While low or decreasing estriol is correlated with an increased risk of poor outcome, the majority of patients with low levels do not have obvious problems. Thus estriol screening is helpful when values are rising, but low or decreasing values are *poor predictors of a bad outcome.* Such abnormal results should be used only as an indication for further evaluation (see following discussion).

Duenhoelter et al. have claimed that monitoring pregnancy by estriol testing does little to decrease perinatal mortality rate.[5] They appropriately suggest that equating a low or falling estriol value with fetal jeopardy may lead to inappropriate premature delivery of a fetus at risk for respiratory distress syndrome. While there are inherent difficulties in estriol determination, we believe that it is useful when integrated into an organized program of perinatal care. Irrespective of the estriol values, there are benefits to be obtained from the existence of supervised urinary collections. The methodology involved ensures close medical supervision and a salutary effect on perinatal outcome.

HUMAN PLACENTAL LACTOGEN

Human placental lactogen (HPL) is a single chain polypeptide of molecular weight 22,000, which is chemically and immunologically similar to growth hormone, being secreted by the syncytiotrophoblast of the placenta. Secretion begins early in pregnancy and progressively rises to reach a plateau in the last 4 to 5 weeks before term. HPL half-life is about 25 minutes, and the amount secreted is roughly proportional to the placental mass present; levels after 30 weeks' gestation are on the order of 4 to 10 μg per ml. Most of the HPL is found in the maternal compartment and very little crosses to the fetus.[6] The ratio of amniotic fluid levels to maternal serum levels is relatively constant throughout pregnancy (approximately 1:8).

The function of HPL seems to be to provide carbohydrate substrate to the fetus from the mother. HPL has a profound effect on maternal carbohydrate metabolism in pregnancy. HPL given to diabetics causes a dramatic increase in blood sugar levels,[7] while nondiabetic patients given a glucose load have a prompt increase in insulin levels.[8] HPL also has a lipolytic effect, mobilizing free fatty acids.[9] Therefore, HPL is diabetogenic, insulinogenic and lipolytic, the effect being to spare maternal glucose for utilization by the fetus, while at the same time increasing fatty acids for use by the mother as an energy substrate.

The control of HPL secretion seems to be largely independent of maternal serum glucose concentration. Small changes in maternal glucose have no appreciable effect, although significant changes in maternal carbohydrate homeostasis or fasting may transiently alter HPL levels.[10-14] There does not seem to be any significant variation in daily levels or any sensitive feedback control. This lack of fluctuation and the ease with which it can be accurately measured by radioimmunoassay techniques would seem to make this placental hormone ideal for use as an indicator of fetal health. Spellacy and co-workers in the United States and Letchworth in England are the most ardent advocates of using HPL as a barometer of fetal well-being. They have

found levels of HPL greater than 4 mg/ml in 95 per cent of pregnancies after 30 weeks' gestation, and describe levels below this as being a "fetal danger zone."[15] Values within this zone are associated with an increased risk of fetal death, ranging from 50 to 80 per cent. Low HPL values are ominous in patients with hypertension.[16] However, others have reported a significant number of false-negative results in which development of fetal hypoxia, acidosis and distress was not anticipated by the use of HPL values.[17]

Sixty to 70 per cent of pregnancies in hypertensive patients with HPL levels in the fetal danger zone will be complicated by intrauterine growth retardation (IUGR).[18, 19] However, this means that at least 30 per cent of these fetuses will not be growth retarded. Therefore, a large false-positive group exists, and our ability to diagnose this problem accurately prior to delivery is not appreciably increased.

It has been suggested that HPL levels are a sensitive indicator of the postmaturity syndrome.[19] However, Berkowitz et al. showed that in a significant number of pregnancies complicated by prolonged gestation, values were above the fetal danger zone, creating a high false-negative rate.[20]

Those conditions that predispose to large placentas such as diabetes mellitus and erythroblastosis fetalis would seem to correlate least with HPL values as a predictor of fetal well-being. The great hazard in antepartum management of the pregnant insulin-dependent diabetic woman is the unanticipated fetal death. In one study of fetal death, HPL levels were low in only 50 per cent.[21] HPL values may correlate better with placental size rather than placental function.

In summary, HPL levels as a predictor of fetal health oxygen appear to be best utilized for evaluation of hypertensive pregnancies with fetal death; they may predict IUGR, but are of limited value in diabetes mellitus and the post-maturity syndrome. Both false-negative and false-positive results do occur, and therefore this parameter cannot be used alone to assess fetal well-being.

Both estriol and HPL values are subject to many interpretative difficulties. When both tests disclose normal values, the false-negative rate is low and the fetus is not likely to be in significant jeopardy. When the values are low or show a drop, the significance is less clear and the interpretation is correspondingly more difficult. In both situations there appears to be an overlap of values between normal and abnormal pregnancies. A low value may or may not identify a fetus at risk, and the degree of risk to the fetus is not a present calculable. The challenge to the obstetrician therefore is to determine in the presence of such low values the real risk to the fetus. When either tests reveals a low value, further testing is warranted.

Biophysical Evaluation

The ability of the fetus to survive and grow within the uterus depends on the transfer of numerous substances across the placenta. The placenta provides for nutritional support of the fetus and for transfer of those nutrients that are essential for its growth. The placenta can also be viewed as being a respiratory organ providing the gas exchange function necessary for the fetus to survive. Any severe change in this function will result in acute asphyxial stress to the fetus and can severely compromise its survival. Estriol is undoubtedly related to nutritional function. Respiratory function is generally assessed by changes in fetal heart rate.

Those conditions that categorize the high-risk pregnancy will either compromise the nutritional status of the placenta or its respiratory capability. Various tests are based on analysis of fetal heart rate and its patterns. In the past, the only means available to the physician to assess this parameter was auscultation. However, for a number of reasons this has not been an accurate predictor of fetal well-being. The procedure is episodic and depends on averaging of heart rate. It tells nothing about the pattern. Past biophysical methods used to measure the respiratory reserve of the placenta were the exercise stress test and the hypoxic stress test. They are not currently being used because of the difficulties in quantifying the amount of stress to the fetus, as well as difficulty in interpretation. The availability of continuous heart rate monitoring by external transducers, and the specificity of patterns found during labor, resulted in development of the contraction stress test and the nonstress test.

CONTRACTION STRESS TEST

The contraction stress test (CST) purports to measure the respiratory reserve of the

TABLE 2. INDICATIONS AND CONTRAINDICATIONS FOR CST

INDICATIONS	CONTRAINDICATIONS
Hypertension	Classic C section scar
Gestational	
Idiopathic	
Renal	
Diabetes mellitus	Incompetent cervix
IUGR	Multiple gestation
Congenital heart disease	Placenta previa
Postmaturity	Premature rupture of
	membranes
Metabolic maternal disease	
(SLE, thyroid, etc.)	
Previous stillbirth	
Low E_3	

placenta. Uterine contractions cause intermittent and transient decreases of uterine blood flow and therefore decrease intervillous space blood flow and maternal-fetal exchange. Consequently, the availability of oxygen to the fetus is decreased in direct proportion to the amplitude and duration of the uterine contractions.[22] This decrease in uteroplacental blood flow is only a transient phenomenon, and if the fetus is doing well this event is well tolerated. However, in those conditions in which uteroplacental insufficiency exists, with diminished functional capacity of the placenta, any further decrease of blood flow and availability of oxygen to the fetus will provoke a characteristic response—the late deceleration (see later discussion).

Indications for the CST include all those conditions in which the potential for uteroplacental insufficiency exists (Table 2). Contraindications to the CST include those conditions in which causing the stress of contractions to the uterus might provoke further complications (Table 2).

TECHNIQUE

Patients are kept in a stretcher bed or in a semi-sitting position to avoid the supine hypotensive syndrome. Initial blood pressure recordings are taken and a heart rate is recorded frequently, and the maternal heart rate is recorded throughout the test. The fetal heart rate pattern and baseline uterine activity recordings are obtained using the fetal electronic monitors presently available. The ultrasound transducers for taking the fetal heart rate have proved to be the best and most reliable means of assessing fetal heart rate patterns. These, however, do not give as clear

TABLE 3. INTERPRETATION OF CST

1. Positive: repetitive late decelerations
2. Negative: no late decelerations
3. Equivocal: late decelerations associated with UC's but not repetitive
4. Hyperstimulation: UC's > q 2 min
5. Unsatisfactory: insufficient contractions, poor recording

a recording as the abdominal wall EKG or microphone.

The goal of the test is to obtain 3 contractions in 10 minutes. This is an attempt to approximate a normal labor pattern. If before starting the oxytocin it is noted that the patient has spontaneous uterine activity that approximates the goal of the test, oxytocin is not started. If spontaneous uterine activity is not present, oxytocin is administered intravenously at a rate of 0.5 milliunits per minute, increasing every 20 minutes until there are 3 contractions in 10 minutes. It is recognized that with the tocodynamometer intrauterine pressure is not accurately determined. However, when the criterion for the test has been met, the test is considered complete and the oxytocin is discontinued. Once the infusion has been stopped, the patient continues to be monitored until contractions have returned to pretest levels.

INTERPRETATION

Interpretation of the CST is done according to Schifrin (Table 3). A vigorous attempt is made to find a "10-minute window," which fulfills the criteria for either a positive or a negative result. A positive window is based only on the presence of periodic late decelerations in the fetal heart rate pattern in relation to the contractions. It should be remembered that late decelerations are uniform, repetitive and reflect the intensity of the waveform of the associated uterine contractions. If both a positive and a negative 10-minute window are found in the same tracing, the positive test takes precedence. If both a negative 10-minute window and an equivocal test are found in the same tracing, the equivocal test is disregarded.

The absence of late decelerations in the face of hypertension is considered a negative test, whereas the presence of late decelerations in this situation cannot be accurately assessed and requires repeat testing. Likewise, equivocal and unsatisfactory tests must be repeated.

RESULTS

Negative. The likelihood of a fetus dying in utero within one week of a negative CST is remote.[23-26] A negative CST thus seems to be a reliable indicator of fetal well-being and suggests that no fetal indication for intervention likely exists. While examples of death within one week of a negative CST have been reported, most are related to trauma or other factors not predictable at the time of the test.

Positive. A positive CST is considered to represent uteroplacental insufficiency and suggests that the fetus is at increased risk. Indeed, in blinded studies about 25 per cent of babies with a positive result have died in the prenatal period. However, when a positive CST is used as an indicator for intervention, few babies die.[27, 28] This has tended to cloud the significance of a positive CST and raise the issue of false-positive results. It is recognized that a substantial rate of false-positive results for the CST does exist and approaches 50 per cent;[29] that is, despite a positive result, late decelerations are absent during labor. This constitutes one of the most serious limitations of the test.

ERRORS IN INTERPRETATION (Table 4)

False-Positive Results. False-positive results occur much more commonly than do false-negative results, and as shown in the table, can be due to several factors. The most common cause is uterine hypertonus produced by oxytocin administration. This can occur by overdosage of the oxytocin. The external transducer may not accurately reflect the actual amount of uterine activity. As the uterus approaches term, it becomes increasingly more sensitive to oxytocin, and there exists a variability from patient to patient in sensitivity of

TABLE 4. ERRORS IN CST INTERPRETATION

FALSE POSITIVES	FALSE NEGATIVES
Uterine hypertonus	Variable decelerations → cord accident
Supine hypotensive syndrome	Sudden maternal deterioration
Variable decelerations	Moribund fetus
Ultrasound "jitter"	Ultrasound "jitter"

the uterus to oxytocin. As a result, the stimulus given during the contraction stress test may be out of proportion to that which is desired to accomplish the goal of the test.

The supine position used for testing is another factor that may cause a false-positive result. The gravid uterus resting on the inferior vena cava diminishes venous return to the heart with subsequent decreased arterial blood pressure. The further stress of uterine contractions added to that of hypotension results in uteroplacental insufficiency and late decelerations. Variable decelerations may also be the cause of false-positive results. These decelerations by definition are variable in frequency, duration and waveform. They occur in 10 to 30 per cent of those patients tested and are more frequent than late decelerations. They may be misread as late decelerations if their waveform closely mimics that of late decelerations. Technical problems with the procedure may simulate a positive test. This is particularly true if the ultrasound transducer is applied so that adjustment of it may cause changes of the heart rate pattern that simulate late decelerations. However, this can usually be recognized by the amount of "jitter" in the tracing.

False-Negative Results. As mentioned previously, false-negative results do occur, albeit rarely.[30-32] These are usually caused by events not reflected in the clinical situation existing during the test. A sudden deterioration in a maternal condition could adversely affect the fetus. For example, in diabetes mellitus the fetus may be surviving at a point below the threshold at which a positive CST result is noted. However, a sudden deterioration in maternal homeostasis may produce fetal asphyxia and the fetus then is compromised in the week following a negative CST.

Rarely, a severely asphyxiated fetus may not show periodic decelerations. This is a paradoxical phenomenon that has several times been observed during labor.[33] It is conceivable that this situation could exist in the antepartum period, during which the fetus is so sick that it no longer has the ability to reset or control its own heart rate. The ultrasound transducer used in the testing procedure may introduce jitter into the signal received and therefore increase the apparent "variability" in the tracing as well as mask late decelerations that may occur with contractions of low amplitude.

The contraction stress test is a valuable tool for surveillance of the high-risk pregnancy. A negative result is a very good indicator of fetal well-being, with few false negatives. A positive result is suggestive of fetal jeopardy, although a high percentage of false positives does occur. Therefore, the challenge has been to further refine our testing techniques to exclude the possibilities of false-positive and false-negative results. A development has been the inclusion of the nonstress test, which can help identify the fetus at risk, into the testing procedure.

NONSTRESS TEST

The nonstress test (NST) was developed in conjunction with the contraction stress test. On the basis of an analysis of the baseline recordings preceding the CST, Lee,[34] Schifrin,[23] and Trierweiler[35] and their colleagues found that the presence of accelerations with fetal movement correlated well with the absence of late decelerations in the CST. It was further shown by Rochard et al.[36] that those fetuses with reactive heart rate patterns—that is, accelerations with fetal movement—tolerated labor well without distress 80 per cent of the time, and 100 per cent survived. This form of testing, which has become increasingly used, has several advantages. Neither stress nor stimuli is applied. It requires less time than the CST and is less inconvenient and less expensive. Like the CST, the results are available immediately and the test can be repeated or continued indefinitely.

With this test there is no attempt to separate the nutrient function from the respiratory function of the placenta; apparently it takes as its end point the effect of overall uteroplacental function on the central nervous system of the fetus. Transient accelerations of fetal heart rate with fetal movement as well as variability in heart rate suggests that the fetus has central nervous system control over those reflex mechanisms controlling heart rate. There is a fine tuning or interplay between the sympathetic and parasympathetic systems exerting control over the heart rate. It is believed that this ability of the fetus to control its heart rate pattern is a measure of the functional reserve of the fetus via its central nervous system. Under conditions of chronic stress, as might occur in hypoxia and acidosis secondary to decreased uteroplacental function, there will be a loss of this control and subsequently a loss of transient fetal accelerations with fetal movement. Physiologic changes such as sleep-like states may also diminish accelerations.

TABLE 5. NST CLASSIFICATION AND INTERPRETATION

	REACTIVE	NONREACTIVE	SINUSOIDAL
Baseline heart rate (bpm)	120–160	120–160	120–160
Accelerations (bpm)	≥15	<15	Absent
With fetal movement	≥2/10 min	<2/10 min	
Variability (bpm)	≥5–15	<10	Absent
Oscillations			
Frequency	—	—	2–5 bpm
Amplitude	—	—	5–15 bpm

Indications for the NST are identical to those in the CST—that is, any high-risk pregnancy in which the potential exists for decreased uteroplacental function, be it either nutritive or respiratory. At present there are no contraindications for the NST, a procedure with no potential for inducing contractions or premature labor.

TECHNIQUE AND INTERPRETATION
(Table 5)

The goal of the test is to obtain any 10-minute window in which there are 2 accelerations with fetal movement. The patient is positioned and the ultrasound transducer and tocodynamometer are applied as in the CST. The test is classified as "reactive" if 2 accelerations more than 15 beats per minute, and longer than 15 seconds in duration, occur with fetal movements in any 10-minute period. If this criterion for a reactive pattern is not met in 40 minutes total recording time, the test is interpreted as having a "nonreactive" pattern. It should be emphasized that the only criterion for a reactive or a nonreactive NST is the presence or absence of fetal accelerations with fetal movements. Although baseline bradycardia, tachycardia, and the presence or absence of presumed variability are noted, they are not taken as criteria for the test.

So-called sinusoidal patterns are occasionally seen, particularly in severe Rh hemolytic disease. Even so, accelerations meeting the goal of the test are classified as "reactive" in the presence of a sinusoidal rhythm.

TABLE 6. ERRORS IN NST INTERPRETATION

FALSE POSITIVES (NRNST)	FALSE NEGATIVES (RNST)
Sleep-wake cycle	Ultrasound "jitter"
Drugs	
Narcotics	
Barbiturates	

False-positive and false-negative results in the nonstress test do occur (Table 6). A false abnormal NST can occur during fetal sleep-like states. It has been observed that fetuses go through sleep-wake cycles that can be 30 to 40 minutes in length. The testing procedure of 40 minutes should overcome this problem, and stimulation of the fetus may wake it from its sleep cycle so that a reactive NST is obtained.

Drugs such as narcotics and barbiturates can depress the fetal central nervous system, producing a false nonreactive NST. It has been our experience that usually one can "read through" the depressive effects of drugs on the fetus to obtain an accurate test. In the majority of instances a nonreactive test *does not* indicate that an abnormality exists. This test result is nondiagnostic and warrants use of other methods of evaluation.

False-negative results—false reactive NST—can occur with the jitter induced by ultrasound transducer. Again this can usually be determined during the testing procedure and corrections made so that an accurate result is obtained. As with the CST, false-normal results are rare, and the majority are related to events that cannot be reasonably predicted at the time of testing.

RESULTS OF NST AND COMBINED TESTING WITH CST (Table 7)

The results of the combined testing procedures are shown in Table 7. This is based on analysis of over 4500 tests performed on 2003 patients.[37] As can be seen, those features with a reactive NST demonstrated the least perinatal morbidity and mortality. Irrespective of the end point chosen (death, respiratory distress syndrome, positive CST) babies demonstrating a reactive pattern have the best correlation with good outcome, and the results would appear to be at least as good as those

TABLE 7. Combined NST/CST Results

	Patients	Late Decelerations		IUGR		RDS		Congenital Anomaly		Death	
		No.	Percentage*	No.	Percentage	No.	Percentage	No.	Percentage	No.	Percentage
Reactive/negative	172	8	5.3	6	3.5	2	1.2	6	3.5	2	1.2
Reactive/positive	4	0	0.0	0	0.0	0	0.0	0	0.0	0	0.0
Nonreactive/negative	82	5	7.0	2	2.4	2	2.4	2	2.4	4	4.9
Nonreactive/positive	8	2	33.3	2	25.0	1	12.5	1	12.5	2	25.0

*Of those monitored.

demonstrating a negative CST. It also is noted that the combination of a nonreactive NST and a positive CST results in more ominous outcome, as these babies fared the worst. Those babies who had a nonreactive NST and a negative CST did worse than those that had just a reactive NST. We think that the combined test procedure can reduce the incidence of false-positive results obtained in the CST with use of the NST prior to its institution, as well as lessen the rate of false-positive results in the NST. A reactive NST is the best indicator of fetal well-being and eliminates the need for a CST. While the nonreactive NST helps identify a large group of fetuses who are at risk for placental insufficiency, it is nondiagnostic and requires confirmation with a follow-up CST. In the event of a nonreactive NST combined with a positive CST, the situation is ominous for the fetus. While this situation further defines the fetus at risk, neither abnormal result alone or in combination is as good a predictor of bad outcome as a reactive NST is of good outcome.

PROTOCOL OF HIGH-RISK PREGNANCY

On the basis of this experience, we use the following protocol for managing a high-risk pregnancy (Fig. 2). The basic premise of this protocol is that those biophysical and biochemical methods used to assess fetal well-being appear to be effective predictors of good outcome, but that any single parameter used is not nearly as good an indicator that the fetus is in jeopardy. We believe that the protocol can be adapted to any pregnancy deemed to be at high risk. Irrespective of which test is used as the initial screening procedure, the very nature of the protocol ensures closer medical supervision, which appears to improve perinatal outcome. Therefore, the scheme of the protocol serves two basic purposes: in the presence of normal tests it reassures the obstetrician that there is no need for intervention, and the combination of these tests helps to decrease the overall incidence of false-positive results, which would demand intervention that could prove unnecessary.

The fetus that has a nonreactive NST and a positive contraction test is delivered if the lecithin/sphingomyelin (L/S) ratio is greater than 2. In the face of an L/S ratio less than 2, indicating pulmonary immaturity, another parameter is used, such as evaluation of plasma or urinary estriol. If these levels are also falling, both parameters are taken as indicative of fetal distress and the fetus is delivered regardless of pulmonary immaturity. However, if the second parameter does not confirm the first, it is elected to wait until pulmonary maturity is achieved.

Summary

With pulmonary immaturity and only one parameter suggesting fetal jeopardy, constant supervision is carried out until either a second parameter supports the first or until pulmonary maturity is obtained. Under this scheme we believe we can more precisely identify those babies that are in jeopardy. Further studies using this particular approach are continuing, in order to further evaluate its effect on improving perinatal outcome.

REFERENCES

1. Scommegna, A.: Clinical uses of estriol essays. *In* Wynn, R. M. (ed.): Obstetrics and Gynecology Annual, Vol. 2. New York, Appleton-Century-Crofts, 1973.
2. Beischer, N. A. and Brown, J. B.: Current status of estrogen assays in obstetrics and gynecology. Obstet. Gynecol. Rev. 27:303, 1972.
3. Goebelsman, U., Freeman, R. K., Mestman, J. H., Nakamura, R. M. and Woodling, B. A.: Estriol in Pregnancy. II. Daily urine estriol assays in the management of the pregnant diabetic women. Am. J. Obstet. Gynecol. 115:795, 1973.
4. Kahn, C. B., White, P. and Younger, D.: Laboratory assessment of diabetic pregnancy; a brief review. Diabetes 21:31, 1972.
5. Duenhoelter, J. H., Whalley, P. J. and MacDonald, P. C.: An analysis of the utility of plasma immunoreactive estrogen measurements in determining delivery time of gravidas with a fetus considered at high risk. Am. J. Obstet. Gynecol. 125:889, 1976.
6. Sprague, A. D., Duhring, J. L., Moser, R. J. and Hollingsworth, D.: Maternal and fetal levels of HCS in preeclampsia. Obstet. Gynecol. 41:770, 1973.
7. Samaan, N., Yen, S. C. C. and Gonzales, D.: Metabolic effects of placental lactogen in man. 48th Annual Meeting of the Endocrine Society, Chicago, 1966.
8. Samaan, N., Yen, S. C., Gonzales D. and Pearson, O. H.: Metabolism effects of placental lactogen in man. J. Clin. Endocrinol. 28:485, 1968.
9. Turtle, J. R. and Kipnus, D. M.: The lipolytic action of human placental lactogen on isolated fat cells. Biochim. Biophys. Acta 144:583, 1967.
10. Prieto, J. C., Cifuentes, I. and Serrano-Rios, M.: HCS regulation during pregnancy. Obstet. Gynecol. 48:297, 1976.
11. Kuhl, C., Gaede, P., Kelbe, J. G. and Pedersen, J.: Human placental lactogen concentration during

physiological fluctuations of serum glucose in normal pregnant and gestational diabetic women. Acta Endocrinol. 80:365, 1975.

12. Gaspard, U., Sandrout, H. and Luyckx, A.: Glucose-insulin interaction and the modulation of human placental lactogen during pregnancy. J. Obstet. Gynecol. Br. Commonwealth 81:201, 1974.

13. Spellacy, W. N., Carlson, K. L. and Birk, S. A.: Dynamics of human placental lactogen. Am. J. Obstet. Gynecol. 96:1164, 1966.

14. Teoh, E. S., Spellacy, W. N. and Buhi, W. C.: Human chorionic somatomammotropin: a new index of placental function. J. Obstet. Gynecol. Br. Commonwealth 78:673, 1971.

15. Spellacy, W. N., Teoh, E. S., Buhi, W. C., Birk, S. A. and McCreary, S. A.: Value of human chorionic somatomammotropin in managing high-risk pregnancies. Am. J. Obstet. Gynecol. 109:588, 1971.

16. Spellacy, W. N., Buhi, W. C. and Birk, S. A.: The effectiveness of human placental lactogen as an adjunct in decreasing perinatal deaths. Am. J. Obstet. Gynecol. 121:835, 1975.

17. Kelly, A. M., England, P., Lorimer, J. D., Ferguson, J. C. and Goran, A. D. T.: An evaluation of human placental lactogen levels in hypertension of pregnancy. Br. J. Obstet. Gynecol. 82:272, 1975.

18. Spellacy, W. N., Buhi, W. C. and Birk, S. A.: Human placental lactogen and intrauterine growth retardation. Obstet. Gynecol. 47:446, 1976.

19. Genazzani, A. R., Cocola, F., Neri, P. and Fioretti, P.: Human chorionic somatomammotropin (HCS) plasma levels in normal and pathological pregnancies and their correlation with placental function. Acta Endocrinol. (Suppl.) 167:5, 1972.

20. Berkowitz, R. L. and Hobbins, J. C.: A re-evaluation of the value of HCS determination in the management of prolonged pregnancy. Obstet. Gynecol. 49:156, 1977.

21. Soler, N. G., Nicholson, H. O. and Malins, J. M.: Serial determinations of human placental lactogen in the management of diabetic pregnancy. Lancet 2:54, 1975.

22. Martin, C. B.: Uterine blood flow and uterine contractions in monkeys. Clin. Res. 20:282, 1972.

23. Schifrin, B. S., Lapidus, M., Doctor, G. S. et al.: Contraction stress test for antepartum fetal evaluation. Obstet. Gynecol. 45:433, 1975.

24. Hayden, B. L., Simpson, J. L., Ewing, D. E. et al.: Can the oxytocin challenge test serve as the primary method for managing high-risk pregnancies? Obstet. Gynecol. 46:251, 1975.

25. Ray, M., Freeman, R., Pine, S. et al.: Clinical experience with the oxytocin challenge test. Am. J. Obstet. Gynecol. 114:1, 1972.

26. Ewing, D. E., Farina, J. R. and Otterson, W. N.: Clinical application of the oxytocin challenge test. Obstet. Gynecol. 43:563, 1974.

27. Cooper, J. M., Soffronoff, E. C. and Bolognese, R. J.: Oxytocin challenge test in monitoring high-risk pregnancies. Obstet. Gynecol. 45:27, 1975.

28. Freeman, R. K.: The use of the oxytocin challenge test for antepartum clinical evaluation of uteroplacental respiratory function. Am. J. Obstet. Gynecol. 121:481, 1975.

29. Freeman, R. K., Goebelsman, U., Nochimson, D. and Cetrulo, C.: An evaluation of the significance of a positive oxytocin challenge test. Obstet. Gynecol. 47:8, 1976.

30. Klapholz, H. and Burke, L.: Intrauterine fetal demise with a negative oxytocin challenge test. J. Reprod. Med. 15:169, 1975.

31. Freeman, R. K. and James, J.: Clinical experience with the oxytocin challenge test. II. An ominous atypical pattern. Obstet. Gynecol. 46:255, 1975.

32. Egley, C. C. and Suzuki, K.: Intrauterine fetal demise after negative oxytocin challenge tests. Obstet. Gynecol. 50 (Suppl. 1):54–57, 1977.

33. Cetrulo, C. L. and Schifrin, B. S.: Fetal heart rate patterns preceeding death in utero. Obstet. Gynecol. 48:523, 1976.

34. Lee, C., Di Loreto, P. C. and Logrand, B.: Fetal activity acceleration determination for the evaluation of fetal reserve. Obstet. Gynecol. 48:19, 1976.

35. Trierweiler, M. W., Freeman, R. K. and James, J.: Baseline fetal heart rate characteristics as an indicator of fetal status during the antepartum period. Am. J. Obstet. Gynecol. 125:618, 1976.

36. Rochard, F., Schifrin, B. S., Sureau, C., Marceau, P. and Vaquier, J.: Non-stressed fetal heart rate monitoring in the antepartum period. Am. J. Obstet. Gynecol. 126:699, 1976.

37. Schifrin, B. S., Foye, G., Amato, J., Kates, R. and McKenna, J.: Routine fetal heart rate monitoring in the antepartum period. Obstet. Gynecol. 54:21, 1979.

Addendum

Recent studies have suggested that real-time ultrasound scanning may add considerable dimension to the dynamic assessment of fetal well-being.[1-6] In addition to facilitating measurement of fetal growth parameters and determining placental location and amniotic fluid volume, high resolution, real-time ultrasound units permit visualization of other fetal activities, such as fetal breathing and body movements, and fetal tone. In addition, we may observe fetal sucking, swallowing, micturition, and periocular or facial movement with repetitive tongue extension. The investigation of these latter activities is still in the research stage, but they give a clue to the enormous potential of contemporary ultrasonic surveillance techniques.

Manning and Schifrin and their colleagues have demonstrated a high correlation between the presence of fetal body movements, fetal breathing movements, fetal tone, normal amniotic fluid volume, and normal fetal outcome.[2-6] Manning and Platt have formalized these five parameters (including accelerations of the fetal heart rate from the NST) into the Biophysical Profile and presented a system for its quantification (Table 7).[3, 4] While these authors have found a progressive deterioration in fetal outcome with decreasing score, Schifrin et al. found that presence of any dynamic parameter is as reliable a predictor of fetal well-being as the reactive NST.[5] Manning et

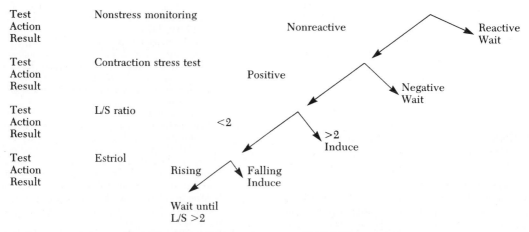

Figure 2. Protocol for management of high-risk pregnancy.

al. consider the Biophysical Profile the primary screening test for high-risk pregnancies, while Schifrin et al. utilize it for evaluation of the nonreactive NST or when other conditions dictate its use (see below). Despite these differences in approach to primary screening, both groups find that perinatal outcome is improved by the addition of Biophysical Profile testing.[2–6]

There is an important theoretical advantage of dynamic testing over other popular tests. Fetal body and breathing movements, like the heart rate response to endogenous or exogenous stimuli, are neither random nor purposeless. Rather, they represent activities and responses modulated by complex, integrated central nervous system mechanisms. As a result, like the reactive NST, normal responses are considered reliable predictors of fetal wellbeing. On the other hand, the absence of a given response or activity may represent asphyxia, but more commonly it represents either sleep state or the effect of medication.

There is a general consensus that assessment of amniotic fluid volume may be of considerable assistance in the evaluation of certain high-risk pregnancies irrespective of the results of dynamic testing.[1, 4–6] Qualitative analysis of amniotic fluid volume has proved useful in detecting intrauterine growth failure and is recommended (1) when uterine size is disproportional to estimated gestational age, (2) when intrauterine growth failure is suspected, (3) when variable decelerations are encountered on the NST or CST, and (4) when pregnancy extends beyond the expected delivery date. Increasingly, the detection of decreased amniotic fluid volume late in pregnancy is considered an indication for termination of pregnancy.

The virtues of ultrasound examination are not limited to the assessment of dynamic parameters and amniotic fluid volume. Indeed, careful ultrasound examination will also provide information on fetal growth, relationship of abdomen to head, placental grade and maturity, and the presence of certain anomalies. While these parameters are not, strictly speaking, included in the Biophysical Profile, they are available with minimal additional effort.

Adoption of the Biophysical Profile has decreased the reliance on both hormonal tests such as estriol and the contraction stress test.[4-6] The ultimate benefits of these tests, especially in low-risk patients, remain to be elucidated.

REFERENCES

1. Manning, F. A., Hill, L. M. and Platt, L. D.: Antepartum detection of IUGR: Use of qualitative amniotic fluid volume. Am. J. Obstet. Gynecol. 139:254, 1981.
2. Manning, F. A., Morrison, I. and Lange, I.: Fetal biophysical profile scoring: A prospective study in 1184 high-risk patients. Am. J. Obstet. Gynecol. 140:289, 1981.
3. Manning, F. A., Platt, L. D. and Sipos, L.: Antepartum fetal evaluation: Development of a fetal biophysical profile score. Am. J. Obstet. Gynecol. 136:787, 1980.
4. Manning, F. A., Morrison, I., Lange, I. R. and Harman, C.: Antepartum determination of fetal health: Composite biophysical profile scoring. Clin. Perinatol. 9:285, 1982.
5. Schifrin, B. S. et al.: The role of real-time scanning in antenatal fetal surveillance. Am. J. Obstet. Gynecol. 140:525, 1981.
6. Eden, R. D., Gersely, R. Z. and Schifrin, B. S.: Comparison of antepartum testing schemes for the management of the postdate pregnancy. Am. J. Obstet. Gynecol. (In press).

Antepartum Fetal Monitoring: The Optimal Method and Role

Roger K. Freeman, M.D.

Thomas J. Garite, M.D.

University of California, Irvine

There are two methods of antepartum evaluation using fetal heart rate monitoring currently in use, the contraction stress test (CST) and the nonstress test (NST). The CST (also known as the oxytocin challenge test [OCT]) came about from the independent observations of Hammacher,[1] Kubli,[2] and Pose,[3] who demonstrated that antepartum patients with late decelerations of the fetal heart rate in response to spontaneous or oxytocin-induced contractions had an increased incidence of fetal asphyxia and fetal death. Subsequently, Ray et al.[4] outlined clearcut methods and end points with the first systematic clinical trial of the CST. They demonstrated that such testing could allow the clinician to prevent antepartum fetal death. Many others have since documented the reliability of this method.[5-19]

During subsequent clinical trials of the CST, various investigators recognized that accelerations of the fetal heart rate in response to fetal movement (called reactivity) indicated fetal well-being and the absence of these accelerations had a high correlation with poor outcome.[2, 13, 20, 21] As a result of these observations, clinical trials have suggested that the NST may be a reasonable primary means of antepartum fetal surveillance with contraction stress testing as a back-up method when the fetus is nonreactive, since sleep-like states may produce a loss of reactivity without fetal distress.[22-27]

The question is which of these tests (CST or NST) serves as a better primary means of antepartum fetal surveillance in the at-risk patient. Specifically, it would be useful to know whether late deceleration is a better end point than loss of fetal reactivity. In this article we discuss the various obvious and noncontroversial advantages and disadvantages of stress as opposed to nonstress testing. A review of the literature and supportive data from our more recent experience are presented, and controversy about advantages and disadvantages is discussed in light of available published studies. We will then attempt to draw conclusions and perhaps pose new questions. Furthermore, an attempt will be made to define the role of antepartum monitoring, since not only the methods of testing but the reasons for it are controversial.

The CST clearly has some disadvantages. It is a time-consuming test, taking an average of 90 minutes to perform. A specially trained nurse or technician must have experience and patience in performing the test, which should be done in a quiet area separate from those of labor and delivery. Oxytocin usually must be given and because there is a theoretical risk of precipitating premature labor, certain situations contraindicate testing (e.g., multiple gestation). In studies in which this problem has been examined, however, there is no evidence of any risk of premature labor from the CST in patients who were not already at high risk for premature labor.[4, 7, 13, 18, 28] With the CST there is a small but significant number of unsatisfactory or equivocal tests, necessitating repeating of the test in 24 hours. Each of these disadvantages makes the test relatively expensive. Late decelerations, the end point of the CST, may at times be subtle and difficult to read or be masked by noisy Doppler tracings. Late decelerations may be caused by other factors, including the maternal supine hypotension syndrome. This last factor and some other unknowns create the problem that causes the CST the most criticism: false-positive results. While the definition is not totally agreed upon, a false-positive result is defined as a positive CST followed by labor that the fetus tolerates without late deceleration. The frequency of this problem is reported to range from 8 to 57 per cent, with an average of about 25 per cent.[11, 14, 18, 19, 28]

Many of these disadvantages are not present with the NST; it takes from one third to one half the time to perform. It does not require experience or patience to perform as is true with stress testing. There are no contraindications to testing, and because no oxytocin is required, there is not even the theoretical risk of causing premature labor. Equivocal results are not generally a problem. Accelerations of the fetal heart rate are not as subtle as late decelerations and are not generally subject to masking by noisy Doppler tracings. Finally,

TABLE 1. Studies Using The CST as Primary Means of Fetal Surveillance

Author	Year	No. Patients Studied	No. With Negative Tests	False Negatives
Spurrett et al.[18]	1971	193	170	0
Ray et al.[4]	1972	68	43	0
Christie and Cudmore[8]	1974	50	35	0
Boyd et al.[7]	1974	41	36	1
Ewing et al.[10]	1974	58	49	0
Cooper et al.[9]	1975	89	66	0
Schifrin et al.[17]	1975	120	101	0
Gaziano et al.[15]	1975	72	64	0
Hayden et al.[16]	1975	105	97	0
Weingold et al.[19]	1975	154	109	0
Freeman et al.[28]	1976	390	324	2
Farahani et al.[11]	1976	333	288	1
Boehm et al.[6]	1976	152	137	2
Fox et al.[13]	1976	209	163	0
Bhakthavathsalan et al.[5]	1976	100	68	0
Garite et al.[14]	1978	430	403	0
*Baskett[35]	1975	Not stated	205	2
*Marcum[36]	1977	Not stated	140	1

False-negative rate = 9/2498 patients with negative tests = 3.6/1000.
*Studies published as case reports in which total number of patients with negative tests are stated.

false-positive results in NST are probably not nearly as serious a problem as false-positive results in contraction stress testing. This is because the nonreactive NST is nearly always checked with a CST; if indeed the CST is positive, one therefore has (by definition) a nonreactive positive, which both Braly[29] and Fox[13] have shown less likely to be falsely positive.

Why then, with all these stated advantages of the NST over the CST, should obstetricians not just use the NST as the primary means of fetal surveillance and keep the CST in reserve for the nonreactive fetus? Several authorities have recommended this approach,[20, 24, 27] and it is our impression that this may be a popular trend.

To determine if there are any overriding advantages to the CST, we surveyed the available literature. The CST is by far the better tested method. Table 1 illustrates the number of reported series and the number of patients tested. The overall experience in the literature is in excess of 2500 patients. The authors reporting their results with few exceptions use a uniform definition for end points and results, conforming to those originally described by Ray and Freeman,[4] and use similar time intervals between tests, i.e., one week between negative and one day between equivocal stress tests. While six or seven years does not mean that the method has stood the test of time, generally reliable and consistent results cer-

tainly substantiate the CST as a valuable means of antepartum monitoring. That the test achieves its primary goal is illustrated in Tables 1 and 2. This goal is to avoid fetal death. In 2498 patients at risk for fetal death secondary to uteroplacental insufficiency (UPI), only 9 deaths (3.6/1000) have been reported with a negative test. Of these 9 instances of fetal death, at least 2 probably involved suspicious tests in retrospect, and at least 4 others had explanations for fetal death other than UPI. The NST, in contrast, is less well evaluated (Table 3), especially considering that in only a few of the studies[24, 26, 30] have

TABLE 2. False-Negative Contraction Stress Tests

Apparent Cause	Time Interval Between CST and Fetal Death
Thrombosis of chroionic vessels	7 days
Tight nuchal cord — several loops	Not specified
Multiple congenital anomalies	Not specified
Multiple congenital anomalies*	7 days
Abruptio placenta	5 days
No apparent cause	5 days
No apparent cause	7 days
No apparent cause (associated with acute lowering of blood pressure with hypotensive agents)	7 days
No apparent cause*	13 hours

*Test probably suspicious in review.

TABLE 3. STUDIES USING NST AS PRIMARY MEANS OF FETAL SURVEILLANCE

Author	Year	No. Patients	No. With Negative Tests	False Negatives	End point of NST	Duration of Test	Frequency of Testing	OCT Backup
Lee et al.[20]	1976	410	406	1	3–4 AFM/15 min	30 min ?	Weekly	Yes
Rochard et al.[25]	1976	125	51	0	HR <120> 160 6 BPM/LTV No AFM Scoring system	30 min ?	Not stated	No
Kubli et al.[31] (low-risk patients only)	1977	1320	1228	1	Scoring system	30 min average	Hours to every 3 weeks	No
Kubli et al.[31] (abnormal tests only)	1977	65	0	NA	Scoring system	30 min average	Hours to every 3 weeks	No
Visser/Huijes[27]	1977	428*	369	0	Absent BL, irregularity or deceleration	20 min ?	Hours to weekly	No
Tushuizen et al.[26]	1977	369	320	1	HR <120> 160 Deceleration of 30 sec + 30 BPM No BTB variability and no AFM	30 min ?	Once or twice/week or daily if abnormal	No
Flynn/Kelly[30]	1977	301	245	0	4 AFM of 15 BPM in 20 min	20–40 min	Weekly if normal	?
Krebs/Petres[22]	1978	253	219	?	5 AFM of 10 BPM in 30 min	30 min ?	Weekly if normal 1 to 3 days if abnormal	No
Nochimson et al.[24]	1978	301	245	0	4 AFM of 15 BPM in 20 min	20–40 min	Not stated	Yes

*Reported an additional 26 patients with "terminal patterns."
Abbreviations: AFM, accelerations with fetal movement; BPM, beats per minute; BL, baseline; LTV, long-term variability; HR, heart rate.

the results systematically been used to manage the patients. Furthermore, since different authors are using such a variety of end points (Table 3) and a different frequency of testing and duration of testing, it is not really valid to collectively compare these various NST studies with the more consistent CST studies. Even so, a normal or reactive NST appears to be similarly reassuring and achieves the same goal as a CST, that of avoiding intrauterine fetal deaths. There have been only 2 fetal deaths in 1380 high-risk patients with reactive tests, as could be gathered from these studies.[23-27, 31]

Certain authors suggest that because the NST correlates better with poor outcome than the CST does, the NST is a more reliable test and because it is simpler, it should be the primary method.[27] Another way of looking at the same facts is that perhaps the CST gives an earlier warning of the fetus in jeopardy and that in waiting for the fetus to become nonreactive, it is more likely that irreversible asphyxic damage has taken place by this time. There are several arguments to support this latter contention and in the following paragraphs we will evaluate them.

First, it is logical from what is known of the physiology of fetal heart rate that late decelerations precede loss of variability. It would seem that in a marginal state, a potentially compromised fetus might show the effects of hypoxia during the stress of uterine contrac-

tions, and the associated diminution in uterine blood flow. This would be analogous to a stress EKG or treadmill. Myers[32] has shown that hypoxia alone can cause late decelerations. Certainly, hypoxia and acidosis will cause late decelerations and make them more pronounced, but Paul[33] has demonstrated that loss of variability of the fetal heart rate, in the presence of late decelerations, may correlate more closely with the degree of fetal acidemia. Therefore, one might reason that loss of reactivity would be a later stage than development of late decelerations without loss of variability or reactivity. It is not clear where fetal heart rate accelerations fit into this picture, but they do seem to go hand-in-hand with variability because often late decelerations are seen with accelerations present, but rarely if ever are accelerations seen with the so-called smooth baseline.

When nonstress testing is the primary means of fetal surveillance, one would do a CST only when the NST is nonreactive, and intervention would be carried out only with a nonreactive NST followed by a positive CST. This is because a reactive NST is interpreted as negative or normal and the CST is not done. Therefore, one would never see the reactive NST and positive CST. Indeed, as Braly[29] has shown, one might eliminate false-positive CST results in this manner but one might also miss earlier warning signs of fetal jeopardy.

TABLE 4. STUDIES REPORTING OUTCOME IN PATIENTS WITH POSITIVE CSTs

PRIMARY AUTHOR	No. PATIENTS	No. POSITIVE TESTS	STILLBIRTHS	NEONATAL DEATHS	5-MINUTE APGAR <7
Spurrett[18]	193	23	2	NR*	13
Ray[16]†	68	15	3	0	5
Christie[8]	50	9	0	0	0
Boyd[7]	41	5	0	1	2
Ewing[10]	58	8	0	1	1
Cooper[9]	89	13	0	0	0
Freeman[28]	390	66	6‡	4	13
Schifrin[17]	120	9	2	0	3
Gaziano[15]	72	7	0	0	2
Hayden[16]	105	8	0	0	0
Weingold[19]	154	14	2§	1	NR
Farahani[11]	333	24	1	1	2
Boehm[6]	152	10	1	0	1
Fox[13]	209	17	0	0	4
Bhakthavathsalan[5]	100	10	1	0	1
Garite[14]	430	10	3	0	NR

*Not reported.
†Blinded study.
‡Three of 6 occurred during blinded portion of study.
§Both occurred 5 days after a positive test.

TABLE 5. STUDIES REPORTING OUTCOME IN PATIENTS WITH NONREACTIVE NSTs

PRIMARY AUTHOR	NO. OF PATIENTS	NO. NONREACTIVE TESTS	STILLBIRTHS	NEONATAL DEATHS	5-MINUTE APGAR <7
Rochard[25]*	125	51	13	3	NR†
Kubli[31] (low-risk patients only)	1320	92	3	4	NR
Kubli[31] (abnormal tests only)	65	65	NR	7	32
Visser[27]	428	59	NR	NR	3
	26‡	26	9	3	NR
Krebs[22]	253	34	"52% perinatal morbidity and mortality"		
Tushuizen[26]	369	49	NR	7	6
Flynn[30]	301	56	4	1	13
Nochimson[24]	421	12	0	0	0

*Partially blinded study.
†Not reported.
‡Additional 26 patients reported with nonreactive tests only.

Comparing outcome in patients managed primarily with CST as opposed to those managed with NST using the available literature is an extremely difficult task. If one examines Tables 4 and 5, showing outcome with nonreactive and positive tests, one can immediately see that authors do not uniformly report outcome. Furthermore, many of these studies were either blinded[4, 25] or the results of the tests not uniformly used for patient management.[27, 31] And as previously mentioned, the NST studies are quite heterogeneous because of differing end points used for positive (or nonreactive) tests. With these limitations in mind, we can compare outcomes in those studies in which (1) high-risk patients only are tested, (2) the number of positive and negative tests are reported, and (3) outcome is stated specifically for positive (or nonreactive) tests. With the criteria in Table 6, the perinatal mortality rates for both the overall populations and specifically for the groups with positive CSTs and nonreactive NSTs are essentially the same. The incidence of low 5-minute Apgar scores in both groups are also similar. However, for the CST studies there is a disproportionately higher stillbirth rate in the positive group. This implies either that the tests were not used for management (as in Weingold's study in which five days elapsed between a positive test and each of the two stillbirths)[19] or that the result was weighed against other factors such as maturity.

Another way of looking at this question is to take studies in which outcome between patients with nonreactive and reactive positive tests were compared. As stated previously, if the NST is used for management, with the CST reserved as a back-up for the nonreactive tests, the nonreactive positive CST group would represent outcome for the NST and the combined nonreactive and reactive positive would represent outcome for the CST. Fox et al.[13] found a 100 per cent (7/7) neonatal morbidity with a nonreactive positive compared to 30 per cent (3/10) with a reactive positive. Braly and Freeman[29] showed a definite higher rate of perinatal mortality, low Apgar scores and intrapartum fetal distress in the nonreac-

TABLE 6. EVALUATION OF OUTCOME:*
POSITIVE CST VS. NONREACTIVE NST

	FOR TOTAL POPULATION	FOR PATIENTS WITH POSITIVE TEST ONLY
OCT		
Perinatal mortality rate†	10	97
Neonatal mortality rate	6	62
Low Apgar rate	16	156
NST		
Perinatal mortality rate	7	74
Neonatal mortality rate	7	68
Low Apgar rate	17	162

*Includes those studies in which:
1. Results were used for patient management
2. Outcome was stated
3. Total number of patients tested was stated
4. High-risk patients were tested only
References:
   CST 4–11, 13–19, 28
   NST 24, 26, 30 (Refer to Tables 4 and 5)
†All rates are per thousand.

tive positive than in the reactive positive group. Farahani[12] found that absence of reactivity in the fetus with a positive CST result was more strongly correlated with stigmata of placental dysfunction, including low Apgar scores, thick meconium and dysmaturity than the group with the reactive positive CSTs.

The final argument that suggests late decelerations may be an earlier warning sign than the loss of reactivity is a rather complex one. If as a fetus becomes compromised in utero it manifests this compromise by late decelerations or by loss of reactivity randomly or variably with the specific variety of pathophysiology, then both nonreactive negative tests and reactive positive tests are seen. Another way of saying this is that loss of reactivity should be seen in the absence of late decelerations equally as frequently as late decelerations in the presence of accelerations are seen. This does not seem to be the case. Nochimson[24] in his article on nonstress testing stated that all patients with a nonreactive NST followed by a negative CST developed fetal reactivity during the CST. He no longer even continues the CST if the fetus becomes reactive with administration of the oxytocin. We reviewed our own data from Women's Hospital, Memorial Medical Center of Long Beach; our findings are similar. The nonreactive negative CST that remains nonreactive during the contraction period is virtually nonexistent. We have seen only two cases: one in which the newborn had multiple neurologic and cardiac congenital abnormalities and one in which the mother was heavily drugged with phenobarbital. The reactive positive CST, on the other hand, is a frequent finding.[12, 13, 29] This suggests that late decelerations precede loss of reactivity and therefore are an earlier sign of fetal jeopardy.

It is clear that evaluation of the antepartum fetal heart rate, whether by CST or NST, is a sensitive but not totally specific means of surveillance. Therefore, abnormal tests are variably predictive while a normal test is highly reliable. It has also been shown that perinatal mortality may be reduced for these high-risk populations by such antepartum testing.[14] The advantages of fetal heart rate testing over biochemical means of fetal evaluation, such as testing HPL or estriol, is that results are immediately available and within the limits of the tests are not subject to laboratory or patient error. What is not clear is which of the methods—CST or NST—shows earlier

signs of fetal jeopardy and therefore should be the primary means of antepartum fetal evaluation.

We have discussed in detail the various advantages and disadvantages of each test. The CST is definitely more cumbersome, time-consuming and expensive and has contraindications not present with the NST. However, the NST has its limitations also. The end points of the NST are not well agreed upon, with some investigators using accelerations of the fetal heart rate, some using variability, or some a combination thereof. The number of accelerations and amplitude of accelerations that are necessary to constitute a reactive test are not universally agreed upon. Frequency of testing is also different from study to study.

There are several factors to suggest that the CST may be an earlier warning sign of the fetus in jeopardy than the NST. This theoretically could allow the clinician to intervene before any permanent or irreversible damage might be done to the fetus. While admittedly many of the positive CSTs may be false, it is a matter of philosophy as to whether one would accept some false-positives as the price to pay for earlier warning. It must be emphasized that the results of any single test must be used in conjunction with the clinical situation. For example, in the patient with postterm pregnancy, one would want the earliest possible warning of fetal jeopardy, since the risk of unnecessary harmful premature intervention is essentially nil. On the other hand, a reactive positive CST in the chronic hypertensive at 28 weeks' gestation might be a warning to perform more frequent NSTs or estriol tests, even on a daily basis, to buy time but to intervene before the fetus is totally nonreactive. This illustrates the concept of using the patient as her own control and watching trends in reactivity. With the CST all the possible fetal heart rate data are available, including late decelerations, reactivity and accelerations evoked by contractions in the previously nonreactive fetus.

The contention that the CST gives an earlier warning sign is admittedly not clearly proved. The theoretical pathophysiology and the fact that nonreactive CSTs are virtually nonexistent as previously described certainly argue in favor of this point. However, outcome data are somewhat unclear if not contradictory. Outcome is not different if NST and CST studies are compared with each other, but if nonreactive positive CST outcome (which is the end point of the NST in essence) is compared with a reactive positive CST, there is clearly poorer outcome in the nonreactive positive group.

One may see a significantly higher incidence of congenital anomalies in patients with non-reactive NSTs or positive CSTs or both. This was first suggested as a possibility of Spurett,[18] and in a recent study, Garite et al.[34] have shown a significantly higher incidence of cesarean section, especially for fetal distress (both antepartum and intrapartum), in mothers of fetuses with major congenital anomalies.

The primary goal of antepartum testing generally agreed upon is to avert fetal death. A recent study by Garite[14] showed that patients who were studied with the CST for high-risk indications had no fetal deaths, while there were 30 fetal deaths among 4920 patients who were not studied but were from the same hospital population. There were no deaths from inappropriate premature intervention. Retrospective analysis revealed that even though the fetal death rate in the patients who were not followed with contraction stress testing was only 5.1/1000, fully one third of these patients had indications for this surveillance. These data suggest that stillbirths may be significantly reduced in a high-risk population if CST surveillance is systematically done. Moreover, while there are no data to indicate a reduction in developmental disabilities in these offspring, it would stand to reason that, if stillbirth is prevented, there may also be a reduction in anoxic morbidity with appropriate intervention as the fetus's condition is deteriorating. It would seem that once the fetus is mature, the test that gives the earlier warning sign would be preferable.

Some authors[11] suggest that the ability of the fetus to tolerate labor should also be a goal because they define failure of a contraction stress test to identify fetuses that develop distress in labor as a false-negative. If the test was used to decide which patient to monitor intrapartum, this might be a reasonable goal. However, since high-risk patients are generally monitored, this is probably not a valid goal.

Finally, and most significantly, it should be the goal of antepartum testing to allow the clinician to avoid inappropriatelytimed intervention. Such conditions as IUGR and the post-term pregnancy have a high percentage of clinical misdiagnosis. Not all patients with diabetes or hypertension or both have fetuses that will succumb in utero. These tests allow the physician to keep "hands off" when the fetus is doing well.

Conclusions

1. There is more extensive experience with the contraction stress test (CST) than with the nonstress test (NST).

2. The methodology and end points of the CST are more uniformly applied and generally agreed upon than those of the NST.

3. Stress testing is more time-consuming, expensive and uncomfortable for the patient.

4. There are more false-positive results with CST than with NST/CST combinations.

5. Loss of reactivity, which is the end point for the NST, appears to be a later change in progressive uteroplacental insufficiency than is the development of late deceleration, which is the end point of the CST.

6. Perhaps the value of the NST is in the fine tuning of management when a positive or equivocal CST is found.

7. Perhaps with more precise quantitation of methodology and interpretation, progressive changes and reactivity (in a given patient studied with adequate frequency) will justify the use of nonstress testing as a primary means of fetal surveillance.

REFERENCES

1. Hammacher, K.: Früherkennung intrauterineo Gefahrenzustände durch Electrophonocardiographie und Focographie. *In* Elert, R., and Hates, K. A. (eds.): Prophylaxe Frundkindlicher Hirnschäden. Stuttgart, George Theime Verlag, 1966.
2. Kubli, F. W., Kaeser, O. and Hinselmann, M.: Diagnostic management of chronic placental insufficiency. *In* Pecile, A. and Finzi, C. (eds.): The Foeto-Placental Unit. Amsterdam, Excerpta Medica Foundation, 1969.
3. Pose, S. V., Escarcena, L. et al.: The influence of uterine contractions on the partial pressure of oxygen of the human fetus. *In* Effects of Labour on the Foetus and Newborn. Oxford, Pergamon Press, 1967.
4. Ray, M., Freeman, R., Pine, S. et al.: Clinical experience with the oxytocin challenge test. Am. J. Obstet. Gynecol. 114:1, 1972.
5. Bhakthavathsalan, A., Mann, L. I., Tejani, N. A. et al.: Correlation of the oxytocin challenge test with perinatal outcome. Obstet. Gynecol. 48:552, 1976.
6. Boehm, F. H., Braun, R. D., Growdon, J. H. et al.:

The oxytocin challenge test. South. Med. J. 69:884, 1976.

7. Boyd, I. E., Chamberlain, G. V. P. and Fergusson, I. L. C.: The oxytocin stress test and the isoxsuprine placental transfer test in the management of suspected placental insufficiency. J. Obstet. Gynecol. Br. Commonwealth 81:120, 1974.

8. Christie, G. B. and Cudmore, D. W.: The oxytocin challenge test. Am. J. Obstet. Gynecol. 118:327, 1974.

9. Cooper, J. M., Soffronoff, E. C. and Bolognese, R. J.: Oxytocin challenge test in monitoring high-risk pregnancies. Obstet. Gynecol. 45:27, 1975.

10. Ewing, D. E., Farina, J. R. and Otterson, W. N.: Clinical application of the oxytocin challenge test. Obstet. Gynecol. 43:563, 1974.

11. Farahani, G., Vasudeva, K., Petrie, R. et al.: Oxytocin challenge test in high-risk pregnancy. Obstet. Gynecol. 47:159, 1976.

12. Farahani, G. and Fenton, N. F.: Fetal heart rate acceleration in relation to the oxytocin challenge test. Obstet. Gynecol. 49:163, 1977.

13. Fox, H. E., Steinbrecher, M. and Ripton, B.: Antepartum fetal heart rate and uterine activity studies. Am. J. Obstet. Gynecol. 126:61, 1976.

14. Garite, T., Freeman, R. K. et al.: Oxytocin challenge test. Achieving the desired goals. Obstet. Gynecol. 51:614, 1978.

15. Gaziano, E. P., Hill, D. L. and Freeman, D. W.: The oxytocin challenge test in the management of high-risk pregnancies. Am. J. Obstet. Gynecol. 121:947, 1975.

16. Hayden, B. L., Simpson, J. L., Ewing, D. E. et al.: Can the oxytocin challenge test serve as the primary method for managing high-risk pregnancies? Obstet. Gynecol. 46:251, 1975.

17. Schifrin, B. S., Lapidus, M., Doctor, G. S. and Leviton, A.: Contraction stress test for antepartum fetal evaluation. Obstet. Gynecol. 45:43, 1975.

18. Spurrett, B.: Stressed cardiotocography in late pregnancy. J. Obstet. Gynecol. Br. Commonwealth 78:894, 1971.

19. Weingold, A. B., DeJesus, T. P. S. and O'Keiffe, J.: Oxytocin challenge test. Am. J. Obstet. Gynecol. 123:466, 1975.

20. Lee, C. Y., Di Loreto, P. C. and Logrand, B.: Fetal activity acceleration determination for the evaluation of fetal reserve. Obstet. Gynecol. 48:19, 1976.

21. Trierweiler, M. W., Freeman, R. K. and James, J.: Baseline fetal heart rate characteristics as an indicator of fetus status during the antepartum period. Am. J. Obstet. Gynecol. 125:618, 1976.

22. Krebs, H. B. and Petres, R. E.: Clinical application of a scoring system for evaluation of antepartum fetal heart monitoring. Am. J. Obstet. Gynecol. 130:765, 1978.

23. Lee, C. Y., Di Loreto, P. C. and O'Lane, J. M.: A study of fetal heart rate acceleration patterns. Obstet. Gynecol. 45:142, 1975.

24. Nochimson, D. J., Turbeville, J. S. and Terry, J. E.: The nonstress test. Obstet. Gynecol. 51:419, 1978.

25. Rochard, F., Schifrin, B. S., Goupil, F. et al.: Nonstressed fetal heart rate monitoring in the antepartum period. Am. J. Obstet. Gynecol. 126:699, 1976.

26. Tushuizen, P. B. T., Stoot, J. E. G. M., and Ubachs, J. M. H.: Clinical experience in nonstressed antepartum cardiotocography. Am. J. Obstet. Gynecol. 128:507, 1977.

27. Visser, G. H. A. and Huisjes, H. J.: Diagnostic value of the unstressed antepartum cardiotocogram. Br. J. Obstet. Gynecol. 84:321, 1977.

28. Freeman, R. K., Goebelsman, U., Nochimson, D. et al.: An evaluation of the significance of a positive oxytocin challenge test. Obstet. Gynecol. 47:8, 1976.

29. Braly, P. and Freeman, R. K.: The significance of fetal heart rate reactivity with a positive oxytocin challenge test. Obstet. Gynecol. 50:689, 1977.

30. Flynn, A. M. and Kelly, J.: Evaluation of fetal wellbeing by antepartum fetal heart monitoring. Br. Med. J. 1:936, 1977.

31. Kubli, F., Boos, R., Rüttgers, H. et al.: Antepartum fetal heart rate monitoring. *In* Beard, R. and Campbell, S. (eds.): The Current Status of FHR Monitoring and Ultrasound Obstetrics. London, Royal College of Obstetricians and Gynecologists, 1977.

32. Myers, R. E., Mueller-Heubach, E. and Adamsons, K.: Predictability of the state of fetal oxygenation from a quantitative analysis of the components of late deceleration. Am. J. Obstet. Gynecol. 115:1083, 1973.

33. Paul, R. H., Suidan, A. K., Sze-Ya, Y. et al.: Clinical fetal monitoring. VII. The evaluation and significance of intrapartum baseline FHR variability. Am. J. Obstet. Gynecol. 123:206, 1975.

34. Garite, T., Linzey, E. M., Freeman, R. et al.: Fetal heart rate patterns and fetal distress in fetuses with congenital anomalies. Obstet. Gynecol. (In press).

35. Baskett, T. F. and Sandy, E.: False negative oxytocin challenge tests. Am. J. Obstet. Gynecol. 123:106, 1975.

36. Marcum, R. G.: False-negative oxytocin challenge test. Am. J. Obstet. Gynecol. 122:894, 1977.

Editorial Comment

Significant and exciting progress has been made during the past decade using biophysical methods to monitor fetal health. The past 15 years has revealed a new era of scientific obstetrics that focuses on determining whether the fetus is ill and the degree of illness. This has culminated, in the past five years, in efforts to determine if the fetus is healthy. Biochemical and biophysical methods of assessing fetal well-being have emerged. Biochemical tests principally involve urinary or serum estriols. The biophysical involve the contraction stress test and nonstress test.

The senior authors in this chapter have pioneered the contraction stress test and the nonstress test in this country. Their contributions indicate the present state of the art in antepartum fetal health evaluation.

The contraction stress test, first presented in this country by Dr. Serafin Pose in 1966 at the Chicago Lying-In Hospital, is known in the Spanish-speaking world as the Pose test. It was designed to stimulate labor. It uses controlled conditions and electronic fetal monitoring and monitors fetal heart rate to evaluate fetal tolerance to labor. There is a 25 per cent false-positive test result; hence, there is no absolute way to assure the obstetrician or the mother that the fetus can completely withstand labor by considering just the fetal heart rate prior to labor.

It is quite clear that the contraction stress test is time-consuming (requiring an average of 90 to 120 minutes to perform) and if cost accounted, is reasonably expensive ($150 to $200). Freeman and his group believe that this test may be an earlier warning sign of fetal jeopardy than the nonstress test. The emerging issue thus concerns whether the present clinical trials of the nonstress test provide sufficient evidence that this test can be used as a primary means of antepartum fetal surveillance, with the contraction stress test as a backup when the nonstress test is nonreactive. More important is determining which of these two tests is appropriate for the individual patient and if she requires even more specific tests for her particular condition. Identification of individuals who need no antepartum fetal surveillance also requires consideration. The primary goal of all antepartum testing is to decrease perinatal morbidity and mortality by eliminating stillbirths and intrapartum deaths.

The proponents of the nonstress test, especially Richard Paul and the University of Southern California group who pioneered its evaluation, agree that any antepartum test should be convenient, noninvasive, technically simple with recognizable end points and relatively inexpensive. (It would be ideal if the test could be done as an office procedure and not just as a hospital evaluation.) The nonstress test comes close to fulfilling these requirements, except that there are times when the results may be equivocal and not absolute. The intrauterine antepartum fetal heart rate variations reflecting fetal movements form the basis of the nonstress test. The pattern is considered reactive when 2 or more accelerations of more than 15 beats per minute and longer than 15 seconds in duration are present in one of two 20-minute observations. The absence of the two accelerations in the two observation periods is considered a nonreactive pattern. The problem with the nonstress test is the different behavior patterns of the intrauterine fetus during deep sleep and REM sleep. Apparently, only during REM sleep does the fetus show heartbeat accelerations during movements. Schifrin and his group think that in the presence of a normal test the obstetrician can be reassured that there is no need for intervention.

Biophysical testing is on the verge of gradually eliminating the need for biochemical monitoring of the fetus. There are some advocates for abandoning biochemical monitoring as unnecessary; however, prudence dictates careful consideration before discarding the well-established estriol evaluations. Estriol evaluation can be a red flag that indicates when uteroplacental insufficiency is present and is useful in postmature pregnancy. It is used more as a screening device rather than for the finer tuning that is seen in the biophysical monitoring.

It appears now that we have screening tools as well as more specific means of fetal assessment in the combination of biochemical and biophysical monitoring used to decrease perinatal mortality and eliminate most stillbirths. Much progress has been made in this area over the past five to seven years, but not all the questions have been answered.

2

The Management of Preterm Labor

Alternative Points of View

by Fernando Arias and Alfred B. Knight
by Robert Landesman and Kathleen Wilson
by Tom P. Barden
by Guy Harbert and Kenneth Spisso
by Joseph Bieniarz, Laurence Burd and
Antonio Scommegna
by Karlis Adamsons

Editorial Comment

Beta-Adrenergic Therapy in the Management of Preterm Labor

Fernando Arias, M.D., Ph.D.
Alfred B. Knight, M.D.
Washington University School of Medicine

The treatment of patients in preterm labor centers heavily on the use of beta-adrenergic agents. Prior to November 1980 the drugs most commonly used for this purpose in the United States were isoxsuprine and terbutaline. At that time another beta agonist, ritodrine, was approved by the Federal Drug Administration (FDA) and quickly became the medication most widely used in this country for the treatment of preterm labor. As of this writing (January 1982), phase III trials are in progress for the eventual FDA approval of another beta-adrenergic drug, fenoterol. In this chapter we will briefly review some pharmacologic and clinical aspects of tocolysis with beta-adrenergic agents using as a model the drug terbutaline. Other agents (isoxsuprine, ritodrine, fenoterol) have similar general prop-

erties, although they vary in their pharmacokinetics and in the extent of their side effects.

Catecholamine Receptors

The variable potencies of different catecholamines to stimulate physiologic processes formed the basis for Ahlquist's proposition[1] that adrenergic drugs be classified by their ability to stimulate alpha or beta receptors. In fact, alpha receptor–mediated functions are stimulated by epinephrine and norepinephrine, but not by isoproterenol. Beta receptor–mediated effects are most strongly stimulated by isoproterenol with epinephrine and norepinephrine less potent. Further pharmacologic differentiation of alpha and beta receptors was provided by the specificity of their respective inhibitors: phentolamine and phenoxybenzamine are selective alpha inhibitors while propranolol is the prototype of the beta blockers. More recently a third type of adrenergic receptor has been described.[2] It is predominantly stimulated by dopamine and has been named dopaminergic receptor. Beta-adrenergic receptors have been further subdivided into β_1 and β_2, depending on the nature of the physiologic responses that they mediate and on their relative potency to stimulate those responses. Isoproterenol is the most potent stimulator of both subtypes of beta receptors and epinephrine and norepinephrine are about $\frac{1}{15}$ to $\frac{1}{10}$ as potent as isoproterenol in activating β_1 receptors (responsible for cardiac stimulation), while they are only $\frac{1}{100}$ to $\frac{1}{1000}$ times as potent in stimulating β_2 receptors (responsible for bronchial and vascular dilatation).[3]

In recent years substantial advances have been made in the identification and characterization of beta receptors using radioactive ligands of high affinity and specificity. For example, beta-adrenergic receptors from frog erythrocytes have been solubilized, quantified (approximately 1000 per cell) and characterized as lipoproteins.[4] Biochemical studies of catecholamine receptors have also produced evidence indicating that most, if not all, of the beta-adrenergic effects appear to follow activation of adenyl cyclase and increased intracellular concentration of cyclic 3'5'-adenosine monophosphate (cAMP).[5]

Mechanism of Action of Beta-Adrenergic Agents on Myometrial Activity

The "in vitro" demonstration of beta receptors in human myometrium has been at best inconsistent. Some investigators,[6-8] using isolated muscle strips, have concluded that the human uterus contains few or no beta receptors while others, using similar techniques, have demonstrated beta activity.[9-11] Results of "in vivo" studies in which motility was inhibited by different types of beta-adrenergic stimulators[12-16] and this effect antagonized by butoxamine (a selective β_2 blocker)[17] confirm the existence of β_2 receptors in human myometrium. These receptors appear to act as mediators of uterine relaxation.

The molecular mechanism of myometrial

relaxation by β_2 adrenergic stimulators has not been completely elucidated. Current data suggest that these receptors indirectly mediate intracellular $Ca++$ concentration. In fact, $Ca++$ is the key intermediate that acts as a coupler between excitation (a membrane phenomenon resulting in the generation of action potentials) and contraction (an intracellular phenomenon resulting from the combination of actin and myosin).[18] Relaxation requires a decrease in intracellular $Ca++$ concentration, achieved by displacement of the ion outside the cell. Extrusion of $Ca++$ is an energy-requiring process that consumes cAMP. Adenyl cyclase stimulated by beta-adrenergic agents will increase intracellular cAMP concentration, thereby activating the $Ca++$ pump and decreasing intracellular $Ca++$ concentration, which, in turn, inhibits myosin light-chain kinase, and phosphorylation of myosin. The contraction mechanism is blocked and the uterus relaxes.[19] Work with turkey erythrocytes supports the concept of interaction between beta-adrenergic receptors, intracellular $Ca++$ and adenyl cyclase activity as key elements in the cellular response to catecholamines.[20]

Terbutaline Sulfate

Terbutaline sulfate is a beta-adrenergic stimulator with predominant β_2 effects. Its chemical structure resembles isoproterenol, except for the presence of an additional methyl group on the amino nitrogen and in the position on the benzene ring of the hydroxyl groups and the side chain (Fig. 1). Subtle differences in the chemical structure of catecholamines are important in determining their pharmacologic behavior. In general, increased

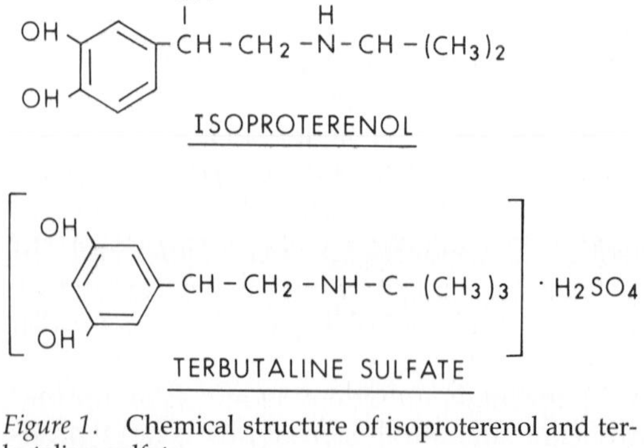

Figure 1. Chemical structure of isoproterenol and terbutaline sulfate.

substitution on the amino group diminishes the affinity of a catecholamine for alpha receptors and enhances its ability to bind beta receptors. The presence of a hydroxyl group on the beta carbon decreases the ability of the compound to bind to dopamine receptors.

Terbutaline not only stimulates β_2 receptors in the myometrium that cause uterine relaxation but also stimulates similar types of receptors in other organs. For example, in bronchial smooth muscle it causes bronchodilatation (its main clinical use); in the peripheral blood vessels, vasodilatation; and in the liver and muscles, increased glycogenolysis. Terbutaline also stimulates β_1 receptors, causing increases in heart rate, relaxation of the intestinal smooth muscle and increases in lipolytic activity, although to a lesser degree than other beta-adrenergic agents. These interactions of terbutaline and other tocolytic agents with β_1 receptors and with extrauterine β_2 receptors cause the side effects that limit their clinical usefulness in the treatment of preterm labor.

Effects of Terbutaline on Mother and Fetus

Acute experiments in pregnant baboons near term demonstrated that maternal and fetal blood pressure, acid-base balance and fetal heart rate were not affected by administration of terbutaline to the mothers. Direct intravascular administration of the drug to the fetus did not change its cardiovascular or acid-base state. Mild maternal tachycardia was observed as a consequence of treatment as well as increases in both maternal and fetal blood glucose concentrations, maternal levels always exceeding those of the fetus.[21] In other animal experiments[22] the effect of terbutaline on the maternal systemic uterine cardiovascular dynamics was studied in chronic preparations of pregnant ewes near term. The authors used doses and rates of administration similar to those known to inhibit spontaneous or induced labor in the ewe, in addition to intravenous bolus injections of 250 μg and 500 μg. No change was found in uterine blood flow and uterine vascular resistance. The maternal systemic cardiovascular effects were limited to mild tachycardia and increased pulse pressure. These findings contradict data from another laboratory[23] showing a decrease in uterine blood flow and a marked increase in cardiac output in chronic animal preparations treated with terbutaline and isoxsuprine.

Studies with human pregnant patients have provided more significant information than animal experiments. All studies report maternal tachycardia as a constant finding following terbutaline administration. The increase in heart rate rarely exceeds 140 beats per minute (bpm) at the dose usually given for inhibition of premature labor. The EKG most commonly shows a sinus tachycardia without arrhythmias or pathologic changes. A slight increase in systolic blood pressure, a decrease in diastolic blood pressure and consequently an increase in pulse pressure are other cardiovascular changes frequently observed in pregnant patients receiving terbutaline. The fetal heart rate either does not change or moderately increases, rarely exceeding 160 bpm.

Two rather dramatic cardiovascular complications have been reported in patients receiving terbutaline, or other beta-adrenergic agents, for the treatment of preterm labor: angina pectoris and pulmonary edema. Patients who develop angina pectoris may do so during intravenous or oral treatment. The initial complaint is a sensation of "tightness" referred to the mid-sternal area. The symptom increases in intensity and eventually becomes a severe retrosternal pain. The EKG may be normal or may show ST segment depression.[24] The pain disappears with nitroglycerin or with discontinuation of the medication.

In 1978 Stubblefield[25] reported in the American literature the sudden and unexpected occurrence of pulmonary edema in a primigravid patient with a twin gestation treated for preterm labor with subcutaneous and oral terbutaline plus intramuscular dexamethasone. This was followed by similar observations by other investigators around the world.[26-30] Recently the FDA alerted physicians in the United States to the possibility of this side effect during beta-adrenergic treatment of patients with preterm labor. Water retention, low hematocrit and twin gestation are commonly associated with this complication. The pathogenesis of this problem is unknown, but direct capillary damage and water retention seem to be important. Discontinuation of beta-adrenergic agents and administration of oxygen and furosemide are the most effective treatments for this complication. Most patients recover and show no evidence of residual cardiovascular lesions.

Terbutaline, as well as other beta-adrenergic agents, may also cause profound metabolic alterations in pregnant patients in preterm labor. The most common laboratory findings are increases in plasma insulin, glucose, glycerol, free fatty acids, beta hydroxybutirate and lactic acid and decreases in hematocrit and potassium concentration.[31-33] These changes are the result of increased hepatic glycogenolysis, increased lipolysis, and direct stimulation of the pancreatic beta cells.[34] The decrease in hematocrit is due to water retention because of the antidiuretic effect of the medication. The decrease in plasma potassium concentration is due to a shift of the ion to the intracellular compartment rather than to a real ion loss. These metabolic alterations are more marked in the insulin-dependent diabetic, are more severe during the intravenous phase of therapy and are additive with the anti-insulinic effect of glucocorticoids.

Terbutaline and Human Labor

The effect of terbutaline on uterine contractility during term labor was initially studied by Andersson et al.[12] These investigators administered the drug to two groups of patients in advanced stages of labor, thus eliminating the possibility of spontaneous cessation of uterine activity that is common in early states of labor. In addition, six patients received intravenous oxytocin throughout the investigation. The authors found that an intravenous infusion of 10 to 20 µg per minute of terbutaline was capable of inhibiting uterine contractions in all patients. The tocolytic effect was immediate and was independent of the stage of labor. A decreased amplitude of contractions was first noted and followed by a reduction in frequency of contractions. No difference in the ability of the drug to decrease uterine activity was found between patients treated or not treated with intravenous oxytocin.[35] After discontinuation of the terbutaline infusion a gradual return of the uterine activity to control levels was observed. Figure 2 is a representative example of the effect of a 250 µg subcutaneous dose of terbutaline on the uterine activity of a patient in spontaneous labor.

The same group of investigators studied the effect of terbutaline in 20 patients undergoing therapeutic abortion in the second trimester of pregnancy with the use of intra-amniotic prostaglandin F2$_\alpha$ or hypertonic saline.[36] They found that an intravenous infusion of 5 to 20 µg per minute caused a decrease in uterine activity from 393 to 214 Montevideo Units

(MU) in the prostaglandin group and from 238 to 68 MU in the hypertonic saline group. They also found a significant decrease in uterine resting pressure after terbutaline administration in both groups of patients.

A double-blind placebo-controlled study of the effect of terbutaline in premature labor was published by Ingemarsson.[37] He selected 30 patients of similar gestational time in premature labor (cervix effaced or almost effaced, with at least 1 to 2 cm but with less than 4 cm of dilatation) and treated them with bed rest, sedation, and intravenous terbutaline or placebo. Premature labor was arrested beyond the treatment period in 80 per cent of the patients receiving terbutaline and only in 20 per cent of those receiving placebo; this difference was significant ($p<0.01$). A similar success rate (78 per cent) was reported in an uncontrolled study[38] carried out in the United States.

Ryden[39] compared the effect of terbutaline and salbutamol on premature labor. Salbutamol arrested labor in 33 of 34 patients and terbutaline in 32 of 34. Delivery was postponed for more than one week in 74 per cent of the salbutamol-treated patients and in 80 per cent of the patients receiving terbutaline.

In the course of our work[40] on the use of terbutaline in the treatment of intrapartum fetal distress, we observed the effect of the drug on the uterine activity of 15 patients who were in the active phase of labor. In six patients labor was monitored with an intrauterine pressure catheter. The subcutaneous or intravenous administration of 250 µg of terbutaline caused a decrease in the intrauterine pressure elicited by contractions from 58.5 mm Hg (range: 30 to 70 mm Hg) to a mean value of 23.5 mm Hg (range: 10 to 40 mm Hg). In three other patients also monitored with intrauterine pressure catheter and in five of six patients monitored with tocodynamometer, there was complete cessation of uterine activity. The last patient monitored externally exhibited a decrease in frequency of contractions followed by complete cessation of uterine activity 20 minutes after terbutaline administration. We also found that the intrauterine resting pressure decreased from a mean value of 15.5 mm Hg (range: 5 to 25 mm Hg) to 7.22 mm Hg (range: 0 to 20 mm Hg). The effect of terbutaline on uterine activity occurred within five minutes of its administration and was still apparent in eight patients who remained undelivered one hour after treatment.

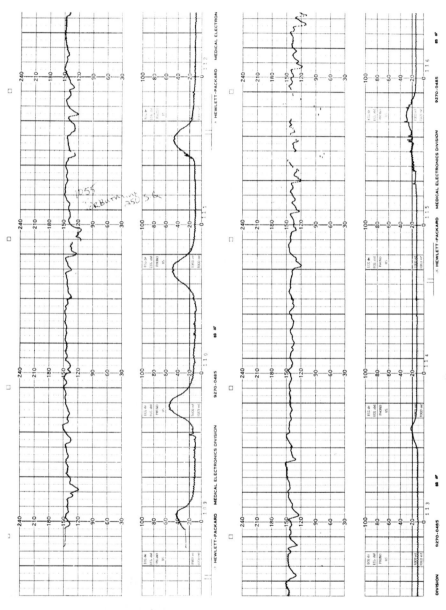

Figure 2. Representative example of the effect of terbutaline on uterine contractility. The monitor trace corresponds to a 24-year-old woman, gravida 2, who developed premature labor at 28 weeks of gestation. Her modified Bishop score on admission was 3. Note the decrease in amplitude and frequency of contractions and the lack of change in fetal heart rate after the subcutaneous injection of 250 mg terbutaline.

Results Obtained with Terbutaline in the Treatment of Preterm Labor

Terbutaline was extensively used at our institution for the treatment of preterm labor from 1976 until FDA approval of ritodrine in 1980. Rapidly terbutaline supplanted isoxsuprine as the primary uterine relaxant because of its effectiveness and its low frequency of significant side effects. Distinct approaches to various problems requiring immediate uterine relaxation were developed gradually and protocols with specific dosages, intervals and indications outlined. The following discussion represents our initial two and a half years' experience with terbutaline and consists of multiple regimens that we have attempted to collate. We believe that our data represent the minimal success that can be expected from this drug, for as our experience with the medication increased so did our success in prolonging gestation.

More than 500 charts of pregnant patients exposed to terbutaline were reviewed. Patients were included in this analysis if their admitting diagnosis was preterm labor (uterine contractions at least once every 10 minutes noted by palpation or recorded by monitoring and/or progressive cervical effacement and dilatation during an observation interval of one hour), and if the clinical estimation of gestational age was 37 weeks or less. Specifically excluded were (1) those patients with preterm rupture of fetal membranes (a complex clinical situation that is the topic of a current prospective protocol), (2) those patients with intrapartum fetal distress in whom terbutaline was used to relax the uterus and allow recovery from fetal acidosis and asphyxia,[40] and (3) those patients in labor in whom terbutaline was utilized to stop uterine activity and allow time for preparations for primary or, more commonly, for repeated cesarean section. All patients included in this study were delivered at our institution. All newborns had an adequate examination to allow the best possible estimation of gestational age. After specific exclusions, 143 patients were found to fulfill the aforementioned criteria. These 143 included both clinic patients on a clinic service managed by residents and private patients of our full- and part-time staff. Figure 3 shows some of the characteristics of this population. Over 60 per cent of the patients were in the age range of 16 to 25 years and half of them were experiencing first or second pregnancy. Over 60 per cent of these patients were at 33 weeks' gestation or less at initiation of therapy based on the evaluation of gestational age of the newborn. Four patients (2.8 per cent) were at

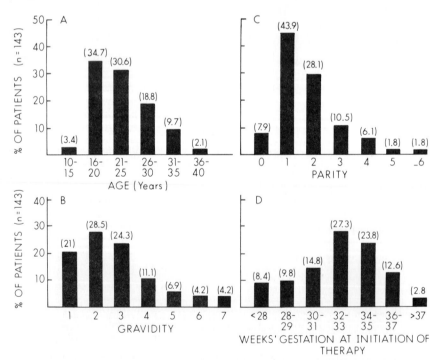

Figure 3. Age, gravidity, pariety and weeks of gestation at initiation of therapy of patients in preterm labor treated with terbutaline.

TABLE 1.   MODIFIED BISHOP SCORE

SCORE	0	1	2	3
Dilatation (cm)	0	1–2	3–4	5 or more
Effacement (%)	0–30	40–50	60–70	80 or more
Station		−3	−2	−1 to 0	+1 or more

term (gestational age equal to or greater than 37 weeks) by newborn examination, and an error in clinical dating of the pregnancy was obvious.

A modified Bishop score[41] was used (Table 1) to evaluate the degree of severity of preterm labor. The modified score is based on dilatation, effacement and station of the presenting part producing a maximum of 9 points. Consistency and position of the cervix are not included because of the high degree of subjective variability involved in these measurements. As shown in Figure 4, panel A, relatively lower scores were predominant in our population. This would suggest that many of these patients were in "false labor" and makes

evident the difficulties in interpreting data in uncontrolled studies. However, we are convinced that excessive uterine activity in early pregnancy is abnormal and that patients exhibiting this phenomenon represent a population at high risk for preterm delivery. These patients were also categorized using the tocolysis index.[42] As with the modified Bishop score, lower numbers predominate, with more than 50 per cent of the population having an index of 3 or less (Fig. 4, panel B).

Significantly, only 21 per cent of the patients had no significant risk factors for preterm labor (Fig. 5). Thirty-one per cent of the patients had delivered a preterm infant previously and 10 per cent had had two or more abortions. In 24.3 per cent of the cases urinary tract infection concomitant with preterm labor was the initial diagnosis (only 10 per cent of these patients had culture-proved infections). Vaginal bleeding (collated in all trimesters) was found among 15 per cent of the patients. Twin gestation represented only 5 per cent of the study group.

Assessment of success in any study of preterm labor is at best difficult. Although main-

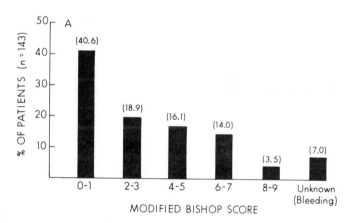

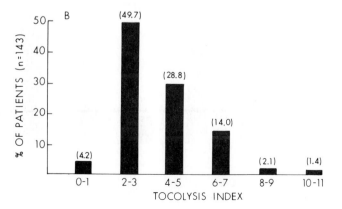

Figure 4. Severity of preterm labor as indicated by the modified Bishop score and the tocolysis index.

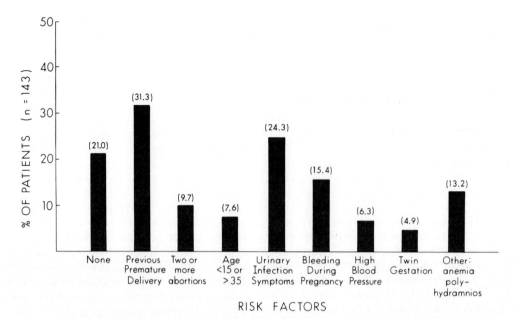

Figure 5. Risk factors for preterm labor found in patients treated with terbutaline.

tenance of intrauterine life until 37 or more weeks of gestation might initially appear to be the ultimate goal of therapy, multiple variables (the presence of hostile intrauterine environment, congenital abnormalities, maternal disease, fetal lung maturation, etc.) militate against such a simplistic approach. Indeed, prolongation of the lag time between onset of premature labor and delivery does not necessarily correlate well with success as measured by fetal lung maturation. For example, a lag time of 4 weeks when therapy was initiated at

28 weeks of gestation is not better than a lag time of 1 week at 34 weeks' gestation if the latter was adequate to achieve lung maturation and the former was not. Neonatal complications with prematurity still center heavily on the morbidity and mortality of the respiratory distress syndrome (RDS). Consequently we have chosen to look at pulmonary maturity of the newborn as our primary index of success. As sophistication of neonatal care grows and the intensive care of premature infants decreases, the complications associated with

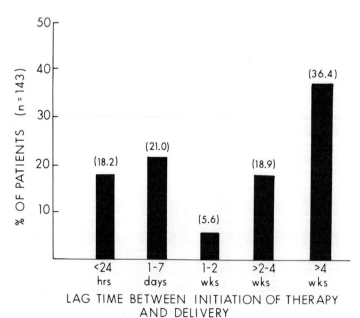

Figure 6. Prolongation of pregnancy achieved with terbutaline treatment.

RDS and other neonatal problems such as apnea, intracranial hemorrhage and sepsis will require re-evaluation of the present index of success.

By standard criteria of lag time (Fig. 6) only 82 per cent of our patients had their parturition delayed more than 24 hours and only 60 per cent delayed more than 1 week. However, a closer look at the group in whom delivery was delayed less than 24 hours shows that in 60 per cent of them the infant had adequate lung maturation. An additional 30 per cent represented nonviable births (birth weight less than 500 g), patients with advanced cervical dilatation, or patients with infants showing congenital malformations incompatible with life. In three cases (10 per cent), physician judgment was inaccurate: Two patients were thought to be in "false labor" and progressed from closed cervix to advanced dilatation in the period of observation. The other patient was a woman with a previous cesarean section who had mild contractions without cervical changes while receiving low-dose terbutaline. Her obstetrician decided to terminate the pregnancy rather than risk dehiscence of the uterine scar. These examples confirm the complexity of any analysis of groups of patients in preterm labor.

The respiratory outcome and the gestational age of the infants delivered after terbutaline treatment of preterm labor is shown in Figure 7. Eighty-four per cent of our population had no evidence of RDS. Three fetuses (2.1 per cent) were not viable (less than 500 g) and two (1.4 per cent) had multiple congenital malformations that were incompatible with life. Eight infants (5.6 per cent) manifested mild and another eight moderate-to-severe RDS. A corrected incidence of adequate pulmonary maturation of 87 per cent is obtained by excluding the nonviable and congenitally malformed infants. Of the remaining 13 per cent, half had mild RDS, which is rarely associated with significant neonatal complications. These results are in contrast with the usual standard index of success—that is, gestational age at delivery. As shown in the lower panel of Figure 7, 54 per cent of our patients delivered at or before 37 weeks of gestation. Table 2 shows the relationship of RDS to gestational age at birth in our study. With the exception of the moderate-to-severe RDS at 32 to 33 weeks, the trend is as one would expect.

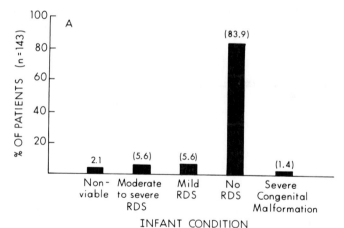

Figure 7. Results of therapy as indicated by the respiratory condition of the infant at birth and the weeks of gestation at delivery.

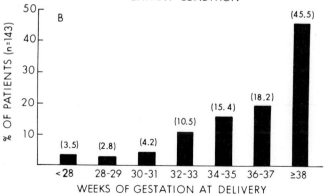

TABLE 2. INCIDENCE AND SEVERITY OF RESPIRATORY DISTRESS SYNDROME IN RELATION TO GESTATIONAL AGE AT BIRTH*

| WEEKS OF GESTATION | RESPIRATORY DISTRESS SYNDROME | | |
	None	Mild	Moderate to Severe
<28	—	1/1 (100%)	—
28–29	1/3 (33%)	—	2/3 (67%)
30–31	5/6 (83%)	—	1/6 (17%)
32–33	10/16 (63%)	1/16 (6%)	5/16 (31%)
34–35	17/21 (81%)	4/21 (19%)	—
36–37	24/26 (92%)	2/26 (8%)	—
>37	65/66 (100%)	—	—

*n = 138. Five patients were excluded (birth weight less than 500 g or severely congenitally malformed).

In an attempt to determine clinical variables that would predict outcome, a comparison of lag time between initiation of treatment and delivery and the modified Bishop score is shown in Table 3. As expected, the greater the modified Bishop score, the more likely the patient will deliver within 1 week after initiation of therapy. However, it is interesting that even if the modified Bishop score is 6 or greater, 40 per cent of the patients can be maintained undelivered for more than 1 week. This somewhat unexpected finding has practical implications in view of the development of therapeutic methods that may improve fetal lung maturation in a relatively short period of time.[43]

The cornerstone of therapy for premature labor has been bed rest. All patients included in this study were counseled to be as inactive

TABLE 3. PROLONGATION OF PREGNANCY IN RELATION TO MODIFIED BISHOP SCORE AT BEGINNING OF TREATMENT

MODIFIED BISHOP SCORE	PERCENTAGE OF PATIENTS WITH LAG TIME LESS THAN 1 WEEK
0–1	9.8
2–3	28.1
4–5	40.9
≥6	60.0

TABLE 4. INCIDENCE OF RDS IN PATIENTS TREATED WITH TERBUTALINE AND 17α-HYDROXYPROGESTERONE CAPROATE AND THOSE TREATED WITH TERBUTALINE ALONE

| | RDS | | |
	None	Mild	Moderate to Severe
Terbutaline	90 (87%)	7 (6.8%)	6 (5.8%)
Terbutaline + 17α-OH-progesterone	36 (92%)	1 (2.5%)	2 (5%)

as possible. Certain highly motivated patients may comply. However, our clinical impression is that the only way to guarantee compliance is for the patient to remain hospitalized, which constitutes a significant financial burden.

The work of Johnson et al.[44] demonstrating the beneficial effect of 17α-hydroxyprogesterone caproate in the prevention of premature labor remains controversial. Twenty-four per cent of our patients received Delalutin in addition to terbutaline in the treatment of premature labor. Table 4 displays the data relative to the frequency and severity of RDS between those patients who received terbutaline alone and those who received terbutaline and this progestin. There are no significant differences between the groups but the numbers are small and the experience was not controlled.

With respect to complications, tremor of the hands, facial flushing because of subcutaneous vasodilatation and palpitations were the most common, although minor, side effects observed with terbutaline treatment. Tachycardia was the single most common objective finding in treated patients. Tachycardia is dose related and can be titrated. Unfortunately, in a few cases, the level of medication necessary for tocolysis is higher than that tolerated by the cardiovascular system. Significant tachycardia (pulse rate equal to or greater than 120 beats per minute) was almost exclusively confined to those patients receiving intravenous bolus or continuous intravenous infusion of terbutaline. Only one patient had the medication discontinued because of tachycardia and two patients because of anginal chest pain; their EKGs did not show changes suggestive of myocardial ischemia. Also, one case of acute appendicitis and another of intra-abdominal bleeding secondary to a ruptured broad ligament varicosity were complicated by erroneous evaluation of the tachycardia; it was thought to be the result of terbutaline treatment of the concomitant premature labor.

We observed four cases of pulmonary edema after completing this review and during our last two years of experience with terbutaline in the treatment of preterm labor.[30] In three cases a combination of terbutaline and glucocorticoid was being used and in the fourth case terbutaline was used alone. None of the patients had demonstrable cardiac disease. In all cases it was possible to demonstrate excessive fluid retention during treatment. All patients recovered quickly and had no sequelae from the therapy.

All our patients receiving intravenous terbutaline treatment and about one third of those in subcutaneous or oral treatment exhibited hyperglycemia. The alteration in carbohydrate metabolism was more marked in patients with gestational diabetes and with insulin-dependent diabetes and in patients who, in addition to terbutaline, were receiving glucocorticoids. Most gestational diabetic patients whose disease was controlled with diet before tocolytic therapy required subcutaneous insulin and patients with insulin-dependent diabetes usually required a continuous intravenous infusion of insulin to regulate their blood sugar levels. Two cases were observed in which the use of terbutaline contributed to a serious metabolic derangement: both patients developed ketoacidosis with relatively normal blood sugar values, probably as a consequence of a marked β_1 lipolytic stimulation. The process was relatively difficult to reverse before delivery, but both patients recuperated easily after parturition.

With respect to the fetus, beta-adrenergic agents seem to be relatively benign and very few reports suggesting fetal toxicity have appeared in the literature in spite of extensive use of these drugs. The occurrence of significant maternal complications, however, has moderated the initial enthusiasm for these agents.

Critical criteria before initiating beta-adrenergic therapy are: (1) to confirm and document the diagnosis of preterm labor, (2) to rule out any fetal or maternal problem that would contraindicate prolongation of gestation, (3) to make certain that the infant is not of a gestational age category that would do better in the neonatal nursery, and (4) to be certain that there is no contraindication to the use of beta-adrenergic agents. Suggested relative and absolute contraindications to the use of beta-mimetics are listed in Table 5.

The best monitor of the tocolytic blood level

TABLE 5. ABSOLUTE AND RELATIVE CONTRAINDICATIONS TO USE OF BETA-ADRENERGIC AGENTS IN TREATMENT OF PRETERM LABOR

A. Absolute
   1. Chronic cardiac disease
   2. High cardiac output situations (hyperthyroidism, sickle cell disease, etc.)
   3. Chorioamnionitis
   4. Patients taking monoaminergic inhibitors

B. Relative
   1. Active internal or external bleeding (abruptio placenta,* placenta previa,* etc.)
   2. Insulin-dependent diabetics
   3. Patients with hypertension

C. High-risk situations
   1. Twin gestation
   2. Hemoglobin concentration under 10 g before therapy
   3. Simultaneous use of glucocorticoids

*In these cases tocolytic therapy may play a role in decreasing the amount of bleeding (previa) or in helping the fetus in distress (abruptio), but this is experimental and its advantages are still to be determined.

is the maternal pulse rate. In fact, the maternal pulse should remain between 100 and 120 bpm during intravenous treatment and between 90 and 100 during oral treatment. Doses that do not raise the pulse rate to these levels are usually ineffective. Doses causing marked tachycardia (more than 140 bpm) are dangerous because the cardiovascular tolerance of the patient is being exceeded.

During treatment it is important to monitor the hematocrit and hemoglobin, the potassium and the glucose levels. We measure the hemoglobin and hematocrit and the potassium concentration before initiation of therapy and every six hours during the intravenous phase of treatment. Measurements of blood glucose are carried out as frequently as necessary. Most insulin-dependent diabetics are treated with continuous intravenous insulin infusion from the beginning of intravenous tocolytic therapy. Nondiabetic patients and gestational diabetics are treated with subcutaneous insulin when the blood sugar concentration exceeds 180 mg/dl.

Our data clearly suggest that the earlier premature labor can be halted, the better the outcome. We think that each case must be individualized, but the more active the labor, as manifested by contractility pattern or cervical changes, the more aggressive must be the therapy. If the modified Bishop score of the cervix is 3 or more, intravenous tocolysis should be instituted. This may be followed by subcutaneous or oral doses on a regular basis after 12 to 18 hours of uterine quiescence. Cervical examination and objective monitoring of uterine activity should take place at daily or more frequent intervals. Fetal pulmonary maturation should be evaluated and steroid therapy instituted when appropriate. The patient must remain confined to the hospital until fetal maturation is confirmed. In patients with a modified Bishop score under 3, the chance of a rapid delivery is less although still significant (greater than 10 per cent in our experience). Initial subcutaneous or oral dosage may be sufficient to inhibit labor, but careful, close monitoring is essential, and hospitalization is necessary for such a purpose. Again, observation of uterine activity and cervical changes are essential for adequate management. Once the acute situation has been adequately treated the patient must be maintained on oral beta-adrenergic therapy until 36 weeks of gestation or until fetal lung maturity is reached.

In this management plan it is recognized that for some patients a goal of delayed delivery for 48 to 72 hours may be all that is realistic, whereas for others many weeks delay of parturition are obtainable. We believe that steroids play an important role in the management of premature labor, and that assessment of fetal lung maturation followed by appropriate treatment is perhaps the optimal management for those patients in whom parturition can be delayed for only a brief period of time.

REFERENCES

1. Ahlquist, R. P.: A study of adrenotropic receptors. Am. J. Physiol. 153:586–600, 1948.
2. Iversen, L. L.: Dopamine receptors in the brain: a dopamine-sensitive adenylate cyclase model synaptic receptors, illuminating antipsychotic drug action. Science 188:1084–1098, 1975.
3. Lands, A. M., Arnold, A., McAuliff, J. P. et al.: Differentiation of receptor systems activated by sympathomimetic amines. Nature 214:597–598, 1967.
4. Makherjee, C., Caron, M. G., Coverstone, M. et al.: Identification of adenylate cyclase-coupled β-adrenergic receptors in frog erythrocytes with (-) [^{3}H]alprenolol. J. Biol. Chem. 250:4869–4876, 1975.
5. Robinson, G. A., Butcher, R. W. and Sutherland, E. W.: Cyclic AMP. Ann. Rev. Biochem. 37:149, 1968.
6. Anadros, M. and Sinha, Y. K.: Action of some drugs on excised human uterus. J. Obstet. Gynecol. Br. Emp. 67:659, 1960.
7. Lehrer, D. N.: Effect of some spasmolytic drugs on

8. Farmer, J. B. and Lehrer, D. N.: The effect of isoprenaline on contraction of smooth muscle produced by histamine, acetylcholine or other agents. J. Pharm. Pharmacol. 18:649, 1966.
9. Landesman, R. and Wilson, K.: The relaxant effect of adrenergic compounds on isolated gravid human myometrium. Am. J. Obstet. Gynecol. 100:969, 1968.
10. Stander, R. W. and Barden, T. P.: Adrenergic receptor activity of catecholamines in human gestational myometrium. Obstet. Gynecol. 28:768, 1966.
11. Andersson, K. E., Ingemarsson, I. and Persson, C. G. A.: Relaxing effects of β-receptor stimulators in isolated, gravid human myometrium. Life Sci. 13:335–344, 1973.
12. Andersson, K. E., Bengtsson, L. Ph., Gustafson, I. et al.: The relaxing effect of terbutaline on the human uterus during term labor. Am. J. Obstet. Gynecol. 121:602–609, 1975.
13. Wesselius-de Casparis, A., Thiery, M., Yo le Sian, A. et al.: Results of double-blind multi-centre study with Ritodrine in premature labour. Br. Med. J. 3:144–147, 1971.
14. Belizan, J. M., Diaz, A. G., Abusleme, C.: Effects of orciprenaline on uterine contractility and maternal heart rate. Obstet. Gynecol. 46:385–388, 1975.
15. Liggins, G. C. and Vaughan, G. S.: Intravenous infusion of salbutamol in the management of premature labor. J. Obstet. Gynecol. Br. Commonwealth 80:29–32, 1973.
16. Csapo, A. I. and Herczeg, J.: Arrest of premature labor by isoxsuprine. Am. J. Obstet. Gynecol. 129:482–491, 1977.
17. Csapo, A. I.: Model experiments and clinical trials in the control of pregnancy and parturition. Am. J. Obstet. Gynecol. 85:359, 1963.
18. Ebashi, S. and Endo, M.: Calcium ion and muscle contraction. Prog. Biophys. Mol. Biol. 18:123, 1968.
19. Marshall, J. M. and Kroeger, E. A.: Adrenergic influences on uterine smooth muscle. Philos. Trans. R. Soc., London (Biol. Sci.) 265:135, 1973.
20. Steer, M. L., Atlas, D. and Levitzki, A.: Interrelations between β-adrenergic receptors, adenyl-ate cyclase and calcium. N. Engl. J. Med. 292:409, 1975.
21. Caritis, S. N., Morishima, H. O., Stark, R. I. et al.: Effects of terbutaline on the pregnant baboon and fetus. Obstet. Gynecol. 50:56, 1977.
22. Caritis, S. N., Mueller-Heubach, E., Morishima, H. O. et al.: Effect of terbutaline on cardiovascular state and uterine blood flow in pregnant ewes. Obstet. Gynecol. 50:603, 1977.
23. Nuwayhid, B. S., Cabalum, M. T., Lieb, S. M. et al.: Hemodynamic effects of isoxsuprine and terbutaline in pregnant and nonpregnant sheep. Am. J. Obstet. Gynecol. 137:25, 1980.
24. Kuang-Hung, T., Desser, K. B. and Benchimol, A.: Angina pectoris associated with the use of terbutaline for premature labor. J.A.M.A. 244:692, 1980.
25. Stubblefield, P. G.: Pulmonary edema occurring after therapy with dexamethasone and terbutaline for premature labor. A Case Report. Am. J. Obstet. Gynecol. 132:341, 1978.
26. Elliot, H. R., Abdulla, U. and Hayes, P. J.: Pulmonary edema associated with ritodrine infusion and

the isolated human myometrium. J. Pharm. Pharmacol. 17:584, 1965.

betamethasone in premature labor. Br. Med. J. 2:799, 1978.

27. Tinga, D. S. and Aarnoudse, J. G.: Postpartum pulmonary edema associated with preventive therapy for premature labor. Lancet 2:1026, 1979.

28. Rogge, P., Young, S. and Goodin, R.: Postpartum pulmonary edema associated with preventive therapy for premature labor. Lancet 2:1026, 1979.

29. Abramovici, H., Lewin, A., Lissak, A. et al.: Maternal pulmonary edema occurring after therapy with ritodrine for premature labor contractions. Acta Obstet. Gynecol. Scand. 59:555, 1980.

30. Jacobs, M. M., Knight, A. and Arias, F.: Maternal pulmonary edema resulting from betamimetic and glucocorticoid therapy. Obstet. Gynecol. 55:56, 1980.

31. Smythe, A. R. and Sakakini, J.: Maternal metabolic alterations secondary to terbutaline therapy for premature labor. Obstet. Gynecol. 57:566, 1981.

32. Borberg, C., Gillmer, M. D. G., Beard, R. W. et al.: Metabolic effects of beta-sympathomimetic drugs and dexamethasone in normal and diabetic pregnancy. Br. J. Obstet. Gynecol. 85:184, 1978.

33. Spellacy, W. N., Cruz, A. C., Buhi, W. C. et al.: The acute effects of ritodrine infusion on maternal metabolism: measurements of levels of glucose, insulin, glucagon, triglycerides, cholesterol, placental lactogen, and chorionic gonadotropin. Am. J. Obstet. Gynecol. 131:637, 1978.

34. Lipshitz, J. and Vimik, I. A.: The effects of hexoprenaline, a β_2-sympathomimetic drug, on maternal glucose, insulin, glucagon and free fatty acid levels. Am. J. Obstet. Gynecol. 130:761, 1978.

35. Andersson, K. E., Ingemarsson, I. and Persson, C. G. A.: Effects of terbutaline on human uterine motility at term. Acta Obstet. Gynecol. Scand. 54:165, 1975.

36. Andersson, K. E., Bengtsson, L. P. and Ingemarsson, I.: Terbutaline inhibition of mid-trimester uterine activity induced by prostaglandin $F_2\alpha$ and hypertonic saline. Br. J. Obstet. Gynecol. 82:745, 1975.

37. Ingemarsson, I.: Effect of terbutaline on premature labor. Am. J. Obstet. Gynecol. 125:520, 1976.

38. Wallace, R. L., Caldwell, D. L., Ansbacher, R. et al.: Inhibition of premature labor by terbutaline. Obstet. Gynecol. 51:387, 1978.

39. Ryden, G.: The effect of salbutamol and terbutaline in the management of premature labor. Acta Obstet. Gynecol. Scand. 56:293, 1977.

40. Arias, F.: Intrauterine resuscitation with terbutaline: a method for the management of acute intrapartum fetal distress. Am. J. Obstet. Gynecol. 131:39, 1978.

41. Bishop, E. H.: Pelvic scoring for elective induction. Obstet. Gynecol. 24:266, 1964.

42. Ritcher, R.: Evaluation of success in treatment of threatening premature labor by betamimetic drugs. Am. J. Obstet. Gynecol. 127:482, 1977.

43. Liggins, G. C. and Howie, R. A.: A controlled trial of antepartum glucocorticoid treatment for prevention of the respiratory distress syndrome in premature infants. Pediatrics 50:515, 1972.

44. Johnson, J. W. C., Austin, K. L., Jones, G. S. et al.: Efficacy of 17α-hydroxyprogesterone caproate in the prevention of premature labor. N. Engl. J. Med. 293:675, 1975.

Management of Preterm Labor

Robert Landesman, M.D.

Kathleen H. Wilson, B.S.

New York, New York

The World Health Organization, in 1972, recommended that the term *preterm labor*[1] rather than premature labor be used to define a pregnancy of less than 37 weeks (less than 259 days), and that the infants under 2500 g be classified as low birth weight infants. The calculation of the duration of pregnancy is not always accurate; unreliability of the history of the last menstrual cycle and the unknown exact date of actual conception result in a high degree of error. This may be compounded by "post-pill amenorrhea," when no reference point for calculation is available. In the past decade, the development of biparietal diameter tables for the measurement of head and abdominal circumference by sonography[2] have helped pinpoint the fetal size to within one to two weeks of true gestational age. However, there are exceptions such as the growth-retarded infant and the macrosomia of diabetes; these cases must be excluded from this computation.

Causes

The recognition of preterm labor has always been a difficult clinical problem and vaginal examination is usually contraindicated because it stimulates uterine contractions. An increase in circulating prostaglandins following vaginal examinations has been reported and would indicate the probable mechanism for the increased uterine contractility.[3] The rate of preterm labor varies from 5 to 8 per cent. A greater frequency occurs in women from poverty areas, in whom poor nutrition and lack of prenatal care are usually associated. Labor is recognized clinically when regular contractions occur under a 10-minute interval with a duration of more than 30 seconds. These contractions may be painful and may produce progressive effacement and dilatation of the cervix. Uterine activity should be monitored with external recording for 30 minutes. If the contractions are maintained or crescendo and are not lessened by the lateral recumbent position, preterm labor may be assumed and treatment instituted. In a number of studies in which groups treated with placebos were observed, one third of the patients so treated who satisfied the aforementioned criteria for labor did not deliver, and the contractions subsided.[4] Spontaneous rupture of the membranes is surprisingly frequent prior to the onset of preterm labor and occurs in approximately one third of cases. The earlier in pregnancy the membranes rupture, the longer is the interval between rupture and the onset of true labor. Gillibrand[5] reported that in 26 per cent of a preterm group, labor had not commenced after 1 week following rupture.

There are causes of preterm labor that complicate the course of pregnancy. Frequently, continuation of gestation may pose serious risk both for mother and infant. If the pregnancy complication could be alleviated, this would be the ideal method for preventing the impending preterm labor that frequently follows. This is usually not possible. Bleeding in pregnancy related to premature separation of the placenta, or placenta previa, occurs with preterm labor three to four times more frequently than in usual term pregnancy.[6] If the bleeding is scanty and does not require transfusion, hospital rest with good nutrition and observation may be sufficient.

If placental separation or hemorrhage or both necessitate blood replacement, delivery should be performed regardless of prematurity. For a maternal indication, preterm delivery may be indicated in spite of fetal growth retardation if the fetus shows evidence of intrauterine distress. This evidence includes lack of fetal growth shown by sonography, reduced serum or urinary estriols, positive contraction stress test and scanty or meconium-stained amniotic fluid. Preterm delivery by cesarean section may be safer for the fetus than continued growth in the uterus.

The incidence of cervical incompetence, effacement and dilatation without pain varies enormously from center to center (0.1 to 7 per cent). If one or two previous pregnancies are associated with painless effacement and premature delivery, the diagnosis of cervical incompetence in a subsequent pregnancy is probably correct. If the membranes are bulging with full effacement and dilatation beyond 3 to 4 centimeters, the cerclage procedure is extremely difficult whether one uses a Shirodkar or a McDonald[7] method. Complications are known to occur in every sizable treatment center from cerclage; these include hemorrhage, infection, rupture of uterus and vesicovaginal fistula. The use of a pharmacologic agent to stop resulting uterine contractions is indicated for at least 24 hours following the procedure. The exact place for the use of these drugs requires additional study.

Congenital anomalies of the uterus play a significant role in preterm labor and comprise about 5 per cent of the total cases. Anomalies include bicornuate and double uterus and, rarely, a pregnancy in a blind uterine horn. A history of preterm labor would indicate that a hysterogram should be performed before a second pregnancy is attempted. Surgical correction of uterine abnormalities may frequently prevent a recurrence of preterm labor. The early onset of hypertensive disorders of pregnancy or toxemia may result in preterm labor and a premature infant. If the syndrome has been sustained for three weeks or more and is associated with chronic hypertension, fetal growth retardation is frequently associated with premature birth. Early recognition and medical therapy may reduce the incidence of prematurity. Unfortunately, clinical control of maternal symptoms and signs does not influence the rate of growth of the fetus. If the criteria for fetal well-being in utero are poor, delivery is indicated after 34 weeks when the fetus usually is over 1500 g. The uterine musculature in hypertensive disease is hyperirritable and spontaneous early labor occurs frequently. The reported incidence of the preterm toxemic infant varies depending on nutrition, medical care and the frequency of hypertensive diseases.

The complications of erythroblastosis will frequently lead to preterm delivery. If the fetus is above 1500 g, with or without exchange transfusions and the disease has advanced as judged by bilirubin analysis, emergency delivery, most frequently preterm, will

TABLE 1. INDICATIONS TO STOP
OR NOT TO STOP PRETERM LABOR

DO NOT STOP	STOP
Toxemia	Unknown causes
Ruptured membranes	Maternal infection
Placenta separation	Multiple pregnancy
Erythroblastosis	Cervical incompetence
Uterine anomaly	Abdominal surgery
Fetal anomaly	Trauma
Medical diseases	Cystitis-pyelonephritis

From Chez, R. A.: Clinical approach to the therapy of premature labor. Intrauterine asphyxia and the developing fetal brain. Gluck, L. (ed.): Modern Prenatal Medicine. Chicago, Year Book Medical Publishers, 1977, p. 139.

be indicated. The uncontrolled diabetic with hydramnios and a diagnosis of fetal macrosomia will require early delivery before or at the 37th week. In these cases, even though the fetus is above 2500 g, it may be considered a premature infant. With recent techniques of close control of gestational diabetes, the hydramnios, macrosomia and evidences of fetal distress do not occur, and a normal-sized infant born at term may be the final result.[8] A severe infection[9] such as pyelonephritis, hepatitis or malaria that is associated with hyperpyrexia results in irritability of the uterine muscle, uterine contractions and labor. Every effort should be made to control the temperature by antipyretics and body cooling and to irradicate the infection by appropriate specific medication.

Multiple gestation will overdistend the uterus and result in preterm labor, causing a high incidence of neonatal deaths in twins. Multiple gestation should be detected as early as possible, and increased rest and reduced activity recommended. Because of the high risk of preterm labor in multiple gestation, pharmacologic agents such as beta-adrenergic agonists have been administered in the second trimester to prophylactically prevent preterm labor. No conclusive data are available as evidence of the effectiveness of such therapy.

A rapid enlargement of the uterus with hydramnios frequently indicates fetal anomalies of the cerebral or renal type and contraindicates therapy to prevent preterm labor. The skillful use of sonography with screening by maternal alpha-fetoprotein may confirm some abnormalities of the fetus.

Therapy is of potential value during preterm labor of unknown origin when the fetus is normal. This category includes 25 to 30 per cent of cases of preterm labor, depending on the highly variable factors specific for any individual hospital. In the presence of a normal-appearing fetus and mother and a uterus without congenital anomalies, active therapeutic agents may be promising. Only 2 to 3 per cent of all obstetric patients comprise this special category. Table 1 lists known causes of preterm labor[11] and identifies those patients who should be permitted to proceed to spontaneous termination (do not stop) and those who may respond to methods to arrest labor (stop).

Beta-Adrenergic Agonists

Because of the limited effectiveness of the available compounds, criteria for their use have been developed to provide a reasonable opportunity for successful therapy. Although these agents have been used in the presence of ruptured membranes and uterine bleeding and when the cervix is dilated over 4 cm and fully effaced, the likelihood of success is limited. The following indications[4] for use of these agents have become standard:

1. Preterm labor of unknown etiology (without excessive uterine bleeding or ruptured membranes).

2. Duration of estimated gestation 20 to 36 weeks and weight of the fetus below 2500 g.

3. Regular painful contractions that occur at intervals of less than 10 minutes monitored with external tomography for a minimum of 30 minutes.

4. Cervix that shows some, but incomplete, effacement and a cervical dilatation of less than 4 cm.

At the present time there are seven different beta-adrenergic agonists that have been used extensively to reverse the onset of labor. These are shown in Table 2.

Lands[12] demonstrated the existence of two different varieties of beta-adrenergic receptors. β_1 receptor stimulation results in tachycardia, relaxation of gut and lipolysis. β_2 re-

TABLE 2. BETA-ADRENERGIC AGONISTS

1. Isoxsuprine
2. Ritodrine
3. Terbutaline
4. Fenoterol
5. Salbutamol
6. Orciprenaline
7. Isoproterenol

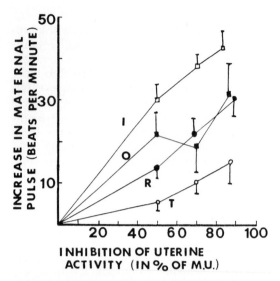

Figure 1. Four beta adrenergic agonists given in comparable effective doses over a period of 20 minutes are compared. During preterm labor, the increase in maternal pulse, a beta 1 effect, is compared to reduction in uterine activity, a beta 2 action. Terbutaline produced the highest uterine muscle inhibition with the least increase in maternal pulse rate. On the other hand, isoproterenol exhibited the highest maternal pulse rate for any given reduction in uterine activity. (Gamissans, O.: Proceedings, 5th Study Group, Royal College of Obstetricians and Gynecologists, 1977, p. 175.)

ceptor stimulation produces relaxation of uterine muscle and bronchi and results in glycogenesis. Gamissans compared the β_1 and β_2 effects of four adrenergic drugs by monitoring the maternal pulse rate, a β_1 modality, against the uterine muscle activity, a β_2 response.[13] The four beta-adrenergic agonists,

isoproterenol, orciprenaline, ritodrine and terbutaline, were infused in patients for 20 minutes in normal labor with 2 to 5 cm dilated cervix. The dose levels ranged between 6 to 18 µg per minute for isoproterenol, 5 to 40 µg per minute for orciprenaline, 100 to 600 µg per minute for ritodrine, and 6 to 24 µg per minute for terbutaline, which are considered to be equally effective doses. Figure 1 shows that at a comparable level of inhibition of uterine activity, terbutaline and ritodrine produced less maternal tachycardia than isoproterenol and orciprenaline. Gamissans in addition studied the effects of the same four beta agonists on the maternal and fetal heart rate.[13] At the prescribed dose range, an increase in maternal pulse rate of up to 40 beats per minute (bpm) was accompanied by an increase of only 10 bpm in the fetal heart rate (Fig. 2). Fetal tachycardia develops with a rise of the heart rate of 20 to 35 per minute only when the dosage of the agents is above the average as shown in six instances.

ISOXSUPRINE

Isoxsuprine is a beta-adrenergic agonist that is given in the United States but not approved for use in preterm labor. Although the tachycardia and hypotension associated with this agent may be serious drawbacks, it is prescribed frequently on many university services. A dose of 500 µg per minute may be given initially and this may be increased to 1250 µg per minute provided that the cardi-

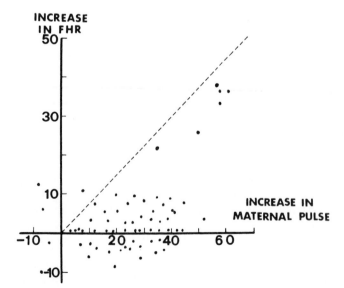

Figure 2. Increase in maternal pulse with the fetal heart rate after the administration of four beta-adrenergic agonists. With average dose of the drugs, the fetal heart rate increased only 10 beats per minute. When extremely high doses were infused (the upper six points) the fetal heart rate rose 20 to 60 per minute. (Gamissans, O..: Proceedings, 5th Study Group, Royal College of Obstetricians and Gynecologists, 1977, p. 177.)

oxascular symptoms are not severe. Once uterine relaxation is obtained, the drug may be continued for an additional 90 minutes. Ten μg of isoxsuprine may be injected intramuscularly every 6 to 8 hours, and this may be followed by 80 mg per day orally in multiple doses. Tolerance to the drug is extremely variable. Severe hypotension may frequently be prevented by good hydration and by turning the patient on the side. Because of the undesirable hypotension and tachycardia and the lack of any good randomized control studies with isoxsuprine, a search for more effective agents has been in progress.

Although experience has indicated that isoxsuprine effect is transient and is complicated by cardiovascular side effects, Csapo and Herczeg[14] treated 36 patients (19 with isoxsuprine and 17 with placebo), all between 26 and 36 weeks of pregnancy. The cervical condition as reflected by the Bishop score[15] averaged about 5. The isoxsuprine was administered with a loading dose of 0.6 mg per minute for 10 minutes and a maintenance level of 0.2 mg per minute for 2 hours followed by isoxsuprine orally 20 mg 4 times a day for 20 days. The placebo group received intravenous dextrose and then oral dextrose orally for an average period of 1 week.

Of the 19 isoxsuprine-treated patients only three delivered prematurely; infants of the remaining 16 weighed over 2500 g. In the placebo group of 17 newborns delivered, only five were over 2500 g and the remaining 12 weighed less. Thus in the isoxsuprine-treated group the incidence of prematurity was 16 per cent, while in the placebo group it was 71 per cent.

These results are far superior to those in other reported studies with this drug. The authors do not indicate the maximum pulse elevations associated with the isoxsuprine administration, which would be an indicator of beta-adrenergic activity. The two groups were not comparable. Nine fetuses of the 19 in the treated group were most likely above 2500 g prior to the isoxsuprine therapy. However, in the placebo group, intravenous therapy was begun at lower fetal weights. The treatment period of isoxsuprine therapy was relatively short, averaging 20 days for pregnancies at 29 to 33 weeks, which did not justify a successful termination of the drug administration. Previous trials, which were not randomized, indicated that isoxsuprine produced relaxation of the uterus, but only in early labor.[16-18]

RITODRINE

Ritodrine was used in this country under an investigational new drug permit until 1980, when it was approved. All who were involved in the program studying its effects were convinced of its value and although it is not ideal, it supplies a useful agent for selected cases and is far more effective than isoxsuprine. The drug has been available in Western Europe for more than seven years, including the United Kingdom, France, Holland, Belgium, Switzerland, Austria and Germany. In many thousands of users, no serious effects in either the mother or the infant have been reported.

Ritodrine trials were begun 14 years ago in the United States and Western Europe under the guidance of Wesselius-de Casparis.[4] Intravenous administration was begun at 100 μg per minute and increased at 10-minute intervals up to 400 μg per minute. The pulse rate is a good criterion of beta-adrenergic effect and toxicity. Pulse rate was tolerable for short periods of 10 to 20 minutes up to 140. Oral dose of 10 to 20 μg every 4 hours was well tolerated. If the criteria as just detailed for use of the beta-adrenergic agonists were fulfilled, about 70 per cent of the preterm labors could be arrested until the 38th week. This level of arrest of preterm labor was two times that found in a control group receiving no therapy. Clinical data on ritodrine may be found in the studies of Coutinho et al.,[19] Gamissans et al.,[20] Wesselius-de Casparis,[4] Barden,[21] Bieniarz et al.,[22] Laursen et al.[23] and Landesman et al.[24]

TERBUTALINE

Ingemarsson,[25] and Andersson et al.[26] have studied the effect of terbutaline on isolated myometrium and the human uterus during term and preterm labor. These authors are most enthusiastic about the excellent results and manageable side effects associated with terbutaline. Thirty patients in preterm labor were selected and 15 in each group were evenly matched so that group 1 received the terbutaline and the other placebo. Terbutaline was given at 10 μg per minute and then increased to 25 μg per minute. When contractions ceased, the rate was reduced until a low maintenance level was reached, which was continued for 8 hours provided that uterine activity had ceased. Then subcutaneous terbutaline was administered for 3 days at 250 μg per six hours followed by drug orally, 5 μg every 8 hours until the 36th week of pregnancy. If labor recurred, intravenous drug administration was repeated.

In the terbutaline group, delivery was postponed in 12 out of 15 patients until after 36 weeks; there were three failures. In the placebo group 10 patients delivered within 24 hours from the start of the infusion, and only 3 delivered term infants. The mean birth weight of infants in the terbutaline-treated group was 3060 g and the placebo group, 2190 g. Terbutaline side effects seem comparable to those of the other beta-adrenergic compounds.

Because preterm labor is frequently associated with ruptured membranes, Ingemarsson[27] attempted to salvage some of these infants with the same terbutaline therapy in a study of 23 patients, with a mean duration of pregnancy of 32.8 weeks. Labor was postponed for a mean of 8 days and no patient delivered within 24 hours; 15 patients delivered in 1 to 7 days and 8 had delivery postponed for more than 7 days. No infants developed infection prior to delivery and there were only three incidents of mild endometritis. This initial study is promising, since no maternal infection occurred and there was successful delay of delivery. At the present time, however, the widespread use of a beta-adrenergic agonist in patients with ruptured membranes is contraindicated because of the danger of intrauterine infection, associated fetal death, and the high probability of failure with this drug therapy.

FENOTEROL

Fenoterol is extensively used in West Germany. It is estimated by Kubli[28] that 1 million ampules of 0.5 mg per year and 6 million 5 mg tablets of fenoterol were administered for the 500,000 deliveries in that country. Eight cases of pulmonary edema have been reported, with one maternal death. All these cases involved fenoterol combined with corticosteroids. The single fatality was associated with clear pathologic evidence of viral myocarditis. In West Germany currently, fenoterol is combined with corticosteroids to postpone labor to permit accelerated maturation of the lungs. To reduce cardiopulmonary complications, careful cardiac screening with weekly electrocardiograms is a routine practice. The combination of the two drugs is now considered by many to be contraindicated. However, even with the many patients receiving the drug in Germany, there has not been a single death related to the beta-adrenergic agonist when used alone. The 6 per cent prematurity rate in West Germany cannot account for the vast amount of fenoterol consumed; indications are broadened to include patients with Braxton Hicks' sign, twin gestations, contractions in the first trimester and even the onset of labor at an inconvenient time or place for the physician or patient. The usual dose of fenoterol[29] for preterm labor is 1 to 4 μg per minute. Once contractions cease, the drug may be continued on a maintenance level for 12 hours. Thereafter, 5 mg may be given sublingually in 6- to 12-hour intervals until the 36th week. The tolerance and effectiveness of the drug may, as in other drugs of its type, be judged by the level of tachycardia in relation to the intensity and frequency of uterine contractions.

SALBUTAMOL

This beta-adrenergic agonist was administered by Liggins to 88 women in preterm labor with and without ruptured membranes.[30] In 88 per cent of the patients labor was postponed for more than 24 hours. When the cervix was dilated more than 4 cm, there was only a 58 per cent success rate. In 14 patients ethanol had been previously prescribed and failed to diminish the contractions. In 9 of these patients salbutamol was successful after ethanol. Salbutamol may be given intravenously and orally. For the parenteral route, 5 mg are diluted in 500 cc of 5 per cent dextrose. The compound is administered from 14 to 48 μg per minute usually for 6 to 12 hours. Salbutamol may be prescribed orally in doses of 4 mg every 6 hours until the 36th week of pregnancy. With increasing dosage, tachycardia, increased pulse pressure and a tremor may be observed.

Alcohol

Ethanol was introduced as a treatment for preterm labor in 1965.[31] A randomized study in 42 patients[32] indicated that ethanol was more effective than a placebo. However, the group was rigidly controlled similarly to the beta-adrenergic groups previously described; not included were patients with ruptured membranes, bleeding, fully effaced cervix and a cervix dilated 4 cm or more. A randomized control study comparing ritodrine and ethanol in three centers including 135 patients in preterm labor indicated that ritodrine was superior to ethanol.[23] Delivery was postponed for more than 72 hours in 49 (73 per cent) patients with ethanol and 61 patients (90 per cent) with ritodrine. Ethanol has serious disadvantages because of maternal intoxication with the loading dose that requires special nursing care. Profound nausea and protracted emesis with the risk of aspiration are frequent side effects of the alcohol; prolonged restlessness and emotional distress are followed by sedation. The ethanol rapidly crosses to the fetus and the fetus does not metabolize the ethanol as fast as the mother. The ethanol must be discontinued as soon as delivery is anticipated. Prior hepatic disease contraindicates its use. Ten per cent ethanol is commercially available. The initial dose is 7.5 ml per kg of body weight of 10 per cent ethanol solution for 2 hours. The maintenance dose is 1.5 ml per kg body weight for 10 hours. If the treatment requires repetition within 10 hours, the dose is reduced 10 per cent for each hour that the interval is less than 10 hours. The alcohol level varies from 0.12 to 0.18 per cent. Although the beta-adrenergic agonists offer the primary mode of therapy, there are numerous instances of an initial trial with these in which they have been unsuccessful and ethanol has promptly blocked the contractions. On the other hand, ethanol may not completely reduce the contractility, and one of the described beta-adrenergic compounds may provide the desired results. Oral ethanol does not provide adequate dose to block concentrations before emesis results. Also, ambulatory patients performing any activity requiring mental alertness may not use ethanol. On the other hand, oral beta-adrenergic agonists have been successfully used for as long as 10 weeks during the third trimester.

Antiprostaglandins

Prostaglandins have been known to be potent myometrial-stimulating agents. In 1972 and 1973 it was demonstrated that aspirin, indomethacin and naproxen prolonged parturition in animals and prolonged the duration

TABLE 3. ANTIPROSTAGLANDIN DRUGS

Aspirin
Indomethacin
Naproxen (Naprosyn)
Ibuprofen (Motrin)
Fenoprofen (Nalfon)
Meclofenamic acid
Flufenamic acid
Phenylbutazone

of second trimester abortion and term labor.[33-36] A group of antiprostaglandin drugs (Table 3) has been synthesized that specifically inhibits the enzyme prostaglandin synthetase. There are serious potential hazards[37] associated with use of these prostaglandin synthetase inhibitors for the treatment of preterm labor, for example:

1. Premature closure of the ductus arteriosus.

2. Increase in bleeding time and inhibition of platelet aggregation.

3. Displacement of bilirubin from its binding sites on albumin resulting in hyperbilirubinemia postpartum.

4. Damage to the cerebral nervous system.

5. Impairment of renal function resulting in oliguria.

6. Increased rate of stillbirth and reduced neonatal weight in chronic users.

Wiqvist[37] reported good control of preterm labor using naproxin in 12 of 14 cases. One infant weighing 2700 g, born in the 37th week, developed mild cardiomegaly and signs of persistent ductus arteriosus. Following a period of digitalization and assisted ventilation, the infant was discharged after eight days. Zuckerman[38] treated 50 patients in preterm labor with indomethacin without controls; 46 infants were considered healthy at birth. According to Wiqvist,[37] the following questions must be answered before prostaglandin synthetase inhibitors may be used for the treatment of preterm labor.

1. Do these drugs have toxic effects too severe to be used in preterm labor?

2. Should their use be limited to a particular stage of pregnancy when fetal death is the alternative?

3. Should these drugs be stopped at least 24 hours before anticipated delivery?

4. Are there levels of the drugs that will reduce uterine contractions and not affect the fetus?

5. Should the drug be limited in dosage and time intervals?

Gamissans[39] and his group in Barcelona went one step further by comparing the effectiveness of ritodrine alone to ritodrine plus indomethacin; 22 patients were evaluated in each group. Ritodrine was maintained in all patients for 24 hours beginning at a dose of 200 μg per minute and then adjusted to the needs of the individual patient. After 24 hours ritodrine at a dose of 10 μg was administered orally every 4 to 6 hours until 36 weeks. In addition, one group received placebo suppositories and the second group received indomethacin suppositories 50 mg every 8 hours for 2 weeks. There was a striking improvement in results with the combined effect of ritodrine and indomethacin as opposed to ritodrine alone. There was a mean increase of 16 days in days gained with ritodrine plus indomethacin and mean additional weight increase of 400 g at delivery. Respiratory distress syndrome occurred in one infant in each group and the final result was favorable. There were four fetal deaths in the placebo group and two in the combined therapy group equally divided between two causes: placental separation and fetal size of under under 650 g. None of the infants whose mothers were treated with indomethacin developed pulmonary hypertension or cardiac failure or showed evidence of premature closure of the ductus arteriosus.

The studies of Wiqvist,[37] Zuckerman[38] and Gamissans[39] have demonstrated the uterine relaxant properties of prostaglandin synthetase inhibitors. When preterm labor occurs prior to fetal weight of 1000 g before 28 to 30 weeks, calculated risks may be necessary to salvage the highly endangered fetus. Gamissans has suggested that ritodrine or any of the beta-adrenergic agonists may block vascular effects of the prostaglandin inhibitors, preventing the early closure of the ductus arteriosus.

Use of Antepartum Glucocorticosteroid Therapy (Betamethasone)

Since 1968, evidence has accumulated indicating that rapid maturation of the fetal lung follows use of glucocorticosteroids (see Chapter 5). In order to determine the possible value of this treatment in prematurity, Liggins and Howie[40] organized a double-blind control trial. Patients with threatened deliveries between 24 and 37 weeks were included. Each woman was given either betamethasone or a control inactive material, cortisone acetate, by the intramuscular route as two injections 24 hours apart. Over 800 premature infants were included in this study. Betamethasone reduced the incidence of respiratory distress syndrome between 30 to 32 weeks but over 34 weeks the special therapy showed no influence on the final result. Treatment must begin at least 24 hours prior to delivery and is not effective after 1 week. The therapy is contraindicated in toxemia of pregnancy. Since available therapy for the prevention of preterm labor is only partially effective and many infants will have a postponed delivery date but will remain in a premature group, a decision must be made as to whether betamethasone should be administered. At present there is a diversity in opinion in university hospitals; some such as Columbia and Harvard Universities use the therapy while others such as Case-Western Reserve and Colorado do not. Those in the latter universities believe that the results in their high-risk premature units are as good as in the centers where the special therapy is advised. The effect of betamethasone, which blocks cellular division as it produces rapid maturation, is at present unknown in other organs such as the brain, liver, intestines and muscle cells. Until follow-up results for 10 to 15 years are known, the steroid therapy should be limited to institutions sponsoring special control studies.

Summary

The exact physiologic mechanism for the onset of preterm and term labor is at present not fully known. There are certain causes of preterm labor that contraindicate the use of drugs to postpone delivery: toxemia, ruptured membranes, placenta separation, erythroblastosis, uterine and fetal anomalies and advanced cardiac disease. Another group of maternal complications may be treated to prevent preterm labor. Every effort should be made to combat infection and block labor. Cervical incompetence, multiple gestation and labor of unknown cause are indications for the use of drugs to block labor. About one third of cases of preterm labor are of unknown cause. These patients have a normal-sized fetus for the duration of pregnancy and intact membranes, and results of all modalities used for evaluating the fetus are normal. It is particularly in this group that pharmacologic agents may benefit the fetus by prolonging the intrauterine period.

The beta-adrenergic agonists are the best available agents to block labor. Ritodrine, fenoterol and terbutaline are approved for use in Western Europe, and ritodrine was approved by the U.S. Food and Drug Administration in 1980. Isoxsuprine, inferior to the other three, is also used in the United States. However, it is doubtful that any of these agents will be successful if labor has progressed beyond the early stages. Membranes must be intact; cervix must be less than 4 cm dilated. Contractions may be only mild or moderate and effacement is to remain only partial if a successful result is to be obtained. Careful antepartum monitoring of the cervix to recognize early signs of change is an essential part of good care. Bishop[15] and Mehta and Shah[41] have devised standards of cervical change and contractility to provide nomenclature to describe the early cervical findings prior to true labor.

If the beta-adrenergic agonists are unsuccessful, intravenous ethanol may be tried. There is no approval in writing by the FDA for its use. The presence of intoxication and severe nausea are serious drawbacks. If the two modalities mentioned are failures, indomethacin may be used in special centers for study, particularly if the fetus is estimated at under 1000 g when the opportunity for salvage in the premature nursery is guarded.

Our understanding of the forces involved in the production of preterm labor is incomplete, and the drugs discussed provide only reversibility at the onset of the process. The high morbidity among survivors under 1000 g and the tremendous costs for the same group in the premature nursery require a redoubling of our efforts to solve this important obstetric problem.

Addendum, February 1982

In 1980, ritodrine was the first drug approved in the United States for the treatment of preterm labor.[42] The complete studies indicated that the drug was well tolerated. The obvious toxicity of β_2 sympathomimetic drugs, the tachycardia, the expanded pulse pressure, and increased glucose levels resulting in larger requirements for insulin demanded that the

initial therapy be given under hospital surveillance. Variability of toxicity was the main factor in determining the optimal and maximum dosages of the drugs. Although the maximum dose was stated to be 350 μg per minute, a dose of 500 μg per minute in an occasional patient produced only mild side effects.[43] If the intravenous administration is successful, intramuscular and oral administration may rapidly follow after a minimum of 12 hours. When at home, the patient may monitor her pulse to determine the quantity absorbed from the gut.

The use of saline solution with the ritodrine further increases the plasma volume and may result in pulmonary edema. To prevent pulmonary congestion with the beta-sympathomimetic drugs, not only is salt solution contraindicated but also intravenous fluid should be curtailed. Serum potassium decreases during intramuscular administration. This decrease has also been noted with intravenous terbutaline.[46] All three beta-adrenergic compounds—ritodrine, terbutaline and salbutamol—produce increases in serum glucose and requirements for insulin. These drugs may have a direct effect on the beta cells of the pancreas. The oral use immediately prior to delivery may produce a sustained hypoglycemia in the infant. Lactic acid acidosis has been reported after intravenous ritodrine; this acidosis rarely results in a reduction in the maternal pH. The hypokalemia as well as the presence of high dose may be additive in the production of toxicity. Because the ideal indications for the use of ritodrine are limited, 11 medical centers were required to study 350 patients over a period of 7 years. Although other drugs, such as terbutaline and fenoterol, are about equally effective and are available in Western Europe, the high cost of such studies and the limitations of the market may discourage approval of other drugs until a more effective agent becomes available.

The serious drawback of these studies was the inability to determine the presence of early preterm labor, which may be as high as 33 per cent.[44] Metabolic and electrolytic changes are produced by the β_2 sympathomimetic drugs, which increase plasma volume with a fall in hemoglobin, hematocrit and serum albumin levels. This was associated with an increase in renin and aldosterone, tachycardia, acidosis that may induce a cardiac arrhythmia, cardiac failure and pulmonary edema. Pregnancy already complicated by cardiac or pulmonary disease usually contraindicates the treatment of preterm labor with the beta-adrenergic stimulants. The danger is that in the haste to treat the preterm labor the cardiopulmonary disease may go unrecognized or disregarded.

At the present time a small group of patients in preterm labor may benefit from available tocolytic agents. The large number of contraindications, including obstetrical and maternal disease, narrows the demand for these agents.[47] Prompt early administration of these tocolytic agents may delay delivery for two to three weeks at the optimal time—for example between 26 to 29 weeks of gestation. This difference may prevent fetal death, limit the severity and frequency of cerebral damage and finally reduce neonatal costs.

REFERENCES

1. Anderson, A. B.: Preterm Labor: Definition. *In* Proceedings of the 5th Study Group, Royal College of Obstetricians and Gynecologists, 1977, p. 2.
2. Campbell, S. and Wilkin, D.: Ultrasonic measurement of fetal abdomen circumference in the estimation of fetal weight. Br. J. Obstet. Gynecol. 82:689, 1975.
3. Flint, A. P. F., Anderson, A. B. M., Patten, P. T. and Turnbull, A. C.: Control of utero-ovarian venous prostaglandin F during labor in the sheep: acute effects of vaginal and cervical stimulation. J. Endocrinol. 63:67, 1974.
4. Wesselius-de Casparis, A., Thiery, M., Yo le Sian, A. et al.: Results of double-blind multicentre study with ritodrine in premature labour. Br. Med. J. 3:144, 1971.
5. Gillibrand, P. N.: Premature rupture of the membranes and prematurity. J. Obstet. Gynecol. Br. Commonwealth 74:678, 1967.
6. Turnbull, E. P. N. and Walker, J.: The outcome of pregnancy complicated by threatened abortion. J. Obstet. Gynecol. Br. Emp. 63:553, 1956.
7. Turnbull, A. C. and Anderson, A. B. M.: Preterm labor. *In* Scarpelli, E. M. and Cosmi, E. V. (eds.): Reviews in perinatal medicine, Vol. 2. New York, Raven Press, 1978, p. 103.
8. Merkatz, I. R. and Adam, P.: Diabetes in pregnancy. Seminars in Perinatology, Vol. 7, No. 4. New York, Grune & Stratton, 1978.
9. Wren, B. G.: Subclinical renal infection and prematurity. Med. J. Aust. 2:596, 1969.
10. Jovanovic, L., Landesman, R. and Saxena, B. B.: Screening for twin pregnancy. Science 198:738, 1977.
11. Chez, R. A.: Clinical approach to the therapy of premature labor. Intrauterine asphyxia and the developing fetal brain. *In* Gluck, L. (ed.): Modern Prenatal Medicine. Chicago, Year Book Medical Publishers, 1977, p. 139.
12. Lands, A. M., Arnold, A., McAulegg, J. P., Luduena, F. P. and Brown, T. G.: Differentiation of receptor

13. Gamissans, O.: Beta adrenergic agonists. *In* Proceedings of the 5th Study Group, Royal College of Obstetricians and Gynecologists, 1977, p. 171.
14. Csapo, A. I. and Herczeg, J.: Arrest of premature labor by isoxsuprine. Am. J. Obstet. Gynecol. 129:482, 1977.
15. Bishop, E. H.: Pelvic scoring for induction. Obstet. Gynecol. 24:266, 1964.
16. Bishop, E. H. and Woutersz, T. B.: Arrest of premature labor. J.A.M.A. 178:812, 1961.
17. Hendricks, C. H., Cibils, L. A., Pose, S. V. and Eskes, K. A. B.: The pharmacologic control of excessive uterine activity with isoxsuprine. Am. J. Obstet. Gynecol. 82:1064, 1961.
18. Briscoe, C. C.: Failure of oral isoxsuprine to prevent prematurity. Am. J. Obstet. Gynecol. 95:885, 1966.
19. Coutinho, E. M., Bomfim de Souza, F., Wilson, K. H. and Landesman, R.: The inhibitory action of a new sympathomimetic amine OV-21220 (ritodrine) on the nongravid uterus. Am. J. Obstet. Gynecol. 104:1053, 1969.
20. Gamissans, O., Esteban-Altirriba, J. and Maiques, V.: Inhibition of human myometrial activity by a new beta-adrenergic drug (OV 21220), ritodrine. J. Obstet. Gynecol. Br. Commonwealth 76:656, 1969.
21. Barden, T. P.: Effect of ritodrine on human uterine motility and cardiovascular responses in term labor and the early postpartum state. Am. J. Obstet. Gynecol. 112:645, 1972.
22. Bieniarz, J., Motew, M. and Scommegma, A.: Uterine and cardiovascular effects of ritodrine in premature labor. Obstet. Gynecol. 40:65, 1972.
23. Laursen, N. H., Merkatz, I. R., Tejani, N., Wilson, K. H., Roberson, D., Mann, L. I. and Fuchs, F.: Inhibition of premature labor: A multicenter comparison of ritodrine and ethanol. Am. J. Obstet. Gynecol. 127:837, 1977.
24. Landesman, R., Wilson, K. H., Cutinho, E. M., Klima, I. M. and Marcus, R. S.: The relaxant action of ritodrine, a sympathomimetic amine, on the uterus during term labor. Am. J. Obstet. Gynecol. 110:111, 1971.
25. Ingemarsson, I.: Effect of terbutaline on premature labor. A double-blind placebo-controlled study. Am. J. Obstet. Gynecol. 125:520, 1976.
26. Andersson, K. E., Bengtsson, L. Ph., Gustafson, I. and Ingemarsson, I.: The relaxing effect of terbutaline on the human uterus during term labor. Am. J. Obstet. Gynecol. 121:602, 1975.
27. Ingemarsson, I.: Premature labour and terbutaline. Proceedings of the 5th Study Group, Royal College of Obstetricians and Gynecologists, 1977, p. 161.
28. Kubli, F.: Discussion of beta-adrenergic agonists in preterm labor. Proceedings of the 5th Study Group, Royal College of Obstetricians and Gynecologists, 1977, p. 218.
29. Cifuentes, J. R., Betitzky, R., Cuadro, S. C., Rios, R. and Caldeyro-Barcia, R.: Effects of adrenoceptor-stimulating drugs on the myometrium and cardiovascular system in nonpregnant women. Physiology and genetics of reproduction, Part B. Coutinho, E. M. and Fuchs, F. (eds.), New York, Plenum Press, 1974.
30. Liggins, G. C. and Vaughan, G. S.: Intravenous infusion of salbutamol in the management of pre-

mature labour. J. Obstet. Gynecol. Br. Commonwealth 80:29, 1973.

31. Fuchs, F.: Treatment of threatened premature labour with alcohol. J. Obstet. Gynecol. Br. Commonwealth. 72:1011, 1965.

32. Zlatnik, F. and Fuchs, F.: A controlled study of ethanol in premature labor. Am. J. Obstet. Gynecol. 112:610, 1972.

33. Aiken, J. W.: Aspirin and indomethacin prolong parturition in rats: evidence that prostaglandins contribute to expulsion of the fetus. Nature 240:21, 1972.

34. Csapo, A. I., Csapo, E. F., Fay, E., Henzel, M. R. and Salan, G.: A delay of spontaneous labor by naproxen in the rat model. Contraception 3:827, 1973.

35. Waltman, R., Tricomi, V. and Palav, A. B.: Midtrimester hypertonic saline induced abortion: effect of indomethacin on indiction/abortion time. Am. J. Obstet. Gynecol. 114:829, 1972.

36. Lewis, R. B. and Schulman, J. D.: Influence of the inhibitor of prostaglandin synthesis by acetyl salicylic acid on the duration of human gestation and labor. Lancet 2:1159, 1973.

37. Wiqvist, N.: Effects of prostaglandins and synthetase inhibitors on the fetal circulation. Proceedings of the 5th Study Group, Royal College of Obstetricians and Gynecologists, 1977, p. 231.

38. Zuckerman, H., Reiss, U. and Rubinstein, T.: Inhibition of human premature labor with indomethacin. Obstet. Gynecol. 44:787, 1974.

39. Gamissans, O., Canas, E., Cararach, V., Ribas, J., Puerto, B. and Edo, A.: A study of indomethacin combined with ritodrine in threatened preterm labor. Europ. J. Obstet. Gynecol. Reprod. Biology 3:123, 1978.

40. Liggins, G. C. and Howie, R. N.: The prevention of respiratory distress syndrome by maternal steroid therapy. *In* Gluck, L. (ed.): Modern Prenatal Medicine. Chicago, Year Book Medical Publishers, 1974, p. 415.

41. Mehta, A. and Shah, P.: Prematurity and cervical status. J. Obstet. Gynecol. India 27:144, 1977.

42. Barden, I. P., Peter, J. B. and Merkatz, I. R.: Ritodrine hydrochloride: a betamimetic agent for use in premature labor. I. Pharmacology, clinical administration, side effects and safety. Obstet. Gynecol. 56:1, 1980.

43. Merkatz, I. R., Peter, J. B. and Barden, T. P.: Ritodrine hydrochloride: a betamimetic agent for use in preterm labor. II. Evidence of efficacy. Obstet. Gynecol. 56:7, 1980.

44. Philipsen, T., Eriksen, P. S. and Lynggard, F.: Pulmonary edema following ritodrine-saline administration in premature labor. Obstet. Gynecol. 58:304, 1981.

45. Schreyer, P., Caspi, E., Snir, E., Herzianiu, E., User, P., Gilboa, Y. and Zaidman, J. L.: Metabolic effects of intramuscular and oral administration of ritodrine in pregnancy. Obstet. Gynecol. 57:730, 1981.

46. Smythe, A. R., III and Sakakini, J.: Maternal metabolic alterations secondary to terbutaline therapy for premature labor. Obstet. Gynecol. 57:566, 1981.

47. Brown, S. M. and Tejani, N. A.: Terbutaline sulfate in the prevention of recurrence of premature labor. Obstet. Gynecol. 57:22, 1981.

The Management of Preterm Labor

Tom P. Barden, M.D.

University of Cincinnati College of Medicine

Premature birth remains the most perplexing problem of modern obstetrics. It is variously described in terms of birth weight less than 2500 grams, or "low birth weight," and of gestation at birth of less than 37 completed weeks, or "preterm birth." The statistics of rates of premature birth and its consequences are often confusing because of the clinical inconsistencies of the two components of prematurity, such as the term but low birth weight infants of patients with hypertensive disease in pregnancy, and the preterm but large for gestational age infants of some diabetics. A review of United States natality statistics from 1968 through 1978 reveals that the incidence of both low birth weight and preterm gestation remained at approximately 7.5 per cent, while the neonatal death rate steadily declined from approximately 16 to 9.5 per 1000 live births during the same period.[166, 179–182, 206] This dramatic improvement of perinatal outcome presumably was due in large part to advances in obstetric and newborn care, along with improved conditions of living, family planning and many other more obscure factors. However, as other causes of perinatal morbidity and mortality are eliminated, the relative importance of premature birth becomes even more obvious. Premature birth remains the major contributing factor to nearly three fourths of all neonatal deaths, and it is strongly implicated in the pathogenesis of physical and neurologic handicaps that so commonly occur among survivors.[62, 168]

Mechanisms of Labor Onset

An understanding of pathophysiology of preterm labor could prove to be useful when its pharmacologic control is considered. Although our knowledge of the exact mechanism of human labor onset remains incomplete, a number of new concepts have emerged from research observations of recent years. There now is conclusive evidence that establishes the role of fetal membranes and decidua in production of prostaglandins and the onset of labor.[6, 92, 128, 162, 171, 188, 210-212] Arachidonic acid is stored in fetal membranes and decidua in its esterified, inactive form as glycerphospholipids. Progesterone serves to stabilize lysosomal phospholipase A_2, located in fetal membranes and uterine decidua. The withdrawal of progesterone or physical stress, as with hyperosmolar conditions or even stretch, serves to labilize lysosomes and causes release of phospholipase A_2 into cytoplasm. This enzyme preferentially hydrolyzes the phosphatidylethanolamines that contain arachidonic acid in the sn-2 position. The liberated arachidonic acid serves as precursor of prostaglandin formation in the decidua. In sheep, there is a rise in the level of prostaglandin $F_{2\alpha}$ in uterine vein blood shortly before the onset of labor.[150] In human pregnancy, Karim and associates[120-122] have reported the appearance of prostaglandins in amniotic fluid and maternal blood at the onset of labor. The increased uterine activity often apparent after manipulation of fetal membranes or with amniocentesis may reflect activation of this system for production of prostaglandins. Kloeck and Jung[132] reported that stretching of in vitro strips of myometrium stimulated their release of prostaglandins. Presumably the attached decidua and membranes may have been their source. Csapo and associates[53] found consistently increased uterine activity in patients at term after injection of as little as 150 ml of isotonic saline to the amniotic fluid volume. The importance of fetal membranes in the mechanism of labor is likely reflected in the frequent development of preterm labor following premature rupture of membranes, amnionitis or uterine manipulation during abdominal surgery.

The role of the human fetus in control of labor onset now appears to be rather minor. In contrast, Liggins and associates[150, 153] reported evidence suggesting an important role for the fetal hypothalamic-pituitary-adrenal system in production of cortisol and initiation of labor in sheep and goats. Also, Drost and Holm[61] observed prolongation of pregnancy in sheep after destruction of the fetal adrenal glands, presumably due to a lack of cortisol production. In contrast to the results reported in sheep, Mueller-Heubach and associates[176] observed that fetal adrenalectomy in a series of rhesus monkeys had no significant influence on the timing of labor onset. Human anencephaly, with its attendant adrenal hypofunction, is associated with premature delivery as often as with prolonged pregnancy.[105, 172] In general, human fetuses with adrenal hypoplasia but no other malformations are usually born at, or close to, term.[149] However, from autopsy studies, Anderson and associates[7] observed that adrenal glands were heavier in a series of premature infants dying soon after birth, when there was no recognizable cause of preterm labor, than those in infants of similar weights in whom an obvious obstetric complication had been associated with early onset of labor.

The possible role of human fetal cortisol production in the mechanism of labor onset has also been investigated by measurement of blood levels. In several reports[41, 85, 146, 177] levels of cortisol in cord blood were higher after spontaneous labor than after oxytocin-induced labor. However, others have found similar levels of cortisol in cord blood in the same two groups of patients.[226, 229] There is further disagreement regarding the level of fetal cortisol following vaginal delivery as opposed to cesarean section. In several studies fetal blood cortisol was higher after vaginal delivery than after cesarean section, with or without labor.[41, 85, 225, 228] However, other observers[227] found no significant difference in levels of cortisol in cord blood of infants born after elective cesarean section when compared with those born after spontaneous onset of labor and vaginal delivery.

In pregnant sheep, the injection of cortisol or dexamethasone is usually followed by preterm labor.[148] In contrast, the administration of large doses of glucocorticoids to pregnant women before term is not associated with preterm labor.[152] However, in studies of postterm human pregnancy, labor was induced in many patients by intra-amniotic injection of hydrocortisone[186] or dexamethasone.[167] Jenssen and Wright[113] reported that uterine sensitivity to oxytocin was enhanced in post-term patients by administration of dexamethasone for four days when compared with a post-term control series. They concluded that there is a relative adrenocortical insufficiency state in the postmature fetus.

Fetal adrenal hypofunction may also be expressed through depression of oxygen production. Evidence now suggests that corticosteroid treatment of patients in late pregnancy depresses estrogen levels by inhibiting fetal adrenal secretion of dehydroepiandrosterone sulfate, but does not appreciably affect maternal pregnanediol excretion or placental metabolism of steroids.[187, 216] However, there is no clear evidence at present that corticosteroid treatment is associated with significant prolongation of human pregnancy. The extremely low estrogen production in a pregnancy complicated by placental sulfatase deficiency is associated with prolonged gestation.[71] In contrast, Raja and associates[199] found higher levels of plasma estradiol in patients who subsequently developed spontaneous preterm labor than in others who delivered at term.

The fetus may further participate in the mechanism of labor onset by its production of oxytocin. Chard and associates[42] found significantly higher levels of oxytocin in cord blood than in maternal blood at delivery. Furthermore, oxytocin levels are higher in umbilical artery blood than in umbilical vein blood; this implies that the fetus is an active source of oxytocin.[42, 57, 58, 138] If fetal production of oxytocin is involved in the mechanism of labor onset, it is not clear how it reaches the myometrium without passing through the maternal circulation and back to the placenta. A more direct route is suggested from the observations of Seppala and associates[214, 215] that the oxytocin content of meconium-stained amniotic fluid is higher than clear fluid, and that the presence of meconium-stained fluid is associated with shorter labors. They also found the oxytocin concentration in fetal urine higher than in amniotic fluid, which suggests that it is excreted by the fetal kidneys.

Research into the role of the placenta in the mechanism of labor onset has focused primarily on its production of progesterone during pregnancy. There is evidence from several species of animals that progesterone is important in maintenance of pregnancy and that its withdrawal is associated with the onset of labor.[49] Csapo[47-49] proposed that placental production of progesterone produces a local block of contractile activity in the myometrium beneath the placental implantation site. The decreasing placental production of progesterone in late pregnancy removes the "block" to permit onset of labor. In support of this hypothesis, Kumar and associates[135] found that the concentration of progesterone was higher in myometrium underlying the placenta than from other sites; however, in a similar study Runnebaum and Zander[205] found the same relationship in first trimester pregnancy, but not at term. In an excellent review of the subject, Liggins and associates[151] proposed that labor onset may be caused by changes in target tissue sensitivity to placental steroids rather than by alterations of their production rates.

There have been rather inconsistent results from attempts to suppress uterine activity in humans by administration of progesterone. From several studies[33, 51, 98, 196, 240] large doses of progesterone or medroxyprogesterone, administered by a variety of routes, failed to inhibit uterine activity. However, Bengtsson[20] reported temporary inhibition of human labor when progesterone was injected directly into the uterine wall. Scommegna and associates[213] observed that human labor was partially inhibited by intravenous infusion of pregnenolone, the immediate precursor of placental progesterone. In a series of patients at risk of preterm labor, Johnson and associates[115, 116] found that prophylactic administration of 17 α-hydroxyprogesterone caproate was highly effective in preventing preterm labor when compared with placebo treatment. They also found significantly lower plasma progesterone levels in patients who later delivered before term than in those whose pregnancy progressed to term.[115]

Pathogenesis of Preterm Labor

Despite our rapidly increasing knowledge of uterine physiology, the exact pathogenesis of preterm labor in an individual patient is often obscure. It has been estimated that 20 to 50 per cent of patients who deliver preterm and/or low birth weight infants have no identifiable risk factors.[55, 195] However, there are many factors that are common to both delivery before term and low birth weight. The most obvious is the striking influence of low socioeconomic status on the incidence of both characteristics of prematurity. Fedrick and Anderson[68] reported the rate of spontaneous preterm births in women in social classes IV and V was about 50 per cent greater than in social classes I and II. Great Britain utilizes the "Registrar-General's classification," in which classes I and II are professional and managerial groups, class III is composed of clerical workers, and classes IV and V are semi-skilled and unskilled workers. They concluded that the risk of spontaneous preterm birth was related to low maternal age, low maternal weight, maternal smoking, illegitimacy, threatened abortion, and a previous history of antepartum hemorrhage, perinatal loss or low birth weight in liveborn infants. Also from Oxford, Fedrick and Adelstein[67] reported that delivery of a low birth weight infant at term was associated with low maternal weight prior to pregnancy, shortness of stature, smoking, primiparity, working during pregnancy, low social class, and history of a previous low birth weight infant, threatened abortion and severe toxemia. They found no association of low birth weight at term with illegitimacy, previous abortion, essential hypertension, mild toxemia or infections.

Using these risk factors, Fedrick devised a scoring system to predict the likelihood of spontaneous preterm birth.[66] The system was relatively ineffective in primigravidous women, but by the addition of previous pregnancy data, the score was very predictive of multigravidous women at risk. Markedly consistently with these findings, D'Angelo and Sokol[55] found that in a series of women with pregnancies that ended in preterm delivery 17.7 per cent had previous borne a premature infant, while only 5.3 per cent of those delivering at term had this risk factor. In other reports[80, 127] the incidence of repeat preterm labor rose to 37 per cent after one and 70 per cent after two previous preterm births. By applying the risk scoring system described by Hobel and associates[104] and validated by their earlier clinical application,[219] D'Angelo and Sokol[55] found that preterm delivery was associated with first or second trimester bleeding, incompetent cervical os, severe preeclampsia, multiple gestation, premature rupture of membranes, pyelonephritis and total placenta previa. They found no apparent association of preterm birth with low maternal age, low or high parity, maternal anemia, smoking or lower urinary tract infection.

Risk factors of premature birth are of particular clinical importance when they are recognized early in pregnancy and amenable to treatment. For example, the recognition and treatment of asymptomatic bacteriuria should reduce the risk of preterm delivery. There is considerable evidence to implicate asymptomatic bacteriuria in pregnancy with the risk of acute pyelonephritis and with both preterm delivery and fetal growth retardation.[1, 95, 123, 124, 238] There also is evidence that amniotic fluid infection is associated with preterm labor. Bobbit and associates[27] found evidence of amniotic fluid infection in 25 per cent of a series of patients in preterm labor with intact membranes. The majority of these patients were asymptomatic. A reduction of premature births due to incompetent cervical os requires early diagnosis and appropriate surgical repair; however, Keirse and associates[127] reported no statistical difference in the incidence of preterm delivery in patients with two or more previous abortions or preterm deliveries or both after placement of a cervical suture early in the current pregnancy.

The influence of smoking on the incidence of premature birth has received considerable attention. There is a well-established association of maternal smoking to low birth weight but a less consistent association with preterm delivery.[1, 145, 170, 174, 178] The available evidence suggests that smoking reduces placental perfusion through effects of nicotine, or from chronic inhalation of carbon monoxide, or both.[145, 178] The importance of nicotine alone is emphasized by the report of Krishna[134] that tobacco chewing during pregnancy, a common habit among women in certain parts of India, produced the same adverse effects on pregnancy as smoking.

Another potentially avoidable factor relating to preterm delivery is coitus during pregnancy. Goodlin and associates[86-88] reported a higher incidence of premature labor in patients who achieve orgasm during late pregnancy. These observations may be of considerable importance considering our current knowledge of the prostaglandins in the mechanism of labor onset, the relatively large amount of prostaglandins in male seminal fluid and the possible role of prostaglandins in the mechanism of orgasm. Also, breast massage is known to stimulate uterine activity during pregnancy. Jhirad and Vago[114] reported 70 per cent of a series of patients at term had successful induction of labor by this technique. The mechanism is thought to involve maternal pituitary release of oxytocin.

From our current knowledge of the pathogenesis of preterm labor, we may logically recommend that patients at risk (1) be placed under careful surveillance for complications and maintenance of good nutrition and rest; (2) be observed for conditions amenable to treatment, such as incompetent cervix and asymptomatic bacteriuria; and (3) be advised to avoid breast massage, coitus, and smoking during their pregnancy. It is imperative that we eliminate iatrogenic prematurity. As recently as 1974, Hack and associates[93] found that 12 per cent of infants with respiratory distress syndrome in their neonatal care unit had been delivered by elective induction of labor or elective cesarean section.

Management

The diagnosis of premature labor is based upon clinical evaluation of uterine activity and cervical change consistent with labor, plus evidence of preterm gestation or small size of fetus or both. Pharmacologic inhibition of labor is usually ineffective when cervical effacement is advanced or dilatation has progressed beyond 4 cm.[19] Our ability to determine gestation by menstrual history, estimated fetal weight or by weight of the uterine fundus is rather limited. In addition, we are interested in the diagnosis of fetal growth retardation, for we assume that it is caused by chronic compromise of intrauterine environment, which in turn may be responsible for triggering premature labor. In this situation, it would be inappropriate to stop labor and prolong the fetal insult. However, even the growth-retarded fetus may be deprived of developmental potential if delivered too early. The ultrasonic determination of total intrauterine volume as described by Gohari and associates[84] is to date the most definitive method for diagnosis of intrauterine growth retardation. These investigators found that only 10 per cent of neonates who were clinically small for dates had intrauterine growth retardation at birth; however, the accuracy of the ultrasonic technique in establishing the diagnosis was extremely high.[103] By the additional measurement of fetal biparietal diameter and ratio of head to body circumference, fetal weight may be predicted to within 106 g per kg.[235] Thus, our initial evaluation of the patient in preterm labor may be greatly facilitated by application of ultrasonic techniques if time permits.

The management of preterm labor is further based upon several other clinical factors that act as absolute or relative contraindications to treatment directed toward inhibition of labor. For example, the presence of intrauterine infection, a major premature separation of the placenta, fetal death or a fetal malformation incompatible with survival are contraindications for our use of a uterine-inhibiting agent. Inhibition of preterm labor associated with premature rupture of membranes remains controversial. Delay of delivery presents an increasing risk of intrauterine infection, but it also permits time for advancement of fetal lung maturity by either endogenous mechanisms or by glucocorticoid drug therapy. The initial work of Liggins and Howie,[152] plus the subsequent widespread clinical experience, has suggested a beneficial effect of glucocorticoid administration in accelerating fetal lung maturity. However, the potential long-term aftereffects of glucocorticoids have not yet been fully evaluated. Although some investigators recommend that preterm labor be delayed for 48 to 72 hours to permit a maximal effect of glucocorticoid treatment upon fetal lung maturation, the ability of most pharmacologic agents to inhibit labor with ruptured membranes is limited, possibly due to the participation of fetal membranes in the mechanism of labor. The management of preterm labor in a pregnancy complicated by placental insufficiency, as with diabetes mellitus or hypertensive disease, should be based upon a judgment of the method that offers the least potential risks to mother and fetus. Zlatnik[24] reported that only 31 of 191 patients who delivered infants weighing less than 2500 g had been candidates for pharmacologic inhibition of preterm labor. Of the 160 excluded, 31 per cent were due to error in judgment of fetal weight, 28 per cent were due to ruptured membranes, and 18 per cent were due to imminent delivery at the time of admission. Many diagnosed cases of preterm labor may appear to have been successfully treated when in fact they would have been diagnosed "false labor" had there been no treatment. From several studies of specific agents in treatment of preterm labor,[40, 237, 242] to be discussed in the following paragraphs, there was from 38 per cent to 71 per cent "success" in the placebo group treated by bed rest and hydration by intravenous infusion of a crystaloid solution. Bed rest, particularly in the lateral decubitus position, where uterine blood flow is maximal,[23, 36, 97] is quite likely the most effective treatment of preterm labor. When we exclude the patients in whom preterm labor ceases with bed rest alone and those in whom inhibition of labor is either contraindicated or likely to fail due to its advanced state, there remains a group of potential candidates for pharmacologic control.

Pharmacologic Inhibition of Premature Labor

The evaluation of efficacy of a drug for treatment of preterm labor is confused by our inability to clearly distinguish true labor from false labor, the many variables of the mechanism of labor as expressed clinically, and the frequent "success" of treatment by only bed rest and supportive care. Historically, the most popular agents were many varieties of sedatives and psycholeptics, hormones, vasodilators and neuromuscular agents. Although sedative and analgesic drugs have enjoyed a reputation as uterine relaxants, quantitative studies of some have revealed a significant increase of uterine activity following drug administration.[59, 69, 202] Several studies[49, 79, 240] have failed to demonstrate an effect of progesterone on established labor; however, Bengtsson[20] reported temporary inhibition of human labor when progesterone was injected directly into the uterine wall. Prior to its withdrawal from clinical availability in the United States, lututrin, an aqueous extract of sow corpus luteum, was rather widely used in treatment of preterm labor. However, the only reports of its clinical application failed to utilize adequate controls to establish potential value.[163, 200, 203] Amyl nitrite, a vasorelaxing agent administered by inhalation, will produce brief uterine relaxation in about 50 per cent of patients in labor at term,[137] but its prolonged use to inhibit preterm labor is no more practical than providing uterine relaxation with inhalation anesthetics such as ethyl ether or fluothane. Not unexpectedly, Iuppa and associates[111] reported that succinylcholine, a skeletal muscle relaxant, had no significant inhibitory effect upon term labor.

Diazoxide, a potent vasodilator structurally related to chlorothiazide, was introduced as an antihypertensive agent but also was found to relax smooth muscle, suppress insulin and elevate blood glucose.[26, 185] Landesman and associates[140, 141] reported that diazoxide relaxed human myometrium in vitro and inhibited contractions of human labor at term. In studies of pregnant baboons, Wilson and associates[239] reported that diazoxide—but not the beta-adrenergic agents ritodrine, isoproterenol and metaproterenol—inhibited prostaglandin uterine activity induced by $F_{2\alpha}$. Morris and associates[175] reported successful management of maternal hypertension in 12 patients with severe preeclampsia or eclampsia. They noted a prompt inhibition of labor in every patient. From our personal experience with diazoxide in 25 patients, 10 in premature labor, we found (1) only moderate uterine relaxing effects, (2) maternal tachycardia, (3) no significant change of maternal blood pressure, and (4) an apparent increase in the occurrence of hypoglycemia in the newborns.[16] The clinical value of diazoxide for treatment of premature labor has not been established; however, it deserves further evaluation.

Magnesium sulfate has gained widespread acceptance in clinical practice for its neurostabilization effects in management of toxemia of pregnancy.[70, 197] From studies in pregnant sheep, Dandavino and associates[54] reported that the continuous infusion of magnesium sulfate in doses of 2 to 4 g per hour produced a slight increase of uteroplacental blood flow but did not alter blood pressure. Several studies[94, 108, 136, 193] have reported inhibition of human uterine activity in spontaneous or oxytocin-induced labor at term during intravenous infusion of magnesium sulfate. Steer and Petrie[222] reported magnesium sulfate more effective than intravenous ethanol for control of preterm labor. In this randomized trial, delay of labor for at least 24 hours was achieved in 24 of 31 patients (77 per cent) treated with magnesium sulfate and 14 of 31 (45 per cent) of those treated with ethanol. Although suggestive, this study did not statistically establish the clinical value of magnesium sulfate for treatment of preterm labor. With further experience and adequately controlled studies, the lack of major side effects of magnesium sulfate at therapeutic levels may prove it better than other forms of treatment for preterm labor.

Aminophylline, a dimethylxanthine derivative used as a bronchial relaxant, also causes relaxation of the uterus. It acts by blocking the action of intracellular phosphodiesterase to prevent degradation of cyclic adenosine monophosphate (cAMP). The accumulation of cAMP in the myometrial cell facilitates movement of calcium to intracellular storage areas or across the cell membrane, resulting in relaxation of the cell.[39] Coutinho and Vieira Lopes[44] reported that intravenous injection of 240 to 480 mg of aminophylline briefly relaxed the spontaneous uterine activity of nonpregnant women. Liu and associates[160, 161] reported delay of premature labor by 24 hours or more in 80 per cent of a series of patients. They administered 250 mg intravenously over 15 minutes, followed by an intravenous infusion of approximately 50 mg per hour for up to 48 hours, and then 100 mg orally every 8 hours. Lipshitz,[155] in a series of patients with oxytocin-induced term labor, reported that intravenous injection of 250 mg of aminophylline over 5 minutes produced a modest decrease of uterine activity with a marked maternal tachycardia. He concluded that aminophylline, compared with the beta-sympathomimetic drugs, has an unfavorable vascular-to-tocolytic ratio. Further studies of aminophylline are needed to establish its potential value in treatment of premature labor.

Aspirin, indomethacin and other nonsteroidal anti-inflammatory drugs inhibit myometrial activity by blocking the synthesis of prostaglandins. Vane[231] reported that these agents block prostaglandin production in rabbit lung preparations by interfering with prostaglandin synthetase, the enzyme necessary for conversion of arachidonic acid to prostaglandin. In addition to aspirin and indomethacin, other compounds with antiprostaglandin activity include naproxen, ibuprofen, fenoprofen, meclofenamic acid, flufenamic acid and phenylbutazone. From studies in rats and primates[3, 50, 117, 184] there was evidence that administration of aspirin, indomethacin and naproxen during pregnancy was followed by a significant delay in onset of labor. Lewis and Shulman[147] reported that labor was delayed in onset and extended somewhat longer in a series of patients who had consumed large doses of aspirin during pregnancy in treatment of arthritis. From Israel, Zuckerman and associates[243] reported successful inhibition of preterm labor in 40 of 50 patients treated with indomethacin, 100 mg by rectal suppository, followed by 25 mg by mouth every six hours for five days. This report stimulated widespread clinical use of indomethacin for treatment of preterm labor in the United States. However, the popularity of this form of treatment soon waned as further studies suggested the potential of dangerous side effects. From numerous observations in both animals and humans[12, 43, 46, 64, 100, 101, 164, 189] it is evident that the antiprostaglandin compounds may cause closure of the fetal duct arteriosus, pulmonary hypertension, congestive heart failure and death. However, indomethacin has been successfully used in treatment of patent ductus arteriosus in newborns.[72, 102] The potential fetal risks of these drugs clearly contraindicate further clinical use for treatment of preterm labor pending the results of carefully designed studies to establish their safety.

Ethanol, administered by intravenous infusion, has been one of the most popular methods for treatment of preterm labor in the United States. From studies in rabbits, Fuchs and associates[73-76] reported evidence that intravenous infusion of ethanol blocks pituitary release of oxytocin. Later, Gibbens and Chard,[83] using a radioimmunoassay technique, reported similar evidence from women in spontaneous labor. They reported a decrease in the frequency of "spurt release" of oxytocin during intravenous infusion of ethanol. In 1967, Fuchs and associates[78] reported on the first clinical studies of intravenous ethanol for treatment of human preterm labor. They reported delay of labor for 3 days or more in 35 of 52 (67 per cent) patients with intact membranes. The treatment was uniformly unsuccessful when membranes had ruptured. The encouraging results of this trial prompted a subsequent controlled study reported by Zlatnik and Fuchs.[242] In this study, 21 patients received intravenous ethanol and 21 received 5 per cent glucose and water. Labor was delayed for at least 72 hours in 17 (81 per cent) of the ethanol group and only 8 (38 per cent) of the control group. The dosage schedule for intravenous ethanol recommended by Fuchs and associates was 7.5 ml of a 9.5 per cent ethanol solution per kg of body weight per hour for two hours as a loading dose, and then 1.5 ml per kg of body weight per hour for 10 hours or more.[77, 244] In contrast, Graff[89] continued the maintenance dose for only one hour after contractions ceased, and all but one of 20 preterm labor patients delivered within 3 days. Also, Watring and associates[236] reported no significant difference between ethanol and control groups.

The most common maternal side effects of intravenous infusion of ethanol are nausea, vomiting, headache, diuresis and restlessness. However, Greenhouse and associates[90] reported a fatal case of aspiration pneumonia after ethanol infusion and Ott and associates[191] reported the development of severe lactic acidosis in a patient during treatment with ethanol. Animal studies[60, 106, 131, 165] have revealed decreased uterine blood flow, fetal asphyxia and fetal cardiac depression during maternal ethanol infusion. However, from clinical evidence in human pregnancy, there is no indication of adverse effects on the fetus or neonate of ethanol infusion during labor. Wagner and associates[232] reported that intravenous infusion of ethanol of six low birth weight infants produced no change in acid-base status, vital signs, or psychomotor behavior. The widespread use of intravenous ethanol for treatment of preterm labor for the past decade has proved it moderately effective but complicated by annoying side effects.

Calcium antagonists, or blockers, are compounds thought to act by interfering with the influx of calcium ions through the cell membrane. One of the most potent of these drugs, nifedipine, has been used in treatment of hypertension and ischemic heart disease. In 1978, Ulmsten and associates[230] reported that nifedipine, 20 to 30 mg orally, rapidly reduced uterine activity of 10 nonpregnant women. The only apparent side effects were a moderate increase of heart rate and a transient facial flushing. Subsequently Andersson and associates[11] observed a marked decrease of the intensity, but not the frequency, of prostaglandin-induced uterine contractions following oral nifedipine in a series of women undergoing induced mid-trimester abortions. To date, there have been no reports of calcium antagonists used in treatment of preterm labor.

Beta-adrenergic receptor active drugs consist of compounds resembling isoproterenol in structure that act to relax smooth muscle of the uterus, bronchial tree and arterioles, to increase heart rate and force of contraction and to produce glycogenolysis and lipolysis. The use of catecholamine-like agents to change uterine activity was suggested as early as 1928, when Bourne and Burn[31] reported that intravenous injection of epinephrine during labor inhibited uterine activity. In contrast, Brown and Wilder[35] reported that intravenous epinephrine stimulated uterine activity. The apparent discrepancy was resolved when further studies[118, 234, 245] revealed that the uterine response to epinephrine is dose dependent, with lower doses producing relaxation and higher doses stimulating activity. Garrett[82] observed that a rebound excitatory response often occurred after stopping the intravenous infusion of epinephrine. This and the dominance of cardiovascular effects of epinephrine precluded its clinical applicability for inhibition of labor.

In 1948, Ahlquist[2] reported evidence that the action of sympathomimetic amines on smooth muscle is mediated through two sets of receptors, the "alpha" and the "beta." Stimulation of beta receptors produces uterine relaxation, while alpha-receptor stimulation results in increased uterine activity. By studying a series of catecholamines, Ahlquist observed that norepinephrine was the prototype of an alpha-receptor stimulating drug, while isoproterenol was the prototype of a beta-adrenergic drug. Epinephrine was intermediate in activity with the ability to stimulate both alpha and beta receptors. Although isoproterenol is a stronger beta-receptor agonist than epinephrine, its side effects disqualify it for treatment of preterm labor.

Sutherland and associates[204, 224] clarified the nature of the beta-adrenergic receptor. "First messenger hormones" such as isoproterenol interact with the target cell membrane to release adenyl cyclase within the cell. Adenyl cyclase serves to catalyze the intracellular formation of cyclic adenosine monophosphate, which serves as a "second messenger" to trigger the cellular action, which in the case of the myometrial cell is relaxation. Lands and associates[143] further clarified the nature of the beta-adrenergic receptor when they described evidence for two populations of beta receptors. The β_1 receptors are responsible for actions such as increase of heart rate and force of contraction, lipolysis and relaxation of intestinal smooth muscle. The β_2 receptors are involved with glycogenolysis and smooth muscle relaxation in arterioles, the bronchi and the uterus. The ideal drug for treatment of preterm labor would stimulate only the β_2 receptors of the uterus. Unfortunately, such an ideal drug has not been identified; however, the use of beta-sympathomimetic drugs has gained widespread acceptance in the treatment of preterm labor.

In 1960, Lish and associates[158] reported that from a series of animal experiments the beta-adrenergic stimulant isoxsuprine hydrochloride has a favorable balance of myometrial versus cardiovascular actions. A year later, Bishop and Woutersz[25] reported that of 120 patients in preterm labor treated with isoxsuprine, delivery in 87 per cent was delayed for more than 24 hours. However, in 10 patients in labor at term, they found almost no effect of isoxsuprine on uterine activity and observed hypotension whenever the intravenous dose was increased to more than 0.5 mg per minute. From another study, Hendricks and associates[99] reported that isoxsuprine inhibited both spontaneous and oxytocin-induced uterine activity. In 1969 Das[56] of India reported on treatment of 50 patients in preterm labor who were entered into a controlled study of isoxsuprine versus bed rest and sedation. Labor was successfully delayed in 72 per cent of the isoxsuprine group, and in only 25 per cent of the controls. Castren and associates[40] reported on a double-blind study of 194 patients with preterm labor treated with isoxsuprine, ethanol, nylidrin or placebo. Nylidrin (Buphenine) is a beta-sympathomimetic agent, structurally similar to isoxsuprine, which is not available in the United States. When success of treatment was defined as birth weight over 2500 g, it was achieved in 86 per cent, 75 per cent, 71 per cent, and 70 per cent of the nylidrin, isoxsuprine, placebo and ethanol groups, respectively. However, when success was defined as delay of labor over 7 days and until 37 or more weeks' gestation, it was achieved in 77 per cent, 73 per cent, 62 per cent and 56 per cent of the nylidrin, placebo, isoxsuprine, and ethanol groups, respectively. Only nylidrin proved statistically more efficient than the placebo. Csapo and Herczeg[52] reported on a prospective study of 36 patients in premature labor treated with isoxsuprine or with placebo. Of the 17 patients treated with placebo, the average delay of delivery was 13.6 days and 5 (29 per cent) delivered infants weighing over 2500 g. In contrast, of the 19 patients treated with isoxsuprine, the average delay of delivery was 46.3 days and 16 (84 per cent) delivered infants weighing over 2500 g.

From the mid 1960s through 1980 isoxsuprine hydrochloride (Vasodilan) was widely used in the United States for treatment of preterm labor. However, the Food and Drug Administration (FDA) did not classify it as effective in treatment of preterm labor but rather as possibly effective for relief of cerebral and peripheral vascular insufficiency. Although never recommended for intravenous administration by the manufacturer, the usual dosage regimen of isoxsuprine for treatment of preterm labor was an intravenous infusion of 0.25 to 0.5 mg per minute, which if successful was continued for 8 to 12 hours, and

followed by oral administration of 5 to 20 mg every 3 to 6 hours. There was no consensus regarding the optimal length of oral maintenance therapy. The intravenous infusion was repeated when preterm labor recurred during oral drug therapy. If labor-like uterine activity persisted during the first hour of the infusion, the dosage was advanced up to 1.0 mg per minute if side effects permitted. When labor persisted at this dosage level, the treatment was discontinued after one hour.

From several early reports[99, 119, 221] there was evidence that up to 10 per cent of patients receiving an intravenous infusion of isoxsuprine developed significant hypotension and evidence of fetal distress. However, further clinical experience revealed that hypotension was unusual when patients were adequately hydrated and strictly maintained in the lateral recumbent rather than the supine position. Other common maternal side effects of isoxsuprine were tachycardia, tremor, restlessness and palpitations. From a study of 70 patients treated with isoxsuprine for preterm labor, Brazy and associates[32] reported that treatment within 2 hours of delivery was strongly associated with neonatal problems including hypoglycemia, hypocalcemia, hypotension, ileus and even death. These authors concluded that isoxsuprine therapy should be discontinued if cervical effacement advances beyond 50 per cent or if dilatation progresses beyond 3 cm. Clinical experience with isoxsuprine and other beta-adrenergic stimulants for treatment of preterm labor has not been associated with subsequent prolonged pregnancy, abnormal labor or postpartum uterine atony.

Terbutaline sulfate was initially described in 1970 by Persson and Olsson[192] as a "selective β_2 receptor stimulator" with effects predominantly upon beta receptors of the bronchi, peripheral vessels and uterus. Clinical studies conducted in Lund, Sweden established that terbutaline effectively inhibits both nonpregnant and pregnant uterine activity with minimal cardiovascular or other side effects.[4, 5, 8-10] Caritis and associates,[37, 38] from observations in pregnant ewes and pregnant baboons, reported that maternal intravenous infusions of terbutaline produced minimal or no changes in maternal blood pressure, no change in uterine blood flow, and no change of fetal cardiovascular or acid-base state, but it effectively relaxed the uterus. Ingemarsson[109] reported on a double-blind placebo-controlled study of terbutaline in a series of 30 patients in preterm labor. The average gestation of patients entering the study was 35 weeks. Terbutaline was administered by intravenous infusion starting at 10 µg per minute and increasing by 5 µg per minute every 10 minutes until contractions ceased or to a maximal dosage of 25 µg per minute. After an hour, the dosage was reduced to 5 µg per minute every 30 minutes to reach the lowest effective dose, which was continued for 8 hours. Then, with continued bed rest, 250 µg of terbutaline was administered subcutaneously every 6 hours for 3 days, and then 5 µg orally every 8 hours with continued bed rest to the end of the 36th week. Of the 15 patients receiving terbutaline, 12 (80 per cent) reached 37 weeks' gestation, while 3 (20 per cent) of the 15 receiving placebo treatment reached 37 weeks. Maternal and fetal side effects were minimal and of no clinical consequence.

Wallace and associates[233] reported on terbutaline treatment of 50 patients, including 7 with multiple gestation, in preterm labor. Terbutaline was administered by intravenous infusion in a dosage range of 10 to 80 µg per minute only until contractions were controlled. Patients were then permitted to ambulate and given terbutaline 250 µg subcutaneously every 4 hours for 24 hours, followed by 2.5 µg orally every 4 hours. Although 47 of 50 patients were initially responsive, there were 11 (22 per cent) treatment failures, 21 (42 per cent) required more than one intravenous infusion, and gestation was prolonged beyond 36 weeks in only 24 (48 per cent). Thus, from this and the previous report we may conclude that terbutaline is more effective when the intravenous infusion is continued well beyond the cessation of contractions and when treatment includes bed rest.

Terbutaline sulfate (Bricanyl or Brethine) became available in the United States during the mid 1970s for use as a bronchodilator for treatment of asthma and reversible bronchospasm associated with bronchitis and emphysema, but it was not approved by the FDA for treatment of preterm labor. Also, the manufacturers recommended only subcutaneous and oral administration. However, as with isoxsuprine, it was widely used for treatment of preterm labor with an initial intravenous infusion usually followed by oral administration. Some clinicians used serial subcutaneous injections rather than an intravenous infusion as the initial therapy.

The usual side effects of terbutaline are similar to those of isoxsuprine and other beta-mimetic drugs, with maternal tachycardia, a widening of pulse pressure, slight elevation of fetal heart rate, and elevation of maternal and fetal blood glucose levels. However, in a study of the metabolic effects of terbutaline after a single intravenous injection during second-stage labor, Ingemarsson and associates[110] observed no differences in maternal blood glucose levels between terbutaline-treated patients and controls. Terbutaline crossed the placenta rapidly with fetal plasma levels up to 55 per cent of maternal plasma levels. Other investigators have reported the development of marked maternal hypokalemia and metabolic acidosis during treatment of preterm labor with terbutaline.[91, 218] The presumed mechanism of these metabolic changes involves hyperglycemia stimulated by beta adrenergics and hyperinsulinemia followed by a shift of glucose and potassium to the intracellular space in exchange for hydrogen ion. In general, these metabolic side effects of terbutaline are transient and of no clinical consequence. However, occasional patients being treated for preterm labor have developed acute pulmonary edema.[112, 125] This very serious complication of terbutaline therapy has usually been associated with concomitant administration of glucocorticoids to enhance fetal pulmonary maturation, with maternal anemia and with excessive intravenous infusion of crystalloid solutions. In the report of Katz and associates[125] an alarming 5 per cent of patients treated with terbutaline for preterm labor experienced cardiovascular complications of pulmonary edema or electrocardiographic signs of myocardial ischemia.

In 1980 ritodrine hydrochloride (Yutopar) became the first drug of any pharmacologic class to be approved by the United States FDA specifically for treatment of preterm labor. The early studies of this agent revealed a favorable balance of uterine relaxant to cardiovascular properties.[81, 142] In 1971, Wesselius-de Casparis and associates[237] of several European countries reported on a double-blind placebo-controlled study of ritodrine in treatment of preterm labor. The treatment consisted of an intravenous infusion for 24 to 48 hours followed by a course of oral administration for 5 to 7 days. Bed rest was enforced for the first 4 days. Maternal side effects were limited to a moderate increase of heart rate and there were no apparent fetal side effects. From data of 63 patients with average gestation of 31.5 weeks, delivery was delayed at least 7 days in 80 per cent of the ritodrine group and 48 per cent of the placebo group. Among the 51 patients with intact membranes, the mean gain per case was 28.2 days in the ritodrine group and 17.4 days in the placebo group. Subsequent studies in the United States confirmed the effectiveness of ritodrine in relaxing the uterus with relatively few side effects in preterm labor[24] and in term labor.[15, 183] Ragni and associates,[198] using a phonocardiographic technique to measure cardiac intervals and plethysmography to record peripheral blood flow, observed that the intravenous infusion of ritodrine, 400 µg per min, caused a significant increase of both cardiac output and peripheral blood flow. From other studies there was evidence of increased cardiovascular sensitivity to ritodrine in patients with hypertensive toxemia.

Brettes and associates[34] observed indirect evidence of increased uterine blood flow during the infusion of ritodrine in patients with hypertension but no change in those who were normotensive. Miller and associates[173] studied 25 toxemia patients in labor during intravenous infusion of ritodrine. They observed four patients with an apparent increase in frequency of premature ventricular contractions during and immediately after the infusion. From fetal scalp blood samples in 24 patients before and after ritodrine there was a mean pH change from 7.30 to 7.28, and a base deficit increase from 3.41 to 4.32. They also observed that the mean fetal serum glucose before and after ritodrine rose from 87.2 to 122.8 mg per cent. In a study of ritodrine treatment of preterm labor, Spellacy and associates[220] observed a rise of maternal blood glucose from approximately 80 to 150 mg per cent during the intravenous infusion period. There was a parallel rise in plasma insulin from about 20 to 100 micro units per milliliter. Borberg and associates[30] observed ketoacidosis in a diabetic treated simultaneously with ritodrine and dexamethasone. They suggested the potential need for insulin therapy of diabetic patients who are given beta-adrenergic stimulants. In a double-blind controlled trial of ritodrine administration during second-stage labor, Humphrey and associates[107] observed that fetal respiratory acidosis during advanced labor was abolished by ritodrine. Kauppila and associates[126] reported that ritodrine was more potent than isoxsuprine in increasing the circulating levels of cAMP, glu-

cose, insulin and triglycerides. They also noted that both drugs caused a significant fall in serum iron and potassium during an intravenous infusion period lasting six hours. Schreyer and associates[208, 209] studied the metabolic effects of intravenous infusion of ritodrine during pregnancy. They observed a highly significant negative correlation between serum and red cell potassium concentrations, suggesting that potassium enters the erythrocyte compartment. In similar studies, Kirkpatrick and associates[130] observed that hypokalemia and other metabolic effects were transient, despite continuation of the infusion of ritodrine. They also observed that the addition of dexamethasone to ritodrine administration had an additive effect on increasing blood glucose levels, but had no additional influence on reduction of potassium concentrations. Osler[190] reported that the metabolic effects of intravenous infusion of ritodrine do not occur when it is administered orally.

As with other beta-adrenergic stimulants, ritodrine has been associated with occasional cases of maternal pulmonary edema. Philipson and associates[194] reported that 7 of 12 patients receiving an intravenous solution of ritodrine in isotonic saline developed pulmonary congestion requiring treatment. In contrast, none of 11 patients receiving equivalent amounts of ritodrine in isotonic glucose solution developed signs of pulmonary edema. These authors recommend that intravenous ritodrine not be administered in isotonic saline solution. Acute pulmonary edema was also reported by Elliott and associates[63] in two patients treated with magnesium sulfate and betamethasone. Both of their patients were anemic and one had twins. Lammintausta and associates[139] observed a significant rise of plasma renin activity during infusions of ritodrine and isoxsuprine in 26 pregnant patients. They suggest that this response may be a compensatory reaction to the vasodilator effect of these agents. Alterations in placental blood flow in response to ritodrine were studied by Suonio and associates[223] using a radionuclide accumulation method. Following maternal intramuscular injection of ritodrine, 10 mg, placental perfusion increased 19 per cent in normotensive patients, 24 per cent in preeclamptic patients, and 45 per cent in patients with chronic hypertension.

Ritodrine was compared to ethanol in treatment of preterm labor in a randomized controlled study among three medical centers in the United States reported by Lauersen and associates.[144] The average gestation of patients entering the study was about 31 weeks. Of the 67 patients who received ethanol, delivery in 49 (73 per cent) was delayed by 72 hours or more, 36 (54 per cent) delivered after 36 weeks' gestation, and the average delay to delivery was 27.6 days. Of the 68 patients treated with ritodrine, delivery in 61 (90 per cent) was delayed by 72 hours or more, 49 (72 per cent) delivered after 36 weeks, and the average delay to delivery was 44.0 days. The authors suggested that the more favorable results with ritodrine were possibly attributable to its continued administration by oral maintenance therapy after discharge from the hospital.

The approval of ritodrine hydrochloride for treatment of preterm labor by the FDA in 1980 followed an analysis of the collaborative data of 13 investigators at 11 university centers in the United States.[17, 169] These studies, conducted from 1972 through 1977, involved 366 women in preterm labor who received parenteral ritodrine (223), intravenous ethanol (77) or an intravenous placebo (66). With the ethanol and placebo treatment designated as the controls, and by considering only the highest risk subgroup of patients who had labor onset prior to 33 weeks of gestation, the mean gestation time gained for infants of mothers treated with ritodrine was 40.9 days as compared to 24.4 days for the controls. In the same subgroup, the incidence of newborn respiratory distress was 13 per cent in the ritodrine group and 29 per cent in the controls, while the incidence of neonatal death was 8 per cent in the ritodrine group and 24 per cent is of an initial intravenous infusion of 50 to 100 μg per minute, which is increased by 50 μg per minute increments every 10 minutes until contractions stop, unacceptable side effects develop or the maximum dose of 350 μg minute is reached. The patient is maintained at bed rest in the lateral decubitus position. Uterine activity, maternal heart rate, maternal blood pressure and fetal heart rate are monitored frequently during the infusion. If unacceptable side effects develop, the dosage is reduced to a tolerable level. The infusion is stopped if labor persists for more than 30 minutes at the maximum dose. If contractions are successfully inhibited, the infusion is maintained for 12 to 24 hours. Oral therapy is started 30 minutes before the infusion is stopped with a dosage of 10 mg and continued

at 10 mg every 2 hours for the next 24 hours (maximum dose 120 mg per day). The oral dose is continued as 10 to 20 mg every 4 to 6 hours until term or earlier if so dictated by obstetric judgment. Ambulation is resumed gradually after 48 hours. If preterm labor recurs and there are no new obstetric or medical contraindications, ritodrine may again be administered by intravenous infusion.

Creasy and associates[45] reported on a trial of continuing treatment with oral ritodrine versus oral placebo in 55 patients who initially had preterm labor inhibited by treatment with intramuscular ritodrine. The number of relapses of preterm labor requiring repeat intramuscular treatment was 1.11 in the ritodrine group as opposed to 2.71 in the placebo group. Also, the mean interval between beginning oral treatment and the first relapse or delivery was 5.8 days in the oral placebo group and 25.9 days among those receiving oral ritodrine.

Other beta-adrenergic agents that have been evaluated in treatment of preterm labor included salbutamol,[133, 154] orciprenaline[14] and fenoterol.[28, 65] In general, they are similar to the beta-adrenergic agents previously discussed. From several comparative studies[13, 156, 157, 207, 217] it can be concluded that fenoterol, orciprenaline and isoxsuprine are less β_2-receptor specific than ritodrine and terbutaline. From South Africa, Lipshitz and associates[156, 157] reported on comparisons of fenoterol, ritodrine, salbutamol and hexoprenaline. By comparing uterine and cardiovascular responses of these agents they concluded that hexoprenaline, which is not yet available in the United States, was the most β_2-selective.

Historically, the administration of glucocorticoids for acceleration of pulmonary maturation prior to premature birth has often involved the concomitant administration of labor-inhibiting drugs. In the initial report by Liggins and Howie[152] an attempt was made to delay delivery for 48 to 72 hours from the time of the first injection of betamethasone by intravenous infusion of ethanol or salbutamol. In their group of patients between 26 and 32 weeks' gestation treated for at least 24 hours, there were 2 of 17 (11.8 per cent) in the betamethasone group and 16 of 23 (69.6 per cent) in the control group whose infants developed respiratory distress syndrome. Others have noted rather similar results in series of infants of mothers who have received uterine-inhibiting agents prior to preterm birth compared with infants of similar weight and gestation who had not been exposed to the drugs. Boog and associates[29] reported the development of respiratory distress syndrome in 5 of 29 (17 per cent) of infants exposed to ritodrine compared to 12 of 13 (35 per cent) in a comparable control group. Similarly, Bergman and Hedner[21] reported respiratory distress syndrome in 1 of 24 infants exposed to terbutaline, as opposed to 5 of 17 controls. Liu[159] observed respiratory distress syndrome in only 3 of 28 infants with average gestation of 30.9 weeks delivered after failed treatment of preterm labor with methylxanthine. Kero and associates[129] found respiratory distress in only 2 of 26 premature infants with average weight of 1720 g and average gestation of 31.6 weeks after maternal treatment of preterm labor with isoxsuprine. Barrada and associates[18] in a series of premature births at 28 to 32 weeks' gestation, reported respiratory distress syndrome in only 6 of 21 infants (28.5 per cent) after failed inhibition of labor with ethanol as opposed to its development in 10 of 15 (66.7 per cent) of those not treated. These observations suggest that uterine-inhibiting agents may exert a protective effect against development of respiratory distress similar to that produced by corticosteroids. The mechanism of this apparent response is not yet understood.

Conclusions

The evaluation of various agents in the management of preterm labor is complicated by the inherent difficulty in its diagnosis, the wide variety of clinical factors that may trigger uterine contractions, the complex mechanism of labor onset, the variables of clinical circumstances when treatment is begun, the dosage schedule of a particular agent, and the ancillary treatment measures such as bed rest and psychologic support that may favorably influence outcome. Baumgarten and Gruber[19] described a "tocolysis index based on contraction frequency, condition of membranes, amount of bleeding and cervical dilatation, for quantitation of the clinical features of premature labor." Richter[201] described a "prolongation index" based on the gestation at onset of treatment and the time from treatment to delivery, which would express the therapeutic effect. However, neither of these calculations

have been widely used in subsequent clinical studies. In a review of 18 trials of various treatments of preterm labor, Hamminki and Starfield[96] noted that of 13 trials comparing placebo and drug, only 2 found the drug better than placebo or "conventional therapy." Obviously, the methodologic deficiencies of many studies distort their relevance to clinical application.

Although the safety of glucocorticoids administered for their effect on fetal pulmonary maturation has not yet been completely established, the tocolytic agents currently available are usually able to delay delivery long enough for the desired effect. Even if glucocorticoids are not used, any delay of preterm delivery is potentially beneficial to the fetus. There is also the possibility that combining low doses of two or more agents with different foci of action will permit inhibition of labor without bothersome side effects. From the report of Bieniarz and associates,[22] who studied the effects of combining several known tocolytic agents, there is a suggestion that a simultaneous attack on several facets of the labor mechanism may be more effective than use of a single agent. In the future, a more complete understanding of the pathogenesis of preterm labor and the role of the fetus and its initiation will undoubtedly permit our more intelligent use of tocolytic agents. Despite the enthusiasm over the clinical availability of ritodrine in the United States, the search for the "ideal" drug for treatment of preterm labor is far from over.

REFERENCES

1. Abramowicz, M. and Kass, E. H.: Pathogenesis and prognosis of prematurity. N. Engl. J. Med. 275:878, 1966.
2. Ahlquist, R. P.: A study of the adrenotropic receptors. Am. J. Physiol. 153:586, 1948.
3. Aiken, J. W.: Aspirin and indomethacin prolong parturition in rats: evidence that prostaglandins contribute to expulsion of fetus. Nature 240:21, 1972.
4. Akerlund, M. and Andersson, K. E.: Effects of terbutaline on human myometrial activity and endometrial blood flow. Obstet. Gynecol. 47:529, 1976.
5. Akerland, M., Andersson, K. E. and Ingemarsson, I.: Effects of terbutaline on myometrial activity, uterine blood flow, and lower abdominal pain in women with primary dysmenorrhea. Br. J. Obstet. Gynaecol. 83:673, 1976.
6. Akesson, G. and Gustavii, B.: Occurrence of phospholipase A_1 and A_2 in human decidua. Prostaglandins 9:667, 1975.

7. Anderson, A. B. M., Lawrence, K. M., Davies, K., Campbell, H. and Turnbull, A. C.: Fetal adrenal weight and the course of premature delivery in human pregnancy. J. Obstet. Gynaecol. Br. Commonwealth 78:481, 1971.

8. Andersson, K. E., Bengtsson, L. Ph., Gustafson, I. and Ingemarsson, I.: The relaxing effect of terbutaline on the human uterus during term labor. Am. J. Obstet. Gynecol. 121:602, 1975.

9. Andersson, K. E., Bengtsson, L. P. and Ingemarsson, I.: Terbutaline inhibition of midtrimester uterine activity induced by prostaglandin $F_{2\alpha}$ and hypertonic saline. Br. J. Obstet. Gynaecol. 82:745, 1975.

10. Andersson, K. E., Ingemarsson, I. and Persson, C. G. A.: Effects of terbutaline on human uterine motility at term. Acta Obstet. Gynecol. Scand. 54:165, 1975.

11. Andersson, K. E., Ingemarsson, I., Ulmsten, U. and Wingerup, L.: Inhibition of prostaglandin-induced uterine activity by nifedipine. Br. J. Obstet. Gynaecol. 86:175, 1979.

12. Archilla, J. A., Thilenius, O. G. and Ranniger, K.: Congestive heart failure from suspected ductal closure in utero. J. Pediatr. 75:74, 1969.

13. Ayala, L. C. and Karchmer, S.: Comparative study of utero-inhibiting action of two β-adrenomimetic drugs. Acta Obstet. Gynecol. Scand. 56:287, 1977.

14. Baillie, P., Meehan, F. P. and Tyack, A. J.: Treatment of premature labour with orciprenaline. Br. Med. J. 4:154, 1970.

15. Barden, T. P.: Effect of ritodrine on human uterine motility and cardiovascular responses in term labor and the early postpartum state. Am. J. Obstet. Gynecol. 112:645, 1972.

16. Barden, T. P. and Keenan, W. J.: Effects of diazoxide in human labor and fetus-neonate. Obstet. Gynecol. 37:631 (Abstr.) 1971.

17. Barden, T. P., Peter, J. B. and Merkatz, I. R.: Ritodrine hydrochloride: a betamimetic agent for use in preterm labor. I. Pharmacology, clinical history, administration, side effects, and safety. Obstet. Gynecol. 56:1, 1980.

18. Barrada, M. I., Virnig, N. L., Edwards, L. E. and Hakanson, E. Y.: Maternal intravenous ethanol in the prevention of respiratory distress. Am. J. Obstet. Gynecol. 129:25, 1977.

19. Baumgarten, K. and Gruber, W.: Tokolyseindex. *In* Dudenhausen, J. W. and Saling, E. (eds.): Perinatale Medizin, vol. 5. Stuttgart, Georg Thieme Verlag, 1974.

20. Bengtsson, L. P.: Experiments on the suppressive effect of a synthetic gestagen on the activity of the pregnant human uterus. Acta Obstet. Gynecol. Scand. 41:124, 1962.

21. Bergman, B. and Hedner, T.: Antepartum administration of terbutaline and the incidence of hyaline membrane disease in preterm infants. Acta Obstet. Gynecol. Scand. 57:217, 1978.

22. Bieniarz, J., Burd, L., Motew, M., Scommegna, A., Lin, S., Winneman, C. and Seals, C.: Inhibition of uterine contractility in labor. Am. J. Obstet. Gynecol. 111:874, 1971.

23. Bieniarz, J., Crottogini, J. J., Curuchet, E., Romero-Salinas, G., Yoshida, T., Poseiro, J. J. and Caldeyro-Barcia, R.: Aortocaval compression by the uterus in late human pregnancy. II. An arteriographic study. Am. J. Obstet. Gynecol. 100:203, 1968.

24. Bieniarz, J., Motew, M. and Scommegna, A.: Uterine and cardiovascular effects of ritodrine in premature labor. Obstet. Gynecol. 40:65, 1972.

25. Bishop, E. H. and Woutersz, T. B.: Isoxsuprine, a myometrial relaxant; a preliminary report. Obstet. Gynecol. 17:442, 1961.

26. Blackard, W. G. and Aprill, C. N.: Mechanism of action of diazoxide. J. Lab. Clin. Med. 69:960, 1967.

27. Bobitt, J. R., Hayslip, C. C. and Damato, J. D: Amniotic fluid infection as determined by transabdominal amniocentesis in patients with intact membranes in premature labor. Am. J. Obstet. Gynecol. 140:947, 1981.

28. Boden, W. and Crabben, H. v. d.: Wehenhemmung mit einer neuen beta-adrenergen Substanz. Med. Welt. 30:1342, 1970.

29. Boog, G., Ben Brahim, M. and Gauder, R.: Beta-mimetic drugs and possible prevention of respiratory distress syndrome. Br. J. Obstet. Gynaecol. 82:285, 1975.

30. Borberg, C., Gillmer, M. D. G., Beard, R. W. and Oakley, N. W.: Metabolic effects of beta-sympathomimetic drugs and dexamethasone in normal and diabetic pregnancy. Br. J. Obstet. Gynaecol. 85:184, 1978.

31. Bourne, A. and Burn, J. H.: The dosage and action of pituitary extract and of the ergot alkaloids on the uterus in labor with a note on the action of adrenalin. J. Obstet. Gynaecol. Br. Emp. 34:249, 1927.

32. Brazy, J. E., Little, V., Grimm, J. and Pupkin, M.: Risk benefit considerations for the use of isoxsuprine in the treatment of premature labor. Obstet. Gynecol. 58:297, 1981.

33. Brenner, W. E. and Hendricks, C. H.: Effect of medroxyprogesterone acetate upon the duration and characteristics of human gestation and labor. Am. J. Obstet. Gynecol. 82:1094, 1961.

34. Brettes, J. P., Renaud, R. and Grander, R.: A double-blind investigation into the effects of ritodrine on uterine blood flow during the third trimester of pregnancy. Am. J. Obstet. Gynecol. 124:164, 1976.

35. Brown, W. E. and Wilder, V. M.: The response of the human uterus to epinephrine. Am. J. Obstet. Gynecol. 54:659, 1943.

36. Caldeyro-Barcia, R., Noriega-Guerra, L., Cibils, L. A. et al.: Effect of position changes on intensity and frequency of uterine contractions during labor. Am. J. Obstet. Gynecol. 80:284, 1960.

37. Caritis, S. N., Morishima, H. O., Stark, R. I., Daniel, S. S. and James, S.: Effects of terbutaline on the pregnant baboon and fetus. Obstet. Gynecol. 50:56, 1977.

38. Caritis, S. N., Mueller-Heubach, E., Morishima, H. O. and Edelstone, D. I.: Effect of terbutaline on cardiovascular state and uterine blood flow in pregnant ewes. Obstet. Gynecol. 50:603, 1977.

39. Carsten, M. E.: Hormonal regulation of myometrial calcium transport. Gynecol. Invest. 5:269, 1974.

40. Castren, O., Gummerus, M. and Saarikoski, S.: Treatment of imminent premature labor. Acta Obstet. Gynecol. Scand. 54:95, 1975.

41. Cawson, M. J., Anderson, A. B. M., Turnbull, A.

C. and Lampe, L.: Cortisol, cortisone, and 11-deoxy-cortisol levels in human umbilical and maternal plasma in relation to the onset of labour. J. Obstet. Gynaecol. Br. Commonwealth 81:737, 1974.

42. Chard, T., Hudson, C. N., Edwards, C. R. W. and Boyd, N. R. H.: Release of oxytocin and vasopressin by the human foetus during labour. Nature 234:352, 1971.

43. Coceani, F. and Olley, P. M.: The response of the ductus arteriosus to prostaglandins. Can. J. Physiol. Pharmacol. 51:220, 1973.

44. Coutinho, E. M. and Vieria Lopes, A. C.: Inhibition of uterine motility by aminophylline. Am. J. Obstet. Gynecol. 110:726, 1971.

45. Creasy, R. K., Golbus, M. S., Laros, R. K., Parer, J. T. and Roberts, J. M.: Oral ritodrine in treatment of preterm labor. Am. J. Obstet. Gynecol. 137:212, 1980.

46. Csaba, I. F., Sulyok, E. and Ertl, T.: Relationship of maternal treatment with indomethacin to persistence of fetal circulation syndrome. J. Pediatr. 92:484, 1978.

47. Csapo, A. I.: Progesterone "block." Am. J. Anat. 98:273, 1956.

48. Csapo, A. I.: Defense mechanism of pregnancy. *In* CIBA Foundation Study Groups; Progesterone and the Defense Mechanism of Pregnancy. Boston, Little, Brown and Co., 1961.

49. Csapo, A. I.: Model experiments and clinical trials in the control of pregnancy and parturition. Am. J. Obstet. Gynecol. 85:359, 1963.

50. Csapo, A. I., Csapo, E. E., Fay, E., Henzl, M. R. and Salav, G.: Delay of spontaneous labor by naproxen in the rat model. Prostaglandins 3:827, 1973.

51. Csapo, A. I., de Sousa, F., de Sousa, J. C. and de Sousa, O.: Effect of massive progestational hormone treatment on the parturient human uterus. Fertil. Steril. 17:621, 1966.

52. Csapo, A. I. and Herczeg, J.: Arrest of premature labor by isoxsuprine. Am. J. Obstet. Gynecol. 129:482, 1977.

53. Csapo, A. I., Jaffin, H., Kerenyi, T., Lipman, J. I. and Wood, C.: Volume and activity of the pregnant human uterus. Am. J. Obstet. Gynecol. 85:819, 1963.

54. Dandavino, A., Woods, Jr., J. R., Murayama, K., Brinkmann, C. R., III and Assali, N. S.: Circulatory effects of magnesium sulfate in normotensive and renal hypertensive pregnant sheep. Am. J. Obstet. Gynecol. 127:769, 1977.

55. D'Angelo, L. and Sokol, R. J.: Prematurity: Recognizing patients at risk. Prenatal Care 10(2):16, 1978.

56. Das, R. K.: Isoxsuprine in premature labor. J. Obstet. Gynaecol. India 19:566, 1969.

57. Dawood, M. Y., Raghaven, K. S., Piciask, C. and Fuchs, F.: Oxytocin in human pregnancy and parturition. Obstet. Gynecol. 51:138, 1978.

58. Dawood, M. Y., Wang, C. F., Gupta, R. and Fuchs, F.: Fetal contribution to oxytocin in human labor. Obstet. Gynecol. 52:205, 1978.

59. DeVoe, S. J., DeVoe, K., Rigsby, W. C. and McDaniels, B. A.: Effect of meperidine on uterine contractility. Am. J. Obstet. Gynecol. 105:1004, 1969.

60. Dilts, P. V.: Effect of ethanol on uterine and umbilical hemodynamics and oxygen transfer. Am. J. Obstet. Gynecol. 108:221, 1970.

61. Drost, M. and Holm, L. W.: Prolonged gestation in ewes after foetal adrenalectomy. J. Endocrinol. 40:293, 1968.

62. Eastman, N. J. and DeLeon, M.: The etiology of cerebral palsy. Am. J. Obstet. Gynecol. 69:950, 1955.

63. Elliott, J. P., O'Keeffe, D. F., Greenberg, P. and Freeman, R. K.: Pulmonary edema magnesium sulfate and betamethasone administration. Am. J. Obstet. Gynecol. 134:717, 1979.

64. Elliott, R. B., Starling, M. B. and Neutze, J. M.: Medical manipulation of the ductus arteriosus. Lancet 1:140, 1975.

65. Eskes, T. K. A. B., Kornman, J. J. C. M., Bots, R. S. G. M., Hein, P. R., Gimbrere, J. S. F. and Vonk, J. T. C.: Maternal morbidity due to beta-adrenergic therapy. Pre-existing cardiomyopathy aggravated by fenoterol. Eur. J. Obstet. Gynaecol. Reprod. Biol. 10:41, 1980.

66. Fedrick, J.: Antenatal identification of women at high risk of spontaneous pre-term birth. Br. J. Obstet. Gynaecol. 83:351, 1976.

67. Fedrick, J. and Adelstein, P.: Factors associated with low birth weight of infants delivered at term. Br. J. Obstet. Gynaecol. 85:1, 1978.

68. Fedrick, J. and Anderson, A. B. M.: Factors associated with spontaneous preterm birth. Br. J. Obstet. Gynaecol. 83:342, 1976.

69. Filler, Jr., W. W., Hall, W. C. and Filler, N. W.: Analgesia in obstetrics. The effect of analgesia on uterine contractility and fetal heart rate. Am. J. Obstet. Gynecol. 98:832, 1967.

70. Flowers, C. E., Easterling, W. E. and White, F. D.: Magnesium sulfate in toxemia of pregnancy. Am. J. Obstet. Gynecol. 19:315, 1962.

71. France, J. T., Seddon, R. J. and Liggins, G. C.: A study of pregnancy with low oestrogen production due to placental sulfatase deficiency. J. Clin. Endocrinol. Metab. 36:1, 1973.

72. Friedman, W. F., Hirschklau, M. J., Printz, M. P., Pitlick, P. T. and Kirkpatrick, S. E.: Pharmacologic closure of patent ductus arteriosus in the premature infant. N. Engl. J. Med. 295:526, 1976.

73. Fuchs, A. R.: Oxytocin and the onset of labor in rabbits. J. Endocrinol. 30:217, 1964.

74. Fuchs, A. R.: The inhibitory effect of ethanol on the release of oxytocin during parturition in the rabbit. J. Endocrinol. 35:125, 1966.

75. Fuchs, A. R., Coutinho, E. M., Xavier, R., Bates, P. E. and Fuchs, F.: Effect of ethanol on the activity of the nonpregnant human uterus and its reactivity to neurohypophyseal hormones. Am. J. Obstet. Gynecol. 101:997, 1968.

76. Fuchs, A. R. and Wagner, G.: The effect of ethyl alcohol on the release of oxytocin in rabbits. Acta Endocrinol. 44:593, 1963.

77. Fuchs, F.: Prevention of prematurity. Am. J. Obstet. Gynecol. 126:809, 1976.

78. Fuchs, F., Fuchs, A. R., Poblete, V. F., Jr. and Risk, A.: Effect of alcohol on threatened premature labor. Am. J. Obstet. Gynecol. 99:627, 1967.

79. Fuchs, F. and Stakemann, G.: Treatment of threatened premature labor with large doses of progesterone. Am. J. Obstet. Gynecol. 79:172, 1960.

80. Funderburk, S. J., Guthrie, D. and Meldrum, D.: Suboptimal pregnancy outcome among women with prior abortions and premature births. Am. J. Obstet. Gynecol. 126:55, 1976.

81. Gamissans, O., Esteban-Altirriba, J. and Maiques, V.: Inhibition of human myometrial activity by a new β-adrenergic drug (DU-21220). J. Obstet. Gynaecol. Br. Commonwealth 76:656, 1969.

82. Garrett, W. J.: Effects of adrenaline and noradrenaline on the intact human uterus in late pregnancy and labor. J. Obstet. Gynaecol. Br. Emp. 61:586, 1954.

83. Gibbens, G. L. D. and Chard, T.: Observations on maternal oxytocin release during human labor and the effect of intravenous alcohol administration. Am. J. Obstet. Gynecol. 126:243, 1976.

84. Gohari, P., Berkowitz, R. L. and Hobbins, J. C.: Prediction of intrauterine growth retardation by determination of total intrauterine volume. Am. J. Obstet. Gynecol. 127:255, 1977.

85. Goldkrand, J. W., Schulte, R. L. and Messer, R. H.: Maternal and fetal plasma cortisol levels at parturition. Obstet. Gynecol. 47:41, 1976.

86. Goodlin, R. C.: Can sex in pregnancy harm the fetus? Contemp. Obstet. Gynecol. 8:21, 1976.

87. Goodlin, R. C., Keller, D. W. and Raffin, M.: Orgasm during late pregnancy. Obstet. Gynecol. 38:916, 1971.

88. Goodlin, R. C., Schmidt, W. and Crewy, D. C.: Uterine tension and fetal heart rate during maternal orgasm. Obstet. Gynecol. 39:125, 1972.

89. Graff, G.: Failure to prevent premature labor with ethanol. Am. J. Obstet. Gynecol. 110:878, 1971.

90. Greenhouse, B. S., Hook, R. and Hehre, F. W.: Aspiration pneumonia following intravenous administration of alcohol during labor. J.A.M.A. 210:2393, 1969.

91. Gross, T. L. and Sokol, R. J.: Severe hypokalemia and acidosis: a potential complication of beta-adrenergic treatment. Am. J. Obstet. Gynecol. 138:1225, 1980.

92. Gustavii, B.: Release of lysosomal acid phosphatase into the cytoplasm of decidual cells before the onset of labor in humans. Br. J. Obstet. Gynaecol. 82:177, 1975.

93. Hack, M., Fanaroff, A. A., Klaus, M. H., Mendelawitz, B. D. and Merkatz, I. R.: Neonatal respiratory distress following elective delivery: a preventable disease? Am. J. Obstet. Gynecol. 126:43, 1976.

94. Harbert, G. M., Cornell, G. W. and Thornton, W. N., Jr.: Effect of toxemia therapy on uterine dynamics. Am. J. Obstet. Gynecol. 105:94, 1969.

95. Harris, R. E., Thomas, V. L. and Shelokov, A.: Asymptomatic bacteriuria in pregnancy: antibody-coated bacteria, renal function, and intrauterine growth retardation. Am. J. Obstet. Gynecol. 126:20, 1976.

96. Hemminki, E. and Starfield, B.: Prevention and treatment of premature labour by drugs: review of controlled clinical trials. Br. J. Obstet. Gynaecol. 85:411, 1978.

97. Hendricks, C. H.: Hemodynamics of a uterine contraction. Am. J. Obstet. Gynecol. 76:969, 1958.

98. Hendricks, C. H., Brenner, W., Gabel, R. and Kerenyi, T.: The effect of progesterone administered intraamniotically in late human pregnancy. *In* Barnes, A. C. (ed.): Brook Lodge Symposium: Progesterone. Brook Lodge Press, pp. 53–64, 1961.

99. Hendricks, C. H., Cibils, L. A., Pose, S. V. and Eskes, T. K. A. B.: Pharmacologic control of excessive uterine activity with isoxsuprine. Am. J. Obstet. Gynecol. 82:1064, 1961.

100. Heymann, M. A. and Rudolph, A. M.: Effects of acetylsalicylic acid on the ductus arteriosus and circulation in fetal lambs in utero. Circ. Res. 38:418, 1976.

101. Heymann, M. A. and Rudolph, A. M.: Ductus arteriosus dilatation by prostaglandin E₁ in infants with pulmonary atresia. Pediatrics 59:325, 1977.

102. Heymann, M. A., Rudolph, A. M. and Silverman, N. H.: Closure of the ductus arteriosus in premature infants by inhibition of prostaglandin synthesis. N. Engl. J. Med. 295:530, 1976.

103. Hobbins, J. C., Berkowitz, R. L. and Grannum, P. A. T.: Diagnosis and antepartum management of intrauterine growth retardation. J. Reprod. Med. 21:319, 1978.

104. Hobel, C. J., Hyvarinen, M. A., Okada, D. M. and Oh, W.: Prenatal and intrapartum high-risk screening. Prediction of the high-risk neonate. Am. J. Obstet. Gynecol. 117:1, 1973.

105. Honnebier, W. J. and Swaab, D. F.: The influence of anencephaly upon intrauterine growth of fetus and placenta and upon gestation length. Br. J. Obstet. Gynaecol. 80:577, 1973.

106. Horiguchi, T., Suzuki, K., Comas-Urrutia, A. C. et al.: Effect of ethanol upon uterine activity and fetal acid-base state of the rhesus monkey. Am. J. Obstet. Gynecol. 109:910, 1971.

107. Humphrey, M., Chang, A., Gilbert, M. and Wood, C.: The effect of intravenous ritodrine on the acid-base status of the fetus during the second stage of labor. Br. J. Obstet. Gynaecol. 82:234, 1975.

108. Hutchinson, H. T., Nichols, M. M., Kuhn, C. R. and Vasicka, A.: Effects of magnesium sulfate on uterine contractility, intrauterine fetus, and infant. Am. J. Obstet. Gynecol. 88:747, 1964.

109. Ingemarsson, I.: Effect of terbutaline on premature labor. A double-blind placebo-controlled study. Am. J. Obstet. Gynecol. 125:520, 1976.

110. Ingemarsson, I., Westgren, M., Lindberg, C., Ahren, B., Lundquist, I. and Carlsson, C.: Single injection of terbutaline in term labor: placental transfer and effects on maternal and fetal carbohydrate metabolism. Am. J. Obstet. Gynecol. 139:697, 1981.

111. Iuppa, J. B., Smith, G. A., Colella, J. J. and Gibson, J. L.: Succinylcholine effect on human myometrial activity. Obstet. Gynecol. 37:591, 1971.

112. Jacobs, M. M., Knight, A. B. and Arias, F.: Maternal pulmonary edema resulting from beta mimetic and glucocorticoid therapy. Obstet. Gynecol. 56:56, 1980.

113. Jenssen, H. and Wright, P. B.: The effect of dexamethasone therapy in prolonged pregnancy. Acta Obstet. Gynecol. Scand. 56:467, 1977.

114. Jhirad, A. and Vago, T.: Induction of labor by breast stimulation. Obstet. Gynecol. 41:347, 1973.

115. Johnson, J. W. C., Austin, K. L., Jones, G. S., Davis, G. H. and King, T. M.: Efficacy of 17 α-hydroxyprogesterone caproate in the prevention of premature labor. N. Engl. J. Med. 293:675, 1975.

116. Johnson, J. W. C., Lee, P. A., Zachary, A. S.,

Calhoun, S. and Migeon, C. J.: High-risk prematurity—Progestin treatment and steroid studies. Obstet. Gynecol. 54:412, 1979.

117. Johnson, W. L., Harbert, G. M. and Martin, C. B.: Pharmacologic control of uterine contractility: in vitro human and in vivo monkey studies. Am. J. Obstet. Gynecol. 123:364, 1975.

118. Kaiser, I. H.: The effect of epinephrine and norepinephrine on the contraction of human uterus in labor. Surg. Gynecol. Obstet. 90:649, 1950.

119. Karim, M.: Isoxsuprine and the human parturient uterus. J. Obstet. Gynaecol. Br. Commonwealth 70:992, 1963.

120. Karim, S. M. M.: Identification of prostaglandins in human amniotic fluid. J. Obstet. Gynaecol. Br. Commonwealth 73:903, 1966.

121. Karim, S. M. M.: Appearance of prostaglandin F_2 in human blood during labour. Br. Med. J. 4:618, 1968.

122. Karim, S. M. M. and Devlin, J.: Prostaglandin content of amniotic fluid during pregnancy and labor. J. Obstet. Gynaecol. Br. Commonwealth 74:230, 1967.

123. Kass, E. H.: Bacteriuria and pyelonephritis of pregnancy. Arch. Intern. Med. 105:194, 1960.

124. Kass, E. H.: Pyelonephritis and bacteriuria: a major problem in preventive medicine. Ann. Intern. Med. 56:46, 1962.

125. Katz, M., Robertson, P. A. and Creasy, R. K.: Cardiovascular complications associated with terbutaline treatment for preterm labor. Am. J. Obstet. Gynecol. 139:605, 1981.

126. Kauppila, A., Tuimala, R., Ylikorkala, C., Haapdlahti, J., Karppanen, H. and Viinikka, L.: Effects of ritodrine and isoxsuprine with and without dexamethasone during late pregnancy. Obstet. Gynecol. 51:228, 1978.

127. Keirse, M. J. N. C., Rush, R. W., Anderson, A. B. M. and Turnbull, A. C.: Risk of pre-term delivery in patients with previous preterm delivery and/or abortion. Br. J. Obstet. Gynaecol. 85:81, 1978.

128. Keirse, M. J. N. C. and Turnbull, A. C.: Metabolism of prostaglandins within the pregnant uterus. Br. J. Obstet. Gynaecol. 82:887, 1975.

129. Kero, P., Hirvonen, T. and Valimaki, I.: Prenatal and postnatal isoxsuprine and respiratory distress syndrome. Lancet 2:198, 1973.

130. Kirkpatrick C., Quenon, M. and Desir, D.: Blood anions and electrolytes during ritodrine infusion in preterm labor. Am. J. Obstet. Gynecol. 138:523, 1980.

131. Kirkpatrick, S. E., Pitlick, P. T., Hirschklau, M. J. and Friedman, W. F.: Acute effects of maternal ethanol infusion on fetal cardiac performance. Am. J. Obstet. Gynecol. 126:1034, 1976.

132. Kloeck, F. K. and Jung, H.: In vitro release of prostaglandins from the human myometrium under the influence of stretching. Am. J. Obstet. Gynecol. 15:1066, 1973.

133. Korda, A. R., Lyneham, R. C. and Jones, W. R.: The treatment of premature labour with intravenously administered salbutamol. Med. J. Aust. 1:744, 1974.

134. Krishna, K.: Tobacco chewing in pregnancy. Br. J. Obstet. Gynaecol. 85:726, 1978.

135. Kumar, D., Goodno, J. A. and Barnes, A. C.: Isolation of progesterone from human pregnant myometrium. Nature 195:1224, 1962.

136. Kumar, D., Zourlas, P. A. and Barnes, A. C.: In vitro and in vivo effects of magnesium sulfate on human uterine contractility. Am. J. Obstet. Gynecol. 86:1036, 1963.

137. Kumar, D., Zourlas, P. A. and Barnes, A. C.: In vivo effect of amyl nitrite on human pregnant uterine contractility. Am. J. Obstet. Gynecol. 91:1066, 1965.

138. Kumaresan, P., Han, G. S., Anandarangam, P. B. and Vasicka, A.: Oxytocin in maternal and fetal blood. Obstet. Gynecol. 46:272, 1975.

139. Lammintausta, R., Erkkola, R. and Katainen, P.: Effect of intravenous infusion of betasympathomimetic agents on plasma renin activity during pregnancy. Br. J. Obstet. Gynaecol. 85:828, 1978.

140. Landesman, R., de Sousa, F. J. A., Coutinho, E. M., Wilson, K. H. and de Sousa, F. M. B.: The inhibitory effect of diazoxide in normal term labor. Am. J. Obstet. Gynecol. 103:430, 1969.

141. Landesman, R. and Wilson, K. H.: Relaxant effect of diazoxide on isolated gravid and nongravid human myometrium. Am. J. Obstet. Gynecol. 101:120, 1968.

142. Landesman, R., Wilson, K. H., Coutinho, E. M., Klima, I. M. and Marcus, R. S.: The relaxant action of ritodrine, a sympathomimetic amine, on the uterus during term labor. Am. J. Obstet. Gynecol. 110:111, 1971.

143. Lands, A. M., Arnold, A., McAuliff, J., Luduena, F. P. and Brown, T. G.: Differentiation of regular systems activated by sympathomimetic amines. Nature 214:597, 1967.

144. Lauersen, N. H., Merkatz, I. R., Tejani, N., Wilson, K. H., Roberson, A., Mann, L. and Fuchs, F.: Inhibition of premature labor: a multicenter comparison of ritodrine and ethanol. Am. J. Obstet. Gynecol. 127:837, 1977.

145. Lehtovirta, P. and Forss, M.: The acute effect of smoking on intervillous blood flow of the placenta. Br. J. Obstet. Gynaecol. 85:729, 1978.

146. Leong, M. K. H. and Murphy, B. E. P.: Cortisol levels in maternal venous and umbilical cord arterial and venous serum at vaginal delivery. Am. J. Obstet. Gynecol. 124:471, 1976.

147. Lewis, R. B. and Schulman, J. D.: Influence of acetylsalicylic acid, an inhibitor of prostaglandin synthesis, on duration of human gestation and labor. Lancet 2:1159, 1973.

148. Liggins, G. C.: Premature delivery of foetal lambs infused with glucocorticoids. J. Endocrinol. 45:515, 1969.

149. Liggins, G. C.: The influence of the fetal hypothalamus and pituitary on growth. *In* Elliott, K. and Knight, J. (eds.): Size at Birth. CIBA Foundation Symposium, No. 27, pp. 165–183. Amsterdam, Elsevier/Excerpta Medica, 1974.

150. Liggins, G. C., Fairclough, R. J., Grieves, S. A., Kendall, J. Z. and Knox, B. S.: Mechanism of initiation of parturition in the ewe. Recent Prog. Horm. Res. 29:111, 1973.

151. Liggins, G. C., Forster, C. S., Grieves, S. A. and Schwartz, A. L.: Control or parturition in Man. Biol. Reprod. 16:39, 1977.

152. Liggins, G. C. and Howie, M. B.: A controlled trial of antepartum glucocorticoid treatment for prevention of the respiratory distress syndrome in premature infants. Pediatrics 50:515, 1972.

153. Liggins, G. C., Kennedy, P. C. and Holm, L. W.:

Failure of initiation of parturition after electroco-agulation of the pituitary of the fetal lamb. Am. J. Obstet. Gynecol. 98:1080, 1967.

154. Liggins, G. C. and Vaughn, G. S.: Intravenous infusion of salbutamol in the management of premature labour. J. Obstet. Gynaecol. Br. Commonwealth 80:29, 1973.

155. Lipshitz, J.: Uterine and cardiovascular effects of aminophylline. Am. J. Obstet. Gynecol. 131:716, 1978.

156. Lipshitz, J. and Baillie, P.: Uterine and cardiovascular effects of beta$_2$-selective sympathomimetic drugs administered as an intravenous infusion. S. Afr. Med. J. 50:1973, 1976.

157. Lipshitz, J., Baillie, P. and Davey, D. A.: A comparison of the uterine beta$_2$-adrenoreceptor selectivity of fenoterol, hexoprenaline, ritodrine, and salbutamol. S. Afr. Med. J. 50:1969, 1976.

158. Lish, P. M., Hillyard, I. W. and Dungan, K. W.: The uterine relaxant properties of isoxsuprine. J. Pharmacol. Exp. Ther. 129:438, 1960.

159. Liu, D. T. Y.: Phosphodiesterase inhibition and respiratory distress syndrome. Lancet 2:378, 1973.

160. Liu, D. T. Y. and Blackwell, R. J.: The value of a scoring system in predicting outcome of preterm labour and comparing the efficacy of treatment with aminophylline and salbutamol. Br. J. Obstet. Gynaecol. 85:418, 1978.

161. Liu, D. T. Y., Measday, B. and Melville, H. A. H.: Premature labour parameters for comparison employing methylxanthine therapy. Aust. N.Z. J. Obstet. Gynaecol. 15:145, 1975.

162. MacDonald, P. C., Schultz, F. M., Duenhoelter, J. H. et al.: Initiation of human parturition: I. Mechanism of action of arachidonic acid. Obstet. Gynecol. 44:629, 1974.

163. Majewski, J. T. and Jennings, T.: Further experiments with the uterine relaxing hormone in premature labor. Obstet. Gynecol. 9:322, 1957.

164. Manchester, D., Margolis, H. S. and Sheldon, R. E.: Possible association between indomethacin therapy and primary pulmonary hypertension in the newborn. Am. J. Obstet. Gynecol. 126:467, 1976.

165. Mann, L. I., Bhaktharaathsalan, A., Liu, M. and Makowski, P.: Placental transport of alcohol and its effect on maternal and fetal acid-base balance. Am. J. Obstet. Gynecol. 122:837, 1975.

166. Manniello, R. L. and Farrell, P. M.: Analysis of United States neonatal mortality statistics from 1968 to 1974, with specific reference to changing trends in major casualties. Am. J. Obstet. Gynecol. 129:667, 1977.

167. Mati, J. K. B., Horrobin, D. F. and Bramley, P. S.: Induction of labor in sheep and in humans by single doses of corticosteroids. Br. Med. J. 2:149, 1973.

168. Mayer, P. S. and Wingate, M. B.: Obstetric factors in cerebral palsy. Obstet. Gynecol. 51:399, 1978.

169. Merkatz, I. R., Peter, J. B. and Barden, T. P.: Ritodrine hydrochloride: a betamimetic agent for use in preterm labor II. Evidence of efficacy. Obstet. Gynecol. 50:7, 1980.

170. Meyer, M. B.: How does maternal smoking affect birth weight and maternal weight gain? Am. J. Obstet. Gynecol. 131:888, 1978.

171. Milewich, L., Gant, N. F., Schwarz, B. E., Chen, G. T. and MacDonald, P. C.: Initiation of parturition. VIII. Metabolism of progesterone by fetal membranes of early and late human gestation. Obstet. Gynecol. 50:45, 1977.

172. Milic, A. B. and Adamsons, K.: The relationship between anencephaly and prolonged pregnancy. Br. J. Obstet. Gynaecol. 76:102, 1969.

173. Miller, F. C., Nochimson, D. J., Paul, R. H. and Hon, E. H.: Effects of ritodrine hydrochloride on uterine activity and the cardiovascular system in toxemic patients. Obstet. Gynecol. 47:50, 1976.

174. Miller, H. C., Hassanein, K. and Hensleigh, P. A.: Fetal growth retardation in relation to maternal smoking and weight gain in pregnancy. Am. J. Obstet. Gynecol. 125:55, 1976.

175. Morris, J. A., Arce, J. J., Hamilton, C. J., Davidson, E. C., Maidman, J. E., Clark, J. E. and Bloom, R. S.: The management of severe preeclampsia and eclampsia with intravenous diazoxide. Obstet. Gynecol. 49:675, 1977.

176. Mueller-Heubach, E., Myers, R. E. and Adamsons, K.: Effects of adrenalectomy on pregnancy length in the rhesus monkey. Am. J. Obstet. Gynecol. 112:221, 1972.

177. Murphy, B. E. P.: Does the human fetal adrenal play a role in parturition? Am. J. Obstet. Gynecol. 115:521, 1973.

178. Naeye, R. L.: Effects of maternal cigarette smoking on the fetus and placenta. Br. J. Obstet. Gynaecol. 85:732, 1978.

179. National Center for Health Statistics: A study of infant mortality from linked records by birth weight, period of gestation, and other variables. United States Vital and Health Statistics, Series 20, No. 12, US DHEW Pub. No. (HSM) 72–1055, Washington, D.C., Health Services and Mental Health Administration, May 1972.

180. National Center for Health Statistics, Vital and Health Statistics, Characteristics of Birth, United States 1973–1975, Series 21, No. 30, US DHEW, Washington, D.C.

181. National Center for Health Statistics: Factors associated with low birth weight, United States, 1976. Vital and Health Statistics, Series 21, No. 37, US DHEW Pub. No. (PHS) 80–1915, April 1980.

182. National Center for Health Statistics: Final Natality Statistics, 1978, Vital and Health Statistics, DHHS Pub. No. (PHS) 80–1120, vol. 29, No. 1, suppl., April 28, 1980.

183. Nochimson, D. J., Riffel, H. D., Yeh, S., Kreitzer, M. S., Paul, R. H. and Hon, E. H.: The effects of ritodrine hydrochloride on uterine activity and the cardiovascular system. Am. J. Obstet. Gynecol. 118:523, 1974.

184. Novy, M. J., Cook, M. J. and Manaugh, L.: Indomethacin block of normal onset of parturition in primates. Am. J. Obstet. Gynecol. 118:412, 1974.

185. Nnwayhid, B., Brinkman, C. R. III, Katchen, B., Symchowicz, S., Martinek, H. and Assali, N. S.: Maternal and fetal hemodynamic effects of diazoxide. Obstet. Gynecol. 46:197, 1975.

186. Nwosu, U. C., Wallach, E. E. and Bolognese, R. L.: Initiation of labor by intra-amniotic cortisol instillation in prolonged human pregnancy. Obstet. Gynecol. 47:137, 1976.

187. Oakey, R. E.: The interpretation of urinary oestro-

gen and pregnanediol excretion in pregnant women receiving corticosteroids. J. Obstet. Gynaecol. Br. Commonwealth 77:922, 1970.

188. Okazaki, T., Okita, J. R., MacDonald, P. C. and Johnston, J. M.: Initiation of human parturition. X. Substrate specificity of phospholipase A_2 in human fetal membranes. Am. J. Obstet. Gynecol. 130:432, 1978.

189. Olley, P. M., Coceani, F. and Bodach, E.: E-type prostaglandins: a new emergency therapy for certain cyanotic congenital heart malformations. Circulation 53:728, 1976.

190. Osler, M.: Side effects and metabolic changes during treatment with betamimetics (Ritodrine). Dan. Med. Bull. 26:119, 1979.

191. Ott, A., Hayes, J. and Polin, J.: Severe lactic acidosis associated with intravenous alcohol for premature labor. Obstet. Gynecol. 48:362, 1976.

192. Persson, H. and Olsson, T.: Some pharmacological properties of terbutaline (INN). 1-(3,5-dihydroxyphenyl)-2-(T-butylamino)-ethanol. A new sympathomimetic β-receptor–stimulating agent. Acta Med. Scand. Suppl. 512:11, 1970.

193. Petrie, R. H., Wu, R., Miller, F. C. et al.: The effect of drugs on uterine activity. Obstet. Gynecol. 48:431, 1976.

194. Philipson, T., Eriksen, P. S. and Lynggard, F.: Pulmonary edema following ritodrine—saline infusion in premature labor. Obstet. Gynecol. 58:304, 1981.

195. Pitkin, R. M.: Assessing the clinical factors in prematurity. Contemp. Obstet. Gynecol. 7:37, 1976.

196. Pose, S. V. and Fielitz, C.: Effects of progesterone on response of the pregnant human uterus to oxytocin. *In* Caldeyro-Barcia, R. and Heller, H. (eds.): Oxytocin. New York, Pergamon Press, 1961, p. 229.

197. Pritchard, J. A. and Pritchard, S. A.: Standardized treatment of 154 consecutive cases of eclampsia. Am. J. Obstet. Gynecol. 123:543, 1975.

198. Ragni, N., Pinto, P. F., Bentivoglio, G., Repetti, F., Peluccod, D. and Muzio, M.: Polyplethysmographic study on the effects of ritodrine on the cardiovascular system of patients in labour. Br. J. Obstet. Gynaecol. 86:866, 1979.

199. Raja, R. L., Anderson, A. B. M. and Turnbull, A. C.: Endocrine changes in premature labor. Br. Med. J. 4:67, 1974.

200. Rezek, G. H.: Lutrexin in the treatment of threatening premature labor by betamimetic drugs. Am. J. Obstet. Gynecol. 127:482, 1977.

201. Richter, R.: Evaluation of success in treatment of threatening premature labor by betamimetic drugs. Am. J. Obstet. Gynecol. 127:482, 1977.

202. Riffel, H. D., Nochimson, D. J., Paul, R. H. and Hon, E. H.: Effects of meperidine and promethazine during labor. Obstet. Gynecol. 42:738, 1973.

203. Rizzolo, E. A.: A uterine relaxant for premature uterine contractions. Clin. Med. 74:53, 1967.

204. Robinson, G. A., Butcher, R. W. and Sutherland, E. W.: Cyclic AMP. Am. Rev. Biochem. 37:149, 1968.

205. Runnebaum, B. and Zander, J.: Progesterone and 20 α-dihydroprogesterone in human myometrium during pregnancy. Acta Endocrinol. 66: Suppl. 150:1, 1971.

206. Rush, R. W., Davey, D. A. and Segall, M. L.: The effect of preterm delivery on perinatal mortality. Br. J. Obstet. Gynaecol. 85:806, 1978.

207. Ryden, G.: The effect of salbutamol and terbutaline in the management of premature labour. Acta Obstet. Gynecol. Scand. 56:293, 1977.

208. Schreyer, P., Caspi, E., Ariely, S., Herziann, P., User, Y., Gilboa, Y. and Zaidman, J. L.: Metabolic effects of intravenous ritodrine infusion during pregnancy. Europ. J. Obstet. Gynecol. Reprod. Biol. 9:97, 1979.

209. Schreyer, P., Caspi, E., Arieli, S., Maor, J. and Modai, D.: Metabolic effects of intravenous ritodrine infusion in pregnancy. Acta Obstet. Gynecol. Scand. 59:197, 1980.

210. Schultz, F. M., Schwarz, B. E., MacDonald, P. C. and Johnston, J. M.: Initiation of human parturition: II. Identification of phospholipase A_2 in fetal chorioamnion and uterine decidua. Am. J. Obstet. Gynecol. 123:650, 1975.

211. Schwarz, B. E., Schultz, F. M., MacDonald, P. C. and Johnston, J. M.: Initiation of human parturition. III. Fetal membrane content of prostaglandin E_2 and $F_{2\alpha}$ precursor. Obstet. Gynecol. 46:564, 1975.

212. Schwarz, B. E., Schultz, F. M., MacDonald, P. C. and Johnstone, J. M.: Initiation of human parturition: IV. Demonstration of phospholipase A_2 in the lysosomes of human fetal membranes. Am. J. Obstet. Gynecol. 125:1089, 1976.

213. Scommegna, A., Burd, L., Goodman, C., Bieniarz, J. and Seals, C.: Effect of pregnenolone sulfate on uterine contractility. Am. J. Obstet. Gynecol. 108:1023, 1970.

214. Seppala, M. and Aho, I.: Physiologic role of meconium during delivery. Acta Obstet. Gynecol. Scand. 54:209, 1975.

215. Seppala, M., Aho, I., Tissari, A. and Ruoslahti, E.: Radioimmunoassay of oxytocin in amniotic fluid, fetal urine, and meconium during late pregnancy and delivery. Am. J. Obstet. Gynecol. 114:788, 1972.

216. Simmer, H. H., Tulchinsky, D., Gold, E. M., Frankland, M., Griepel, M. and Gold, A. S.: On the regulation of estrogen production by cortisol and ACTH in human pregnancy at term. Am. J. Obstet. Gynecol. 119:283, 1974.

217. Sims, C. D., Chamberlain, G. V. P., Boyd, I. E. and Lewis, P. J.: A comparison of salbutamol and ethanol in the treatment of preterm labour. Br. J. Obstet. Gynaecol. 85:761, 1978.

218. Smythe, A. R., II and Sakakini, J., Jr.: Maternal metabolic alterations secondary to terbutaline therapy for premature labor. Obstet. Gynecol. 57:566, 1981.

219. Sokol, R. J., Rosen, M. G., Stojkov, J. and Chik, L.: Clinical application of high risk scoring on an obstetric service. Am. J. Obstet. Gynecol. 128:652, 1977.

220. Spellacy, W. N., Cruz, A. C., Buhi, W. C. and Birk, S. A.: The acute effects of ritodrine infusion on maternal metabolism: measurements of levels of glucose, insulin, glucagon, triglycerides, cholesterol, placental lactogen, and chorionic gonadotropin. Am. J. Obstet. Gynecol. 131:637, 1978.

221. Stander, R. W., Barden, T. P., Thompson, J. F., Pugh, W. R. and Werts, C. E.: Fetal cardiac

effects of maternal isoxsuprine infusion. Am. J. Obstet. Gynecol. 89:792, 1964.

222. Steer, C. M. and Petrie, R. H.: A comparison of magnesium sulfate and alcohol for prevention of premature labor. Am. J. Obstet. Gynecol. 129:1, 1977.

223. Suonio, S., Oikkonen, H. and Lahtinen, T.: Maternal circulatory response to a single dose of ritodrine hydrochloride during orthostasis in normal and hypertensive late pregnancy. Am. J. Obstet. Gynecol. 130:745, 1978.

224. Sutherland, E. W. and Rall, T. W.: Relation of adenosine 3'5'-phosphate and phosphorylase to the actions of catecholamines and other hormones. Pharm. Rev. 12:265, 1960.

225. Sybulski, S., Goldsmith, W. J. and Maughan, G. B.: Cortisol levels in fetal scalp, maternal and umbilical cord plasma. Obstet. Gynecol. 46:268, 1975.

226. Sybulski, S. and Maughan, G. B.: Cortisol levels in umbilical cord plasma in relation to labor and delivery. Am. J. Obstet. Gynecol. 125:236, 1976.

227. Talbert, L. M., Easterling, W. E. and Potter, H. D.: Maternal and fetal plasma levels of adrenal corticoids in spontaneous vaginal delivery and cesarean section. Am. J. Obstet. Gynecol. 117:554, 1973.

228. Talbert, L. M., Pearlman, W. H. and Potter, H. D.: Maternal and fetal serum levels of total cortisol and cortisone, unbound cortisol, and corticosteroid-binding globulin in vaginal delivery and cesarean section. Am. J. Obstet. Gynecol. 129:781, 1977.

229. Tuimala, R. J., Kauppila, A. J. I. and Haapalahti, J.: Response of pituitary-adrenal axis on partal stress. Obstet. Gynecol. 46:275, 1975.

230. Ulmsten, U., Andersson, K. E. and Wingerup, L.: Treatment of premature labor with the calcium antagonist nifedipine. Arch. Gynecol. 229:1, 1980.

231. Vane, J. R.: Inhibition of prostaglandin synthesis as a mechanism of action for aspirin-like drugs. Nature (New Biol) 231:232, 1971.

232. Wagner, L., Wagner, G. and Guerrero, J.: Effect of alcohol on premature newborn infants. Am. J. Obstet. Gynecol. 108:308, 1970.

233. Wallace, R. L., Caldwell, D. L., Ansbacher, R. and Otterson, W. N.: Inhibition of premature labor by terbutaline. Obstet. Gynecol. 51:387, 1978.

234. Wansbrough, H., Nakanishi, H. and Wood, C.: Effect of epinephrine on human uterine activity in vitro and in vivo. Obstet. Gynecol. 30:779, 1967.

235. Warsof, S. L., Gohari, P., Berkowitz, R. L. and Hobbins, J. C.: The estimation of fetal weight by computer-assisted analysis. Am. J. Obstet. Gynecol. 128:881, 1977.

236. Watring, W. G., Benson, W. L., Wiebe, R. A. and Vaughn, D. L.: Intravenous alcohol—a single blind study in the prevention of premature delivery: a preliminary report. J. Reprod. Med. 16:35, 1976.

237. Wesselius-de Casparis, A., Thiery, M., Yo Le Sian, A. et al.: Results of double-blind, multicentre study with ritodrine in premature labour. Br. Med. J. 3:144, 1971.

238. Whalley, P. J., Martin, F. G. and Peters, P. C.: Significance of asymptomatic bacteriuria detected during pregnancy. J.A.M.A. 193:879, 1965.

239. Wilson, K. H., Lauersen, N. H., Raghaven, K. S., Fuchs, F. and Niemann, W. H.: Effects of diazoxide and beta-adrenergic drugs on spontaneous and induced uterine activity in the pregnant baboon. Am. J. Obstet. Gynecol. 118:499, 1974.1974.

240. Wood, C., Elstein, M. and Pinkerton, J. H. M.: Effect of progestogens upon uterine activity. J. Obstet. Gynaecol. Br. Commonwealth 70:839, 1963.

241. Zlatnik, F. J.: Applicability of labor inhibition to the problem of prematurity. Am. J. Obstet. Gynecol. 113:704, 1972.

242. Zlatnik, F. J. and Fuchs, F.: A controlled study of ethanol in threatened premature labor. Am. J. Obstet. Gynecol. 112:610, 1972.

243. Zuckerman, H., Reiss, U. and Rubinstein, I.: Inhibition of human premature labor by indomethacin. Obstet. Gynecol. 44:787, 1974.

244. Zuspan, F. P., Barden, T. P., Bieniarz, J. et al.: Premature labor; its management and therapy. J. Reprod. Med. 9:93, 1972.

245. Zuspan, F. P., Cibils, L. A. and Pose, S. V.: Myometrial and cardiovascular responses to alterations in plasma epinephrine and norepinephrine. Am. J. Obstet. Gynecol. 84:841, 1962.

The Management of Preterm Labor: Use of Magnesium Sulfate

Guy M. Harbert, Jr., M.D.
Kenneth R. Spisso, M.D.
University of Virginia School of Medicine

Despite advances in other aspects of prenatal care, immature births have comprised between 7.4 per cent and 7.6 per cent of the total births in the United States each year since 1970.[1] Due in part to the referral nature of patient population at the University of Virginia Hospital, over 10 per cent of infants born here in the past 10 years have weighed 2499 g or less. Latest mortality statistics report that immature births account for 16.3 per cent of perinatal deaths in the country.[2] There is no doubt that immaturity remains a leading cause of perinatal morbidity and mortality and that preterm labor continues to be one of the major complicating factors in obstetrics. The continuing controversy in the management of the patient with preterm labor is exemplified by the more than 14 pharmacologic agents advocated for its treatment in current literature. However, development of a panacea for arresting preterm labor will not eliminate this reproductive hazard. In many instances, both the prematurity and the perinatal loss are related to some other underlying pathophysiologic process that engenders the immature birth. The clinician's task in the management of preterm labor is to define the situations in which delay will enhance the infant's probability of attaining maximal adult potential, as well as to attempt to prevent delivery in these patients.

Patient Selection

Before a patient is considered a candidate for attempts at pharmacologic control of preterm labor, specific maternal and fetal risk factors associated with an increased incidence of immature birth must be evaluated. Conditions associated with premature births at the University of Virginia Hospital are listed in Table 1. Patients may be excluded from treatment when maternal conditions such as bleeding, hypertension or diabetes compromise the intrauterine environment and make premature birth the lesser risk. Patients may also be excluded when attempts to pharmacologically suppress uterine activity appear futile. Molecular changes in the myometrium and in the collagen of the cervix are occurring throughout pregnancy and during labor.[3, 4] Although the changes have not been precisely defined, clinical experience justifies the assumption that during labor these processes eventually reach an irreversible point. When the cervix is dilated more than 3 or 4 cm, attempts to stop labor are generally unsuccessful.

Fetal conditions that may either favor early delivery or make attempts to stop preterm labor meaningless include erythroblastosis fetalis, severe congenital abnormalities, abnormal presentation and intrauterine growth retardation resulting from such factors as toxoplasmosis or rubella. In our patient population about 8 per cent of low birth weight neonates display these complications. Premature rupture of the amniochorionic membranes also complicates the gestation of more than 10 per cent of low birth weight infants at the University of Virginia Hospital. In these patients, the risk of prematurity versus the risk of maternal and fetal infection must be weighed. While many clinicians consider rupture of the membranes as an absolute contraindication to therapeutic attempts to stop labor, current methods of high-risk pregnancy management challenge this concept. The occurrence of amnionitis makes the risk of prematurity secondary regardless of the duration of gestation. After those patients in whom attempts to arrest labor may be either contraindicated or deemed futile are excluded, approximately 20 per cent of our low birth weight group remain. The next critical judgment of management is to identify infants in this group in whom the degree of prematurity warrants attempting therapy. With no identifiable contraindication, attempts should be made to stop all labors that occur prior to the end of the 34th week of gestation. Pregnancies in the gestational period between 34 and 37 weeks present a clinical dilemma that necessitates careful evaluation, sound judgment and individualization of care. Clinical estimates of fetal size and maturity, aided by ultrasonic

TABLE 1. CONDITIONS ASSOCIATED WITH DELIVERY OF 1000 INFANTS WEIGHING 2499 G OR LESS*

CONDITION	NO. INFANTS
A. Maternal	
1. Bleeding (abruptio placenta, placenta previa)	58
2. Chronic hypertensive, cardiovascular, renal disease	20
3. Pregnancy-induced hypertension	181
4. Diabetes and other severe maternal diseases	31
5. Cervix dilated more than 4 cm on admission	112
B. Fetal	
1. Isoimmunization	15
2. Known severe congenital abnormality	11
3. Abnormal presentation	29
4. Intrauterine growth retardation or fetal distress from fetal causes or both	21
5. Product of multiple gestation (167 sets of twins, one set of triplets at risk)	205
6. Ruptured amniochorionic membranes	107
7. Amnionitis	
a. With ruptured amniochorionic membranes	10
b. Without ruptured amniochorionic membranes	6
C. Other	194

*At the University of Virginia Hospital.

cephalometry and amniotic fluid indices of fetal maturation,[5] may help determine the approach to management.

Management

Effective therapy to arrest preterm labor should be based on sound physiologic principles. Unfortunately, development of a rational pharmacodynamic approach has been handicapped by lack of precise knowledge of the mechanisms that initiate labor. Many attempts at pharmacologic suppression of labor are based upon principles of interfering with processes that form links in the hypothetical chain of events considered responsible for the onset of parturition. Other forms of therapy have their genesis in empirical observations of how drugs affect the uterus.

At the University of Virginia Hospital, the primary agent used for pharmacologic suppression of uterine activity has been magnesium sulfate. Elevated serum levels of magnesium decrease acetylcholine release, reduce the motor end-plate sensitivity and depress the amplitude of the motor end-plate potential by competitive displacement of calcium ions.[6] Calcium, in turn, appears to be a major intercellular mediator for controlling electromechanical coupling and effecting muscle contraction,[7, 8] with the release of calcium ions into the cytoplasm activating the regulatory proteins of the myofibril.[9] Selection of mag-

nesium sulfate for the treatment of preterm labor is based upon both in vitro investigation and in vivo clinical studies. In vitro investigations, in which myometrial strips excised from pregnant uteri were used, have demonstrated a dose-response decrease in frequency and amplitude of contraction.[10] Clinically, the observation was made that intravenous administration of magnesium sulfate in concentrations sufficient to prevent or control convulsions in the treatment of preeclampsia and eclampsia resulted in prolongation of labor.[11] Serum magnesium concentrations of 6 to 8 mEq per liter result in reductions of frequency, amplitude and duration of contraction and a decrease in tonus of baseline resting pressure that combine to cause a reduction in average intra-amniotic pressure.[12]

The method of therapy consists of preparing 20 g of magnesium sulfate ($MgSO_4 \cdot 7 H_2O$) in 1000 ml 5 per cent dextrose in distilled water, and administering this medication as a continuous intravenous drip infusion. The prepared solution is given at a rate of:

7 ml (0.14 g) per minute for 60 minutes—total 8.4 g;

4 ml (0.08 g) per minute for 60 minutes—total 4.8 g;

2 ml (0.04 g) per minute, 2.4 g per hour, as maintenance dosage for the duration of therapy.

The infusion is maintained for several hours after cessation of uterine contractions. The patient's respiratory rate, blood pressure, pulse rate, urinary output and deep tendon reflexes are monitored. Prior to discontinuing intravenous therapy, the majority of the patients are given a beta-mimetic agent orally every 4 to 6 hours. Reduced activity along with bed rest are integral parts of continued management. If contractions recur, magnesium sulfate infusion therapy may be reinstituted.

Magnesium toxicity is judged clinically by the deep tendon reflexes that may be completely suppressed at serum concentrations approximating 10 mEq per liter.[13] In general, toxicity is avoided if the patient's urinary output is greater than 30 ml per hour. However, a calcium salt should be available to reverse immediately any toxicity seen in either mother or infant. Since magnesium crosses the placenta by simple diffusion, serum levels in the fetus are in the same range as those of the mother.[14] Continuous infusion for more than 72 hours has produced no serious side effects for either mother or fetus even when attempts to prevent preterm labor have been unsuccessful.

Initiation of therapy is based upon the clinical status of the patient. Specific attention is given to the status of the cervix and the presence of regular uterine contractions noted by both the patient and the examiner. Documentation by external electronic monitoring of uterine contractility is recommended. The primary goal of therapy is to prevent delivery until the fetus has reached greater maturity as evidenced by a postmenstrual age beyond 37 weeks, amniotic fluid indices of maturity[5] and a birth weight of more than 2500 g. A secondary goal, in selected cases, is to delay delivery for sufficient time to permit complete evaluation of fetal status or to allow maximal response to corticosteroids administered in an effort to accelerate fetal pulmonary maturity.[15]

Comment

There is no replacement for good prenatal care and early identification, and control of high-risk situations is the first step in the management of preterm labor. However, certain maternal and fetal complications of pregnancy are known to be associated with an increased incidence of immature births and may preclude efforts to prevent premature delivery. Inability to correct all pregnancy complications leading to preterm labor necessitates evaluation of the patient for pharmacologic management.

The tocolytic efficacy of magnesium sulfate is demonstrated in a review of 108 patients, including 10 women with multiple gestation, who received this agent in an effort to arrest uterine contractions considered clinically to constitute preterm labor. Seventy of the patients were white and 38 were black. Parity ranged from 0 to 5 with 46 of the patients being pregnant for the first time. In 76 patients, the presence of regular uterine contractions was documented by external electronic monitoring. The majority of the patients (75 per cent) also received isoxsuprine hydrochloride administered orally. Fifty-six patients received betamethasone as a potential method of facilitating fetal pulmonary maturation.[15]

For the purpose of review, patients were divided into four groups based on outcome of pregnancy (Table 2). Group 1 was composed of patients with intact amniochorionic membranes who had preterm labor and birth despite therapy or who were allowed to deliver because it was believed that maximal therapeutic benefit had been achieved. Premature birth was defined as delivery of an infant weighing from 500 to 2499 g and having a gestational age of less than 37 weeks. Group 2 contained 14 patients who had experienced premature rupture of the membranes prior to admission, 2 for more than 24 hours, and had delivered prematurely. This group of patients reflects the continuing philosophy of the University of Virginia Department of Obstetrics that in the absence of fetal maturity and overt signs of maternal or fetal sepsis, premature rupture of the membranes does not mandate prompt delivery. None of the patients with ruptured membranes received prophylactic antibiotics. Of the patients with amniochorionic membranes intact (Group 1), 59 per cent did not deliver for more than 48 hours after admission, while 57 per cent of the patients who had experienced spontaneous rupture of the membranes (Group 2) delivered more than 48 hours following admission. Fourteen of the 15 patients in Group 1 and 4 of the 6 in Group 2 delivering within 48 hours of admission failed to respond to magnesium sulfate infusion.

Group 3 contained the 24 patients in whom intercurrent complications necessitated termination of therapy and subsequent delivery of infants weighing less than 2499 g, earlier than the 37th week of gestation. Fifty-four per cent of these patients were not delivered for at least 48 hours after admission. Obstetric indications necessitated abdominal delivery in

TABLE 2. COMPARISON OF PREGNANCY OUTCOME BASED ON STATUS OF CERVIX
AND TIME FROM ADMISSION TO DELIVERY

No. Patients and Cervical Dilatation on Admission	Time: Admission to Delivery						
	≤24 hr	24–48 hr	48–72 hr	≥72 hr	≥1 wk	≥2 wk	≥3 wk
GROUP I — PREMATURE BIRTH (Membranes intact)							
Gravidas at risk	9	6	6	9	3		4
Cervical dilatation							
≤1 cm	1	1	2	3	1		3
1–2 cm		1	1	6	1		
2–3 cm	2	2	1		1		1
3–4 cm	4		1				
>4 cm		2					
Not examined	2		1				
GROUP II — PREMATURE BIRTH (Membranes ruptured)							
Gravidas at risk	4	2	4	3	1		
Cervical dilatation							
≤1 cm		1	2	3			
1–2 cm	2	1	1		1		
2–3 cm	1		1				
3–4 cm	1						
GROUP III — PREMATURE BIRTH (Treatment terminated)							
Gravidas at risk	9	2	7	3		1	2
Cervical dilatation							
≤1 cm	4	1	4			1	
1–2 cm			1				
2–3 cm	2	1		1			1
3–4 cm	2						
>4 cm			1				
Not examined	1		1	2			1
GROUP IV — BIRTH AT TERM							
Gravidas at risk	3	2	2	1	4	3	18
Cervical dilatation							
≤1 cm		1	1	1	2	2	11
1–2 cm	1		1		1		5
2–3 cm		1					
3–4 cm	1				1		
>4 cm							
Not examined	1					1	2

15 patients, including three patients with placenta previa in whom cervical dilatation was not determined on admission. The other 9 patients had treatment terminated and labor augmented by intravenous oxytocin infusion because of elevated maternal temperature (4 patients), evidence of fetal distress (2 patients), abruptio placenta (2 patients) and loss of fetal heart tones (1 patient).

Group 4 was composed of patients who subsequently delivered infants weighing more than 2500 g. All 33 patients were thought to have pregnancy of 36 weeks or less and to be in danger of delivering a premature infant at the time of admission and initiation of therapy. Twenty-five of these 33 patients (75.7 per cent) delivered more than 1 week after initiation of therapy and 18 (54.5 per cent) more than 3

weeks after. The greatest degree of success in all groups was seen when cervical dilatation was less than 2 cm. There was no difference in outcome related to percentage effacement of the cervix at any diameter of dilatation. In contrast with the experience of other investigators in the use of magnesium sulfate for the prevention of preterm labor,[16] no difference was noted in response between primiparous and multiparous patients. Febrile morbidity occurred in 13 mothers (12 per cent), of whom 5 were delivered abdominally. One patient in Group 2, admitted with ruptured membranes and delivering a premature infant, developed postpartum endometritis.

Successful treatment, if defined as delay of delivery for greater than 48 hours after admission, was accomplished in 71 (65.8 per cent) of the 108 patients treated with magnesium sulfate. However, because of the difficulty in distinguishing between actual preterm labor and the Braxton-Hicks sign, the effectiveness of tocolytic agents is more accurately measured by comparing the number of patients who delivered within 48 hours after admission. Of the 37 patients (34.2 per cent) who delivered within 48 hours of admission, parturition occurred in 23 patients in the presence of continued magnesium sulfate infusion, a specific drug failure rate of 21.2 per cent. Intravenous administration of ethanol is another protocol that has been reported to arrest preterm labor, but it did not postpone delivery beyond 48 hours in 48.5 per cent[17] and beyond 24 hours in 27.5 per cent[18] of the women treated. Others have found alcohol of even more limited value and its fetal effects discouraging.[19]

The use of beta-adrenergic agents in attempts to stop preterm labor has also produced varying success. Reported results using intravenous isoxsuprine hydrochloride indicate that between 25[20] and 38.4 per cent[21] of the patients still delivered within 48 hours. Other adrenergic agents used, with which at least 1 in 5 patients delivered within 48 hours, include mesuprine hydrochloride, a derivative of isoxsuprine, 47.0 per cent,[22] and terbutaline, an agent that exerts preferential effect on β_2 receptors, 20 per cent[23] to 22 per cent.[24] Ritodrine, another beta-mimetic agent with a formula quite similar to isoxsuprine, appeared to be among the more effective of this group of agents, with 23.4 per cent of patients delivering within 48 hours[25] and 13 per cent within 24 hours.[26] Compared to the other beta-adrenergic agents, the cardiovascular effects of ritodrine, including maternal and fetal tachycardia, are less severe.[27] The prostaglandin synthetase inhibitor indomethacin appears to be among the most effective of tocolytic drugs, with only 12.0 per cent of the patients treated with it delivering in 48 hours.[28] Although preliminary data on this agent look promising, use of the drug for prolonged periods demands further evaluation of its potential severe adverse effects on the fetus.

While the 34.2 per cent of patients who received magnesium sulfate and delivered within 48 hours is comparable to the failure rates of many of the other agents, the potential adverse maternal and fetal effects are significantly less.[14, 29, 30] No maternal or fetal toxicity resulted from magnesium sulfate therapy and

there were no maternal deaths. Safety of magnesium sulfate infusion is verified by its use in patients with pregnancy-induced hypertension, in whom the drug has been given continuously for as long as 144 hours.[31] In contrast to most other agents,[32] magnesium sulfate may have the additional potential of increasing uterine blood flow.[12]

Success of management must be judged also by perinatal outcome. Infant mortality and morbidity among our patients are tabulated in Table 3. The death of 11 of the 118 infants delivered yielded an uncorrected mortality of 9.3 per cent. The 3 infant deaths in Group 1 occurring between 24 and 48 hours of admission were directly related to treatment failure. All 3 infants weighed 1200 g or less. The other 3 deaths in this group were infants weighing less than 1100 g. The mothers of 2 of these infants had received a full course of corticosteroids. The third delivered after removal of a cervical cerclage following 3 magnesium sulfate infusions performed over several weeks. No perinatal deaths occurred in Group 2 patients admitted with premature rupture of the membranes. Of the 5 perinatal deaths in Group 3, 2 were associated with severe congenital abnormalities, 2 with abruptio placenta, and 1, in an infant delivered within 24 hours of admission because of maternal fever, with severe respiratory distress and sepsis.

Morbidity due to respiratory or septic factors occurred in 23.3 per cent of the surviving infants and reflects in part the low mean birth weights of the population delivered prematurely. However, only 3 of 44 surviving infants whose mothers received corticosteroids at least 48 hours prior to delivery developed moderate or severe respiratory distress. Only 1 surviving infant, delivered of a treated patient with intact membranes within 48 hours of admission (Group 1), required specific treatment for sepsis. All 35 infants in Group 4, including one product of a multiple gestation that weighed 2270 g, did well.

The possibility of reducing the incidence of severe respiratory distress by administration of corticosteroids to the mother has directly contributed to the large percentage of patients treated with magnesium sulfate in our hospital. As with the use of alcohol, beta-adrenergic agents and prostaglandin synthetase inhibitors in the management of preterm labor, the potential long-term effects of corticosteroid administration are not evident. However, the alternatives of severe respiratory distress and

TABLE 3. Comparison of Perinatal Mortality, Respiratory and Febrile Morbidity and Mean Birth Weights in Relation to Pregnancy Outcome and Time from Admission to Delivery

No. Infants, Perinatal Outcome and Mean Birth Weights	Time: Admission to Delivery						
	≤24 hr	24–48 hr	48–72 hr	≥72 hr	≥1 wk	≥2 wk	≥3 wk
GROUP I — PREMATURE BIRTH (Membranes intact)							
Infants at risk	10	6	6	11	5		5
Perinatal deaths		3	1	2			
Respiratory distress							
Mild*	2			3	1		
Moderate to severe†	1	1			1		
Sepsis							
Birth weight (Mean g ± SD)	1790 ± 370	1212 ± 416	1483 ± 526	1433 ± 476	1344 ± 364		2158 ± 171
GROUP II — PREMATURE BIRTH (Membranes ruptured)							
Infants at risk	4	2	4	4	2		
Perinatal deaths							
Respiratory distress							
Mild*	1	1	1	1			
Moderate to severe†	1			1			
Sepsis							
Birth weight (Mean g ± SD)	1877 ± 448	1500– 2235	1718 ± 341	1305 ±4110	1780 1080		
GROUP III — PREMATURE BIRTH (Treatment terminated)							
Infants at risk	9	2	7	3		1	2
Perinatal deaths	1		2	2			
Respiratory distress							
Mild*	3	1	2				
Moderate to severe†	2		1				
Sepsis							
Birth weight (Mean g ± SD)	1638 ± 473	1730– 1560	1381 ± 559	1783 ± 444		2350	2040– 1405
GROUP IV — BIRTH AT TERM							
Infants at risk	3	2	2	1	5	3	19
Perinatal deaths							
Respiratory distress							
Mild*							
Moderate to severe†							
Sepsis							
Birth weight (Mean g ± SD)	2980 ± 230	2570– 3020	2860– 2870	2650	2988 ± 706	3486 ± 809	3265 ± 416

*Received O_2 only.
†Required assisted ventilation.

hyaline membrane disease are considered to support the use of steroids in selected patients. Justification of treatment of Group 2 patients is evidenced by the absence of antepartum and intrapartum maternal or neonatal septic morbidity in patients delivered more than 48 hours after admission for premature rupture of the membranes. A conservative philosophy regarding selective management in an effort to prolong fetal intrauterine maturation also is the basis for attempts at uterine suppression in patients with documented placenta previa.[33]

Summary

A major limitation in the management of preterm labor is the difficulty in deciding which patients are in actual preterm labor at a time when a treatment protocol will be most effective. No matter which agent is chosen for therapy, success is variable and the clinician still has the difficult decision of whether labor can and should be arrested. Delaying therapy until cervical dilatation and effacement are present may jeopardize treatment, especially when the cervix becomes dilated more than 3 to 4 cm. Difficulty in evaluating the difference between actual premature labor and Braxton-Hicks contractions may at times be unresolved despite the best of clinical judgment and laboratory facilities. Success in some instances may be on the basis of a clear instance of missed diagnosis. However, if the therapy is safe for both mother and infant, the tendency should be to treat more patients as long as the results can justify therapy and the outcome is the desirable one: delivery of an infant that survives without permanent compromise.

Our experience indicates that magnesium sulfate administered by continuous intravenous infusion is a safe and satisfactory agent for arresting preterm labor. Its use is justified also for delaying delivery to allow further evaluation and maturation of the fetus, and in selected patients, enhancement of fetal lung maturity by specific therapy. As in all aspects of obstetrics, the eventual pregnancy outcome of the patients managed for preterm labor depends upon sound clinical judgment and individualization of care.

REFERENCES

1. Statistical Annual Report of the Virginia State Department of Health, Richmond, 1977, Commonwealth of Virginia.
2. Vital Statistics of the United States, Mortality, Washington, D.C., 1976, United States Government Printing Office, vol. II, Part A.
3. Theobald, G. W.: Nervous control of uterine activity. Clin. Obstet. Gynecol. 11:15, 1968.
4. Danforth, D. N., Veis, A., Breen, M., Weinstein, H. G., Buckingham, J.C. and Manalo, P.: The effect of pregnancy and labor on the human cervix: changes in collagen, glycoproteins, and glycosaminoglycans. Am. J. Obstet. Gynecol. 120:641, 1974.
5. Harbert, G. M.: Evaluation of fetal maturity. Clin. Obstet. Gynecol. 16:171, 1973.
6. Hubbard, J. I.: Microphysiology of vertebrate neuromuscular transmission. Physiol. Rev. 53:674, 1973.
7. Carsten, M. E.: Hormonal regulation of myometrial calcium transport. Gynecol. Invest. 5:269, 1974.
8. Ebashi, S. and Endo, M.: Calcium ion and muscle contraction. Prog. Biophys. Molec. Biol. 18:123, 1968.
9. Marshall, J. M.: Effects of catecholamines on the smooth muscle of the female reproductive tract. Ann. Rev. Pharmacol. 13:19, 1973.
10. Bueno-Montano, M.: Species variation in contractile response of excised mammalian uterine tissues. Am. J. Obstet. Gynecol. 94:1062, 1966.
11. Hall, D. G., McGaughey, H. S., Corey, E. L. and Thornton, W. N.: The effects of magnesium therapy on the duration of labor. Am. J. Obstet. Gynecol. 78:27, 1959.
12. Harbert, G. M., Cornell, G. W. and Thornton, W.

13. Goodman, L. S. and Gilman, A.: The Pharmacological Basis of Therapeutics, 5th ed. New York, Macmillan, 1975, p. 787.
14. Stone, S. R. and Pritchard, J. A.: Effect of maternally administered magnesium sulfate on the neonate. Obstet. Gynecol. 35:574, 1970.
15. Liggins, G. C. and Howie, R. N.: A controlled trial of antepartum glucocorticoid treatment for prevention of the respiratory distress syndrome in premature infants. Pediatrics 50:515, 1972.
16. Steer, C. M. and Petrie, R. H.: A comparison of magnesium sulfate and alcohol for the prevention of premature labor. Am. J. Obstet. Gynecol. 129:1, 1977.
17. Fuchs, F., Fuchs, A. R., Poblete, V. F. and Risk, A.: Effect of alcohol on threatened premature labor. Am. J. Obstet. Gynecol. 99:627, 1967.
18. Fuchs, F.: Prevention of prematurity. Am. J. Obstet. Gynecol. 126:809, 1976.
19. Graff, G.: Failure to prevent premature labor with ethanol. Am. J. Obstet. Gynecol. 110:378, 1971.
20. Bishop, E. H. and Woutersz, T. B.: Arrest of premature labor. J.A.M.A. 178:812, 1961.
21. Hendricks, C. H., Cibils, L. A., Pose, S. V. and Eskes, T. K. A. B.: The pharmacologic control of excessive uterine activity with isoxsuprine. Am. J. Obstet. Gynecol. 82:1064, 1961.
22. Barden, T. P.: Inhibition of premature labor by mesuprine hydrochloride. Obstet. Gynecol. 37:98, 1971.
23. Ingemarsson, I.: Effect of terbutaline on premature labor: a double-blind placebo-controlled study. Am. J. Obstet. Gynecol. 125:520, 1976.
24. Wallace, R. L., Caldwell, D. L., Ansbacher, R. and Otterson, W. N.: Inhibition of premature labor by terbutaline. Obstet. Gynecol. 51:387, 1978.
25. Wesselius-de Casparis, A., Thiery, M., Yo Le Sian, A. et al.: Results of double-blind, multicentre study with ritodrine in premature labour. Br. Med. J. 3:144, 1971.
26. Renaud, R., Irrmann, M., Gandar, R. and Flynn, M. J.: The use of ritodrine in the treatment of premature labour. J. Obstet. Gynecol. Br. Commonwealth 81:182, 1974.
27. Bieniarz, J., Motew, M. and Scommegna, A.: Uterine and cardiovascular effects of ritodrine in premature labor. Obstet. Gynecol. 40:65, 1971.
28. Zuckerman, H., Reiss, U. and Rubinstein, I.: Inhibition of human labor by indomethacin. Obstet. Gynecol. 44:787, 1974.
29. Babaknia, A. and Niebyl, J. R.: The effect of magnesium sulfate on fetal heart rate baseline variability. Obstet. Gynecol. 51:2s, 1978.
30. Hutchinson, H. T., Nichols, M. M., Kuhn, C. R. and Vasicka, A.: Effects of magnesium sulfate on uterine contractility, intrauterine fetus, and infant. Am. J. Obstet. Gynecol. 88:747, 1964.
31. Andersen, W. A. and Harbert, G. M.: Conservative management of preeclamptic and eclamptic patients: a re-evaluation. Am. J. Obstet. Gynecol. 129:260, 1977.
32. Johnson, W. L., Harbert, G. M. and Martin, C. B.: Pharmacologic control of uterine contractility. Am. J. Obstet. Gynecol. 123:364, 1975.
33. Williams, T. J.: The expectant management of placenta previa. Am. J. Obstet. Gynecol. 55:1, 1948.

N.: Effect of toxemia therapy on uterine dynamics. Am. J. Obstet. Gynecol. 105:94, 1969.

Management of Preterm Labor

Joseph Bieniarz, M.D.

Laurence Burd, M.D.

Antonio Scommegna, M.D.

Michael Reese Hospital and the Pritzker School of Medicine, University of Chicago

Importance of the Problem

Prematurity is the foremost problem in obstetrics and perinatology, responsible for almost 80 per cent of perinatal mortality, 10 times the rate expected from the average per cent incidence of preterm labor. Of greater importance are survivors of preterm labor who are left with permanent neurologic or behavioral abnormalities. Even with perfect application of all current knowledge, 10 to 25 per cent of preterm babies are left with major handicaps requiring lifelong institutional care. They impose a major emotional stress and economic burden upon the family and society.

A delay in the onset of labor even for a few days could spell the difference between life and death and could improve the quality of the human life at the time of birth. Prolongation of intrauterine life by 1 week only, between the 26th and 30th week of pregnancy, could improve the chances of the infant's survival by 15 per cent (Fig. 1) and give the baby better prospects of developing its full genetic capacity in life. However, this aim is not easy to attain because maintenance of pregnancy and the onset of labor are complex biologic phenomena, controlled by multiple regulatory mechanisms that are only partly known and are poorly understood. Differences in regulatory mechanisms between species preclude any universal explanation and make virtually impossible any extrapolation of results obtained in experimental animals to other species, including humans.

Furthermore, the compounds used to treat preterm labor, to reduce uterine contractility or accelerate maturation of fetal lungs may not be as innocuous as initially thought; the harm caused may outweigh the advantages expected. Finally, complications that predispose to prematurity may compromise fetal growth and development so that further prolongation of intrauterine life might be more dangerous than premature delivery and care in a modern intensive care nursery (ICN). At each stage of pregnancy the dangers of intrauterine life must be assessed and weighed against the dangers for the newborn in the ICN.

An unresolved problem of such magnitude has inspired organization of special symposia[1-5] and publication of many articles on the subject.[1-55] It would be redundant to write another of these articles. Our aim is to review critically the main controversies concerning this complex problem in order to recognize the limits of our capabilities and to outline the most practical approach to a safe and effective treatment.

Control of Uterine Contractility

A concise review of regulatory mechanisms controlling uterine contractility (Fig. 2) may facilitate the search for the most effective pharmacologic control of prematurity.[4, 21] These mechanisms are grouped into: (1) hypothalamohypophyseal neurosecretory factors, (2) hormonal factors of fetoplacental origin and (3) endogenous factors of tissue origin, affecting directly the myometrial cell. Maintenance of pregnancy or prevention of the onset of labor depends ultimately on the balance of factors inhibiting and activating uterine contractility.[4, symp. 1]

The central nervous system control is probably exerted through release of oxytocin, an octapeptide similar to antidiuretic hormone (ADH). Ethanol, a known inhibitor of ADH release, has been reported by Fuchs et al.[20-22] to block oxytocin release as well, thus curbing uterine contractility. Fluid volume expansion has also been shown to block ADH release through the Henry-Gauer reflex from the distended left auricle.[26] A similar inhibition of oxytocin release by rapid fluid infusion is possible.[4] Oxytocin of fetal origin may also be involved in onset of labor.[8]

Hormonal factors of fetoplacental origin seem to play a major role in regulatory mechanisms controlling uterine contractility. Estrogens have principally metabolic effects, increasing synthesis of RNA, proteins and enzymes; this results in myometrial hypertrophy. Estrogens affect contractile action through the actomyosin-ATP-ase system. Inversely, progesterone decreases the sensitivity

80

PERINATAL AND NEONATAL MORTALITY RATE
BY BIRTH WEIGHT

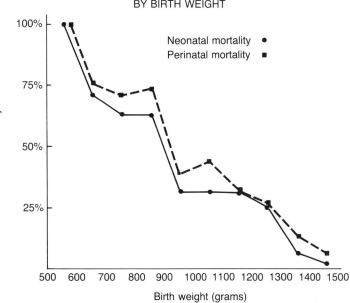

Figure 1. The crucial period for reduction of mortality from 75 to 25 per cent is the prolongation of pregnancy between 26th and 30th week of pregnancy. (Perinatal and neonatal mortality rates plotted by 100 g birth weight increments.) (From Bowes, W. A.: Intensive perinatal management of very low birth weight infants (501–1500 gm). *In* Pre-term Labor, Proc. 5th Study Group, Royal College of Obstetrics & Gynecology, London, 1978, p. 334.)

of the myometrial cell by hyperpolarization and conduction blocking.[12]

However, progesterone has been unsuccessful in inhibiting contractility once preterm labor has already started. To explain the striking ineffectiveness of progesterone in the treatment of preterm labor in women, Csapo[12, 13] introduced the concept of a local myometrial block by progesterone at the placental site. There, such high progesterone concentration gradient exists that it cannot be surpassed by systemic administration of this steroid. Labor starts when placental progesterone block is withdrawn. Recently, Johnson et al.[28] reported apparent success using 17α-hydroxyprogesterone caproate in the prevention of preterm labor in patients with repeated instances of preterm labor.

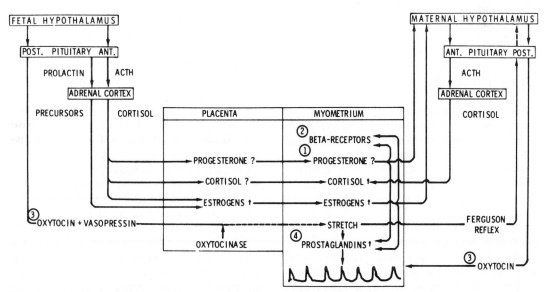

Figure 2. Schematic illustration of the factors assumed to play a role in the mechanism of human labor. The numbers refer to factors which may be influenced by pharmacological agents to arrest threatened premature labor. (From Fuchs, F.: Prevention of prematurity. Am. J. Obstet. Gynecol. 126:809, 1976.)

The ratio of estrogen to progesterone also appears to influence uterine contractility.[50] Increased levels of plasma estradiol have been found in patients who develop spontaneous preterm labor.

There is increasing evidence that the fetus itself may contribute to the timing of delivery by increasing the activity of its pituitary-adrenal axis, as shown by successful labor inductions in sheep with ACTH or cortisol infusion to the fetus.[32, 49] Normally, fetal corticosteroids increase prior to labor and may trigger labor onset in this species. Inversely, anencephalic fetuses with underdeveloped pituitary and adrenal glands tend to be postmature. While labor starts spontaneously in the woman with a dead fetus, the precise tuning of the term labor is usually lost.

The ultimate target of all these regulatory mechanisms is the myometrial cell. These cells are activated through changes in extracellular and intracellular ionic equilibrium affecting cell membrane permeability with discharge of an action potential.[12] Propagation of the action potential results in a uterine contraction. Adrenergic amines influence these cellular mechanisms, activating uterine contractility through alpha-receptor stimulation and inhibiting it through beta-receptor stimulation. These events are calcium dependent and are associated with increased tissue levels of cyclic AMP. Marshall and Kroeger postulated that adrenergic mechanisms may involve an electrogenic calcium pump activated by cyclic AMP.[39] On the other hand, calcium antagonists may have an inhibitory effect on uterine contractility.[symp. 4, 5b]

Estimation of Fetal Gestational Age

The term premature has been replaced by preterm because babies are described in terms of either gestational age or birthweight and not maturity.[symp. 5a] Such definition presupposes certainty of the duration of pregnancy. This is difficult to assess because of irregularity of the menstrual cycle and lack of knowledge of the conception date. Hence, the importance of clinical information such as the date of quickening and the objective documentation by the physician of the date when the fetal heart tones were first heard by a nonelectronic fetoscope (about 20 weeks). This is the simplest, most reliable, safest, least expensive and most noninvasive way to determine gestational age.

Other corroborative evidence of gestational age includes either of the following: (1) the date when the pregnancy test becomes positive (7 weeks of pregnancy if done by a standard immunologic method, 5 weeks if done by a radioreceptor assay); (2) serial measurement of the fetal biparietal diameter between 20 and 30 weeks of gestation; (3) at a later stage of pregnancy fetal thoracic diameters and real-time scan of a single transverse section of the fetal abdomen's circumference.[symp. 5h] Also, a lecithin/sphingomyelin (L/S) ratio higher than 2.0 and the presence of phosphatidylglycerol suggest maturation of fetal lungs and good prognosis for respiratory distress syndrome (RDS).[symp. 5j]

Early Diagnosis and Treatment of Preterm Labor

Evidence obtained by others[22, 25] and confirmed by us suggests that the efficiency of pharmacologic control of uterine contractility decreases rapidly with the progress of labor. If treatment starts with less than 1 cm cervical dilatation, 80 per cent of preterm labors are stopped. Results become rapidly worse with further cervical dilatation. Early recognition of preterm labor is essentially the patient's own diagnosis and depends on her antenatal education. After the 20th week of pregnancy each woman must be informed that true preterm labor contractions are painful and regular, gradually increasing in intensity and frequency (1 to 3 contractions per 10 minutes). They start in the back and spread around the belly, resulting in expulsion of a mucus plug mixed with blood from the vagina. If untreated, they lead invariably to delivery. The informed patient will recognize them, will arrive at the hospital and will be treated early. Conversely, false labor contractions are irregular, localized anteriorly and wane with bed rest and reassurance, without treatment.

The obstetrician recognizes true labor by repeated vaginal examinations, finding progress of labor, effacement and dilatation of the cervix and descent of the presenting part. For research purposes, it is essential to exclude from treatment false labors that would stop without treatment, biasing the results. This is evidently not easy, even for experienced investigators: in three recent clinical trials 40 per cent of patients, 25 of 65, had not yet been delivered although the diagnosis of true labor had been made and placebo treatment initiated a week earlier.[symp. 5a] In practice it is more rewarding to start treatment early than to miss the right time and risk failure in a futile effort to exclude false labors from treatment.[7, symp. 1]

Routine work-up of a premature labor starts with history and physical examination, special attention being paid to the following points: (1) estimation of gestational age and fetal weight; (2) monitoring of uterine tone, tenderness and irritability; (3) estimation of fetal heart rate by auscultation; and (4) speculum examination for leakage of amniotic fluid or blood. Progress of labor is assessed by cervical effacement, dilatation and descent of presentation. However, vaginal examinations predispose to prostaglandin release and should be limited to a minimum, as should intercourse in women predisposed to preterm labor.[24, 51]

Routine laboratory data should include (1) hematocrit, blood glucose, electrolytes; (2) fibrinogen and coagulation profile if occult abruptio placentae is suspected; (3) complete urinalysis with culture and sensitivity; (4) electronic monitoring of contractions and fetal heart rate; (5) ultrasound if needed for determination of gestational age, diagnosis of multiple pregnancy, location of placenta; and (6) amniocentesis for L/S ratio as well as for identification of amniotic infection from presence of white blood cells, bacteria in fluid sediment and culture.

Excluded from treatment are women with pregnancy complications that may endanger the mother or the fetus more than prematurity, such as severe forms of the following complications: preeclampsia and eclampsia, chronic hypertension, heart disease, renal diseases, abruptio placentae, life-threatening hemorrhage from placenta previa, ruptured membranes and amnionitis. Excluded also are conditions in which prolongation of pregnancy is pointless: advanced active labor with cervix 80 per cent effaced and dilated more than 4 cm; congenital anomalies incompatible with life and fetal death.

Bed rest and an intravenous infusion of 500 cc of lactated Ringer's solution in 60 minutes are the first steps to be taken in treating preterm labor. If contractions do not space out and stop, intravenous infusion of the FDA-approved beta-adrenergic agent ritodrine is started, monitored by an external cardiotocograph if possible. Blood pressure and pulse rate are checked every 15 minutes. Two ampules of Yutopar containing 100 mg of ritodrine are dissolved in 250 cc of fluid, and

infused with a controlled device such as an IVAC pump with a minidropper through a standard intravenous infusion (one half normal saline, one half 5 per cent dextrose 100 cc per 8 hr) starting from 100 μg (16 drops per minute). The rate of infusion is increased by 50 μg (7 drops per minute) every 10 minutes until contractions stop, unacceptable side effects develop or the maximum dose of 350 μg per minute (52 drops) is reached. The infusion is maintained at the lowest rate that suppresses uterine contractions. Once the infusion has reached a stable, effective level, it will be maintained for a minimum of 12 hours.

Vital signs and uterine contractility are checked every 30 minutes for the next 4 hours and then every hour until 1 hour after discontinuing intravenous treatment. Fluid is ordered to avoid overhydration if prolonged intravenous treatment is necessary; if arrhythmias or chest pain develop, an EKG and electrolyte studies are requested and any abnormalities such as hypopotassemia are corrected.

One half hour before discontinuation of intravenous therapy, ritodrine oral therapy is instituted and continued with 1 tablet (10 mg) every 2 hours for at least 1 day, and 2 tablets every 4 hours the next day, during which time the patient remains in the hospital. At discharge the dose is reduced to 1 tablet or 2 tablets every 4 to 6 hours depending on uterine activity and unwanted effects until 36 weeks of gestation are attained.

Repeat courses of intravenous therapy will be necessary if there is a recurrence of preterm labor.

A similar beta-adrenergic agent, fenoterol (Partusisten), is at present undergoing clinical evaluation for FDA approval. Preliminary observations suggest an action similar to ritodrine, with less subjective cardiac symptoms, palpitation or chest pain. The solution is prepared and administrated as is ritodrine, but the concentration used is 100 times lower (1 mg per 250 cc fluid).

The high cost of ritodrine treatment compared with compounds not approved by the FDA has resulted in the use of less expensive beta-mimetics available on the market for nonobstetric indications. Terbutaline has been used with good efficiency, although a high incidence of pulmonary edema has been reported, 5 per cent of 160 patients.[29a] The most striking sign accompanying subjective symptoms was maternal tachycardia to 160 to 180 beats per min. Discontinuation of terbutaline infusion, oxygen breathing and diuretics was followed by resolution of the problem within 4 to 6 hours.

Another beta-mimetic agonist, which is available on the market and has been used extensively in pioneering studies,[25, 35] is isoxsuprine (Vasodilan). Two ampules of this drug (4 cc = 20 mg) dissolved in 200 cc of 5 per cent dextrose connected to the intravenous infusion should secure a constant rate of 0.25 mg per minute with a pump. The infusion rate is increased every 20 minutes to 0.5 per minute, 0.75 per minute, rarely up to 1 mg per minute, until the uterus relaxes completely. Then the infusion rate is lowered to 0.1 to 0.3 mg per minute for 24 hours. Left lateral position and good hydration prevent supine hypotension. If marked tachycardia or hypotension develop, the infusion rate must be decreased or discontinued. Isoxsuprine may be also given by intramuscular 10 mg injections q 4 to 6 hours and maintained by oral administration, 1 to 2 tablets (10 to 20 mg) every 4 to 6 hours.

Our results confirm the observation that maternal pulse rate is a simple clinical indicator of the beta-mimetic serum level (Fig. 3). The pulse can be easily used to check the adequacy of treatment; heart rate between 90 and 140 beats per minute indicates this. Whenever the maternal pulse decreases below 90 beats per minute preterm labor may recur and the rate of infusion should be increased. Inversely, maternal tachycardia (over 140 beats per minute) suggests developing circulatory insufficiency. The beta-mimetic infusion rate should be lowered to avoid the danger of pulmonary edema.

Intravenous alcohol administration enjoyed great popularity in treating preterm labor with the aim of inhibiting oxytocin release.[20-22] While it is highly unlikely that in the second half of gestation, a short exposure to ethanol can cause the fetal alcohol syndrome, the psychologic effect of using alcohol in treating women who have been told to avoid it in pregnancy is obvious.[21a] It is not an ideal agent, since it may increase the risk of RDS in the newborn when alcohol fails to arrest labor. We use alcohol rarely when beta-mimetics are contraindicated or to support their relaxing action when they fail. Combined administration of various agents acting on multiple targets is more efficient in inhibiting uterine contractility than a single compound acting on one regulatory mechanism only.[4, 5, 7]

We use a rapid venous infusion of 5 per cent ethanol solution (1000 cc = 50 g in 60 minutes) followed by the same amount infused at a slower rate over 6 hours. If contractions disappear completely, the patient is placed on bed rest and observed for 24 to 48 hours and discharged with instructions for gradual mobilization and immediate rehospitalization for repeated treatment if painful contractions reappear.

Recently, magnesium sulfate has been used to inhibit uterine contractility in preterm labor. We have no personal experience with this modality of treatment and refer to a recent publication in which results are reviewed.[42a] It seems to be successful as a preventive rather than as a therapeutic measure when used before cervical effacement and dilatation take place. Its potential value in combined multitarget approach in treatment of preterm labor requires further exploration.

In treating preterm labor it is usually not difficult to inhibit uterine contractility with gradually increasing rates of beta-mimetic

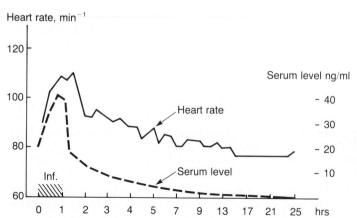

Figure 3. Close correlation between maternal heart rate and serum ritodrine level permits use of the pulse as an easy indicator of biological betanimetic activity. Mean heart rates and serum ritodrine levels in six healthy females during and following one hour infusion of 0.15 mg/min. (From Post, L. C.: Pharmacokinetics of beta-adrenergic agonists. *In*: Pre-term Labour, Proc. 5th Study Group, Royal College of Obstetrics & Gynecology, London, 1977, p. 148).

drugs. The main difficulty involves maintaining uterine relaxation, when toxic effects oblige us to reduce the rate of infusion when oral treatment starts or preterm labor recurs. The strategy of treatment has to be adjusted to these realities. The aim to carry the pregnancy to term has to be replaced by the less ambitious but still desirable aim to reach over 33 weeks of gestation, a time at which perinatal mortality and morbidity clearly are lower. Finally, a short-term prolongation of pregnancy for 24 to 48 hours is also desirable for the purpose of transferring the patient with a viable fetus at less than 26 weeks of gestation to a tertiary center or to allow further maturation of fetal lungs after premature rupture of membranes.

Management of Preterm Labor in Multiple Pregnancy[7]

The single most important cause of high perinatal morbidity and mortality in multifetal pregnancy is prematurity. With an increase in the number of fetuses in a single gestation, the incidence and degree of prematurity increases as well. The perinatal mortality rates of single, twin, triplet and quadruplet gestations have been reported to be 39, 152, 309 and 509 per 1000, respectively.[19] It is the production of many small infants of reduced viability that is mainly responsible for the high death rate in multiple pregnancy.

The progressively shorter duration of gestation and earlier onset of labor with multiple fetuses has been attributed to earlier uterine distension[40] and increase in local prostaglandin formation. We have used ritodrine in a small series of multifetal pregnancies with the goal of increasing uterine tolerance to distension. Different criteria of care must be used to treat preterm labor in multifetal pregnancy as compared with those used in pregnancy with one fetus.[7]

It is much more difficult to distinguish between true and false labor in multifetal than in singleton pregnancy: cervical dilatation, effacement and descent of the presenting part may be observed long before the onset of labor, due to marked uterine distension. This predisposes to an almost asymptomatic progress into an irreversible active phase of labor. Since the onset of active labor is so insidious, we believe that to avoid this danger the patient

should be treated when any type of regular contractions appear.

Also, the criteria of failed treatment accepted for singleton preterm labor (i.e., cervical dilatation over 4 cm and 80 per cent effacement) are not valid in multiple pregnancy. We have been able to delay delivery for 3 weeks with combined ritodrine and ethanol treatment in a triplet pregnancy with cervical dilatation of 6 to 7 cm and 60 to 80 per cent effacement, until membranes ruptured at 35 weeks.

Once controlled, preterm labor tends to recur frequently in multiple pregnancies. Immediate, repeated intravenous ritodrine administration is the most efficient form of treatment. To ensure prompt treatment, prolonged hospitalization may be required. The cost for several weeks of hospitalization of the mother is still less than the cost of treating three to four premature infants in an ICN. Although it is relatively easy to inhibit uterine contractility in preterm labor, the tendency to recurrences requires progressively increasing doses of medication, while maternal pulse rate is monitored (see Fig. 3).

Conduct of Uncontrollable Preterm Labor

If contractions continue in spite of treatment and labor progresses, use of further medication is pointless and should be discontinued. A premature infant is more susceptible to the dangers of hypoxia, analgesia, trauma, cooling and infection than a term one. Oxygen administration, epidural or pudendal conduction anesthesia, large episiotomy and an outlet primi-forceps should be used routinely. The smaller the fetus, the larger should be the episiotomy. All maneuvers during preterm labor should be carried out very gently, without haste. Unattended, sudden delivery in bed is a medical error. By the time the infant is 1 to 2 minutes of age, prompt and efficient resuscitation must be initiated if spontaneous ventilation is not established.

Immediate and continuing attention to the maintenance of the newborn's body temperature is imperative. This is attained by drying the newborn with warm towels and placing it under an overhead heat source to minimize radiant heat loss. If these precautions are not taken, small premature infants can decrease their body temperature by 0.25° C per minute in the delivery room and on the way to the ICN. The premature infant's body temperature on admission is a major determinant of its mortality rate.

The major purpose of the first hour of care in the infant having a short gestation is to prevent or minimize the severity of RDS. Birth asphyxia and hypothermia predispose to acidemia, which is a crucial component of the pathophysiology of surfactant deficient RDS. Surfactant synthesis is pH dependent, and it is very important to minimize intrapartum asphyxia and acidemia and assure immediate postnatal care.

Preterm labor is a high-risk condition requiring intensive care during labor and during the first hours of life. To deliver low birth weight infants somewhere other than appropriately equipped and staffed perinatal centers is irresponsible. Antenatal transfer of the mother is preferable to postnatal transportation of the infant. The best incubator for the transport of a low birth weight baby is the womb of its mother.

With the increased emphasis on maternal (in utero) transport of high-risk infants, the number of low birth weight babies treated at the University of Colorado increased dramatically from around 30 per year to over 90 per year, as reported by Bowes.[symp. 5g] Total births at the hospital did not increase. Intensive perinatal care, both intrapartum and in the immediate neonatal period, was responsible for a significant decrease in neonatal mortality from 90 to 55 per cent for infants < 1000 g, and from 40 to 20 per cent for those with birth weights 1001 to 1500 g (see Fig. 1). The success of this program was assured also by inclusion of the most qualified obstetricians and neonatologists.

Bowes attributes his improved results partly to lowering the minimal gestational weight and age criteria (less than 26 weeks and less than 600 g) at which cesarean section would be performed in the presence of fetal distress. Such strict criteria have been accepted because of routine underestimation of the fetal weight by 250 g in the 500 to 1000 g group and by 450 g in the 1001 to 1500 g groups. Cesarean section was also used for breech presentations to avoid trauma of the aftercoming head or prolapse of the umbilical cord. However, some authors cite a high incidence of major congenital anomalies (up to 20 per cent) in infants in breech presentation and the

risks of higher maternal morbidity and mortality. They support the view that only "footlings" are to be delivered by cesarean section, while infants in frank and complete breech presentation may be delivered vaginally.[29]

The question of the minimal gestational age at which cesarean section should be performed for fetal indications still generates controversy. Steward[symp. 5q] thought that if a baby weighs more than 1000 g (27 weeks), it is advantageous to deliver it by cesarean section. Kubli[symp. 5l] considered that this depends not only on gestational age but also on the quality of a given ICN. On the basis of data collected from 72 departments in European institutions he found a median value at 33 weeks, with a rather large scatter from 29 weeks on, from which cesarean sections are being performed in Europe for fetal indications. Beard criticized the use of a cesarean section in early prematurity because of the possible complications for the mother. He suggested double-blind, randomized studies to reach an accurate, honest answer as to the best route of delivery.

The Risks of Beta-mimetic Treatment

The use of beta-adrenergic agonists as potent inhibitors of uterine contractility in premature labor[25, 33-35, symp. 1-5] has been limited by maternal hypotension and tachycardia, which might reduce placental blood flow and endanger the fetus. However, the second generation of beta-mimetic drugs such as ritodrine, fenoterol and terbutaline is largely devoid of these undesirable effects. We found that hypotension is not manifested with ritodrine, because an increase in cardiac output compensates for it. However, the markedly increased workload on the heart dictates exclusion of patients with heart disease, circulatory insufficiency and tendency to stenocardia from treatment with beta-mimetics.[6, symp. 5f]

Kubli[symp. 5m] reported 8 cases of maternal pulmonary edema in approximately 200,000 women treated in 3 years since 1974 with fenoterol, all in combination with corticosteroids. One death occurred two weeks after delivery in a patient with a subvalvular pulmonary stenosis and was not attributed to beta-mimetic treatment discontinued much earlier. However, a policy has been introduced that patients to be treated with beta-mimetics be screened by EKG and checked for a history of cardiac diseases. Promising synergistic effects have been reported of beta-mimetics with highly active spasmolytics and calcium antagonists, e.g., isoptin or nifedipine.[symp. 4, 5b] They cause coronary vasodilation, reduce myocardial oxygen requirement and reinforce the tocolytic effects of beta-mimetic drugs.

Chez,[symp. 5i] weighing the risk-to-benefit ratio, considered the following conditions as absolute contraindications to treatment with beta-mimetic drugs: (1) hyperthyroidism, a hyperbeta-adrenergic activity state that could develop into thyroid storm; (2) asthma already treated by beta agonists that may be at risk from excess beta stimulation; and (3) poorly controlled juvenile diabetes in patients who experience hyperglycemia without a compensatory hyperinsulinemia. The list of absolute contraindications to the use of beta-mimetic drugs includes also myotonia dystrophica (a rare familial disease), hypertrophic outlet cardiomyopathies and narrow-angled glaucoma.

Beta-mimetic drugs have, undoubtedly, a glucogenic effect.[3] However, the carbohydrate intolerance induced by intravenous ritodrine administration gradually diminishes after 24 hours and disappears completely by 48 hours, due to reactive hyperinsulinemia. If this reaction compensates for hyperglycemia, it is safe to use beta-mimetics in diabetes, provided that the blood sugar is monitored frequently and hyperglycemia is corrected with insulin.[symp. 5e] It seems likely that the glucogenic effect of beta-sympathomimetics and steroids is additive. In combination they may lead to the loss of diabetic control and ketoacidosis. Large amounts of insulin are necessary to reestablish control.

Acceleration of Fetal Lung Maturation

There are more than 20 experimental studies and clinical observations confirming that antenatal administration of glucocorticoids to the mother can accelerate fetal lung maturation by way of cytoplasmic and nuclear receptor systems and enzyme induction. The large type 2 cells produce a mixture of lipids and proteins, which allows the alveoli to open easily and prevents their collapse in respiration. Thus RDS, the major cause of neonatal morbidity and mortality in preterm babies,

could be considerably reduced. This effect occurs only just before the time at which surfactant synthesis would occur normally. Very immature cells are incapable of a response, while mature cells already have the capacity to synthesize surface active lecithins.

However, because of the wide occurrence of glucocorticoid receptors in fetal tissues, early enzymatic maturation of other cells and organs may be induced. Administration of pharmacologic doses of corticoids to pregnant animals has interfered with the proliferative phase of organ growth, resulting in reduced brain weight, reduced content of CNS deoxyribonucleic acid and impaired CNS function in fine motor control. Placental mitoses may be reduced, with accelerated senescence, fetal intrauterine growth retardation, increased incidence of cleft palate and higher perinatal mortality. In most of these animal studies the dosages of steroids used have been large and the treatment prolonged.

These adverse effects have not been documented in infants born to mothers who received corticoids in therapeutic doses for a variety of conditions. The short-term effects on maturation of fetal lungs, as well as the long-term effects of physiologic dosages of glucocorticoids administered during the third trimester, remain to be determined in well-designed double-blind studies. Liggins and Howie from New Zealand have the widest experience in this field.[32, symp. 5k] The infant's chances of survival were considerably improved by reducing the incidence of RDS (from 29 to 9 per cent), hyaline membrane disease, cerebral hemorrhage and possibly pneumonia. However, there are certain limitations of therapy.

Treatment must be started at least 24 hours before delivery and effectiveness of therapy is only apparent in infants delivered between 1 and 7 days after entry to the trial. Therapy should not be repeated in less than 7 days, or after 32 weeks, and treatment should not be started after 34 weeks. Because of an increased risk of fetal death, treatment is contraindicated in the presence of hypertension sufficiently severe to warrant delivery. Using various tests including psychological examinations at 4 years, Liggins and Howie found no other evidence of short-term or long-term harm to mother or baby but long-term studies of the development of the children are still in progress. Similar results have been reported by others.[2]

A fervent plea against the use of glucosteroids for maturation of fetal lungs was expressed by Gluck.[symp. 5j] The greatest danger of corticoid treatment in women is not the fact that early induction of enzymes results in a runted animal. What preoccupied him most was that this treatment gives the obstetrician license to deliver premature infants that are exposed to other serious disorders besides RDS: apnea, bradycardia, bleeding, problems of digestion and necrotizing enterocolitis, plus the possibility of infection.

Avery[1] called attention to the fact that any infant with RDS has three or four times the concentration of cortisol present in the non-stressed infant without RDS. The levels required for prenatal lung maturation are no higher than the levels the baby generates 24 hours later on its own when it has the disease. Since fetal glucocorticoid production increases normally in the last few weeks of pregnancy and concentrations rise in amniotic fluid, it is probable that a relatively high cortisol milieu is a physiologic state for the near-term fetus.[symp. 5c, d] Cortisol, even in physiologic concentrations, would appear to be a means of accelerating lung maturity and indeed would appear to be the critical timer of lung maturation in preterm onset of labor. Giving such medications is doing for the baby what it would do for itself in terms of an endogenous glucocorticoid surge if it had been allowed the privilege of remaining in utero for the full gestation.

A recent report of a Collaborative Group on Antenatal Steroid Therapy[10a] presented the results of a study to ascertain the effects of antenatal dexamethasone administration on prevention of RDS. The incidence of RDS was different between control subjects (18.0 per cent) and infants of steroid-treated mothers (12.6 per cent) $P = 0.05$). The effect was, however, mainly attributable to discernible differences among singleton female infants, whereas no treatment effect was observed in male infants. Dexamethasone does cross the placenta and has no demonstrable short-term effect, but the answer in respect to the potential long-term effects will have to wait until full evidence is obtained in follow-up studies.

Role of Prostaglandin Synthetase Inhibitors (PGSI)

A rapidly growing bulk of evidence[41] indicates that prostaglandins, 20-carbon derivatives of fatty acids generated locally in the cells, play a vital role as a final link in the multiple regulatory mechanisms mediating the onset of labor. Zuckerman et al.[55] and Wiqvist et al.[54] reported spectacular results in halting premature labor by administration of indomethacin, a known inhibitor of prostaglandin synthesis. However, similar clinical investigations have not been published since, because of the risks related to the use of PGSI during pregnancy. It was Rudolph et al.[27, symp. 5p] who supplied experimental proof in sheep that the high prostaglandin levels in fetal circulation, rising toward the end of gestation, fulfill an important role in normal fetal circulatory regulation: they maintain the ductus arteriosus open. The rapid fall in prostaglandin levels in the newborn to very low levels of adults coincides with ductus arteriosus constriction and conversion of fetal to adult circulation.

Untimely lowering of prostaglandin levels in fetal circulation by administration of PGSI to the mother may result in dramatic constrictions of the ductus arteriosus. Chronic prostaglandin synthetase inhibition probably results in pulmonary hypertension in some infants. An FDA advisory panel on the use of aspirin during pregnancy enumerated further following complications: increased bleeding time and inhibited platelet aggregation, bleeding tendency before and after delivery, increased stillbirth rate and reduced neonatal birth weight in chronic users, hyperbilirubinemia postpartum.

Although this list appears horrifying, if we exclude those ill effects that may occur in chronic users there is only one complication that is confirmed clinically—namely, premature closure of the ductus arteriosus. Wiqvist from Stockholm stressed[symp. 5r] that this complication has been reported in only a few instances, although millions of women have taken anti-inflammatory drugs during pregnancy. He administered indomethacin 250 mg q 6 hours to women at 25 to 32 weeks' gestation whose preterm labor was not responding to beta-mimetics. In 12 of 14 cases, treatment inhibited premature labor and fetal heart rate remained normal. Postnatal circulatory adaptation was normal as judged from blood gas studies, arterial blood pressure, EKG and respiratory function. Coagulation profile was normal. Only three neonates had bilirubin elevated, one requiring phototherapy.

In Israel, Lindner et al.[symp. 5n] reported 18

women in preterm labor at 28 to 36 weeks, treated with flufenamic acid 0.5 to 1 g over a period of 4 hours in divided doses, later maintained with daily doses of 5 to 10 g divided in four parts. In three women admitted with 4 cm dilatation and 80 per cent effacement the treatment failed, while 15 patients had a mean delay of 21 days between admission and delivery. There was one stillbirth due to abruptio placentae that had not been recognized in time because there was no uterine hypertension and very little abdominal pain. The obstetrician has to be alert in looking for such complications, since the clinical picture may be somewhat masked. The other newborns were in good condition, except for one who developed symptoms suggestive of pulmonary hypertension but recovered fully under oxygen treatment.

Both the Swedish and Israeli investigators admit that further experimental studies in animals are necessary. However, they think that carefully controlled clinical studies in a few centers with special resources are justified. The clinical studies should be limited to early periods of pregnancy when the dangers of ductal closure are remote.

It is clear that a multitude of questions remain unanswered in the diagnosis and management of the patient with preterm labor. There is an urgent need to further our understanding of the physiologic mechanisms surrounding the initiation of labor, myometrial contractility and fetal organ maturation. All aspects of well-designed basic and clinical research must be encouraged so that our knowledge of the factors that cause prematurity can become complete. Until then, the physician must weigh the benefits of various therapeutic programs against their risks to both mother and infant. At all times, care should be individualized in an attempt to maximize results. The underlying aim is to provide obstetric and newborn care that will avoid the major hazard of prematurity, birth asphyxia. With this in mind, the outcome for the premature infant should be greatly improved.

REFERENCES
SYMPOSIA

1. Zuspan, F. P. (coord.): Premature labor: The management and therapy. J. Reprod. Med. 9:93, 1972.
2. Reid, D. E. and Christian C. D. (eds.): Controversy in Obstetrics and Gynecology, Vol. 2. Philadelphia, W. B. Saunders Co., 1974.
   a. Barden, T. P.: The management of impending labor prior to the thirty-fifth week, p. 75.
   b. Cibils, L. A.: The management of impending labor prior to the thirty-fifth week, p. 88.
   c. Landesman, R.: The management of impending labor prior to the thirty-fifth week, p. 103.
3. Chez, R. A. (moder.): Therapeutic approaches to premature labor. Contemp. Obstet. Gynecol. 8:58, 1976.
4. Weidinger, H. (ed.): Labour Inhibition: Betamimetic Drugs in Obstetrics. New York, G. Fisher Verlag, 1976.
5. Anderson, A., Beard, R., Brudenell, J. M. and Dunn, P. M. (eds.): Pre-term Labour. Proceedings of the Fifth Study Group of the Royal College of Obstetricians and Gynaecologists, London, 1977.
   a. Anderson, A. M. B.: Pre-term labour: Definition, p. 3.
   b. Andersson, K. E.: Inhibition of uterine activity by the calcium antagonist nifedipine, p. 101.
   c. Avery, M. E.: Mechanisms and drugs accelerating fetal pulmonary maturation, p. 273.
   d. Avery, M. E.: Discussion, p. 405.
   e. Beard, R. W.: The effect of beta-sympathomimetic drugs on carbohydrate metabolism in pregnancy, p. 203.
   f. Bieniarz, J.: Cardiovascular effects of beta-adrenergic agonists, p. 188.
   g. Bowes, W. A.: Results of the intensive perinatal management of very low birth weight infants (501–1500 gm), p. 331.
   h. Campbell, S.: Discussion, p. 363.
   i. Chez, R.: Discussion, p. 215.
   j. Gluck, L.: Discussion, p. 294.
   k. Howie, R. N.: Clinical trial of antepartum betamethasone therapy for prevention of respiratory distress in preterm infants, p. 281.
   l. Kubli, F.: Discussion, p. 356.
   m. Kubli, F.: Discussion, p. 218.
   n. Lindner, H.: Discussion, p. 249.
   o. Roberton, N. R. C.: Immediate management of the pre-term newborn infant, p. 315.
   p. Rudolph, A. M.: Effects of prostaglandins and synthetase inhibitors on the fetal circulation, p. 231.
   q. Stewart, A.: Follow-up of pre-term infants, p. 372.
   r. Wiqvist, N.: Discussion, p. 243.

OTHERS

1. Avery, M. E.: Pharmacological approach to the acceleration of fetal lung maturation. Br. Med. Bull. 31:13, 1975.
2. Ballard, R. A., Ballard, P. L., Granberg, J. P. and Sniderman, S.: Prenatal administration of betamethasone for prevention of respiratory distress syndrome. Pediatrics 94:97, 1979.
2a. Barden, T. P., Peter, J. B. and Merkatz, I. R.: Ritodrine hydrochloride: a betamimetic agent for use in preterm labor. I. Pharmacology, clinical history, administration, side effects, and safety. Obstet. Gynecol. 56:1, 1980.
3. Bergstein, N. A. M. and Flynn, M. J.: An analysis of studies of carbohydrate metabolism in patients receiving ritodrine during pregnancy. Report No. 56638/1369/73. Amsterdam, Philips-Duphar, 1973.
4. Bieniarz, J., Burd, L., Motew, M. and Scommegna, A.: Inhibition of uterine contractility in labor. Am. J. Obstet. Gynecol. 111:874, 1971.

5. Bieniarz, J., Burd, L. and Scommegna, A.: Multitarget approach to prevention of prematurity. Obstet. Gynecol. 37:632, 1971.

6. Bieniarz, J., Ivankovich., A. and Scommegna, A.: Cardiac output during ritodrine treatment in premature labor. Am. J. Obstet. Gynecol. 118:910, 1974.

7. Bieniarz, J., Shah, N., Dmowski, W. P., Rao, R. and Scommegna, A.: Premature labor treatment with ritodrine in multiple pregnancy with three or more fetuses. Acta Obstet. Gynecol. Scand. 57:25, 1978.

8. Chard, T., Hudson, C. N., Edwards, C. R. W. and Boyd, N. R. H.: Release of oxytocin and vasopressin by the human fetus during labor. Nature 234:352, 1971.

9. Cibils, L. A. and Zuspan, F. P.: Pharmacologic control of premature labor. Clin. Obstet. Gynecol. 16:199, 1973.

10. Clifford, S. H.: High-risk pregnancy. I. Prevention of prematurity, sine qua non for reduction in mental retardation and other neurologic disorders. N. Engl. J. Med. 271:243, 1964.

10a. Collaborative Group on Antenatal Steroid Therapy: Effect of antenatal dexamethasone administration on the prevention of respiratory distress syndrome. Am. J. Obstet. Gynecol. 141:276, 1981.

11. Cohen, W. R. and Friedman, E. M.: Etiology and management of premature labor. *In* Kistner, R. W. (ed.): Current Problems in Obstetrics and Gynecology, Vol. 1, No. 9. Chicago, Year Book Medical Publishers, 1978.

12. Csapo, A. and Takeda, H.: Effect of progesterone on the electric activity and uterine pressure of pregnant and parturient rabbits. Am. J. Obstet. Gynecol. 91:221, 1965.

13. Csapo, A. I., Pohanka, P. and Kaihola, H. L.: Progesterone deficiency and premature labor. Br. Med. J. 1:137, 1974.

14. Csapo, A. I. and Herczeg, J.: Arrest of premature labor by isoxsuprine. Am. J. Obstet. Gynecol. 129:482, 1977.

15. Eskes, T. K. A. B.: Prevention and management of early labour. *In* Proceedings of the Second European Congress of Perinatal Medicine. Basel, S. Karger AG, 1971, p. 210.

16. Fanaroff, A. A. and Merkatz, I. R.: Modern obstetrical management of the low birth weight infant. Clin. Perinatol. 4:215, 1977.

17. Federick, J. and Anderson, A. M. B.: Factors associated with spontaneous preterm birth. Br. J. Obstet. Gynaecol. 83:342, 1976.

18. Fitzhardinge, P. M.: Early growth and development in low birth weight infants following treatment in an intensive care nursery. Pediatrics 56:162, 1975.

19. Friedman, E. A. and Little, W. A.: The twin delivery: factors influencing twin mortality. Obstet. Gynecol. Survey 13:611, 1958.

20. Fuchs, A. R.: The inhibitory effect of ethanol on the release of oxytocin during parturition in the rabbit. J. Endocrinol. 35:125, 1966.

21. Fuchs, F.: Prevention of prematurity. Am. J. Obstet. Gynecol. 126:809, 1976.

21a. Fuchs, A. R. and Fuchs, F.: Ethanol for prevention of preterm birth. Semin. Perinatol. 5:236, 1981.

22. Fuchs, F., Fuchs, A., Poblete, V. F. and Risk, A.: Effect of alcohol on threatened premature labor. Am. J. Obstet. Gynecol. 99:627:1967.

23. Fuller, W. E.: Management of premature labor. Clin. Obstet. Gynecol. 21:533, 1978.

24. Goodlin, R. C. K.: Orgasm and premature labor. Lancet 2:646, 1969.

25. Hendricks, C. H., Cibils, L. A., Pose, S. V. and Eskes, T. K. A. B.: The pharmacologic control of excessive uterine activity with isoxsuprine. Am. J. Obstet. Gynecol. 82:1064, 1961.

26. Henry, J. P., Gauer, O. H. and Reeves, J. L.: Evidence of the atrial location of receptors influencing urine flow. Circ. Res. 4:85, 1956.

27. Heymann, M. A., Rudolph, A. M. and Silverman, N. H.: Closure of the ductus arteriosus in premature infants by inhibition of prostaglandin synthesis. N. Engl. J. Med. 295:530, 1976.

28. Johnson, J. W. C., Austin, K. L. and Jones, G. S.: Efficacy of 17α-hydroxyprogesterone caproate in the prevention of premature labor. N. Engl. J. Med. 293:675, 1976.

29. Karp, L. E., Doney, J. R., McCarthy, T., Meis, P. J. and Hall, M.: The premature breech: trial of labor or cesarean section. Obstet. Gynecol. 53:88, 1979.

29a. Katz, M., Robertson, P. A. and Creasy, R. K.: Cardiovascular complications associated with terbutaline treatment for preterm labor. Am. J. Obstet. Gynecol. 139:605, 1981.

30. Korda, A. R.: The prevention of prematurity. Med. J. Aust. 2:671, 1977.

31. Lauerson, N. H., Merkatz, I. R., Tejani, N., Wilson, K. H., Roberson, A., Mann, L. I. and Fuchs, F.: Inhibition of premature labor: a multicenter comparison of ritodrine and ethanol. Am. J. Obstet. Gynecol. 127:837, 1977.

32. Liggins, G. L. and Howie, R. N.: The prevention of RDS by maternal steroid therapy. *In* Gluck, L. (ed.): Modern Perinatal Medicine. Chicago, Year Book Medical Publishers, 1974, p. 415.

33. Lipshitz, J., Baillie, P. and Davey, D. A.: A comparison of uterine β₂ adrenoreceptor selectivity of feneterol, hexoprenaline, ritodrine and salbutamol. S. Afr. Med. J. 50:1969, 1976.

34. Lipshitz, J.: Use of a β₂-sympathomimetic drug as temporizing measure in the treatment of acute fetal distress. Am. J. Obstet. Gynecol. 129:31, 1977.

35. Lish, P. M., Hillyard, I. W. and Dungan, K. W.: The uterine relaxant properties of isoxsuprine. J. Pharmacol. Exp. Ther. 129:438, 1960.

36. Lubchenco, L. O., Bard, H., Goldman, A. L., Coyer, W. E., McIntyre, C. and Smith, D. V.: Newborn intensive care and long-term prognosis. Dev. Med. Child. Neurol. 16:421, 1974.

37. Lubchenco, L. O., Delivoria-Papadopoulos, M. and Searls, D.: Long-term follow-up studies of prematurely born infants. II. Influence of birth weight and gestational age on sequelae. J. Pediatr. 80:509, 1972.

38. Mann, L. I., Bhakthavathsalan, A., Liu, M. and Makowski, P.: Effect of alcohol on fetal cerebral function and metabolism. Am. J. Obstet. Gynecol. 122:845, 1975.

39. Marshall, J. M. and Kroeger, E. A.: Adrenergic influences on uterine smooth muscle. Philos. Trans. R. Soc. Lond. (Biol.) 265:135, 1973.

40. McKeown, T. and Record, R. G.: Observations on foetal growth in multiple pregnancy in man. J. Endocrinol. 8:386, 1952.

40a. Merkatz, I. R., Peter, J. B. and Barden, T. P.: Ritodrine hydrochloride: a betamimetic agent for use in preterm labor. Obstet. Gynecol. 56:7, 1980.

41. Niebyl, J. R., Blake, D. A., Johnson, J. W. C. and

King, T. M.: The pharmacologic inhibition of premature labor. Obstet. Gynecol. Survey 33:507, 1978.

42. Papiernik, E.: L'accouchement premature et sa prevention. Arch. Fr. Pediatr. 34:488, 1977.

42a. Petrie, R. H.: Tocolysis using magnesium sulfate. Semin. Perinatol. 5:266, 1981.

43. Pitkin, R. M.: Assessing the clinical factors in prematurity. Contemp. Obstet. Gynecol. 7:38, 1976.

44. Pose, S. V., Cibils, L. A. and Zuspan, F. P.: Effect of 1-epinephrine infusion on uterine contractility and cardiovascular system. Am. J. Obstet. Gynecol. 84:297, 1962.

45. Richter, R.: Evaluation of success in treatment of premature labor by betamimetic drugs. Am. J. Obstet. Gynecol. 127:482, 1977.

46. Rush, R. W., Keirse, M. J. N. C., Howat, P., Baum, J. D., Anderson, A. M. B. and Turnbull, A. C.: Contribution of pre-term delivery to perinatal mortality. Br. Med. J. 2:965, 1976.

47. Scommegna, A., Burd, L., Goodman, C., Bieniarz, J. and Sears, C.: The effect of pregnenolone sulfate on uterine contractility. Am. J. Obstet. Gynecol. 108:1023, 1970.

48. Scommegna, A., Burd, L. and Bieniarz, J.: Progesterone and pregnenolone sulfate in pregnancy plasma. Am. J. Obstet. Gynecol. 113:60, 1972.

49. Takahashi, K. and Burd, L: Initiation of labor. *In* Sciarrra, J. J. (ed.): Obstetrics and Gynecology, Vol. 3, New York, Harper and Row, 1979.

50. Tamby-Raja, R. L., Anderson, A. M. B., and Turnbull, A. C.: Endocrine changes in premature labor. Br. Med. J. 4:67, 1974.

51. Wagner, N. N., Butler, J. C. and Sanders, J. P.: Prematurity and orgasmic coitus during pregnancy: data on a small sample. Fertil. Steril. 27:911, 1976.

52. Wallenburg, A. C. S., Mazer, J. and Hutchinson, D. L.: Effects of a β-adrenergic agent (metaproterenol) on uteroplacental circulation. Am. J. Obstet. Gynecol. 117:1067, 1973.

53. Wesselius-de Casparis, A., Thiery, M., Yo Le Sian, A. et al.: Results of a double-blind multicentre study with ritodrine in premature labour. Br. Med. J. 3:144, 1971.

54. Wiqvist, N., Lundstrom, V. and Green, K.: Premature labor and indomethacin. Prostaglandins 10:515, 1975.

55. Zuckerman, H., Reiss, U. and Rubinstein, I.: Inhibition of human premature labor by indomethacin. Obstet. Gynecol. 44:787, 1974.

Diazoxide in the Management of Preterm Labor

Karlis Adamsons, M.D., Ph.D.
Susan A. Arnold, M.D.
University of Puerto Rico School of Medicine

General Considerations

Traditionally the discussion of agents used in the management of preterm labor consists of review of pharmacologic properties of substances capable of suppressing myometrial activity and discussion of clinical experience with them. Such an approach might appear unduly confined in view of the fact that modern therapy seeks the elimination of causes rather than simply treatment of symptoms of a disorder. In preterm labor this approach might be justified because in a large proportion of cases the cause is thought to be unknown. Furthermore, irrespective of the predisposing or precipitating factor of preterm labor, suppression of myometrial activity might be essential to prevent irreversible changes from occurring in the excitability of the uterine musculature, which in itself would sustain labor.

From the clinician's point of view, it is desirable to divide preterm labor in two categories. The first category encompasses conditions in which the predisposing factor is transient or subject to iatrogenic resolution. Examples include transient catecholamine release secondary to anxiety or hypovolemia, fever, small and nonprogressive separation of the placenta, and conditions that are or might be associated with release of substances with oxytocic properties, such as ADH and prostaglandins. The second category consists of a group of disorders in which the initiating factor is progressive and potentially capable of endangering the health of the fetus or even that of the mother. Examples include placental separation, choriodeciduitis or chorioamnionitis, progressive reduction in uterine perfusion as seen with pregnancy-induced hypertension, and fetal hyperthyroidism. On theoretic grounds tocolytic therapy for the first category of disorders is necessary for the period during which the initiating factor is operational, and the management should include, if possible, steps to eliminate the predisposing factor. The argument in favor of the prompt use of tocolytic agents instead of expectant management during the period of increased uterine activity is that the latter, even if effective, is more likely to result in shortening and widening of the cervical canal, which in turn would predispose the patient to ascending choriodeciduitis.

The principal objective of tocolytic therapy in the second group of patients in preterm labor is to prolong gestation in the presence of adverse factors for a sufficiently long period of time to allow the fetus to mature without jeopardizing its health or that of the mother.

The properties of an ideal tocolytic agent should include (1) selective action on uterine muscle, (2) beneficial effect on uterine perfusion without production of disruptive high pressures in the terminal portion of the spiral arterioles, (3) distribution of action limited to the maternal compartment with no action on other maternal organs, (4) prompt reversibility of action, (5) ease of administration and (6) low cost.

Myometrium is not known to have organ-specific receptors the activation of which would lead to the relaxation of the uterus. Hence, all currently used tocolytic drugs lack selectivity of action. The choice of the clinician is presently limited chiefly to three classes of agents. The first consists of drugs that are nonspecific suppressors of smooth muscle activity (fluorinated hydrocarbons, magnesium, diazoxide), while the second group, commonly referred to as beta-mimetic drugs, encompasses agents that lead to relaxation of smooth muscle through activation of β_2 receptors (orciprenaline, terbutaline, ritodrine, hexoprenaline). The third class comprises drugs that interfere with the biosynthesis of prostaglandins (aspirin, indomethacin). They would be particularly applicable to clinical conditions in which the presumed cause of increased uterine activity is an increased production and release of prostaglandins either locally or systemically. In addition, reduction in myometrial prostaglandin concentration might lower conductivity of that tissue, and thus impart to prostaglandin synthetase inhibitors a more general capacity as suppressors of uterine contractility.

PHARMACOLOGY OF DIAZOXIDE

The history of this antihypertensive, hyperglycemic and tocolytic benzothiadiazine is intricate. It began in the 1930s when the antibacterial properties of sulfonamides were first discovered. A decade later this led to the synthesis of the first orally active carbonic anhydrase–inhibiting diuretic, acetazolamide. The discovery of chlorothiazide with its antihypertensive properties followed shortly, and it was thought that the antihypertensive action of this thiazide diuretic was independent of changes in plasma volume. To confirm this theory, certain benzothiadiazines without diuretic properties were studied. It was during these experiments that the hypotensive properties of diazoxide were first discovered.[1] When diazoxide was administered with a benzothiadiazine with diuretic properties, a synergistic action involving hyperglycemia was observed.[2] When diazoxide was administered intravenously the salt-retaining properties were minimal, not requiring the use of a sodium diuretic. Hyperglycemia was also infrequent. Thus diazoxide was used chiefly as a parenteral hypotensive agent and for the treatment of chronic hypoglycemia.

The potency of this compound in the management of hypertensive crisis provided impetus for scientists to characterize more completely its mode of action. Animal models showed that spinal cord transection or blockade of autonomic ganglia or of adrenergic, histaminic or cholinergic receptors did not alter the hypotensive response.[3] It was further shown that diazoxide could inhibit spontaneous contractions of isolated rabbit intestine and human myometrium.[4, 5] These findings suggested that diazoxide acts directly upon the contractile function of smooth muscle cells of all types, and that its hypotensive action is achieved by lowering peripheral vascular resistance mainly through a relaxation of smooth muscle cells of the arterioles.

The tocolytic properties of diazoxide were first noted when it was used in the management of severe pregnancy-induced hypertension.[6-8] However, the initial prospects of this agent to become a clinically useful tocolyticum were poor because of the profound hypotension that nearly always followed the rapid ("bolus") administration of the drug to the normotensive pregnant patient. It was not until 1970 that our studies, using the pregnant rhesus monkey, demonstrated that it was possible by administering diazoxide through slow infusions to minimize the hypotensive effect while preserving the tocolytic action.[9] Slow administration increases the amount of diazoxide bound to albumin and hence decreases the amount of free drug that can instantaneously bind to arteriolar receptors.[10] Since the ratio of blood flow to receptor sites per unit of time for myometrium is much smaller than that for arterioles, more circulation cycles are necessary to produce saturation of myometrial receptors comparable to that of arterioles.

When diazoxide was first used in the management of pregnancy-induced hypertension, fetal bradycardia was a frequently occurring phenomenon.[11] This was correctly interpreted as signifying fetal hypoxia due to the fall in uterine blood flow, because transplacentally acquired diazoxide in the well-oxygenated fetus was expected to elicit reflexly mediated tachycardia. The explanation for this observation is that in pregnancy venous capacitance is markedly increased. Hence, a further increase in the diameter of venous channels in pregnancy will produce a proportionally larger increase in venous capacitance (volume) than that seen in a nonpregnant patient. This change will be expressed in a fall in central venous pressure and in right atrial filling, leading to a fall in cardiac output in spite of a reduction in arteriolar resistance. This effect will be particularly marked in the presence of relative hypovolemia such as in patients with toxemia or those dehydrated by ethanol infusion. When diazoxide is given slowly and the intravascular volume is adequately expanded or the patient is placed in a Trendelenburg position, cardiac output is likely to be increased and uterine perfusion will be maintained. It appears that these considerations were not given sufficient attention during the initial period of obstetric use of diazoxide, accounting for the unfavorable assessment of this compound as a potential tocolyticum.

Diazoxide is a chlorine and methyl-substituted benzothiadiazine, a close congener to the widely used diuretic thiazide. It is water soluble and possesses high affinity for binding sites of plasma and tissue proteins. It has been determined by ultrafiltration that at a concentration of about 20 mg per liter, about 90 per cent of diazoxide is bound to plasma proteins. The high protein-binding and tubular resorption (due to a pK^a of 8.5) account for the plasma half-life of about 24 hours. The pharmacologic effect on the arteriolar smooth muscle is, however, only of 6 to 8 hours' duration.[10] At present there is no explanation for the discrepancy between the half-life and duration of the therapeutic effect. Accurate information pertaining to myometrial suppression in humans is not yet available because of the difficulties in obtaining a constant excitability of the myometrium over prolonged periods of time. Diazoxide is metabolized by the liver and about 50 per cent is excreted unchanged by the kidneys.

The exact mechanism of action by which diazoxide inhibits smooth muscle is unknown. It has been suggested that it involves the activation of cyclic AMP, ultimately resulting in a decrease in cytoplasmic calcium concentration and of myosin light-chain phosphorylation.[12]

Diazoxide has multiple pharmacologic actions aside from its effect on smooth muscle cells. These include a hyperglycemic action, stimulation of hair growth and salt and water retention. Diazoxide-induced hyperglycemia is the result of multiple actions of the drug, some of which still remain to be elucidated. There is agreement that diazoxide inhibits insulin secretion; it might also affect cellular glucose uptake without affecting the response to exogenous insulin.[13] With intravenous administration of diazoxide the hyperglycemic response is transient, and correction with insulin might be necessary only in patients with diabetes mellitus.[14] The effect on glucose concentration of plasma might be of significance to the newborn because diazoxide crosses the placenta. When given shortly before delivery diazoxide can cause transient neonatal hyperglycemia of sufficient magnitude and duration to cause osmotic diuresis and thus dehydration of the newborn.[15] This is readily corrected by administration of insulin.

Clinical Experience

During the initial phase of the clinical studies with diazoxide at Mt. Sinai Hospital in New York it was appreciated that adequate expansion of intravascular volume, either with solutions of normal saline or with albumin prior to administration of diazoxide, eliminated any adverse cardiovascular effects in the mother. There was also no evidence, as detectable by fetal heart rate monitoring, of impairment in fetal oxygenation. This was true for patients for whom the rate of administration of diazoxide did not exceed 0.5 mg per kg per minute. Marked maternal hypotension with systolic blood pressure as low as 50 torr was occasionally observed when the drug was given by bolus injection as is recommended in the treatment of hypertension. In the patient who has expanded blood volume and who is lying on her side even such a reduction in perfusion pressure produces remarkably few symptoms. This observation is consistent with the contention that the venous system of the expanded intravascular compartment is not measurably affected by diazoxide. Thus, venous return and cardiac output are maintained at preinjection levels, and the low perfusion pressure merely reflects a fall in arteriolar resistance and not a reduction of organ blood flow.

Because of the effectiveness of the drug as a tocolyticum and the ease of administration and absence of significant side effects, diazoxide became the principal agent in the treatment of preterm labor at Women and Infants Hospital of Rhode Island in Providence, Rhode Island, from 1975 to 1979.[16] Experience over the initial three years as summarized by Vigliani and coworkers comprised 68 patients with gestations ranging from 25 to 35 weeks. Unlike in most studies, patients with ruptured membranes were included, provided that there was no evidence of chorioamnionitis; minimal vaginal bleeding and cervical dilatation of more than 4 cm were not considered contraindications for tocolytic therapy. The following protocol was employed:

1. Uterine activity and fetal heart rate were recorded for 30 minutes with the patient in the left lateral position.

2. Expansion of intravascular volume was attained with 500 cc of normal saline or 250 cc of 10 per cent albumin solution.

3. Diazoxide was infused, 5 mg per kg, at a rate not exceeding 0.5 mg per minute.

4. Uterine activity, fetal heart rate, maternal heart rate and maternal blood pressure were continuously monitored.

5. In case of recurrence of uterine contractions within 2 hours of administration, no further tocolytic therapy was administered.

6. If uterine contractions recurred after 4 hours of initial therapy, the steps outlined in items 2 to 4 were repeated for a maximum of 3 consecutive doses.

Administration of diazoxide resulted in ces-sation of uterine contractions in all patients within 10 to 15 minutes. The decrease in maternal blood pressure averaged 15 per cent and was accompanied by a 10 to 20 per cent increase in heart rate. In no instance was fetal bradycardia observed. A transient increase in fetal heart rate by about 10 per cent was observed in some instances.

The efficacy of diazoxide therapy, when measured in prolongation of gestation, was similar to that reported by other investigators as characterizing beta-mimetic agents or magnesium sulfate. In the group of patients without ruptured membranes, vaginal bleeding or cervical dilatation of more than 4 cm, the success rate in delaying delivery by 72 hours or more was 83 per cent (14/18). In cases in which a single dose of diazoxide eliminated uterine contractions for at least 12 hours, the probability of the pregnancy reaching term was 40 per cent.

In contrast, in the group of patients with overt predisposing factors of preterm labor such as ruptured membranes or vaginal bleeding or in those with cervical dilatation of more than 4 cm, the success rate in postponing delivery by more than 72 hours was 36 per cent (18/50).

Subclinical chorioamnionitis or partial separation of the placenta appeared to be the main factors to account for the short duration of the tocolytic effect of diazoxide. Histologic evidence of these conditions was found in about 80 per cent of cases in which delivery could not be delayed by more than 72 hours.

In reviewing the neonatal outcome among patients with complications such as premature rupture of membranes or vaginal bleeding, it was noted that survival rates were higher, and frequency and severity of respiratory distress syndrome (RDS) were less than those seen in a control population. All neonates, including one weighing only 850 g, were breathing room air by 48 hours.

In addition to transient hypotension, the adverse effects associated with use of diazoxide included nausea, vomiting, chest pain, shortness of breath and headache. These effects occurred infrequently (less than 10 per cent) and were of short duration. The only serious adverse effect with diazoxide was pulmonary edema, which developed in 2 cases (3 per cent). In both instances the patient had received more than 1000 ml of normal saline over a 4-hour period, and in both diazoxide had been administered repeatedly. In one of the patients the symptoms developed immediately after delivery. Both patients responded promptly to diuretic therapy and other supportive measures.

Pulmonary edema is a known complication of tocolytic therapy with beta-mimetic drugs, particularly when they are combined with sodium-retaining steroids. Most of the reports have appeared in the European literature. A recent United States study gives a relative frequency of this side effect of 10 per cent.[17] Although experimental data regarding the causation of pulmonary edema are limited, the sequence of events is rather predictable from the general knowledge of the pharmacology of the agents involved and of the circumstances under which they are employed. Because of their action on the pulmonary arterioles, diazoxide and beta-mimetic compounds are expected to increase the hydrostatic pressure within the pulmonary capillaries.[18] The net filtration pressure is further increased by the low oncotic pressure of plasma that results from rapid expansion of its volume by electrolyte solutions given before or during the administration of these tocolytic agents. Slow administration of diazoxide and replacement of saline by albumin solutions for prophylactic expansion of plasma volume have eliminated this potentially serious adverse effect.

Over the last three years the experience with diazoxide in management of preterm labor at the University of Puerto Rico Medical Center, San Juan, has been similar to that gained at Mt. Sinai Hospital and at Women and Infants Hospital in Providence. The total number of patients treated at the time of preparation of this report exceeds 100. Significant hypotension has been observed only when the recommended rate of infusion was exceeded. The efficacy in prolonging pregnancy has been contingent upon the underlying condition of preterm labor. We have also confirmed the original findings that diazoxide is not able to suppress uterine activity for an extended period of time in the presence of subclinical chorioamnionitis.

The untoward reactions that are commonly attributed to diazoxide such as sodium retention, thrombocytopenia, damage of beta cells of the pancreas, hyperuricemia and hypertrichosis have been observed only with chronic use of diazoxide, and hence are not relevant to the discussion of contraindications to diazoxide as a short-term tocolyticum. The transient hyperglycemia did not produce any clinical problems in our series. Nevertheless, it is recognized that in the presence of diabetes, a transient increase in plasma ketones could occur. Such a side effect could be readily prevented by administration of appropriate doses of insulin.

Comparison of Diazoxide with Other Tocolytic Agents

Growing experience in the management of preterm labor with different classes of tocolytic agents appears to substantiate the contention that the effects of therapy, at least as measured by prolongation of gestation, are similar. Whenever substantial or statistically significant differences between different compounds or treatment regimens are reported, they seem to be traceable to the different criteria applied in the selection of patients.[19] In reviewing our own experience, as well as that of other investigators, we noted that the underlying or predisposing conditions of preterm labor, rather than the mode of therapy, appeared to determine the outcome. In our own series a high success rate (86 per cent) characterized the group of patients with intact membranes, no vaginal bleeding and cervical dilatation less than 4 cm, while a low success rate (36 per cent) was recorded in patients with overt complications or cervical dilatation greater than 4 cm. In view of these considerations it seems more productive to concentrate on evaluation of side effects of the different classes of tocolytic agents, rather than on determination of the tocolytic superiority of one agent over another.

If emphasis is placed on the examination of side effects, substantial differences are encountered among the various classes of tocolytic agents. In the case of ethanol a major side effect is depression of the central nervous system of the mother and also of the fetus with only minimal direct effect on the smooth muscle. Prostaglandin synthetase inhibitors, at least theoretically, can have an adverse effect on the fetus by reducing the diameter of the ductus arteriosus and by interfering with platelet functions. There is no evidence that their use has an unfavorable effect on uterine blood flow.

On theoretic grounds, the principal drawback of beta-adrenergic agents as tocolytic drugs is the distribution pattern of beta receptors in the vasculature. Beta-adrenergic receptors are not present in the vascular beds supplying the uterus but are present in those supplying skeletal musculature and lungs. Thus, administration of beta-mimetic agents might result in reduction in uterine perfusion in spite of an increase in cardiac output. Indeed, such has been found to be the case in pregnant Rhesus monkeys and in sheep.[20, 21] In addition, activation of receptors in the pulmonary circulation of the mother and fetus will cause an increase in conductance, which in the case of the fetus will lead to a diversion of the right ventricular output from the ductus arteriosus to the lung and a resultant fall in oxygen tension in the cephalic circulation. Prolonged exposure of the adrenergic receptors of the fetus to beta-mimetic agents might create an additional problem. In vitro studies have demonstrated that beta-receptor density decreases upon sustained exposure of a given system to beta-mimetic agents and creates an apparent increase in the sensitivity to alpha-adrenergic agonists.[22] Assuming that this principle is applicable to the receptors of the pulmonary circulation of the newborn, the sudden withdrawal of the agonist at the time of delivery could lead to a less-than-needed increase in pulmonary vascular conductance. In this context it is of note that in one large collaborative study a disproportionate number of near-term newborns with symptoms suggestive of RDS has been observed.[23]

The side effects of diazoxide as described earlier are largely preventable. However, the potency of this agent mandates a thorough understanding of its pharmacologic actions and limits its use and administration to experienced individuals. Based on available information regarding chronic use of diazoxide in the management of patients with hypoglycemic or hypertensive disorders, diazoxide is not a suitable agent for maintenance therapy if such were indicated.

We have also learned that suppression of labor in the presence of ruptured membranes improves neonatal outcome without jeopardizing maternal health. Therapy with diazoxide as described in this article prolonged gestation but could not prevent the recurrence of labor in the presence of subclinical chorioamnionitis.

Conclusion

Based on clinical experience gathered over the past decade, we conclude that diazoxide is an effective drug to suppress uterine con-tractions. The previously cited serious adverse effect, namely profound maternal hypotension, can be eliminated with expansion of the intravascular volume prior to therapy and with slow infusion of drug. The potential advantage of diazoxide over other tocolytic agents such as magnesium or beta-mimetic drugs is not effectiveness in prolonging gestation but rapidity of action, paucity of adverse responses, ease of administration, and good tolerance of the patient to the minor side effects. Our data also suggest that delaying the delivery of the preterm infant by suppression of labor for as short a period as 48 to 72 hours considerably improves the ventilatory performance and prospects for survival of the newborn.

REFERENCES

1. Rubin, A. A., Roth, F. E. et al.: New class of antihypertensive agents. Science 133:2067, 1961.
2. Okun, R., Russell, R. P. and Wilson W. R.: Use of diazoxide with trichlormethiazide for hypertension. Arch. Intern. Med. 112:882, 1963.
3. Golden, M. G.: Diazoxide and the treatment of hypoglycemia. Ann. N.Y. Acad. Sci. V150:464, 1968.
4. Preziosi P., Bianchi, A. et al.: On the pharmacology of chlorothiazide, with special regard to its diuretic and anti-hypertensive effects. Arch. Int. Pharmacodyn. Ther. 118:467, 1959.
5. Landesman, R. and Wilson, K. H.: The relaxant effect of diazoxide on isolated gravid and nongravid human myometrium. Am. J. Obstet. Gynecol. 101:120, 1968.
6. Finnerty, F. A., Kakviatos, N. and Tuchman, J.: Clinical evaluation of diazoxide. Circulation 28:302, 1963.
7. Morris, J. A., Arce, J. J., Hamilton C. J. et al.: The management of severe preeclampsia and eclampsia with intravenous diazoxide. Obstet. Gynecol. 49:675, 1977.
8. Neumann, J., Weiss, B., Rabello, Y. L. et al.: Diazoxide for the acute control of severe hypertension complicating pregnancy: a pilot study. Obstet. Gynecol. 53:50A, 1979.
9. Adamsons, K. and Myers, R.: Unpublished data.
10. Sellers, E. and Koch-Weser, J.: Influence of intravenous injection rate on protein binding and vascular activity of diazoxide. Ann. N.Y. Acad. Sci. 226:319, 1973.
11. Barr, P. A. et al.: Effect of diazoxide on the antepartum cardiotocography in severe pregnancy associated hypertension. Aust. N.Z. J. Obstet. Gynaecol. 21:11, 1981.
12. Johansson, S., Andersson, R. and Wikberg, J.: Mechanical and metabolic effects of diazoxide on rat uterus. Acta Pharmacol. Toxicol. 41:328, 1977.
13. Fajans, S. S., Floyd, J. C. et al.: Benzothiadiazine suppression of insulin release from normal and abnormal islet tissue in man. J. Clin. Invest. 45:481, 1966.

14. Tabachnick, IIA, Gulberkian, A. and Seidman, F.: The effect of a thiadiazine, diazoxide, on carbohydrate metabolism. Diabetes 13:408, 1964.
15. Boulos, B. M., Davis, L. E. et al.: Placental transfer of diazoxide and its hazardous effects on the newborn. J. Clin. Pharmacol. 11:206, 1971.
16. Bert, J. and Adamsons, K.: Clinical use of diazoxide in premature labor. Soc. Gynecol. Invest. Prog. Abs. 1978.
17. Katz, M., Robertson, P. and Creasy, R.: Cardiovascular complications associated with terbutaline treatment for preterm labor. Am. J. Obstet. Gynecol. 139:605, 1981.
18. Hyman, A.: Pulmonary vasodilator responses to catecholamines and sympathetic nerve stimulation in the cat. Circ. Res. 48:407, 1981.
19. Hemminki, E. et al.: Prevention and treatment of premature labour by drugs. review of controlled clinical trials. Br. J. Obstet. Gynecol. 85:411, 1978.
20. Myers, R. E., Joelsson, I. and Adamsons, K.: The effects of isoproterenol on fetal oxygenation. Acta Obstet. Gynecol. Scand. 57:317, 1978.
21. Siimes, A. S. I. and Creasy, R.K.: Cardiac and uterine hemodynamic responses to ritodrine hydrochloride administration in pregnant sheep. Am. J. Obstet. Gynecol. 133:20, 1978.
22. Tothill, A.: Investigation of adrenaline reversal in the rat uterus by the induction of resistance to isoprenaline. Br. J. Pharmacol. Chemother. 29:291.
23. Larsen, F., Hansen, K., Hesseldahl H. et al.: Ritodrine in the treatment of preterm labour. Br. J. Obstet. Gynecol. 87:949, 1980.

Editorial Comment

The greatest single problem in perinatology today is the patient who delivers a low birth weight infant. The more premature the infant, the worse the prognosis. Understanding the cause of labor and using this knowledge to develop therapy to prevent preterm labor will make an impact on perinatal morbidity and mortality. The National Institute of Child Health and Human Development, and private foundations, have not identified this as a high priority item in health care. It is indeed unfortunate that the assault on our major problem in obstetrics is on the periphery and not at the heart of current health care considerations. It is known that there is a higher incidence of low birth weight babies among patients in low socioeconomic groups and in those who seek care in the latter part of the second trimester and in the third trimester. The incidence of prematurity in Ohio is three to four times higher in women who have no prenatal care or are first seen in the last trimester of pregnancy than in those who seek care in the first or early part of the second trimester. The unanswered questions are: Why does this occur? Is this a result of the patient as an individual or is it related to prenatal care?

The authors for this Controversy chapter were chosen because of their special interest in a drug to prevent premature labor or because of their perspective on the problem: Fernando Aries' studies on terbutaline, Guy Harbert's work with magnesium sulfate, Richard Landesman's interest in multiple drugs, Tom Barden's work with ritodrine and Karlis Adamsons' use of diazoxide.

Several common denominators exist in all these articles. Primary is our incomplete understanding of the causes of labor. Each author also emphasizes the importance of determining whether or not labor should be stopped, since this is an essential decision in the management of the mother with preterm labor. Next, if labor can be prevented, the pulmonary maturity of the fetus should be determined. Another vital decision then needs to be made: whether glucocorticoids are an appropriate modality for the enhancement of pulmonary maturity. A separate chapter in this book is devoted to the evaluation of these drugs.

A prominent issue concerning preterm labor is how to make the diagnosis. This is essential if clinical investigations of methods are to be evaluated. The effects of bed rest, sedation and hydration on a patient with preterm labor will yield a success rate of approximately 40 per cent. All medications are judged against this. Thus, successful clinical investigation of any drug must achieve results of at least 70 per cent or 30 per cent above baseline control levels.

It is important to rule out associated conditions that cause increased uterine activity, such as acute cystitis or pyelonephritis, and other acute pelvic or thermogenic catastrophes during pregnancy. If therapy is withheld too long in the patient in preterm labor the tocolytic agent has less of a chance for success and if used too early, labor may have stopped without it.

It was our observation in 1958 when epinephrine was infused into women in labor or in oxytocin-stimulated labor that uterine activity was decreased and remained decreased for at least 20 to 30 minutes, at which time there was a recurrence of uterine activity. If the dosage of epinephrine is further increased, uterine activity again decreases. Eventually the problem of side effects from high doses of epinephrine and the natural tendency for the uterus to rebound to its original activity limited its use.

Many of the tocolytic drugs that have been developed since then are modifications of the dihydroxyphenylethylamine nucleus (epinephrine) that functions through beta receptors. The problem with most of these drug derivatives has been the pronounced cardiovascular effects from large doses. The development of tocolytic drugs has led to the production of drugs with less β_1 receptor activity (cardiovascular) and more β_2 receptor activity (uterus).

Maintenance dose therapy after acute tocolysis is in order if best results are to be achieved. The Food and Drug Administration to date has approved only one drug for premature labor and this is ritodrine (Yutopar). The drug was developed by Philips-Duphar in Holland and has been leased to Merrell-National Laboratories in this country for manufacture. As of 1981, it is readily available in both parenteral and oral form.

The contributions in Chapter 3 on Preterm Labor bear reading and rereading, as this essentially is the state of the art as of 1982. The major issue concerns the decision of whether or not to treat the patient and if glucocorticoids are indicated. More basic and clinical research is essential if we are to conquer the problem of preterm labor.

The discussion by Adamsons on the use of diazoxide adds another tocolytic agent for use in preterm labor. Its use, like that of other agents, involves efficacy, side effects, interaction with other drugs as well as physician familiarity with the drug. All enter into decision making. One added concern has to do with cost and availability of drug—a problem seldom encountered in the United States but a point of serious consideration for some areas of the world. The same precautions and pretherapy considerations for diazoxide hold for most other tocolytic agents; that is, keep the patient on her side, hydrate before therapy with 750 ml of lactated Ringer's solution or normal saline, then infuse diazoxide over a 10- to 15-minute period. If these precautions are followed, problems of transient pulmonary congestion and hypotension are usually avoided. The problem with diazoxide is that no oral maintenance regimen is available and this may be a problem, since preterm labor may often be recurrent.

3
Treatment of Patients With Premature Rupture of Fetal Membranes

Alternative Points of View

by Eberhard Mueller-Heubach, Hugh M. MacDonald and Steve N. Caritis
by Philip B. Mead and Patrick M. Catalano
by William C. Scott

Editorial Comment

Treatment of Patients with Premature Rupture of the Fetal Membranes

Eberhard Mueller-Heubach, M.D.

Hugh M. MacDonald, M.D.

Steve N. Caritis, M.D.

University of Pittsburgh School of Medicine

Rupture of the fetal membranes before the onset of uterine contractions has remained one of the most difficult management problems in obstetrics. Difficulty in management is greatest in preterm patients, in whom the risk of maternal and fetal infection that can accompany expectant treatment has to be weighed against the potential improvement in neonatal outcome that comes with greater maturity of fetal organ systems. Large patient populations are necessary to assess the risk of prematurity against the risk of infection. Considerations in determining the risk of infection are gestational age, time elapsed between rupture and delivery and socioeconomic status of the mother. Risk assessments have to be continuously re-evaluated because advances in neonatology improve the chances of intact survival in prematurely delivered neonates. Nevertheless, presently at our institution 83 per cent of neonatal deaths occur in neonates with birth weights of less than 2500 g, although newborns with such birth weights represent only 8.6 per cent of our total deliveries. Therefore management of premature rupture of the fetal membranes is particularly difficult when the fetus is preterm with a birth weight of less than 2500 g.

Initial Evaluation of Patients with Premature Rupture of Fetal Membranes

The patient with possible premature rupture of the membranes should be examined by an experienced physician in order to avoid the need for multiple pelvic examinations. A careful obstetric history with detailed description of the vaginal fluid leakage is mandatory. Rupture of membranes suggested by the patient's history should be verified by sterile speculum examination. Presence of amniotic fluid in the posterior vaginal vault provides evidence of rupture of membranes. When no amniotic fluid is seen in the vagina it is frequently possible to see drainage of fluid from the cervix when the patient coughs or when the examiner slightly elevates the presenting fetal part by abdominal manipulation. A nitrazine test and an amniotic fluid crystallization test are performed on the amniotic fluid present in the vagina. The combination of history, positive nitrazine test and amniotic fluid crystallization is 93 per cent accurate in diagnosing rupture of membranes.[1] A cervical culture is taken. Speculum and manual examination also allow the diagnosis of umbilical cord prolapse, which occasionally accompanies premature rupture of the membranes. The amniotic fluid is examined for turbidity and odor, since both are signs of intrauterine infection. Uterine tenderness on abdominal palpation is sometimes present in cases of intrauterine infection. In addition, maternal temperature is taken and a complete blood count with differential as well as urinalysis are performed. This evaluation permits the clinical diagnosis of amnionitis and rules out other sources of infection.

In recent years a number of attempts have been made to diagnose subclinical amnionitis by examining amniotic fluid. Presence of polymorphonuclear leukocytes in amniotic fluid was reported in a study by Larsen et al. to reliably predict intrauterine infection.[2] However, other investigators did not find the presence of leukocytes predictive of infection.[3, 4] Although bacterial colony counts of amniotic fluid have been reported by Bobitt and Ledger as helpful in predicting intrauterine infection,[5] in two other studies bacteria in amniotic fluid did not indicate a high risk of infection.[2, 3] In the aforementioned studies, amniotic fluid was obtained during labor. In a preliminary report of a small series of patients between 27 and 35 weeks of gestation without labor, amniotic fluid was obtained by amniocentesis.[6] The results of this study suggest that transabdominally obtained amniotic fluid after premature rupture of membranes can be used to predict presence or absence of infection. However, the number of patients in this preliminary report is too small to permit valid conclusions. A reliable indicator of subclinical amnionitis has not yet been identified and further work in this area is needed.

Assessment of fetal status is mandatory before a decision about treatment of premature rupture of the membranes can be made. Gestational age is assessed by careful history and physical examination and, in cases of uncertainty, by ultrasonographic determination of fetal biparietal diameter. Ultrasonographic examination is also done when the fetal presentation cannot be clearly assessed by initial pelvic and abdominal examinations. External fetal heart rate monitoring gives information about baseline fetal heart rate, the presence of accelerations and, in patients in labor, the presence of decelerations in relationship to uterine contractions. The presence of fetal heart rate accelerations with fetal movement is an indication of fetal well-being, whereas late decelerations of fetal heart rate or absence of beat-to-beat variability suggests fetal distress. Occasionally we have observed persistent fetal tachycardia above 160 beats per minute (bpm) without any symptom or sign of infection; however, at delivery it became apparent that chorioamnionitis had been present. Therefore we include persistent fetal tachycardia above 160 bpm in our list of indicators of infection.

In all patients in whom fetal distress has been diagnosed, delivery by cesarean section is necessary. The diagnosis of intrauterine infection is also an indication for delivery. Patients with infection undergo induction of labor with intravenous infusion of a dilute solution of oxytocin by Harvard pump while the fetus is continuously monitored for signs of distress.

Risk of Infection After Premature Rupture of Membranes

Following premature rupture of membranes the risk of maternal and fetal infection is directly related to the time interval between rupture and delivery. The time interval between rupture of membranes and spontaneous onset of labor is related to gestational age. The younger the fetus by gestational age, the longer will be the interval.[7] Thus, the more immature fetus that will potentially benefit most from remaining in utero for further organ maturation has also the greater chance of not being expelled prematurely. On the other hand, with increasing duration of ruptured membranes the risk of fetal and maternal infection will become greater.[7-13] Based upon this fact a number of authors have recommended that the fetus be delivered promptly after rupture of the membranes.[7-13] In these studies the risks of maternal, fetal and neonatal morbidity and mortality from infection were evaluated but no comparison was made with the risk of neonatal death from prematurity alone. The potential reduction in the neonatal death rate resulting from greater fetal maturity if an expectant approach is used has not been examined in any of these studies.

The assessment of the risks from infection becomes very difficult when an attempt is made to relate this risk to gestational age, since large patient populations are required. In Figure 1 we have illustrated the risk of neonatal infection with rupture of fetal membranes of less or more than 24 hours' duration. These data represent over 33,000 consecutive deliveries at our institution between 1970 and 1975. Neonatal infection is defined as culture-proved septicemia or meningitis, or autopsy-

proved pneumonia. Our data indicate that there is a slightly higher risk of infection when the time elapsed between membrane rupture and delivery exceeds 24 hours. A marked decrease in the rate of neonatal infection is seen with advancing gestational age. The highest rate of infection is less than 15 per cent and occurs at gestational ages between 27 and 30 weeks. Time elapsed between rupture and delivery is a far less important factor than gestational age for the risk of neonatal infection.

Intrauterine infection after rupture of membranes not only carries a risk for the fetus but also a certain risk for the mother. The risk to the mother has been used as an additional argument for aggressive management of premature rupture of the membranes. Webb[14] reported on 54 maternal deaths associated with premature rupture of the membranes in 2,943,863 deliveries occurring in California between August 1957 and December 1964. This gives an incidence of 0.18 maternal deaths per 10,000 deliveries. At Magee-Womens Hospital between 1959 and 1978 only one patient died from infection following premature rupture of one gestational sac in a twin pregnancy at 36 weeks and delivery at term. During this period there were about 126,000 deliveries, giving a maternal death rate of only 0.08 per 10,000 deliveries related to premature rupture of the membranes. If the data of Webb are analyzed for maternal deaths follow-

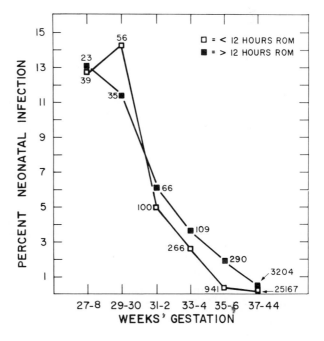

Figure 1. Risk of neonatal infection (%) in patients with premature rupture of membranes of less than 24 hours' duration (open squares) and more than 24 hours' duration (closed squares) at various weeks of gestation. Numbers next to squares indicate total number of patients in each group.

ing rupture of membranes, between 26 and 35 weeks' gestation only 10 maternal deaths are found (only 18.5 per cent of the total number of deaths, or 0.033 per 10,000). Since the debate concerning aggressive as opposed to expectant management of premature rupture of membranes centers mostly on gestational ages between 26 and 35 weeks, Webb's data should be evaluated for the maternal mortality rate during these specific gestational ages. It would appear that the risk of maternal death is extremely small at this period of gestation.

The use of prophylactic antibiotics to decrease the risk of fetal and maternal infection following rupture of the fetal membranes has been investigated by several authors.[8, 15-18] There is general agreement that the risk of fetal and neonatal infection is not reduced with the use of prophylactic antibiotics irrespective of the choice of antibiotic or the route of administration; however, with antibiotics the incidence of puerperal endometritis appears to be lower.[15, 18]

Risks From Premature Delivery Following Premature Rupture of Membranes

The risks of fetal and neonatal infection can be reduced by induction of labor and vaginal delivery or cesarean section promptly after rupture of the membranes. On the other hand, premature delivery is frequently followed by neonatal morbidity and mortality due to immaturity of fetal organ systems—in particular, immaturity of the fetal lungs. In Figure 2 the risk of neonatal mortality is illustrated for various gestational ages. In preterm infants respiratory distress syndrome (RDS) is the most common cause of death. The risk of neonatal death due to lung immaturity is greater with cesarean section than with vaginal delivery.[19] There has been considerable debate whether premature rupture of membranes accelerates fetal lung maturation and reduces the risk of neonatal RDS.[20-28] Several authors have reported a decreased incidence of neonatal RDS with premature rupture of the membranes when membranes had been ruptured for at least 24 hours.[20-22, 24-28] In contrast, Jones et al.[23] could not find such a correlation. Unpublished data from our institution[29] essentially corroborate the data of Jones et al.[23]

Since fetal lung maturity is one of the most crucial factors in terms of survival of the premature infant, the use of amniocentesis and the lecithin-sphingomyelin (L/S) ratio of amniotic fluid has become important in obstetrics. According to the data of Gluck et al.,[30] an L/S ratio above 2.0 predicts the absence of neonatal RDS. We, as well as many others, have used the L/S ratio extensively whenever premature delivery was anticipated and found it to be reliable except in diabetic pregnancies, in which neonatal RDS may occur with L/S ratios above 2.0.[31] An L/S ratio of 2.0 or above is usually present at 35 to 36 weeks' gestation.[32]

Amniocentesis between 32 and 35 weeks' gestation in patients with premature rupture of membranes can be of benefit when a decision between aggressive or expectant management has to be made. Generally, amniocentesis is an innocuous procedure with a very small risk of fetal injury or death. Following rupture of membranes and drainage of most of the amniotic fluid it can be technically rather difficult to find a pocket of amniotic fluid when amniocentesis is attempted, even with the aid of ultrasonography. Recently it has been demonstrated that L/S ratios done on amniotic fluid from vaginal pools after rupture of membranes reliably predict fetal lung maturity.[33, 34] Determination of phosphatidylglycerol in vaginally obtained amniotic fluid has also been shown to accurately reflect fetal lung maturity.[35] Since bloody contamination of amniotic fluid does not interfere with phosphatidylglycerol determination, this test may be particularly helpful when maternal blood from the cervix has been mixed with vaginally pooled amniotic fluid.[36] We perform amniotic fluid analysis for assessment of fetal lung maturity in all patients with premature rupture of membranes between 32 and 35 weeks' gestation. Patients with documented fetal lung maturity are delivered, whereas an expectant approach is taken in patients with immature fetal lungs. After 35 weeks of gestation the risk of neonatal RDS is so low that amniotic fluid analysis is not indicated. However, in diabetic pregnancies a certain percentage of fetuses between 35 and 37 weeks' gestation still has immature lungs.[31] Therefore, in diabetic mothers with premature rupture of the membranes between 35 and 37 weeks' gestation amniotic fluid analysis for L/S ratio determination may be justified.

Acceleration of fetal lung maturation by means of pharmacologic agents prior to preterm delivery has become a field of major interest since Liggins and Howie[37] reported initially on their success in reducing neonatal morbidity and mortality from RDS by administration of betamethasone to the mother. Since the initial report, Liggins has vastly expanded his series[38] and found a consistent reduction in neonatal RDS with betamethasone therapy when gestational age was 34 weeks or less. Based on these data, administration of betamethasone in 2 doses of 12 mg each, 24 hours apart, and delay of delivery for at least 12 hours after the second dose is desirable prior to preterm delivery in patients with premature rupture of membranes. A major concern with steroid therapy is the masking of maternal and fetal infection. However, Liggins[38] as well as Mead and Clapp[39] have found similar rates of infectious morbidity for mothers and infants in their steroid-treated and control groups. The long-term effects of betamethasone on infants whose mothers were treated with this drug are not clear,[40] but follow-up of infants for 6 years with IQ tests did not reveal any difference between steroid-treated and control infants, according to Liggins.

Glucocorticoid therapy will produce leukocytosis for up to 48 hours after the last dose of steroid. Many obstetricians follow patients with premature rupture of the membranes with daily white blood cell counts in order to discover the onset of infection. The obstetrician has to realize that he loses this indicator of infection for about 48 hours after betamethasone administration to the pregnant patient with premature rupture of the membranes. Leukocytosis should not be misinterpreted as a sign of infection when it is in fact due to glucocorticoid administration. Conversely, it is of extreme importance to assess whether a patient with ruptured membranes is infected before glucocorticoid therapy is initiated. Our studies in pregnant sheep have delineated the changes in total leukocytes, neutrophils, lymphocytes, eosinophils and monocytes in mother and fetus after glucocorticoid administration.[41]

The pregnant patient with toxemia and premature rupture of membranes represents a special situation as far as betamethasone therapy is concerned. Liggins has reported a somewhat higher intrauterine fetal death rate following betamethasone therapy in patients with severe hypertension, edema and proteinuria. The reason for this is uncertain. In our experimental studies in pregnant sheep we were unable to demonstrate a change in uterine blood flow following glucocorticoid administration[42] or a change in vascular response to vasoactive substances (norepinephrine and angiotensin).[43] In patients with mild hypertension, edema and proteinuria betamethasone may be administered if the fetal heart rate is continuously monitored for signs of fetal distress throughout the 36-hour period following the first dose of the steroid. In cases of severe hypertension, edema and proteinuria the disease probably imposes such stress on the fetus that lung maturation is accelerated due to endogenous glucocorticoid release by the fetus in response to stress.

Although it has been well demonstrated that the incidence of neonatal RDS is decreased following prenatal glucocorticoid administration, it has remained less clear whether the acceleration of fetal lung maturation can be documented by determination of the L/S ratio. In a small series of our Rh-sensitized patients we have not seen a marked rise in the L/S ratio after betamethasone therapy.[44] Therefore, we do not perform amniocentesis for L/S ratio determination following steroid therapy.

Management of Premature Rupture of Fetal Membranes

The aforementioned considerations play an important role when decisions about management of premature rupture of fetal membranes are made. However, the ultimate choice between an aggressive therapeutic approach and an expectant one involves evaluating the risk of infection versus potential improvement in neonatal outcome. The rationale for prompt delivery of the premature fetus is prevention of infection, whereas the rationale for expectant management is improvement in neonatal outcome from increased fetal maturity.

In order to examine these alternatives, it is necessary to compare the risk of death at birth in uninfected neonates at various gestational ages with the risk of neonatal death resulting from infection that can develop when fetal membranes have been ruptured for a prolonged period. In Figure 2 we have made this comparison on our own patient population over a 5-year period. The bars represent the risk of neonatal death from noninfectious causes in uninfected neonates compared with the risk of neonatal death from infection when fetal membranes have been ruptured less than

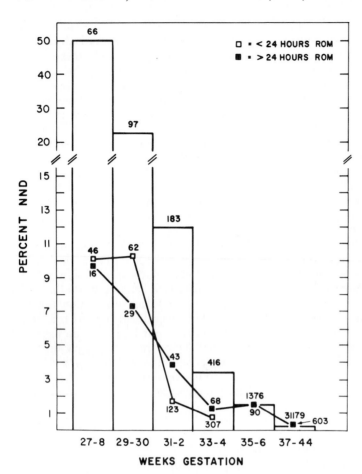

Figure 2. Risk of neonatal death at various weeks of gestation without neonatal infection (open bars) and risk of neonatal death from infection following premature rupture of membranes of less than 24 hours' duration (open squares) and more than 24 hours' duration (closed squares). Numbers next to squares indicate total number of patients in each group.

or more than 24 hours (solid lines) before delivery. For example, in a pregnant patient with premature rupture of the membranes at 27 to 28 weeks' gestation immediate delivery of an uninfected fetus will result in neonatal death from prematurity in 50 per cent of cases. The risk of an infant dying *from infection* at this gestational age is about 10 per cent. If an attempt is made to maintain this pregnancy until 29 to 30 weeks, the overall risk of neonatal death is decreased to 22.7 per cent, while the risk of neonatal death due to infection remains around 10 per cent during this period of time. At 35 weeks' gestation and more, the risk of death in neonates from infection is slightly higher than the risk of death in neonates without infection. Therefore, in patients with premature rupture of membranes at 35 weeks' gestation or more, delivery should be accomplished without delay. In patients with premature rupture of membranes between 27 and 34 weeks' gestation our data support an expectant approach, since the risk of death in newborn infants from

infection is less than the risk of death from prematurity. The data illustrated in Figure 2 depict risks of neonatal death at our institution prior to the institution of betamethasone therapy. Therefore it is likely that neonatal outcome is even more favorable using an expectant approach and betamethasone therapy because decreased morbidity and mortality from neonatal RDS without increased morbidity and mortality from infection can be expected with betamethasone treatment.

Out current approach to management of premature rupture of fetal membranes is based on our own experience just described as well as the cited studies from the literature. This therapeutic approach is summarized in the form of a flow chart in Figure 3. Our recent use of amniotic fluid studies for assessment of fetal lung maturity has been incorporated. If the patient is found to be without infection and in early labor (4 cm or less cervical dilatation) or if labor starts within 36 hours following the first dose of betamethasone, we try to inhibit labor. Thirty-six hours

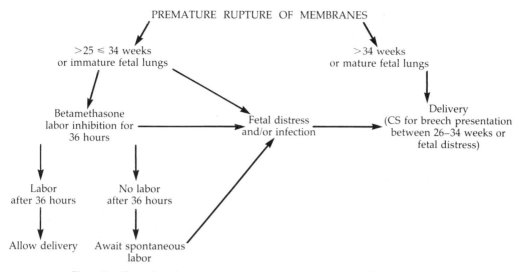

Figure 3. Flow chart for management of premature rupture of fetal membranes.

after the first betamethasone dose we allow the patient to continue in labor if this occurs spontaneously or, if labor is not present, we await spontaneous onset of uterine contractions. Labor is induced only when infection is present.

Until recently labor inhibition for 36 hours was carried out at our institution using intravenous magnesium sulfate[45-48] or ethanol.[49-51] Magnesium sulfate has been and occasionally still is administered initially in a 4-g dose as a slow intravenous push followed by continuous infusion of 2 g per hour by means of a mechanical pump. Ethanol has been given according to the protocol described by Fuchs.[42] In recent years beta-mimetic drugs have been used for labor inhibition. We have used terbutaline on an experimental basis because this agent has been shown to be an effective labor inhibitor in a double-blind placebo-controlled study.[52] We have found that terbutaline inhibits labor more effectively than ethanol[53] and, as a result, have abandoned the use of ethanol for labor inhibition. Since the approval of ritodrine by the Food and Drug Administration, this drug has been widely used to inhibit preterm labor.[54, 55] Side effects of various beta-mimetic agents (ritodrine, terbutaline, fenoterol, salbutamol) are similar and consist of maternal tachycardia, hypokalemia, hyperglycemia and rarely pulmonary edema.[54] As a result of these side effects we still prefer to use magnesium sulfate for labor inhibition in patients with cardiac problems or diabetes mellitus.

Our approach to management of premature rupture of the membranes before 35 weeks' gestation requires obstetric resources in terms of personnel and equipment that are available only at tertiary centers of obstetric care. In addition, care of the newborns delivered prematurely at varying intervals after premature rupture of membranes requires a nursery with considerable expertise. Such experience is generally only available to a sufficient degree in tertiary neonatal centers. The transfer of the pregnant patient with the fetus in utero to a tertiary center for obstetric and neonatal care is indicated whenever premature rupture of membranes occurs before 35 weeks' gestation. This "in utero transfer" is far better in terms of neonatal outcome than the hurried emergency transfer of a premature baby that has been delivered in a small hospital and is suffering from complications of prematurity. There is probably no area in obstetrics in which the concept of regionalization of obstetric care pays greater dividends than in the case of the patient with premature rupture of fetal membranes before 35 weeks' gestation.

REFERENCES

1. Friedman, M. L. and McElin, T. W.: Diagnosis of ruptured fetal membranes. Clinical study and review of the literature. Am. J. Obstet. Gynecol. 104:544–550, 1969.
2. Larsen, J. W., Golkrand, J. W., Hanson, T. M. and Miller, C. R.: Intrauterine infection on an obstetric service. Obstet. Gynecol. 43:838–843, 1974.

3. Listwa, H. M., Dobek, A. S, Carpenter, J. and Gibbs, R. S.: The predictability of intrauterine infection by analysis of amniotic fluid. Obstet. Gynecol. 48:31–34, 1976.

4. Gibbs, R. S., Listwa, H. M., Read, J. A., Carpenter, J. and Dobek, A. S.: Amniotic fluid neutrophils prior to cesarean section and intrauterine infection. Obstet. Gynecol. 50:102–103, 1977.

5. Bobitt, J. R. and Ledger, W. J.: Amniotic fluid analysis—its role in maternal and neonatal infection. Obstet. Gynecol. 51:56–62, 1978.

6. Platt, L. D., Schmidt, P. L., Manning, F. A. and Ledger, W. J.: Amniocentesis can influence the management of patients with premature rupture of the membranes. Soc. Gynecol. Invest. (Abstr. 9), 1979.

7. Shubeck, F., Benson, R. C., Clark, W. W., Berendes, H., Weiss, W. and Deutschberger, J.: Fetal hazard after rupture of the membranes. A report from the collaborative project. Obstet. Gynecol. 28:22–31, 1966.

8. Burchell, R. C.: Premature spontaneous rupture of the membranes. Am. J. Obstet. Gynecol. 88:251–255, 1964.

9. Lanier, L. R., Scarbrough, R. W., Fillingim, D. W. and Baker, R. E.: Incidence of maternal and fetal complications associated with rupture of the membranes before onset of labor. Am. J. Obstet. Gynecol. 93:398–404, 1965.

10. Webster, A.: Management of premature rupture of the fetal membranes. Obstet. Gynecol. Surv. 24:485–496, 1969.

11. Gunn, G. C., Mishell, D. R. and Mortan, D. G.: Premature rupture of the fetal membranes. Am. J. Obstet. Gynecol. 106:469–483, 1970.

12. MacVicar, J.: Chorioamnionitis. Clin. Obstet. Gynecol. 13:272–290, 1970.

13. Martin, J. E.: Management of premature rupture of the membranes. Clin. Obstet. Gynecol. 16:213–225, 1973.

14. Webb, G. A.: Maternal death associated with premature rupture of the membranes. An analysis of 54 cases. Trans. Pac. Coast Obstet. Gynecol. Soc. 34:12–19, 1966.

15. Lebherz, T. B., Hellman, L. P., Madding, R., Anctil, A. and Arje, S. L.: Double-blind study of premature rupture of the membranes. A report of 1896 cases. Am. J. Obstet. Gynecol. 87:218–225, 1963.

16. Brelje, M. C. and Kaltreider, D. F.: The use of vaginal antibiotics in premature rupture of the membranes. Am. J. Obstet. Gynecol. 94:889–897, 1966.

17. Habel, A. H., Sandor, G. S., Conn, N, K. and McCrae, W. M.: Premature rupture of membranes and effects of prophylactic antibiotics. Arch. Dis. Child. 47:401–404, 1972.

18. Huff, R. W.: Antibiotic prophylaxis for puerperal endometritis following premature rupture of the membranes. J. Reprod. Med. 19:79–82, 1977.

19. Usher, R. H., Allen, A. C. and McLean, F. H.: Risk of respiratory distress syndrome related to gestational age, route of delivery and maternal diabetes. Am. J. Obstet. Gynecol. 111:826–832, 1971.

20. Yoon, J. J. and Harper, R. G.: Observations on the relationship between duration of rupture of the membranes and the development of idiopathic respiratory distress syndrome. Pediatrics 52:161–168, 1973.

21. Bauer, C. R., Stern, L. and Colle, E.: Prolonged rupture of membranes associated with a decreased incidence of respiratory distress syndrome. Pediatrics 53:7–12, 1974.

22. Richardson, C. J., Pomerance, J. J., Cunningham, M. D. and Gluck, L.: Acceleration of fetal lung maturation following prolonged rupture of the membranes. Am. J. Obstet. Gynecol. 118:1115–1118, 1974.

23. Jones, M. D., Burd, L. I., Bowes, A. W., Battaglia, F. C. and Lubchenco, L. O.: Failure of association of premature rupture of membranes with respiratory distress syndrome. N. Engl. J. Med. 292:1253–1257, 1975.

24. Chiswick, M. L.: Prolonged rupture of membranes, pre-eclamptic toxaemia, and respiratory distress syndrome. Arch. Dis. Child. 51:674–679, 1976.

25. Berkowitz, R. L., Bona, B. W. and Warshaw, J. E.: The relationship between premature rupture of the membranes and the respiratory distress syndrome. Am. J. Obstet. Gynecol. 124:712–718, 1976.

26. Sell, E. J. and Harris, T. R.: Association of premature rupture of membranes with idiopathic respiratory distress syndrome. Obstet. Gynecol. 49:167–169, 1977.

27. Worthington, D., Maloney, A. H. A. and Smith, B. T.: Fetal lung maturity. I. Mode of onset of premature labor. Influence of premature rupture of the membranes. Obstet. Gynecol. 49:275–279, 1977.

28. Thibeault, D. W. and Emmanouilides, G. C.: Prolonged rupture of fetal membranes and decreased frequency of respiratory distress syndrome and patent ductus arteriosus in preterm infants. Am. J. Obstet. Gynecol. 129:43–46, 1977.

29. Stinson, D. A. and Allen, A. C.: Unpublished observations.

30. Gluck, L., Kulovich, M. V., Borer, R. C., Bremer, P. H., Anderson, G. G. and Spellacy, W. N.: Diagnosis of the respiratory distress syndrome by amniocentesis. Am. J. Obstet. Gynecol. 109:440–445, 1971.

31. Mueller-Heubach, E., Caritis, S. N., Edelstone, D. I. and Turner, J. H.: Lecithin/sphingomyelin ratio in amniotic fluid and its value for the prediction of neonatal respiratory distress syndrome in pregnant diabetic women. Am. J. Obstet. Gynecol. 130:28–34, 1978.

32. Gluck, L. and Kulovich, M. V.: Lecithin-sphingomyelin ratios in amniotic fluid in normal and abnormal pregnancies. Am. J. Obstet. Gynecol. 115:539–546, 1973.

33. Goldstein, A. S., Mangurten, H. H., Libretti, J. V. and Berman, A. M.: Lecithin/sphingomyelin ratio in amniotic fluid obtained vaginally. Am. J. Obstet. Gynecol. 138:232–233, 1980.

34. Sbarra, A. J., Blake, G., Cetrulo, C. L., Selvaraj, R. J., Herschel, M. J., Delise, C., Kennedy, J. L. and Mitchell, G. W.: The effect of cervical/vaginal secretions on measurements of lecithin/sphingomyelin ratio and optical density at 650 nm. Am. J. Obstet. Gynecol. 139:214–216, 1981.

35. Stedman, C. M., Crawford, S., Staten, E. and Cherny, W. B.: Management of preterm premature rupture of membranes: assessing amniotic fluid in the vagina for phosphatidylglycerol. Am. J. Obstet. Gynecol. 140:34–38, 1981.

36. Bustos, R., Kulovich, M. V., Gluck, L., Gabbe, S.

G., Evertson, L., Vargas, C. and Lowenberg, E.: Significance of phosphatidylglycerol in amniotic fluid in complicated pregnancies. Am. J. Obstet. Gynecol. 133:899–903, 1979.

37. Liggins, G. C. and Howie, R. N.: A controlled trial of antepartum glucocorticoid treatment for prevention of the respiratory distress syndrome in premature infants. Pediatrics 50:515–525, 1972.

38. Liggins, G. C.: Prenatal glucocorticoid treatment: Prevention of respiratory distress syndrome. *In* Lung Maturation and the Prevention of Hyaline Membrane Disease, Report of the Seventieth Conference on Pediatric Research, Ross Laboratories, Columbus, 1976, pp. 97–103.

39. Mead, P. B. and Clapp, J. F.: The use of betamethasone and timed delivery in management of premature rupture of the membranes in the preterm pregnancy. J. Reprod. Med. 19:3–7, 1977.

40. Taeusch, H. W.: Glucocorticoid prophylaxis for respiratory distress syndrome: a review of potential toxicity. J. Pediatr. 87:617–623, 1975.

41. Edelstone, D. I., Mueller-Heubach, E. and Caritis, S. N.: Effects of dexamethasone on leukocyte counts in pregnant sheep and fetal lambs. Am. J. Obstet. Gynecol. 131:677–681, 1978.

42. Edelstone, D. I., Mueller-Heubach, E. and Caritis, S. N.: Effects of dexamethasone on maternal and fetal hemodynamic states and fetal oxygenation. Am. J. Obstet. Gynecol. 127:273–277, 1977.

43. Edelstone, D. I., Botti, J. J., Mueller-Heubach, E. and Caritis, S. N.: Response of the circulation of pregnant sheep to angiotensin and norepinephrine before and after dexamethasone. Am. J. Obstet. Gynecol. 130:689–692, 1978.

44. Caritis, S. N., Edelstone, D. I. and Mueller-Heubach, E.: Effect of betamethasone on analysis of amniotic fluid in the rhesus-sensitized pregnancy. Am. J. Obstet. Gynecol. 127:529–532, 1977.

45. Kumar, D., Zourlas, P. A. and Barnes, A. C.: In vitro and in vivo effects of magnesium sulfate on human uterine contractility. Am. J. Obstet. Gynecol. 86:1036–1040, 1963.

46. Hutchinson, H. T., Nichols, M. M., Kuhn, C. R. and Vasicka, A.: Effects of magnesium sulfate on uterine contractility, intrauterine fetus, and infant. Am. J. Obstet. Gynecol. 88:747–758, 1964.

47. Harbert, G. M., Cornell, G. W. and Thornton, W. N.: Effect of toxemia therapy on uterine dynamics. Am. J. Obstet. Gynecol. 105:94–104, 1969.

48. Steer, C. M. and Petrie, R. H.: A comparison of magnesium sulfate and alcohol for the prevention of premature labor. Am. J. Obstet. Gynecol. 129:1–4, 1977.

49. Fuchs, F., Fuchs, A-R., Poblete, V. F. and Risk, A.: Effect of alcohol on threatened premature labor. Am. J. Obstet. Gynecol. 99:627–637, 1967.

50. Zlatnik, F. J. and Fuchs, F.: A controlled study of ethanol in threatened premature labor. Am. J. Obstet. Gynecol. 112:610–612, 1972.

51. Fuchs, F.: Prevention of prematurity. Am. J. Obstet. Gynecol. 126:809–820, 1976.

52. Ingemarsson, I.: Effect of terbutaline on premature labor: a double-blind placebo-controlled study. Am. J. Obstet. Gynecol. 125:520–524, 1976.

53. Caritis, S. N., Carson, D., Greebon, D., McCormick, M., Edelstone, D. I. and Mueller-Heubach, E.: A comparison of terbutaline and ethanol in the treatment of preterm labor. Am. J. Obstet. Gynecol. 142:183–190, 1982.

54. Barden, T. P., Peter, J. B. and Merkatz, I. R.: Ritodrine hydrochloride: A betamimetic agent for use in preterm labor. I. Pharmacology, clinical history, administration, side effects, and safety. Obstet. Gynecol. 56:1–6, 1980.

55. Merkatz, I. R., Peter, J. B. and Barden, T. P.: Ritodrine hydrochloride: A betamimetic agent for use in preterm labor. II. Evidence of efficacy. Obstet. Gynecol. 56:7–12, 1980.

Management of the Patient With Premature Rupture of the Membranes

Philip B. Mead, M.D.

Patrick M. Catalano, M.D.

University of Vermont College of Medicine

Introduction

Premature rupture of the membranes, defined classically as rupture of the membranes prior to the establishment of regular uterine contractions, is a common event occurring in approximately 10 per cent of all pregnancies.

There is little controversy concerning management of the condition when it occurs after 34 weeks, when the majority of fetuses can be presumed to have attained pulmonary maturity. Several studies have clearly shown that when premature rupture of the membranes occurs in the last six weeks of pregnancy, prolongation of the latent period is associated with increased incidences of intrapartum fever, perinatal deaths (not necessarily related to infection), and maternal endometritis.[1] Because of these well-documented risks of a prolonged interval after membrane rupture near term, and because most fetuses can be presumed to have obtained pulmonary maturity by this time, most authorities recommend that patients with premature rupture after 34 to 36 weeks' gestation be delivered within 24 hours of membrane rupture.[2] There is no benefit to the fetus from delaying delivery, and there are serious potential maternal and fetal complications.

Tremendous controversy exists concerning the management of premature rupture of membranes in the preterm pregnancy. Low birth weight and prematurity, from whatever cause, are the major challenges to today's perinatologist. Premature rupture of membranes contributes disproportionately to the problem of prematurity. At the Medical Center Hospital of Vermont, premature rupture is the presenting symptom of one third of patients subsequently delivering low birth weight infants and is the prime etiologic event in fully one quarter of all low birth weight deliveries. In the remainder of this chapter we will attempt to place in perspective the debate surrounding management of premature rupture of membranes in the preterm pregnancy.

Risk of Membrane Rupture in Preterm Pregnancy: Prematurity vs. Infection

Designing management strategies for preterm pregnancies complicated by premature rupture of membranes forces one to judge whether infection or prematurity poses the more serious risk for the fetus. A gradually enlarging body of data now convincingly argues that the leading cause of neonatal morbidity and mortality in the preterm gestation complicated by premature membrane rupture is respiratory distress syndrome (RDS), presumably on the basis of prematurity. (The interrelationships between presence or absence of premature rupture, gestational age and duration of latency are complex. Failure to consider all of these variables when evaluating outcome data [i.e., RDS as opposed to infection] render many of the conclusions re-

garding premature rupture from the older literature invalid. It is beyond the scope of this article to outline these complex interrelationships in detail, but a brief summary, particularly focusing on infection-related outcomes, might be as follows: While it has been shown that the incidences of perinatal death [overall] and perinatal death due to infection, neonatal infection, intrapartum fever and maternal endometritis are increased in patients delivering preterm compared to those delivering at term, these risks due solely to premature rupture of membranes are insignificant compared with the risk associated with preterm delivery per se. Moreover, in the preterm gestation, the incidences of these complications do not increase with prolonged latency provided that differences in gestational ages are taken into account.[1, 3]) The compelling evidence that prematurity poses the greatest risk in preterm pregnancies associated with premature membrane rupture has served to stimulate efforts to prolong pregnancy or prevent or ameliorate neonatal RDS in patients with premature rupture. Before such strategies are considered, it is important to consider two subgroups of patients with rupture of membranes in preterm pregnancy, namely those with already established infection, and those in whom the fetus has attained pulmonary maturity.

Amniotic Fluid Analysis in Patients With Premature Rupture of Membranes

While the risk of infection due solely to premature rupture of membranes is insignificant compared with the risk attributable to preterm birth, nonetheless it has been shown that the incidence of RDS, perinatal death and overall neonatal infection is increased in newborns delivered in the presence of intrauterine infection.[4] Thus it is desirable to predict that group destined to develop clinical infection so that appropriate steps can be taken to prevent such infection, ensure early diagnosis or minimize morbidity. The classicial clinical findings of chorioamnionitis—including maternal fever, maternal and fetal tachycardia, leukocytosis, uterine tenderness and purulent, foul-smelling discharge—are late-appearing signs indicating a well-established infection.

Efforts at prolonging pregnancy in the preterm patient with premature rupture of membranes must be aimed at ruling out occult intrauterine infection rather than well-established infection. In the absence of maternal fever, Gram stain and culture of amniotic fluid are the only reliable predictors of occult or incipient chorioamnionitis. Several authors have documented the statistically significant association of positive Gram stains or cultures from amniotic fluid with subsequent chorioamnionitis.[5, 6] Thus the finding of bacteria on Gram stain of uncentrifuged amniotic fluid obtained either by amniocentesis or aspirated through an intrauterine pressure catheter appears to be a rapid, practical and precise technique for identifying patients with early chorioamnionitis. Despite early reports to the contrary, the finding of leukocytes in amniotic fluid does not accurately predict subsequent chorioamnionitis. Therefore, whenever possible, amniocentesis should be included in the evaluation of the preterm patient with premature membrane rupture in whom a delay in delivery is considered as part of the management. With evidence of frank or occult infection, management should include parenteral antibiotic therapy and expeditious delivery. However, there is no currently available evidence that indications for cesarean section or duration of labor allowed should be altered by the presence of chorioamnionitis.[7]

A second important subgroup of patients with early membrane rupture in preterm pregnancy are those whose fetus has achieved functional pulmonary maturity despite early gestational age. Identification of such fetuses greatly simplifies management decisions, arguing for early delivery and thus avoidance of potential complications of intrauterine infection and unnecessary use of corticosteroids. Depp et al., in a study of 439 women at risk to deliver prior to 37 weeks, found that approximately 19 per cent of their fetuses at less than 34 weeks have mature lung function as measured by L/S ratios.[8] In studies utilizing the technique of amniocentesis in preterm pregnancies complicated by premature rupture of membranes, amniocentesis has been successfully performed approximately 50 per cent of the time.[5] Moreover, two recent studies suggest that absence of RDS in the neonate can be reliably predicted by the presence of phosphatidylglycerol in vaginal pool samples of amniotic fluid.[12, 13] If additional reports corroborate the reliability of this simple, noninvasive procedure, it will become a most useful tool for identifying those fetuses that can and should be delivered immediately.[9]

Assuming that one has documented the occurrence of premature membrane rupture, is certain of a gestational age between 26 and 34 weeks and has by amniotic fluid analysis excluded those patients with frank or incipient chorioamnionitis and those fetuses with demonstrable pulmonary maturity, one must next select a management strategy. It is here that the controversy occurs between advocates of conservative management (expectant watchful waiting with the hope that the fetus will gain sufficient time in utero for pulmonary maturity to develop) and advocates of aggressive management (generally implying the use of maternal glucocorticoids followed by delivery within 24 to 48 hours).

Conservative Management

Although concern for the development of infection is commonly stated as the greatest risk of a conservative approach to premature membrane rupture in the preterm patient, this is not a legitimate fear. While seldom expressed, a far more serious consideration relates to the anticipated length of the latent period following premature membrane rupture in the preterm pregnancy. Obviously, protocols advocating expectant management must include the fact that a latent period that is long enough to enhance fetal maturity significantly will regularly occur. Table 1 shows that such is not the case. In the series reported to date, only approximately one fifth of patients with premature rupture in a preterm pregnancy failed to spontaneously enter labor in a period of less than seven days. Data such as these offer little encouragement for expectant management with the hope that sufficient time will pass for the fetus to become mature. A critical piece of information that we presently lack is the latent period for each gestational week of the preterm period. Knowledge of this might allow selective use of expectant management if substantial latency could be demonstrated at certain gestational ages.

An additional concern inevitably associated with expectant management is the nagging feeling that an occasional stillbirth might have been prevented by earlier delivery. While such might be the case in isolated instances, review of most series involving expectant management suggests that policy changes needed to deliver these infants and all in similar situations at an earlier gestational age might well have resulted in no overall reduction in

TABLE 1. LATENT PERIOD AFTER PREMATURE RUPTURE OF THE MEMBRANES IN PRETERM PREGNANCY AS DOCUMENTED IN 10 STUDIES

AUTHOR	GESTATION AGE OR BIRTH WEIGHT	PER CENT WITH LATENT PERIOD > 7 DAYS
Guilbeau (1955)	1000–2500 g	7.6
Breese (1961)	500–2500 g	24.1
Buemann and Lange (1962)	1000–2500 g	33.0
Gillibrand (1967)	<34 weeks	26.0
Mead and Clapp (1978)	27–33 weeks	15.0
Fayez et al. (1978)	27–33 weeks	20.0
Kappy et al. (1978)	<34 weeks	20.0
Schreiber and Benedetti (1980)	<2500 g	26.0
Johnson et al. (1981)	<32 weeks	13.0
Wilson et al. (1982)	<36 weeks	19.0
Average of all authors		20.4

mortality. In summary, expectant management of premature membrane rupture in the preterm pregnancy does not appear to have adverse effects on the incidence of maternal or neonatal morbidity, but seems to us relatively effectual in achieving significant extensions of intrauterine time.

Corticosteroids and Early Delivery

In a landmark paper published in 1972, Liggins and Howie showed a significant reduction in RDS in newborns of women treated with intramuscular betamethasone in whom delivery was between 28 and 32 weeks and the interval between treatment and delivery was more than 1 day but less than 7 days.[10] No adverse effects on neonates or mothers were noted. Despite the fact that additional well-controlled studies attempting to confirm or refute these findings have appeared, it has been difficult to precisely determine the benefit of glucocorticoid therapy in the clinical situation of premature membrane rupture in preterm pregnancy for the following reasons: (1) most of these studies deal with all causes of threatened premature delivery, not specifically premature membrane rupture; (2) standard regimens have not been used; (3) in many instances numbers available for analysis of subsets of preterm patients with premature membrane rupture are too small to achieve statistical significance; (4) standard definitions of RDS and hyaline membrane disease (HMD) have not always been used; (5) it is often difficult to make a clear distinction between neonatal RDS secondary to HMD and respiratory disease of infectious etiology; and (6) none of the studies differentiate between small for gestational age (SGA) and appropriate for gestational age (AGA) infants, a critical risk factor for development of RDS. Table 2 summarizes those studies in which the effect of corticosteroids on the prevention of RDS were evaluated in the preterm pregnancy complicated by premature rupture. It is obvious that no clear trend is suggested by these contradictory results.

One of the greatest surprises in comparing the results of glucocorticoid therapy with expectant management has been the extreme variation in the reported incidence of RDS. Despite the fact that most of these studies deal with similar gestational ages and use similar criteria for the diagnosis of RDS, incidences of RDS ranging from 8 to 81 per cent have been reported. Admitting differences between populations, variations in experimental design and difficulties in precise clinical diagnosis, this extreme range of RDS incidence is nonetheless inexplicable, and renders comparison of the efficacy of different trials most difficult.

Although concerns about short-term effects of the use of glucocorticoids have centered on increasing the risk of maternal or neonatal infection, such problems have not materialized, especially if delivery is performed within 48 hours of steroid administration. Documentation of any possible long-term effects on the fetus await the completion of collaborative follow-up studies now in progress.[11]

TABLE 2. CLINICAL STUDIES OF STEROIDS IN PREMATURE MEMBRANE RUPTURE
IN PRETERM PREGNANCY

AUTHOR, GESTATIONAL AGE (NO. PATIENTS)	INCIDENCE OF RDS (%)			PERINATAL MORTALITY (%)		
	Control	Steroid	p Value	Control	Steroid	p Value
Mead and Clapp 1977 27–32 wks (43)	85	20	<.001	45	16	<.01
Block 1977 <37 wks (51)	19	12	ns	Not available		—
Kappy et al. 1979 <34 wks (89)	8	14	ns	Not available		—
Quirk et al. 1979 27–34 wks (170)	14	16	ns	13	12	ns
Young et al. 1980 28–33 wks (113)	71	45	<.05	Not available		—
Garite et al. 1980 <34 wks (160)	Not available		ns	Not available		ns
Collaborative 1981 <34 wks or L/S <2.0 (326)	13	10	ns	Not available		—
Garite et al. 1981 28–34 wks (51)	21	17	ns	6	3	ns

ns = Difference not significant.

Accuracy of Previous Predictions

It is interesting to review retrospectively the comments of contributors to previous editions of Controversy in Obstetrics and Gynecology regarding management of premature membrane rupture in preterm pregnancy. From the first edition (1969): Lebherz's suggestion that "prematurity is the primary culprit" has been clearly proved to be correct. Burchell's conclusion that perinatal mortality was associated directly with the length of the latent period probably reflects the fact that 77 per cent of the infants in his series weighed more than 2500 g. Therefore he was not really addressing the problem of premature membrane rupture in preterm pregnancy. Swartz expressed the thought, "If there were an infallible method of determining fetal maturity. . . ." Perhaps the determination of phosphatidylglycerol levels in vaginally obtained amniotic fluid following premature rupture in preterm pregnancy will fulfill this wish.

From the 1974 edition, David Charles' suggestion that the most serious complication of premature membrane rupture is sepsis has not proved to be true, at least in the preterm pregnancy. Gordon and Weingold correctly predicted the difficulty of performing prospective studies of this complex and multifaceted problem. They also documented the infrequency of perinatal deaths due to fetal or maternal infection. Russell and Cheung advocated aggressive management because of concern about maternal and fetal infection, a fear that has been documented for the term infant but not for the preterm newborn. Finally, Scott introduced suggestions for use of L/S ratios in determining fetal maturity and for management with glucocorticoids.

The closing sentence of the editorial comment for this section in the 1974 edition of Controversy in Obstetrics and Gynecology was quoted by the editor from a contributor's letter: "I don't think that the right study of premature rupture of the fetal membranes has been done yet." I seriously question whether such a study can ever be successfully carried off. Assume that an investigator wanted to make what would appear to be the relatively simple comparison of glucocorticoid therapy and expectant management in pregnancies between 26 and 33 weeks complicated by premature membrane rupture. Other than careful assessment of gestational age and performance of L/S ratio on amniocentesis fluid or phosphatidylglycerol determination on vaginally obtained fluid when possible, no additional diagnostic measures are taken. Assume also that from 26 to 29 weeks the incidence of RDS is approximately 75 per cent, and from 30 to 33 weeks the incidence of RDS is approximately 25 per cent. Given these assumptions (all conservative and reasonable), it would take a minimum of 1528 evaluable cases to give a 90 per cent chance of identifying a 33 per cent decrease in RDS at the 95 per cent confidence level! This figure is more than twice the number of patients in the largest trial reported to date. It appears to us that those waiting for the definitive clinical study to identify the optimal management of preterm membrane rupture in the preterm pregnancy will not soon be rewarded. We would hope that progress will instead be made as individual institutions provide greater understanding of component parts of the problem (e.g., surfactant analysis of amniotic fluid, prediction of occult chorioamnionitis, optimal glucocorticoid regimen, profiles of patients expected to benefit from expectant management and so forth.) In the meantime, the clinician should approach the patient with a history of this problem with four admonitions in mind: (1) Carefully document the occurrence of premature membrane rupture, lest unnecessary intervention in a patient who does not have ruptured membranes precipitate an iatrogenic misadventure. (2) Meticulously assess gestational age, since specific therapy will ultimately be determined largely by this parameter. (3) Utilize surfactant analysis of amniotic fluid obtained from the vaginal pool or by amniocentesis whenever possible to identify the fetus with mature pulmonary function that can be safely delivered immediately. (4)

Whether the treatment selected be expectant or aggressive, officials of a service should develop a precise protocol, adhere to it strictly and keep prospective and regularly reviewed records so as to be clearly aware of the success or failure of the chosen method of management.

REFERENCES

1. Johnson, J. W. C., Daikoku, N. H., Niebyl, J. R. et al.: Premature rupture of the membranes and prolonged latency. Obstet. Gynecol. 57:547, 1981.
2. Mead, P. B.: Management of the patient with premature rupture of the membranes. Clin. Perinatol. 7:243, 1980.
3. Daikoku, N. H., Laktreider, D. F., Johnson, T. R. B. et al.: Premature rupture of membranes and preterm labor: neonatal infection and perinatal mortality risks. Obstet. Gynecol. 58:417, 1981.
4. Garite, T. J. and Freeman, R. K.: Chorioamnionitis in the preterm gestation. Obstet. Gynecol. 59:539, 1982.
5. Garite, T. J., Freeman, R. K., Linzey, E. M. et al.: The use of amniocentesis in patients with premature rupture of membranes. Obstet. Gynecol. 54:226, 1979.
6. Miller, J. M., Hill, G. B., Welt, S. I. et al.: Bacterial colonization of amniotic fluid in the presence of ruptured membranes. Am. J. Obstet. Gynecol. 137:451, 1980.
7. Gibbs, R. S., Castillo, M. S. and Rodgers, P. J.: Management of acute chorioamnionitis. Am. J. Obstet. Gynecol. 136:709, 1980.
8. Depp, R., Boehm, J. J., Nosek, J. A. et al.: Antenatal corticosteroids to prevent neonatal respiratory distress syndrome: risk versus benefit considerations. Am. J. Obstet. Gynecol. 137:338, 1980.
9. Dombroski, R. A., Mackenna, J. and Brame, R. G.: Comparison of amniotic fluid lung maturity profiles in paired vaginal and amniocentesis specimens. Am. J. Obstet. Gynecol. 140:461, 1981.
10. Liggins, G. C. and Howie, R. N.: A controlled trial of antepartum glucocorticoid treatment for the prevention of the respiratory distress syndrome in premature infants. Pediatrics 50:515, 1972.
11. Collaborative group on antenatal steroid therapy: Effect of antenatal dexamethasone administration on the prevention of respiratory distress syndrome. Am. J. Obstet. Gynecol. 141:276, 1981.
12. Stedman, C. M., Crawford, S., Staten, E. et al.: Management of preterm premature rupture of membranes: assessing amniotic fluid in the vagina for phosphatidylglycerol. Am. J. Obstet. Gynecol. 140:34, 1981.
13. Yambao, T. J., Clark, D., Smith, C. et al.: Amniotic fluid phosphatidylglycerol in stressed pregnancies. Am. J. Obstet. Gynecol. 141:191, 1981.

Treatment of Patients With Premature Rupture of the Fetal Membranes

William C. Scott, M.D.

University of Arizona Health Sciences Center

Among the more perplexing problems of the specialty of obstetrics and gynecology is the unabating incidence of premature rupture of the membranes. The application of our burgeoning knowledge within the field of perinatology is steadily reducing mortality within the liveborn infant class. However, prematurity is still responsible for roughly half of all infant deaths, with 40 per cent of these being brought about following spontaneous or induced labor after premature rupture of the membranes. The removal of nature's normal barrier to intrauterine infection surprisingly is of little consequence to the mature infant, but many times is disastrous to the younger fetus. This discussion will outline the present status of knowledge of the management of premature rupture of the membranes for the improvement of results in the immature infant.

A compilation of several large reported series (Table 1) reveals some variation in incidence, undoubtedly resulting from known difficulties in establishing the exact time of rupture in relation to onset of labor. The majority of reports accept a one-hour latent period as proper definition. Eastman[38] included all cases of rupture before labor, disregarding the latent period, and reported a 13 per cent incidence, as opposed to the lower figures in Table 1.

No satisfactory solution to the etiology of this condition has yet been presented. Taylor and associates[151] have shown that many of these patients display markedly increased uterine irritability throughout pregnancy. Polishuk and his colleagues[123] claim to show an ethnic predisposition in women of European origin on the basis of decreased membrane tensile strength, while Danforth and his co-workers[34] demonstrated tensile strength in American women far above normal intra-amniotic pressures. Artal et al.[3] confirmed the lack of statistically significant stress-strain differences between prematurely and spontaneously ruptured membranes. However, they found that the membrane thickness was reduced near the rupture site, suggesting an inherent difference between those membranes that rupture prematurely and those that do not. Of unknown relationship to these findings are the findings of Wideman and colleagues,[162] who recorded the incidence of premature rupture of the membranes to be 15 per cent in patients with severe ascorbic acid deficiency compared with only 1 per cent in those with normal levels of this vitamin. Speculations on the relationships of infection, congenital defects, maternal age, parity, trauma and numerous other possibilities seem to be of declining importance as suggested etiologic factors. As with toxemia, preventive treatment awaits further elucidation of an etiology not yet understood but of vital importance for reducing perinatal mortality rate.

Diagnosis

The diagnosis of premature rupture of the membranes is in most instances obvious from the sudden release of clear amniotic fluid from the vagina and its continued dribbling thereafter. Confirmation is needed and is most important, since management depends on positive knowledge. Differentiation between amniotic fluid and urine or endocervical mucus is most practically made by the tests listed in Table 2.

The manner of diagnosis is of utmost importance, most particularly as the time from estimated date of confinement increases. All of these diagnostic maneuvers should be carried out in such a fashion as to keep to a minimum introduction of pathogenic organisms into the vagina and cervix, or through the cervix and into the uterus. That amniotic fluid is exuding from the cervix can be confirmed by tests or possibly by obtaining enough fluid to demonstrate fetal squames at the vaginal orifice. When the vagina needs to be examined, only a sterile speculum under aseptic conditions should be used. The cervix may be visualized, the presenting part displaced, and the presence of fluid release con-

TABLE 1. INCIDENCE OF SPONTANEOUS PREMATURE RUPTURE OF THE MEMBRANES

	TOTAL DELIVERIES	PREMATURE RUPTURE OF MEMBRANES	PERCENTAGE
Sacks[135]	6269	415	6.6
Lanier[83]	7637	473	6.2
Breese[17]	44,723	2887	6.4
Clark[26]	32,022	1009	2.1
Gunn[57]	17,562	1884	10.7
Rovinsky[131]	30,336	3800	12.5
	138,549	10,468	7.5

firmed. Introducing gloved fingers into the vagina and cervix adds nothing to the diagnosis, rarely affects management and may markedly increase the risk of infection. Furthermore, attempts to sterilize the vagina with antibiotics and thus prevent ascending infection, such as those of Brelje and Kaltreider,[18] have proved futile.

After the diagnosis of premature membrane rupture is established, certain immediate and delayed complications may be anticipated. Prolapse of the umbilical cord surprisingly is infrequent, with an average incidence of 0.3 to 0.6 per cent, rising to 2 to 3 per cent in infants with shorter gestations.[58, 136, 139] Fetal mortality in these few cases, however, especially with vertex presentation, is horrendous, reaching 60 per cent.[17] With breech presentation, as might be expected, occult prolapse during labor is a constant concern. Breech presentation in itself is of ominous significance when the membranes rupture early (Table 3). Occurring in about 6.3 per cent of all cases of premature rupture of the membranes, with a perinatal mortality rate of about 25 per cent,

the incidence of breech is much higher (16 to 18 per cent) in the fetus under 2500 g, and these have a mortality rate of 36 to 40 per cent.[58] The perinatal mortality risk for the fetus under 1500 g is almost double when a breech rather than vertex presentation exists. The trend toward abdominal delivery has raised cesarean section rates but lowered perinatal morbidity and mortality associated with breech presentation.

Risks to Fetus and Mother

Perhaps the greatest immediate risk to the fetus is prematurity itself. Two reviews of 4771 cases of premature rupture of the membranes reported 786 babies weighing less than 2500 g, an incidence of 18 per cent.[17, 58] This is approximately three times the incidence of premature infants in the total newborn population. Since the perinatal mortality rate rises sharply as fetal weight declines, obviously this factor alone weighs heavily in infant loss. When the latent period between rupture of membranes and onset of labor is considered, it will be seen that the addition of infection to prematurity is often the coup de grace leading to fetal death (Fig. 1).

The invasion of the uterus by pathogens not only causes amnionitis and deciduitis, but may also present as endometritis and parametritis. Wilson and his colleagues[164] reported maternal

TABLE 2. DIAGNOSIS OF RUPTURED MEMBRANES

TEST	PERCENTAGE OF REPORTED ACCURACY
Nitrazine	94–97
Amniotic fluid crystallization	75–98
Nile blue	98
Nitrazine yellow (Mills)	92
Diamine oxidase (Elmfors)	99

Modified from Elmfors, B. Tryding, N. and Tufesson, G.: The diagnosis of ruptured fetal membranes by measurement of the diamine oxidase (DAO) activity in vaginal fluid. J. Obstet. Gynecol. Br. Commonwealth 81:361, 1974; and Mills, A. M. and Garrioch, D. B.: Use of nitrazine yellow swab test in diagnosis of ruptured membranes. Br. J. Obstet. Gynecol. 49:38, 1977.

TABLE 3. FETAL MORTALITY BY PRESENTATION

	PERCENTAGE BREECH	PERCENTAGE VERTEX
2000–2500 g	17.8	13.1
1500–1999 g	60	32.3
1000–1499 g	86.2	45.7
500–999 g	89	100

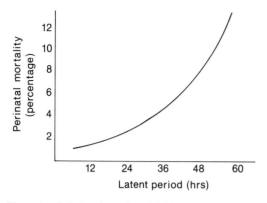

Figure 1. Relationship of perinatal mortality to duration of latent period. (From Gunn, G. C., Mishell, D. R., Jr., and Morton, D. G.: Premature rupture of the fetal membranes. Am. J. Obstet. Gynecol. 106:477, 1970.)

infection associated with one in two infected infants. Other studies[26, 45, 126, 135, 139, 143] indicate an overall maternal morbidity rate of up to 18 per cent, either intrapartum or postpartum. Maternal mortality, on the other hand, is exceedingly rare but cases exist in sufficient numbers to warrant serious consideration. Webb,[157] analyzing California statistics, calculated maternal deaths secondary to rupture of the membranes as 1 in 5551, but Webster,[158] in reporting Cook County Hospital 10-year statistics of 226,878 deliveries, found 13 maternal deaths from sepsis associated with premature rupture of the membranes. With the same method of calculation as Webb used, this gives an incidence of 2.4 per 5000. Thus, even though the risk to the fetus is far greater, we cannot disregard the safety of the mother in the management decision.

The Latent Period

Numerous studies[6, 58, 65, 126] have repeatedly stressed the importance of the latent period in the development of ascending infection and the increasing hazards with time to both mother and baby. The mature fetus enjoys a significantly lesser risk, for while the latent period totals less than 24 hours in 50 to 54 per cent, in the term pregnancy it varies from 81 to 95 per cent.[17] Howard and Bauer[65] report perinatal mortalities of 0.28 to 0.5 per cent in the term pregnancy in which the infant is delivered within 24 hours of rupture of the membranes. Spontaneous onset of labor in

these cases will nearly always solve the problem in the last four weeks of pregnancy and when necessary and not obstetrically contraindicated, induction with pitocin is now almost universally standard procedure for the few not in labor at the end of 12 to 24 hours. Hellman and Pritchard[63] recommend cesarean delivery for the occasional patient not in labor in 12 hours. The aggressive management of Russell and Anderson,[136] using cesarean section to ensure termination of all pregnancies within 24 hours after rupture of the membranes, raised their rate of cesarean sections from 4.5 to 12 per cent but reduced fetal deaths by two thirds.

Since it is obvious that the neonatal death rate rises in a linear fashion with the length of the latent period, the percentage associated with premature rupture of the membranes doubles from 14 to 30 between 24 and 48 hours.[58, 84] Therefore the disagreement over management between the "conservatives" and the "activists" has involved primarily the premature infant. Not being able to accurately assess the fetal size or ability to survive extrauterine existence, the clinician was always tempted to believe that the additional intrauterine time was worth the risk of infection. Indeed, Pryles and his associates[126] found that 59 per cent of infants born to mothers whose latent periods were over 24 hours were premature, and all authors agree that there is an inverse relationship between length of gestation and latent period.

After a 24-hour latent period, the incidence of amnionitis rises to involve from 10 to 30 per cent of pregnancies. Breese,[17] in addition, has correlated the rising mortality rate with both diminishing fetal size and increasing latent period (Table 4). Bryans (Lanier et al.[84]) also detected a marked rise from 8 per cent

TABLE 4. PERINATAL MORTALITY BY WEIGHT AND LATENT PERIOD

	LATENT PERIOD	
WEIGHT	*Percentage Under 48 Hr*	*Percentage Over 48 Hr*
2000–2500 g	9.6	20.6
1500–1999 g	31.2	42.8
1000–1499 g	60.8	63.1
500–999 g	55	100

Modified from Breese, M. W.: Spontaneous premature rupture of the membranes. Am. J. Obstet. Gynecol. 81:1086, 1961.

TABLE 5. MORTALITY IN PREMATURE INFANTS OF PATIENTS WITH
PREMATURE RUPTURE OF MEMBRANES

	MORTALITY		
INTERVAL UNTIL DELIVERY	RDS	Infection	Both
16 hr	70/455 (15%)	8/455 (2%)	2/455 (0.4%)
<24	159/879 (18%)	20/825 (2%)	
>24	12/120 (10%)	7/84 (8%)	
All	241/1454 (17%)	35/1364 (3%)	

Data taken from references 4, 9, 10, 24, 36, 79, 106, 114, 130, 142, 152, 165.

to 46.19 per cent infant mortality when maternal infection coexists. These figures have led to the conclusion that the infant over 2000 g is best treated similarly to the mature infant, with prompt delivery.

A reappraisal of the mortality risks associated with premature delivery began with the report by Richardson et al.[130] in 1973. They studied 64 infants with premature rupture of the membranes and found in those infants with time elapsed between premature rupture of the membranes and delivery of less than 24 hours, 13 times as many died of idiopathic respiratory disease as of infection. Numerous other authors since that time have corroborated this, and in Table 5 the overall mortality rate in preterm infants with premature rupture of the membranes is found to be 17 per cent due to respiratory distress syndrome (RDS) as compared to 2 per cent from infection. However, these studies still show a rise in the infection rate to 8 per cent after a latent period of 24 hours. Bada[4] and Knudsen[79] also showed a fetal infection rate of from 3 to 8 per cent and a neonatal mortality rate of 4.5 per 100; 53 per cent of deaths were due to RDS. It seems obvious then that when addressing fetal mortality, the problem of RDS is much more important than that of infection. As seen in Table 5, mortality from RDS dropped from 15 to 18 per cent for those who had less than 24 hours elapse between rupture and delivery to roughly 10 per cent in those who had a time lapse of over 24 hours. Thus some protection may result as the duration of time increases between membrane rupture and delivery.

Premature Membrane Rupture and the Respiratory Distress Syndrome

The effect of premature rupture of the membranes on the development of RDS has been the subject of a number of studies in the past three years, a compilation of which is seen in Tables 6 and 7. In both those studies by fetal weight as well as by week of gestation, a decreased incidence of RDS is seen in the infant coming from a pregnancy with premature rupture of the membranes. However, the two significant variables, length of gestation and length of time elapsed between membrane rupture and delivery, are addressed in several other studies. Berkowitz et al.[9] in 1978 found a statistically significant reduction in the incidence of RDS in infants of 33 weeks' gestational age and older when time between premature membrane rupture and delivery was in excess of 16 hours. Miller et al.[142] found the incidence of RDS to be less in infants of 1000 to 1500 g after a delay of 48 hours between rupture of membranes and delivery. Sell and Harris[142] from the Arizona Health Sciences Center found significantly fewer cases of RDS in patients of all gestational ages when the time elapsed between rupture of membranes and delivery was longer than 24 hours (Table 8). They concluded the benefit

TABLE 6. EFFECT OF PREMATURE MEMBRANE
RUPTURE ON INCIDENCE OF RDS
BY FETAL WEIGHT

	RDS	
FETAL WEIGHT	No Premature Rupture	Premature Rupture Present
501–1000 g	32/67 (48%)	13/17 (71%)
1001–1500	84/141 (54%)	40/113 (35%)
1501–2000	137/378 (36%)	47/292 (16%)
2001–2500	63/265 (24%)	24/226 (11%)
>2500	214/673 (32%)	76/572 (13%)

Modified from Lee, K. S. et al.: Respiratory distress syndrome of the newborn and complications of pregnancy. Pediatrics 58:675, 1976; and Miller et al.: Premature labor and premature rupture of the membranes. Br. J. Obstet. Gynecol. 132:1, 1978.

TABLE 7. EFFECT OF PREMATURE MEMBRANE RUPTURE ON RDS INCIDENCE BY WEEK OF GESTATION

	RDS	
GESTATION	No Premature Rupture	Premature Rupture Present
20–27 wks	6/8 (75%)	2/3 (66%)
29	20/51 (39%)	4/21 (19%)
29–31	29/65 (45%)	5/21 (24%)
32	64/143 (45%)	11/45 (24%)
32–34	50/166 (30%)	11/64 (17%)
28–36	21/60 (35%)	7/62 (11%)
33–37	3/25 (12%)	
All	138/394 (35%)	34/137 (25%)

Data taken from references 7, 8, 9, 10, 25, 42, 69, 142, 152, 154, 165.

to the premature infant in the form of reduced risk of developing RDS is possible if the mother is allowed 24 hours after premature rupture of membranes before delivery is initiated. These reports agreed with results reported by Lee et al.[86] in 1976. The major study to disagree with these observations has been that reported by Jones and colleagues in 1975.[69] Their retrospective study, done some 7 to 20 years after delivery, concluded that there was no protective effect from allowing time to elapse between premature rupture of the membranes and delivery. It has been criticized on the grounds that gestational age was established only by menstrual history and by the failure to further evaluate the effect of respiratory failure in the infants involved.

The majority of studies seem to indicate that the major risk to the premature infant delivered after rupture of the membranes is idiopathic respiratory distress syndrome; however, the incidence of this syndrome varies with both infant size and duration of time between membrane rupture and delivery. Estimates as to fetal size through clinical examination have always been grossly inaccurate, and many decisions made on that basis were later regretted. Ultrasonography has now changed this. Thompson[153] has calculated a formula by which he has been able to determine fetal size within 300 g using the B-scan and chest circumference. The biparietal diameter of the fetal head may also be measured to within a 2 mm accuracy, adding a second dimension for the assessment of fetal growth. The experiences of our ultrasonography laboratory support the view that the combined results of these two measurements are indeed correlating well with gestational age and fetal size. In studies in various parts of the country a variety of charts have been developed to predict gestational age from biparietal diameter. Sabbagha and Hughey[138] have compiled a chart showing the composite mean biparietal values of all studies and suggest that it be used universally for the prediction of fetal age. Ultrasonography is a standard procedure prior to the planned induction of any labor and is extremely valuable when infant size is borderline or questionable.

Postnatal Risks

The major threat to extrauterine existence of the premature infant is respiratory distress syndrome, or hyaline membrane disease. The pioneering work of Gluck and his associates[55] has given us a means of accurately assessing fetal lung maturity. Adequate amounts of surfactant in the alveolar lining ensure alveolar stability during respiration and thus are necessary for normal respiratory function. This surfactant, produced by the type 2 epithelial

TABLE 8. EFFECT OF LENGTH OF PREMATURE MEMBRANE RUPTURE ON INCIDENCE OF RDS BY WEEK OF PREGNANCY

	RDS Premature Rupture of Membranes		
GESTATION	<12 Hrs	<16 Hrs	>16 Hrs
<28 wks		17/33 (52%)	9/24 (38%)
<32	125/196 (64%)	286/461 (62%)	22/74 (30%)
<36	125/196 (64%)	361/642 (56%)	33/133 (25%)
<37	251/809 (31%)	436/823 (53%)	44/192 (23%)
All	251/809 (31%)	440/830 (53%)	44/202 (22%)

Data taken from references 7, 8, 9, 10, 25, 42, 142, 152, 165.

cells of the alveoli, is a complex lipoprotein containing 90 per cent dipalmital lecithin.[78, 105] This substance is synthesized from phosphatidyl ethanolamine by transmethylation via the enzyme N-methyl-transferase.[111] Concentrations of this enzyme are high in the microsomal fractions of lung extract. Brumley[19] has shown a markedly lowered pulmonary synthesis of phosphatidyl choline, with low fetal Po_2 and acidosis, especially in the premature infant.

There is a rapid increase in amniotic fluid lecithin after weeks 32 to 34. By amniocentesis, measurements of lecithin phosphate directly or comparatively, as the lecithin/sphingomyelin (L/S) ratio, have proved to be of great value in predicting lung maturity.[11, 160] The L/S ratio technique was developed to avoid potential errors caused by variation in amniotic fluid volumes affecting lecithin concentration.

Additional evidence of fetal liver maturity may easily be obtained, using the same specimen, by determining the creatinine level. Zwirek and Pitkin[168] in 1969 showed a progressive rise in creatinine level concentration in late gestation, and a level of 2 mg per dl or over is comforting corroborating evidence for a prediction of viability in extrauterine existence.[37] In the small for gestational age infant, however, the creatinine concentration does not correlate well and lecithin levels are a better guide.[109, 110]

In the original work of Kittrich[74] the fetal squames in amniotic fluid could be identified when stained by Nile blue sulfate. Husain and Sinclair[67] developed a method yielding equally good results with hematoxylin and eosin or Papanicolaou staining techniques. However, predictability of fetal maturity with this method is considered by some to be less reliable than with the methods using creatinine and lecithin concentrations.[37]

When ultrasonography confirms the size and creatinine and lecithin levels indicate maturity, there is no difficulty in deciding management if the membranes are ruptured. In the smaller infant, not yet mature and subject to RDS, perinatal mortality rates can be improved only by attempts to produce pulmonary maturity.

Enhancement of Pulmonary Maturity

Enhanced pulmonary maturity with its protective effects against RDS occurs in the premature infant following an interval after rupture of the membranes until delivery that is prolonged over 16 hours[9, 10] and in the fetal rabbit subjected to heroin,[149] Bromhexametabolite 8[95] and the injection of thyroxine into the amniotic fluid.[101] Gould et al.[57] in 1977 studied the effects of chronically stressed pregnancy on the infant. Twenty-five infants under 32 weeks' gestation had an L/S ratio over 2 and all 25 showed neurologic scores 3 to 8 weeks beyond that expected from their gestational age. These investigators concluded that acceleration of clinical neurologic maturation was secondary to the high-stress pregnancy and may have resulted from endogenously elevated levels of corticosteroids.

The classic work of Liggins[92] in studying adrenal corticosteroid-related maturational events in the fetus showed that glucocorticoids have the general action of inducting enzyme activity. This stimulates functional lung maturation, as shown by cytodifferentiation of the type 2 cells as well as modification of the structural elements of the alveolus to improve compliance. This work made possible the understanding of studies of amniotic fluid cortisol and its levels in normal pregnancy and labor as well as its relationship to the L/S ratio. Hayden et al.[62] showed increased lecithin and L/S ratio with a decrease in phosphorylcholine transferase activity in the fetal lung of the rabbit fetus at 26 to 27 days' gestation. Peltonen et al.[120] found that both L/S ratio and palmitate and cortisol rose in the amniotic fluid from 25 to 38 weeks, while Roopnarinesingh et al.[133] reported a plasma corticoid rise at the 33rd week of pregnancy. In addition, others have found a correlation between amniotic fluid cortisol levels and the L/S ratios when the cortisol levels were over 40 nanograms per ml.[42, 148] Whittle and Hill[161] and Nwosu et al.[118] found that the early rise in the L/S ratio induced by labor brought the ratio in the premature up to the range of a fetus from a normal term pregnancy as labor continued. They concluded that there was either a rise in surfactant release or an increase in surfactant production. Zuspan and colleagues[167] and Kotas et al.[81] have both shown a rise in L/S ratio following the administration of corticoids. Lefebvre et al[87] injected 9 patients with 500 mg of hydrocortisone 48 hours before cesarean section and found increased cortisol in the maternal component in 4 hours as well as an increase in amniotic fluid cortisol and increased L/S ratio with positive foam test. These effects on amniotic fluid cortisol parallel those reported by Cohen et

TABLE 9. EFFECT OF GLUCOCORTICOIDS ON RDS INCIDENCE

	By Week of Gestation			By Fetal Weight			
	<32	*32–36*	*>36*	*1000 g*	*1001–1500*	*1501–2000*	*2001–2500*
Control	55/97 (57%)	122/287 (43%)	40/164(24%)	8/8 (100%)	41/82 (50%)	36/86 (42%)	105/273 (38%)
Corticoid	21/99 (21%)	18/200 (9%)	0/11	12/17 (71%)	8/60 (13%)	5/88 (9%)	5/53 (9%)

Data taken from references 12, 91, 104, 114, 154.

al.[28] and Bauer et'al.[8] who reported increased amniotic fluid cortisol and total blood corticoids in infants from pregnancies in which the interval after premature rupture of the membranes exceeded 16 hours. Studies illustrated in Table 9 of the effect of glucocorticoids on the incidence of RDS by week of pregnancy reveal a marked decrease in RDS incidence following administration of glucocorticoids to the mother, particularly in gestations of 32 weeks and over. Kotas and Avery,[82] using rabbits, and Knelson,[78] working with lambs, have been able to accelerate lung surfactant synthesis by the administration of hydrocortisone and prednisolone. Ewerbeck and Helwig[41] in Germany treated with prednisolone 10 premature infants who had RDS. Five of these infants died, but none as a result of hyaline membrane disease. Provenzano[125] reported preliminary beneficial results without side effects in pioneer work between 1950 and 1953.

Even though the transfer of betamethasone across the placenta is rapid, its induction effect upon the fetal enzyme system in the lung seems to take over 24 hours to afford the infant protection from RDS,[2, 5] a time sequence similar to those reported from studies on the effect of premature rupture of the membranes. Preliminary studies at our institution seem to indicate a role for prolactin in this sequence of events that has not yet been elucidated. Thus time becomes important in the management of the patient with premature rupture of the membranes. If possible, the onset of labor should be delayed for 24 hours after the onset of either preterm labor or premature rupture of the membranes.

Effects of Antibiotics (Table 10)

Rovinsky and Shapiro,[135] Lebherz and associates,[85] and Russell and Anderson[136] have all demonstrated the lack of effectiveness of prophylactic antibiotic therapy following rupture of the membranes in decreasing perinatal mortality rate. Maternal morbidity rates for endometritis, parametritis and pyelitis are all reduced by antibiotic treatment during labor and the postpartum period, because with labor there may be hematogenous spread mediated by the contractile forces of the uterus. Breese[17] reports a lowering of the fetal mortality rate from 37 to 29 per cent with antibiotics administered in labor.

All antibiotics in use today rapidly cross the placental barrier, and the obstetrician must therefore consider the effect upon the fetus whenever medication is given to the mother during pregnancy or labor, or upon the newborn during lactation.[16, 23, 73, 75, 97, 115] That these agents may have effects not immediately recognized is demonstrated by the nine-year lag between Scott and Taylor's[141] advocating chloramphenicol in obstetric infections to Kent and Wideman's[71] reporting of its toxicity, and Burns and his colleagues' description of the "gray syndrome."[21]

The fetal liver has a marked deficiency of oxidative enzymes necessary for detoxification of drugs in utero. The principal metabolic pathway is either acetylation or conjugation with uridine diphosphoglucuronic acid by the enzyme glycuronyl transferase.[1] The practical implications are impaired acetylation of sulfonamides and decreased conjugation of other antibiotics.[84, 96, 108] The sulfonamides reduce binding of proteins, resulting in an increased fraction of diffusible bilirubin, and when they are administered near the time of birth, the fetus may be delivered before the placenta

TABLE 10. EFFECT OF DRUGS ON FETUS AND NEONATE

Streptomycin	Deafness
Tetracyclines	Bone anomalies
	Dental staining
Nitrofurantoin	Hemolysis
Novobiocin	Hyperbilirubinemia
Chloramphenicol	Cardiovascular collapse
	"Gray syndrome"
Sulfonamides	Kernicterus
Kanamycin	Possible neurotoxicity
Gentamicin	Possible ototoxicity

can aid in clearance, resulting in neonatal kernicterus.[96]

Penicillin and streptomycin become highly concentrated in the fetus because of the low clearance capacity of the kidney for organic acids.[1] So far, no tolerance limits for penicillin have been exhibited, but Conway and Birt[30] report fetal deafness associated with administration of streptomycin to the mother.[108, 132] The tetracyclines pose special problems because of deposition of analogues in the tooth crown when fetal teeth are undergoing mineralization during late pregnancy, as well as deposition of tetracycline phosphorus in the skeleton and resulting growth retardation.[29, 75, 83, 128] The "gray syndrome" of chloramphenicol toxicity is secondary to the high fetal concentration of this agent and develops from the resulting inhibition of protein synthesis. This inhibition, an interference with the attachment of RNA to ribosomes, precludes the synthesis of enzymes so necessary for extrauterine existence—an effect that continues after birth.[108, 159] Novobiocin also is implicated in competitive interference with bilirubin conjugation, while the cephalosporins so far have not been shown to be toxic.[1, 20, 94, 146]

Dailey[33] has recently shown the increasing antibiotic resistance of coliform organisms in neonatal infections. Thirty-eight per cent of the species or strains were resistant to ampicillin, streptomycin and the tetracyclines, but fewer were resistant to cephalothin and kanamycin. Our preferred mode of maternal therapy in infection is large doses of penicillin (30 to 60 million units per day intravenously) in the nonallergic patient, or keflin in doses of 1 to 2 g every 4 hours in cases in which sensitive organisms are resistant to penicillin. Kanamycin has a wider spectrum of effectiveness, but its fetal nephrotoxicity and neurotoxicity are unproved. Gentamicin has potential ototoxicity but is effective when Proteus and Pseudomonas infections are superimposed.[76, 103] Clindamycin and metronidazole complete the triad covering both the aerobes and anaerobes involved. The drugs mentioned are effective primarily against the major pathogenic organisms that may invade the uterus following premature rupture of the membranes. Selection of the drug with maximum effectiveness and minimum fetal risk can therefore be made intelligently. Other modalities of therapy may be added in severe maternal infections, such as septic shock.

Preserving the immature fetus within the uterus following premature rupture of the membranes deserves not only the careful sterile diagnostic handling previously described but also isolation from the hospital environment with its virulent pathogens. Most obstetricians would prefer to maintain the patient at home, without intravaginal manipulations, recording the temperature twice daily and restricting activity. As long as the patient is afebrile and without purulent vaginal discharge this management is continued, with weekly sonograms, until fetal pulmonary maturity is diagnosed.

Diagnosing Intrauterine Infections

The diagnosis of intrauterine infection is fraught with potential danger.[45] To make sense out of the bacteriologic findings in the vagina is nearly impossible because, as Prystowsky[127] says, the microbiologic findings in specimens from the cervix, placenta and vagina are "a big sea of ignorance." Prevedourakis and his co-workers[124] found 7.8 per cent positive amniotic fluid cultures without fetal or maternal morbidity and identical organisms in both the fetal throat and urine as in the vagina and cervix, even without rupture of the membranes. Barbaro[6] found pathogens in 45 of 96 patients, 77 per cent of which were anaerobic Streptococcus or gram-negative organisms. Even the initial cultures following rupture of the membranes were positive in 33 per cent, but in only 3 per cent was actual infection established. Bobitt and Ledger[14, 15] studied amniotic fluid obtained by intrauterine catheter from 24 patients believed to be at increased risk of maternal or neonatal infectious morbidity. Their qualitative laboratory determinations of the fluid revealed fever to be a late sign of amnionitis, with heavy bacterial contamination of amniotic fluid present for many hours in the absence of fever. Gibbs et al.,[51] obtaining amniotic fluid intra-abdominally at the time of cesarean section, were unable to discriminate between the groups at high and low risk for intrauterine infection by the numbers of polymorphonuclear leukocytes per microscopic field. Wilson and his co-workers[164] found the cord to show inflammation in 39 per cent, with only 8 per cent of infants actually infected. Mandsley and associates,[99] analyzing 3000 samples from 494 cases of premature rupture of the membranes, found maternal deciduitis in 89 per cent and chorioamnionitis in 27 per cent, yet 50 per cent of the uterine cultures were negative. In studies of Hosmer and Sprunt[64] cord blood, gastric aspirate and infant blood cultures were 50 to 80 per cent negative or misleading. Pryles and his colleagues,[126] after examining 358 cases, reported that 80 per cent of infants with umbilical cord vasculitis did well without treatment; therefore they concluded that antibiotic therapy needed additional justification.

Both Listwa et al.[93] and Gassner and Ledger[50] found postpartum maternal infection in less than 10 per cent of women delivering vaginally who had evidence of intrauterine infection. Studies by the latter group showed a tenfold increase in incidence of severe infection in the patient delivering by cesarean section. Prophylactic antibiotic therapy in this group has been advocated and may be the important benefit of intra-abdominal amniotic fluid analysis before delivery.

The febrile patient, particularly with purulent or foul-smelling amniotic fluid and uterine tenderness, presents a much more ominous picture, as well as making possible a much more positive diagnostic conclusion. When amnionitis is present, Bryans and Lanier have reported 50 per cent fetal loss.[84] Pryles and his co-workers[126] found 57 per cent of babies to be ill when maternal fever was present, and Clark and Anderson[27] report 17 per cent of stillbirths and 14.4 per cent of all neonatal deaths occurring in the presence of amnionitis. The presence of infection may be difficult to document bacteriologically, but when clinically present it demands immediate uterine evacuation, in spite of the size of the infant. Procrastination at this point could well lead to severely prejudicing the mother's health while not improving fetal chances of survival. The choice of obstetric delivery is that which is most expedient.[119] Willson and colleagues[163] justify cesarean section if effective labor cannot be induced and delivery expected within 24 hours. Cesarean hysterectomy often should be the choice where induction fails and gross infection exists, particularly when further childbearing is not a factor.

Upon arrival at the delivery room, the patient whose premature rupture of the membranes has been confirmed needs confirmation of fetal gestational age by ultrasonography and, if possible, confirmation of fetal pulmonary maturity and the presence or absence of leukocytosis and positive bacterial infection by analysis of amniotic fluid either by intrauterine monitoring catheter or by amniocentesis of the uterine cavity through the abdomen. In addition, the mother needs to be evaluated for the presence or absence of fever, leukocytosis, uterine tenderness or any other sign that would lead to the diagnosis that intrauterine infection is present.

Managing the Immature Infant

That the presence of premature rupture of the membranes induces a stress acceleration of surfactant production or release has been shown by numerous authors.[8, 28, 57] The concomitant decrease in the incidence of RDS in the fetus results in an associated decreased mortality rate (see Table 6). When infants are studied by birth weight, beneficial effects of premature rupture of the membranes seem limited to those over 1000 g. Studies of Sell[142] and Berkowitz[9] indicate that a duration of ruptured membranes of 16 to 24 hours is necessary before the protective effect is maximally observed. For the patient with a preterm pregnancy who is admitted with premature rupture of the membranes, observation for that length of time needed to allow normal sequential development of an increased L/S ratio may well be considered. Fayez et al.[42] followed 74 patients observed for over 72 hours and found that 16 per cent developed intrapartum amnionitis or postpartum infection or both. They found infection in only 3 neonates but no neonatal mortality. Four of the infants under 31 weeks' gestation developed RDS. They concluded that despite the infection rate, the severity of the RDS militated against early delivery in the absence of actual intrauterine infection for the best possible result in neonatal survival.

For the patient in whom the diagnosis of premature rupture of the membranes is suspected but not proved, a latent period between admission and delivery in the uninfected case gives the opportunity to take advantage of the fact that maternal administration of corticosteroids may induce life-saving pulmonary maturity. Morrison[114] and Thornfelt[154] studied the effect of maternal glucocorticoids by week of gestation and found a marked reduction in the incidence of RDS in the infant over 32 weeks' gestation. Glucocorticoids need to be administered to have a 24-hour lag time or latent period for maximum effect.[48, 91] Meade et al.,[104] giving 6 mg of betamethasone initially and again 16 hours later, were able to reduce their neonatal mortality from 50 to 15 per cent, an effect almost entirely due to the decreased frequency and severity of RDS. Gluck et al.[53] studied 128 premature infants whose mothers had received 12 mg of betamethasone. In the 33 infants with L/S ratios under 2, the incidence of RDS dropped from 70 to 25 per cent. In the 25 patients, however, in whom premature rupture of the membranes was present, they found no appreciable additional decrease in the incidence of RDS. They concluded that betamethasone was of no significant help when premature rupture of the membranes was present.

To ensure the latent period necessary for maturation of fetal lung surfactant in the patient with premature rupture of the membranes or in the patient treated with glucocorticoids in the hope of enhancing fetal maturity, use of drugs to inhibit preterm labor may be necessary. Since the report by Fuchs et al.[49] in 1967, maternal intravenous ethanol has been used for this purpose. Barrada et al.[7] studied 89 infants whose mothers had received alcohol in the antenatal period. At the gestational interval of from 28 to 32 weeks, the infant of the alcohol-treated mother showed a significantly lower incidence of RDS, with an even greater decrease in the incidence of severe form of the disorder. Beyond 32 weeks, the same effect was not observed in the alcohol-treated group with premature rupture of the membranes. The numbers of infants developing RDS was so small that the small decrease in incidence was not thought to be significant. Recently, intravenous isoxsuprine, which seems to have an equal or greater degree of control of premature labor without the side effects of maternal alcohol intoxication, has become popular. Similar decreases in the incidence of RDS following inhibition of labor with isoxsuprine have been reported.[32, 40, 155] Currently, inhibiting labor to allow a prolonged latent period with the additive effect of premature rupture of the membranes and perhaps increased surfactant production or release secondary to the inhibiting agent is proper management of the uninfected immature infant.

Summary

Since at the present time the obstetrician is unable to effectively prevent spontaneous rupture of the membranes, his management of the patient with this condition must be im-peccable. Prompt confirmation of the diagnosis by sterile speculum examination and analysis of the leaking fluid should be followed by evaluation of fetal size corroborated by ultrasonography and fetal lung maturity by amniotic fluid analysis by L/S ratio. Culture and microscopic analysis of the fluid are also indicated for diagnosis of intrauterine infection. Induction of labor when not obstetrically contraindicated should be initiated within 12 to 24 hours in the uninfected, mature fetus, with cesarean section or cesarean hysterectomy when induction fails. The immature fetus may be allowed to remain in the uterus until it reaches pulmonary maturity, using isoxsuprine or ethanol to ensure an adequate latent period as appropriate, or until clinical infection supervenes, at which time rapid delivery with antibiotic coverage in labor is indicated.[44] At delivery, aerobic and anaerobic cultures of infant blood from two different sites should be obtained for intelligent neonatal and postpartum therapy. It is hoped that such management will result in maintaining as low a perinatal loss as is possible at the present state of our knowledge of this perplexing obstetric problem.

REFERENCES

1. Adamsons, K., Jr. and Joelsson, I.: The effects of pharmacologic agents upon the fetus and newborn. Am. J. Obstet. Gynecol. 96:437, 1966.
2. Anderson, A. M., Gennser, G., Jeremy, J. Y., Ohrlander, S., Sayers, L. and Turnbull, A. C.: Placental transfer and metabolism of betamethasone in human pregnancy. Obstet. Gynecol. 49:471, 1977.
3. Artal, R., Sokol, R. J., Neuman, M., Burnstein, A. H. and Stonkov, J.: The mechanical properties of prematurely and non-prematurely ruptured membranes: methods and preliminary results. Am. J. Obstet. Gynecol. 125:655, 1976.
4. Bada, H. S., Alojipan, L. C. and Andrews, B. F.: Premature rupture of the membranes and its effect on the newborn. Pediatr. Clin. North Am. 24:491, 1977.
5. Ballard, P. C., Granberg, P. and Ballard, R. A.: Glucocorticoid levels in maternal and cord serum after prenatal betamethasone therapy to prevent respiratory distress syndrome. J. Clin. Invest. 56:1548, 1975.
6. Barbaro, C. A.: Foetal prognosis after spontaneous premature rupture of the membranes. Med. J. Aust. 2:57, 1967.
7. Barrada, M. I., Virnig, N. L., Edwards, L. E. and Hakanson, E. Y.: Maternal syndrome. Am. J. Obstet. Gynecol., 129:25, 1977.
8. Bauer, C. R., Stern, L. and Colle, E.: Prolonged rupture of membranes associated with a decreased incidence of respiratory distress syndrome. Pediatrics 53:7, 1974.

9. Berkowitz, R. L., Kantor, R. D., Beck, G. J. and Warshaw, J. B.: The relationship between premature rupture of the membranes and the respiratory distress syndrome. Am. J. Obstet. Gynecol. 131:503, 1978.

10. Berkowitz, R. L., Bonta, B. W. and Warshaw, J. B.: The relationship between premature rupture of the membranes and the respiratory distress syndrome. Am. J. Obstet. Gynecol. 124:712, 1976.

11. Bhagwanani, S. G., Fahmy, D. and Turnbull, A. C.: Prediction of neonatal respiratory distress by estimation of amniotic fluid lecithin. Lancet 1:159–635, 1972.

12. Block, M. F., Kling, O. R. and Crosby, W. M.: Antenatal glucocorticoid therapy for the prevention of respiratory distress syndrome in the premature infant. Obstet. Gynecol. 50:186, 1977.

13. Blumenfeld, T. A., Stark, R. I. and James, L.: Determination of fetal lung maturity by fluorescence polarization of amniotic fluid. Am. J. Obstet. Gynecol. 130:782, 1978.

14. Bobitt, J. R. and Ledger, W. J.: Amniotic fluid analysis. Its role in maternal and neonatal infection. Obstet. Gynecol. 51:56, 1978.

15. Bobitt, J. R. and Ledger, W. J.: Unrecognized amnionitis and prematurity: a preliminary report. J. Reprod. Med. 19:8, 1977.

16. Bray, R. E.: Transfer of ampicillin into fetus and amniotic fluid from maternal plasma in late pregnancy. Am. J. Obstet. Gynecol. 96:938, 1966.

17. Breese, M. W.: Spontaneous premature rupture of the membranes. Am. J. Obstet. Gynecol. 81:1086, 1961.

18. Brelje, M. D. and Kaltreider, D. F.: The use of vaginal antibiotics in premature rupture of the membranes. Am. J. Obstet. Gynecol. 94:889, 1966.

19. Brumley, G. W.: Lung development and lecithin metabolism. Arch. Intern. Med. 127:413, 1971.

20. Burland, W. L., Simpson, K. and Samuel, P. D.: Combining caphaloride and streptomycin for the treatment and prophylaxis of neonatal infections. Postgrad. Med. J. (Suppl.) 46:85, 1970.

21. Burns, L. E., Hodgman, J. and Cass, A. B.: Fatal circulatory collapse in premature infants receiving chloramphenicol. N. Engl. J. Med. 261:1318, 1959.

22. Caspi, E., Schreyer, P., Weinraub, Z., Bukovsky, I. and Tamir, I.: Changes in amniotic fluid lecithin-sphingomyelin ratio following maternal dexamethasone administration. Am. J. Obstet. Gynecol. 122:327, 1975.

23. Charles, D. J.: Placental transmission of antibiotics. J. Obstet. Gynecol. Br. Emp. 61:750, 1954.

24. Chiswick, M. L.: Prolonged rupture of membranes, pre-eclamptic toxaemia, and respiratory distress syndrome. Arch. Dis. Child. 51:674, 1976.

25. Christensen, K. K., Christensen, P., Ingemarsson, I., Mardh, P. A. et al.: A study of complications in preterm deliveries after prolonged premature rupture of the membranes. Obstet. Gynecol. 48:670, 1976.

26. Clark, D. M. and Anderson, G. V.: Perinatal mortality and amnionitis in a general hospital population. Obstet. Gynecol. 31:714, 1968.

27. Clark, D. M., Anderson, G. V. and Burchell, R. C.: Premature spontaneous rupture of the membranes. Am. J. Obstet. Gynecol. 88:251, 1964.

28. Cohen, W., Fencl, M. M. and Tulchinsky, D.: Amniotic fluid cortisol after premature rupture of membranes. J. Pediatr. 88, 1007, 1976.

29. Cohlan, S. P., Bevelander, G. and Tiamsic, T.: Growth inhibitions of prematures receiving tetracycline. Am. J. Dis. Child. 105:453, 1963.

30. Conway, N. and Birt, B. D.: Streptomycin in pregnancy, effect on the foetal ear. Br. Med. J. 2:260, 1965.

31. Copeland, Jr., W. Stempel, L. and Lott, J. A.: Assessment of a rapid test on amniotic fluid for estimating fetal lung maturity. Am. J. Obstet. Gynecol. 130:225, 1978.

32. Czapo, A. I. and Herczeg, J.: Arrest of premature labour of isoxsuprine. Am. J. Obstet. Gynecol. 129:482, 1977.

33. Dailey, K. M.: Incidence of antibiotic resistance and R factors among gram-negative bacteria isolated from the neonatal intestine. J. Pediatr. 80:198, 1972.

34. Danforth, D. N., McElin, T. W. and Stites, M. N.: Studies on fetal membranes: I. Bursting tension. Am. J. Obstet. Gynecol. 65:480, 1953.

35. Delamos, R. A., Shermeta, D. W., Knelson, J. H., Kotas, R. J. and Avery, M. D.: The induction of the pulmonary surfactant in the fetal lamb by the administration of corticosteroids. Pediatr. Res. 3:505, 1969.

36. Dluholuck, Y. S., Babic, J. and Taufer, I.: Reduction of incidence and mortality of respiratory distress syndrome by administration of hydrocortisone to mother. Arch. Dis. Child. 51:420, 1976.

37. Droegemueller, W., Jackson, C., Makowski, E. L. and Battaglia, F. C.: Amniotic fluid examination as an aid in the assessment of gestational age. Am. J. Obstet. Gynecol. 104:424, 1967.

38. Eastman, N. J.: Editorial discussion of Roth, N. E.: Early rupture of the membranes: significance, etiology and prognosis. Obstet. Gynecol. Surv. 10:14, 1955.

39. Elmfors, B., Tryding, N. and Tufesson, G.: The diagnosis of ruptured fetal membranes by measurement of the diamine oxidase (DAO) activity in vaginal fluid. J. Obstet. Gynecol. Br. Commonwealth. 81:361, 1974.

40. Enhorning, G., Chamberlain, D., Contreras, C., Burgoyne, R. and Robertson, B.: Isoxsuprine-induced release of pulmonary surfactant in the rabbit fetus. Am. J. Obstet. Gynecol. 129:197, 1977.

41. Ewerbeck, H. and Helwig, H.: Treatment of idiopathic respiratory distress with large doses of corticoids. Pediatrics 49:467, 1972.

42. Fayez, J. A., Hasan, A. A., Jones, H. S. and Miller, G. L.: Management of premature rupture of the membranes. Obstet. Gynecol. 52:17, 1978.

43. Fencl, M. and Tulchinsky, D.: Total cortisol in amniotic fluid and fetal maturation. N. Engl. J. Med. 292:133, 1975.

44. Flowers, C. E.: The obstetric management of infants weighing 1000–2000 grams. J. Reprod. Med. 20:51–55, 1978.

45. Franciosi, R. A.: Fetal infection via the amniotic fluid. Rocky Mountain Med. J. 67:32, 1970.

46. Frantz, I. D., Adler, S. M., Thach, B. T., Wyzogrodski, I., Fletcher, B. D., Taeusch, H. W. and Avery, M. E.: The effect of amniotic fluid removal on pulmonary maturation in sheep. Pediatrics 56:474, 1975.

47. Freidman, M. D. and McElin, T. W.: Diagnosis of ruptured fetal membranes. Am. J. Obstet. Gynecol. 104:544, 1969.

48. Frosolono, M. F. and Roux, J. F.: Surface-active material in human amniotic fluid. Am. J. Obstet. Gynecol. 130:562, 1978.

49. Fuchs, F., Fuchs, A., Poblete, V. F. and Risk, A.: Effect of alcohol on threatened premature labor. Am. J. Obstet. Gynecol. 99:627, 1967.

50. Gassner, G. B. and Ledger, W. J.: The relationship of hospital acquired maternal infection to invasive intrapartum monitoring techniques. Am. J. Obstet. Gynecol. 126:33, 1976.

51. Gibbs, R. S., Listwa, H. M., Read, J. A., Carpenter, J. and Dobeck, A. S.: Amniotic fluid neutrophils prior to cesarean section and intrauterine infection. Obstet. Gynecol. 50:102, 1977.

52. Gilbert, J. M., Taylor, N. F. and McFadyen, I. R.: A comparison between the lecithin/sphingomyelin ratio and the nile blue sulphate test in the estimation of fetal maturity. Acta Obstet. Gynecol. Scand. 56:491, 1977.

53. Gluck, L.: Administration of corticosteroids to induce maturation of fetal lung. Am. J. Dis. Child. 130:976, 1976.

54. Gluck, L., Julovich, M. D., Borer, R. C. and Keidel, W. N.: The interpretation and significance of the lecithin-sphingomyelin ratio in amniotic fluid. Am. J. Obstet. Gynecol. 120:142, 1974.

55. Gluck, L., Kulovich, M. V., Borer, R. C., Jr., Brenner, P. H., Anderson, G. G. and Spellacy, W. N.: Diagnosis of the respiratory distress syndrome by amniocentesis. Am. J. Obstet. Gynecol. 109:440, 1971.

56. Goldkrand, J. W., Varki, A. and McClurg, J. E.: Rapid prediction of pulmonary maturity by amniotic fluid lipid globule formation. Obstet. Gynecol. 50:191, 1977.

57. Gould, J. B., Gluck, L. and Kulovich, M. D.: The relationship between accelerated pulmonary maturity and accelerated neurological maturity in certain chronically stressed pregnancies. Am. J. Obstet. Gynecol. 127:181, 1977.

58. Gunn, G. C., Mishell, D. R., Jr. and Morton, D. G.: Premature rupture of the fetal membranes. Am. J. Obstet. Gynecol. 106:469, 1970.

59. Gusdon, J. P. and Waite, B. M.: A colorimetric method for amniotic fluid phospholipids and their relationship to the respiratory distress syndrome. Am. J. Obstet. Gynecol. 112:62, 1972.

60. Habel, A. H., Sandor, G. S., Conn, N. K. and McCrae, W. M.: Premature rupture of membranes and effects of prophylactic antibiotics. Arch. Dis. Child. 47:401, 1972.

61. Harrison, R. F., Roberts, A. P. and Campbell, S. A.: A critical evaluation of tests used to assess gestational age. Br. J. Obstet. Gynecol. 84:98, 1977.

62. Hayden, W., Olsen, Jr., E. B. and Zachman, R. D.: Effect of maternal isoxsuprine on fetal rabbit lung biochemical maturation. Am. J. Obstet. Gynecol. 129:691, 1977.

63. Hellman, L. M. and Pritchard, J. A.: Williams Obstetrics, 14th ed. New York, Appleton-Century-Crofts, 1971.

64. Hosmer, M. E. and Sprunt, K.: Screening method for identification of infected infant following premature rupture of maternal membranes. Pediatrics 49:283, 1972.

65. Howard, P. J. and Bauer, A. R.: Infection in the newborn infant and its association with prolonged rupture of the amniotic membranes. Henry Ford Hosp. Med. J. 15:161, 1967.

66. Huff, R. W.: Antibiotic prophylaxis for puerperal endometritis following premature rupture of the membranes. J. Reprod. Med. 19:79, 1977.

67. Husain, O. A. N. and Sinclair, L.: Studies on the cytology of amniotic fluid and of the newborn infant's skin in relation to maturity of the infant. Proc. R. Soc. Med. 64:1213, 1971.

68. Johnson, J. W. C., Mitzner, W., London, W. T., Palmer, A. E., Scott, R. and Kearney, K.: Glucocorticoids and the rhesus fetal lung. Am. J. Obstet. Gynecol. 138:8, 1978.

69. Jones, M. D., Jr., Burd, L. I., Bowes, W. A., Jr., Battaglia, F. C. and Lubchenco, L. D.: Failure of association of premature rupture of membranes with respiratory distress syndrome. N. Engl. J. Med. 292:1253, 1975.

70. Kauppila, A., Simila, S., Ylokorkala, O., Koivisto, M., Makela, P. and Haapalahti, J.: ACTH levels in maternal, fetal and neonatal plasma after short-term prenatal dexamethasone therapy. Br. J. Obstet. Gynecol. 84:124, 1977.

71. Kent, S. P. and Wideman, G. L.: Prophylactic antibiotic therapy in infants born after premature rupture of membranes. J.A.M.A. 171:1199, 1959.

72. Kero, P., Hirvonen, T. and Valimaki, I.: Prenatal and postnatal isoxsuprine and respiratory distress syndrome. Lancet 2:198, 1973.

73. Kiefer, L.: The placental transfer of erythromycin. Am. J. Obstet. Gynecol. 69:174, 1955.

74. Kittrich, M.: Editorial. Lancet 1:132, 1972 (Geburtsh. Frauenheilkd. 26:156, 1963).

75. Klein, J. O. and Marcy, S. M.: Infection in the newborn. Clin. Obstet. Gynecol. 13:321, 1970.

76. Klein, J. O., Herschel, M., Therakan, R. M. and Ingall, D.: Gentamicin in serious neonatal infections: absorption, excretion, and clinical results in 25 cases. J. Infect. Dis. (Suppl.) 124:224, 1971.

77. Kline, A. H., Blattner, R. J. and Zunin, M.: Transplacental effect of tetracyclines on teeth. J.A.M.A. 188:178, 1964.

78. Knelson, J. H.: Environmental influence on intrauterine lung development. Arch. Intern. Med. 127:421, 1971.

79. Knudsen, F. U. and Steinrud, J.: Septicaemia of the newborn, associated with ruptured foetal membranes, discoloured amniotic fluid or maternal fever. Acta Paediatr. Scand. 65:725, 1976.

80. Korda, A. R., Lyneham, R. C. and Jones, W. R.: The treatment of premature labor with intravenously administered salbutamol. Med. J. Aust. 1:744, 1974.

81. Kotas, R. V., Kling, O. R. and Block, M. F.: Response of immature baboon fetal lung to intra-amniotic betamethasone. Am. J. Obstet. Gynecol. 130:712, 1978.

82. Kotas, R. V. and Avery, M. D.: Accelerated appearance of pulmonary surfactant in the fetal rabbit. J. Appl. Physiol. 30:358, 1971.

83. Kutscher, A. H., Zegarelli, E. V., Tovell, A. M., Hochberg, B. and Hauptman, J.: Discoloration of deciduous teeth induced by administration of tet-

racycline ante partum. Am. J. Obstet. Gynecol. 96:291, 1966.

84. Lanier, L. R., Jr., Scarbrough, R. W., Jr., Fillingim, O. W. and Baker, R. E., Jr.: Incidence of maternal and fetal complications associated with rupture of the membranes before onset of labor. Am. J. Obstet. Gynecol. 93:398, 1965.

85. Lebherz, J. B., Hellman, L. M., Madding, R., Anctil, A. and Arje, S. L.: Double-blind study of premature rupture of the membranes. Am. J. Obstet. Gynecol. 87:218, 1963.

86. Lee, K. S., Eidelman, A. I., Tseng, P. I., Kandall, S. R. and Gartner, E. M.: Respiratory distress syndrome of the newborn and complications of pregnancy. Pediatrics 58:675, 1976.

87. Lefebvre, Y., Marier, R., Amyot, G., Bilodeau, R., Hotte, R., Raynalut, P., Durocher, J. G. and Lanthier, A.: Maternal, fetal and intra-amniotic hormonal and biologic changes resulting from a single dose of hydrocortisone injected in the intra-amniotic compartment. Am. J. Obstet. Gynecol. 125:609, 1976.

88. Levitz, M., Jansen, V. and Dancis, C.: The transfer and metabolism of corticosteroids in the perfused human placenta. Am. J. Obstet. Gynecol. 132:363, 1978.

89. Lewis, J. F., Johnson, P. and Miller, P.: Evaluation of amniotic fluid for aerobic and anaerobic bacteria. Am. J. Clin. Pathol. 61:58, 1976.

90. Lipshitz, J.: Use of a beta 2-sympathomimetic drug as a temporizing measure in the treatment of acute fetal distress. Am. J. Obstet. Gynecol. 129:31, 1977.

91. Liggins, G. C. and Howie, R. N.: The prevention of respiratory distress syndrome by maternal steroid therapy. *In* Gluck, L. (ed.): Modern Perinatal Medicine. Chicago, Year Book Medical Pub., 1974, pp. 415–424.

92. Liggins, G. C.: Adrenocortical-related maturational events in the fetus. Am. J. Obstet. Gynecol. 126:931, 1976.

93. Listwa, H. M., Dobek, A. S., Carpenter, J., et al.: The predictability of intrauterine infection by analysis of amniotic fluid. Obstet. Gynecol. 48:31–34, 1976.

94. Lokietz, H., Dowben, R. M. and Hsia, D. Y-Y.: Studies on the effect of novobiocin in glycuronyl transferase. Pediatrics 32:47, 1963.

95. Lorenz, U., Ruttgers, A., Fux, G. and Kubli, F.: Fetal pulmonary surfactant induction by bromhexine metabolite VIII. Am. J. Obstet. Gynecol. 119:1126, 1974.

96. Lucey, J. F. and Driscoll, T. J.: Hazard to newborn infants of administration of long-acting sulfonamides to pregnant women (letter to editor). Pediatrics 24:498, 1959.

97. MacAulay, M. A., Abou-Sabe, M. and Charles, D.: Placental transfer of ampicillin. Am. J. Obstet. Gynecol. 96:943, 1966.

98. MacDonald, H. N. and Isherwood, D. M.: Assessment of gestational age from amniotic fluid. Lancet 1:321, 1972.

99. Mandsley, R. F., Brix, G. A., Hinton, N. A., Robertson, E. M., Bruans, A. M. and Haust, M. D.: Placental inflammation and infection. Am. J. Obstet. Gynecol. 95:648, 1966.

100. Martin, J. E.: Management of premature rupture of

the membranes. Clin. Obstet. Gynecol. 16:213, 1973.

101. Mashiach, S., Barkae, G. and Sack, J.: Enhancement of fetal lung maturity by intra-amniotic administration of thyroid hormone. Am. J. Obstet. Gynecol. 130:289, 1978.

102. McCracken, G. H., Jr.: Changing pattern of the antimicrobial susceptibilities of *Escherichia coli* in neonatal infections. Pediatrics 78:942, 1971.

103. McCracken, G. H., Jr. and Jones, L. C.: Gentamicin in the neonatal period. Am. J. Dis. Child. 120:524, 1970.

104. Meade, P. B. and Clapp, J. F.: The use of betamethasone and timed delivery in management of premature rupture of the membranes in the preterm pregnancy. J. Reprod. Med. 19:3, 1977.

105. Menzel, D. B.: Perspective and conclusions: symposium on pollution and lung biochemistry. Arch. Intern. Med. 127:373, 1971.

106. Miller, J. M., Pupkin, M. D. and Crenshaw, C.: Premature labor and premature rupture of the membranes. Br. J. Obstet. Gynecol. 132:1, 1978.

107. Mills, A. M., and Garrioch, D. B.: Use of nitrazine yellow swab test in the diagnosis of ruptured membranes. Br. J. Obstet. Gynecol. 49:38–39, 1977.

108. Mirkin, B. L.: Effects of drugs on the fetus and neonate. Postgrad. Med. 47:91, 1970.

109. Moore, W. M. O.: Assessment of gestational age from amniotic fluid. Lancet 1:493, 1972.

110. Moore, W. M. O., Murphy, P. J. and Davis, J. A.: Creatinine content of amniotic fluid in cases of retarded fetal growth. Am. J. Obstet. Gynecol. 110:908, 1971.

111. Morgan, T. E.: Biosynthesis of pulmonary surface–active lipid. Arch. Intern. Med. 127:401, 1971.

112. Morrison, J. C., Whybrew, W. D. and Bucovaz, E. T.: The L/S ratio and shake test in normal and abnormal pregnancies. Obstet. Gynecol. 52:410, 1978.

113. Morrison, J. C., Whybrew, W. D., Bucovaz, E. T., Wiser, W. L. and Fish, S. A.: Amniotic fluid tests for fetal maturity in normal and abnormal pregnancies. Obstet. Gynecol. 49:21, 1977.

114. Morrison, J. C., Whybrew, W. D., Bucovaz, E. T. and Schneider, J. M.: Injection of corticosteroids into the mother to prevent neonatal respiratory distress syndrome. Am. J. Obstet. Gynecol. 131:358, 1978.

115. Morrow, S. J., Jr., Palmisano, P. and Cassady, G.: The placental transfer of cephalothin. Pediatrics 73:262, 1968.

116. Murphy, B. E.: Cortisol and cortisone levels in the cord blood at delivery of infants with and without the respiratory distress syndrome. Am. J. Obstet. Gynecol. 119:1112, 1974.

117. Murphy, B. E. P., Patrick, J. and Denton, R. L.: Cortisol in amniotic fluid during human gestation. J. Clin. Endocrinol. Metab. 40:164, 1975.

118. Nwosu, E. C., Bolognese, R. J., Allach, E. E. and Bongiovanni, A. M.: Amniotic fluid cortisol concentrations in normal labor, premature labor and postmature pregnancy. Obstet. Gynecol. 49:715, 1977.

119. Overstreet, E. W. and Romney, S. L.: Premature rupture of the membranes—consultation. Am. J. Obstet. Gynecol. 96:1037, 1966.

120. Peltonen, J., Viinikka, L. and Laatikainen, T.: Amniotic fluid cortisol during gestation and its relation to fetal lung maturation. J. Steroid Biochem. 8:1155, 1977.

121. Perry, L. A., Isherwood, D. M. and Oakley, R. E.: Comparisons of the concentrations of palmitate and cortisol in amniotic fluid for the prediction of pulmonary maturity. Clin. Chim. Acta 83:171, 1978.

122. Plunkett, G. D.: Neonatal complications. Obstet. Gynecol. 41:467, 1973.

123. Polishuk, W. Z., Kohane, S. and Wiznitzer, N.: Premature rupture of membranes in different ethnic groups. Israel J. Med. Sci. 1:450, 1965.

124. Prevedourakis, C. N., Strigou-Charalambis, E., St. Michalas and Alvanou-Iakovakis, M.: Intrauterine bacterial growth during labor. Am. J. Obstet. Gynecol. 113:33, 1972.

125. Provenzano, R. W.: Editorial comment on Ewerbeck, H. and Helwig, H.: Treatment of idiopathic respiratory distress with large doses of corticoids. Pediatrics 49:468, 1972.

126. Pryles, C. V., Steg, N. L., Nari, S., Gellis, S. S. and Tenny, B.: A controlled study of the influence on the newborn of prolonged premature rupture of the amniotic membranes and/or infection in the mother. Pediatrics 31:608, 1963.

127. Prystowsky, H.: Management of premature rupture of membranes. Northwest Med. 64:124, 1965.

128. Rendle-Short, T. J.: Tetracycline in teeth and bone. Lancet 1:1188, 1962.

129. Reynolds, J. W.: Comment on H. Ewerbeck's letter to editor on treatment of idiopathic respiratory distress with large doses of corticoids. Pediatrics 49:467, 1972.

130. Richardson, C. J., Pomerance, J. J., Cunningham, M. D. and Gluck, L.: Acceleration of fetal lung maturation following prolonged rupture of the membranes. Am. J. Obstet. Gynecol. 118:1115, 1974.

131. Rivkind, J., and Pisani, B. J.: Premature rupture of fetal membranes. Postgrad. Med. 42:52, 1967.

132. Robinson, G. C. and Cambon, K. G.: Hearing loss in infants of tuberculous mothers treated with streptomycin during pregnancy. N. Engl. J. Med. 271:949, 1964.

133. Roopnarinesingh, S., Alexis, D., Lendore, R. and Morris, D.: Fetal steroid levels at delivery. J. Obstet. Gynecol. 50:442, 1977.

134. Roux, J. F., Nakamura, J., Brown, E. and Sweet, A. Y.: The lecithin-sphingomyelin ratio of amniotic fluid: an index of fetal lung maturity? (Letter to editor). Pediatrics 49:464, 1972.

135. Rovinsky, J. J. and Shapiro, W. J.: Management of premature rupture of membranes: I. Near term. Obstet. Gynecol. 32:855, 1968.

136. Russell, K. P. and Anderson, G. V.: The aggressive management of ruptured membranes. Am. J. Obstet. Gynecol. 89:930, 1962.

137. Ryden, G.: The effect of salbutamol and terbutaline in the management of premature labour. Acta Obstet. Gynecol. Scand. 56:293, 1977.

138. Sabbagha, R. E. and Hughey, M.: Standardization of sonar cephalometry and gestational age. Obstet. Gynecol. 52:402, 1978.

139. Sacks, M. and Baker, T. H.: Spontaneous premature rupture of the membranes. Am. J. Obstet. Gynecol. 97:888, 1967.

140. Sbarra, A. J., Michelwitz, H. and Selvaraj, R. J.: Relations between optical density at 650 nm and L/S ratios. Obstet. Gynecol. 50:723, 1977.

141. Scott, W. C. and Taylor, E. S.: The use of chloramphenicol in obstetric infections. West. J. Surg. Obstet. Gynecol. 60:36. 1952.

142. Sell, E. J. and Harris, T. R.: Association of premature rupture of membranes with idiopathic respiratory distress syndrome. Obstet. Gynecol. 49:167, 1977.

143. Shubeck, F., Benson, R., Clark, W. W., Berendes, H., Weiss, W. and Duetschberger, J.: Fetal hazard after rupture of the membranes. Obstet. Gynecol. 28:22, 1966.

144. Sivakumaran, T., Duncan, M. L. and Effer, S. B.: Relationship between cortisol and lecithin/sphingomyelin ratios in human amniotic fluid. Am. J. Obstet. Gynecol. 122:291, 1975.

145. Spellacy, W. N., Gelman, S. R. and Wood, S. D.: Comparison of fetal maturity evaluation with ultrasonic biparietal diameter and amniotic fluid lecithin-sphingomyelin ratio. Obstet. Gynecol. 51:109, 1978.

146. Sutherland, J. M. and Keller, W. H.: Novobiocin and neonatal hyperbilirubinemia. An investigation of the relationship in an epidemic of neonatal hyperbilirubinemia. Am. J. Dis. Child. 101:447, 1961.

147. Sybulski, S.: Umbilical cord plasma cortisol levels in association with pregnancy complications. J. Obstet. Gynecol. 50:308, 1977.

148. Szabo, I., Tenyi, I., Nemuth, M., Drozgyik, I. and Novak, P.: Cortisol concentrations and lecithin/sphingomyelin ratios in amniotic fluid. Lancet 1:282, 1978.

149. Taeusch, H. W., Jr., Carson, S. H., Nai San Wang and Avery, M. D.: Heroin induction of lung maturation and growth retardation in fetal rabbits. J. Pediatr. 82:869, 1973.

150. Tan, S. Y., Gewolb, L. H. and Hobbins, J. C.: Unconjugated cortisol in human amniotic fluid. J. Clin. Endocrinol. Metab. 43:412, 1976.

151. Taylor, E. S., Morgan, R. L., Bruns, P. D. and Drose, V. E.: Spontaneous rupture of the fetal membranes. Am. J. Obstet. Gynecol. 82:1341, 1961.

152. Thibeault, D. W. and Emmanouilides, G. C.: Prolonged rupture of fetal membranes and decreased frequency of respiratory distress syndrome and patent ductus arteriosus in preterm infants. Am. J. Obstet. Gynecol. 129:43, 1977.

153. Thompson, H. E.: Diagnostic Ultrasound. New York, Plenum Press, 1966.

154. Thornfeldt, R. E., Franklin, R. W., Pickering, W. A., Thornfeldt, C. R. and Arnell, G.: The effect of glucocorticoids on the maturation of premature lung membranes. Am. J. Obstet. Gynecol. 131:143, 1978.

155. Van Iddekinge, B. and Hughes, E. A.: The effect of intrauterine transfusion and a β-sympathomimetic substance on the lecithin/sphingomyelin ratio in human amniotic fluid. Br. J. Obstet. Gynecol. 84:669, 1977.

156. Warsof, S. L., Gohari, P., Berkowitz, R. L. and Hobbins, J. C.: The estimation of fetal weight by computer-assisted analysis. Am. J. Obstet. Gynecol. 128:881, 1977.

157. Webb, G. A.: Maternal death associated with premature rupture of the membranes. Am. J. Obstet. Gynecol. 98:594, 1967.

158. Webster, A.: Management of premature rupture of the fetal membranes. Obstet. Gynecol. Surv. 24:485, 1969.
159. Weiss, C. F.: Chloramphenicol in the newborn infant. N. Engl. J. Med. 262:787, 1962.
160. Whitfield, C. R. and Sproule, W. B.: Prediction of neonatal respiratory distress. Lancet 1:382, 1972.
161. Whittle, M. J. and Hill, C. M.: Effect of labour on the lecithin-sphingomyelin ratio in serial samples of amniotic fluid. Br. J. Obstet. Gynecol. 84:500, 1977.
162. Wideman, G. L., Baird, G. H. and Balding, O. T.: Ascorbic acid deficiency and premature rupture of fetal membranes. Am. J. Obstet. Gynecol. 88:592, 1964.
163. Willson, J. R., Beecham, C. T. and Carrington, E. D.: Obstetrics and Gynecology, 4th ed. St. Louis, C. V. Mosby Co., 1971.
164. Wilson, M. D., Armstrong, D. H., Nelson, R. C. and Boak, R. A.: Prolonged rupture of fetal membranes. Am. J. Dis. Child. 107:138, 1964.
165. Worthington, D., Maloney, A. H. and Smith, B. T.: Fetal lung maturity. 1: Mode of onset of premature labor. Influence of premature rupture of the membranes. Obstet. Gynecol. 49:275, 1977.
166. Yoon, J. J. and Harper, R. G.: Observations on the relationship between duration of rupture of membranes and the development of idiopathic respiratory distress syndrome. Pediatrics 53:166, 1973.
167. Zuspan, F. P., Corders, L. and Semchyshyn, S.: The effects of hydrocortisone on lecithin-sphingomyelin ratio. Am. J. Obstet. Gynecol. 128:571, 1977.
168. Zwirek, S. J. and Pitkin, R. M.: Direct spectrophotometric estimation of amniotic fluid volume. Am. J. Obstet. Gynecol. 101:934, 1968.

Editorial Comment

One of the perplexing problems that confronts the tertiary care center is the patient between 27 and 34 weeks of gestation with premature rupture of membranes. Fortunately, this occurs in but 10 per cent of pregnancies. Eighty per cent of neonatal mortality occurs in the infant less than 2500 g in weight; this category constitutes but 8 per cent of the total obstetric population. The majority of these situations involve the problem of prematurely ruptured membranes. Premature rupture of membranes is causally related to 10 per cent of all perinatal deaths irrespective of gestational age and roughly 25 per cent of all low birth weight deliveries. This chapter identifies the particular advantages and disadvantages of different management protocols. The final decision is individualization of therapy on the basis of specific findings in each patient.

The risks of delivery for the premature newborn include respiratory distress syndrome and death. These must be weighed against continuation of the pregnancy and the possibility of fetal infection that may also kill the baby or cause serious morbidity. The uterus is a marvelous organ that protects the mother from rather profound degrees of amnionitis; hence, it may be difficult to diagnose amnionitis. The key to management is an accurate assessment of gestational age, pulmonary maturity and the presence or absence of sepsis.

There is reasonable disagreement as to whether or not amniocentesis performed under ultrasound to localize a pocket of fluid should be done. Some investigators believe that vaginal amniotic fluid is generally satisfactory for maturity studies and that amniocentesis is not necessary. (Fluid collected at amniocentesis can be used for maturity studies, culture and Gram stain.)

A major point in treatment of a patient with premature ruptured membranes is to realize that the "infection clock" begins once a vaginal examination is done. Most physicians insert a sterile speculum; however, if they do not prep the vulva and perineum, the sterile speculum may introduce the bacterial flora of the labia and vestibule into the vagina, which then starts the infection clock.

Fetal age and pulmonary maturity are more significant factors in outcome than the time elapsed since rupture of membranes. Antibiotics do not seem to decrease sepsis when given prophylactically. There does not appear to be a decrease in the incidence of respiratory distress syndrome with premature rupture of membranes. One question yet to be answered concerns the use of glucocorticoids (betamethasone, dexamethasone or hydrocortisone) in the patient with premature rupture of membranes between 27 and 34 weeks of gestation. Do the glucocorticoids decrease RDS or increase the incidence of fetal sepsis or both?

The following questions should be answered in developing the management profile for each patient:

1. Are membranes ruptured?
2. Has an internal examination been done?
3. If membranes are ruptured, can the patient be observed?
4. Is the rupture a low or high leak?
5. Is the gestational age accurate? How can it be documented?
6. If amniotic fluid is available, can pulmonary maturity be identified by an L/S ratio, O.D. 650 or phosphatidylglycerol? If the fetus is mature, should the patient be delivered and by what route?
7. If there is a lack of pulmonary maturity, will glucocorticoids be used to enhance maturity?
8. If glucocorticoids are used and the patient begins in labor, should a tocolytic agent be used to postpone delivery 24 hours after completion of therapy?
9. Once a decision is made for delivery, can cesarean section be done if needed?
10. If the patient is not in labor and gestational age is less than 36 weeks, should delivery be avoided?

The best way to handle premature rupture of membranes is prevention, since answers to questions about management and therapy are far from precise and are steeped with anecdotal medicine.

4
How to Deliver the Under 1500-Gram Infant

Alternative Points of View

by Karlis Adamsons and William J. Cashore
by Watson Bowes
by Carlyle Crenshaw, Jr. and Joseph M. Miller, Jr.
by D. V. I. Fairweather and Ann L. Stewart
by J. A. Low and D. Worthington

Editorial Comment

How to Deliver the Under 1500-Gram Infant

Karlis Adamsons, M.D., Ph.D.
University of Puerto Rico School of Medicine

William J. Cashore, M.D.
Brown University Program in Medicine

Recent years have witnessed a substantial increase in the survival rate of premature infants in virtually all weight categories. Particularly gratifying have been the results for the category of infants whose birth weights approach 1500 grams. In a number of tertiary care centers the survival rates for such infants exceed 85 per cent. This percentage increases if infants born with malformations incompatible with prolonged extrauterine survival are eliminated. These developments have focused more attention on the obstetric management of patients in preterm labor to ensure maximal protection of the fetus from adverse events during the intrapartum period.

The care of a patient in preterm labor begins with a detailed explanation of the prevailing circumstances and the likely plan of management. Often the patient is referred from another institution and is meeting the medical professionals now in charge of her care for the first time. We have found it highly desirable to repeat ultrasonographic evaluation of the fetus and amniocentesis even if these tests have been performed at the referring hospital. We make every effort to ascertain the attitude of the patient toward the fetus and her willingness to accept cesarean section in case it becomes medically indicated.

Discussion regarding the prospects for the

newborn is best carried out by the neonatologist rather than the obstetrician. The predelivery period is an opportune time for the neonatologist to be introduced to the patient and her family, and also to confer with the obstetrician in charge about anesthesia and medications likely to be given during the course of labor and delivery and about mode of delivery. The majority of patients, even unmarried teenagers, will more than willingly comply with the recommendations of the physician and accept delivery by cesarean section. We have, however, encountered situations in which the patient has explicitly declined cesarean section in delivery involving prematurity and breech presentation or has not consented to fetal monitoring.

Because infants weighing about 1500 g at birth constitute less than 1 per cent of all those delivered, even institutions with large obstetric services have rarely been in the position to evaluate statistically specific management protocols. The issue has been further complicated by the nonhomogeneity of the maternal and fetal cohorts and the complex, often interdependent actions of various pharmacologic agents upon the fetus and the newborn, notably tocolytic drugs, antihypertensives, anticonvulsants, and glucocorticoids. It is noteworthy that in contrast to the voluminous literature dealing with causation and suppression of preterm labor, as well as the iatrogenic facilitation of maturation of fetal lungs, coverage of the intrapartum period from the clinical and experimental points of view is scant, particularly if one excludes the topic of delivery of the premature infant in breech presentation. This, however, should not be interpreted as implying that events during labor might not play an important or even a decisive role on outcome of the newborn. The purpose of this communication is to discuss the considerations at our institutions that currently govern the management of patients anticipated to deliver a fetus weighing approximately 1500 g.

The onset of labor before the 31st to 32nd week of gestation, at which time the fetus normally attains a weight of 1500 g, is often associated with other abnormalities of pregnancy such as maternal infection, toxemia, incompetent cervix, partial separation of placenta, multiple gestation, polyhydramnios and premature rupture of membranes. With the exceptions of clinically significant placental separation, increasing bleeding from placenta previa and progressive toxemia with or without uncontrollable seizures, such maternal conditions rarely necessitate active intervention to terminate pregnancy prematurely. Effort is directed toward correcting the underlying maternal condition in the anticipation that improvement of it may prolong the gestation and create more favorable conditions for the fetus. Emphasis is placed on correction of functional hypovolemia if such is present or is likely to be present, restoration of normal oncotic pressure of plasma by administration of albumin, reduction in maternal temperature if pyrexia is present, use of tocolytic agents and expectant management of the patient if premature rupture of membranes is not associated with clinically detectable chorioamnionitis.

Morphologic and Morphometric Considerations of the Fetus

The average singleton fetus of a healthy nonsmoking mother living at sea level reaches a body weight of 1500 g at about 31 weeks. A more rapidly growing fetus (97th percentile) will reach this body mass at 29 weeks, whereas a more slowly growing fetus (3rd percentile) will not weigh 1500 g until the conclusion of the 34th week. Since intrapartum morbidity and mortality (particularly neonatal morbidity and mortality), is a function of age of the fetus rather than its mass, it is evident that rather discrepant clinical courses are likely to be observed within this category. The mean biparietal diameter of the 1500 g fetus by ultrasonographic measurements in utero is about 7.5 to 7.9 cm. It is appreciated that at this stage of gestation, knowledge of the biparietal diameter of the fetus enables a better estimate of the gestational age than when pregnancy approaches term. The mean circumference of the head at 31 weeks is about 28.7 cm. This is 4.7 cm more than the circumference of the thorax, according to the data provided by Usher and McLean.[1] Depending on the gestational age and nutritional status of the 1500 g fetus, the difference between the circumference of the head and that of the thorax can be as much as 6.5 cm and as little as 2.5 cm. These measurements are of significance when vaginal delivery is contemplated for a fetus in breech presentation. From a small series of newborns from our experience weighing between 940 and 1380 g, we have estimated that the difference between the head circumference and that of the breech was 2.9 cm for a group of infants of appropriate weight for gestational age in contrast with a difference of 4.7 cm for a group of infants designated as "small for gestational age."

Determination of biparietal diameter by ultrasonography and careful scanning of the fetus and placenta constitute an essential evaluation of all patients in preterm labor. This procedure is recommended for all patients assumed to be more than 24 weeks from the last menstrual period, because underestimation of true fetal age and size, both by history and external measurement of the uterus, is not uncommon. It should be recalled that late in the second trimester the volume of the amniotic fluid approximately equals that of the fetus, and that even partial loss of the fluid following rupture of membranes may lead to a substantial reduction in uterine 'size. Perinatal morbidity and mortality is known to be significantly increased among infants judged to be "previable" during the intrapartum period and managed in the so-called "hands-off" manner, but found to be 1200 to 1500 g upon delivery.[2]

If hydrocephalus is suspected, efforts are made to determine the thickness of the brain cortex by ultrasonography or by computerized tomographic scanner. The fetal trunk is examined for morphologic abnormalities such as spina bifida, and the sex of the fetus is determined if technically feasible. Placenta is scanned for location and for evidence of retroplacental clots in cases of suspected partial separation of placenta. In our experience, ultrasonographic diagnosis of placental separation has been difficult. There have been sufficient instances of "false positives" to cause us not to change the course of clinical management in the absence of other findings indicative of placental separation.

Functional Maturity of the Fetus

Estimate of functional maturity of the lungs plays a major role in evaluation of any fetus to be delivered before the 35th or 36th week. The concentration of several substances in the amniotic fluid has been related to gestational age or the probability for the newborn to develop respiratory distress syndrome. Among constituents of the fluid, phosphatidylglycerol appears to predict maturation of the lung best in fetuses less than 30 weeks of age whose lung maturation has been accelerated by either prolonged interval after rupture of membranes, maternal vascular disease or

administration of beta-mimetic drugs to suppress preterm uterine contractions.[3] Determination of phosphatidylglycerol is done by chromatography. The chromatogram used for determination of lecithin/sphingomyelin (L/S) ratio is rotated by 90 degrees and different solvents are used. After the 30th week of gestation, the conventional L/S ratio, or the so-called shake test, has more than satisfactory predictive value of pulmonary maturity.[4]

The initial amniocentesis is performed with the assistance of ultrasonography to avoid the placenta and, in cases of ruptured membranes and the resultant oligohydramnios, to minimize risk of penetrating the fetus or the umbilical cord. Fetal heart rate is always recorded electronically prior to and following amniocentesis. The amniotic fluid is also examined for the presence of hemoglobin, red blood cells, white cells and microorganisms. Hemoglobin can be expected to be present in amniotic fluid after prolonged partial separation of the placenta or dissection of blood from spiral arterioles between the decidua and the chorioamnion. The presence of polymorphonuclear leukocytes even in the absence of bacteria is strongly suggestive, if not diagnostic, of at least subclinical chorioamnionitis.

Prior to the withdrawal of the needle we recommend injection of 1 g of aqueous penicillin into the amniotic cavity in all cases in which the presumed cause of preterm onset of labor is suspected to be chorioamnionitis and in which the mother is not allergic to penicillin. The concentration of penicillin in the amniotic fluid is likely to be sufficiently high to be bactericidal not only for gram-positive organisms but also for gram-negative ones.

Prenatal Use of Glucocorticoids

Liggins and Howie state that administration of glucocorticoids in conjunction with beta-mimetic drugs to suppress preterm labor reduces the relative frequency of respiratory distress syndrome, provided that a minimum of 24 hours and up to 7 days elapse between initiation of treatment and delivery.[5, 6] Beneficial effects of this treatment were most noticeable in the gestational age group from 30 to 32 weeks. Liggins and Howie's findings also indicate a reduction in intraventricular cerebral hemorrhage and possibly neonatal pneumonia. No unusual side effects were observed, with the exception of patients with severe hypertension and proteinuria in whom administration of betamethasone was associated with an increase in fetal death from 7 per cent to 25 per cent.

Administration of betamethasone to the mother leads to suppression of production of adrenal steroids both by the mother and fetus. Judged from the estriol excretion, fetal adrenal steroid production is likely to be suppressed for as long as three weeks.[7] Without disputing the findings of Liggins and Howie, we have, however, limited the use of betamethasone or other glucocorticoids to cases in which preterm delivery is decided upon for fetal or maternal indications in the absence of preterm labor or ruptured membranes, and in which analysis of amniotic fluid prior to initiation of therapy yields an L/S ratio of less than 2, or an intermediate or negative "shake test." In a few instances we have administered glucocorticoids directly into the amniotic fluid to minimize their effect on the mother, without achieving a change in L/S ratio or shake test.

The principal reason for omitting glucocorticoid treatment at our hospital has been the low frequency of respiratory distress syndrome (RDS) even among infants of 28 to 29 weeks of gestation in cases in which preterm labor had been delayed for 48 to 72 hours by administration of diazoxide. Beta-mimetic drugs have not been used as tocolytic agents except in isolated instances. The need for glucocorticoid-facilitated maturation of the fetal lung might also have been reduced at our institution owing to expectant management of patients with premature rupture of membranes and without clinical or laboratory evidence of chorioamnionitis.

We refer to the data by Gluck and his co-workers to support the contention that a minimum of 48 hours and preferably 72 hours must elapse between rupture of membranes and the evolution of pulmonary maturity of the fetus.[3] We do consider, however, using glucocorticoids if the loss of amniotic fluid after the rupture of membranes has been minimal and there has been no increase in myometrial activity. This would be particularly employed by physicians who prefer to deliver their patients routinely within 72 hours after documentation that membranes have ruptured.

Breech Presentation

The relative frequency of breech presentation early in third trimester when the fetus reaches a weight of about 1500 grams is about 12 per cent, or 3 to 4 times that observed at term. Breech presentation at 30 to 32 weeks in itself indicates higher probability of other unfavorable factors. The data of Brenner and co-workers indicate that the weight of the breech fetus at 30 weeks is only 80 per cent of the fetus in vertex presentation and that the relative frequency of congenital abnormalities is increased by a factor of 2 to 3. A breech pregnancy at 31 weeks has the probability of preterm delivery 10 times greater than that for vertex (23 versus 2.3 per cent). The fetus in breech presentation is also far more likely to die in utero prior to onset of labor than its counterpart in vertex presentation. This pertains particularly to the age group between 28 to 35 weeks. According to the same authors, the probability of stillbirth of a breech fetus between 20 and 31 weeks is 26 per cent, in contrast to only 6 per cent for the same category in the vertex presentation.[8]

There is ample documentation that vaginal delivery of the preterm breech fetus is accompanied by disproportionately higher intrapartum and neonatal morbidity and mortality than that observed following delivery by cesarean section. Principal risk factors to the fetus during vaginal delivery are compression of the umbilical cord during the negotiation of the head with resultant asphyxia and trauma to the neck and head. The head requires a 3 to 5 cm larger circumference of the cervix than that needed for passage of the thorax. Liver injuries secondary to pressure applied to the fetal abdomen during extraction of the fetus are also not uncommon. Thus, delivery of the premature infant in breech presentation in most institutions today is by cesarean section, exceptions being cases in which labor has progressed so rapidly as to make it technically impossible. Such cases may have a more favorable outcome than the group as a whole, particularly if the fetus is born in an intact amniotic sac.

The declining popularity and acceptance of external or bimanual version of the breech fetus early in the third trimester precludes one from assessing the safety and efficacy of this maneuver with any degree of precision. It appears that under select circumstances—characterized by a relaxed nonresponsive uterus, ample amount of amniotic fluid, relaxed abdominal wall of the mother, availability of continuous electronic fetal monitoring, opportunities for prompt delivery by cesarean section if necessary—version of the fetus may constitute a reasonable alternative to the traditional cesarean section. Unfortunately, such criteria are rarely present for delivery at 30 to 32 weeks.

Electronic Surveillance of the Fetus During Labor

Continuous monitoring of fetal heart rate constitutes, in our opinion, an essential component in optimal management of the premature fetus during labor. The theoretic reason for using the surveillance system is that several factors that predispose to or cause preterm labor are simultaneously at work reducing fetal oxygenation and, hence, fetal tolerance to further interruption in oxygen supply. Examples would include toxemia of pregnancy, markedly elevated body temperature, influx of certain pyrogens, partial separation of placenta and polyhydramnios. Although it has been well documented in animal experiments that at midgestation the central nervous system is more tolerant to oxygen deprivation than it is during the later part of gestation, this constitutes no advantage for the physician who wishes to depend on fetal heart rate recording to assess the state of fetal oxygenation. On the contrary, the less well-developed vasomotor reflexes of the immature fetus are less likely to permit an early identification of problems such as compression of the umbilical cord than would be expected in the case of fetuses near term. It has been suggested that hypoxic bradycardia, "late deceleration," appears in premature infants at somewhat lower hydrogen ion concentrations (higher pH) than in those near or at term.[2, 9] This might be due to the fact that the rate of rise in hydrogen ion concentration (or the rate of fall in pH) is more gradual in premature fetuses than in those near or at term; this introduces a systemic sampling error. Failure to monitor the premature fetus during labor is likely to significantly increase both fetal and neonatal mortality. In one of the larger studies on this subject, neonatal mortality of very low birth weight newborns (larger than 1000 g, however) was about two times higher in the non-monitored group than in the monitored.[2]

Baseline heart rate of 160 to 180 beats per minute is not uncommon among preterm fetuses and does not appear to indicate reduced fetal oxygenation unless combined with reduced baseline variability (a fluctuation of heart rate 3 to 6 times per minute not related to uterine contractions), or other specific heart rate patterns characteristic of hypoxia. Martin and co-workers[10] found in their detailed examination of fetal heart rate patterns in low birth weight infants that death from RDS in this moderate tachycardia group was less than that of infants with lower heart rates (less than 160 bpm), while death from other causes was increased. Marked hypoxic bradycardia, either in the form of severe late decelerations or severe variable decelerations, signals a grave prognosis for the neonate. In the aforementioned study of the 18 fetuses who exhibited such heart rate patterns, 12 developed RDS of which 7 died.

It is our practice to perform analysis of fetal blood for pH, Po_2, Pco_2, and base deficit whenever there is a substantial reduction in the variability of fetal heart during labor or when late deceleration or severe variable deceleration, irrespective of the magnitude, appears. When an experienced individual is unable to obtain a fetal blood sample in the presence of hypoxic bradycardia or loss of baseline variability, this is indicative of peripheral vasoconstriction secondary to asphyxia, and prompt delivery of the fetus is carried out by cesarean section if vaginal delivery by forceps is not applicable.

A low pH value (less than 7.20) in itself does not constitute indication for immediate delivery of the fetus unless there is additional evidence from fetal heart rate recording that fetal oxygenation is progressively declining. We take the position that after restoration of oxygen supply, which could have been temporarily curtailed by a tetanic contraction, transient maternal hypotension or adverse drug reaction, the fetus will recover more readily in utero than otherwise. We have been able to document full recovery of the fetus (pH over 7.30) after a transient episode of hypoxia during which fetal blood pH had fallen below 7.20.

Vaginal Delivery

According to earlier studies, the course of labor in preterm delivery closely resembles that of labor at term. In a sample of 480 preterm labors the duration of the first, second and third stages was essentially identical with the corresponding phases of labor in 525 term deliveries. The only distinction between the two populations was in the magnitude of postpartum blood loss. Nine per cent of patients in the premature delivery group were judged to have blood loss in excess of 600 ml or more in contrast to only 3 per cent in the term cohort.[11]

Management of labor of a preterm fetus is basically identical with that of the fetus near or at term. We do not hesitate to treat dysfunctional labor with oxytocin, provided that fetal monitoring indicates a satisfactory state of fetal oxygenation. The need for augmentation of labor, however, is infrequent even in patients who have received diazoxide previously. It is possible that augmentation of labor is required more often when the patient has received large doses of magnesium ion for treatment of toxemia or eclampsia.

Analgesics, sedatives and tranquilizers are used sparingly in preterm labor, if at all. Although well-controlled clinical studies are not available to incriminate them as hazardous if used appropriately, the obvious theoretic concerns are suppression of the cardiovascular and respiratory activity in the newborn, reduction in thermal stability, and saturation of a proportion of binding sites of protein molecules required in neonatal life for unconjugated bilirubin. Often the fetus has already been exposed to a variety of pharmacologic agents used in the treatment of the maternal condition or specifically for suppression of preterm labor. Ethanol is known to potentiate substantially the depressant properties of phenothiazines and barbiturates. When pain relief becomes necessary we recommend the use of epidural analgesia,[12] emphasizing that the agent selected has either exceedingly short half-life time in maternal plasma (2-chloroprocaine [Nesacaine]) or is firmly bound to plasma proteins and hence not readily transmitted to the fetus (bupivacaine [Marcaine]).[13, 14] This disqualifies lidocaine, which is readily transmitted to the fetus and upon delivery will remain in the newborn for a prolonged period because of its slow metabolic degradation by the immature newborn liver. A low spinal analgesia ("saddle block") is an acceptable substitute to epidural analgesia during the delivery. It does not, however, offer the flexibility of dosage and extent of sensory and motor block that epidural analgesia does. Prior to administration of either epidural or spinal analgesia it is essential that the patient be normovolemic. This is often not the case with transfer patients who might have become dehydrated as a result of transport or as a result of previously receiving medications such as diuretics and ethanol.

Pudendal block or even simple local infiltration of the perineum provides satisfactory analgesia. Neither of them, however, produces relaxation of the levator ani and produces bulbocavernous muscles, which is highly desirable to reduce soft tissue resistance of the lower birth canal. General anesthesia is rarely used in the management of patients in preterm labor to eliminate depression of the fetus by pharmacologic agents. There is also statistical evidence from earlier reports that perinatal mortality has increased by as much as 50 per cent in patients delivered under general anesthesia in comparison with those delivered under conduction anesthesia. It is difficult to ascertain what role, if any, is played by the anesthetics themselves because of the retrospective nature of most studies and the nonhomogeneity of the cohorts. No analgesia or anesthesia has also been associated with poor neonatal outcome. Since very low birth weight infants are characteristically delivered without analgesia or anesthesia, it is incorrect to infer from the data that omission of analgesia or anesthesia per se doubles or triples neonatal mortality.

Although it is probable that the principal force acting in a nonhomogeneous manner on the fetal head is transmitted by the cervix rather than the lower birth canal, it is generally agreed that episiotomy is indicated in the vaginal delivery of a premature infant. In the earlier reports, neonatal mortality for infants weighing 1500 to 2000 g was 50 per cent higher (26 as opposed to 18 per cent) if delivery took place without episiotomy.[15] It is of note that this discrepancy was even more marked in the group weighing 2001 to 2500 g, in which the perinatal mortality for patients delivered without episiotomy was 13 as opposed to 4 per cent in those delivered after episiotomy. We recommend that episiotomy be performed before the fetal vertex begins to distend the perineum. Although it may require additional effort to secure adequate hemostasis prior to its repair, it facilitates the delivery process and minimizes the need for outlet forceps.

Controversy regarding the merit of forceps in the delivery of the low birth weight infant remains unresolved. It is likely that other factors operating either during labor or delivery influence neonatal outcome more than the use of forceps. Midforceps rotation in particular can be distinctly injurious to the calvarium and its contents. Data by Brisco on 2000 premature deliveries analyzed in cohorts of 500-g increments are often referred to as validating the claim that forceps delivery is safer to the fetus than spontaneous delivery.[16] Specifically, among the 56 infants in the 1500- to 2,000-g category delivered by "prophylactic low forceps," the perinatal mortality was 5.4 per cent in contrast to 9.5 per cent among 158 infants in the same weight category delivered spontaneously. Paradoxically, in the same data the difference was smaller in the weight cohort 1000 to 1500 g, in which the alleged protective effect of the forceps should have been more discernible. The performance of a forceps delivery by necessity calls for more preparation and administration of analgesia. This inevitably introduces a systematic bias in favor of the larger infants and excludes the precipitated deliveries associated with partial separation of placenta or abnormal uterine contractions or both, which are known to increase probability of perinatal morbidity and mortality. Since we do not share the notion that the head of the 1500-g fetus benefits from forceps "protection" during its passage through the lower birth canal after an appropriate episiotomy and adequate relaxation of the muscles of the pelvic floor, we prefer not to use forceps unless there is a need to shorten the second stage of labor.

Clamping of the umbilical cord is performed after the nose and oropharynx of the infant have been carefully cleared of mucus and meconium, if these are present. No particular effort is made to clamp the cord as soon as possible in view of the fact that during the initial inspiratory efforts there is little pulmonary uptake of oxygen. It is doubtful that delaying the clamping of the umbilical cord for 1 to 2 minutes after delivery can lead to circulatory overloading of the newborn secondary to influx of blood from the placenta. Taylor and co-workers, however, noted increased frequency of tachypnea and retraction in a large group of premature infants in which cord clamping was delayed for 1 to 3 minutes compared with a group of premature infants in which cord clamping was performed immediately after delivery.[17]

Delivery by Cesarean Section

We prefer to perform cesarean section under regional analgesia rather than general anesthesia. The choice is usually between a single injection, epidural using 0.25 per cent of bupivacaine, or spinal anesthesia. Due to the relatively small size of the uterus at 30 to 32 weeks, the compression of the vena cava in supine position produces fewer circulatory problems following the administration of regional analgesia than with patients who are at term. Nevertheless, we maintain the patient in an oblique position on the operating room table prior to draping and displace the uterus manually to the left of midline once the patient is supine. We prefer to enter the abdominal cavity via a Pfannenstiel's incision, even in cases in which a fundal incision in the uterus might be necessary. The choice of Pfannenstiel's incision is not only preferable from the cosmetic point of view but it also seems to minimize postoperative discomfort and creates less strain on the wound closure during coughing and deep inspiration. Midline incision in the abdominal wall is usually reserved for emergency situations such as prolapse of the umbilical cord, marked and persistent fetal bradycardia, or profuse vaginal bleeding due to placental separation or placenta previa.

When cesarean section is performed for breech presentation, it is important to assess whether the lower uterine segment possesses sufficient width for a transverse incision to permit easy delivery of the aftercoming head. Since most of these patients have not been in labor at all or have been in labor for a short period only, the lower uterine segment is often poorly developed and essentially unsuited for a transverse or elliptical incision for breech delivery. Under such circumstances we recommend a vertical incision either in the lower half of the uterus or in the fundus, depending on the localization of the placenta. Occasionally it is possible with good uterine relaxation and an ample amount of amniotic fluid to convert the fetus from breech presentation into vertex presentation just prior to making the uterine incision. With the uterus exposed and the fetus to be delivered within minutes after such maneuver, customary reservations regarding version of the breech are unlikely to apply.

In case the obstetrician chooses to extract the fetus from breech presentation, the uterine incision must be about 15 cm in length in order to provide sufficient aperture for the aftercoming head, which is likely to have a circumference of 27 to 29 cm. We discourage the practice of beginning with a smaller incision that then requires extension either by blunt dissection or the use of scissors. These maneuvers are often difficult to perform because the trunk of the fetus fills the uterine opening. Unlike in vertex presentation, umbilical circulation is interrupted during that phase of the operative procedure, predisposing the fetus to gasping and aspiration of amniotic fluid and its contents. It has been our experience that inadequate length of the uterine incision in the delivery of the premature infant in breech presentation may constitute a serious problem for safe extraction of the head and may, on occasion, lead to a more traumatic delivery than would have occurred during delivery of the fetus via the vaginal route.

Clinical Outcome

During 1976 and 1977 there were 10,600 live births at Women & Infants Hospital of Rhode Island. These included 154 infants weighing between 500 and 1500 g, of whom 99 were delivered vaginally and 55 by cesarean section. There were 51 neonatal deaths (33.1 per cent), with 34 deaths following vaginal delivery (34.4 per cent) and 17 following cesarean section (31 per cent). Chi-square analysis showed no significant difference in mortality related to mode of delivery. Mean values for 1- and 5-minute Apgar scores and the incidence of severe asphyxia (as judged by Apgar scores of 3 or less) were likewise not related to route of delivery. The incidence of RDS was approximately 50 per cent in both groups (50 of 99 for vaginal delivery and 27 of 55 for cesarean section), but 20 of the 27 infants delivered by cesarean section required assisted ventilation, compared with 27 of 50 infants delivered vaginally. These results suggest that cesarean section per se does not increase the survival of very low birth weight infants and may instead contribute to an increased severity of neonatal respiratory distress. These latter findings are consistent with the observations of Leviton et al.[18] and also with the observed increase in respiratory distress among infants delivered by cesarean section.

Since there is no clear survival advantage conferred by cesarean section, we suggest that the vaginal route is the preferred route of delivery for infants of very low birth weight. Carefully monitored and properly managed normal labor followed by vaginal delivery should not be unduly traumatic for the preterm fetus and should allow maximum opportunity for its physiologic adaptation. Infants delivered vaginally are less likely to require mechanical ventilatory support than infants born by cesarean section. The hypothetical advantages of an "atraumatic" delivery by cesarean section may be nullified by a higher incidence of severe respiratory distress syndrome requiring assisted ventilation—conditions known to be associated with a high incidence of neonatal intracranial hemorrhage.

Cesarean section is indicated for acute fetal distress and for the usual maternal indications, properly diagnosed and documented. We recognize that certain maternal or placental complications may appear proportionately more frequently in association with preterm labor than they would at term, making cesarean section in some of these situations the best of several undesirable alternatives. We also believe that when the gestational age, properly documented, is less than 26 completed weeks, or fetal size is estimated at less than 750 to 800 g, the chances of neonatal survival are so slim as to constitute a relative contraindication to cesarean section unless maternal factors make it necessary. Finally, we think that one additional indication for cesarean delivery may be found in the small for dates fetus presenting as a breech with a malnourished body and a disproportionately large head.

REFERENCES

1. Usher, R. and McLean, F.: Intrauterine growth of live-born caucasian infants at sea level: standards obtained from measurements in 7 dimensions of infants born between 25 and 44 weeks of gestation. J. Pediatr. 74:901, 1969.
2. Paul, R. H.: Fetal heart rate monitoring and low birth weight. *In* Anderson, A., Beard, R., Brudenell, J. M. and Dunn, P. M. (eds.): Pre-term Labour. London, Royal College of Obstetricians and Gynecologists, 1978, pp. 308–314.
3. Gluck L.: *In* Anderson, A., Beard, R., Brudenell, J. M. and Dunn, P. M. (eds.): Pre-term Labour. London, Royal College of Obstetricians and Gynecologists, 1978, p. 296.
4. Gluck, L. and Kulovich, M. V.: Lecithin/sphingomyelin ratios in amniotic fluid in normal and abnormal pregnancy. Am. J. Obstet. Gynecol. 115:539, 1973.
5. Liggins, G. C. and Howie, R. N.: A controlled trial of antepartum glucocorticoid treatment for prevention of respiratory distress syndrome in premature infants. Pediatrics 50:515, 1972.
6. Howie, R. N. and Liggins, G. C.: Clinical trial of antepartum betamethasone therapy for prevention of respiratory distress in preterm infants. *In* Anderson, A., Beard, R., Brudenell, J. M. and Dunn, P. M. (eds.): Pre-term Labour. London, Royal College of Obstetricians and Gynecologists, 1978, p. 281.
7. Ohrlander, S. A. V., Gennser, G. M. and Grennert, L.: Impact of betamethasone load given to pregnant women on endocrine balance of fetoplacental unit. Am. J. Obstet. Gynecol. 123:228, 1975.
8. Brenner, W. E., Hendricks, C. H., and Bruce, R. D.: The characteristics and perils of breech presentation. Am. J. Obstet. Gynecol. 118:700, 1974.
9. Kubli, F. W., Hon, E. H., Khazin, A. F. et al.:

Observations on heart rate and pH in the human fetus during labor. Am. J. Obstet. Gynecol. 104:1190, 1969.

10. Martin, C. B., Siassi, B. and Hon, E. H.: Fetal heart rate patterns and neonatal death in low birth weight infants. Obstet. Gynecol. 44:503, 1974.

11. Cavanagh, D. and Sandberg, J.: Prematurity and urinary tract infection. II: A clinical study of 270 patients. Am. J. Obstet. Gynecol. 96:579, 1966.

12. Hodgkinson, R., Marx, G., Kim, S. et al.: Neonatal neuro-behavioral tests following vaginal delivery under ketamine, thiopental, and extradural anesthesia. Anesth. Analg. 56:548, 1977.

13. Bromage, P. R.: An evaluation of bupivacaine in epidural analgesia for obstetrics. Can. Anaesth. Soc. J. 16:46, 1969.

14. Brown, W. U., Bell, G. C., Lurie, A. O. et al.: Newborn blood levels of lidocaine and mepivacaine in the first postnatal day following maternal epidural anesthesia. Anesthesiology 42:698, 1975.

15. Cavanagh, D.: *In* Cavanagh, D. and Talisman, M. R. (eds.): Prematurity and the Obstetrician. New York, Appleton-Century-Crofts, 1969, p. 383.

16. Brisco, C. C.: Delivery of the premature infant. Clin. Obstet. Gynecol. 7:695, 1964.

17. Taylor, P. M., Bright, N. H. and Birchard, E. L.: Effect of early versus delayed clamping of the umbilical cord on the clinical condition of the newborn infant. Am. J. Obstet. Gynecol. 86:893, 1963.

18. Leviton, A., Gilles, F. H. and Strassfeld, R.: Cesarean section and the risk of neonatal intracranial hemorrhage. Trans. Am. Neurol. Assoc. 101:121, 1976.

Intensive Obstetric Management of the Very Low Birth Weight Infant

Watson Bowes, M.D.

University of Colorado Medical Center

Perinatal mortality is due predominantly to preterm births, with 85 per cent of neonatal deaths occurring in the small proportion of infants born at less than 37 weeks' gestation.[1] Helen Chase, statistician in the Office of Research and Statistics of HEW, writing about the current trends in perinatal mortality, states that physicians, parents, hospitals and the government must join in an effort to reduce the 100,000 annual perinatal deaths that occur in this country each year.[2] She suggests that this endeavor must focus on two areas: prevention of low birth weight in infants and improvement of medical care required for infants weighing 2500 grams or less. Without belittling the importance of prevention, this paper will deal with some of the questions about intrapartum and immediate neonatal management of low birth weight preterm infants, especially those very small infants weighing 1500 g or less.

All patients who are pregnant should be carefully evaluated for abnormalities that forewarn of potential preterm births.[3-6] Remediable conditions such as anemia, urinary tract infection, hyperthyroidism and incompetent cervix should be identified and corrected wherever possible. Intercurrent conditions associated with preterm deliveries such as diabetes, preeclampsia, renal disease and cigarette smoking should be treated meticulously to prolong gestation to its maximum without incurring serious fetal jeopardy. Women who are experiencing increased uterine activity should be treated with limitation of movement, increased recumbency in the lateral decubitus position or pharmacologic agents to prevent or control premature dilatation of the cervix. Patients with one or more previous preterm births or those who have had second trimester abortions are particularly susceptible to recurrent delivery of low birth weight infants and must be evaluated extremely closely throughout pregnancy for any conditions that might be amenable to change or treatment.

When preterm labor occurs spontaneously or must be induced because of fetal jeopardy, two important issues that are discussed in other chapters must be faced by the patient's physician.

1. Should corticosteroids be given to the mother in an effort to enhance lung maturity

and reduce the risk of hyaline membrane disease?[7] With rare exceptions, corticosteroids have not been used on the obstetric service at the University of Colorado Medical Center. (The risks and benefits of this therapy are discussed elsewhere in this volume.)

2. Should labor be inhibited with tocolytic drugs?[8,9] A small proportion of patients will be candidates for and respond to labor inhibition of this kind, and we advocate the use of these drugs in selected cases. However, we do so with reservation, realizing the paucity of well-controlled prospective studies and long-term follow-up of the infants to document the effectiveness and safety of these agents. When the appropriate contraindications are invoked, only 25 per cent of patients who enter a hospital in preterm labor are candidates for tocolytic therapy[10, 11] and of those, about 20 to 30 per cent will not respond to the treatment.

Even if optimal prenatal screening and labor inhibition practices are followed, there will be a significant group of patients who will inevitably deliver a low birth weight infant. Such patients are characterized by one of the following situations:

1. Spontaneous idiopathic preterm labor in which the patient does not respond to tocolytic therapy.

2. Premature rupture of membranes followed by the onset of labor.

3. Amnionitis that may occur with fetal membranes intact or may follow a prolonged time lapse after rupture of membranes.

4. Third trimester placental hemorrhage from either placenta previa or premature separation of the placenta.

5. Multiple pregnancy.

6. Intercurrent illness in which labor ensues and the mother is too ill to tolerate treatment with tocolytic agents; for example, acute infectious diseases, cardiac disease, severe respiratory distress and so forth.

7. Intercurrent illness in which the infant must be delivered because the maternal condition is worsening or because fetal tests indicate uncorrectable uteroplacental insufficiency; for example, severe preeclampsia, diabetes mellitus, severe erythroblastosis fetalis and so forth.

It is to the patients who will have an inevitable preterm birth that the following discussion applies. More specifically, the discussion will deal with those patients in whom the fetal birth weight is expected to be less than 1500 g and the gestational age less than 32 weeks. Larger premature infants (1500 to 2500 g) have had good enough survival rates for long enough to encourage obstetricians and pediatricians to treat mothers and infants in this situation with all of the intensive care resources, fully expecting survival to occur in most cases. However, in very low birth weight infants (less than 1500 g) the attitude and expectation about survival and long-term outcome are not so clear-cut; thus the perinatal management is much less easily formulated. Management is often determined by a certain perinatal pessimism that is characterized by some long-held beliefs. One such belief is that most babies whose birth weights are less than 1500 g do not survive regardless of the obstetrical and neonatal effort expended. It is believed that if they do survive, they are subject to such high risks of long-term developmental handicap as to make intervention that carries risks to the mother (e.g., fetal monitoring or operative delivery) not worthwhile. Another belief is that patients in preterm labor with a very low birth weight infant should be given a guarded (often dismal) prognosis about their infant to forewarn them of the inevitably poor outcome and, in some measure, to explain why more vigorous obstetric and neonatal efforts should not be invoked. There is often a sense of relief when the fetus or neonate dies because of the suffering (financial and emotional) that would otherwise have occurred with the prolonged hospitalization and expense of neonatal intensive care, not to mention the burden of a handicapped child.

More recent literature about the survival and long-term follow-up of infants weighing less than 1500 g hardly supports such a negative attitude. Data from several institutions demonstrate the gradually improving trend of neonatal survival in very low birth weight infants.[12–18] Perhaps even more encouraging is improvement in long-term development in the survivors, which is reported by a number of studies that are documented in Table 1.[19–27] Whereas original studies by Lubchenco and her colleagues reported a 70 per cent incidence of severe developmental handicaps in very low birth weight survivors born in the 1950s,[28] Stewart and her colleagues are now finding up to 90 per cent normal survivors in preterm infants of similar birth weight born

TABLE 1. FOLLOW-UP STUDIES OF LOW BIRTH WEIGHT INFANTS

AUTHOR AND LOCATION	YEARS OF BIRTH AND WEIGHT OF INFANTS	NUMBER		TESTS AND EXAMINATIONS	FOLLOW-UP PERIOD	% NORMAL	REFERENCE
Lubchenco U. Colorado Medical Center, Denver	1947–1953 1500 g or less	Admitted Survived Studied	446 254 133	Physical Neurologic Ophthalmologic Audiologic Intelligence and Developmental	10 yr	32	19
Janus-Kukulska Warsaw Medical Academy, Poland	1950–1958 1250 g or less	Admitted Survived Studied	542 140 67	Physical Neurologic Ophthalmologic Audiologic Intelligence and Developmental	3 to 12 yr	37	20
Drillien U. Edinburgh, Scotland	1955–1960 1360 g or less	Admitted Survived Studied	? 50 48	Intelligence and Developmental	5 yr or more	42	21
Wright U. Chicago	1952–1956 1500 g or less	Admitted Survived Studied	159 70 67	Physical Neurologic Ophthalmologic Audiologic Intelligence and Developmental	10 yr	46 (IQ > 90)	22
Fitzhardinge Royal Victoria Hospital	1960–1966 880– 1250 g	Admitted Survived Studied	118* 39 32	Physical Neurologic Ophthalmologic Audiologic Intelligence and Developmental	5 yr	31	23
Francis-Williams Hammersmith Hospital, London	1961–1968 1500 g or less	Admitted Survived Studied	? 123 105	Intelligence and Developmental	4 to 12 yr	72 IQ 90 or more 49 IQ 100 or more	24
Stewart U. College Hospital, London	1966–1970 501– 1500 g	Admitted Survived Studied	197 98 95	Physical Ophthalmologic Audiologic Intelligence and Developmental	2 yr 10 mo to 7 yr 10 mo	90	25
Fitzhardinge Montreal Childrens Hospital, Quebec	1970–1972 1500 g or less	Admitted Survived Studied	153 80 67	Neurologic Intelligence and Developmental	12 mo	87	26
Hommers Coventry Maternity Hospital, England	1973–1974 1500 g or less	Admitted Survived Studied	103 47 42	Physical Developmental	9 to 31 mo	98	27

*Only average for gestational age infants.

TABLE 2. RELATIONSHIP OF BIRTH INJURY AS SHOWN BY 1–MINUTE APGAR SCORE TO NEONATAL MORTALITY IN LOW BIRTH WEIGHT INFANTS (UNIVERSITY OF COLORADO MEDICAL CENTER 1970–1974)

BIRTH WEIGHT (G)	NEONATAL MORTALITY	
	Apgar < 5	Apgar 5 or More
501–1000	29/32 (90%)	3/9 (33%)* p = < .01
1001–1500	24/48 (50%)	11/42 (26%)* p = < .05
501–1500	53/80 (66%)	14/51 (27%)* p = < .01

*p values were derived from chi-square determinations with correction for continuity.
Birth injury included one or more of the following: intracranial, spinal cord, bone or nerve injury, significant hematomas including cephalohematomas and rupture of viscera.

in the 1970s.[25] One might surmise that this improvement has resulted from the increasing sophistication of neonatal intensive care.

In the period from July 1, 1970 to June 30, 1974 at the University of Colorado Medical Center, during which time there were 9263 live births, there were 131 infants born weighing between 501 to 1500 g. The overall neonatal mortality of these infants was 54 per cent. Both low Apgar score at 1 minute and birth trauma were found to be associated with increased neonatal mortality as documented in Tables 2 and 3, respectively. It is possible that the high mortality and morbidity of the tiny preterm infant may be related in some way to intrapartum asphyxia or trauma and that measures to minimize the hazards of labor and delivery might result in additional improvements in survival potential for these infants.

Intensive Perinatal Management of Very Low Birth Weight Infants

A policy of intensive intrapartum and immediate neonatal management was instituted on the perinatal service at the University of Colorado Medical Center in January 1975, for all very low birth weight infants (1500 g or less). This included first the presence of an experienced staff obstetrician and neonatologist at the delivery of every infant whose expected birth weight was less than 1500 g. A second requirement was continuous fetal heart monitoring during labor whenever possible, with cesarean section being utilized for fetal distress in a manner similar to its use in term infants, and whenever possible for all noncephalic presentations. Also part of the policy was vigorous resuscitation of all infants born with any evidence of life. Present at each delivery was a resuscitation team headed by a staff neonatologist and including a pediatric resident and neonatal intensive care nurse. Prompt endotracheal intubation and ventilatory support with the Gregory C-PAP apparatus was accomplished in all infants who were significantly depressed or in whom adequate ventilation could not be maintained with a bag and mask. The prevailing philosophy and operating protocol was that all of these babies were potential survivors and undue trauma or asphyxia was avoided whenever possible.

Neonatal and perinatal mortality data in this two-year period are shown by 100-g birth weight groups in Figure 1. There were no survivors among infants weighing 501 to 600

TABLE 3. EFFECT OF BIRTH INJURY AS SHOWN BY APGAR SCORE ON NEONATAL MORTALITY IN LOW BIRTH WEIGHT INFANTS (UCMC 1970–1974)

BIRTH WEIGHT (G)	NEONATAL MORTALITY	
	Birth Injury	No Birth Injury
501–1000	2/2 (100%)	35/39 (90%)* ns
1001–1500	11/15 (73%)	24/85 (28%)* p = < .01
501–1500	13/17 (76%)	59/124 (48%)* p = < .05

*p values were derived from chi-square determinations with correction for continuity.

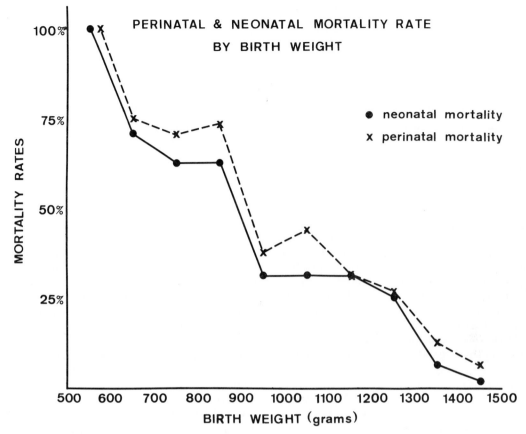

Figure 1. Neonatal and perinatal mortality rates by 100-g birth weight increments for infants with birth weights of 501 to 1500 g born at University of Colorado Medical Center during the two-year period 1975–1976.

g, but one third of those infants between 601 to 900 g lived, as did two thirds of those weighing 901 to 1300 g. When these data were compared with data from two previous periods at the same hospital (1958 to 1968 and 1970 to 1974) a substantial improvement in mortality was found for infants weighing 1500 g or less (Tables 4, 5 and 6).

In the 1958 to 1968 period, a premature infant nursery was part of the facility, and intravenous therapy, oxygen support and temperature maintenance were utilized, but only occasionally was ventilator support used. During this period there was no electronic monitoring of high-risk patients in labor. In the 1970 to 1974 period the intensive care nursery was fully operational with complete ventilatory support available and widely used. Intrapartum continuous fetal heart monitoring and fetal scalp sampling were standard procedures in the delivery unit, and intravenous alcohol was used to inhibit contractions in preterm

TABLE 4. NEONATAL MORTALITY RATES OF ALL INFANTS WITH BIRTH WEIGHTS < 1500 GRAMS (UCMC)

PERIOD		NEONATAL MORTALITY RATES
1958–1968	n = 299	60%
		NS
1970–1974	n = 131	55%
		*p = < .01
1975–1976	n = 166	32%

*p values were derived from chi-square determinations with correction for continuity.
The number of very low birth weight infants in the first 2 years was 30 per year and in 1975–1976, 80 per year.

TABLE 5. COMPARATIVE NEONATAL MORTALITY RATES IN INFANTS
WITH BIRTH WEIGHTS 1001–1500 GRAMS (UCMC)

PERIOD		NEONATAL MORTALITY RATES	
1958–1968	n = 190	44%	
			NS
1970–1974	n = 90	37%	
			*p < .01
1975–1976	n = 110	20%	

*p values were derived from chi-square determinations with correction for continuity.

Significant improvement in neonatal mortality in the 1975–1976 period was associated with an increase in number of births from 20 to 55 per year.

labor before 35 weeks' gestation. However, meticulous fetal monitoring and vigorous intervention was not the practice in babies under 1500 g, and deliveries were attended by first- or second-year members of the obstetric and pediatric house staff without neonatal nursing or staff support in the delivery room. It is interesting that there was no significant difference in survival rates between the 1958 to 1968 period and the 1970 to 1974 period. Yet, when very experienced individuals committed to intensive support of the fetus and newborn were present in the perinatal situation in the 1975 to 1976 period, there was a dramatic and statistically significant improvement in neonatal survival. Long-acting corticosteroids were not administered to the patients in preterm labor in any of the three study periods; consequently, the improved neonatal survival figures were achieved without the use of pharmacologic measures to accelerate pulmonary maturation. This suggests that attitudes and experience, not simply facilities and equipment, play a strong role in improving the outcome of the very small infant. Data in the medical literature and from our institution provide some clues to explain the improved outcome in very low birth weight infants when a more aggressive perinatal management is used.

INTRAPARTUM ASPHYXIA

Intrapartum asphyxia is regarded as dangerous to a full-term infant, and there is some evidence that fetal heart rate patterns suggestive of umbilical cord compression (severe variable decelerations) or uteroplacental insufficiency (late decelerations) are predictive of a high incidence of hyaline membrane disease in low birth weight infants. Studies at Harbor General Hospital (UCLA) by Hobel and his colleagues[30] and at Los Angeles County Hospital (USC) by Martin and his associates[31] document a higher incidence of hyaline membrane disease in infants who had "ominous" fetal heart rate patterns in labor. Both of these studies were confined largely to infants with birth weights in excess of 1500 g. Paul, reporting a more recent study from Los Angeles County Hospital, has confirmed the improved neonatal survival in very low birth weight preterm infants achieved with continuous fetal monitoring in labor.[32] In New London, Ontario, Low and his co-workers have reported that low birth weight infants are more likely to demonstrate fetal heart rate patterns associated with intrapartum asphyxia than are larger, full-term infants.[33] The same study also showed a significant relationship between abnormal heart rate patterns and fetal asphyxia

TABLE 6. COMPARATIVE NEONATAL MORTALITY RATES IN INFANTS
WITH BIRTH WEIGHTS 501–1000 GRAMS (UCMC)

PERIOD		NEONATAL MORTALITY RATES	
1958–1968	n = 108	90%	
			NS
1970–1974	n = 41	91%	
			*p < .01
1975–1976	n = 56	55%	

*p values were derived from chi-square determinations with correction for continuity.

Significant improvement in neonatal mortality in the 1975–1976 period was associated with an increase in the number of births from 10 to 28 per year.

as determined by measurements of umbilical artery buffer base. Worthington and Smith at Queen's University, Kingston, Ontario, studied the effect of intrapartum fetal asphyxia on the incidence of respiratory distress syndrome (RDS) in premature infants.[34] They found that when the lecithin/sphingomyelin (L/S) ratio was more than 2, RDS developed in 6 of 18 infants, while no RDS developed in the preterm infants with L/S ratios more than 2 when there was no intrapartum asphyxia. Kenny and his associates from Baylor College of Medicine related cord blood gas data and lactic acid concentrations to the subsequent development of hyaline membrane disease.[35] Those infants born after 31 weeks' gestation who developed hyaline membrane disease had significantly higher hydrogen ion concentrations than those infants who did not develop the disease. In the 34 infants between 26 and 31 weeks, however, cord blood hydrogen ion concentrations bore no relationship to the development of hyaline membrane disease.

Finally, autopsies in newborns suggest a correlation between birth asphyxia and subependymal and subarachnoid hemorrhage, which are frequent complications in low birth weight infants.[36] There is, therefore, evidence that intrapartum hypoxia and asphyxia lead to higher perinatal morbidity and mortality in low birth weight infants, and current methods of fetal monitoring in labor can identify the patient with significant fetal distress.

INTRAPARTUM TRAUMA

What part birth trauma due to mechanical factors plays in the high mortality and morbidity of preterm birth is not a settled issue. Nor is there any consensus about the best method of protecting the low birth weight infant from mechanical birth trauma. In 1977, Goldenberg and Nelson reviewed the outcome of vaginal breech delivery in infants weighing less than 2500 g.[37] They concluded that morbidity and mortality in these infants was higher than could be accounted for on the basis of prematurity and suggested that prophylactic cesarean section should be considered for all premature breech fetuses when delivery is anticipated. Cruikshank and Pitkin, in a later article, emphasized that there were no data proving conclusively that cesarean section is safer than vaginal delivery for the premature infant in breech presentation or that the benefits of prophylactic cesarean section for premature breech infants outweigh the added maternal morbidity that would result from such a policy.[38] More recently a study from Lund, Sweden, compared 42 preterm infants in breech presentation delivered by cesarean section with 48 infants delivered vaginally as breeches.[39] Evaluating the mortality and the long-term morbidity, the vaginally delivered infants had a significantly higher incidence of poor outcomes. Specifically, there was a greater frequency of babies who died of intracranial hemorrhage or who survived with cerebral palsy among those delivered vaginally than among those delivered by cesarean section. Stewart, reporting from University College Hospital in London, documented the improvement in survival among infants weighing less than 1500 g. She states that the most significant obstetric factor to be correlated with the improved outcome is a higher cesarean section rate in the survivors than in the nonsurvivors.[40]

The relationship between method of delivery and perinatal mortality at the University of Colorado Medical Center during the 1975 to 1976 period of intensive perinatal management of very low birth weight infants is shown in Table 7. The lower mortality of infants in noncephalic presentation (largely breeches), delivered by cesarean section, is consistent with the findings of other authors mentioned previously; but because this was not a prospectively controlled study, it cannot be used as proof of the superiority of cesarean section

TABLE 7. EFFECT OF PRESENTATION AND DELIVERY METHOD ON NEONATAL MORTALITY OF VERY SMALL PREMATURE INFANTS (UCMC 1975–1976)

Weight (G)	Cephalic Presentation		Noncephalic Presentation	
	Vaginal Del.	*C Section*	*Vaginal Del.*	*C Section*
501–1000	14/28 (50%)	3/7 (43%)	7/8 (88%)*	5/14 (36%)*
1001–1500	10/63 (16%)	6/18 (33%)	3/8 (37%)	3/19 (16%)

*p < .025.

p values were derived from chi-square determinations with correction for continuity.

as a means of delivering the small preterm infant. Although there is no conclusive study demonstrating that cesarean section protects the preterm infant from the trauma of vaginal delivery, it is our feeling that the weight of the evidence at this time justifies, if it does not dictate, a liberal use of abdominal delivery, especially in the case of breech presentations. It should be emphasized that even cesarean section must be done with special expertise and the small infant delivered in the most gentle manner to avoid undue trauma.

NEONATAL RESUSCITATION

Important in the continuum of intensive perinatal care is the immediate resuscitation of low birth weight infants. Ranck and Windle demonstrated the permanent central nervous system lesions that occur in newborn monkeys subjected to birth asphyxia in a controlled experimental situation.[41] Retrospective studies at the Princess May Hospital, Newcastle

upon Tyne, showed that preterm infants weighing between 1000 and 2000 g had a significantly improved survival rate if prompt resuscitation occurred in the delivery room prior to transfer to the neonatal intensive care unit.[42] It is frequently difficult to assess the "survivability" of small preterm infants by their appearance immediately after birth. The Apgar score, which depends to a great extent on muscle tone, is often low in small preterm infants. Figure 2, illustrating the 1-minute Apgar score of infants born during the 1975 to 1976 period, demonstrates that 39 per cent of the survivors had Apgar scores of 3 or less at 1 minute.[27] Figure 3 shows that 11 per cent of the survivors had an Apgar score of 3 or less even at 5 minutes. This suggests that predictions about survival based on the infant's immediate appearance can be quite deceptive.

We believe that the condition of the infant in the first few minutes of life is so poorly predictive of eventual survival that babies with any sign of life should be resuscitated and decisions about viability postponed until ad-

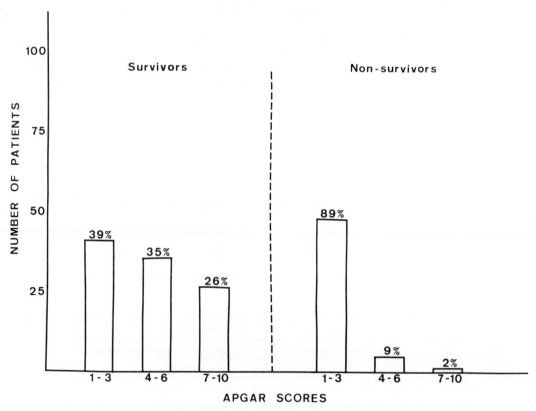

Figure 2. Distribution by one-minute Apgar scores of infants with birth weights of 501 to 1500 g born at the University of Colorado Medical Center in the two-year period 1975–1976.

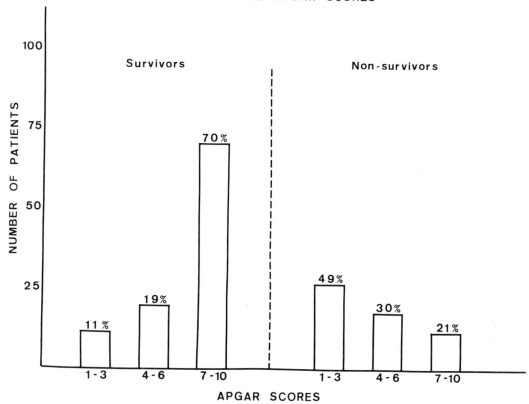

Figure 3. Distribution by five-minute Apgar scores of infants with birth weights of 501 to 1500 g born at the University of Colorado Medical Center in the two-year period 1975–1976.

ditional data about accurate birth weight, response to ventilation and so forth can be assessed. Moreover, it is important to have very skilled pediatricians conduct the resuscitation of small preterm infants and to have immediately available the proper equipment to support ventilation (Gregory C-PAP apparatus, proper endotracheal tubes), maintain body temperature, evaluate blood pressure and augment blood volume. This policy will not needlessly prolong survival in babies who will ultimately die but will save some infants who would otherwise succumb without resuscitation.

Figure 4 is a histogram showing data on those babies between 501 and 1500 g who died in the neonatal period; the vast majority (75 per cent) did so within the first 72 hours after birth.[27] Only 13 per cent of the deaths occurred after the 12th day. Moreover, long-term follow-up studies of premature infants with birth weights of less than 1500 g currently

being conducted at the University of Colorado Medical Center by Lubchenco have so far demonstrated no greater incidence of handicaps in those infants born during the period of intensive perinatal management (1975 to 1976) than in those born in the year before that.

Limits of Intensive Perinatal Management

Results achieved by a policy of intensive perinatal management of very low birth weight infants raise the question of the low limit of gestational age or birth weight in which vigorous obstetric and immediate neonatal intervention should be employed. We have selected 26 weeks' gestation and estimated fetal weight of 600 g. We have found that we consistently underestimate fetal weight (250-g

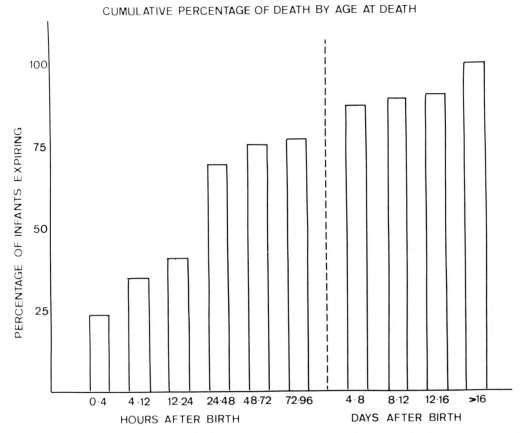

Figure 4. This histogram illustrates the cumulative percentage of all deaths by hour of death among infants with birth weights 501 to 1500 g born at the University of Colorado Medical Center in the two-year period 1975–1976.

error below 1000 g and 400-g error between 1000 and 1500 g), even when real-time ultrasonography is used. Rarely was a baby's actual weight in excess of the estimated fetal weight. A 200-g difference in fetal weight below 1000 g can make a substantial difference in prognosis.

Survivors below 26 weeks' gestation and below 500 g are extraordinarily rare. In our series, during the two-year period, no baby below 600 g survived. Pulmonary and central nervous system development prior to this time in almost all cases appears not to have progressed enough for even the most sophisticated supportive measures to be useful. The survival data reported in this study were achieved without the use of corticosteroids to enhance fetal pulmonary maturation. It remains to be seen what the improvements in technology or measures to enhance maturity in utero with pharmacologic agents will mean to survival in the very low birth weight infant.

Cost of Intensive Perinatal Care

The cost of intensive perinatal care is high and is sometimes used as an excuse to withhold care from very low birth weight infants in hopes of sparing a family undue financial indebtedness. Pomerance and his colleagues at Cedars-Sinai Medical Center (UCLA) have recently published data about the cost of intensive care of premature infants weighing 1000 g or less.[43] These are the preterm infants who are most likely to have a multitude of complications of prematurity, very prolonged hospitalizations and, as a consequence, the most extraordinary expenses. Those infants who survived had average daily costs of $450 while those who died had costs of $825. A comparison of total costs per patient for those admitted to a neonatal intensive care unit with costs for severely ill patients admitted to an adult intensive care unit is illustrated in Table 8 and puts the matter in somewhat clearer

TABLE 8.   COMPARATIVE COSTS OF ADULT AND NEONATAL INTENSIVE CARE

	NEONATAL INTENSIVE CARE INFANTS 1000 G OR LESS[40]	ADULT INTENSIVE CARE CLASS 4 (SEVERELY ILL) PATIENTS[41]
No. patients studied	75	226
No. survivors (1 yr)	30 (40%)	62 (27%)
No. normal survivors	19 (63%)	27 (43%)
Cost per patient	$24,656.	$ 17,037.
Cost per normal survivor	$88,058.	$142,606.

Data from Pomerance, J. J., et al.[40] and Cullen, D. J., et al.[41]

Cost figures of intensive care of infants weighing 1000 g or less at Cedars-Sinai Hospital in Los Angeles are compared with costs of adult intensive care at Massachusetts General Hospital. Class 4 includes primarily postoperative patients who were critically ill prior to or as a result of a surgical procedure, excluding cardiopulmonary bypass operations.

perspective.[44] Not only does the neonatal intensive care unit result in a higher percentage of normal survivors (63 as opposed to 43 per cent), but it does so at a lower cost per normal survivor ($88,058 as opposed to $142,606).

Summary

There are now data to suggest that very small preterm infants (birth weight 1500 g or less) will benefit from an intensive approach to perinatal management. Measures that have been utilized to protect larger infants from birth asphyxia and trauma, such as fetal heart monitoring, judicious use of cesarean section and vigorous but expert resuscitation of all infants born with signs of life, should be employed for infants with expected birth weights as low as 600 g. It is essential that the most experienced and talented physicians and nurses supervise and participate in the care of these infants with the highest perinatal risk. With such a program of intensive perinatal care, one can expect the survival of one third of infants weighing 601 to 900 g, two thirds of those weighing 901 to 1300 g, and 90 per cent of those weighing more than 1300 g.

REFERENCES

1. Rush, R. W., Keirse, M. J. N. C., Howat, P. et al.: Contribution of preterm delivery to perinatal mortality. Br. Med. J. 2:965, 1976.
2. Chase, H. C.: Perinatal mortality: overview and current trends. Clin. Perinatol. 1:3, 1974.
3. Papiernik-Berkhauer, E. and Kaminski, M.: Multifactorial study of the risk of prematurity at 32 weeks of gestation. I. A study of the frequency of 30 predictive characteristics. J. Perinatal Med. 2:30, 1974.
4. Donahue, C. L. and Wan, T. T. H.: Measuring obstetric risks of prematurity: A preliminary analysis of neonatal death. Am. J. Obstet. Gynecol. 116:911, 1973.
5. Johnson, J. W. C., Austin, K. L., Jones, G. S. et al.: Efficacy of 17 alpha-hydroxyprogesterone caproate in the prevention of premature labor. N. Engl. J. Med. 293:675, 1975.
6. Keirse, M. J. N. C., Rush, R. W., Anderson, A. B. M. et al.: Risk of pre-term delivery in patients with previous pre-term delivery and/or abortion. Br. J. Obstet. Gynecol. 85:81, 1978.
7. Liggins, G. C. and Howie, R. N.: A controlled trial of antepartum glucocorticoid treatment for prevention of the respiratory distress syndrome in premature infants. Pediatrics 50:515, 1972.
8. Zlatnik, F. J. and Fuchs, F.: A controlled study of ethanol in threatened premature labor. Am. J. Obstet. Gynecol. 112:610, 1972.
9. Niebyl, J. R., Blake, D. A., Johnson, J. W. C. et al.: The pharmacological inhibition of premature labor. Obstet. Gynecol. Surv. 33:507, 1978.
10. Zlatnik, F. J.: The applicability of labor inhibition to the problem of prematurity. Am. J. Obstet. Gynecol. 113:704, 1972.
11. Baillie, P., Malan, A. F., Saunders, M. C. et al.: The active management of pre-term labour and its effect on fetal outcome. Aust. N.Z. J. Obstet. Gynaecol. 16:94, 1976.
12. Behrman, R. E., Babson, G. S. and Lessel, R.: Fetal and neonatal mortality in white middle-class infants. Mortality risks by gestational age and weight. Am. J. Dis. Child. 121:486, 1971.
13. Lubchenco, L. O., Searles, D. T. and Brazie, J. V.: Neonatal mortality rate: relationship to birth weight and gestational age. J. Pediatr. 81:814, 1972.
14. Alden, E. R., Mandelkorn, T., Woodrum, D. E. et al.: Morbidity and mortality of infants weighing less than 1000 grams in an intensive care nursery. Pediatrics 50:40, 1972.
15. Kitchen, W. N. and Campbell, D. G.: Controlled trial of intensive care for very low birth weight infants. Pediatrics 48:711, 1971.
16. Malan, A. F., Vader, C. and Knutzen, V. K.: Fetal and early neonatal mortality. S. Afr. Med. J. 49:1079, 1975.
17. Lee, K., Tseng, Po-I., Eidelman, A. I. et al.: Determinants of neonatal mortality. Am. J. Dis. Child. 130:842, 1976.
18. Usher, R.: Changing mortality rates with perinatal intensive care and regionalization. Sem Perinatol. 1:309, 1977.

19. Lubchenco, L. O., Delivoria-Papadopoulos, M. and Searles, D.: Long-term follow-up studies of prematurely born infants. I. Relationship of handicaps to nursery routines. J. Pediatr. 80:501, 1972.

20. Janus-Kukulska, A. and Lis, S.: Developmental peculiarities of prematurely born children with birthweight below 1250 grams. Dev. Med. Child Neurol. 8:285, 1966.

21. Drillien, C. M.: The incidence of mental and physical handicaps in school age children of very low birth weight. Pediatrics 39:238, 1967.

22. Wright, F. H., Blough, R. R., Chamberlin, A. et al.: A controlled follow-up study of small prematures born from 1952 through 1956. Am. J. Dis. Child. 124:506, 1972.

23. Fitzhardinge, P. M. and Ramsay, M.: The improving outlook for the small prematurely born infant. Develop. Med. Child Neurol. 15:447, 1973.

24. Francis-Williams, J. and Davies, P. A.: Very low birth weight and later intelligence. Develop. Med. Child Neurol. 16:709, 1974.

25. Stewart, A. L. and Reynolds, E. O. R.: Improved prognosis for infants of very low birth weight. Pediatrics 54:724, 1974.

26. Fitzhardinge, P. M.: Early growth and development in low birth weight infants following treatment in an intensive care nursery. Pediatrics 56:162, 1975.

27. Homers, M. and Kendall, A. C.: The prognosis of the very low birth weight infant. Dev. Med. Child Neurol. 18:745, 1976.

28. Lubchenco, L. O., Horner, F. A., Reed, L. H. et al.: Sequelae of premature birth: evaluation of premature infants of low birth weights at 10 years of age. Am. J. Dis. Child. 106:101, 1963.

29. Bowes, W. A., Jr., Halgrimson, M. and Simmons, M. A.: Results of the intensive perinatal management of very low birth weight infants (501–1500 grams). *In* Anderson, A., Beard, R., Brudenell, J. M. et al. (eds.): Pre-Term Labour: Proceedings of the Fifth Study Group of the Royal College of Obstetricians and Gynaecologists, 1977. London, 1977, pp. 331–355.

30. Hobel, C. J., Hyvarinen, M. A. and Oh, W.: Abnormal fetal heart rate patterns and fetal-acid base balance in low birth weight infants in relation to respiratory distress syndrome. Obstet. Gynecol. 39:83, 1972.

31. Martin, C. B., Jr., Siassi, B. and Hon, E. H.: Fetal heart rate patterns and neonatal death in low birth weight infants. Obstet. Gynecol. 44:503, 1974.

32. Paul, R. H.: Fetal heart rate monitoring and low birth weight. *In* Anderson, A., Beard, R., Brudenell, J. M. et al. (eds.): Pre-Term Labour: Proceedings of the Fifth Study Group of the Royal College of Obstetricians and Gynaecologists, 1977. London, 1977, pp. 308–314.

33. Low, J. A., Pancham, S. R. and Worthington, D.: Fetal heart deceleration patterns in relation to asphyxia and weight—gestational age percentile of the fetus. Obstet. Gynecol. 47:14, 1976.

34. Worthington, D. and Smith, B. T.: Relationship of amniotic fluid lecithin/sphingomyelin ratio and fetal asphyxia to respiratory distress syndrome in premature infants. Can. Med. Assoc. J. 118:1384, 1978.

35. Kenny, J. D., Adams, J. M., Corbet, A. J. J. et al.: The role of acidosis at birth in the development of hyaline membrane disease. Pediatrics 58:184, 1976.

36. Wigglesworth, J. S., Davies, P. A., Keith, I. H. et al.: Intraventricular hemorrhage in the preterm infant without hyaline membrane disease. Arch. Dis. Child. 52:447, 1971.

37. Goldenberg, R. L. and Nelson, K. G.: The premature breech. Am. J. Obstet. Gynecol. 127:240, 1977.

38. Cruikshank, D. P. and Pitkin, R. M.: Delivery of the premature breech. Obstet. Gynecol. 50:367, 1977.

39. Ingemarsson, I., Westgren, M. and Svenningsen, N. W.: Long-term follow-up of preterm infants in breech presentation delivered by cesarean section. Lancet 2:172, 1978.

40. Stewart, A.: Follow-up of pre-term infants. *In* Anderson, A., Beard, R., Brudenell, J. M. et al. (eds.): Pre-Term Labour: Proceedings of the Fifth Study Group of the Royal College of Obstetricians and Gynaecologists, 1977. London, 1977, pp. 372–384.

41. Ranck, J. B., Jr. and Windle, W. F.: Brain damage in the monkey macaca mulatta by asphyxia neonatorum. Exp. Neurol. 1:130, 1959.

42. Omer, M. I. A., Robson, E. and Neligan, G. A.: Can initial resuscitation of preterm babies reduce the death rate from hyaline membrane disease? Arch. Dis. Child. 49:219, 1974.

43. Pomerance, J. J., Ukrainski, C. T., Tara Ukra, D. et al.: Cost of living for infants weighing 1000 grams or less at birth. Pediatrics 61:908, 1978.

44. Cullen, D. J., Ferrara, L. C., Briggs, B. A. et al.: Survival, hospitalization charges and follow-up results in critically ill patients. N. Engl. J. Med. 294:982, 1976.

How to Deliver the Less Than 1500-Gram Infant

Carlyle Crenshaw, Jr., M.D.
Joseph M. Miller, Jr., M.D.
Duke University Medical Center

Even five years ago the answer to this question might have been "vaginally unless maternal indications dictate abdominal delivery." At that time the majority of babies weighing less than 1500 g died of hyaline membrane disease and survivors had an exceedingly high incidence of major central nervous system dysfunction. The fact that this question is again being raised is an indication of the increasing expertise of neonatologists in resuscitating these babies and providing them with the proper respiratory, metabolic and nutritional support. It is also an indication of the concern for the fetus that the obstetrician has developed in the past few years, an indication of increased ability through technologic advances to estimate better the health, size and maturity of the fetus in utero, and an indication that obstetricians and patients now view certain types of deliveries with more apprehension for mother and fetus than in years past and view cesarean section with less alarm than previously. Today, if the obstetrician can give his neonatology colleagues an infant weighing less than 1500 g that is non-asphyxiated and nontraumatized, that infant's chances of surviving with an intact central nervous system are great. Unfortunately, our technology has not advanced sufficiently to determine always, in utero, the size and maturity of the fetus and the presence or absence of fetal anomalies. Moreover, our technology and expertise have not advanced sufficiently to justify the "routine" attempt to salvage the less than 1000-g infant by major obstetric surgery. Insufficient numbers of these very small infants have been followed long enough to determine their long-term emotional, motor and intellectual performance. To be blunt, each time we are faced with the question of how to deliver a very small baby we must ask ourselves, "Can we justify to this patient, her family and society these very expensive perinatal heroics because we can deliver an infant who ultimately will be a productive citizen?" Also, we must consider the subsequent reproductive consequences to the mother of any type of operative delivery that we choose. Whereas cesarean section is a safe procedure today, there is greater febrile morbidity than with vaginal delivery: the earlier in gestation that one does a cesarean section, the greater the febrile morbidity.

Until well-controlled studies with long-term follow-up of mother and infant are performed, it will be impossible to answer scientifically the question of how to deliver the less than 1500-g infant. The obstetrician must rely upon the few studies that do exist and upon clinical judgment of the individual patient, the precipitating event requiring delivery, and the perinatal personnel and facilities available. This discussion is based upon the following:

1. The need for early delivery of such an infant.

2. Whether or not labor can be delayed or prevented.

3. Presentation of the fetus.

4. Status of the cervix.

5. Health of the fetus during labor and delivery.

6. The potential risk of one type of delivery or another.

7. The care of the infant following delivery.

If there is time prior to delivery, transportation of those patients with fetuses of less than 1500 g to a perinatal center capable of providing a full range of pulmonary, metabolic and nutritional support will ultimately lead to the most favorable outcome for the newborn. Because such transportation is not always available, and since transfer is inadvisable many times because of imminent delivery, it behooves all physicians taking care of pregnant patients to remain proficient in the techniques of newborn resuscitation and support.

Factors Necessitating Very Early Delivery

Identifiable factors necessitating early delivery can be broken down into maternal, uteroplacental and fetal. However, as seen in

TABLE 1. FACTORS AFFECTING DELIVERY OF THE LESS THAN 1500-G INFANT*

Preterm labor and delivery	45
Premature rupture of the membranes	36
Toxemia	12
Bleeding	11
Incompetent cervix	8
Amnionitis	4
Urinary tract infection	3
IUGR > 36 weeks	3
Uterine anomaly	1
Uterovaginal fistula	1
Sickle cell disease	1
Auto accident	1
Adult RDS	1
Retroperitoneal mass	1
	129

*At Duke University Medical Center, 1976–1977.

Table 1, idiopathic premature rupture of the membranes and idiopathic preterm labor have been among the most frequent reasons for delivery of a less than 1500-g baby at our institution.

At this time there are few maternal factors that mandate delivery prior to 32 weeks' gestation. Severe, uncontrollable preeclampsia, severe preeclampsia superimposed upon chronic hypertensive vascular disease and eclampsia are the most common illnesses that require early delivery for the sake of the mother and the fetus. Those illnesses plus acute pyelonephritis, sickle cell disease, diabetes mellitus, hyperthyroidism, maternal cyanotic heart disease, collagen diseases and any severe, prolonged maternal febrile illness may precipitate preterm labor.

Uteroplacental factors lead to a number of deliveries of babies weighing less than 1500 g. Uncontrollable maternal and fetal bleeding from premature separation of the placenta and placenta previa mandate delivery for both maternal and fetal reasons. Such abnormalities of the uterus as leiomyomas, uterine anomalies and an incompetent cervix are fairly frequently associated with preterm labor. A uterus overdistended from polyhydramnios or multiple gestation also is frequently associated with preterm labor.

Fetal factors leading to delivery of a less than 1500-g infant include severe Rh isoimmunization and intrauterine growth retardation. With the advent of intrauterine transfusion, rarely is the delivery of a small, "affected" baby indicated; however, the disease process itself may precipitate preterm labor. Severe growth retardation is associated with spontaneous preterm labor but is often found in more advanced gestations, necessitating active intervention.

Can Delivery be Delayed or Prevented?

Management of preterm labor and premature rupture of the membranes have been discussed in previous chapters; however, we think that a brief discussion here will be helpful.

At our institution those patients who are prone to preterm labor are started on intramuscular 170 H progesterone caproate 250 mg weekly beginning at about 14 weeks' gestation and continuing until 37 weeks.[9] We so treat those patients who have a uterine anomaly, leiomyomas, incompetent cervix or history of previous idiopathic preterm labor.

Patients admitted in preterm labor prior to 34 weeks' gestation are treated with intravenous isoxsuprine after rapid hydration with 500 ml of lactated Ringer's solution.[7] If any cervical change has been observed while isoxsuprine therapy was initiated or if the cervix is dilated 4 cm or more before isoxsuprine is started, we treat our patients following the protocol of Liggins with intramuscular betamethasone 12 mg, repeated in 24 hours. If after 24 hours of intravenous isoxsuprine treatment labor has stopped, the patient is started on oral isoxsuprine 10 to 20 mg every 4 to 6 hours. If labor does not resume, the oral isoxsuprine is continued until 37 weeks' gestation.

Those patients admitted with premature rupture of the membranes between 26 and 34 weeks' gestation are also treated with betamethasone. If labor begins in these patients less than 24 hours after receiving the first dose of betamethasone, we attempt to delay labor with intravenous isoxsuprine for at least 24 hours after the betamethasone dose, in the event that there is no evidence of chorioamnionitis. If labor does not occur by 48 hours after the first dose of betamethasone, delivery is effected.

Data from our institution (1971 to 1975), obtained from patients with no other obstetric complications who delivered infants weighing 1000 to 1500 g, revealed that the incidence of the idiopathic respiratory distress syndrome decreased significantly the longer the period of time between rupture of membranes and onset of labor. However, amnionitis developed in 13 per cent of the patients who went into labor when more than 24 hours had elapsed after rupture of the membranes.[13]

Presentation of the Fetus

Transverse position, compound presentations and breech presentation are more frequently encountered in the less than 1500-g infant than in the general population. The uncompromised fetus lying in transverse position should be delivered by cesarean section if gestation has lasted 27 weeks or more. Likewise, the uncompromised fetus with a compound presentation or a breech presentation and no indications of labor should be delivered by cesarean section when delivery is indicated.

Status of the Cervix at the Time Delivery is Contemplated

Frequently in those preterm patients with maternal or fetal indications for delivery the cervix is firm, thick, located posteriorly and closed. Induction of labor under such circumstances usually is long and difficult. Frequently the best obstetric judgment is to proceed with delivery by cesarean section rather than attempt induction of labor and vaginal delivery because the maternal-fetal condition dictates immediate delivery and because adequate fetal monitoring may be impossible.

Fetal Health During Labor and Delivery

Once labor has begun or induction of labor is planned, every effort should be made to ensure the healthiest infant possible. Although work by Cibils[4] suggests that the premature fetus can withstand distress longer than the term fetus, we believe that these infants are more susceptible to hypoxia and are more subject to central nervous system damage. This damage is different in the term infant and is present in the center of the hemisphere and located in the germinal matrix of the periventricular region, with relative sparing of the cortical mantle. The routine use of external electronic fetal monitoring is indicated in order to serve as an early warning signal for the development of acute fetal distress. The membranes should be left intact as long as possible. An internal electrode should be applied if there is a question concerning the reliability of the external fetal heart monitoring. Intrauterine pressure catheters should be avoided because of increased likelihood of ascending infection with their use.[19] Secondary arrest of labor should not be allowed to persist and should be corrected using a carefully regulated oxytocin infusion.[2]

The patient should be placed in the lateral recumbent position and oxygen administered by mask. Little analgesia, if any, should be administered. A conduction anesthetic, either epidural or caudal block, provides good relief of pain as well as relaxation of soft parts of the birth canal for labor and delivery. If a regional anesthetic is not available or if it is contraindicated (for example, by maternal bleeding), a pudendal nerve block will suffice for delivery. If such evidence of fetal distress (as severe variable decelerations, persistent late decelerations, persistent tachycardia greater than 180 or bradycardia less than 100 develops and the condition fails to respond to change of position and administration of oxygen, cesarean section should be considered. It should be remembered that loss of beat-to-beat variability of the fetal heart (a usual sign of fetal distress of the mature infant) may be absent and tachycardia may be present in the healthy premature infant. Biochemical confirmation of fetal status generally should be obtained; however, technically this method of fetal monitoring is more difficult and potentially more dangerous in the less than 1500-g fetus.

Every effort should be made to keep the delivery atraumatic. A generous episiotomy is indicated, in an attempt to shorten the second stage of labor and decrease the resistance of maternal tissues. Data from Jackson Memorial Hospital[3] show a decrease in the perinatal mortality rate with use of episiotomy (Table 2).

The use of forceps is debatable. Excessive compression with forceps may arrest cerebral circulation to the point of asphyxia, and malfitting forceps may tear the falx or tentorium or fracture the fetal skull, although shortening of the second stage of labor and protection of the fragile head from the resistancy of the maternal soft parts are desirable. More important is ease and control in the delivery to prevent rapid decompression of the head and consequent intracranial bleeding.

TABLE 2.   EFFECT OF EPISIOTOMY ON PERINATAL MORTALITY

INFANT BIRTH WEIGHT	EPISIOTOMY	NUMBER	PERCENTAGE PERINATAL MORTALITY
501–1500	Yes	28	54
	No	82	79
<2500	Yes	247	13
	No	208	42

The management of breech presentations in patients with preterm labor and delivery is controversial, although a major text advocates cesarean section with a healthy but premature fetus of more than 1000 g.[16] However, as pointed out by Cruikshank and Pitkin,[5] before cesarean section should be considered for a delivery, it is necessary to show the following:

1. A decrease in perinatal morbidity and mortality with routine abdominal delivery.

2. A failure of improvement with alternate approaches.

3. A favorable risk-to-benefit ratio in which perinatal outcome outweighs the hazards of cesarean section.

Several recent studies suggest that the perinatal outcome of the vaginally delivered breech can be significantly improved by careful attention to the management of the labor. Three factors are important: fetal monitoring,[17] conduction anesthesia[6] and forceps delivery of the aftercoming head.[14]

As in the term infant in breech presentation, another factor—type of breech presentation—is important. Infants in frank breech presentation have the same incidence of cord prolapse as those in vertex presentation but comprise only one third of infants in breech if less than 1500 g. Infants in complete breech presentation have a higher incidence of cord prolapse and those in footling presentation, the highest.

The infant in single or double footling breech presentation, if otherwise healthy (no radiologic or sonographic anomalies) and more than 26 weeks' gestational age, probably should be delivered by cesarean section. Those in other breech presentations, if labor is adequate and the maternal pelvis is suffi-ciently large, should be delivered vaginally with care and with fetal monitoring. Epidural anesthesia, enough to help prevent early pushing against an incompletely dilated cervix but not enough to block motor function, is desirable. Forceps delivery of the aftercoming head is useful, as shown in Table 3.

One must also consider that the anomaly rate for breech infants of 32 weeks or less is approximately 8 per cent.[1] Since most of these anomalies are unsuspected, aggressive use of cesarean section will result, at times, in the delivery of a seriously compromised and perhaps nonviable infant; therefore, routine use of cesarean section in delivery of premature breech infants has not yet been proved to be the method of choice.

As in pregnancies with fetuses of greater than 1500 g, we do not use oxytoxin induction or oxytocin augmentation when a fetus patient of less than 1500 g is in breech presentation.

The Potential Risk of One Type of Delivery or Another

The early and more liberal use of cesarean section, particularly for problems such as premature separation of the placenta and placenta previa, and perhaps for the extremely brittle diabetic, may help reduce maternal morbidity and mortality. However, cesarean section in the less than 1500-g infant in the face of overt uterine infection, coagulopathies or serious medical illnesses is relatively contraindicated.

Although cesarean section is now viewed as one of the safest major surgical procedures, the risk involved is considerable and includes early complications such as hemorrhage and injury to other organs or later problems including wound infection, herniation and bowel obstruction. Additionally, there is the possibility that subsequent cesarean section will be necessary or that labor in subsequent pregnancies may be complicated by uterine rupture.

As far as the fetus is concerned, the delivery may be difficult with some entrapment of the

TABLE 3.   NEONATAL MORTALITY RATES AND USE OF FORCEPS IN VAGINAL BREECH DELIVERIES

INFANT BIRTH WEIGHT	NO FORCEPS	FORCEPS
<1000	47/55 (88%)	3/3 (100%)
1000–1499	41/87 (47%)	3/18 (22%)

head if the uterine incision is not long enough. An infant delivered by cesarean section is more likely to develop the respiratory distress syndrome.[9]

If abdominal delivery of the less than 1500-g fetus is elected, usually a low transverse uterine incision is best; however, a low vertical section may be desirable if the lower uterine segment is not well developed and not wide enough to permit an ample transverse incision. The low vertical incision has the advantage of allowing upward extension as needed.

Care of the Infant Following Delivery

Once the infant is delivered, oropharyngeal suction should be performed. Although the umbilical cord should not be "milked," neither should it be rapidly clamped. The small extra volume of blood flowing into the premature infant may help prevent hypovolemia.

It is essential to have pediatric coverage for the delivery of the less than 1500-g infant. Early and aggressive management will improve neonatal morbidity and mortality.

An overly pessimistic attitude is not warranted, particularly in view of the improved prognosis of very low birth weight infants.[18] At the University College Hospital, London, follow-up of survivors from the period 1966 to 1970 was obtained; 197 infants weighed 1500 g or less and 98 survived. Follow-up on 95 infants ranging from age 2 years, 10 months to 7 years, 10 months revealed 86 (90.5 per cent) with no detectable handicap, 4 (4.2 per cent) with physical handicaps only, and 5 (5.3 per cent) with mental handicaps.

Pape et al.[15] pointed out in a two-year follow-up study of infants of less than 1000 g that CNS defects were closely associated with a neonatal history of intrauterine hemorrhage or seizures in addition to growth retardation.

The overly pessimistic approach may lead to a "vulnerable child syndrome" in later years.[8] The obstetrician should be aware of the neonate's condition and be appropriately reassuring and supportive to the family. The mother should be allowed and encouraged to see, touch and if possible hold her infant after birth. Lactation should not be suppressed.

Since the less than 1500-g infant will be cared for in a nursery setting instead of a mother's bedside, it is important to promote an environment for optimal maternal-infant interaction. Preliminary data suggest that the IQs of premature infants who have had early contact with their mothers are significantly higher than those of infants who have experienced delayed contact.[11]

REFERENCES

1. Brenner, W. E. et al.: The characteristics and perils of breech presentation. Am. J. Obstet. Gynecol. 118:700, 1974.
2. Briscoe, C. C.: Delivery of the premature infant. Clin. Obstet. Gynecol. 7:695, 1964.
3. Cavanaugh, D. and Talisman, M. R.: Prematurity and the Obstetrician. New York, Appleton-Century-Crofts, 1969, p. 383.
4. Cibils, L.: Clinical significance of fetal heart rate patterns during labor. Am. J. Obstet. Gynecol. 129:833, 1977.
5. Cruikshank, D. and Pitkin, R.: Delivery of the premature breech. Obstet. Gynecol. 50:367, 1977.
6. Crawford, J. S.: An appraisal of lumbar epidural blockades in patients with singleton fetus presenting in the breech. J. Obstet. Gynecol. Br. Commonwealth 81:867, 1974.
7. Csapo, A. I. and Herczey, J.: Arrest of premature labor by isoxsuprine. Am. J. Obstet. Gynecol. 129:482, 1977.
8. Green, M. and Sulmit, A. J.: Reactions to the threatened loss of a child: a vulnerable child syndrome. Pediatrics 34:58, 1964.
9. Hine, R. M. F. et al.: Association between maternal diabetes and the respiratory distress syndrome in the newborn. N. Engl. J. Med. 294:357, 1976.
10. Johnson, J. W. C. et al.: Efficacy of 17α-hydroxy-progesterone caproate in the prevention of premature labor. N. Engl. J. Med. 293:675, 1975.
11. Klaus, M. H. and Kevnell, J. H.: Maternal-Infant Bonding. St. Louis, C. V. Mosby Co., 1976, p. 114.
12. Liggins, G. C.: Prenatal glucocorticoid treatment: Prevention of respiratory distress syndrome. In Lung Maturation and the Prevention of Hyaline Membrane Disease. Columbus, Ross Laboratories, 1976, pp. 97–103.
13. Miller, J. M., Jr., Pupkin, M. J. and Crenshaw, M. C., Jr.: Premature labor and premature rupture of the membranes. Am. J. Obstet. Gynecol. (in press).
14. Milner, R. D. G. Neonatal mortality of breech deliveries with and without forceps to the aftercoming head. Br. J. Obstet. Gynecol. 82:783, 1975.
15. Pape, K. E. et al.: The status at two years of low birth weight infants born in 1974 with birth weights of less than 1001 grams. J. Pediatr. 92:253, 1978.
16. Pritchard, J. A. and MacDonald, P. C.: Williams' Obstetrics, 5th ed. New York, Appleton-Century-Crofts, 1977, pp. 666–676.
17. Rovinsky, J. J., Miller, J. A. and Kaplan, S.: Management of the breech presentation at term. Am. J. Obstet. Gynecol. 115:497, 1973.
18. Stewart, A. L. and Reynolds, E. O. R.: The improved prognosis of very low birth weight infants. Pediatrics 54:724, 1974.
19. Thadepalli, H. et al.: Amniotic fluid contamination during internal fetal monitoring. J. Reprod. Med. 20:93, 1978.
20. Towbin, A.: Central nervous system damage in the human fetus and newborn: mechanical and hypoxic injury incurred in the fetal-neonatal period. Am. J. Dis. Child. 119:259, 1970.

How to Deliver the Under 1500-Gram Infant

D. V. I. Fairweather

Ann L. Stewart

University College Hospital, London

Twenty years ago prognosis for the survival of infants with a birth weight of 1500 g or less was so poor (less than 20 per cent) that obstetricians were not inclined to consider special measures or additional care for their delivery. Indeed, there was considerable reluctance to even contemplate the delivery of very small premature infants by cesarean section. It was argued that the poor prognosis did not justify operative delivery with its small additional risk to the mother. The philosophy then was "Let them take their chance."

In practice, however, a number of these infants survived, despite the fact that they were often born in extremely poor condition and received minimal attention at birth. It was not surprising, therefore, that pediatricians reported highly unfavorable results from long-term follow-up studies. For example, Lubchenco and colleagues reported that up to 70 per cent of very low birth weight survivors had significant developmental handicaps.[14] Drillien also reported that 83 per cent of the few surviving infants in her survey weighing less than 1250 g at birth proved abnormal at follow-up.[5] Additionally, Drillien[4] and later Holt[7] suggested that measures taken to increase the survival rate of infants of very low birth weight would result only in increasing numbers of handicapped children who would burden their families and society.

Only after research into fetal and neonatal physiology allowed insight into the hazards that immature infants have to overcome was consideration given to improving their outcome. It was argued that if homeostasis could be maintained in the perinatal period or deviations rapidly and adequately corrected, potentially lethal or damaging complications would be avoided and both mortality and morbidity among the survivors reduced.[16] In the early 1960s these considerations began to be applied to specialist centers, and, as a result

of collaboration between obstetricians and pediatricians, regimens of intensive perinatal management were introduced. Almost immediately, mortality rates fell among high-risk infants, particularly for those of very low birth weight.[23] More recent follow-up studies of survivors have indicated a much improved long-term prognosis.[2, 19, 23]

The concept of perinatal intensive care is now well established. Management of this kind pays particular attention to early identification of the high-risk pregnancy and to careful management of the pregnancy and delivery. In addition, it includes the provision of facilities for prompt resuscitation of the newborn and a high standard of neonatal care for all infants born after complications of pregnancy and labor, particularly those of very low birth weight (less than 1500 g).

The influence of delivery method on survival of very low birth weight infants managed with modern methods was highlighted by Stewart and Reynolds.[19] Reporting on a follow-up study of 197 infants weighing 1500 g or less at birth admitted to the neonatal unit at University College Hospital, London (UCH), during 1966 to 1970, they showed that the chance of survival was greatest for infants delivered by cesarean section (69 per cent) and least among infants delivered vaginally in breech presentation (47 per cent). They later reported that among the smallest infants who weighed 1000 g or less, 64 per cent survived after cesarean section, whereas only 27 per cent survived among those who were delivered vaginally.[20] From these results, they concluded that the method of delivery of very low birth weight infants was crucial to their survival and subsequent development, and that cesarean section deserves serious consideration as the preferred method in some circumstances. In order to further support this view we have reviewed the outcome of 497

TABLE 1. REASONS FOR PREMATURE DELIVERY IN LIVEBORN INFANTS 500–1500 G*

	SINGLETON No. (Percentage)	MULTIPLES No. (Percentage)	TOTAL No. (Percentage)
Spontaneous onset	303 (77)	96 (93)	399 (80)
Induced or elective cesarean	89 (22)	7 (7)	96 (19)
No information	2 (0.5)	—	2 (0.5)
Total	394 (100)	103 (100)	497 (100)

*Statistics in Tables 1–8 from University College Hospital, London, 1971–1977.

liveborn infants weighing 500 to 1500 g at birth and delivered at UCH or transferred during 1971 to 1977.

Results

Of the 497 infants in the study group, 394 (79 per cent) resulted from singleton and 103 from multiple pregnancies (83 were members of twin sets, 9 of triplet, 6 of quadruplet and there was 1 set of quintuplets). The distribution of birth weight among the singleton infants was similar to that of the infants from multiple pregnancies: about 30 per cent weighed 500 to 1000 g and 70 per cent 1001 to 1500 g. There were 250 male and 247 female infants.

Table 1 shows the reason for the premature delivery; in 80 per cent (399 cases) the onset of labor was spontaneous. In these cases, there was associated maternal hypertension in 10 per cent and antepartum hemorrhage in just under 40 per cent. Infants from multiple pregnancies were much more likely (p<0.001) to have had mothers with hypertensive complication in the pregnancy than were the singletons. In the 96 cases in which labor was induced or in which elective cesarean section was undertaken, the principal indication (73

per cent [69 cases]) was maternal hypertension (including toxemia, eclampsia and renal disease). The other two notable indications were antepartum hemorrhage (14 per cent) or suspected intrauterine growth retardation (12 per cent).

The overall 28-day mortality rate for the 497 infants was 38 per cent, and mortality fell significantly as both birth weight (p<0.0005) and length of gestation (p<0.0005) increased (Tables 2 and 3). For example, 55 per cent of infants who weighed 751 to 1000 g died, whereas the mortality was 76 per cent among the smallest infants who weighed less than 751 g. For infants who weighed more than 1000 g the mortality was much lower. Similar differences were noted in both singleton infants and those resulting from multiple pregnancies. Likewise, the mortality rate for infants born before 28 completed weeks of gestation was 60 per cent or more, whereas it fell to 44 per cent at 28 weeks and 30 per cent or below at 29 weeks. The 28-day mortality

TABLE 2. 28-DAY MORTALITY AND BIRTH WEIGHT OF LIVEBORN INFANTS 500–1500 G

BIRTH WEIGHT	NO. CASES	28-DAY MORTALITY PERCENTAGE
500–750	33	76
751–1000	119	55
1001–1250	179	36
1251–1500	166	20.5
Total	497	38

Overall significance p<0.0005.

TABLE 3. 28-DAY MORTALITY AND WEEK OF GESTATION OF LIVEBORN INFANTS 500–1500 G

GESTATION IN WEEKS	NO. CASES	28-DAY MORTALITY PERCENTAGE
22	2	100
23	2	100
24	7	86
25	10	90
26	45	62
27	59	64
28	91	44
29	76	26
30	77	30
31	41	15
32	40	17.5
33	12	17
34 and over	35	17
Total	497	38

Overall significance p<0.0005.

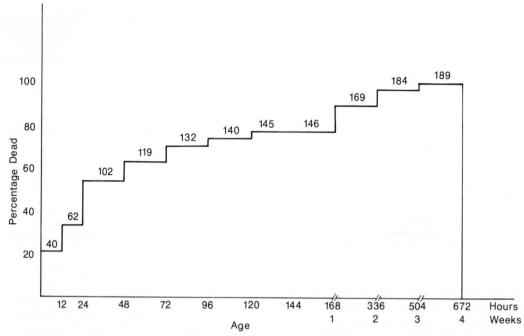

Figure 1. Cumulative 28-day mortality by time of death for 189 low birth weight infants, 1971 to 1977.

for females (32 per cent) was significantly (p <0.025) less than that for males (44 per cent).

Figure 1 shows, in the form of a histogram, the cumulative 28-day mortality by time of death. It indicates that nearly 80 per cent of the deaths had occurred by the end of 5 days and 90 per cent by the end of 2 weeks.

Two hundred and fifteen (43 per cent) of the 497 infants in the study were born in UCH and, of those, 28 were transferred from other units before birth because of anticipated problems of low birth weight. The 28-day mortality for those infants transferred to UCH after delivery was 43 per cent compared to 32 per cent for infants delivered in UCH, and this difference was statistically significant (p <0.025). The 28-day mortality (29 per cent) was significantly lower in the 187 infants who had both antenatal care and delivery (booked cases) in UCH, than in the 282 infants who were transferred after delivery (43 per cent) (p<0.025). This difference occurred in spite of the fact that referred infants were "selected" by their ability to live long enough for transfer.

Of all infants born in UCH in the years 1971 to 1977, the 215 live births and 35 stillbirths of infants weighing 500 to 1500 g represented 1.55 per cent. In 1971 to 1976 in England and Wales this weight group contributed 0.65 to 0.7 per cent of all births.[15] During the study period in UCH the total perinatal mortality (stillbirths plus first-week deaths) for this weight group was 36 per cent. Infants weighing 1000 g or less had a perinatal mortality rate of 65 per cent, while those weighing 1001 to 1500 g had a rate of only 24 per cent. The adverse effect of very low birth weight was also evident among stillborn infants: 21 per cent among infants who weighed 1000 g or less compared with 11 per cent in infants who weighed 1001 to 1500 g.

Among booked cases, or those transferred in utero, attempts were made to stop preterm labor when the membranes were intact and fetal or maternal conditions were favorable, using drugs including isoxsuprine and, more recently, salbutamol. However, steroids were not used routinely to enhance lung maturation. Consequently, only a small proportion of the total study group received this treatment, including just three infants delivered at UCH (one neonatal death and two survivors).

Fifty-two per cent (258) of the 497 infants in the study were born vaginally with the vertex presenting, while 26 per cent (128) were delivered by cesarean section and 21 per cent (106) were born vaginally by the breech. Table 4 shows the overall 28-day mortalities by method of delivery. The difference between the mortalities in spontaneous and for-

TABLE 4.   28-Day Mortality by Method of Delivery and Birth Weight of
Liveborn Infants 500–1500 G

Presentation and Method of Delivery	Percentage 28-Day Mortality (n)		
	Weight 500–1000 g	*Weight 1001–1500 g*	*Weight 500–1500 g*
Vertex			
spont.	62 (60)	·27 (103)	40 (163)
forceps	62.5 (24)	34 (70)	41 (94)
ventouse	— —	0 (1)	0 (1)
Breech			
spont.	71 (34)	46 (50)	56 (84)
FACH	60 (5)	41 (17)	45 (22)
All breech	69 (39)	45 (67)	54 (106)
Brow/face spont.	100 (2)	67 (3)	80 (5)
CS in labor	50 (10)	14 (43)	21 (53)
CS elective	23.5 (17)	15.5 (58)	17 (75)
All CS	33 (27)	15 (101)	19 (128)
Total	59 (152)	29 (345)	38 (497)

(n) = total number of cases in each group.

ceps deliveries involving vertex presentation was not significant; neither was that between forceps deliveries of vertex presentations and vaginal deliveries of breech presentation infants. There was no difference either in mortalities between cases involving elective and emergency cesarean section. However, there were markedly significant differences between the mortalities among cesarean section deliveries and unassisted vaginal deliveries of infants in vertex ($p < 0.0005$), vaginal deliveries of vertex infants using forceps ($p < 0.0005$) and all breech deliveries ($p < 0.0005$). The difference between the mortalities for spontaneous vertex compared with all breech deliveries was also significant ($p < 0.05$). Only five infants with abnormal presentations (face and brow) were delivered vaginally. Four of these five infants died.

Considering the 28-day mortality for each method of delivery, we found that whatever the method, the mortality of infants weighing 1000 g or less was significantly higher than that of the group weighing more than 1000 g. Table 4 also gives the breakdown by the two weight groups. In the 500 to 1000 g group the mortality for vaginal delivery in infants in vertex ($p < 0.025$) and breech presentations ($p < 0.01$) was significantly higher than among infants delivered by cesarean section. In the 1001 to 1500 g group vaginal delivery mortality of the breech infant was again significantly higher ($p < 0.0005$) than that for all cesarean section deliveries. In this heavier group, vaginal delivery using forceps was also signifi-

cantly ($p < 0.01$) more hazardous than cesarean section.

Further subdivision of birth weight into 4 groups showed that even among the smallest infants who weighed 500 to 750 g those delivered by cesarean section had a lower mortality than breech deliveries. It also showed that vaginal breech delivery was the only method for which the 28-day mortality did not fall progressively as birth weight increased.

Table 5 shows the 28-day mortality for all methods of delivery according to the period of gestation. In order to give adequate numbers for analysis, period of gestation is shown in two-week groups in this table. No infants survived before 24 weeks of gestation and no cesarean sections were performed before 26 weeks. Thereafter, for every two-week period until 34 weeks the mortality for infants delivered by cesarean section was lower than that for all vaginal deliveries of breech infants. What is more, mortality for vaginal vertex deliveries and cesarean sections fell progressively ($p < 0.0005$ and $p < 0.025$) as length of gestation increased. In contrast, mortality among vaginal deliveries of breech infants did not improve as length of gestation increased from 26 to 34 weeks and did not appear to be gestation-dependent.

Ninety-two (18.5%) of the 497 infants in the study had birth weights below the 10th percentile for their period of gestation (SGA), according to Lubchenco's criteria.[14] The 28-day mortality for these infants was 23 per cent and was significantly lower ($p < 0.0005$) than

TABLE 5. PERCENTAGE OF 28-DAY MORTALITY BY WEEKS OF GESTATION AND METHOD OF DELIVERY OF LIVEBORN INFANTS 500–1500 G

GESTATION IN WEEKS	SPONT. VERTEX % (n)	FORCEPS VENTOUSE % (n)	BREECH % (n)	FACE/ BROW % (n)	CS % (n)	TOTAL % (n)
22–23	100 (2)	100 (1)	100 (1)	—	—	100 (4)
24–25	78 (9)	100 (3)	100 (3)	100 (2)	—	88 (17)
26–27	62 (55)	86 (14)	60 (30)	—	40 (5)	63 (104)
28–29	26 (54)	32.5 (40)	57 (35)	100 (2)	31 (36)	36 (167)
30–31	19 (26)	42 (24)	33 (24)	0 (1)	14 (43)	25 (118)
32–33	10 (10)	0 (9)	71 (7)	—	11.5 (26)	17 (52)
34 and over	28.5 (7)	0 (4)	33 (6)	—	11 (18)	17 (35)
Total	40 (163)	41 (95)	54 (106)	80 (5)	19 (128)	38 (497)
Overall significance at 22–33 weeks	$p<0.0005$	$p<0.0005$	ns	—	$p<0.025$	—

(n) = total number of cases in each group.

that among the 405 infants whose birth weight was appropriate for their gestational age (AGA) (41 per cent). Within the SGA group, the numbers in the individual vaginal delivery categories were too small to allow comparison with those in the AGA group. However, considering all infants delivered vaginally, the mortality for the 44 SGA infants (32 per cent) was lower than that among the 325 AGA infants (46 per cent), but this difference was not statistically significant. Likewise, the mortality for the 48 SGA infants delivered by cesarean section (15 per cent) did not differ from that among the 80 AGA infants delivered by cesarean section (21 per cent). Thus it is unlikely that the significantly different proportions ($p<0.0005$) of SGA infants among cesarean (37.5 per cent) and vaginal deliveries (12 per cent) affected the mortalities in the different delivery categories in the group as a whole.

Table 6 shows, for singletons only, the 28-day mortality of infants in vertex presentation compared with other presentations at the time of delivery. This clearly indicates the adverse loading for other than vertex presentation in the case of vaginal delivery.

Among singleton infants weighing 1001 to 1500 g delivered spontaneously per vaginum following spontaneous onset of labor, the 28-day mortality was significantly higher in instances in which the membranes remained intact to within an hour of delivery than among those in which the membranes ruptured earlier in the labor. This difference was not noted in the case of infants weighing 1000 g or less. As can be seen from Table 7, however, the significant effect of time of membrane rupture in labor of spontaneous onset was present regardless of method of delivery in the total group of singleton infants.

Table 7 also shows that when the onset of

TABLE 6. 28-DAY MORTALITY BY PRESENTATION AND DELIVERY METHOD OF LIVEBORN SINGLETONS 500–1500 G

| | VERTEX | | OTHER THAN VERTEX | | |
	Vaginal	*CS*	*Vaginal*	*CS*	TOTAL
28-day survivors	129	69	34	15	247
Neonatal deaths	78	18	46	4	146
Total	207	87	80	19	393
Percentage 28-day mortality	38%[x]	21%	57.5%[x][y]	21%[y]	37%

Significant difference x $p<0.005$ y $p<0.01$.

TABLE 7. PERCENTAGE OF 28-DAY MORTALITY BY MODE OF ONSET AND METHOD OF DELIVERY OF LIVEBORN SINGLETONS 500–1500 G

		METHOD OF DELIVERY			
MODE OF ONSET OF LABOR	*Total* n (n_1)	*CS in Labor* n (n_1)	*Spont. Vag.* n (n_1)	*Assist. Vag.* n (n_1)	*Percentage 28-Day Mortality*
Spontaneous ⎱ Membranes ⎱ <1 hr	105 (55)	11 (6)	69 (34)	25 (15)	52 x
onset ⎰ ruptured ⎰ >1 hr	192 (65)	13 (2)	115 (39)	64 (24)	34 x
Subtotal	297 (120)	24 (8)	184 (73)	89 (39)	40 z
Elective cesarean section	70 (14)	—	—	—	20 y
Induction of labor	19 (3)	13 (2)	2 (0)	4 (1)	16 y
Subtotal	89 (17)	13 (2)	2 (0)	4 (1)	19 z

n (n_1) = number of cases (including number of 28-day mortalities).
Significant difference x $p<0.01$ y ns.   z $p<0.001$

labor was spontaneous (77 per cent), the majority of infants were delivered vaginally (92 per cent), including 62 per cent spontaneously and only 8 per cent by cesarean section. The remaining 23 per cent of all singleton births had either elective cesarean section (79 per cent) or induction of labor, and of that latter group 68 per cent ended with cesarean section. Thus only 7 per cent of patients who did not go into labor spontaneously had a vaginal delivery.

Induction of labor was undertaken in only 21 cases (Table 8) in this series, including in one set of twins with delivery induced because of maternal hypertension (both survived after vaginal delivery). Of the 19 singleton pregnancies in which labor was induced, 13 ended in cesarean section. In 10 of these pregnancies the indication for induction was maternal hypertension (8 infants survived); in 2, severe intrauterine growth retardation and in 1, severe Rh disease (all 3 infants survived). The remaining 6 singletons were delivered vaginally. In 2, the indication for induction was

maternal hypertension (both survived). In 2, there was severe intrauterine growth retardation (1 survived); in the remaining 2, both of whom survived, induction was necessary because of Rh disease in one and antepartum hemorrhage in the other. The overall 28-day infant survival for induced labor cases was 86 per cent.

Although the differences in 28-day mortality between vertex infants with spontaneous and forceps deliveries were not statistically significant, it is interesting to note than in the 1001 to 1500 g group the mortality was lower for the spontaneously delivered group (27 per cent) than in those deliveries involving forceps (34 per cent). Among infants who weighed 1000 g or less, there was no difference in the mortality of vertex infants spontaneously delivered (62 per cent) and with forceps-assisted deliveries (62.5 per cent). In the case of breech presentation application of forceps to the aftercoming head appeared to reduce the mortality in both weight groups. However, possibly because of small numbers, none of these

TABLE 8. INDICATIONS FOR PREMATURE INDUCTION AND OUTCOME OF LIVEBORN INFANTS 500–1500 G*

		OUTCOME			
INDICATION	N	VAGINAL DELIVERY	CS	28-DAY SURVIVOR	PERCENTAGE SURVIVING
Maternal hypertension	14*	4	10	12	86%
IUGR	4	2	2	3	75%
Rh	2	1	1	2	100%
APH	1	1	–	1	100%
Total	21	8	13	18	86%

*Included 1 set of twins—both survived.

differences were statistically significant. Thus we found no evidence to support the belief that the application of forceps was advantageous in the delivery of these very low birth weight infants.

In all, 130 infants were in the breech presentation at delivery, including 106 (84 per cent) who were delivered vaginally. Among those delivered by cesarean section the 28-day mortality was 17 per cent compared with 54 per cent for those delivered vaginally (p <0.0005). Only 14 infants (including 9 from multiple pregnancies) were delivered electively by cesarean section because of breech presentation after labor had commenced spontaneously. A further 10 had cesarean section in labor for other reasons when the breech presentation was an incidental feature.

Of the 128 cesarean sections performed, 75 (58 per cent) were elective and of those 55 (74 per cent) were undertaken because of associated maternal hypertension. In 12 others (16 per cent) there was associated antepartum hemorrhage and in 7 (9 per cent) the delivery was undertaken because of suspected serious intrauterine growth retardation. In the remaining case the indication was not recorded.

In the 13 cases in which cesarean section followed induction of labor, the cesarean in 8 was indicated because of failure of labor to progress and in 4 because fetal distress developed. The other cesarean section was performed because of maternal hypertension. There were only 2 infants in this group who died within 28 days. Both weighed less than 1000 g and induction was undertaken because of maternal hypertension.

Of the remaining 40 infants where delivery ended in cesarean section and in whom labor commenced spontaneously, 14 had cesarean undertaken because of the fetal presentation (breech) and the associated prematurity, 11 because of antepartum hemorrhage and 6 because of fetal distress. Four cesarean deliveries were performed because of maternal hypertension, 3 for other associated maternal distress (diabetes and severe Rh disorders) and 2 because of failure of labor to progress.

The 28-day infant mortality for elective cesarean section was 17 per cent and was not significantly different from that for emergency cesarean section (21 per cent). The worst outcome (36 per cent mortality) was in infants delivered by cesarean section in labor in association with antepartum hemorrhage. When elective cesarean section was undertaken in cases of antepartum hemorrhage before the

onset of labor the mortality was only 15 per cent. In cases involving maternal hypertension there was no difference in 28-day infant mortality between those in which delivery by cesarean section was elective and those in which cesarean section was performed in labor.

The median birth weight of the whole group of 497 patients was 1145 g (range 500 to 1500 g) and the median length of gestation was 29 weeks (range 22 to 42 weeks). The medians of both birth weight and gestation were greatest among infants delivered by cesarean section (1242 g [range 570 to 1494 g]; 30 weeks [range 26 to 38 weeks]) and least among the vaginal breech deliveries (1103 g [range 510 to 1498 g]; 28 weeks [range 22 to 39 weeks]).

The condition of the infants at birth differed according to the method of delivery. For example, 60 per cent of the vertex infants delivered vaginally (both spontaneously and assisted) had an apex beat of greater than 80 per minute at birth, whereas this was noted in 47 per cent of the infants delivered by cesarean section and only 33 per cent of those breech infants delivered vaginally. Likewise, the onset of spontaneous respirations was delayed for more than 30 minutes in 18 per cent of infants in breech delivered vaginally compared with 11 per cent of infants delivered by cesarean section and 8 per cent of vertex infants delivered vaginally.

Measurements of H^+ ion concentration and negative base excess made within 2 hours of birth were available for 258 (52 per cent) of the 497 infants in the study. The mean value of H^+ ion concentration was highest among breech infants delivered vaginally (70.13, pH equivalent, 7.15) and lowest among infants delivered by cesarean section (62.20, pH equivalent, 7.21). These values differed significantly (p<0.05). A similar trend was noted for the mean values of negative base excess, with significantly lower values (p<0.01) among vaginal breech deliveries (−12.6 mEq per L) than among infants delivered by cesarean section (−9 mEq per L).

These observations suggest that the condition of breech presentation infants delivered vaginally was worse than that of infants delivered by cesarean or of vertex infants delivered vaginally. From the biochemical measurements available on 258 of the 497 study infants, we inferred that this was because breech infants delivered vaginally had suffered a greater degree of anoxia at the time of birth.

In contrast to the findings relating to the

condition of the infants at birth, the incidence of illnesses later in the neonatal period differed according to the method of delivery in only a few respects. For example, 46 per cent of the vaginally delivered infants and 50 of the infants delivered by cesarean section developed hyaline membrane disease; the percentages of infants who developed apneic spells due to immature control of breathing were 34 and 26, respectively. Although these proportions did not differ significantly, the number of infants who required mechanical ventilation for the management of apneic spells was significantly less (p<0.0005) among infants delivered by cesarean section (9 per cent) than among the vaginally delivered infants (28 per cent). In addition, it is interesting to note that the incidence of respiratory distress during the first 24 hours of life due to delay in the clearance of lung liquid was greatest among infants delivered by cesarean section (11 per cent) and least among vaginal breech deliveries (3 per cent) (p<0.05).

Follow-up was conducted on 280 of the 284 surviving infants. Thirty (11 per cent) aged 2 years or more had handicaps likely to affect, in the long term, their ability to lead a normal life. These included 13 children with multiple handicaps; 5 children with sensory neural deafness, 6 with cerebral palsy, 3 who were intellectually dull and 3 with retrolental fibroplasia, without additional problems. The incidence of these handicaps among vertex infants in spontaneous and assisted deliveries was 11 per cent, among breech infants it was 15 per cent and among infants delivered by cesarean section it was 8 per cent. Although these figures suggest that the prognosis for breech infants delivered vaginally was worse than other methods, the differences were not statistically significant.

Discussion

From the results of the study reported here, in addition to others reported previously,[23] it appears that infants of very low birth weight or short gestation now often live, and that the majority of the survivors are capable of developing without serious handicaps. Thus obstetricians are faced with decisions concerning the optimal management of the fetus as well as the mother in complicated pregnancies. Consideration of fetal outcome must be included in decisions on the best time and method of delivery when perinatal complications make preterm birth inevitable.

When Walsh surveyed the subsequent development of 100 children born prematurely with birth weights of 3 lbs (1360 g) or less, he noted that there was no association between a particular type of delivery and the follow-up findings.[25] More recent studies[11] have shown that cesarean section in cases of low birth weight infants with abnormal positions in utero helped to reduce mortality rates. Fuller, reporting experience from the University of Colorado Medical Center, also cited a reduction in neonatal mortality from 54 to 32 per cent in infants weighing 1500 g or less at birth.[6] He attributed this change to the policy during labor of managing all patients in whom the estimated fetal weight was 600 g or more or the gestational age was 26 weeks or more with intensive perinatal care, monitoring, liberal use of cesarean section to avoid fetal trauma or asphyxia, and immediate neonatal resuscitation by an experienced neonatologist. We previously described the important influence of method of delivery on mortality among even the smallest infants (less than 1000 g), and the significant advantage conferred by cesarean section,[20] and this was also noted by Smith et al.[17] for infants under 2000 g. The further study reported now confirms the importance of the method of delivery in terms of survival and late development of these very small infants.

Obviously many factors are determinants of neonatal mortality. Lee and co-workers[10] noted that annual neonatal mortality rate in their center in the Bronx bore a direct relationship to the annual incidence of infants with a birth weight of 1500 g or less. They suggested that three quarters of the improvement might be attributable to public health factors and only one quarter to either improvement in neonatal care or the improved health status of the newborn. Thus they argued that public health, socioeconomic factors and the institution of specific services (abortion programs and family planning) reduced the actual number of high-risk infants, including those of very low birth weight. Nevertheless, although such socioeconomic factors are important, there is good evidence to suggest that neonatal mortality may be affected by both intrauterine factors causing premature birth or immaturity of the infant and management during delivery and the neonatal period.[22]

Bishop et al.[1] noted that the difference in outcome dependent on the presentation of the infant at delivery was accentuated by low birth weight. They took a birth weight of 2000 g or less as the critical level and showed that when an infant of this weight presented as other than cephalic there was a considerably increased risk of subsequent abnormal development (mental or neurologic) among survivors. Krause and colleagues[9] also noted that the perinatal mortality of underweight fetuses was five times higher in those in breech presentation delivered vaginally than in those delivered by cesarean section.

Our recent study again highlights the hazard to very low birth weight (less than 1500 g) infants presenting abnormally and clearly supports the value of cesarean section for delivery of these infants to ensure the highest survival rates and the best long-term prognosis. Ingemarsson et al.[8] stated that delivery by cesarean section significantly reduced the frequency of severe prolonged asphyxia. The results of our study support the observation. Like us Ingemarsson also reported that cesarean section reduced the neonatal mortality in their series of infants in premature breech presentations. However, they noted that data from 71 European departments showed only a minority of obstetricians prepared to perform cesarean section for fetal reasons before 30 weeks' gestation. In their series cerebrospinal fluid hemorrhage was less common in infants delivered by cesarean section (9 per cent) than in vaginally delivered infants (39 per cent). Recent studies using real-time ultrasound to scan the brains of newborn infants also indicate that intraventricular hemorrhage (IVH) occurs most frequently among infants delivered vaginally in breech presentation and least in infants delivered by cesarean section.[3, 12] In our own study[12] the mean gestation of infants delivered vaginally in breech presentation was significantly shorter than that of the infants delivered by cesarean section. However, because the incidence of IVH decreases as length of gestation increases,[12] it seems likely that gestation rather than mode of delivery was responsible for these differences. Ingemarsson et al.[8] argued, and we would certainly support their statement, that routine cesarean section performed because of impending preterm breech delivery improves neonatal mortality and morbidity and also reduces long-term neurologic sequelae. Furthermore, this approach seems to be justified (as shown in our series) even in extremely early delivery provided that adequate obstetric and neonatal intensive care is available. It seems important,

however, to emphasize that we are advocating cesarean section to avoid all the hazards associated with vaginal breech delivery and not specifically to prevent IVH.

The provision of adequate obstetric and neonatal intensive care is vital and is one of the reasons we support the referral of these patients to special centers. Usher[24] also emphasized referral of patients in whom imminent delivery appeared prematurely. His Canadian experience showed that regionalized perinatal intensive care markedly reduced perinatal mortality. Analyzing neonatal mortality from birth to day 7 for very low birth weight infants according to the type of hospital in which the infants were delivered, he found that hospitals providing neonatal intensive care facilities had a neonatal mortality for infants weighing 1001 to 1500 g of 15 per cent. Hospitals that systematically transferred cases to a referral center had a mortality rate of 25 per cent, while those that provided neither intramural nor postnatal referral lost 48 per cent.

Conclusions and Recommendations

From the experience reported here, we can draw the following conclusions. Provided that they received skilled management throughout the perinatal period, premature infants are potentially viable, even when their birth weights are as low as 750 g and the period of gestation is only 26 weeks. The majority of the survivors are capable of developing without handicaps. Among infants weighing 500 to 1500 g, 28-day mortality falls as birth weight rises. It also falls as length of gestation increases until 29 weeks. Thereafter, there is no significant improvement in mortality for this birth weight range. At all birth weights within this range and at gestations between 26 and 34 weeks, the 28-day mortality is significantly lower for all infants delivered by cesarean section than for those in breech presentation delivered vaginally. This is true, irrespective of whether the infant is presenting by the vertex or the breech at the time of operation. In addition, breech infants delivered vaginally are in a worse condition at birth, probably because they have suffered a greater degree of anoxia, than infants delivered otherwise. They also have a higher incidence of neurodevelopmental handicaps at follow-up. The routine application of forceps in vaginal deliveries of very low birth weight infants, either when the vertex is presenting or to the after-coming head in breech presentations, does not significantly reduce mortality or improve the condition of the infant at birth and should probably be abandoned.

We therefore suggest the following management routines when the estimated fetal weight is more than 500 g or the gestation is 26 weeks or more.

When preterm labor cannot be stopped or when delivery of a very low birth weight infant (less than 1500 g) has to be undertaken because of either maternal or fetal factors, the mother should be transferred to a special unit in which are available expert obstetric care facilities and a neonatal intensive care unit staffed and equipped to treat high-risk infants. If this is impossible, adequate facilities for resuscitation of the infant must be provided, with an experienced neonatologist present, and arrangements made for immediate transfer of the infant to a neonatal intensive care unit. Where delivery is to take place electively it is helpful to carry out an ultrasound examination in order to try to establish whether the fetal weight is under or over 700 g.

FOR SPONTANEOUS LABOR

Delivery by emergency cesarean section should be considered when:

1. There is any presentation other than vertex;

2. There is associated APH,

3. Labor is not progressing as judged by cervical dilatation or lack of descent of presenting part in the presence of regular contractions,

4. Fetal distress develops and the estimated fetal weight is 750 g or more, or gestation is more than 26 weeks.

Vaginal delivery should be anticipated when:

1. The vertex is presenting,

2. There is steady progress of cervical dilation,

3. There is no fetal distress,

4. The maternal condition is satisfactory.

The membranes should be ruptured once labor is definitely established and cervical dilatation is proceeding (beyond 3 cm). Delivery should be spontaneous with an episiotomy and controlled delivery of the head unless there is obvious delay in the second stage, when forceps should be used.

FOR ELECTIVE DELIVERY

Cesarean section should be considered when:

1. There is any presentation other than vertex,

2. Estimated fetal weight is less than 1000 g,

3. There is associated APH,

4. Condition of the cervix is unfavorable for induction (long/posterior),

5. Other conditions apart from prematurity causing fetal compromise are present.

Induction of labor by artificial rupture of the membranes and oxytocin stimulation should be considered only when:

1. The vertex is presenting,

2. Estimated fetal weight is over 1000 g,

3. The cervix is favorable for induction.

The labor should be monitored and, if progress is poor or there is evidence of fetal distress or deterioration of the maternal condition, emergency cesarean section should be undertaken. If progress is satisfactory, delivery should be aided by episiotomy and controlled delivery of the head.

REFERENCES

1. Bishop, E. H., Israel, S. L. and Briscoe, C. C.: Obstetric influence on the premature infant's first year of development. Obstet. Gynecol. 26:628–635, 1965.

2. Câlame, A., Prod'hom, L. S. and Van Melle, G.: Outcome of very low birth weight infants treated in an intensive care unit. Rev. Epidemiol. Sante Publique 25:21–32, 1977.

3. de Lemos, R. A., Tomasovic, J. J. and Null, D. M.: The role of postnatal factors in the pathogenesis of subependymal and intraventricular hemorrhage in the premature infant. Perinatal Intracranial Hemorrhage Conference, Washington, D. C. Syllabus, Columbus, Ross Laboratories, 1980.

4. Drillien, C. M.: Growth and development in a group of children of very low birth weight. Arch. Dis. Child. 33:10–18, 1958.

5. Drillien, C. M.: Incidence of mental and physical handicaps in school age children of very low birth weight. Pediatrics 27:452–464, 1961.

6. Fuller, W. E.: Management of premature labor. Clin. Obstet. Gynecol. 21:2, 542, 1978.

7. Holt, K. S.: The quality of survival. *In* Occasional Papers, 2, 3 and 4. Institute of Research into Mental Retardation. London, Butterworth, 1972.

8. Ingemarsson, I., Westgren, M. and Svenningsen, N. W.: Long-term follow-up of pre-term infants in breech presentation delivered by cesarean section. Lancet 2:172–175, 1978.

9. Krause, W., Michels, W. and Kunath, H.: Supervision and delivery in immature breech presentation. Zentralbl. Gynakol. 100:1062–1067, 1978.

10. Lee, K., Tseng, P., Im Eidelman, A. I., Kandall, S.

R. and Gartner, L. M.: Determinants of the neonatal mortality. Am. J. Dis. Child. 130:842–845.

11. Lehmann, W. D., Jonatha, W. and Forstner, H. A.: Progress in diagnosis and treatment of pregnancies with low birth weight infants. Geburt. Frauenh. 38:606–618, 1978.

12. Lipscomb, A. P., Thorburn, R. J., Blackwell, R. J. et al.: Detection of brain damage in newborn infants by ultrasound and other objective techniques. Perinatal Intracranial Hemorrhage Conference, Washington, D.C. Syllabus, Columbus, Ross Laboratories, 1980.

13. Lubchenco, L. O., Hansman, C., Dressler, M. and Boyd, E.: Intrauterine growth as estimated from liveborn birth weight data at 24–32 weeks of gestation. Pediatrics 32:793–800, 1963.

14. Lubchenco, L. O., Horner, F. A., Reed, L. H. et al.: Sequelae of premature birth. Am. J. Dis. Child. 106:101–115, 1963.

15. Pharoah, P. O. D. and Alberman, E. D.: Mortality of low birth weight infants in England and Wales 1953 to 1979. Arch. Dis. Child. 56:86–89, 1981.

16. Rawlings, G., Reynolds, E. O. R., Stewart, A. L. and Strang, L. B.: Changing prognosis for infants of very low birth weight. Lancet 1:516–519, 1971.

17. Smith, M. L., Spencer, S. A. and Hull, D.: Mode of delivery and survival in babies weighing less than 2000 G at birth. Br. Med. J. 281:1118–1119, 1980.

18. Starte, D. R., Jones, R. A. K., Hall, M. A. and

Harvey, D. R.: Survival of preterm babies. Lancet 2:639–640, 1980.

19. Stewart, A. L. and Reynolds, E. O. R.: Improved prognosis for infants of very low birth weight. Pediatrics 54:724–735, 1974.

20. Stewart, A. L.: Follow-up of preterm infants. *In* Pre-Term Labor. Proceedings of the Fifth Study Group of the Royal College of Obstetricians and Gynaecologists, pp. 372–384, 1977.

21. Stewart, A. L., Turcan, D. M., Rawlings, G. and Reynolds, E. O. R.: Prognosis for infants weighing 1000 G or less at birth. Arch. Dis. Child. 52:97–104, 1977.

22. Stewart, A. L., Turcan, D. M., Rawlings, G., Hart, S. and Gregory, S.: Outcome for infants at high risk of major handicap. *In* CIBA Foundation Symposium No. 59 (New Series). Major Mental Handicap: Methods and Costs of Prevention. pp. 151–164, 1978.

23. Stewart, A. L., Reynolds, E. O. R. and Lipscomb, A. P.: Outcome for infants of very low birth weight: survey of world literature. Lancet 1:1038–1041, 1981.

24. Usher, R.: Changing mortality rates with perinatal intensive care and regionalization. Semin. Perinatol. 1:309–319, 1977.

25. Walsh, H.: Development of children born prematurely with birth weight of 3 lbs or less. Med. J. Austr. 1:108–114, 1969.

How to Deliver the Under 1500-Gram Infant

J. A. Low, M.D.

Queen's University, Kingston, Ontario

D. Worthington, M.D.

The Medical College of Wisconsin

A better understanding of problems presented by the baby who is less than 1500 g at delivery is essential for a rational approach to management. Two major questions arise at this time: Can perinatal mortality rates and handicap rates in children who survive be reduced? What are the perinatal mechanisms relevant to the intrapartum period that contribute to this mortality and subsequent handicap? Data will be presented to indicate that outcome in both areas has improved in the last two decades. Evidence will be reviewed indicating that pulmonary immaturity, perinatal asphyxia, birth trauma and intracranial hemorrhage are mechanisms of mortality and morbidity that should be of concern to the obstetrician during the intrapartum period. On the basis of this background, a plan for

management of labor and delivery of the very low birth weight infant will be developed.

The Problem

INCIDENCE OF PERINATAL MORTALITY AND SUBSEQUENT HANDICAPS

Trends in perinatal mortality rates and survival rates of liveborn infants less than 1500 g at birth are demonstrated by the statistics reported for England and Wales between 1956 and 1974[1] (Table 1). The important observation here is that the modest decrease of fetal and early neonatal deaths has not been associated with an increase of deaths later in the neonatal period.[2]

TABLE 1. PERINATAL MORTALITY AND SURVIVAL
RATES OF INFANTS 500–1500 G
IN ENGLAND AND WALES

	1956	1966	1974
Percentage of perinatal deaths	80.1	76.8	67.7
Percentage of fetal deaths	40.4	37.5	32.2
Percentage of live births– survival rate	33.4	37.1	47.7

Trends in regard to the incidence of handicap in later life are expressed by a number of excellent studies in surviving very low birth weight infants born in the decade 1950 to 1960 in United States, Britain and Europe.[3-11] These provide a basis for comparison for subsequent long-term follow-up studies from the decade 1960 to 1970[12-16] and short term follow-up studies of children born 1970 to 1975.[17-20] The spectrum of handicaps that may occur singly or in combination include neurologic handicaps, sensory system defects and mental retardation.

The incidence of major neurologic handicap, which during 1950 to 1960 usually exceeded 20 per cent, is now less than 10 per cent (Table 2). This decrease is due principally to a decrease of spastic diplegia.[21] However, a new element was added in the 1970s with the introduction of mechanical ventilation in the management of recurrent apnea and severe respiratory distress syndrome (RDS) during the neonatal period—with again an increased incidence of major neurologic handicap in children so treated. It remains to be seen whether this increased incidence of neurologic handicap in children who required mechanical ventilation can be further reduced by a better understanding and improved management of the relevant perinatal events.

Common sensory system defects include loss of vision due to retrolental fibroplasia and hearing defects due to a moderate or severe high-frequency hearing loss. The trends in regard to these defects are outlined in Table 3. Although the incidence of retrolental fibroplasia has decreased with awareness of the importance of oxygen toxicity, it continues to occur in those patients with difficult management problems requiring mechanical ventilation during the neonatal period. The incidence of hearing defects has similarly decreased in recent years.

Trends of severe and particularly borderline mental retardation in very low birth weight infants in relation to the general population are more difficult to establish. During 1950 to 1960, the incidence of IQ less than 90 (40 to 60 per cent) was consistently greater than in available "control" children (8 to 10 per cent). Additionally, McDonald reported an incidence of severe mental retardation—that is, an IQ less than 50—in 2.7 per cent of their very low birth weight infants in relation to an expected incidence of 0.4 per cent in the general population. Initial long-term follow-up studies of very low birth weight infants born since 1960 suggest a decreasing incidence of severe mental retardation and borderline IQ scores[13, 15] and an improved mean IQ for the very low birth weight group.[16]

TABLE 2. INCIDENCE OF NEUROLOGIC HANDICAP IN VERY LOW BIRTH WEIGHT INFANTS*

	DATE	BIRTH WEIGHT	NO. IN STUDY	NO. WITH HANDICAPS	PERCENTAGE
A					
Lubchenko	1948–1953	<1500	133	58	43%
Wright	1952–1956	<1500	65	23	35%
McDonald	1951–1953	<1800	1081	70	7%
Drillien	1948–1960	<1360	91	20	21%
Janus Kukulska	1950–1958	<1250	67	12	21%
B					
Fitzhardinge	1960–1966	<1250	32	2	6%
Davies	1961–1970	<1500	165	7	4%
Stewart	1966–1970	<1500	95	4	4%
Drillien	1966–1971	<1500	88	7	8%
C					
Fitzhardinge	1970–1972	<1500	44	9	20%
Fitzhardinge	1970–1973	<1500	73	21	29%
Marriage	1966–1973	<1500	24	3	12%

*A, born in the decade 1950–1960; B, born in the decade 1960–1970; C, treated with mechanical ventilation.

TABLE 3. INCIDENCE OF RETROLENTAL FIBROPLASIA AND HEARING HANDICAP IN
VERY LOW BIRTH WEIGHT INFANTS*

	DATE	STUDY Birth Weight	No.	VISUAL HANDICAP No.	%	HEARING HANDICAP No.	%
A							
Lubchenko	1947–1953	<1500	133	33	25%	14	18%
Wright	1952–1956	<1500	65	7	11%	6	9%
McDonald	1951– 1953	<1800	1081	40	4%	19	2%
Drillien	1948–1960	<1360	98	25	24%	9	9%
B							
Fitzhardinge	1960–1966	<1250	32	4	12%	1	3%
Davies	1961–1970	<1500	165	4	2.5%	5	3%
Stewart	1966–1970	<1500	95	1	1%	1	1%
C							
Fitzhardinge	1970–1973	<1500	73	4	5%		

*A, born in the decade 1950–1960; B, born in the decade 1960–1970; C, treated with mechanical ventilation.

MECHANISMS OF PERINATAL MORTALITY AND SUBSEQUENT HANDICAP

Some mortality and subsequent handicap is caused by specific prenatal fetal problems such as major central nervous system malformations, chromosomal and metabolic abnormalities or specific fetal infections. Such fetal problems are infrequent but should be identified as a separate category because of their relative importance, particularly in regard to subsequent handicap. For example, of the 90 children in the National Collaborative perinatal project with severe handicaps, the conditions of 27 (30 per cent) were caused by such specific problems.[27]

Perinatal mortality increases with degree of prematurity, and this relationship is important in the very low birth weight infant. The fact of mortality, particularly that due to RDS in the neonatal period, has demonstrated the importance of pulmonary maturity in very low birth weight infants. Pulmonary immaturity underlies many of the major problems encountered by the newborn infant during the neonatal period; similarly, the incidence of subsequent handicap increases with shorter gestation periods. However, in studies of very low birth weight infants, Fitzhardinge[12] observed no association between birth weight or gestational age and subsequent handicap; and Francis Williams[13] saw no correlation between birth weight or gestational age and IQ. Recent follow-up studies of children less than 1000 g at birth[22, 23] have demonstrated an incidence of handicap in keeping with results of the very low birth weight group as a whole. These observations in regard to subsequent handicap suggest that the same priority is justified to improve survival in those infants less than 1000 g in relation to those 1000 to 1500 g at birth.

In experimental studies, perinatal asphyxia with cerebral hypoxia has been identified as a cause of cerebral injury that comes about from changes in the hemodynamics of the cerebral circulation.[24, 25] Assessment of this factor in clinical studies reported to date has been based on the correlation of clinical events assumed to be associated with cerebral hypoxia. The evidence from such clinical studies is somewhat contradictory but would support this conclusion. Lubchenco[5] and Davies[14] did not, while McDonald[9] and Fitzhardinge[12] did demonstrate an association between birth asphyxia or apneic episodes and neurologic handicap. Data from the National Collaborative Perinatal Project similarly led to different conclusions. Churchill,[26] in 44 preterm infants with spastic diplegia, observed no correlation with birth asphyxia; however, Nelson and Broman,[27] in 50 severely handicapped children, demonstrated a significant correlation to the clinical signs of perinatal asphyxia. Two recent studies[15, 23] with acid-base confirmation of metabolic acidosis have demonstrated a significant correlation with neurologic handicap.

Intraventricular hemorrhage, which may in many instances be a result of perinatal asphyxia, is a common observation at autopsy of very low birth weight infants, and there is increasing evidence that this is a significant factor in the subsequent neurologic handicaps in these children. Nelson and Broman[27] have demonstrated that intracranial hemorrhage and neonatal seizures are the most potent predictors in the perinatal period of subsequent major handicap. Churchill,[26] in preterm children with spastic diplegia, concluded that the low hematocrit observed in these children was caused by hemorrhage, particularly intracranial hemorrhage. Fitzhardinge,[19] in children requiring mechanical ventilation, demonstrated a strong correlation between intracranial hemorrhage and neonatal seizures and subsequent neurologic handicap. The importance of intraventricular hemorrhage is being clarified with improved diagnosis by real-time ultrasonography and computerized tomography.

That birth injury may occur in the very low birth weight infant is well demonstrated by occasional experience involving the "trapped" aftercoming head in the precipitate breech delivery. A relationship between birth injury and subsequent handicap in the very low birth weight infant is difficult to establish because of the absence of a specific clinical marker of birth injury. Neither Churchill[26] or Davies[14] could establish a relationship between birth trauma or abnormal delivery and neurologic handicap. However, birth injury must continue to be viewed as a potential mechanism of central nervous system injury until more definitive information is available.

The magnitude of this problem deserves comment. Very low birth weight infants, 500 to 1500 g, account for only 1.0 to 1.2 per cent of total births. Although the incidence is low, it is a matter of national significance. Annual births in this category of three representative countries are outlined in Table 4. The very low birth weight infants in these countries will account for approximately 32,000 deaths annually, while the quality of approximately 16,000 surviving children will be a matter of

TABLE 4. ESTIMATES OF THE ANNUAL NUMBER OF VERY LOW BIRTH WEIGHT INFANTS BASED ON AN INCIDENCE OF 1.0 TO 1.2% OF TOTAL BIRTHS

		TOTAL BIRTHS	BIRTHS <1500 G
United States	1973	3,100,000	37,000
England and Wales	1975	600,000	7,200
Canada	1973	350,000	4,200

concern to society. A second issue arising from the infrequent occurrence of such births relates to the delivery of health care. The average obstetric service with 2000 to 3000 annual deliveries will be responsible for approximately 25 to 30 very low birth weight infants, while the individual physician will encounter only two to three such problems each year. A regional policy for this pregnancies is mandatory in light of the current perinatal mortality and the potential for subsequent handicap, and the complexity of the perinatal health care resources necessary to manage the spectrum of problems that occur in these patients.

The Management

In obstetric management of the very low birth weight infant during labor and delivery, the following general principles should be recognized on the basis of present understanding of the problem:

1. Mortality and subsequent handicap in children who survive can be reduced. Optimal management to attain this objective requires a regional policy and the resources of a perinatal intensive care unit.

2. Those responsible for intrapartum management should strive to assure optimal pulmonary maturity of the newborn, avoid perinatal asphyxia, avoid birth trauma and prevent intracranial hemorrhage.

The first major area of controversy in the management of labor and delivery involves attitudes toward the prenatal administration of glucocorticoids to accelerate pulmonary maturity of the fetus. The second area involves attitudes toward the aggressive management, as opposed to a "hands-off" policy, in patients in labor with a fetus whose estimated birth weight is under 1500 g, and particularly under 1000 g. The third area involves the question of the mode of delivery: Should cesarean section or vaginal delivery be used? Addressing these three issues in general terms, it can be stated that: (1) There is good evidence to show the beneficial effects of prenatal glucocorticoid administration. However, each case must be individually assessed and the benefits and potential risks balanced. (2) An aggressive approach to the management of labor and delivery is justified when the estimated birth weight of the live normal infant is equal to or greater than 750 g. Delivery per vaginum is optimal if this can be accomplished without fetal asphyxia or trauma.

In ideal circumstances the delivery of a low birth weight infant should be conducted in a center with access to appropriate diagnostic and therapeutic resources. Facilities for x-ray, ultrasonography, assessment of fetal pulmonary maturity and intrapartum electronic fetal monitoring may influence the handling of the fetus. The presence of qualified personnel equipped to handle the newborn will optimize care of these small infants. Further, it is likely that most regional centers will have established guidelines for the management of preterm labor and delivery and for the handling of the low birth weight infant based on significant experience.

The obstetrician's first responsibility in regard to successful management of labor and delivery is attention to maternal and fetal factors relevant to and reflecting the heterogenous nature of this group of patients. Although the common clinical situation involving delivery of the under 1500 g baby is the patient in spontaneous labor or with ruptured membranes prior to a gestational length of 32 weeks, there will be instances in which delivery is required. Maternal factors such as severe preeclamptic toxemia, hemorrhage due to placenta previa or abruptio placentae, infection due to chorioamnionitis and disseminated intravascular coagulation due to retained dead fetus will force delivery. Fetal factors associated with a deteriorating intrauterine environment such as severe growth retardation, erythroblastosis fetalis, effect of maternal diabetes mellitus and ultimate deterioration in cases of fetal death may also require delivery. Therefore, fetal assessment should identify multiple pregnancy, differentiate the normal from the congenitally malformed fetus (ultrasonography and x-ray) and assess the well-being of the fetus with the aid of tests of fetoplacental function (serum or urinary estriol levels, serum human placental lactogen [HPL], nonstressed fetal heart rate monitoring and so forth).

Estimation of the gestational age and fetal weight must be carried out in each pregnancy. A careful review of the gestational data and landmarks established during antenatal care is mandatory. Often in preterm labor the gestational data are insecure so that estimation should also include physical examination by an experienced observer supplemented by an ultrasonographic assessment of the fetus. Conflict may further be generated by the possibility of intrauterine growth retardation, and

again ultrasonography will be of value in the estimation of fetal weight.

Following initial assessment, a decision must be made as to whether delivery should be delayed. There are two aspects to this: the first is the question of long-term delay. In the absence of factors necessitating delivery—that is, when the fetal membranes are intact, the cervix is less than 4 cm dilated and there are no contraindications to the use of tocolytic agents—long-term delay may well obviate the problems of the very low birth weight infant. The second aspect is the question of postponement long enough to allow administration of glucocorticoids in an effort to reduce the risk of the newborn infant developing RDS. Liggins has shown that such treatment is associated with a decreased risk for the development of RDS.[28] However, potential risks should be borne in mind. Experiments in which glucocorticoids were administered to newborn mice demonstrated subsequent reduced DNA content in the central nervous system with impairment of brain growth. In the clinical situation there may be an increased incidence of intraventricular hemorrhage when steroids are used to treat newborn infants with RDS.[29] The prenatal administration of glucocorticoids may predispose to an increased risk for maternal infection.[30] For these reasons and because there are situations in which the fetal lungs may have spontaneously accelerated maturity, we believe that each case must be assessed individually. For instance, a reduced incidence of RDS has been shown to be associated with premature rupture of the membranes after a gestational age of 28 weeks or birth weight of 1000 g,[31] and fetal pulmonary maturity may be accelerated in association with severe preeclampsia, recurrent antepartum hemorrhage and fetal growth retardation.[32]

If delivery can be realistically and safely delayed by tocolytic agents to allow assessment of fetal pulmonary maturity, amniotic fluid should be obtained by amniocentesis after ultrasonographic localization of the placenta or aspiration from the cervical canal in cases of premature membrane rupture. The fluid should be submitted for estimation of the lecithin/sphingomyelin (L/S) ratio. If the L/S ratio suggests maturity of the fetal lungs, continuation of tocolytic therapy in cases in which delivery is imminent is not necessary. However, if the L/S ratio suggests the possibility of severe RDS, therapy is continued to allow the administration of the glucocorticoid. We have used the regimen of betamethasone, 12 mg every 12 hours for 2 doses.

In cases of premature rupture of the membranes without labor, each center must review its own experience. Severe intrauterine infection has not been a problem in this center, so that a conservative policy has usually been adopted. Confirmation of rupture is established by direct inspection of the cervix and cultures taken from the cervix and amniotic fluid. In the absence of clinical evidence of chorioamnionitis, the patient is kept in the hospital, vaginal examinations minimized and the onset of spontaneous labor awaited. Maternal assessment includes attention to the nature of the vaginal discharge, recording of temperature and pulse four times daily and evaluation of the white cell count every other day. A white cell count above 15,000 is considered to be indicative of developing infection. Prophylactic antibiotics are not used until the onset of labor. Induction of labor is reserved for those cases in which there is unequivocal evidence of developing infection.

The second controversial question at this time is: What is the minimal gestational age at which an aggressive attitude to the management of labor and delivery is pursued? By an aggressive attitude we mean (1) intensive intrapartum surveillance of the fetus by internal electronic monitoring of the fetal heart rate with fetal capillary acid-base assessment, (2) cesarean section performed in the presence of signs of fetal asphyxia and (3) a commitment to resuscitation of the newborn infant. Again, each center must review its own experience, looking not only at survival but at significant handicap in follow-up of these infants. We would agree with the point of view expressed by Goldenberg and Nelson[33] that an aggressive attitude is certainly justified when 28 weeks of gestation have elapsed (1000 g) and in some cases even earlier. Bowes, for instance, pursues this policy for patients in preterm labor with a fetus whose estimated birth weight is 600 g and gestational age 26 weeks.[34]

In established labor with inevitable delivery, when an aggressive attitude appears justified, internal monitoring of the fetal heart rate is initiated. In the presence of suspicious fetal heart rate patterns, fetal capillary blood is obtained to confirm the diagnosis of fetal asphyxia. Although the primary cause of death in the neonatal period of the low birth weight infant is RDS,[35] fetal asphyxia may set the

stage for the severity of the disease[36] and for intraventricular hemorrhage or necrotizing enterocolitis. Therefore, the purpose of internal fetal monitoring is the early recognition and confirmation of the signs of developing fetal asphyxia. Should these be present and vaginal delivery is not imminent, cesarean section should be performed in an effort to deliver an infant in good condition at birth.

The third controversial area relates to the mode of delivery. If fetal asphyxia does not occur or occurs terminally during labor and if obstetric indications for cesarean section (prolapsed cord, hemorrhage and so forth) are not present, vaginal delivery may be anticipated. The principal is to avoid trauma. Analgesics are best withheld in order to avoid a depressant action in the newborn infant. The labor of low birth weight infants may be so rapid that analgesic agents are not cleared by the time of delivery. Maternal psychological support is necessary and pain relief may be obtained safely by regional techniques such as epidural anesthesia. The delivery should be spontaneous with careful control of the head or the head protected by outlet forceps over a liberal episiotomy. If the infant is born without immediate ventilatory problems, delayed cord clamping for 60 seconds is recommended, since Usher et al. showed mortality from RDS to be reduced in association with higher red cell volumes in the infant.[37] A neonatologist should be present in the delivery room for immediate assessment and management of the infant.

Obstetricians have felt some reluctance to perform cesarean section for the very low birth weight infant. This reluctance is based on a concern for maternal morbidity, on the possibility of an increased risk for the development of RDS in the newborn infant[38] and an unwillingness to be aggressive when chances for survival of the newborn infant are deemed slim. While concern for maternal morbidity should always be kept in mind, the data of Stewart would suggest that delivery by cesarean section, when necessary, may improve the chance of survival. For infants delivered by cesarean section, neonatal mortality fell from 31 per 1000 in 1966 to 1970 to 14 per 1000 in 1970 to 1976, whereas neonatal mortality for all other modes of delivery showed no improvement.[39]

With regard to premature delivery of the infant in breech presentation, an attitude is developing that this is best performed by cesarean section. Cruikshank and Pitkin point out that proof demonstrating that cesarean section represents the optimal mode of delivery for the premature breech does not exist.[40] Rather, close intrapartum surveillance by internal electronic monitoring of the fetus may obviate the need for cesarean section for some very low birth weight infants in breech presentation.

The psychological impact on the parents of a labor involving a low birth weight fetus should be kept in mind. The techniques involved in management of the labor must be carefully explained to both parents, and the parents must be involved in decision-making. Once delivery has occurred the staff of the neonatal intensive care nursery should obviously be sensitive to the issues of maternal-infant bonding in situations in which by necessity the mother must be separated from the infant.

REFERENCES

1. Committee on Child Health Services, Fit for the Future. Vol. 2, Cmnd. 6684, London, H.M.S.O., 1976.
2. Alberman, E.: Stillbirths and neonatal mortality in England and Wales by birthweight, 1953–1971. Health Trends 6:14, 1974.
3. Harper, P. A., Fischer, L. K. and Rider, R. V.: Neurological and intellectual status of prematures at 3 to 5 years of age. J. Pediatr. 55:679–690, 1959.
4. Lubchenco, L. O., Horner, F. A., Reed, L. H. et al.: Sequelae of premature birth. Am. J. Dis. Child. 106:101–115, 1963.
5. Lubchenco, L. O., Delivoria-Papadopoulos, M., Butterfield, L. J. et al.: Long term follow-up studies of prematurely born infants. I. Relationship of handicaps to nursery routines. J. Pediatr. 80:501–508, 1972.
6. Wright, F. H., Blough, R. R., Chamberlin, A. et al.: A controlled follow-up study of small prematures born from 1952 through 1956. Am. J. Dis. Child. 124:506, 1972.
7. Drillien, C. M.: The incidence of mental and physical handicaps in schoolage children of very low birth weight. Pediatrics 27:452–464, 1961.
8. Drillien, C. M.: The incidence of mental and physical handicaps in schoolage children of very low birth weight. II. Pediatrics 39:238–247, 1967.
9. McDonald, A.: Children of very low birth weight. M.E.I.U. Research Monograph Vol. 1. London, Spastics Society and Heineman, 1967.
10. Janus-Kakulska, A. and Lis, S.: Developmental peculiarities of prematurely born children with birth weight below 1250 gm. Dev. Med. Child Neurol. 8:285, 1966.
11. Dargassies, S. S.: Long-term neurological follow-up study of 286 truly premature infants. 2. Neurological sequelae. Dev. Med. Child Neurol. 19:462–478, 1977.
12. Fitzhardinge, P. M. and Ramsay, M.: The improving outlook for the small prematurely born infant. Dev. Med. Child Neurol. 15:447–459, 1973.
13. Francis-Williams, J. and Davies, P. A.: Very low birth weight and later intelligence. Dev. Med. Child Neurol. 16:709–728, 1974.
14. Davies, P. A. and Tizard, J. P. M.: Very low birth weight and subsequent neurological defect. Dev. Med. Child Neurol. 17:3–17, 1975.
15. Stewart, A. L. and Reynolds, E. O. R.: Improved prognosis for infants of very low birth weight. Pediatrics 54:724–735, 1974.
16. Blake, A., Stewart, A. and Tuscan, D.: Perinatal intensive care. J. Psychosomat. Res. 21:261–272, 1977.
17. Drillien, C. M.: Etiology and outcome in low birth weight infants. Dev. Med. Child Neurol. 14:563–574, 1972.
18. Fitzhardinge, P. M.: Early growth and development in low birth weight infants following treatment in an intensive care nursery. Pediatrics 56:162–172, 1975.
19. Fitzhardinge, P. M., Pape, K., Arstikaites, M. et al.: Mechanical ventilation of infants less than 1501 gram birth weight: health, growth, and neurologic sequelae. J. Pediatr. 88:531–541, 1976.
20. Marriage, K. J. and Davies, P. A.: Neurological sequelae in children surviving mechanical ventilation in the neonatal period. Arch. Dis. Child. 52:176–182, 1977.
21. Hagberg, B., Hagberg, G. and Olow, I.: The changing panorama of cerebral palsy in Sweden 1954. 1. Analysis of the general changes. Acta Paediatr. 64:187–192, 1975.
22. Pape, K. E., Buncic, R. J., Ashby, S. and Fitzhardinge, P. M.: The status of two years of low birth weight infants born in 1974 with birth weights less than 1001 grams. J. Pediatr. 92:253–260, 1978.
23. Stewart, A. L., Tiereau, D. M., Rawlings, G. and Reynolds, E. O. R.: Prognosis for infants weighing 1000 grams or less at birth. Arch. Dis. Child. 52:97–104, 1977.
24. Myers, R. E.: Two patterns of perinatal brain damage and their conditions of occurrence. Am. J. Obstet. Gynecol. 112:246, 1972.
25. Braun, A. W. and Myers, R. E.: Central nervous system findings in the newborn monkey following severe in utero partial asphyxia. Neurology 25:327, 1975.
26. Churchill, J. A., Masland, R. S., Naylor, A. A. and Ashworth, M. R.: The etiology of cerebral palsy in prematures. Dev. Med. Child Neurol. 14:114, 1972.
27. Nelson, K. B. and Broman, S. H.: Perinatal risk factors in children with serious motor and mental handicaps. Am. Neurol. 2:371–377, 1977.
28. Liggins, G. C.: Prenatal glucocorticoid treatment: prevention of respiratory distress syndrome. In Moore, T. D. (ed.): Lung Maturation and the Prevention of Hyaline Membrane Disease. Seventieth Conference on Pediatric Research, Columbus, Ross Laboratories, pp. 97–103, 1976.
29. Taeusch, H. W., Jr.: Glucocorticoid prophylaxis for respiratory distress syndrome: a review of potential toxicity. J. Pediatr. 87:617–723, 1975.
30. Taeusch, H. W., Jr., Frigoletto, F., Kitzmiller, J., et al.: Risk of respiratory distress syndrome and maternal infection after prenatal dexamethasone treatment. Pediatr. Res. (Abstract, in press).
31. Worthington, M. D., Maloney, A. and Smith, B. T.:

Fetal lung maturity 1. Mode of onset of premature labor. Influence of premature rupture of the membranes. Obstet. Gynecol. 49:275–279, 1977.

32. Gould, J. B., Gluck, L. and Kulovich, M. V.: The relationship between accelerated pulmonary maturity and accelerated neurological maturity in certain chronically stressed pregnancies. Am. J. Obstet. Gynecol. 127:181–186, 1977.

33. Goldenberg, R. L. and Nelson, K. G.: Viability of the premature fetus in distress. Lancet 1:764–765, 1978.

34. Bowes, W. A.: Results of the intensive perinatal management of very low birth weight infants (501–1500 grams). *In* Anderson, A., Beard, R., Brudenell, J. M. and Dunn, P. M. (eds.): Preterm Labour. Proceedings of the Fifth Study Group of the Royal College of Obstetricians and Gynaecologists, 1977.

35. Rush, K. W., Keirse, M. J., N. C., Howat, P. et al.: Contribution of preterm delivery to perinatal mortality. Br. Med. J., 965–968, 1976.

36. Worthington, D. and Smith, B. T.: Relation of amniotic fluid lecithin/sphingomyelin ratio and fetal asphyxia to respiratory distress syndrome in premature infants. Can. Med. Assoc. J. 118:1384–1389, 1978.

37. Usher, R. H., Saigal, S., O'Neil, A. et al.: Estimation of red blood cell volume in premature infants with and without respiratory distress syndrome. Biol. Neonatol. 26:241–248, 1975.

38. Usher, R., McLean, F. and Maughan, G. B.: Respiratory distress syndrome in infants delivered by cesarean section. Am. J. Obstet. Gynecol. 88:806, 815, 1964.

39. Stewart, A.: Follow-up of preterm infants. *In* Anderson, A., Beard, R., Brudenell, J. M. and Dunn, P. M. (eds.): Preterm Labour. Proceedings of the Fifth Study Group of the Royal College of Obstetricians and Gynaecologists, 1977.

40. Cruikshank, D. P. and Pitkin, R. M.: Delivery of the premature breech. Obstet. Gynecol. 50:367–369, 1977.

Editorial Comment

Many exciting advances in health care have occurred in the area of perinatology and one of these is the special consideration for the very low birth weight baby. Not too many years ago the outcome for the baby under 1500 g was considered with guarded prognosis. It is an accepted fact in the 1980s that any baby over 1500 g should have at least a 90 per cent chance of survival and the under 1500-g baby has an extraordinarily good chance of survival and productivity with major handicaps occurring in less than 10 per cent.

The contributors to this significant chapter have made major contributions in the area of perinatology. One would consider the challenge of obstetric and neonatal care for the under 2500-g fetus as the most significant in perinatology.

The major consideration is that perinatal mortality and morbidity rates, and the major handicap problems in children under 2500 g who survive, can now be kept to a minimum. The most significant intrapartum factors that contribute to problems of morbidity and mortality in these small babies are pulmonary immaturity, perinatal asphyxia and birth trauma with associated intracranial hemorrhage. The challenge is to discover how these problems can be averted and neurologic handicaps, as seen in the decades from 1950 to 1980, reduced to below 10 per cent.

Low and Worthington point out that intrapartum management should strive to (1) ensure optimal pulmonary maturity of the newborn, (2) avoid perinatal asphyxia, (3) avoid birth trauma and (4) prevent intracranial hemorrhage. One major area of controversy deals with the prenatal administration of glucocorticoids to accelerate pulmonary maturity of the fetus. We have been proponents of utilizing hydrocortisone (Codero and Semchyshyn) in a dose of 1 g every 8 hours for a total of 4 g, then waiting 24 hours after the last dose before delivery is effected. (Eighty per cent of patients had an increased L/S.) Most physicians who use glucocorticoids, however, utilize betamethasone in two doses, 12 to 14 hours apart. The critical issue is that the lowest dosage to achieve fetal pulmonary maturity has yet to be determined.

A most critical issue for the small baby is to determine gestational age and fetal weight with a high degree of accuracy. The laying on of hands is reasonable to estimate fetal weight, but we have the impression that the baby's weight is usually underestimated instead of overestimated. Ultrasonography is most helpful and great advances have been made in this area to assist in decision-making. Our group at Ohio State has been able to calculate fetal weights to within 6 to 8 per cent of actual weights utilizing real-time ultrasonography. This has been a major breakthrough in decision making. Once membranes rupture, it is difficult to get an accurate reading and estimation of fetal weight.

The history should be relied upon and evaluated in relation to estimation of fetal weight, then this should be confirmed with ultrasonography. The physician should evaluate all parameters, such as status of membranes, condition of cervix, labor, pulmonary maturity and reaction of fetus by fetal heart studies.

The next question that emerges is how and when the baby should be delivered. How can you offer the baby the maximum protection against birth trauma and intrapartum asphyxia? Most obstetricians in the 1980s will undoubtedly do a cesarean section for the premature infant in breech presentation, and this is substantiated by the contribution from Fairweather and Stewart in which they evaluate the weeks of gestation and survival by method of delivery. They report the outcome of 490 liveborn infants weighing between 500 to 1500 g delivered at University College Hospital in London during the years 1971 to 1977. This group has had extensive experience with the small baby and have afforded us evidence of a good follow-up and outcome. They point out the extreme significance of weight and that the baby over 1000 g has a considerably better chance of survival than that under 1000 g; hence, the distribution within the group of the 500- to 1500-g baby will determine results. They did not utilize steroids except in three patients. Significant differences were noted between the mortalities among the cesarean section deliveries, vaginal deliveries involving forceps and all deliveries of breech infants. Their studies clearly indicate that the low birth weight baby of less than 1500 g that presents abnormally benefits from cesarean section. Further, in 71 European departments of obstetrics it was shown that only a minority of obstetricians were prepared to perform cesarean section for fetal reasons before 30 weeks of gestation; I think that this would be in keeping with the current practice in the United States. It would appear that this is where our thinking must be altered.

All authors re-emphasize the significance of electronic monitoring of the small baby and the necessity of an atraumatic delivery utilizing a generous episiotomy, shortening the second stage of labor by use of forceps and using good anesthesia for perineal relaxation. Crenshaw and Miller advocate an atraumatic delivery of a nonasphyxiated infant with a neonatologist present. They state that it is impossible to scientifically answer the question of precisely how to deliver each individual patient.

Adamsons and Cashore, at Women & Infants Hospital, Rhode Island, were unable to demonstrate a difference in survival of the 500- to 1500-g infant, whether delivered vaginally or by cesarean section. Furthermore, infants in both delivery groups had an incidence of RDS of approximately 50 per cent; these authors believe that there is no clear survival advantage conferred by cesarean section.

Bowes, from the University of Colorado Medical Center, reiterates what others have said and states that they do not use glucocorticoids for the small infant. At each delivery a resuscitation team headed by a staff neonatologist, which also includes pediatric residents and a neonatal intensive care nurse, was available in the delivery room along with a staff obstetrician experienced in care of the under 1500-g baby. What Bowes is saying is that if the effort that needs to be put into the care of the small baby is going to be made, it should be made by the first team from the beginning. If having a staff neonatologist and obstetrician present is not a matter that is disagreed on, then why don't other institutions do the same thing? Is the focus of controversy the neonatologist, the obstetrician or the under 1500-g baby? The Colorado investigators feel that they do not have conclusive evidence that cesarean section protects the preterm infant from the trauma of a vaginal delivery; however, the literal use of abdominal delivery, especially in breech presentations, is emphasized. They point out the work of others and follow this themselves in believing that the most significant time for the baby certainly is the first hour of life and often the first five minutes, and that first team efforts are necessary to achieve higher salvage.

When all is said and done, the points of significance in this chapter deal with a philosophy of care, in which there are areas of controversy. It is important to put full effort into the salvage of the small baby and the first team should be present to institute this therapy, which begins from the time the patient is admitted to the obstetric unit. Abnormal presentations are probably best handled by abdominal delivery. The most important thing to offer the infant, whether delivered via abdominal or vaginal route, is an atraumatic delivery with the absence of intrapartum hypoxia and an excellent neonatal intensive care unit in which to reside. This interest in the survival of the small baby has rattled the chains of conventional thinking in obstetrics today.

5
Administration of Steroids for Acceleration of Fetal Lung Maturity

Alternative Points of View

by Edward H. Bishop
by Allen P. Killam and L. L. Penney
by Leandro Cordero and Stefan Semchyshyn
by Jack M. Schneider and John C. Morrison
by A. E. Seeds

Editorial Comment

Administration of Steroids for Acceleration of Fetal Lung Maturity: Yes or No?

Edward H. Bishop, M.D.
University of North Carolina School of Medicine

Pulmonary complications of the premature infant continue to be a major and largely unsolved problem for both obstetricians and pediatricians. The etiology of preterm labor is multifaceted and, even when a cause is recognized, too often unresponsive to the best preventive or therapeutic practices of the obstetrician. Under some circumstances indicated preterm labor may be the best solution in the face of many maternal and fetal complications of pregnancy. In such situations the obstetrician is often obliged to balance the risks to the mother or the fetus or both of continued intrauterine existence in a less than optimal, even dangerous, environment against the risk of pulmonary problems in the neo-nate, which may result from premature termination of pregnancy.

The presumption that respiratory distress syndrome (RDS) and hyaline membrane disease result from a deficiency or absence of surfactant in the fetal or neonatal lung is well accepted. A potential response to this problem has been evoked by the observation, first in animals and later in human subjects, that antenatal administration of corticosteroids to the mother can diminish the expected incidence and severity of neonatal pulmonary problems. The impelling need for a method of reduction of these complications stimulated investigators in the obstetric and pediatric specialties to quickly and enthusiastically act on the suggestion that administration of exogenous steroids appears to accelerate fetal pulmonary maturity. The value of this new procedure has been supported by many, questioned by some, and approached with an attitude of caution or even rejection by others. The apparent rapid and widespread acceptance of this method of management has given rise to several controversial issues.

Does the administration of steroids result in a reduction in the frequency and the severity of RDS and a decrease in the associated perinatal mortality rate? The first portion of this question hardly remains a controversial issue. Although the effectiveness of therapy depends on many factors—including gestational age, type and dosage of drug, interval from treatment to delivery and reason for preterm labor—there appears to be a uniformity of opinion in both published and anecdotal reports that the antenatal administration of steroids markedly reduces the expected frequency of neonatal pulmonary problems. This is particularly evident for those infants delivered with a gestational age between 28 and 32 weeks and for whom the incidence of RDS is reduced to approximately one quarter of that of control groups. There is less uniformity of opinion regarding the beneficial effects to those outside of these time limits. The effect of numerous variables other than treatment has made it difficult to judge whether therapy reduces the severity of the disease when it does occur. In spite of many favorable reports there is no consistently accepted opinion that the overall perinatal mortality rate is decreased by this method of therapy.

What is the mechanism of action? Steroids apparently act as a stimulant to lung maturity in several ways. Accumulated evidence indicates the presence of binding sites or receptors specific for glucocorticoids in the nuclei and cytoplasm of fetal lung cells. It is a reasonable conclusion that glucocorticoids induce local enzymatic activity, which in turn promotes morphologic and functional differentiation of the type II alveolar cells. These maturational changes eventually result in the synthesis and release of surfactant. If these suppositions are correct they provide a physiologic justification for the antepartum prevention and treatment of RDS.

Johnson[1] using the rhesus monkey as an experimental model, reached somewhat different conclusions. His work indicated that the administration of a steroid produces an increase in maximum fetal lung volumes and subsequent improved respiratory function by connective tissue alterations. He was unable to demonstrate a significant increase in alveolar surfactant following therapy. As yet this divergent point of view has not been confirmed by others.

What are the indications for use? A majority of experiences have indicated that the prospect of a planned or threat of an unplanned delivery occurring between 28 and 32 weeks of gestational age is an indication for the use of steroid therapy. It appears that before 28 weeks the fetal lungs are insufficiently developed to respond to these agents, while after 32 weeks there is ordinarily sufficient physiologic response and spontaneous production of surfactant to make exogenous medication of little value. Two problems exist with this position. First, it is often difficult to accurately estimate gestational age. Therefore, it has been the policy at my institution to err on the side of giving a steroidal agent, possibly even when it is neither needed nor beneficial, rather than subject the unexpectedly small fetus to the risk of pulmonary problems without the benefit of preventive treatment. Contrary to the majority opinion, at least one group of investigators[2] has demonstrated to its satisfaction that this method of therapy may be of value in selected circumstances even up to 37 weeks' gestational age. Under such circumstances we prefer—and it seems more rational—to determine the lecithin/sphingomyelin (L/S) ratio first and utilize steroid therapy only when unfavorable functional pulmonary maturity is indicated in spite of apparently advanced gestational age. Our present criteria for selection of suitable candidates are as follows:

1. Delivery is anticipated or planned after 28 weeks but prior to 32 weeks' gestational age.

2. Delivery can be safely deferred for at least 24 hours.

3. Delivery is anticipated after 32 weeks' gestational age but with an L/S ratio indicating prematurity.

4. There are no contraindications for administration of steroids or continuation of pregnancy.

What agent should be used? Numerous compounds have been used and demonstrated to be effective, including betamethasone, dexamethasone, cortisol, prednisone, prednisolone and hydrocortisone.

Betamethasone (a combination of betamethasone acetate and betamethasone sodium phosphate), as originally recommended by Liggins,[3] remains the most commonly used and apparently preferable agent. It has the main advantage that relatively small amounts can be used to accomplish the desired end result. The only potential advantage of some of the more potent agents is a possible decrease in the time between administration and attainment of maximal effectiveness. At least this appears true when the drug effectiveness is measured by the rate of suppression of maternal estriol excretion rates. This slight advantage does not appear to warrant the use of either more potent drugs or larger dosages.

What is the optimum dosage? The original schedule proposed by Liggins[3] (6 mg of betamethasone acetate combined with 6 mg of betamethasone phosphate), given intramuscularly and repeated in 24 hours, seems to be the most efficacious schedule. A controversial issue is the question of repeating the medication if delivery does not occur within a reasonable period of time but while the gestational age is still within the critical period. If it is possible to accurately judge the effectiveness by measurement of maternal plasma cortisol levels, it would appear that the effects of steroid therapy begin within 24 hours and continue for approximately 4 days. However, even with the use of controls there is relatively little documented evidence that repeated administration improves outcome. On the other hand, it probably does not appreciably increase risk.

What are the contraindications? Although documented unfavorable side effects are few, there is little justification for the use of this method of management outside the limits of gestational age for which effectiveness has been demonstrated. In a similar vein, it must be emphasized that there is no indication or justification for unnecessary delivery of a premature infant merely because it has been "protected" by the use of steroids.

It has been repeatedly suggested that steroid therapy should not be used in those pregnancies complicated by hypertensive disorders, particularly toxemia of pregnancy. This is based on the premise that the use of exogenous steroids may result in a further deterioration of placental function already impaired by the complication of pregnancy. Conclusions are primarily based on a small experience reported in the original work of Liggins.[3] Up to the present time we at the University of North Carolina have not hesitated to use steroids under these circumstances when the benefits apppear to outweigh the risks. The presence of maternal diabetes is a relative contraindication, which must be evaluated for each particular instance. The presence of either maternal or intrauterine infections is ordinarily considered as a major contraindication.

Does the prenatal administration of a steroid result in a favorable change in the L/S ratio? The majority of investigators[3-5] who have measured L/S ratios both in animals and human subjects—before and after the administration of steroids—have observed a significant increase in the rise of the L/S ratio. Johnson,[1] using rhesus monkeys, noted only a trend in this direction. Liggins,[3] in his original publication, reported that the L/S ratio was unchanged but supportive data were not supplied. However, if it is accepted that this method of management is clinically effective, it is of only academic interest whether the salutary effects can be demonstrated by laboratory means.

Is it justifiable to delay delivery by inhibiting labor until the steroid therapy becomes effective? It is a consensus that little benefit can be expected before a lapse of 12 hours after the first administration of the drugs, with maximal effectiveness occurring 12 to 24 hours after the second dose. This conclusion frequently provokes attempts to delay delivery by the use of pharmacologic agents. However, such a delay may be associated with some risks: the risk of continuation of the disease that is provoking preterm labor as well as, particularly in the situation of premature rupture of the membranes, the increased risk of infection. Obviously this point remains controversial and each case must be evaluated on its own merit to ensure that the benefits exceed the risks.

Are there dangers or disadvantages for the mother? The pharmacologic effects of glucocorticoids on adult human subjects are well known.[6] However, few undesirable major side effects can be expected resulting from the short-term low-dosage schedule ordinarily used for this purpose. An increase in the incidence of sepsis might be expected but is seldom reported. A masking of the manifestations of potential or early infections remains a possibility. An acceleration of the risk of the hypertensive disorders of pregnancy exists as a possibility as well. Possible association with episodes of maternal gastrointestinal bleeding has been reported.[7] One practical advantage of steroid therapy during pregnancy results in the associated diminished maternal urinary excretion of estriol, which precludes use of this method of assessment of fetoplacental integrity.

In summary, it appears that at this time the potential fetal benefits outweigh any theoretical or actual maternal risks, except under particular circumstances.

Are there dangers or disadvantages for the infant? At the present time it appears that sufficient data have been collected to indicate that, in respect to pulmonary complications, the neonatal course of the premature infant is ordinarily improved by antenatal administration of corticosteroid compounds to the mother. Nevertheless, almost without exception, every author who has published material on this subject has included some words regarding concerns and fears for the fetus—fears of growth retardation, potential alteration of the central nervous system function, increased chance of amnionitis, risk of impaired placental function and numerous other concerns. It is known that many maturational processes can be accelerated by the administration of corticosteroids and this acceleration also implies the possibility of simultaneous limitation of growth. In spite of the recognized undesirable side effects of these agents in adults, and in spite of documentation of adverse effects in experimental animals, up to this time no serious deleterious effects have been noted in surviving human subjects. However, it must be recognized that insufficient time has elapsed since the institution of this program to evaluate the possibility of occurrence of late toxic effects, many of which cannot be recognized or elucidated until the subjects reach school age. Therefore, in spite of the many favorable reports, steroid therapy should not be instituted without serious consideration of the benefits and risks and only after full explanation to the parents.

REFERENCES

1. Johnson, J. W. C., Mitzner, W., London, W. T., Palmer, A. E., Scott, R. and Kearney, K.: Glucocorticoids and the rhesus fetal lung. Am. J. Obstet. Gynecol. 130:905, 1978.
2. Thornfeldt, R. E., Franklin, R. W., Pickering, N. A., Thornfeldt, C. R. and Amell, G.: The effect of glucocorticoids on the maturation of premature lung membranes. Am. J. Obstet. Gynecol. 131:143, 1978.
3. Liggins, G. C. and Howie, R. N.: A controlled trial of antepartum glucocorticoid treatment for prevention of the respiratory distress syndrome in premature infants. Pediatrics 50:515, 1972.
4. Spellacy, W. N., Buhi, W. C., Riggall, F. C. and Holsinger, K. L.: Human amniotic fluid lecithin/sphingomyelin ratio changes with estrogen or glucocorticoid treatment. Am. J. Obstet. Gynecol. 115:216, 1973.
5. Caspi, E., Schryeyer, P., Weinraub, Z., Reif, R., Levi, I. and Mundel, G.: Prevention of the respiratory distress syndrome in premature infants by antepartum glucocorticoid therapy. Br. J. Obstet. Gynecol. 83:187, 1976.
6. Taeusch, H. W., Jr.: Glucocorticoid prophylaxis for respiratory distress syndrome: a review of potential toxicity. Pediatrics 87:617, 1975.
7. Brown, B. J., Gabert, H. A. and Stenchever, M. A.: Respiratory distress syndrome, surfactant biochemistry and acceleration of fetal lung maturity: a review. Obstet. Gynecol. Surv. 30:71, 1975.

Administration of Steroids for Hastening Fetal Lung Maturity

Allen P. Killam, M.D.
Duke University Medical Center

L. L. Penney, M.D.
William Beaumont Army Medical Center, El Paso, Texas

In 1972 Liggins and Howie reported that newborns of 28 to 32 weeks' gestational age born 1 to 7 days following betamethasone administration to their mothers had significantly less respiratory distress syndrome (RDS) and lower mortality rates than a corresponding group whose mothers had received cortisone.[41] Subsequent reports have also indicated substantial clinical improvement in premature infants related to antepartum corticosteroid treatment.

To date, serious side effects of these drugs

have not materialized; however, it is not possible to conclude that untoward reactions will not occur. The potential for long-term complications is unknown; therefore, this potential, particularly with the spectre of incidents involving such drugs as antepartum diethylstilbestrol ever present, demands caution in assuring patients of the safety of antepartum corticosteroids. The Food and Drug Administration has not, to our knowledge, authorized any manufacturer to claim efficacy of a corticosteroid for the purpose of hastening maturity in fetal lung.

The physician must make the difficult decision of whether to deny therapy to a fetus at high risk, therapy that may improve the chances of survival 50 per cent with potential side effects. The physician is in jeopardy of litigation, whether or not he administers one of these drugs, if he delivers a premature infant who dies or suffers a major complication. The purpose of this chapter is to review the literature pertaining to antepartum corticosteroid and to discuss the pros and cons of its use in several common clinical situations.

Animal Research

Major impetus in the steroid aspect of RDS prevention resulted from Liggins' observation in 1969 of increased survival in prematurely delivered fetal lambs that had received dexamethasone injections.[40] Multiple corticosteroid preparations of differing potency, duration of action, ability to cross the placenta unchanged and affinity to cortisol-binding globulin and cell receptors have been administered by several routes experimentally in numerous animal species at variable periods of gestation. Their effects on many parameters of fetal lung maturity have been quantitated by many techniques. These in vivo experiments and related studies are summarized in Table 1. Types of preparations, dosages, routes of administration, and periods of gestation are available in each instance in the listed reference as are the number of animals and method of control. The danger of extrapolating animal data, primate or other species, to the human should be recognized.

Human Research

Numerous corticosteroids have been evaluated in regard to human RDS. In vitro, lungs from human fetuses at 17 to 24 weeks respond to cortisol by increasing lecithin production and choline incorporation into lecithin.[18] Lung tissue from fetuses at 10 to 20 weeks shows enhanced growth, as monitored by DNA accumulation, if cortisol is added to the culture media.[60] Cortisol inhibited the growth of fetal larynx, trachea, esophagus and skin fibroblasts. Lung cells were capable of converting cortisone to cortisol. Clinical investigations have been conducted with betamethasone, dexamethasone, methylprednisolone and cortisol. Additional studies directed at determining placental transfer have been reported that have involved prednisone, prednisolone, hydrocortisone and cortisone.

PLACENTAL STUDIES

Metabolic clearance rates and transplacental passage of prednisone, prednisolone, cortisone and cortisol in near-term pregnancy have been investigated.[6, 7] Intravenous maternal cortisone yields approximately the same concentration of fetal cortisol as maternal cortisol infusion, even though maternal cortisol infusion yields higher maternal cortisol concentration than maternal cortisone infusion. Cortisone, which is loosely bound to protein, would be expected to cross the placenta more readily than cortisol. Cortisol is converted to cortisone by placental dehydrogenase activity. This may account for some of the higher levels of cortisone in cord plasma. The same situation exists with maternal prednisone and prednisolone infusion. Equal infusions of both yield higher fetal levels of prednisone, presumably by a combination of less protein binding of prednisone and the conversion of prednisolone to prednisone by placental dehydrogenase activity as it crosses the placenta.

Ballard and associates studied 43 infants whose mothers had received doses of 6 mg each betamethasone phosphate and acetate and 22 infants of mothers treated with placebo.[5] Highest cord blood betamethasone levels were 14.3 μg cortisol equivalents at 1 hour and were undetectable 2 days after a second dose at 24 hours. Mean cord blood cortisol levels following the second dose were 5.9 μg per dl compared with 13.05 μg per dl in untreated premature infants. Betamethasone was either bound to albumin or was unbound. The unbound glucocorticoid activity in treated infants delivered 1 to 10 hours after the second

TABLE 1. Parameters Investigated

	Lung SA and/or Total PC	AW, TF and/or AF SA PC	Lung and/or AW ST	L/S Ratio	Lung Dist	Lung DNA Content and/or Syn	Histologic Lung Maturation	PD and/or FD	Ref and Misc
Dexamethasone									
Baboon				I				No	35, IA
Rat	I	I							47, M
Guinea Pig	I	I						Yes	47, M
						D*		Yes	55, F
Sheep	I	I				U			49, F
μP									
Sheep			U		U		U	Yes	66, F
9-FP									
			U		I				38, F, IA
Rabbit			D		I				39, F, IA†
			D				I		74, F, IA
									24, Enzymatic study
Betamethasone									
Rhesus									21, F‡
	U		U	U, I	I	U			30, M
Baboon	I		D	I	U				37, IA (I Lung stability)
Cortisol									
			D		I			Yes	16, F
Sheep			D		I			Yes	37, F
	U		U						29, F
			U					Yes	46, M
			D				I		46, F
								No	64, F (I Lung stability)
Rabbit	U		D			U			54, F¶
	(PG changes)	I					I		50, 52F¶
Metapirone									
Baboon				D	U			No	35, M
Rat	D								47, M
Corticotropin									
Rabbit					§		‖		15, F

*Also decreased in brain, adrenal, kidney and heart.
†No change in ossification centers.
‡Evidence of neuronal brain injury in steroid treated animals.

§No change in stability following decapitation.
‖Treatment restored pre-decapitation appearance
¶Enzymatic studies. See also Ref 18 and Ref 19, M.

I = Increased or improved, D = decreased, U = unchanged, MP = Methylprednisolone, 9-FP = 9-Fluoroprednisolone, PC = Phosphatidylcholine, PG = Phosphatidylglycerol, TF = Tracheal fluid, AW = Alveolar wash, AF = Amniotic fluid, SA = Surface active, ST = Surface tension, DIST = Distensibility, SYN = Synthesis, PD = Premature delivery, FD = Fetal death, REF = Reference, MISC = Miscellaneous, M,F, or IA = Maternal, fetal, or intra-amniotic administration.

dose was similar to unbound cortisol levels after birth in untreated premature infants who develop RDS. Ballard's associates commented that second doses should be considered at 18 hours and third doses 24 hours after the second and concluded that "serum glucocorticoid levels in the physiologic stress range can induce lung maturation in the human, and antenatal treatment with this dose of betamethasone does not expose the human fetus to potentially harmful pharmacologic levels of steroid."[5]

Intravenous pharmacologic doses of cortisol (1000 mg at 0, 8, 16 and 24 hours) produce a more rapid and profound suppression of maternal serum unconjugated estriol in preterm pregnancies than 12 mg of intramuscular betamethasone at 0 and 24 hours.[75] Compared to a retrospective control group there was less RDS with either drug and, compared to untreated peer infants with and without RDS, no adverse effects were detectable up to 2 years of age.[34] Growth rates of height, weight and head circumference were included in the comparison.

Blanford and Murphy have shown 67 and 51 per cent conversion respectively of cortisol and prednisolone to inactive 11-keto metabolites after 2 hours of in vitro incubation with minced human placenta.[8] Comparable figures for dexamethasone and betamethasone were 1.8 and 7.1 per cent.

EFFECTS OF CORTICOSTEROIDS ON THE L/S RATIO

The effects of various corticosteroids on the L/S ratio of amniotic fluid have been studied by several investigators.[12, 13, 19, 42, 58, 61, 77] No consistent increase in the L/S ratio was found within a week of starting therapy. This is notable in view of the fact that clinical improvement of lung function is reported after only 24 hours of therapy.

RDS INCIDENCE AND MORTALITY RATES

The intramuscular combination of 6 mg betamethasone phosphate and 6 mg betamethasone acetate on entry to the trial, with a second dose 24 hours later if delivery had not occurred, was used by Liggins and Howie in 289 patients with unplanned preterm labor.[41] Control patients received 6 mg cortisone acetate as placebo and 266 were treated. Due to a reduction in early neonatal deaths, the treated infants' perinatal mortality was 10.4 per cent as opposed to 17.7 per cent in the controls. Occurrence of RDS was less frequent in treated infants from 26 to 32 weeks of gestational age (21.2 as opposed to 63.2 per cent) and in those 1 to 7 days from institution of therapy (8.7 and 26.3 per cent). Also noted was a decrease of neonatal deaths with intraventricular cerebral hemorrhage in treated infants. However, in planned deliveries prior to 36 weeks, for hypertension-edema-proteinuria syndrome, there were more perinatal deaths in treated infants. This was not significant at $p < 0.1$ using the chi-squared test with Yates's correction. One might also be more suspicious of a higher incidence of RDS subsequent to ethanol treatment to inhibit labor. Doubling the dose of betamethasone does not appear to improve results.[42] Presumably the choice of cortisone as the control treatment is not detrimental. This trial now includes at least 884 infants, and the results are as just cited, with the added finding of benefit to infants of 32 to 34 weeks' gestational age.[43]

Fargier et al. injected 2 doses of 12 mg betamethasone 24 hours apart. He compared a group of 42 infants born to treated mothers with 397 control infants of untreated mothers chosen in a nonblind manner. Both groups had a mean gestational age of 33 weeks. RDS was reduced from a control of 20 per cent to 4.4 per cent and a concomitant decrease in neonatal mortality was noted.[23]

In another study using betamethasone, Block et al. administered a 1 cc volume containing either saline, 6 mg each betamethasone phosphate and acetate, or 125 mg methylprednisolone.[6] A second injection 24 hours later was given in the absence of delivery. All treatment schedules were blinded. Alcohol was used to delay labor. There were 57 live births and 3 stillbirths in the betametasone infants and 53 live births and 1 stillbirth in the saline controls. Methylprednisolone did not affect the RDS incidence but betamethasone lowered the figures to 8.7 per cent compared to 22.6 per cent in the saline group when all live births were considered. This was true with all premature infants less than 37 weeks, and a differential effect at less than 32 weeks was not appreciated. There was no increased efficacy if more than 24 hours elapsed from institution of therapy. Interestingly, the infants who did not develop RDS in the methylprednisolone and control groups averaged 2 to 3 days more "treatment time" than those with RDS, and those who did not develop RDS in the betamethasone group about 2 days less "treatment time." Intact membranes also seemed to be important in achieving desired treatment results, but it is not clear whether the betamethasone is less effective with premature rupture of the membrane or the controls have less RDS with premature rupture. Overall perinatal mortality rates were lowest in the betamethasone group but the data were not statistically significant.

From 179 infants born to mothers treated with Liggins and Howie's regimen, Kennedy studied the 41 who were between 27 and 34 weeks' gestation, weighed less than 2000 g and had a treatment-delivery interval of 1 to 7 days.[33] They were retrospectively matched randomly to infants of similar birth weight and gestational age born in the same time frame to untreated mothers. A reduction of 56 to 14.6 per cent in the prevalence of RDS occurred with treatment. A 50 per cent reduction in related deaths (from 8 to 4) was not statistically significant. There were 28 with premature membrane rupture in the treated group and 7 among the controls. No untoward effects were reported.

Caspi et al. treated a group of 55 mothers (5 sets of twins) between 28 and 36 weeks' gestation with isoxsuprine to delay labor when necessary and intramuscular dexamethasone 4 mg tid for up to 7 days.[13] Their control group of 62 patients (9 sets of twins or 71 infants) received no treatment. They reported significant differences in incidence of RDS and neonatal death rates with reductions from 35.2 to 8.3 and 38 to 6.6 per cent, respectively. Among the treated group "the few patients in whom delivery occurred less than 24 hours after admission were omitted from the study."

A further reduction (continuing a 13-year trend) in crude incidence rates of RDS and related mortality rates following broad use of betamethasone in mothers whose fetuses were believed more than 1000 g in weight has been published.[48]

In another study, nonblind, using untreated controls, dexamethasone was administered in a dose of 8 mg a day for 2 days with a repeat dose in 1 week if delivery had not occurred. Reductions in incidence of RDS in 26 infants less than 32 weeks' gestation and in 84 infants 32 to 36 weeks' gestation were cited.[70]

In a small series of patients compared with controls "chosen at random," a reduction in RDS at less than 37 weeks' gestation was reported, if a single intramuscular dose of 100 mg hydrocortisone preceded delivery by more than 24 hours.[17] Morrison[45] reported increased survival with antenatal hydrocortisone and Young[76] reported reduced perinatal mortality with dexamethasone.

Clinical Situations

PREMATURE RUPTURE OF THE FETAL MEMBRANES

In theory, there are at least two reasons not to give corticosteroids to patients with ruptured membranes. Under some circumstances, corticosteroids may increase a patient's susceptibility to infection and at the same time obscure the clinical evidence of infection if it occurs. Secondly, rupture of the fetal membranes may be associated with elevated fetal cortisol levels[5] and may in itself accelerate fetal lung maturation. In Liggins' study, there was no evidence of increased morbidity from infection in the treated as opposed to the control group with ruptured fetal membranes. There are conflicting reports concerning the effect of prolonged ruptured fetal membranes on fetal lung maturation. Many newborns who have had ruptured fetal membranes for 24 hours or more have significant RDS. In our opinion, the data on corticosteroids in patients with prolonged rupture of the fetal membranes has not proved the efficacy or the safety of the drugs. Although we may in the future make occasional exceptions, as in multiple births, we have not routinely used tocolytic drugs, antibiotics or corticosteroids on patients who have ruptured fetal membranes.

HYPERTENSION

Initially Liggins reported an increase of antepartum fetal deaths in hypertensive patients receiving betamethasone. Although this increase was not statistically significant, it is a cause for caution against delaying delivery to treat with corticosteroids if preeclampsia becomes severe. Chronic hypertension appears to accelerate fetal maturation. If the clinical situation, in terms of fetal well-being, maternal blood pressure, proteinuria, creatinine clearance, and symptoms of headache, visual changes, or abdominal pain indicates prompt delivery, an L/S ratio is usually superfluous and corticosteroids would not, in our opinion, be indicated. There are times in which the hypertension is relatively stable, but it is anticipated that the fetus will need to be delivered within a week. If the L/S ratio or other indicators of fetal maturity predict a high risk of death or RDS, then corticosteroids may be justified.

THIRD TRIMESTER BLEEDING

If a patient is bleeding heavily and her condition cannot be stabilized quickly, then the fetus must be delivered before corticosteroids have time to become effective. If a patient is believed to have placenta previa and the bleeding is not a threat to maternal or fetal well-being, corticosteroids may be indicated. After the 34th week we would use them only if the L/S ratio was known to be immature. When there is chronic abruption, the internal stress may have already matured the fetal lungs, and the additional stress of the steroids could be both unnecessary and harmful. When there is definitive evidence of placental separation, such as altered blood clotting factor, hypovolemia or fetal distress, we do not give steroids. In the majority of cases of mild intermittent vaginal bleeding, we hesitate to use tocolytic drugs or corticosteroids. We may use them if it appears fairly certain that the fetus is not compromised and that delivery will most likely occur when the fetus is at high risk for RDS.

DIABETES

If one realizes that corticosteroids may make the control of diabetes more difficult, that an ill patient may react adversely to the corticosteroids and that high fetal insulin levels may blunt the effect of the steroids on the fetal lungs,[48] the decision as to when to give corticosteroids to a pregnant diabetic is not too different from the decision for the nondiabetic. We do not advocate the elective use of corticosteroids, since most diabetics can be delivered after lung maturation has occurred spontaneously without undue risk of fetal death. We realize that lung maturation may be delayed in the gestational or class B diabetic, but we are not convinced that these fetuses will respond appropriately to the exogenous corticosteroids. The most efficacious treatment revolves around good medical management of the patient's blood glucose and careful monitoring of the fetal well-being. There may be unusual cases in which delivery is indicated prior to fetal pulmonary maturity. Corticosteroids could be used if it appears the neonatal unit would not be able to save the newborn if the corticosteroids were not used.

Rh AND OTHER BLOOD GROUP ISOIMMUNIZATION

When a patient has significant titers of erythrocyte antibodies and the optical density analysis of the amniotic fluid is fast approaching or is in Liley's zone III, after 34 weeks, we use corticosteroids if the L/S ratio is immature. In general, 30 per cent of patients may not have RDS when the L/S ratio is immature, but in our experience, fetuses with erythroblastosis and an immature L/S ratio rarely survive if delivered within 48 hours of the amniocentesis. When the gestational age exceeds 34 weeks, and one is reluctant to do an intrauterine fetal transfusion, then the other option is to accept the risk for fetal death or worsening erythroblastosis until the L/S ratio becomes mature. Corticosteroids are not proved to be effective in the erythroblastotic fetus but they have been used with generally good results. When corticosteroids are given antenatally to a fetus with erythroblastosis, the delta OD may fall, producing a false impression of clinical improvement, presumably by aiding the excretion of bilirubin without helping the fetal anemia.

ACUTE FEBRILE ILLNESSES

Acute pyelonephritis, pneumonia or viremia may precipitate preterm labor. Oxygen consumption by the fetus is increased and the fetus may become infected by the agent infecting the mother. Beta-mimetic drugs might increase the tachycardia associated with the illness to the point that cardiac output is compromised. The combination of tocolytic drugs and corticosteroids in a patient with an acute febrile illness has the potential for considerable harm and should be used cautiously and only if the infection is under control.

Summary and Conclusion

Antepartum corticosteroid treatment clearly accelerates pulmonary maturity in several animal species. Numerous factors, in addition to species variability, affect outcome. These include gestational length, the agent chosen, method of administration, dose, length of administration and to a certain extent the choice of lung maturity parameters monitored. In no instance is the site, or sites, of drug action unequivocally established. There is evidence supporting effects on several enzymes involved in surfactant synthesis,[53] effects on surfactant release[1] and effects on lung connective tissue.[22, 30] Deleterious fetal effects, particularly with pharmacologic doses, are not uncommon.[68] Premature delivery may be induced in nonprimate species.[40]

In humans the issue may be further compounded by the presence or absence of complications of pregnancy, by the use of therapies to arrest labor, by concurrent medications[32, 50] or drug abuse.[65] The highest benefit seems to be in fetuses 30 to 32 weeks of gestation in whom delivery can be delayed 24 hours or more. Betamethasone and dexamethasone seem effective, as might be expected, in the physiologic concentration range. Hydrocortisone may require higher doses but more data are needed. Methylprednisolone and cortisone do not appear to be effective. Occasional reports of maternal morbidity[10] associated with antepartum corticosteroid therapy emphasize the need for careful scrutiny of conditions that would be affected by the diverse actions of corticosteroids. Using corticosteroids in the presence of premature rupture of the membranes has not resulted in the anticipated problems with infections. Fetal complications thought most likely to occur, such as adrenal insufficiency, preterm labor, growth retardation impaired immune mechanism with increased susceptibility to infection, hypoglycemia and hyperbilirubinemia, have not shown an increase in treated infants. Finally, complications not known to exist on the basis of current animal or human experimentation may occur.[44, 67, 68]

If the patients have other complicating factors such as obstetric problems in addition to preterm labor, we agree with advocates who advise caution.[21, 26, 43] Thorough patient counseling is, of course, imperative and a written, informed consent is desirable.

The FDA has published an announcement (40FR15392), reiterated on 17 March 1978 (43FR11207), regarding the use of approved drugs for indications that have not been approved that is applicable:

". . . the labeling is not intended either to preclude the physician's use of his best judgement in the interest of the patient or to impose liability if he does not follow the package insert. The (FDA) Commissioner clearly recognizes that the labeling of a marketed drug does not always contain all the most current information available to physicians relating to the proper use of the drug in good medical practice. Advances in medical knowledge and practice inevitably precede labeling revision by the manufacturer and formal label approval by the Food and Drug Administration. Good medical practice and patient interests thus require that physicians be free to use drugs according to their best knowledge and judgement. Certainly, where a physician uses a drug for use not in the approved labeling, he has the responsibility to be well informed about the drug and to base such use on a firm scientific rationale or on sound medical evidence, and to maintain adequate medical records of the drug's use and effects, but such usage in the practice of medicine is not in violation of the Federal Food, Drug and Cosmetic Act. . ."

Finally, the incidence of mortality and morbidity from RDS will improve as modalities and drugs for the prevention of premature labor improve.[30] If perinatal asphyxia[11] is avoided and neonatal intensive care units become more available to the sick neonate,[31] morbidity and mortality will be further decreased. Newer drugs for acceleration of fetal lung maturation may be developed. Surfactant may be applied to the newborn lung through its trachea.[20, 27] Assessment of the relative efficacy of corticosteroids remains extremely difficult in spite of massive efforts to control all the factors that affect pregnancy outcome, including fetal sex.[4] For these reasons the use of corticosteroids for the purpose of accelerating fetal lung maturation will likely remain controversial for some time to come.

REFERENCES

1. Anderson, G., Lamden, M., Cidlowski, J. A. and Ashikaga, T.: Comparative pulmonary surfactant-inducing effect of three corticosteroids in the near-term rat. Am. J. Obstet. Gynecol. 139:562, 1981.
2. Arias, F. and Pineda, J.: Failure of glucocorticoid administration in inducing the production of a mature L/S ratio. Gynecol. Invest. 8:63, 1977.
3. Ballard, R. B., Ballard, P. L., Goanberg, P. and Sniderman, S.: Prenatal administration of beta-methasone for prevention of respiratory distress syndrome. J. Pediatr. 94:97, 1979.
4. Ballard, P. L., Gluckman, P. D., Liggins, G. C., Kaplan, S. L. and Grumbach, M. M.: Steroid and growth hormone levels in premature infants after prenatal bethamethasone therapy to prevent respiratory distress syndrome. Pediatr. Res. 14:122, 1980.
5. Ballard, P. L., Granberg, P. and Ballard, R. A.: Glucocorticoid levels in maternal and cord serum after prenatal betamethasone therapy to prevent respiratory distress syndrome. J. Clin. Invest. 56:1548, 1975.
6. Beitins, I. Z., Bayard, F., Ances, I. G., Kowarski, A. and Migeon, C. J.: The transplacental passage of prednisone and prednisolone in pregnancy near term. J. Pediatr. 81:936, 1972.
7. Beitins, I. Z., Bayard, F., Ances, I. G. et al.: The metabolic clearance rate, blood production, interconversion and transplacental passage of cortisol and cortisone in pregnancy near term. Pediatr. Res. 7:509, 1973.
8. Blanford, A. T. and Murphy, B. E. P.: In vitro metabolism of prednisolone, dexamethasone, betamethasone, and cortisol by the human placenta. Am. J. Obstet. Gynecol. 127:264, 1977.
9. Block, M. F., Kling, O. R. and Crosby, W. M.: Antenatal glucocorticoid therapy for the prevention of respiratory distress syndrome in the premature infant. Obstet. Gynecol. 50:186, 1977.
10. Brown, G., Gobert, H. and Stenchever, A.: Respiratory distress syndrome. Obstet. Gynecol. Surv. 30:71, 1975.
11. Brumley, G. W. and Crenshaw, C.: Fetal lamb lung phosphatidylcholine: response to asphysia and recovery. J. Pediatr. 97:631, 1980.
12. Caspi, E., Schreyer, P. and Tamir, I.: Amniotic-fluid lecithin/sphingomyelin ratios and dexamethasone. Lancet 2:575, 1975.

13. Caspi, E., Schreyer, P., Weinraub, Z. et al.: Prevention of the respiratory distress syndrome in premature infants by antepartum glucocorticoid therapy. Br. J. Obstet. Gynaecol. 83:187, 1976.

14. Chiswick, M. L., Ahmed, A., Jack, P. M. B. et al.: Control of fetal lung development in the rabbit. Arch. Dis. Child. 48:709, 1973.

15. Comroe, J. H.: Premature science and immature lungs. Part III. The attack on immature lungs. Am. Rev. Resp. Dis. 116:497, 1977.

16. DeLemos, R. A., Shermeta, D. W., Knelson, J. H. et al: Acceleration of appearance of pulmonary surfactant in the fetal lamb by administration of corticosteroids. Am. Rev. Resp. Dis. 102:459, 1970.

17. Dluholucky, S., Babic, J. and Taufer, I.: Reduction of incidence and mortality of respiratory distress syndrome by administration of hydrocortisone to mother. Arch. Dis. Child. 51:420, 1976.

18. Ekelund, L., Arvidson, G. and Astedt, B.: Cortisol-induced accumulation of phospholipids in organ culture of human fetal lung. Scand. J. Clin. Lab. Invest. 35:419, 1975.

19. Ekelund, L., Arvidson, G., Ohrlander, S. et al.: Changes in amniotic fluid phospholipids on treatment with glucocorticoids to prevent respiratory distress syndrome. Acta Obstet. Gynecol. Scand. 55:413, 1976.

20. Enhorning, G., Hill, O., Sherwood, G., Cutz, E., Robertson, B. and Brogan, C.: Improved ventilation of prematurely delivered premature following tracheal deposition of surfactant. Am. J. Obstet. Gynecol. 132:529, 1978.

21. Epstein, M. F., Farrell, P. M. and Sparks, J. W.: Maternal betamethasone and fetal growth and development in the monkey. Am. J. Obstet. Gynecol. 127:261, 1977.

22. Frank, L., Summerville, J. and Massaro, D.: The effect of prenatal dexamethasone treatment on oxygen toxicity in the newborn rat. Pediatrics 65:287, 1980.

23. Fargier, P., Salle, B., Baud, M. et al.: Prevention du syndrome de detresse respiratoire chez le premature. Nouv. Presse Med. 3:1595, 1974.

24. Farrell, P. M. and Zachman, R. D.: Induction of choline phosphotransferase and lecithin synthesis in the fetal lung by corticosteroids. Science 179:298, 1973.

25. Gilen, C., Sevanian, A., Tierney, D. F. et al.: Regulation of fetal lung phosphatidyl choline synthesis by cortisol: role of glycogen and glucose. Pediatr. Res. 11:845, 1977.

26. Gluck, L.: Administration of corticosteroids to induce maturation of fetal lung. Am. J. Dis. Child. 130:978, 1976.

27. Hallman, M., Schneider, H. and Gluck, L.: Human fetus, a potential surfactant donor: isolation of lung surfactant from amniotic fluid. Pediatr. Res. 15:663, 1981.

28. Howie, R. N. and Liggins, G. C.: Prevention of respiratory distress syndrome in premature infants by antepartum glucocorticoid treatment. *In* Villee, C. A., Villee, D. B. and Zuckerman, J. (eds.): Respiratory Distress Syndrome. New York, Academic Press, 1973, pp. 369–380.

29. Johnson, J. W. C., Lim, H. S., Kearney, K. C. et al.: Effect of cortisone administration on fetal lung surfactant activity. (Abst) Gynecol. Invest. 7:95, 1976.

30. Johnson, J. W. C., Mitzner, W., London, W. T. et al.: Glucocorticoids and the rhesus fetal lung. Am. J. Obstet. Gynecol. 130:905, 1978.

31. Kappy, K. A., Certrallo, C. I., Knuppel, R. L. et al.: Premature rupture of the membranes: a conservative approach. Am. J. Obstet. Gynecol. 134:655, 1979.

32. Karotkin, E. H., Kido, M., Redding, R. et al.: The inhibition of pulmonary maturation in the fetal rabbit by maternal treatment with phenobarbital. Am. J. Obstet. Gynecol. 124:529, 1976.

33. Kennedy, J. L., Jr.: Prenatal glucocorticoid treatment: prevention of respiratory distress syndrome. *In* Lung Maturation and the Prevention of Hyaline Membrane Disease. Report of the 70th Ross Conference on Pediatric Research, Columbus, Ross Laboratories, p. 105, 1976.

34. Killam, A. P.: Prenatal glucocorticoid treatment: effect on surviving infants. *In* Lung Maturation and the Prevention of Hyaline Membrane Disease. Report of the 70th Ross Conference on Pediatric Research, Columbus, Ross Laboratories, p. 110, 1976.

35. Kling, O. R. and Kotas, R. V.: Endocrine influences on pulmonary maturation and lecithin/sphingomyelin ratio in the fetal baboon. Am. J. Obstet. Gynecol. 124:664, 1975.

36. Knelson, N. H.: Environmental influence on intrauterine lung development. Arch. Intern. Med. 127:421, 1971.

37. Kotas, R. V., Kling, O. R., Block, M. F. et al.: Response of immature baboon fetal lung to intra-amniotic betamethasone. Am. J. Obstet. Gynecol. 130:712, 1978.

38. Kotas, R. V. and Avery, M. E.: Accelerated appearance of pulmonary surfactant in the fetal rabbit. J. Appl. Physiol. 30:358, 1971.

39. Kotas, R. V., Fletcher, B. D., Torday, J. and Avery, M. E.: Evidence for independent regulators of organ maturation in fetal rabbits. Pediatrics 47:57, 1971.

40. Liggins, G. C.: Premature delivery of foetal lambs infused with glucocorticoids. J. Endocrinol. 45:515, 1969.

41. Liggins, G. C. and Howie, R. N.: A controlled trial of antepartum glucocorticoid treatment for prevention of the respiratory distress syndrome in premature infants. Pediatrics 50:515, 1972.

42. Liggins, G. C. and Howie, R. N.: The prevention of RDS by maternal steroid therapy. *In* Gluck, L. (ed.): Modern Perinatal Medicine. Chicago, Year Book Medical Publishers, p. 415, 1974.

43. Liggins, G. C.: Prenatal glucocorticoid treatment: prevention of respiratory distress syndrome. *In* Lung Maturation and the Prevention of Hyaline Membrane Disease. Report of the 70th Ross Conference on Pediatric Research. Columbus, Ross Laboratories, p. 97, 1976.

44. Liggins, G. C.: Adrenocortical-related maturational events in the fetus. Am. J. Obstet. Gynecol. 126:931, 1976.

45. Morrison, J. C., Whybrew, W. D., Bacovaz, E. T. and Schneider, J. M.: Injection of corticosteroids into the mother to prevent neonatal respiratory distress syndrome. Am. J. Obstet. Gynecol. 131:358, 1978.

46. Motoyama, E. K., Orzalesi, M. M., Kikkawa, Y. et al.: Effect of cortisol on the maturation of fetal rabbit lungs. Pediatrics 48:547, 1971.

47. Nelson, G. H., Eguchi, K. and McPherson, J. C.: Effects of gestational age, dexamethasone, Metopirone, and chronic hypoxia on lecithin concentration in fetal lung tissue and amniotic fluid. Gynecol. Invest. 6:55, 1975.

48. Newfeld, N. D., Sevanian, A., Barrett, C. T. and Kaplan, S. A.: Inhibition of surfactant by insulin in fetal rabbit lung slices. Pediatr. Res. 13:752, 1979.

49. Platzker, A. C. G., Kitterman, J. A., Mescher, E. J. et al.: Surfactant in the lung and tracheal fluid of the fetal lamb and acceleration of its appearance by dexamethasone. Pediatrics 56:554, 1975.

50. Redding, R., Douglas, W. H. J. and Stein, M.: Thyroid hormone influence upon lung production. Science 197:194, 1972.

51. Rooney, S. A., Gross, J., Gassenheimer, N. G. et al.: Stimulation of glycerolphosphate phosphatidyltransferase activity in fetal rabbit lung by cortisol administration. Biochim. Biophys. Acta 298:433, 1975.

52. Rooney, S. A., Gobran, L., Gross, I. et al.: Studies on pulmonary surfactant: effects of cortisol administration to fetal rabbits on lung phospholipid content, composition, and biosynthesis. Biochim. Biophys. Acta 450:121, 1976.

53. Rooney, S. A., Gobran, L. I., Marino, P. A. et al.: Effects of betamethasone on phospholipid content, composition and biosynthesis in the fetal rabbit lung. Biochim. Biophys. Acta 572:64, 1979.

54. Russell, B. J., Nugent, L. and Chernick, V.: Effects of steroids on the enzymatic pathways of lecithin production in fetal rabbits. Biol. Neonate 24:306, 1974.

55. Sanfacon, R., Possmayer, F. and Harding, P. G. R.: Dexamethasone treatment of the guinea pig fetus: its effects on the incorporation of 3H-thymidine into deoxyribonucleic acid. Am. J. Obstet. Gynecol. 127:745, 1977.

56. Schneider, A., Hallman, M., Benirchke, K. and Gluck, L.: Human surfactant: a therapeutic trial in premature rabbits. Pediatr. Res. 15:730, 1981.

57. Schutte, M. F., Treffers, P. E., Koppe, J. G. and Breur, W.: The influence of betamethasone and orciprenaline on the incidence of respiratory distress syndrome in the newborn after preterm labor. Br. J. Obstet. Gynaecol. 87:127, 1980.

58. Schwenzel, W., Jung, H. and Lahmann, H. et al.: Erste Erfahrungen mit der praenatalen Beeimflussung der Kindlichen Lungenreife durch Betamethasone. Z. Geburtshilfe Perinatol. 179:45, 1975.

59. Sevanian, A., Gilden, C., Kaplan, S. A. and Barrett, C. T.: Enhancement of fetal lung surfactant production by aminophylline. Pediatr. Res. 13:1336, 1979.

60. Smith, B. T., Torday, J. S. and Giround, C. J. P.: The growth promoting effect of cortisol on human fetal lung cells. Steroids 22:515, 1973.

61. Spellacy, W. N., Buhi, W. C. and Rigall, F. C.: Human amniotic fluid lecithin/sphingomyelin ratio changes with estrogen or glucocorticoid treatment. Am. J. Obstet. Gynecol. 115:216, 1973.

62. Stocker, J.: Prenatal glucocorticoid treatment. Reduction in neonatal deaths. *In* Lung Maturation and the Prevention of Hyaline Membrane Disease. Report of the Seventieth Ross Conference on Pediatric Research. Columbus, Ross Laboratories, p. 115, 1976.

63. Sybulski, S. and Maughan, G. B.: Relationship between cortisol levels in umbilical cord plasma and development of the respiratory distress syndrome in premature newborn infants. Am. J. Obstet. Gynecol. 125:239, 1973.

64. Taeusch, H. W., Heitner, M. and Avery, M. E.: Accelerated lung maturation and increased survival in premature rabbits treated with hydrocortisone. Am. Rev. Resp. Dis. 105:971, 1972.

65. Taeusch, H. W., Carson, S. and Wang, N. S.: The effects of heroin on lung maturation and growth in fetal rabbits. Pediatr. Res. 6:335, 1972.

66. Tauesch, H. W., Avery, M. E. and Sugg, J.: Premature delivery without accelerated lung development in fetal lambs treated with long-acting methylprednisolone. Biol. Neonate 20:85, 1972.

67. Taeusch, H. W.: Glucocorticoid prophylaxis for respiratory distress syndrome: a review of potential toxicity. J. Pediatr. 87:6, 1973.

68. Taeusch, H. W., Frigoletto, F., Kitzmiller, J. et al.: Risk of respiratory distress syndrome after prenatal dexamethasone treatment. Pediatrics 63:64, 1979.

69. Taeusch, H. W. and Tulchinsky, D.: Obstetric factors affecting risk of respiratory distress syndrome. Premature Labor Meadow Johnson Symposium on Perinatal and Developmental Medicine, No. 15, Vail, Colorado, June 7–10, 1979.

70. Thornfeldt, R. E., Franklin, R. W. and Pickering, N. A.: The effect of glucocorticoids on the maturation of premature lung membranes. Am. J. Obstet. Gynecol. 131:143, 1978.

71. Teramo, K., Hallman, M. and Raivio, K.: Maternal glucocorticoid in unplanned premature labor. Controlled study on the effects of betamethasone phosphate on the phospholipids of the gastric aspirate and on the adrenal cortical function of the newborn infant. Pediatr. Res. 14:326, 1980.

72. Tyden, O., Berne, C. and Eriksson, U.: Lung maturation in fetuses of diabetic rats. Pediatr. Res. 14:1192, 1980.

73. Demottaz, V., Epstein, M. F. and Frantz, I. D., III: Phospholipid synthesis in lung slices from fetuses of alloxan diabetic rabbits. Pediatr. Res. 14:47, 1980.

74. Wang, N. S., Kotas, R. V., Avery, M. E. et al.: Accelerated appearance of osmiophilic bodies in fetal lungs following steroid injection. J. Appl. Physiol. 30:362, 1971.

75. Whitt, G. G., Buster, J. E., Killam, A. P. et al.: A comparison of two glucocorticoid regimens for acceleration of fetal lung maturation in premature labor. Am. J. Obstet. Gynecol. 124:479, 1976.

76. Young, B. K., Klein, S. A., Katz, M. et al.: Intravenous dexamethasone for prevention of neonatal respiratory distress: a prospective controlled study. Am. J. Obstet. Gynecol. 138:203, 1980.

77. Zuspan, F. P., Cordero, L. and Semchyshyn, S.: Effects of hydrocortisone on lecithin-sphingomyelin ratio. Am. J. Obstet. Gynecol. 128:571, 1977.

Administration of Glucocorticoids to the Pregnant Patient

Leandro Cordero, M.D.,
Ohio State University, College of Medicine

Stefan Semchyshyn, M.D.
St. Barnabas Medical Center,
Livingston, New Jersey

It was only a few years ago that Liggins reported his observations on the experimental induction of preterm labor in sheep.[1] He demonstrated that dexamethasone could induce preterm labor when injected into the fetus but not when administered to the mother. Almost incidentally, he observed that prenatally treated lambs survived longer than their placebo-treated counterparts and at autopsy had partial aeration of the lungs. These unexpected histologic findings were even more remarkable considering that the animals were delivered as early as 115 days of gestation (gestation in the ewe is 140 days). The speculation that a glucocorticoid could have altered the biological timer of pulmonary surfactant production initiated one of the most fascinating therapeutic adventures in discovery of modern times.

Liggins's experimental observations correlated very well with the studies of Mogg,[2] who established that glucocorticoids were capable of enhancing alkaline phosphatase activity in the intestinal mucosa of suckling mice, and those of Buckingham,[3] who demonstrated that activity of the same enzyme was present in the fetal lung and increased with advancing gestational age. Since the intestine and the lung derived from the same embryologic pouch (foregut), these authors suggested the possibility that pharmacologic enzymatic induction could also be possible in the latter.[3]

Further support for this theory was later produced by DeLemos et al.,[4] who reported that the infusion of cortisol in utero to one of twin lambs advanced lung maturation on the treated animal but not in the twin control. Soon thereafter Kotas et al.[5] and Motoyama et al.[6] reported similar results while working with fetal rabbits. That endogenously produced cortisol could also affect organ development was demonstrated by Chiswick et al.[7] and Blackburn et al.[8] These authors observed that decapitation in utero of fetal rats resulted in delayed lung development and also that this effect could be reversed or prevented by an injection of cortisol at the time of surgery. It was not until a few years later, however, that similar inhibition of lung growth was produced by the administration of Metopirone to does and fetal rabbits.[9]

In all mammals so far studied, anatomic and physiological pulmonary maturation intensifies at about 85 to 90 per cent of the duration of gestation (the equivalent in humans to 34 weeks). In the rat and the rabbit this maturational event is preceded by a rise in fetal serum cortisol, and in the human larger amounts of cortisol are detected in amniotic fluid shortly before the rise in lecithin concentration. Direct and indirect evidence lead to the idea that a "corticosteroid surge" was a mandatory step before readiness for extrauterine life could be expected.[10] However, the developmental sequence seen in rats and rabbits does not occur in fetal lambs, where surfactant is detected in tracheal fluid before rises in fetals serum cortisol begin. In light of these facts, it is very likely that endogenously produced cortisol is not the only stimulus for pulmonary surfactant production.

Effects of Corticosteroids on the Mammalian Lung

Alveolarization and increased aeration of the lungs of treated lambs have been demonstrated histologically. Changes in inflation-pressure curves after the administration of dexamethasone were readily documented by DeLemos et al.[4] Large amounts of osmophilic granules and increased number of lamellar bodies were detected in the lungs of fetal rabbits prenatally treated with glucocorticoids.[6] In vitro and in vivo studies have demonstrated an increased rate of choline incorporation following the administration of corticosteroid. In vitro experiments with cell lines of human[11] and rabbit lungs[12] also demonstrated an increased incorporation of radioactive cytidine diphosphocholine (CDP-choline). All this would suggest that glucocorticoids act by inducing activity of enzymes involved in the biosynthesis of lecithin. Which specific enzyme activity is more critical remains unclear, but most of the available evidence points to choline phosphotransferase[13] and phosphatidic acid phosphatase.[12] It is worth noting that all the changes just described occur in the presence of minuscule amounts of glucocorticoid.

MECHANISM OF ACTION

Two major theories have evolved regarding the mechanism of action by which glucocorticoids enhance lung development. Barrett et al.[14] have postulated that the effect is mediated by cyclic AMP (cAMP) and is caused by either local increase in production or a decrease in biodegradation. This theory is supported by the fact that pharmacologic induction of pulmonary maturity by different agents (cortisol, aminophylline, thyroxine, and so forth) occurs simultaneously with the detection of increased tissue levels of cAMP. Ballard et al.[15] postulated a more direct action of glucocorticoids on the type II pneumocytes. The glucocorticoids would bind to cytoplasmic and nuclear receptors and then generate messenger RNA to form new protein (enzyme). Whatever the mechanism, it is important to remember that the effect of glucocorticoids is not specific and does affect other rapidly dividing cells, mainly by reducing the activity of thymidine kinase and subsequently DNA proliferation.[16] This nonspecificity of the glucocorticoid action is the reason for concern in terms of short-term and long-term side efects.

Prenatal Administration of Glucocorticoids to the Human Fetus

Liggins and Howie[17] were the first to report results of a double-blind clinical trial of betamethasone for the induction of pulmonary maturation. They documented a significant decline in the incidence of RDS and a decrease in the neonatal mortality among treated infants. More recently Liggins[18] reported on the outcome of 884 infants and stated that only 6.8 per cent of those prenatally treated died in the first week of life, compared with 11.6 per cent of the controls. He attributed the decreased mortality to reduction in the incidence of respiratory distress syndrome (RDS) (15.6 per cent in the control and 10 per cent in the group of treated infants). Liggins further explained that if one considers only those infants born between 1 and 7 days following the onset of treatment, the incidence of RDS was reduced from 23.7 per cent in the controls to 8.8 per cent in the treated group.[18]

In the years that followed Liggins and Howie's initial report, numerous articles were written describing therapeutic trials from around the globe.[18-36] Unfortunately, only a handful of them were double-blind trials, and in most cases the information was neither standardized nor detailed enough to allow rigorous comparisons. Tabulation of some of these data was made in an effort to obtain an overview and draw some general comments (Table 1). Information about drug choice and dosage was easily found, but patient selection criteria and diagnostic working definitions (RDS, premature rupture of the membranes and so forth) were not consistently described. Some investigators included a variety of high-risk pregnancies, while others carefully excluded cases of pregnancy-induced hypertension and other hypertensive disorders of pregnancy. In terms of neonatal outcome, definitions of RDS and method of assessing gestational age created significant difficulties in the interpretation of the data. Entities such as transient tachypnea of the newborn, hypothermia and aspiration syndromes could conceivably have been included in the diagnosis of RDS. Surprisingly, very few authors made reference to this critical issue. Gestational age was frequently mentioned, but investigators seldom explained if it referred to time of treatment or delivery. As is known, even a few days could play a significant role in the developmental sequence of lung maturation.

Except for the placebo groups in the double-blind studies, no patients could justifiably be termed controls. We chose to refer to the comparison group as the "untreated" and consider it a reference group rather than a true control. We believe that its inclusion in the table is valid as long as the reader understands that it was the reference group (perhaps the only available choice) selected by the authors.

Data from double-blind trials were pooled and are presented in Table 2. It can be seen that the incidence of RDS was three times lower for infants prenatally treated when compared with the placebo group. These obser-

TABLE 1. PRENATAL ADMINISTRATION OF GLUCOCORTICOID TO THE HUMAN

				NEONATAL OUTCOME		
AUTHORS	DRUG	ROUTE	DOSAGE	Gest. Age (Weeks)	Untreated RDS/Tot.	Treated RDS/Tot.
Liggins and Howie[17, 18]	B	IM	12 mg QID × 2 doses	<30	15/26	10/36*
				30–32	14/25	2/23
				≥33	8/105	4/123
Fargier et al.[19]	B	IM	12 mg QID × 2 doses	<37	80/396	2/42
Kennedy[20, 21]	B	IM	12 mg QID × 2 doses	<37	23/41	6/41
Bureau et al.[22]	D	IM	12 mg QID × 2 doses	25–32	12/26	1/8
				33–36	8/68	2/12
Taeusch[23]	H	IM	4 mg TID × 6 doses	26–33	14/65	7/50
Killam[52]	B	IV	500 mg TID × 4 doses	≤32		0/13
				33–35	78/217	1/9
Schwenzel et al.[26]	D	IM	10.5 mg QID × 2 doses	26–32	7/7	1/2
				33–37	7/17	1/17
Caspi et al.[27]	H	IM	4 mg TID up to 7 days	28–32	19/28	5/26
				33–36	6/43	0/34
Dluholucky et al.[28]	P	IV	100 mg × 1 dose	<37	18/40	5/31
Ballard et al.[30]	B	IM	12 mg QID × 2 doses	(B. wgt. <1750 g)	70/138	14/56
Block et al.[31]	B	IM	12 mg QID × 2 doses	<37	12/53	5/57
Mead and Clapp[32]	H	IM	6 mg QI2 h × 2 doses	27–32	13/16	6/27
Morrison et al.[33]	B	IV	500 mg QID × 2 doses	<36	14/59	6/67*
Papageorgiou et al.[34]	D	IM	12 mg QID × 2 doses	<35	18/32	7/28*
Thornfeldt et al.[36]	D	IM	8 mg QID × 2 doses	<32	18/24	9/26
				32–36	117/202	14/84
				>36	40/164	0/1

*Double-blind studies
B = bethamethasone, D = dexamethasone, H = hydrocortisone, P = prednisolone.

vations provided early and definite evidence of the beneficial effects of prenatally administered corticosteroid (see addendum).

In an effort to estimate the time during gestation that corticosteroids are the most effective, a breakdown by gestational age of the population reported in Table 1 was conducted. Patients were grouped into those delivered at or before 32 weeks and those delivered at or between 33 and 37 weeks of gestation (Fig. 1). Display of these data in this fashion gives a good idea of the incidence of RDS for treated and untreated patients. It can be seen that under 32 weeks the incidence of RDS was 64 and 21 per cent for the untreated and treated groups, respectively. The influence of treatment on the incidence of RDS for infants in the 33- to 37-week group was also remarkable (30 per cent for the untreated and 10 per cent for the treated group). For reference purposes, data on the natural incidence of RDS in infants born vaginally[37] are also presented in Figure 1. The interval between 33 and 37 weeks encompasses too large a

TABLE 2. INCIDENCE OF RDS FOLLOWING PRENATAL GLUCOCORTICOID TREATMENT*

AUTHORS	GESTATIONAL AGE (WEEKS)	CONTROL RDS/Total	TREATED RDS/ Total
Liggins and Howie[17, 18]	<30	15/26	10/36
	30–32	14/26	2/23
	>33	8/105	4/123
Tauesch[23]	<37	14/65	7/50
Block et al.[31]	<37	18/40	5/31
Morrison et al.[33]	<36	14/59	6/69
Papageorgiou et al.[34]	<35	18/32	7/28
All patients	<37	101/353	41/350
Percentage with RDS		30	11

*Double-blind studies.

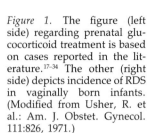

Figure 1. The figure (left side) regarding prenatal glucocorticoid treatment is based on cases reported in the literature.[17-34] The other (right side) depicts incidence of RDS in vaginally born infants. (Modified from Usher, R. et al.: Am. J. Obstet. Gynecol. 111:826, 1971.)

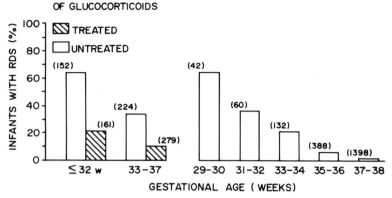

PRENATAL ADMINISTRATION
OF GLUCOCORTICOIDS

period of critical developmental events to allow meaningful comments. Untreated patients seem to have an RDS incidence more like the one of patients of younger gestational age.

Above all, the fact that prenatal glucocorticoid treatment alters the incidence of RDS can no longer be disputed. It seems clear that major benefits would be obtained for those infants born at or about 32 weeks of gestation; but how beneficial the treatment below 28 weeks would be cannot be determined at present (Tables 1 and 2). Beyond 34 weeks the incidence of RDS is low enough that the magnitude of the beneficial effects of glucocorticoid treatment is extremely difficult to determine.

Liggins[17, 18] repeatedly confirmed his earlier observations that infants delivered less than 24 hours or more than 7 days after onset of therapy derived little or no benefit from the glucocorticoid treatment. The time lapse between treatment and clinical response has been repeatedly documented by most investigators.[20-21, 23, 27-29, 36] To our knowledge only Block et al.[31] did not support the notion that time between treatment and delivery was a significant variable.

Ballard and associates[30] recently reported that the incidence of RDS in treated and untreated patients who delivered within 24 hours from the beginning of treatment was similar (55 and 51 per cent, respectively).

The occurrence of premature rupture of the membranes in patients prenatally treated with corticosteroids is so common that many have questioned whether the benefits from this form of treatment were indeed a reflection of the duration of time elapsed from rupture of membranes. Several articles have dealt with the subject[39-51] and yet the controversy continues. However, evidence seems to minimize the importance of prolonged time after rupture of membranes as a protective factor.[44-50] Liggins and associates[17, 18, 52] have repeatedly reported that the incidence of RDS was reduced only if membranes have been ruptured for more than 3 days. Years ago we observed that the duration of time from membrane rupture until delivery did not alter the incidence of hyaline membrane disease in a group of 259 very small premature infants.[51] Recently Ballard et al.[30] produced more data supporting this observation.

Most authors[24, 29, 31, 34] involved in therapeutic trial of glucocorticoids have concluded that the time elapsed after rupture of membranes until delivery does not influence significantly the incidence of RDS in either treated or untreated patients.

That glucocorticoids could exert beneficial effects in terms of pulmonary maturation even in the absence of rupture of the membranes was clearly demonstrated by Caspi et al.[27] These investigators found that the incidence of RDS in the treated group was about four times lower than that in the untreated "controls." This observation seems to be supported by our studies, in which we demonstrated that lecithin/spingomyelin (L/S) ratio changes occurred later than 48 hours from the onset of the glucocorticoid treatment in patients with intact membranes.

Tocolytic Agents and Pulmonary Maturation

Preliminary reports suggest that uterine inhibitors per se may reduce the incidence of RDS.[53-56] Kero and associates[53] reported that no case of RDS was seen among the offspring of 12 isoxsuprine-treated mothers. Those infants weighed between 1250 and 2080 g and were born from 28 to 35 weeks of gestation. In their brief report Kero et al. did not detail their cases or explain the discrepancies between birth weight and length of gestation. No reference was made to the natural incidence of RDS in their population and to the need for a control group. In spite of this the investigators stated "that according to these preliminary experiments it seems justified to consider the use of this agent prenatally."

Caspi and associates[27] analyzed data from 34 women treated with isoxsuprine and dexamethasone and 26 patients who received dexamethasone alone. They concluded that antepartum isoxsuprine had no apparent effect on the incidence of RDS. A few years later similar conclusions were reached by Papageorgiou et al.,[35] who studied 146 women treated with isoxsuprine in the course of a double-blind study on the effects of glucocorticoid. Almost simultaneously Ballard and Ballard[30, 57] reviewed their experience and reported that uterine inhibitors per se did not produce changes in the incidence of RDS.

In a retrospective study conducted in France, Bogg et al.[54] reported that 5 of 29 ritodrine-treated fetuses and 8 of 18 nontreated "controls" developed RDS. Birth weight of these infants ranged from 900 to 2700 g, and the authors claimed that the difference in RDS was significant only if infants who weighed less than 2300 g were compared. The limitation of these observations became quite noticeable when, using the data presented by Bogg et al., we compared infants who weighed under 1600 g and found that ritodrine did not have any influence on the incidence of RDS, because 4 out of 8 treated and 8 out of 16 untreated infants developed such complications.

Intravenous infusion of alcohol has been reported to lower the risk of RDS in infants born between 28 and 32 weeks.[55] This finding was in marked contrast with the earlier observations of Liggins,[17, 18, 52] which had shown that neither salbutamol nor alcohol modified the incidence of RDS. Among the limitations of the work of Barrada et al.[55] is the fact that alcohol-treated women had 2 per cent incidence of cesarean section in comparison with 20 per cent of the so-called untreated controls, and as the authors readily admitted the potential influence of this factor certainly cannot be overlooked.

Dluholucky et al.[28] routinely used orciprenaline to treat preterm labor and discounted any effect of the beta-adrenergic agent on pulmonary function. Specifically they reported that RDS occurred in 25 per cent of cortisone-treated and in 45 per cent of untreated patients even when all patients received tocolytic agents.

Experimental work done by Enhorning et al.[56] had recently shown that the injection of isoxsuprine in fetal rabbits at term resulted in dehydration of the fetal lung and caused release of the surfactant stored in type II pneumocytes. The clinical significance of this observation is far from clear, and at present most evidence seem to indicate that uterine inhibitors do not play a significant role in the incidence of RDS.

Prenatal Glucocorticoid Treatment and Neonatal Morbidity and Mortality

Many authors[17-21, 26-28, 31-34] have addressed the subject of neonatal mortality but not much information on the causes of death is available. Data taken from current literature are presented in Table 3. It can be seen that treated infants represent about one third the neonatal mortality of the untreated "control." These figures are very similar to those reported by Ballard et al.[30] of a lower overall mortality (8.6 per cent) for prenatally treated than for the untreated controls (23 per cent).

From these data one can only assume that the change in neonatal mortality is due to a decline in the incidence and severity of RDS. Tauesch et al.[24] in a recent report stated that severe RDS and/or death due to RDS occurred in 1 of 30 liveborn infants whose mothers received 6 doses of steroids and in 11 of 65 whose mothers received at least 1 dose of placebo.

The problem of neonatal morbidity remains extremely complex. At least one group of investigators[34] reported a greater incidence of hypoglycemia in infants prenatally treated. These authors described early blood glucose levels of less than 40 mg in 38 per cent of dexamethasone-treated and in 15 per cent of control infants. These observations were made when patients were admitted to the NICU and before an intravenous infusion of glucose could have been started.

Decreased resistance to infection in the

TABLE 3. PRENATAL GLUCOCORTICOID TREATMENT: EFFECTS ON NEONATAL MORTALITY

AUTHORS	DRUG	GEST. AGE (WEEKS)	UNTREATED #Dead/Total	TREATED #Dead/Total
Liggins and Howie[17, 18]	B	<37	29/16	16/186
Fargier et al.[19]	B	<37	64/396	3/42
Kennedy[20, 21]	B	<37	10/41	5/41
Schwenzel et al.[26]	B	<37	11/109	1/76
Caspi et al.[27]	B	<36	27/71	4/60
Dhulolucky et al.[28]	H	<37	14/40	3/31
Block et al.[31]	B	<37	5/44	1/49
Mead and Clapp[32]	B	27–32	8/16	4/27
Morrison et al.[33]	H	<36	7/59	3/67
Papageorgiou et al.[34]	B	<35	6/32	0/28
		<37	181/824	40/607
Percentage neonatal mortality			21.9	6.5

B = betamethasone, H = hydrocortisone.

mother or the fetus or both has been a long-standing source of concern for those involved in glucocorticoid treatment. Liggins et al.[18] and later Mead et al.[32] examined the question in detail and concluded that no association of infection and prenatal steroid treatment could be established. Among the authors involved in clinical trials,[19-36] only Tauesch et al.[24] presented data to the contrary. The latter found that steroid treatment in women with premature rupture of membranes of more than 48 hours' time lapse until delivery was associated with an increased number of maternal infections. This complication occurred in 5 of 10 treated women and in only 1 of the 17 placebo patients. Owing to the experimental design no patient with signs of infection was admitted to the study, and it was assumed that this complication developed after the onset of therapy.

Many of those who did not observe an increase in maternal infection are quite liberal in the use of antibiotic therapy, and that was thought to be a possible explanation. Papageorgiou et al.[34] did not use antibiotic prophylaxis and yet did not find an increase in maternal, fetal or neonatal infections.

FETAL LOSSES FOLLOWING USE OF GLUCOCORTICOIDS

The question of fetal jeopardy following this mode of therapy was first raised by Liggins et al.[18] in reference to patients with hypertensive disorders. They originally reported that 12 of 46 treated hypertensive patients and 3 out of 42 untreated controls experienced fetal death.

They expressed a word of caution and speculated that glucocorticoids may have further compromised placental function. These early observations had a profound impact on other workers and for years patients with hypertensive disorders of pregnancy have been excluded from similar therapeutic trials.

Semchyshyn and associates[58] administered prenatal glucocorticoid treatment to 50 hypertensive pregnant patients in labor and recorded only 3 perinatal deaths (1 antepartum, 1 in labor and 1 neonatal). The incidence of perinatal loss was similar to that reported by Liggins[18] for the untreated glucocorticoid group, and although the incidence is high, this fact must be taken in the context of the extremely high-risk population. Semchyshyn et al.[58] also reported that the administration of 1000 mg of hydrocortisone succinate intravenously did not result in significant changes in maternal blood pressure or further compromise of renal function. Liggins[59] reanalyzed the original data on preeclamptic patients and found that perinatal losses were closely related to the severity of the proteinuria. He reported that for patients excreting more than 3 g of protein the perinatal mortality was 43 per cent while for those with less proteinuria it was only 14 per cent. Furthermore, he added that no untoward effects were seen in over 100 hypertensive pregnant women recently treated and attributed the success to a more aggressive medical management and the rarity of massive proteinuria.

As stated, following Liggins' initial comments on fetal jeopardy most investigators decided to exclude patients with hypertensive

TABLE 4. FETAL LOSSES FOLLOWING PRENATAL GLUCOCORTICOID TREATMENT

AUTHORS	DRUG	GEST. AGE (WK)	#SB/# FETUSES
Fargier et al.[19]	B	<37	0/42
Gennser et al.[60]	B	≤37	0/34
		<27	7/9
Kennedy[21]	B	27–34	0/127
Killam et al.[25]	H	27–32	0/28
Stocker et al.[61]	B	<36	0/?
Tauesch et al.[24]	D	26–33	0/24
Ballard et al.[29]	B	26–34	0/40
Caspi et al.[27]	D	28–36	0/55
Dluholucky et al.[27]	H	≤37	0/120
Block et al.[31]	B	<37	3/49
Mead and Clapp[32]	B	27–32	0/27
Morrison et al.[33]	H	<36	0/67
Papageorgiou et al.[34]	B	<35	0/28
Thornfeldt et al.[36]	D	<33	0/121
Liggins and Howie[18]	D	≤37	12/443
Total		<37	22/1214

B = betamethasone, H = hydrocortisone, D = dexamethasone.

disorders from glucocorticoid prenatal trials.[60, 61] Pooling of these data has been used to produce Table 4, in which it can be seen that only 22 of 1214 treated fetuses died. This represents a 2 per cent mortality that is not surprisingly high considering the maternal risk factors involved. It is worth mentioning that in one study seven of nine very small fetuses below 27 weeks died antepartum.[21] The authors did not offer any explanation for those losses and not enough information was available to shed light on the subject.

DRUG CHOICE, DOSAGE AND LENGTH OF TREATMENT

Table 5 contains a list of the different regimens proposed as of this writing. Few investigators have discussed reasons for the given choice of glucocorticoids and most of them have merely followed Liggins' recommendation.[17] Block et al.[31] in 1976 reported on the effects of methylprednisolone, betamethasone and placebo in a prospective double-blind study. They found that the incidence of RDS was 9 per cent in the betamethasone-treated patient and 23 per cent in both placebo and methylprednisolone groups. Their results suggested that methylprednisolone either failed to cross the placenta or if it did was insufficient to induce pulmonary maturation to a significant degree.

Valuable information came also from the work of Whitt et al.,[64] who measured the efficiency of betamethasone and hydrocortisone and the promptness of its pharmacologic action in terms of the fetal adrenocortical-axis suppression. This effect was manifested by the percentage changes in the concentration of urinary estriol. These investigators concluded that the intravenous infusion of hydrocortisone produced a more rapid effect than intramuscularly injected betamethasone, and they speculated that an earlier response such as that could be useful in cases of imminent delivery.

In a more recent publication Tauesch et al.[24] explained their preference for dexamethasone based on the following reasons: (1) the acetate salt (betamethasone) is poorly absorbed and may give prolonged exposure; (2) betamethasone phosphate has not been readily available in the United States; (3) dexamethasone and betamethasone have similar biologic potency with regard to glucocorticoid-binding receptors in the fetal lung; and (4) dexamethasone promptly crosses the placenta and is associated with fetal adrenal suppression. Available evidence seems to indicate that dexamethasone, betamethasone and hydrocortisone are all efficacious in the prevention of RDS. Trials with dexamethasone and hydrocortisone continue. According to Ballard and Ballard[57] it is likely that once optimal dose

TABLE 5. PRENATAL GLUCOCORTICOID TREATMENTS

DEXAMETHASONE		
Tauesch et al.[24]	IM	4 mg Q 8 hr × 6 doses
Caspi et al.[27]	IM	4 mg Q 8 hr × 7 days
Thornfeldt et al.[36]	IM	8 mg Q 24 hr × 2 doses
Spellacy et al.[62]	PO	0.5 mg Q 6 hr × 14 days
BETAMETHASONE		
Liggins and Howie[17, 18]	IM	12 mg Q 24 hr × 2 doses
Fargier et al.[19]	IM	12 mg Q 24 hr × 2 doses
Kennedy[20, 21]	IM	12 mg Q 24 hr × 2 doses
Ballard et al.[30]	IM	12 mg Q 24 hr × 2 doses
Block et al.[31]	IM	12 mg Q 24 hr × 2 doses (weekly up to 34 wks)
Papageorgiou et al.[34]	IM	12 mg Q 24 hr × 2 doses
Gennser et al.[65]	IM	12 mg Q 24 hr × 3 doses
Schwenzel et al.[26]	IM	10.5 mg Q 24 hr × 2 doses
Stocker[61]	IM	12 mg Q 12 hr × 2 doses × 7 days
Ekelund et al.[63]	IM	12 mg Q 24 hr × 3 doses
Mead and Clapp[32]	IM	6 mg Q 12 hr × 2 doses
HYDROCORTISONE		
Killam[25]	IV	500 mg Q 8 hr × 4 doses
Dluholucky et al.[28]	IV	100 mg once
Morrison et al.[33]	IV	500 mg Q 12 hr × 5 doses
Zuspan et al.[38]	IV	1000 mg Q 6 hr × 4 doses
Whitt et al.[64]	IV	1000 mg Q 8 hr × 4 doses

regimens are established hydrocortisone (natural glucocorticoid) will be the drug of choice.

A collaborative double-blind randomized clinical trial sponsored by the National Heart, Lung and Blood Institute is continuing; it was designed to test the efficacy of dexamethasone in the prevention of RDS (see addendum).

In terms of dosages and regimens, it is evident that the minimum effective dosage has yet to be determined. Ballard et al.[57] estimated that high doses of hydrocortisone[25, 33, 38] have produced fetal exposures of 17 to 67 mg of hydrocortisone per kg of body weight in contrast to the 5 mg kg produced by a 12-mg dose of betamethasone. Considering that the clinical results with both types of regimens are similar, we agree that there are no benefits from excessive dosage of cortisol but that there are dangers involved.

It would seem that until final information from the ongoing collaborative studies becomes available the drugs and dosages to be considered are:

1. Betamethasone (acetate/phosphate) 12 mg Q 24 hr × 2 doses IM.
2. Dexamethasone (phosphate) 4 mg Q 8 hr × 6 doses IM.
3. Hydrocortisone (succinate) 500 mg Q 12 hr × 2 doses IV.

The need for repeated treatment is related to the possibility that acceleration of lung maturation would be extremely transient, and some of Liggins' observations would seem to indicate so.[17, 18] In our opinion, these matters are still unclear and there is no justification for repeated treatment unless follow-up amniotic fluid studies still show pulmonary immaturity.

Ballard and associates[65] demonstrated that betamethasone levels in the mother peak at about one hour after the injection and then decline rapidly. The half-life of the drug is about six hours and little remains in the circulation two days after the injection. Endogenous cortisol activity declines about two hours after injection, remains low and returns to normal range by about four days. Combined cortisol activity following the injection of betamethasone is about three times that of the endogenously produced hormone in the untreated pregnant woman.

Ballard's data also suggest that fetal serum cortisol is lower than maternal and that it peaks about one hour following administration of betamethasone to the mother. A second injection has been shown to produce a greater rise in fetal serum betamethasone, and by 72

hours after injection such serum glucocorticoid activity is undetectable. Endogenous production of cortisol remains low for about four days but the potential for response has not been completely abolished, since severe stress is known to produce sharp elevations in serum cortisol activity. Ballard[29] also reported that the combined glucocorticoid activity measured in fetal serum of treated infants (cord specimens) is quite similar to that observed in the serum of nontreated newborns who developed RDS.

An indirect way to assess glucocorticoid potential usefulness is through an evaluation of glucocorticoid receptors activity in the fetal lung.[65] Another interesting observation is that based on maternal and fetal plasma glucocorticoid levels. It has been established that the maternal-fetal gradient for cortisol is twice as large as that of betamethasone, this suggests that to produce the same fetal serum activity twice as much exogenous cortisol would be required. Since the half-life of cortisol is shorter, a higher dosage at closer intervals would be required.

CONTRAINDICATIONS

Review of the available literature does not reveal any uniform criteria for contraindications to the treatment. We have tabulated only those that have more often been agreed upon (Table 6). The absolute contraindications are clear enough that no further comment is needed. On the other hand, the relative contraindications have not been sufficiently defined.

While hypertension poses a relative contraindication, Semchyshyn et al. found no statistically significant difference in blood

TABLE 6. CONTRAINDICATIONS

ABSOLUTE
Amnionitis
Maternal infections (Herpes)
Severe bleeding
Hyperthyroidism
Peptic ulcers
Imminent delivery
Mature: L/S ratio, OD 650, shake test
Inability to continuously monitor mother and fetus

RELATIVE
Hypertensive disorders
Diabetes
Placental insufficiency

pressure changes in their hypertensive patients while under therapy.[58]

Since delay of delivery even in the presence of a prolonged interval since rupture of membranes is critical for the efficacy of steroid treatment, the possibility of maternal and fetal infection cannot be ignored. Only an active and intelligent plan of detection can prevent situations of catastrophic potential. It has been our policy to obtain serial maternal white blood cell counts and differentials, Gram stain and cultures of the amniotic fluid as well as to carefully monitor vital signs—especially the maternal and fetal heart rate.

It has been observed that the use of glucocorticoids in pregnant diabetics produces increased insulin requirements, particularly at the beginning of the therapy. Once the adequate dosages have been determined, at least in our experience, we have not found other problems.

Efforts should be made to stop preterm labor for the duration of treatment to at least 24 hours past the first dose. Alcohol, salbutamol, ritodrine, isoxsuprine, terbutaline and more recently magnesium sulfate have all been used with a certain degree of success.

A case report of pulmonary edema following therapy with dexamethasone and terbutaline alerted us to a potentially serious complication.[66] It is unlikely that dexamethasone contributed to the pulmonary edema seen in that patient. Prolonged exposure to a high dose of the adrenergic superimposed on the hypervolemic status of the laboring pregnant patient could have precipitated that emergency.

PATIENT SELECTION CRITERIA

Review of the literature and our own experience has allowed the drawing of general and

TABLE 7. GUIDELINES FOR PATIENT SELECTION FOR PRENATAL GLUCOCORTICOID TREATMENT

GENERAL
Premature labor with or without PROM
Planned premature termination of pregnancy
Anticipate delivery later than 24 hours
Prolongation of pregnancy for 48 hours safe for mother and fetus

SPECIFIC (According to Gestational Age)
At ≤32 Weeks
  Shake test negative or unavailable
  L/S immature or unavailable
  OD 650 immature or unavailable

At 33–34 Weeks
  Shake test negative
  L/S immature or OD 650 immature
  L/S and OD 650 unavailable in *Rh* or *diabetes*

At 35–36 Weeks
  Shake test negative or unavailable
  Only when L/S or OD 650 immature

specific guidelines of patient selection for glucocorticoid therapy (Table 7).

Patients eligible for glucocorticoid therapy should be those with estimated fetal weight less than 5 pounds (2300 g) or those with gestations less than 34 weeks. Since dates (LMP) are often questionable and clinical estimation of weight may be in error, ultrasonography can be of great help. The value of amniocentesis for analysis of lung-produced phospholipids cannot be overemphasized. It is of particular importance in cases of intrauterine growth retardation, in which the fetal size could be deceivingly small.

TOXIC EFFECTS OF PRENATAL GLUCOCORTICOID TREATMENT

The issues of side effects and drug toxicity have to be examined in light of available information. For the sake of simplicity we

TABLE 8. TOXIC EFFECTS OF GLUCOCORTICOIDS ADMINISTERED TO PREGNANT ANIMALS

AUTHOR*	ANIMAL	DRUG	DOSAGE	DURATION % OF GESTATION	EFFECTS
Glauback et al.[70]	Rat	C	10 mg/kg/d (6–20 d)	27–90	↑ Fetal and neonatal death, ↓ growth
Faunstat et al.[71]	Rabbit	C	60 mg/kg/d (4–5 d)	13–60	Cleft palate
Lee and Ring[72]	Rabbit	C	4 mg/kg/d (7 d)	22	Pancreatic inlet degeneration
Wong and Burton[73]	Mouse	D	1–4 mg/kg/d (1 d)	5	↓ Maternal glucose transfer
Motoyama et al.[6]	Rabbit	c	30 mg/kg/d (3 d)	10	↓ Fetal body and lung
Wellman and Volk[74]	Rabbit	C	4 mg/kg/d (2–7 d)	6–22	↓ Placental unitosis
Van Geijn et al.[75]	Rat	H	57 mg/kg/d (1 d)	5	Normal brain amine development

*Chronological listing.
C = cortisone, D = dexamethasone, c = cortisol, H = hydrocortisone.

TABLE 9. TOXIC EFFECTS OF GLUCOCORTICOID ADMINISTERED TO ANIMAL FETUSES

AUTHOR	ANIMAL	DRUG	DOSE	RESULTS
Motoyama et al.[6]	Rabbit	C	1 mg	↓ lung growth
Carson et al.[76]	Rabbit	C	2 mg	↓ somatic and lung growth
Kotas et al.[77]	Rabbit	H	2 mg	reversible effects
DeLemos[78]	Monkey	D	1–3 mg	↓ lung growth, transient, brain growth

C = cortisol, D = dexamethasone, H = hydrocortisone.

have organized the information according to type of study and length of prenatal or neonatal exposure or both.

First, we shall consider studies dealing with prenatal glucocorticoid administration (Table 8). It is safe to assume that most of the treatments were given at the later stages in pregnancy and in amounts that can hardly be compared to those used in the human. Ballard[15] in a recent publication estimates that dosages used in animals were up to 300 times greater per kilogram of body weight than those used in humans by Liggins and Howie.[17] The potential for toxicity exists, and extreme caution should be exercised when interpreting these results.

That glucocorticoid directly injected into animal fetuses produces somatic and lung growth retardation can no longer be disputed (Table 9). Neither can the reversibility of some of these developmental delays be disputed.

It has been almost axiomatic that toxic effects are related to dosage and duration of therapy. The latter is particularly important if one considers the timing of the treatment and the species involved in these experimental models. According to the data presented in Table 10, it can be seen that most treatments had a relatively short duration and yet they produced significant effects. The data in rats show clearly that dendritic and synaptogenic growth were considerably altered, but one must remember that unlike the laboratory animal cortex the human cortex is well assembled long before term. Neuronal multiplication in the developing brain is followed by migration to the outer cortical zones. This migratory process occurs up to 24 weeks of gestation; it is unlikely that many new neurons will enter the cerebral cortex beyond that time. This developmental event is followed by dendritic growth, which continues to about 35 to 36 weeks, and by synaptogenesis, which extends probably through term. Glial development and myelinization complete the developmental sequence extending well into the second year of postnatal life.

It is likely that the temporal pattern of brain development in the human may not be subject to some of the detrimental effects of glucocorticoid treatment seen in the rat. The data accumulated on humans is presented in Table 11. Relative to the human, a note of caution should be made, since not all the cortical areas develop simultaneously and the dendritic and synaptogenic processes would be extremely critical for neurobehavioral competency in later years.

TABLE 10. EFFECTS OF GLUCOCORTICOID TREATMENT ON ANIMALS DURING NEONATAL PERIOD

AUTHOR	ANIMAL	DRUG	DOSE-ROUTE	EFFECTS
Branceni et al[79]	Rat	P	15,000 mg/kg/d	↓ immune response; ↑ thymic involution
Howard and Granoff[80]	Mouse	Cc	Pellets	↓ CNS DNA; CNS malfunction
Shapiro[81]	Rat	c	1 mg/kg/d	↓ somatic growth; ↓ myelinization; ↓ immunity
Winnick[82]	Rat	C	100 mg/kg/d	runting; ↓ organ DNA
Shapiro et al. [83]	Rat	c	0.5 mg/kg/d	↓ onset of swimming; ↑ purposeless movement
Taylor and Howard[84]	Rat	Cc	210 mg/kg/d	↓ abnormal glucose metabolism
Cotterrell et al.[85]	Rat	c	0.2 mg/kg/d	↓ somatic, thymus and brain growth
Krieger[86]	Rat	D	0.1 mg/kg/d	↑ pulmonary susceptibility to O_2 toxicity
De Souza and Adlard[87]	Rat	D	1–20 µg/kg/d	↓ somatic, brain and thymus growth
Gumbinas[88]	Rat	M	0.8 mg/kg/d	↓ somatic, brain growth; ↓ myelinization
Weischel[16]	Rat	c	0.6 mg/kg/d	↓ somatic and brain growth

P = prednisolone, Cc = corticosterone, c = cortisol, C = cortisone, D = dexamethasone, M = methylprednisolone.

TABLE 11. Effects of Glucocorticoids in the Human Neonate

Author	Drug	Route	Dosage	Effect
Silverman et al.[89]	ACTH	IM	14–20 mg/kg/d × 9–27 d	↓ growth (temporary)
Altman[90]	C	IM	25–50 mg Q 6 hr	none
DeLemos[91]	M	IV	40 mg QID × 3 d	↑ residual CNS damage
Ewerbeck[92]	P	IV	20–40 mg/kg/d	↑ incidence of CNS damage
Baden et al.[93]	H	IV	15 mg/kg × 1 d	none
Tauesch et al.[94]	H	IV	12.5 mg/kg Q 12 hr × 2 d	↑ incidence intraventricule bleeding
Fitzhardinge[95]	H	IV	12.5 mg/kg Q 12 hr × 1 d	minor neurologic findings

C = cortisone, M = methylprednisolone, P = prednisolone, H = hydrocortisone.

Conclusions

Yes: Glucocorticoids prenatally administered accelerate lung maturation, although they will *not* prevent RDS in every infant.

Yes: The incidence of RDS and even neonatal mortality can be decreased by the use of steroids, but it will *not* eliminate the other major problems associated with prematurity.

Yes: Maximum benefits from this mode of therapy would be obtained if delivery could be delayed for at least 24 hours after the initial dose. *No* treatment should be initiated unless there is a good chance that this will occur.

Yes: Most impressive results would be obtained if treatment is given to patients at or below 32 weeks of gestation, but there is *no* hard data that demonstrate similar benefit to fetuses below 28 weeks.

Yes: An occasional premature infant of 35 to 36 weeks' gestation benefits from the glucocorticoid treatment, but this mode of prophylaxis should *not* be used unless laboratory data are consistent with pulmonary immaturity.

Yes: Toxic effects have been documented in laboratory animals but these findings *cannot* be freely extrapolated to humans because of differing drug dosage, duration of treatment, life span and above all temporal differences in the neurobiological development of different species.

Yes: This mode of therapy should be initiated only after informed consent has been obtained from the parents. It should *not* be instituted carelessly or injudiciously.

Yes: Prenatal glucocorticoid treatment commits the physician and the institution to a carefully planned long-term follow-up that is *not* usually available outside tertiary care level facilities.

Yes: The most commonly recommended glucocorticoids are dexamethasone and hydrocortisone, but minimum effective dosages and drug of choice have *not* yet been determined.

Yes: There is some indication that the effect on lung maturation may be temporary, but there is *no* justification for repeated courses of therapy without laboratory evidence consistent with pulmonary immaturity.

Yes: Short-term benefits of this mode of therapy are real, but the potential for long-term toxicity has *not* yet been ruled out.

Yes: Glucocorticoid treatment of the unborn fetus represents a remarkable advance, but the search for a more effective and less potentially dangerous agent should *not* stop.

Addendum

The response of the fetal lung to antenatally administered glucocorticoids seems to be greater in females than in males. Cord blood betamethasone and the degree and duration of the adrenocortical axis suppression seems to be similar in treated infants disregarding sex;* therefore, the reason for the difference in responsiveness still remains obscure.

Preliminary results from the antenatal glucocorticoid collaborative study† recently documented the overall effectiveness of the treatment, the absence of maternal and neonatal complications and the lack of neurologic abnormalities in treated infants when tested at 40 weeks of gestation.

---

*Ballard, P. et al.: Fetal sex and prenatal betamethasone therapy. J. Pediatr. 97:451, 1980.

†Collaborative Group on Antenatal Steroid Therapy. Am. J. Obstet. Gynecol. 141:276, 1981.

REFERENCES

1. Liggins, G. C.: Premature delivery of fetal lambs infused with glucocorticoids. J. Endocrinol. 45:515, 1969.
2. Moog, F. and Richardson, D.: The functional differentiation of the small intestine. IV. The influence of adrenocortical hormones on differentiation and phosphatase synthesis in the duodenum of the chick embryo. J. Exp. Zool. 130:29, 1955.
3. Buckingham, S., McNary, W. F., Sommers, S. C. et al.: Is lung on analog of Moog's intestine? Phosphatase and pulmonary alveolar differentiation in fetal rabbits. (Abstr.) Fed. Proc. 27:328, 1968.
4. DeLemos, R., Shermeta, D., Knelson, J. et al.: Acceleration of appearance of pulmonary surfactant in the fetal lamb by administration of corticosteroids. Am. Rev. Resp. Dis. 102:459, 1970.
5. Kotas, R. V. and Avery, M. R.: Accelerated appearance of pulmonary surfactant in the fetal rabbit. J. Appl. Physiol. 30:358, 1971.
6. Motoyama, E. K., Orzalesi, M. M., Kikkawa, Y. et al.: Effect of cortisol on the maturation of fetal rabbit lungs. Pediatrics 48:547, 1971.
7. Chiswick, M. L., Ahmed, A., Jack, P. M. B. et al.: Control of fetal lung development in the rabbit. Arch. Dis. Child. 48:709, 1973.
8. Blackburn, W. R., Kelly, J. S., Dickman, P. S. et al.: The role of the pituitary-adrenal-thyroidaxes in lung differentiation. II. Biochemical studies of developing lung in anencephalic fetal rats. Lab. Invest. 28:352, 1973.
9. Vidyasagar, D. and Chernick, V.: Effect of metopirone on the synthesis of lung surfactant in does and fetal rabbits. Biol. Neonate 27:1, 1975.
10. Liggins, G. C.: Adrenocortical-related maturational events in the fetus. Am. J. Obstet. Gynecol. 126:931, 1976.
11. Ekelund, L., Arvidson, G. and Astedt, B.: Cortisol-induced accumulation of phospholipids in organ culture of human fetal lung. Scand. J. Clin. Lab. Invest. 35:419, 1975.
12. Brehier, A., Benson, B. J., Williams, M. C. et al.: Corticosteroid-induction of phosphatidic acid phosphatase in fetal rabbit lung. Biochem. Biophys. Res. Commun. 77:883, 1977.
13. Farrell, P. M. and Zachman, R. D.: Induction of choline phosphotransferase and lecithin synthesis in the fetal lung by corticosteroids. Science 179:297, 1973.
14. Barrett, C. T., Sevanian, A., Phelps, D. L. et al.: Effects of cortisol and aminophylline upon survival, pulmonary mechanics, and secreted phosphatidylcholine of prematurely delivered rabbits. Pediatr. Res. 12:38, 1978.
15. Ballard, P., Benson, B. and Brehier, A.: Glucocorticoid effects in the fetal lung. Am. Rev. Resp. Dis. 115 (suppl.):29, 1977.
16. Weichsel, M.: Glucocorticoid effect upon thymidine kinase in the developing cerebellum. Pediatr. Res. 8:361, 1974.
17. Liggins, G. C. and Howie, R. N.: A controlled trial of antepartum glucocorticoid treatment for prevention of the respiratory distress syndrome in premature infants. Pediatrics 50:515, 1972.
18. Liggins, G. C.: Prenatal glucocorticoid treatment: prevention of respiratory distress syndrome. Proceedings of the 70th Ross Conference on Pediatric Research. Columbus, Ross Laboratories, 1975, pp. 97–105.
19. Fargier, P., Salle, B., Band, M. et al.: Prevention du syndrome de detresse respiratoire chez le premature. Nouv. Presse Med. 3:1595, 1974.
20. Kennedy, J. L.: Antepartum betamethasone in the prevention of RDS. (Abstr.) Pediatr. Res. 8:447, 1974.
21. Kennedy, J. L.: Prenatal glucocorticoid treatment: prevention of respiratory distress syndrome. Proceedings of the 70th Ross Conference on Pediatric Research. Columbus, Ross Laboratories, 1975, pp. 105–110.
22. Bureau, M., Stocker, J., DeLeon, A. et al.: Utilisation de la betamethasone dans la prevention du syndrome de detresse respiratoire du nouveau-ne premature. Union Med. Can. 104:99, 1975.
23. Taeusch, H. W.: Catecholamines, insulin, glucocorticoids and respiratory distress syndrome: tribulations of controlled trials. Proceedings of the 70th Ross Conference on Pediatric Research. Columbus, Ross Laboratories, 1975, pp. 92–97.
24. Taeusch, H. W., Frigoletto, F., Kitzmiller, J. et al.: Risk of respiratory distress syndrome after prenatal dexamethasone treatment. Pediatrics 63:64, 1979.
25. Killam, A. P.: Prenatal glucocorticoid treatment: effect on surviving infants. Proceedings of the 70th Ross Conference on Pediatric Research. Columbus, Ross Laboratories, 1975, pp. 110–115.
26. Schwenzel, W., Jung, H., Lahmann, H. et al.: Erste erfahrungen mit der praenatalen beeinflussung der kindlichen lungenreife durche betamethason. Z. Geburtshilfe Perinatol. 179:45, 1975.
27. Caspi, E., Schreyer, P., Weinraub. Z. et al.: Prevention of the respiratory distress syndrome in premature infants by antepartum glucocorticoid therapy. Br. J. Obstet. Gynecol. 83:187, 1976.
28. Dluholucky, S., Babic, J. and Taufer, I.: Reduction of incidence and mortality of respiratory distress syndrome by administration of hydrocortisone to mother. Arch. Dis. Child. 51:420, 1976.
29. Ballard, R. A. and Ballard, P. L.: Use of prenatal glucocorticoid therapy to prevent respiratory distress syndrome. Am. J. Dis. Child. 130:982, 1976.
30. Ballard, R. A., Ballard, P. L., Granberg, J. P. et al.: Prenatal administration of betamethasone for prevention of respiratory distress syndrome. J. Pediatr. 94:97, 1979.
31. Block, M. F., Kling, O. R. and Crosby, W. M.: Antenatal glucocorticoid therapy for the prevention of respiratory distress syndrome in the premature infant. Obstet. Gynecol. 50:186, 1977.
32. Mead, P. B. and Clapp, J. F., III: The use of betamethasone and timed delivery in management of premature rupture of the membranes in the preterm pregnancy. J. Reprod. Med. 19:3, 1977.
33. Morrison, J. C., Shybrew, W. D., Bucovaz, E. T. et al.: Injection of corticosteroids into mother to prevent neonatal respiratory distress syndrome. Am. J. Obstet. Gynecol. 131:358, 1978.
34. Papageorgiou, A. N., Desgranges, M. F., Masson, M. et al.: A controlled double-blind study of antenatal betamethasone. Pediatr. Res. 12:531, 1978.
35. Papageorgiou, A. N., Desgranges, M. F., Masson,

M. et al.: The antenatal use of betamethasone in the prevention of respiratory distress syndrome: a controlled double-blind study. Pediatrics 63:73, 1979.

36. Thornfeldt, R. E., Franklin, R. W., Pickering, N. A. et al.: The effect of glucocorticoids on the maturation of premature lung membranes. Am. J. Obstet. Gynecol. 131:143, 1978.

37. Usher, R., Allen, A. C. and McLean, F. H.: Risk of RDS related to gestational age, route of delivery and maternal diabetes. Am. J. Obstet. Gynecol. 111:826, 1971.

38. Zuspan, F. P., Cordero, L. and Semchyshyn, S.: Effects of hydrocortisone on lecithin-sphingomyelin ratio. Am. J. Obstet. Gynecol. 128:571, 1977.

39. Alden, E. R., Mandelkorn, T., Woodrum, D. E. et al.: Morbidity and mortality of infants weighing less than 1,000 grams in an intensive care nursery. Pediatrics 50:40, 1972.

40. Yoon, J. J. and Harper, R. G.: Observations on the relationship between duration of rupture of the membranes and the development of idiopathic respiratory distress syndrome. Pediatrics 51:161, 1973.

41. Chiswick, M. L. and Burnard, E.: Respiratory distress syndrome. Lancet 1:1060, 1973.

42. Bauer, C. R., Stern, L. and Colle, E.: Prolonged rupture of membranes associated with a decreased incidence of respiratory distress syndrome. Pediatrics 53:7, 1974.

43. Richardson, C. J., Pomerance, J. J., Cunningham, M.D. et al.: Acceleration of fetal lung maturation following prolonged rupture of the membranes. Am. J. Obstet. Gynecol. 118:1115, 1974.

44. Jones, M. D., Burd, L. L., Bowes, W. A. et al.: Failure of association of premature rupture of membranes with respiratory distress syndrome. N. Engl. J. Med. 292:1253, 1975.

45. Berkowitz, R. L., Bonta, B. W. and Warshaw, J. E.: The relationship between premature rupture of the membranes and the respiratory distress syndrome. Am. J. Obstet. Gynecol. 124:712, 1976.

46. Thibeault, D. W. and Emmanouildes, G. C.: Prolonged rupture of fetal membranes and decreased frequency of respiratory distress syndrome and patent ductus arteriosus in preterm infants. Am. J. Obstet. Gynecol. 129:43, 1977.

47. Christensen, K. K., Christensen, P., Ingemarsson, I. et al.: A study of complications in preterm deliveries after prolonged premature rupture of the membranes. Obstet. Gynecol. 48:670, 1976.

48. Zachman, R. D.: Premature rupture of the membranes and the incidence of respiratory distress syndrome. Perinatal Press. 1:4, 1976.

49. Sell, E. J. and Harris, T. R.: Association of premature rupture of membranes with idiopathic respiratory distress syndrome. Obstet. Gynecol. 49:167, 1977.

50. Mead, P. D.: Does prolonged rupture of the membranes protect against respiratory distress? Perinatal Press. 1:4, 1977.

51. Cordero, L. and Urrutia, J.: Premature rupture of membranes: influence on the incidence of HMD. Revista Argentina de Perinatologia (in press).

52. Liggins, G. C. and Howie, R. N.: The prevention of RDS by maternal steroid therapy. Gluck, L. (ed.): Neonatal Perinatal Medicine. Year Book Medical Publishers, 1974, p. 415.

53. Kero, P., Hirvonen, T. and Valimaki, I.: Prenatal and postnatal isoxsuprine and respiratory distress syndrome. Lancet 2:198, 1973.

54. Boog, G., Brahem, M. D. and Gandar, R.: Beta-mimetic drugs and possible prevention of respiratory distress syndrome. Br. J. Obstet. Gynecol. 82:285, 1975.

55. Barrada, M. J., Virnig, N. L., Edwards, L. E. et al.: Maternal intravenous ethanol in the prevention of respiratory distress syndrome. Am. J. Obstet. Gynecol. 129:25, 1977.

56. Enhorning, G., Chamberlain, D., Contreras, C. et al.: Isoxsuprine-induced release of pulmonary surfactant in the rabbit fetus. Am. J. Obstet. Gynecol. 129:197, 1977.

57. Ballard, P. L. and Ballard, R. A.: Corticosteroid and respiratory distress syndrome: status 1979. Pediatrics 63:163, 1979.

58. Semchyshyn, S. et al.: Cardiovascular response and complications of glucocorticoid therapy in hypertensive pregnancies. In press.

59. Liggins, G. C.: Personal communication, 1980.

60. Gennser, G., Ohrlander, S. and Eneroth, P.: Cortisol in amniotic fluid and cord blood in relation to prenatal betamethasone load and delivery. Am. J. Obstet. Gynecol. 124:43, 1976.

61. Stocker, J.: Prenatal glucocorticoid treatment: reduction in neonatal death. Proceedings of the 70th Ross Conference on Pediatric Research. Columbus, Ross Laboratories, 1975, pp. 115–119.

62. Spellacy, W. N., Buhi, W. E., Riggall, F. C. et al.: Human amniotic fluid lecithin-sphigomyelin ratio changes with estrogen or glucocorticoid treatment. Am. J. Obstet. Gynecol. 115:216, 1973.

63. Ekelund, L., Arvidson, G., Ohrlander, S. et al.: Changes in amniotic fluid phospholipids on treatment with glucocorticoids to prevent respiratory distress syndrome. Acta Obstet. Gynecol. Scand. 55:413, 1976.

64. Whitt, G. G., Buster, J. E., Killam, A. P. et al.: A comparison of two glucocorticoid regimens for acceleration of fetal lung maturation in premature labor. Am. J. Obstet. Gynecol. 124:479, 1976.

65. Ballard, P. L., Granberg, P. and Ballard, R. A.: Glucocorticoid levels in maternal and cord serum after prenatal betamethasone therapy to prevent respiratory distress syndrome. J. Clin. Invest. 56:1548, 1975.

66. Stubblefield, P. G.: Pulmonary edemia occurring after therapy with dexamethasone and terbutaline for premature labor. A case report. Am. J. Obstet. Gynecol. 132:341, 1978.

67. Gluck, L. and Kulovich, M. V.: Lecithin-sphingomyelin ratio in amniotic fluid in normal and abnormal pregnancies. Am. J. Obstet. Gynecol. 115:539, 1973.

68. Sbarra, A. J., Michlewitz, H., Selvaraj, R. J. et al.: Relation between optical density at 650 mm and L/S ratios. Obstet. Gynecol. 50:723, 1977.

69. Copeland, W. Jr., Stempel, L., Loh, J. A. et al.: Assessment of a rapid test on amniotic fluid for estimating fetal lung maturity. Am. J. Obstet. Gynecol. 130:225, 1978.

70. Glauback, S., Antopol, W. and Graff, S.: Excessive doses in cortisone in pregnant mice: Effect on development and survival of the fetus and newborn, and on maternal breast tissue. Bull. N.Y. Acad. Med. 27:398, 1951.

71. Fainstat, T.: Cortisone-induced congenital cleft palate in rabbits. Endocrinology 55:502, 1954.

72. Lee, J. and Ring, P.: The effect of maternally administered cortisone and ACTH upon the pancreas of the fetus. J. Endocrinol. 14:284, 1956.

73. Wong, M. and Burton, A. F.: Inhibition by corticosteroids of glucose incorporation into fetuses of several strains of mouse. Biol. Neonate 18:146, 1971.

74. Wellman, K. and Volk, B.: Fine structure changes in the rabbit placenta induced by cortisone. Arch. Pathol. 94:147, 1972.

75. Van Geijn, H., Copeland, K., Vorys, A. et al.: The effects of hydrocortisone on the development of the amine systems in the fetal brain. (Abstr.) Soc. for Gynecol. Invest., 1979.

76. Carson, S. H., Tauesch, H. W., Jr. and Avery, M. E.: Inhibition of lung cell division after hydrocortisone injection into fetal rabbits. J. Appl. Physiol. 34:660, 1973.

77. Kotas, R. V., Mims, L. C. and Hart, L. K.: Reversible inhibition of lung cell number after glucocorticoid injection into fetal rabbits to enhance surfactant appearance. Pediatrics 53:358, 1974.

78. DeLemos, R. A.: Glucocorticoid effect: Organ development in monkeys. Proceedings of the 70th Ross Conference on Pediatric Research. Columbus, Ross Laboratories, 1975, pp. 77–80.

79. Branceni, D. and Arnason, B.: Thymic involution and recovery: Immune responsiveness and immunoglobulins after neonatal prednisolone in rats. Immunology 10:35, 1966.

80. Howard, E. and Granoff, D.: Increased voluntary running and decreased motor coordination in mice after neonatal corticosterone implantation. Exp. Neurol. 22:661, 1968.

81. Schapiro, S.: Some physiological, biochemical, and behavioral consequences of neonatal hormone administration: Cortisol and thyroxine. Gen. Comp. Endocrinol. 10:214, 1968.

82. Winnick, E.: Cellular growth of the fetus and placenta. *In* Waisman, H. and Kerr, G. (eds.): Fetal Growth and Development. New York, McGraw-Hill Book Co. Inc., 1968, p. 19.

83. Schapiro, S., Salas, M. and Vukovich, K.: Hormonal effects on the ontogeny of swimming ability in the rat: assessment of CNS development. Science 168:147, 1970.

84. Taylor, M. and Howard, E.: Impaired glucose homeostasis in adult rats after corticosterone treatment in infancy. Endocrinology 88:1190, 1971.

85. Cotterrell, M., Balazs, R. and Johnson, A. L.: Effects of corticosteroids on the biochemical maturation of rat brain: Postnatal cell formation. J. Neurochem. 19:2151, 1972.

86. Krieger, D.: Circadian corticosteroid periodicity: critical period for abolition by neonatal injection of corticosteroid. Science 178:1205, 1972.

87. De Souza, S. W. and Adlard, B. P.: Growth of suckling rats after treatment with dexamethasone or cortisol. Arch. Dis. Child. 48:519, 1973.

88. Gumbinas, M., Oda, M. and Huttenlocher, P.: The effect of corticosteroids on myelination of the developing rat brain. Biol. Neonate 22:255, 1973.

89. Silverman, W. A., Day, R. L. and Blodi, F. C.: Effects of ACTH in premature infants. Pediatrics 8:177, 1951.

90. Altman, H.: The RDS of the newborn. S. Afr. Med. J. 39:746, 1965.

91. DeLemos, R. A. and Haggerty, R. J.: Corticosteroid as an adjunct to treatment in bacterial meningitis. Pediatrics 44:30, 1969.

92. Ewerbeck, H. and Helwig, H.: Treatment of idiopathic respiratory distress syndrome with large doses of corticoids. Pediatrics 49:467, 1972.

93. Baden, M., Bauer, C. R., Colle, E. et al.: A controlled trial of hydrocortisone therapy in infants with respiratory distress syndrome. Pediatrics 50:526, 1972.

94. Taeusch, H. W., Wang, N. S., Baden, M. et al.: A controlled trial of hydrocortisone therapy in infants with RDS: II. Pathology. Pediatrics 52:850, 1973.

95. Fitzhardinge, P. M., Eisen, A., Lejtenyi, C. et al.: Sequelae of early steroid administration to the newborn infant. Pediatrics 53:877, 1974.

Administration of Steroids for Acceleration of Fetal Lung Maturity: Yes or No?

Jack M. Schneider, M.D.
John C. Morrison, M.D.
The University of Tennessee Center for the Health Sciences

Complications of prematurity are the primary cause of perinatal mortality. Respiratory distress syndrome (RDS) with attendant hyaline membrane disease (HMD) heads the list of complications contributing to neonatal mortality.

The most important advances in the past decade toward a solution of the problem of preterm birth have been development and refinement of tests to assess fetal lung maturity. At this time the most important potential advance in the prevention of RDS with HMD is maternally administered corticosteroid with its effect on fetal pulmonary maturity. This discussion offers an approach to glucocorticoid usage in patients at risk for preterm delivery.

Background: RDS and Steroids

Victims of HMD appear to have the common physiologic factor of a deficiency of surface-active material (surfactant) in the saccules (alveoli) of the lung. Surface-active material was first described approximately 20 years ago by Pattle.[1, 2] He also proposed a direct relationship with HMD in noting that animals born after a certain length of gestation attained enough surfactant to allow them to breathe spontaneously.

The infant's first inspiration must overcome a high intrathoracic pressure. Expansion of the saccules from this inspiration is unequal. If surface tension is unaltered by some factor, the Laplace equation indicates that the pressure (retractive force) in the smaller alveoli would be greater than that of the larger ones, and thus smaller alveoli would collapse. However, surfactant lowers surface tension, thus enabling the lung to retain up to 40 per cent of its volume on expiration and preventing overdistention on inspiration. Hence subsequent breaths require far lower inspiratory pressure.[3]

Deficiency of this surface-active material in the preterm infant precludes adequate stabilization of the saccules and thereby prevents retention of a functional residual volume. The collapsed alveoli require repetitive high inspiratory pressures to overcome the elevated intrathoracic pressure. Such effort soon exhausts the infant. Suffering from acidosis and hypoxia from a poor ventilation-to-perfusion ratio, the infant soon develops RDS with hyaline membrane formation.

The surface-active material is composed predominately of phospholipids, of which the most abundant is lecithin or phosphocholine. Gluck has shown that disaturated (dipalmitoyl) lecithin, an acetone-insoluble fraction of lung phospholipids, is the predominating surface-active agent.[4] Further, two acidic phospholipids, phosphatidyl inositol (PI) and phosphatidyl glycerol (PG), are necessary to stabilize lecithin in the surfactant.

Lecithin appears to be produced, stored and secreted by the type II lining cells in the pulmonary saccules, while the site of production remains controversial. Although dipalmitoyl lecithin appears to be the major type produced by the fetus near term, the type of lecithin produced depends on the stage of gestation and milieu of the fetus. For instance, in humans until about 35 weeks' gestation the lung produces small amounts of the dipalmitoyl lecithin. However, after this time the CDP pathway becomes the major source of lecithin production, and the disaturated compound increases in amount.[5] Maternal and fetal complications may accelerate this maturation process, while it may be reduced by hypothermia, hypoxia and acidosis.[6, 7]

Physiochemical and biochemical studies of the origin, properties and composition of surfactant, stimulated by the postulation that the absence of surface-active material in the lung of premature infants was the underlying cause of hyaline membrane disease, led investigators to search for methods to enhance surface-active material production or secretion. Buckingham suggested that earlier work showing selective maturation of the fetal liver by steroids might be applicable to the developing pulmonary system.[8] While performing experiments on the role of glucocorticoids in the initiation of parturition, Liggins observed an increased survival rate of immature fetal lambs delivered after maternal steroid injection.[9] This result was unexpected, since others had observed uniformly fatal RDS because of lack of surface-active material in lambs delivered before 130 days of gestation. Liggins postulated that the glucocorticoids caused premature enzyme induction and early surfactant biosynthesis with subsequent release into the fetal lung. Confirmation of accelerated pulmonary maturity was produced by DeLemos, who infused one of twin premature lamb fetuses with hydrocortisone.[10] When the lungs were compared with those in a control group, pulmonary maturity, as indicated by reduction of surface tension, was shown to be enhanced in the treated group. Additional data from several animal species treated with corticosteroids indicated that fetuses exposed to corticosteroids were viable earlier in gestation and had increased lecithin production in the lung when compared with controls.[11-14]

The mechanism and site of action of these steroids were demonstrated by Giannopoulos and colleagues, who defined specific lung receptor sites as well as competitive binding by a variety of steroid compounds.[15] Moreover, they indicated that nuclear incorporation of cortisone increased markedly in the last trimester, implying a physiologic role for endogenous fetal cortisol in normal lung development. This work was substantiated by the Ballards, who showed that fetal rabbit lung tissue, in contrast to other organs studied, bound tritiated dexamethasone with greater affinity and had 40 to 80 per cent more abundant cortisol receptors.[16]

Observations that humans follow similar patterns with regard to premature development of lecithin production by steroids is provided by several sources. Naeye and his associates, in an autopsy study of 387 neonates, found that the adrenal glands were of lower weight in infants dying of HMD than those dying of other disorders.[17] Furthermore, the lungs of anencephalic neonates had 45 per cent fewer intracellular inclusion bodies in the pulmonary alveolar Type II cells than did the lungs of normocephalic newborns. Finally, they showed that intrauterine bacterial infection was associated with an increased adrenal weight and a decreased incidence of RDS. Other investigators have shown that a prolonged interval after rupture of the fetal membranes results in higher blood levels of glucocorticoid after birth and a decreased incidence of RDS.[18]

Liggins and Howie, giving bethamethasone to women in preterm labor, tested whether exogenous steroids were clinically effective in preventing RDS.[19] Twelve per cent of the infants treated prior to 32 weeks of gestation developed RDS compared with 70 per cent of the infants receiving placebo. Other series also showed a decrease in incidence of RDS and an increase in neonatal survival when steroids were given as opposed to placebo.[20–25] In a greatly expanded study, Liggins reported similar results in 1976.[26] In each of these studies, the incidence of RDS was significantly reduced in those fetuses under 32 weeks of gestation. Moreover, in all the studies, the greatest benefit seemed to be derived over 24 hours after initial treatment with steroids. The recently reported collaborative study showed the positive effect of antenatal dexamethasone administration on the prevention of RDS to be mainly attributable to the effect on singleton female infants.[22] Although several different agents were used in these various investigations, in each, amelioration of RDS was obtained if the infant was less than 32 weeks of gestation and the mother was treated with steroids for more than 24 hours. These findings are consistent with Solomon's concept that the steroid receptor in the fetal Type II alveolar cell should recognize any corticosteroid.[27] Such recognition reflects receptor-steroid binding at that part of the steroid molecule common to all of the corticosteroids utilized.

Baden and co-workers have shown that the administration of corticosteroids to newborn infants with RDS had no benefit,[28] and therefore its use after birth is not recommended.

Questions on Steroid Action

Although in human studies no pattern of adverse effect of the steroid on the mother or developing fetus is reported, a number of questions remain unanswered. Since many of the treated patients had otherwise uncomplicated preterm labor, experience with one or more additional disease processes in most series is quite small—thus, the risk-to-benefit ratio in these patients cannot be stated. The effect of the steroid on fetal amniotic fluid tests of lung maturation is not well defined, yet an accurate gauge of fetal maturity is often needed prior to delivery, particularly in certain maternal-fetal disease states associated with intrauterine growth retardation (IUGR). Morrison and Zuspan have shown that hydrocortisone increases the L/S ratio, although further work must be done.[29, 30] Endocrinologic studies to assess influences of the compound on the placental-fetal unit and short-term or long-term risk, if any, to the mother as well as the infant are required. These questions should necessarily be answered before the use of steroids to prevent RDS can be endorsed without qualification.

Because the mode of administration, vehicle, dosage and route of administration has often varied, it is difficult to determine which steroid is best in a given situation and how it should be used. Hydrocortisone, dexamethasone, betamethasone and fluorinated compounds have all been used, as have other corticosteroid analogs, in combination with various preparation vehicles. The lowest effective dose of any of these compounds has yet to be established, since each investigator continues to use the amount that has been effective in the past. At the present time, there are no controlled (or uncontrolled) studies comparing various dosages, routes of administration or preparations of corticosteroids with the exception of a recent work with animals. In this study it was observed that perhaps larger doses than those currently used might be more effective. In contrast, if excess hydrocortisone was given, the entire beneficial effect could be lost. Much more investigation is needed in this area. Betamethasone 12 mg per 24 hours for 2 intramuscular doses has been widely used. Hydrocortisone given intravenously has been used in dosages of 250 to 500 mg every 12 hours for 4 doses. Most of the newer studies report the use of dexamethasone in dosages of 5 to 8 mg every 12 hours intramuscularly for a total of 4 doses. A 5-mg dose of dexamethasone was used in a large collaborative study in this country supported by the National Heart, Lung and Blood Institute.[22] From the current data, although there is confusion, it appears that all the compounds are effective in any of the dosages used.

The effect of the steroids on fetal lung maturity assessments remains controversial. Liggins states that there was no effect on the lecithin/sphingomyelin (L/S) ratio measured after betamethasone therapy. However, Spellacy et al.[32] as well as Caspi et al.[20] have shown increases with dexamethasone; whereas Kennedy,[23] Morrison et al.[29] and Zuspan[30] have shown increases in the L/S ratio after hydrocortisone therapy. It would appear, as shown in Table 1, that most investigators agree that the L/S ratio is changed after therapy with corticosteroids. This change would be reasonable as shown by the previously cited concept of Solomon.[27] It would follow that if the receptor recognizes the steroid, increases the synthesis of lecithin and then extrudes the compound into the saccules of the lung, this should appear in the tracheal effluent. Indeed, Morrison et al. showed that the L/S ratio may begin to change in as few as 24 to 36 hours after treatment.[25] Although the L/S ratio did not consistently change during this time, the lecithin may indeed have been secreted into the alveoli of the fetal lung and simply had not made its way in sufficient quantity into the amniotic fluid. Since this study was conducted on a small number of patients and many of the patients were "stressed" by maternal-fetal disease, confirmation must be awaited. Also, it has recently been demonstrated that male infants are not as well stimulated as females with regard to the L/S ratio.[22] Further, it is not known if the L/S ratio reverts to its pretreatment levels after a period of time has elapsed and delivery has not occurred. There is some suggestion that this happens 7 to 10 days after treatment, as evidenced by Liggins' data[26] as well as Morrison's[25] study, which showed a decrease in the L/S ratio in those patients having amniocentesis after treatment on a weekly basis shortly before delivery.

While the controversy regarding steroid influence on L/S ratio remains unsettled, it is of the utmost importance, since it has direct bearing on obstetric practice. If the obstetrician is delaying delivery in a patient in preterm labor, the delivery could be effected once the steroids had matured the L/S ratio. The time at which the L/S ratio matures is not clear, however.

The effect of steroids on the endocrinologic system of the mother and fetus has been more thoroughly studied. Whitt gave bethamethasone to mothers who were in preterm labor (induced or spontaneous).[30] Other investigators have also studied the effects of steroids on the fetal-placental unit.[31, 32] It appears that maternal ACTH and cortisol are decreased. This decrease has been shown not to be deleterious to the mother. Moreover, Migeon et al. have shown by radioactive studies that the corticosteroid compounds cross the placenta and concentrate in the cord blood at between 20 and 50 per cent of the levels found in maternal plasma.[37] The infant shows no discernible adverse effect from the exogenous steroid but, as expected, the endogenous production of cortisol is suppressed until the infant's adrenal gland recovers.[35-37] Moreover, metabolites of the maternal-placental-fetal unit, such as estriol, are depressed. Liggins is presently conducting a trial to determine whether the simultaneous administration of dehydroepiandrosterone to the mother will prevent alterations in steroid production.[38]

In summary, the following conclusions seem warranted: (1) the etiology of RDS with HMD involves a deficiency of surface-active material, principally lecithin; (2) lecithin production increases as the fetus matures, and this increase in lecithin appears to be mediated by endogenous produced fetal corticosteroids; (3) lung maturity owing to premature production of lecithin may be produced by the action of exogenously administered corticosteroids on receptors in the fetal lungs; (4) the presence of such steroid receptors suggests that the effect is caused by a primary action rather than a secondary event triggered by the steroid; and (5) the "best" steroid, its appropriate dosage and its acute effect on amniotic fluid surfactant components have not been adequately defined.

TABLE 1. EFFECT OF MATERNAL STEROID ON L/S RATIO

PRINCIPAL INVESTIGATOR	REFERENCE	DRUG	EFFECT ON L/S RATIO
Spellacy	Am J Obstet Gynecol 115:216, 1973	Dexamethasone	Increased
Caspi	Am J Obstet Gynecol 122:327, 1975	Dexamethasone	Increased
Fargier	Nouv. Presse Med 22:1595, 1975	Dexamethasone	Increased
Kennedy	Pediatr Res 8:447, 1974	Hydrocortisone	Increased
Morrison	Am J Obstet Gynecol 131:4, 358–366, 1978	Hydrocortisone	Increased
Lefebvre	Am J Obstet Gynecol 125:5, 609–612, 1976	Hydrocortisone	Increased
Zuspan	Am J Obstet Gynecol 128:5 571–574, 1977	Hydrocortisone	Increased
Ekelund	Acta Obstet Gynecol. Scand 55:413, 1976	Betamethasone	Increased
Liggins	70th Ross Conference on Pediatric Research 97–105, 1976	Betamethasone	Unchanged
Cartis	Am J Obstet Gynecol 127:5, 529–532, 1977	Betamethasone	Unchanged

For Steroid Administration

We believe that the data currently available supports the use of corticosteroids to facilitate adequate surfactant production by the preterm fetal lung. Appropriate patient selection is a requirement, and commitment to long-term follow-up of the infant is essential. However, the significant decrease in occurrence or severity of RDS with HMD when steroid is administered must be weighed against the hazards of steroid use to the mother or fetus or to the newborn.

Against Steroid Administration

The most difficult problem to solve is the physiologic or pathophysiologic long-term effect of the glucocorticosteroids on the mother or infant or both. One may reasonably assume that if contraindications to steroid administration in the mother are excluded (Table 2) there should be little maternal risk in taking small amounts of steroids for a short period of time. Certainly adults take steroids in much

TABLE 2. MATERNAL CONTRAINDICATIONS TO STEROID USE

ABSOLUTE
  Keratitis: viral
  Peptic ulcer disease: active within past 6 months
  Active tuberculosis

RELATIVE
  Inactive tuberculosis, still on suppressive therapy
  Previous history peptic ulcer disease (>6 months prior)
  Acute systemic infection

larger dosages and for much longer periods of time without developing any sequelae of steroid toxicity. Moreover, patients ingesting moderate amounts of steroids for prolonged periods of time (if they do not develop toxicity) have been seen not to have any permanent damage.

The hazards or complications of this prenatal treatment for the infant, however, is a much more complex issue. Steroids are widely used in the management of many diseases during pregnancy, but double-blind studies have not been performed to determine the effects of such therapy on the fetus and the neonate. First, there have been reports of teratologic effects, including cleft palate and resorption of the fetus in hamsters, mice and sheep.[39-41] All of these effects occurred with large doses administered early in the gestation. In humans, infants born to cushingoid mothers (secondary to high doses of glucocorticoids) have developed normally and reports of women with other diseases taking steroids in high doses usually do not show severe fetal teratologic effects.[42, 43] On the other hand, untreated Cushing's disease has a markedly high perinatal mortality rate in pregnancy.

The effects of steroids on the growth of the fetus and newborn have been well studied by Schlesinger,[44] who demonstrated runting in neonatal mice exposed to cortisol. The etiologic mechanisms that have been proposed for growth retardation related to steroids are inhibition of growth hormone releasing factor, infection, increased utilization of essential amino acids, interference with cartilage differentiation and direct effect on cell mitosis.[45] However, it would appear that growth retardation related to steroids appears to occur directly at the peripheral tissue level and not centrally.[46] Worrisome are studies in rabbits by Kotas,[47] which showed that decrease in cell size, number and DNA content occurred first and was most pronounced in those organs responsive to corticosteroid differentiation. He thought that this change, however, was reversible. Studies also showed that the brain (which contains corticosteroid receptors) was affected in animals given steroids.[44] This should cause great concern to those recommending the use of steroids for maturation of the fetal lungs. In animal studies the brain weight was decreased, lower ratios of cholesterol to DNA were found and clinical associations were made between these findings and decreased performance of fine motor control and purposeful activity, which persisted into adulthood.[45-49] More disconcerting is the work of Beck et al.,[50] who with similar dosages as used in the animal studies showed many abnormal fetal effects in rhesus monkeys. Therefore, there is increasing concern about the safety of steroids for newborn infants when administered to the mother.

No human studies, controlled or otherwise, have substantiated these findings in primates. There is genuine concern, however, that the premature maturation by steroids of the liver, gut and lung would include premature growth and function of the glial cells in the fetal cerebrum. Since the glial cells do not regenerate, this early somatic maturity might lead to reduction in cerebral growth potential, as noted in animals. Serious but subtle neurologic effects could occur, and although this has not been observed in humans, no sensitive neurologic assessment has been done in infants of mothers who have ingested corticosteroids. Additionally, there is the report of Liggins' earlier study[19] and the work by Taeusch[51] that perinatal intraventricular hemorrhage, particularly in hypertensive patients, might be associated with steroid administration. This relationship, however, was not borne out in Liggins' later study[26] and was not noted in other studies.[20, 25, 52]

As indicated by the data of Schlesinger,[44] the runting syndrome caused by steroids results from the effects of the steroid on the thymus and spleen. The immunologic consequences of this type of therapy in animals have been previously described by Howard[53] and resulted in impairment of the immunologic response that persisted in adulthood. This would suggest that while steroids mature some organs, they cause retarded development in others; therefore, the immaturity of the animal

at birth from the "medical thymectomy" may be the deciding factor in determining permanency of the immunologic deficit. This is particularly true because most of the animals were premature and were immunologically deficient at least at physiological levels. Hence the effect of the steroids appeared to be additive. In humans, the major maturation of immune responses obtainable in a term infant takes place *after* 26 weeks of gestation—a time when steroids would be used.

Other possible risks of prenatal administration of the corticosteroids include neonatal adrenal cortical insufficiency, hypoglycemia and hypocalcemia.[54] Experimental work also suggests that the placenta undergoes morphologic changes that resemble premature aging of this organ when exposed to corticosteroids, at least in high doses. The placenta may be affected by a syndrome of placental insufficiency presenting as IUGR or as a hypoxic acidotic episode during labor or both.

It must be remembered that the most damaging evidence of adverse effects on the neonate from prenatal maternal corticosteroid administration has been developed from animal experiments and has not been demonstrated in humans. Moreover, any teratologic effect of the steroid should not be a factor since it is given after embryogenesis. The dosage and length of time of steroid administration to promote human fetal lung maturity and to control maternal disease are much less when compared with the experimental models. Acute and chronic physiologic drug effects, however, are not directly corroborative.

Clinical Issues

The main problem in appropriate patient selection for steroid use relates to the vagaries in assessing fetal maturity and defining preterm labor. Table 3 lists the available assessors of fetal maturity. None of these consistently predicts maturity. While it can be said that a fetus at 37 weeks or more of gestational age in a normal pregnancy is at almost no risk of developing RDS, the incidence of iatrogenic RDS at greater than 10 per cent speaks to the limitation of clinical fetal maturity assessments. Furthermore, ultrasonograms need to be performed serially to be particularly helpful, and they are most difficult to use when the issue is IUGR versus prematurity. Estriols are generally unreliable in this situation.

TABLE 3. FETAL MATURITY ASSESSORS

TEST	DETERMINANT	PREDICTIVE OF WEEKS' GESTATION	USEFUL < 34 WEEKS' GESTATION	PREDICTIVE OF LUNG MATURITY
Menstrual history	Regular in quantity, duration and interval prior to pregnancy; LMP *not* related to oral contraceptive use	Yes, *if* accurate	Yes, *if* accurate	No
Uterine size	Exam 14–18 weeks and repeat on admission compatible with date	Yes, if subsequent growth between exams correlates	Yes, if subsequent growth between exams correlates	No
Fetal heart tones	Unaided FHT heard in mid trimester and projected 18 weeks forward	Yes, if FHT heard at 18–22 weeks	No	No
Quickening	Fetal movements perceived by patient	No	No	No
Estimated fetal weight	Naegele's rule or clinical estimate	No	No	No.
X-rays	Distal femoral or proximal epiphyses	No	No	No.
Estriol determination	Significant estriol production begins at 26–30 weeks' gestation	No	No	No
Serial ultrasound (USG)	Growth adjusted sonographic age	Yes, if USG done at 18–20 weeks and repeated at 28–32 weeks	Yes, if USG done at 18–20 weeks and repeated at 28–32 weeks	No
Single USG	Biparietal diameter	Yes, if BPD > 8.7 cm with normal BPD-thoracic diameter ratio	Yes, if BPD > 8.7 cm with normal BPD-thoracic diameter ratio	No
Amniotic fluid assessors				
Bilirubin	Absent at 450 mμ	No, too many false positives	No	No
Creatinine	> 2.0 mg/dl	Yes, if fetal somatic growth normal	No	Not directly
Fat staining cells (FSC)	> 10% positive FSC = 37 weeks' gestation	Yes, if correct procedure used	No	Not directly
Optical density	Variable	Yes, but new technique (unsubstantiated)	No	Not directly
Micro-viscosity	Variable	Yes, but new technique (unsubstantiated)	No	Not directly
Shake test	Stable meniscus of bubbles	Yes, but caution in fetomaternal disease	No	Yes
L/S ratio	≥ 2.0	Yes, but caution in fetomaternal disease	Yes	Yes
Lung profile	Phosphatidylglycerol present	Yes, but caution in fetomaternal disease	Yes	Yes
Disaturated lecithin	≥ 60%	Yes, but caution in fetomaternal disease	Yes	Yes
Foam stability index	≥ 0.47	Yes, but caution in fetomaternal disease	Yes	Yes

Only the bubble stability,[55] the L/S ratio and, when appropriate, the lung profile[56] and the percentage of disaturated lecithin[56] provide essential information on fetal lung maturity. Although false-positive results are rare, false-negative ones—that is, adequate lung maturity associated with a test result suggesting lung immaturity—are common with the bubble stability and the L/S ratio assessments. While the presence of phosphatidylglycerol (PG) essentially negates any risk of RDS,[57] this acidic phospholipid is not predominant until 35 weeks' gestation or later, a time when steroid administration is not a useful clinical approach.[26] The recently described foam stability index (FSI) test may prove to be the assessment of choice for the determination of fetal lung maturity, particularly when IUGR is suspected.[58]

A few of the clinical assessments are helpful in assuring that a pregnancy has advanced 34 weeks or more—a time when steroid administration is no longer recommended. Early, careful uterine sizing, which at 14 to 18 weeks into pregnancy reveals a normal uterine configuration compatible with gestational dating by history and associated with subsequent normal uterine growth (Fig. 1), is reliable within a range of approximately 2 weeks in the last trimester. Thus if uterine size as defined herein is compatible with 36 weeks' gestation, the woman is not a candidate for steroid administration. If the date the fetal heart is first detected by fetoscope (not Doppler) is projected 18 weeks forward, the date obtained assures at least a gestational age of 34 weeks. We advocate listening for the fetal heart weekly starting at 16 weeks' gestation by uterine size. This procedure is at least as reliable as dating a pregnancy as equal to or more than 34 weeks' gestation on the basis of a single last trimester ultrasonogram; it is less costly than ultrasonography, amniocentesis or amniotic fluid assessments and is noninvasive. An ultrasonogram showing a normal ratio of the biparietal and thoracic diameters and a biparietal diameter exceeding 8.7 cm is predictive of a pregnancy of at least 34 weeks, again precluding use of exogenous steroid at this time, but not excluding attempts to stop preterm labor, if appropriate. None of the other assessments in Table 3 (except L/S ratios and perhaps the FSI) are discriminating at 34 weeks' gestation. In summary, early gestation (at less than or equal to 16 weeks) and continuous confirmation of appropriate for gestational age growth of the uterus, attainment of

the date after first detection of the fetal heart (fetoscope) plus 18 weeks, and/or a single ultrasonogram showing a biparietal diameter more than 8.7 cm with a normal biparietal/thoracic diameter ratio almost always assure attainment of at least 34 weeks. These three assessments then can be used to exclude the use of exogenous steroids but *not* to assure lung maturity.

A most difficult problem facing the obstetrician treating the patient between 26 and 34 weeks of gestation is whether the pregnancy is complicated by prematurity or by intrauterine growth retardation (IUGR). At this time of rapid fetal somatic growth, none of the tests are useful as a single assessment of fetal maturity except those evaluating fetal lung maturation. Unfortunately, these tests, while having a few false-positive indicators, commonly produce a negative (many of which are false-negative) or a "transitional" result, which may or may not be associated subsequently with RDS. Finally, it must be noted that steroids administered to the mother influence surfactant in the neonate's lung; they do not prevent other life-threatening risks of prematurity and they do not assure the availability of appropriate personnel and services necessary for neonatal intensive care. If the obstetrician's concern is one of delivery of an infant under 33 weeks' gestation in the 24 to 72 hours after initiation of a steroid, he must deliver the infant in a facility where required expertise for neonatal intensive care is at hand.

Recommendations On Steroid Administration

Essential to any scheme for administration of steroids to influence fetal lung maturity are the following considerations that the clinician must recognize and appropriately weigh:

1. Premature delivery is to be avoided, *not* permissively endorsed, because of the availability of steroids; a premature newborn with mature lungs may still have formidable problems related to prematurity.

2. The animal data cited earlier, particularly those related to neurologic development, preclude casual, indiscriminate use of steroids.

3. Several maternal-fetal conditions alter the rate of fetal lung maturation.

4. The sex of the fetus may influence the effectiveness of antenatal steroids.

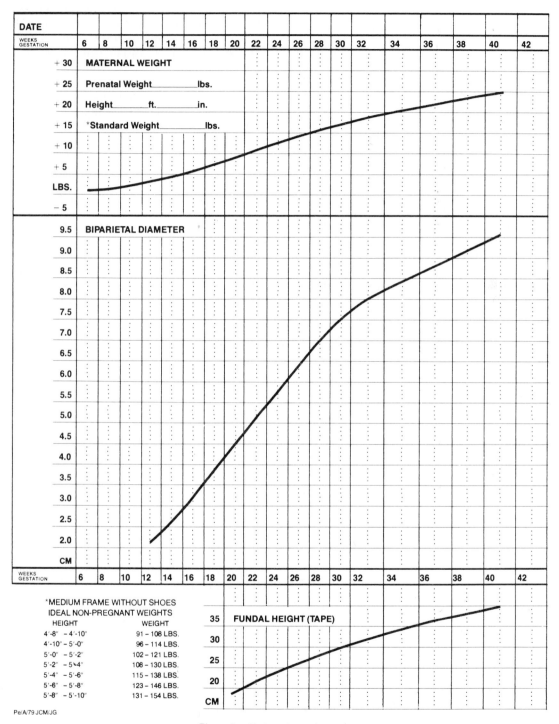

DATE																			
WEEKS GESTATION	6	8	10	12	14	16	18	20	22	24	26	28	30	32	34	36	38	40	42

MATERNAL WEIGHT (+30 to −5 LBS.)

Prenatal Weight_____lbs.

Height_____ft._____in.

*Standard Weight_____lbs.

BIPARIETAL DIAMETER (9.5 to CM)

*MEDIUM FRAME WITHOUT SHOES
IDEAL NON-PREGNANT WEIGHTS

HEIGHT	WEIGHT
4'-8" – 4'-10"	91 – 108 LBS.
4'-10" – 5'-0"	96 – 114 LBS.
5'-0" – 5'-2"	102 – 121 LBS.
5'-2" – 5'-4"	108 – 130 LBS.
5'-4" – 5'-6"	115 – 138 LBS.
5'-6" – 5'-8"	123 – 146 LBS.
5'-8" – 5'-10"	131 – 154 LBS.

FUNDAL HEIGHT (TAPE) (35 to CM)

Pe/A/79 JCM/JG

Figure 1. Perinatal graphics chart.

5. The only assessments of fetal maturity useful at 26 to 34 weeks of gestational age are accurate gauges of surfactant in the amniotic fluid.

6. Informed consent should be acquired before administration of steroids, since the potential risks and hazards of these drugs are not adequately defined.

7. Mothers receiving steroids should be supportive of the need for long-term evaluation of the child by both neurologic as well as behavioral assessment tools. (Prospective approaches to case finding are more successful and far less expensive than retrospective methods.)

The usual situation the clinician faces involves differentiating gestational maturity (prematurity as opposed to intrauterine growth retardation in the fetus), the presence or absence of labor and the presence or absence of ruptured membranes. Figure 2 outlines our approach to these determinants as

they affect the decision to administer steroids to the mother. We believe that an assessment of amniotic fluid surfactant should be performed before the administration of steroids until future studies show that the steroid does not have an adverse long-term effect for the child. Approximately 25 per cent of our patients screened for administration of steroids are excluded on the single criterion of an L/S ratio greater than or equal to 1.8, even though assessment of gestational age greater than 34 weeks' fetal size, uterine measurement and biparietal diameter measurement by ultrasonography are compatible with prematurity rather than the intrauterine growth retardation that pertains.[52]

Patients should be repeatedly advised that premature rupture of membranes constitutes an emergency for which prompt evaluation is necessary. Labor should not be awaited at home. Early diagnosis of prolapsed cord and not allowing labor to advance beyond the stage that would preclude appropriate operative in-

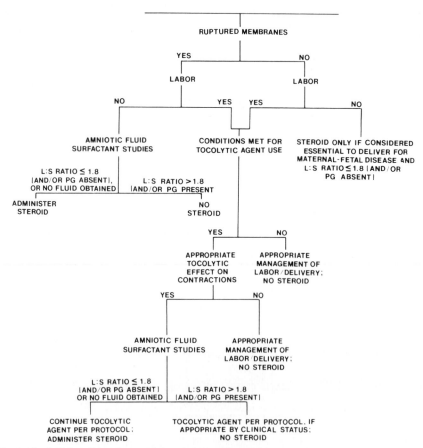

Figure 2. Prenatal administration of steroid (weeks' gestation unknown or considered less than or equal to 34 weeks). L/S ratio by the modification by Morrison et al.[63] of Gluck's technique.

tervention or the use of tocolytic agents are obvious advantages. Early evaluation of amniotic fluid for surfactant determination can be done on the fluid pooled within the vagina. Ultrasonography and amniocentesis with attendant delay in initiation of therapy are thereby avoided. With regard to L/S ratio determinations, this fluid, if free-flowing, is representative of intraamniotic fluid.[59] It is important to note that only a sterile speculum examination is performed with avoidance of pelvic manipulation, which could introduce infection. In those cases in which fluid cannot be obtained vaginally, amniocentesis directed with real-time ultrasonography should be performed. Even when little fluid accumulation is expected after membrane rupture, small pockets sufficient for amniocentesis may be identified by ultrasonography.

The diagnosis of preterm labor poses a major dilemma. Patients who note a change in the character (frequency, duration or severity) of uterine contractile activity should come to the hospital. The assumption, without personal assessment, that the patient is not in labor because it is "too early" is no longer tenable; in preterm labor, drugs are available to suppress uterine contractions. Because many patients will report that the contractions were "stronger" or "closer" when at home, the patient should be observed for an adequate period of time (2 to 3 hours) in the hospital before being sent home with a diagnosis of "false premature labor." This may prevent the patient's returning in advanced labor some hours later. We commonly employ an external fetal heart rate monitor and a tocodynanometer, not because the machine can better assess contractions than the patient or the nurse or both, but because many of our patients are at risk for abruptio placentae and we are also seeking evidence of fetal distress.

With initial evidence of changes in cervical effacement or dilatation, progressive effacement or dilatation of the cervix or both during observation, or increasing frequency or strength of contractions into a regular pattern (generally of 2 or more contractions in any 15-minute period), a tocolytic agent is begun to suppress uterine activity. We now use ritodrine or magnesium sulfate or both for this purpose. Amniocentesis is usually performed only after the effect of the tocolytic agent is assessed (usually in 1.5 to 2 hours) to avoid delay in starting of the tocolytic agent, aggravation of uterine contractility and, perhaps most importantly, an unnecessary risk if labor cannot be abated. Suprapubic amniocentesis following elevation of the presenting part is advised if ultrasonography is not immediately available. Indications for use of a tocolytic agent are outlined in Table 4.

We do not believe that rupture of the membranes (without evidence of fetal or maternal infection) precludes use of either a tocolytic agent or a steroid. At 28 to 33 weeks' gestation, the risk of serious neonatal infection at 48 hours after rupture of the membranes is far exceeded by the possibility of RDS. Liggins[26] and Miller et al.[60] did not record an increased risk of neonatal infection in the steroid-treated group. Further, many of the newborns with severe infection following ruptured membranes are probably infected at or soon after rupture.

Many have emphasized the factors accelerating or delaying lung maturity.[51] While most authors agree that hypertensive disorders, use of heroin, certain hemoglobinopathies, diabetes with vascular involvement and use of such drugs as isoxsuprine and steroids accelerate lung maturation, there is much controversy regarding the influence of ruptured membranes and classes A, B and C (White) diabetes. Do ruptured membranes produce acceleration of lung maturity after 48 hours? Do these classes of diabetes produce delay of fetal lung maturation? A prospective study is required to adequately resolve both issues. Recent studies by Curet et al,[61] Gabbe et al.,[62] and Morrison[29] may explain the difference of opinion in the literature regarding diabetes. Indeed, it is not our experience that patients with class B and class C diabetes benefiting

TABLE 4. INDICATIONS FOR TOCOLYTIC SUPPRESSION OF LABOR

1. Absence of fetal maturity with a live fetus (stop labor, then investigate if there is any question regarding fetal maturity).
2. Absence of maternal or fetal conditions precluding continuation of pregnancy.
3. Absence of the maternal conditions of severe hypertension, severe preeclampsia, moderate-to-marked blood loss, intrauterine infection, or sepsis.
4. Cervical dilatation of 4 cm or less.
5. Intact amniotic membranes *unless* afebrile, fetal heart rate <180 beats per minute and trial of lung maturation is to be done (steroids and/or 48–72 hour period before delivery).
6. Availability of personnel and equipment necessary to assess mother.
7. Availability of personnel and equipment necessary to assess fetus, including fetal lung maturity assessment.
8. Availability of rapid blood typing and cross-match if needed.

from long-term as well as intrapartum blood glucose–insulin homeostasis need be managed differently with regard to the L/S ratio. As preterm intervention in the patient with well-controlled class A diabetes is not appropriate, RDS in the newborns of this group of patients should be a moot consideration except when tocolytic management of preterm labor is contemplated.

In the past three years, we have used a study protocol incorporating dexamethasone, but experience already cited, including our own work,[25] suggests that choice of steroid and efficacy of RDS amelioration are not the prime considerations. Safety is the unresolved issue.

Conclusions

Investigations relating prenatal corticosteroid therapy to a decreased incidence and severity of RDS with HMD in premature infants offer exciting promise in reducing the leading cause of mortality for these newborns. However, until questions related particularly to long-term infant sequelae are definitely answered, we recommend that the drugs be used under thoroughly controlled conditions. The data presently being collected in a large collaborative study by the National Heart, Lung and Blood Institute may answer questions regarding short-term and long-term risks attendant to steroid use.[22]

Many investigators, because of the positive relationship of steroid therapy and decreased incidence of RDS, would argue that the use of steroids is justified and no further study is required. However, medical history is replete with examples of agents that were not prospectively evaluated with subsequent tragic consequences. Certainly, diethylstilbestrol and neonatal ocular oxygen toxicity might not have engendered as much controversy had a large prospective double-blind study been undertaken to define risk-to-benefit factors before general use was advocated. Much animal data suggest growth and development risk to the progeny of mothers receiving steroids. It must be noted that the effects of diethylstilbestrol were documented in animal studies in the early 1940s.

REFERENCES

1. Pattle, R. E.: Properties, function and origin of the alveolar lining layer. Nature 175:1125, 1955.
2. Pattle, R. E.: Properties, function and origin of the alveolar lining layer. Proc. R. Soc. Lond. (Biol.) 148:217, 1958.
3. Gribetz, I., Frank, N. R. and Avery, M. E.: Static volume pressure relations of excised lungs of infants with hyaline membrane disease. Newborn and stillborn infants. J. Clin. Invest. 38:2168, 1959.
4. Gluck, L., Kulovich, M. V., Borer, R. C., Brenner, P. H., Anderson, G. G. and Spellacy, W. N.: The diagnosis of respiratory distress syndrome (RDS) by amniocentesis. Am. J. Obstet. Gynecol. 109:440, 1971.
5. Gluck, L., Kulovitch, M. V., Eidelman, A. I., Cordero, L. and Khazin, A. F.: Biochemical development of surface activity in mammalian lung IV. Pulmonary lecithin synthesis in the human fetus and newborn and etiology of the respiratory distress syndrome. Pediatr. Res. 6:81, 1972.
6. Gluck, L., Stribney, M. and Kulovich, M. V.: The biochemical development of surface activity in mammalian lung. II. The biosynthesis of phospholipids in the lung of the developing rabbit fetus and newborn. Pediatr. Res. 1:247, 1967.
7. Gluck, L., Landowne, R. A. and Kulovich, M. V.: Biochemical development in lung lecithin during development of rabbit fetus and newborn. Pediatr. Res. 4:352, 1970.
8. Buckingham, S., McNary, W. F., Sommers, S. C. and Rothschild, J.: Fed. Proc. 27:328, 1968.
9. Liggins, G.: Premature delivery of fetal lambs infused with glucocorticoids. J. Endocrinol. 45:515, 1969.
10. DeLemos, R., Shermata, D., Knelson, J., Kotas, R. and Avery, M. E.: Acceleration of appearance of pulmonary surfactant in the fetal lamb by administration of corticosteroids. Am. Rev. Resp. Dis. 102:459, 1970.
11. Platzker, A., Kitterman, J., Clements, J. et al: Surfactant appearance and secretion in fetal lamb lungs in response to dexamethasone. Pediatr. Res. 6:406, 1972.
12. Kotas, R. and Avery, M. E.: Accelerated appearance of pulmonary surfactant in the fetal rabbit. J. Appl. Physiol. 30:359, 1971.
13. Kotas, R. V., Fletcher, B. D., Avery, M. E. and Torday, J.: Evidence for independent regulators of organ maturation in fetal rabbits. Pediatrics 47:57, 1971.
14. Taeusch, H. W., Heitner, M. and Avery, M. E.: Accelerated lung maturation and increased survival in premature rabbits treated with hydrocortisone. Am. Res. Resp. Dis. 105:971, 1972.
15. Giannopoulos, G., Mulay, S. and Solomon, S.: Cortisol receptors in rabbit fetal lung. Biochem. Biophys. Res. Commun. 47:411–418, 1972.
16. Ballard, P. L. and Ballard, R. A.: Glucocorticoid receptors and the role of glucocorticoids in fetal lung development. Proc. Natl. Acad. Sci. 69:2668, 1972.
17. Naeye, R. L., Hartke, H. T., Jr. and Blanc, W. A.: Adrenal gland structure and the development of hyaline membrane disease. Pediatrics 47:650, 1971.
18. Bauer, C. R., Stern, L. and Colle, R.: Prolonged rupture of membranes associated with a decreased incidence of respiratory distress syndrome. Pediatrics 53:7, 1974.
19. Liggins, G. C. and Howie, R. N.: A controlled trial of antepartum glucocorticoid treatment for prevention of the respiratory distress syndrome in premature infants. Pediatrics 50:515, 1972.
20. Caspi, E., Schreyer, P., Weinraub, Z., Reif, R., Levi, I. and Mandel, G.: The prevention of the

respiration distress syndrome in premature infants by antepartum glucocorticoid therapy. Br. J. Obstet. Gynecol. 83:187–193, 1976.

21. Young, B. K., Klein, S. A., Katz, M., Wilson, S. J. and Douglas, G. W.: Intravenous dexamethasone for prevention of neonatal respiratory distress: A prospective controlled study. Am. J. Obstet. Gynecol. 138:203–209, 1980.

22. Collaborative Group on Antenatal Steroid Therapy: Effect of antenatal dexamethasone administration on the prevention of respiratory distress syndrome. Am. J. Obstet. Gynecol. 141:276–287, 1981.

23. Kennedy, J. L.: Antepartum betamethasone in preventing respiratory distress syndrome. Pediatr. Res. 8:447, 1974.

24. Caspi, E., Schreyer, P., Weinraub, Z., Lifshitz, Y. and Goldberg, M.: Dexamethasone for prevention of respiratory distress syndrome: Multiple perinatal factors. Obstet. Gyncol. 57:41–47, 1981.

25. Morrison, J. C., Whybrew, W. D., Bucovaz, E. T. and Schneider, J. M.: Infection of corticosteroids into the mother to prevent neonatal respiratory distress syndrome. Am. J. Obstet. Gynecol. 131:358–366, 1978.

26. Liggins, G. C.: Prenatal glucocorticoid treatment: prevention of respiratory distress syndrome. 70th Conference on Pediatric Research. Columbus, Ross Laboratories, 1976.

27. Solomon, S. A.: Personal Communication.

28. Baden, M., Bauer, C. R., Colle, E., Klein, G., Papageorgiou, A. and Stern, L.: Plasma corticosteroids in infants with respiratory distress syndrome. Pediatrics 52:782, 1973.

29. Morrison, J. C., Schneider, J. M., Whybrew, W. D. and Bucovaz, E. T.: Effect of corticosteroids and fetomaternal disorder on the L:S ratio. Obstet. Gynecol. 56:583–590, 1980.

30. Zuspan, F. P., Cordero, L. and Semchyshyn, S.: Effects of hydrocortisone on lecithin-sphingomyelin ratio. Am. J. Obstet. Gynecol. 128:571, 1977.

31. Morrison, J. C.: Which corticosteroid should I use? Unpublished abstract, May, 1981.

32. Spellacy, W. N., Buhi, W. C., Riggall, F. C. and Holsinger, K. L.: Human amniotic fluid lecithin/sphingomyelin ratio changes with estrogen or glucocorticoid treatment. Am. J. Obstet. Gynecol. 115:216–218, 1973.

33. Ruvinsky, E. D., Morrison, J. C., Farnell, P. M., McKay, M. L.: Changes in the amniotic fluid phospholipid content after maternal dexamethasone administration. Meeting of Society of Gynecologic Investigation, March, 1981.

34. Whitt, G. G., Buster, J. E., Killam, A. P. and Scragg, W. H.: A comparison of two glucocorticoid regimens for acceleration of fetal lung maturation in premature labor. Am. J. Obstet. Gynecol. 124:479–482, 1976.

35. Lauritzen, C., Shackleton, C. H. L. and Mitchell, F. L.: The effect of exogenous corticothrophin on steroid excretion in the newborn. Acta Endocrinol. 58:655–663, 1968.

36. Ohrlander, S. A., Gennser, G. M. and Grennert, L.: Impact of betamethasone load given to pregnant women on endocrine balance of fetoplacental unit. Am. J. Obstet. Gynecol. 123:228–236, 1975.

37. Migeon, C. J., Bertrand, J. and Wall, P. E.: Physiological disposition of 4-^{14}C-cortisol during late pregnancy. J. Clin. Invest. 36:1350, 1957.

38. Liggins, G. C. and Howie, R. N.: The prevention of

RDS by maternal steroid therapy. Modern Perinatal Medicine, 422, 1974.

39. Saxen, I.: Effects of hydrocortisone on the development in vitro of the secondary palate in two inbred stains of mice. Arch. Oral Biol. 18:1469, 1973.

40. Chaudhry, A. P. and Shah, R. M.: Estimation of hydrocortisone dose and optimal gestation period for cleft palate induction in golden hamsters. (Abstract) Teratology 8:139–142, 1973.

41. Halliday, R. and Bottle, H. R.: The effects of cortisone acetate on the length of the gestation period and the survival of fetal Scottish blackface lambs. J. Endocrinol. 41:447, 1968.

42. Yackel, D. B., Kempers, R. D. and McConahey, W. M.: Adrenocorticosteroid therapy in pregnancy. Am. J. Obstet. Gynecol. 96:985, 1966.

43. Walsh, S. D. and Clark, F. R.: Pregnancy in patients on long-term corticosteroid therapy. Scot. Med. J. 12:302, 1967.

44. Schlesinger, M. and Mark, R.: Medical thymectomy using HC in newborn rats runting similar to surgical thymectomy. Science 143:965, 1963.

45. Sereni, F.: Effects of steroids. XII International Congress of Pediatrics 1:299, Mexico, 1968.

46. Sereni, F. and Principi, N.: Developmental pharmacology. Ann. Rev. Pharmacol. 8:453, 1968.

47. Kotas, R. V., Mims, L. C. and Hart, L. K.: Reversible inhibition of lung cell number after glucocorticoid injection into fetal rabbits to enhance surfactant appearance. Pediatrics 53:358, 1974.

48. Mosier, H. C., Jr.: Failure of compensating (catch-up) growth in the rat. Pediatr. Res. 5:59, 1971.

49. Howard, E. and Granoff, D.: Increased voluntary running and decreased motor coordination in mice after neonatal corticosteroid implantation. Exp. Neurol. 22:661, 1968.

50. Beck, J. C. Johnson, J. W. C., Mitzner, W., Lee, P. A., London, W. T. and Sly, D. L.: Glucocorticoids, hyperinsulinemia, and fetal lung maturation. Am. J. Obstet. Gynecol. 139:465–470, 1981.

51. Taeusch, H. W., Wang, N. S., Baden, M., Bauer, C. R. and Stern, L.: A controlled trial of hydrocortisone in infants with respiratory distress syndrome. II. Pathology. Pediatrics 52:850, 1973.

52. Nochimson, D. J. and Petrie, R. H.: Glucocorticoid therapy for the induction of pulmonary maturity in severely hypertensive gravid women. Am. J. Obstet. Gynecol. 133:449–451, 1979.

53. Howard, E.: Effects of corticosterone and food restriction on growth and on DNA, RNA and cholesterol content of brain and liver in infant mice. J. Neurochem. 12:181, 1965.

54. Klevit, H. D.: Corticosteroid therapy in the neonatal period. Ped. Clin. N. Am. 17:1003, 1970.

55. Clements, J. A., Platzker, A. C. G., Tierney, D. F. et al.: Assessment of the risk of the respiratory distress syndrome by a rapid test for surfactant in amniotic fluid. N. Engl. J. Med. 286:1077, 1972.

56. Gluck, L.: Evaluating functional fetal maturation. Clin. Obstet. Gynecol. 21:55, 1978.

57. Hallman, M., Feldman, B. H., Kirkpatrick, E. and Gluck, L.: Absence of phosphatidylglycerol (PG) in respiratory distress syndrome in the newborn: Study of the minor surfactant phospholipids in newborns. Pediatr. Res. 11:714, 1977.

58. Sher, G., Statland, B. E. and Knutzen, V. K.: Diagnostic reliability of the lecithin/sphingomyelin ratio assay and the quantitative foam stability index test. J. Reprod. Med. 27:51, 1982.

59. Schneider, J. M., Morrison, J. C., Anderson, G. D. et al.: Prediction of neonatal RDS based on vaginal-amniotic fluid pulmonary maturity studies. In press.

60. Miller, J. M., Brazy, J. E., Gall, S. A., Crenshaw, M. C. and Jelovsek, F. R.: Premature rupture of the membranes: Maternal and neonatal infectious morbidity related to betamethasone and antibiotic therapy. J. Reprod. Med. 25:173, 1980.

61. Curet, L. B., Olsen, R. W., Schneider, J. M., Henderson, P. A. and Zachman, R. D.: Effect of diabetes mellitus on amniotic fluid lecithin/sphingomyelin ratio and respiratory distress syndrome. Am. J. Obstet. Gynecol. 135:10, 1979.

62. Gabbe, S. G., Lowensohn, R. I., Mestman, J. H. et al: Lecithin/sphingomyelin ratio in pregnancies complicated by diabetes mellitus. Am. J. Obstet. Gynecol. 128:757, 1977.

63. Morrison, J. C., Wiser, W. L., Arnold, S. W., Whybrew, W. D., Morrison, D. L. and Fish, S. A.: Modification of the lecithin/sphingomyelin assay for fetal development. 120:1087–1091, 1974.

Antenatal Prevention of Respiratory Distress Syndrome With Maternal Glucocorticoid Administration

A. E. Seeds, M.D.*

University of Cincinnati Medical Center

Neonatal respiratory distress syndrome following premature labor and delivery remains one of the major causes of perinatal mortality and morbidity. Antenatal maternal administration of glucocorticoids has recently become increasingly popular as a means of lowering the incidence of respiratory distress in the premature newborn. This new therapeutic regimen is in large part based on a well-controlled double-blind study by Liggins, wherein a significant reduction in neonatal respiratory distress was reported prior to 34 weeks' gestational age, following the administration of 12 mg of betamethasone to the mother at least 24 hours before delivery.[1]

Additional clinical trials with betamethasone and other glucocorticoids have also indicated significant decreases in neonatal morbidity and mortality from respiratory distress problems following antepartum maternal administration.[2-6] These more recent reports involved small case numbers and most were not well-controlled double-blind studies. Nevertheless, a majority of perinatologists have become convinced that maternal antepartum glucocorticoid administration is effective in reducing the risk of respiratory distress syndrome in the premature newborn, and this procedure has been adopted in many centers throughout the country. Obstetricians in a significant number of equally highly regarded perinatal units are still not routinely using glucocorticoids for this condition because of great concern about potential toxic side effects to the mother (and particularly the newborn) resulting from exposure to such a potent hormonal agent.

Retardation in growth of brain, CNS, lung, kidney and overall growth and development have been reported in animal studies.[7-13] Few, if any, adverse effects have been definitely documented in the human.[1, 3, 7, 14, 15] However, the still relatively limited time span that this therapeutic regimen has been used in human pregnancy makes it impossible to absolutely refute the possibility of damage to the offspring. This, together with the devastating late sequelae discovered following routine clinical use of that potent steroid diethylstilbestrol (DES) in pregnancy, adds weight to the position of some skeptics. They are reluctant to expose the fetus to any potent biologic compound until the risk-to-benefit ratio is clearly established.

Role of Endogenous Corticoids in Fetal Lung Maturity

In further examining this complex therapeutic problem, it is reasonable to review some of the clinical and basic experimental data providing evidence that glucocorticoids in vivo contribute to fetal lung maturation.

Several lines of evidence indicate that en-

---

*Dr. Seeds died May 12, 1980.

dogenous cortisol levels play a significant role in fetal lung maturation in utero.

1. It has been recognized for some time that fetuses exposed to chronic in utero stress experience accelerated pulmonary maturation.[16] The offspring of pregnancies complicated by severe diabetes, hypertension, intrauterine growth retardation, chronic abruption of the placenta (i.e., significant stress that could possibly elevate endogenous fetal glucocorticoid levels) have a reduced occurrence of respiratory distress syndrome compared with those in control groups of the same gestational age.

2. Amniotic fluid cortisol levels increase in pregnancy and this increase parallels the elevation in lecithin/sphingomyelin (L/S) ratios in fetal lung maturation.[17] Cortisol is present in the amniotic fluid (mainly in its conjugated form as cortisol sulfate) and is assumed to be deposited in this cavity primarily from fetal sources. This is because amniotic fluid over the last part of pregnancy is principally a product of exchanges with the fetal rather than maternal circulation. The sharp rise in amniotic fluid cortisol occurring after the 34th week of pregnancy corresponds to increases in cord blood corticosteroid levels as well as fetal adrenal weight increases over the last few weeks in pregnancy. Furthermore, this evidence for increased fetal corticosteroid production corresponds to increases in amniotic fluid L/S ratio that parallel fetal lung maturation. It is also of interest to note that in women with severe preeclampsia, in whom the fetus is exposed to severe stress in utero, higher than normal L/S ratios have been observed, together with increased amniotic fluid cortisol levels (Fig. 1).[17]

3. Metyrapone inhibits betahydroxylase in the adrenal gland, thereby blocking cortisol production. Chernik et al. injected metyrapone into pregnant rabbits at various gestational ages and demonstrated significantly elevated minimum surface tension in fetal lung extracts. This indicates a probable negative effect on fetal pulmonary maturity by this agent.[18]

4. Smith reported increased lecithin synthesis by fetal lung cell cultures following the addition of glucocorticoids to the preparation.[12] This investigator compared the effect of several steroids on the formation of saturated lecithin and found that the effectiveness of the individual steroids in reducing lecithin synthesis paralleled their binding to fetal lung receptors. Steroids that did not bind to receptor sites had little or no effect on saturated lecithin production. Smith's work provided strong evidence that endogenous glucocorti-

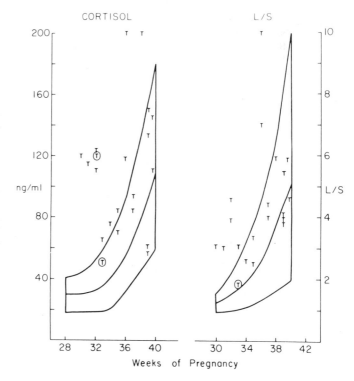

Figure 1. Amniotic fluid L/S ratios and amniotic fluid cortisol concentrations of patients with hypertensive disease of pregnancy. Women whose infants developed RDS are circled (T). The solid boundaries represent the 95 per cent confidence limits and the middle solid lines the mean values of normal pregnant patients. (From Tulchinsky, D.: *In* Moore, T. D. (ed.): Lung Maturation and the Prevention of Hyaline Membrane Disease. Report of the Seventieth Ross Conference on Pediatric Research, Columbus, Ohio, Ross Laboratories, 1976, p. 82.)

coids binding to fetal lung receptor sites stimulate lecithin production in the fetal lung.

5. There have been several studies in animals[19, 20] wherein direct ACTH administration to the fetus reduced respiratory distress syndrome in the newborn or gave some other indication of fetal lung maturity. The implication from these studies is that the beneficial effect of ACTH was mediated through fetal cortisol production.

6. There are clinical data indicating some protection from fetal respiratory distress syndrome by labor regardless of the route of delivery.[21] There is evidence that maternal and fetal cord blood cortisol levels are higher in labor; cord blood cortisol levels are elevated in infants born vaginally over those of infants delivered by elective cesarean section or section with no labor.[22, 23] However, cesarean section following labor results in cord blood cortisol levels comparable to those of infants delivered vaginally. These higher cord blood cortisol levels would correspond then to fetuses seemingly having some protection from respiratory distress.

Mechanism of Steroid Action in Accelerating Fetal Lung Maturity

It is widely believed that an increase in fetal lung surfactant activity is a major in utero event determining fetal pulmonary maturity and resistance to respiratory distress. Furthermore, although fetal lung surfactant represents a complex lipoprotein with a total composition still somewhat controversial, it is clear that a major portion of this complex is phospholipid, and the principal, essential phospholipid is a disaturated lecithin or phosphatidyl choline molecule. Therefore, it appears that biosynthesis of disaturated lecithin by the fetal lung is the key step in providing a surface-active stabilizing capability to the phospholipid fraction of fetal lung surfactant.

Hydrocortisone and aminophylline have been shown by Barrett and co-workers to augment cyclic AMP (cAMP) production and incorporation of precursors into phosphatidyl choline in fetal rabbit lung in vitro.[24, 25] These investigators cited evidence that the two agents acted through a common metabolic pathway; that is, by inhibiting phosphodiesterase activity and thus augmenting lung cAMP concentration (Fig. 2). There apparently are two possible pathways for lecithin synthesis in fetal lung (Fig. 3): choline incorporation or pathway I and methylation or pathway II. It has been proposed that cAMP increases the rate of phosphatidyl choline production via the choline incorporation pathway. Barrett and co-workers showed a significant increase in precursor uptake by both the choline incorporation and the methylation pathways in response to hydrocortisone and aminophylline treatment. A possible mechanism of action for other compounds thought to increase phosphatidyl choline production results from the observation that thyroxine, epinephrine and ACTH have been shown to augment the formation of tissue-cAMP by increasing the adenylate cyclase enzyme activity. This enzyme increases the concentration of cAMP, thus increasing production of phosphatidyl choline.

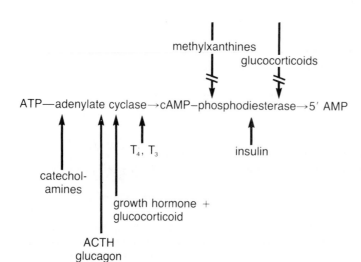

Figure 2. Mechanism by which agents can effect formation of cyclic AMP. (From Barrett, C. T.: *In* Moore, T. D. (ed.): Lung Maturation and the Prevention of Hyaline Membrane Disease. Report of the Seventieth Ross Conference on Pediatric Research, Columbus, Ohio, Ross Laboratories, 1976, p. 41.)

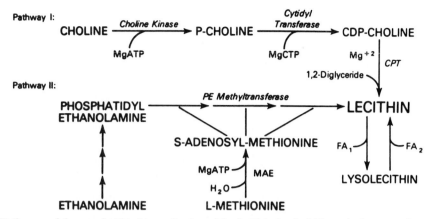

Figure 3. Pathways of de novo lecithin biosynthesis and the lecithin-lysolecithin cycle that may play an important role in determining the fatty acid substructure of the phospholipid. (From Farrell, P. M.: *In* Moore, T. D. (ed.): Lung Maturation and the Prevention of Hyaline Membrane Disease. Report of the Seventieth Ross Conference on Pediatric Research, Columbus, Ohio, Ross Laboratories, 1976, p. 29.)

Glycogen has been proposed as a precursor of surfactant and has been shown to be depleted in the presence of increased synthesis of phosphatidyl choline.[25] There is evidence that prior to incubation with C_{14}-labeled glucose, lung glycogen content of fetuses treated with cortisol in utero was lower than that of controlled fetuses. After incubation, higher concentrations of the C_{14} label were found in lung slice glycogen from cortisol-treated animals than in controls, indicating an increased rate of turnover of glycogen in these animals. In addition, specific activities of phosphatidyl choline were higher in tissue slices from cortisol-treated animals. These findings suggest an increased glycogen turnover and utilization, leading to formation of phosphatidyl choline in fetal lungs after administration of cortisol in vivo.

Fetal rabbit lung choline phosphotransferase was significantly increased after injection with glucocorticoids by Ferrell.[26] Choline phosphotransferase is believed by some to be the rate-limiting enzyme in the choline incorporation pathway synthesis of disaturated lecithin, as shown in Figure 3. This enzyme mediates a conversion of CPD choline to dipalmitoyl lecithin. Acceleration of this enzyme pathway could be extremely important in the overall regulation of lecithin synthesis, since choline phosphotransferase is apparently a very low activity enzyme in the pathway. It seems clear from Ferrell's studies that although some phosphatidyl choline production in the fetal lung results from the methylation pathway, by far the major source production of this disaturated phospholipid is via the choline incorporation pathway.

Other biochemical effects observed after fetal lung exposure to exogenous glucocorticoids include increased concentrations of disaturated phosphatidyl choline and increased activities of other enzymes such as glycerol phosphate phosphatidyl transferase, and lipoprotein lipase. Thus, in addition to stimulating the synthesis of phosphatidyl choline, apparently the biosynthetic capacity to produce phosphatidyl glycerol is also accelerated. Phosphatidyl glycerol has also been shown to be an important phospholipid in the formations of stable adult surfactant. An increase in amniotic fluid phosphatidyl glycerol over the last few weeks in pregnancy has been described.[27] This compound may be an essential component in addition to the disaturated (Fig. 4) lecithin in stabilizing fetal lung surfactant and avoiding respiratory distress syndrome.

In vivo studies have shown that not only was the net rate of formation of disaturated lecithin increased by dexamethasone administration, but the rate of secretion of this compound into the airways was even further enhanced.[28]

Possible Toxicity of Antenatal Maternal Steroid Administration

The role of glucocorticoids in the perinatal maturation of enzymatic systems in extrapulmonary tissue has been previously recognized.[7, 29] A marked effect in late gestation on

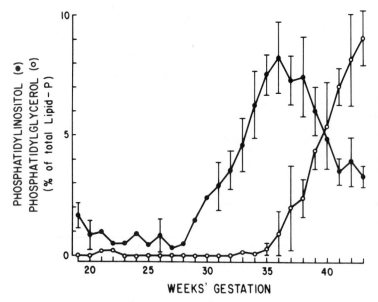

Figure 4. The content of phosphatidylinositol (●) and phosphatidylglycerol (○) in amniotic fluid during normal gestation. The phospholipids were quantified by measuring the phosphorus (P) content and expressed as percentages of total lipid phosphorus. Means ± standard deviations of 3 to 5 samples are shown for each point. (From Hallman, M. M., Kulovich, M. V., Kirkpatrick, R. G., Sugarman, G. and Gluck, L.: Phosphatidylinositol (PI) and phosphatidylglycerol (PG) in amniotic fluid: indices of lung maturity. Am. J. Obstet. Gynecol. 125:616, 1976.)

several enzymes involved in glycogen synthesis and during the first neonatal week on enzymes such as ornithine-aminotransferase, alanine-aminotransferase, and arginase has been demonstrated. The activity of all of these enzymes is increased by glucocorticoids. Exogenous glucocorticoids have also been shown to have a significant effect on maturation of endodermal structures, such as small intestine, pancreas and on brain and cerebellar enzyme systems. This information emphasizes the multiple activity of glucocorticoids in regulating perinatal enzymatic differentiation in many organs in addition to the lung. It seems reasonable to consider the possibility that such a biologically active compound in excess concentrations could adversely affect fetal development. Again, largely based on animal studies, there is significant reason for concern about possible toxicity of these agents in utero as follows: Numerous studies have indicated that perinatal exposure to exogenous glucocorticoids in animals resulted in significant in utero and neonatal growth retardation and occasionally in runting.[7] Multiple explanations for the growth retardation have been suggested, including inhibition of release of growth hormone releasing factor, direct inhibition of cell mitosis, interference with chondrocyte growth and differentiation, loss of thymic growth factor, increased consumption of amino acids by the liver, and increased susceptibility to infection. Timing of in utero exposure to glucocorticoids has also been indicated as critical, since organs near the end

of a critical growth period when stressed would be least capable of catch-up growth. Most of these studies have employed glucocorticoid or steroid doses considerably in excess of the physiologic stress range or the exogenous therapy range used in human studies.

Decreased growth in specific organ systems has been demonstrated following fetal exposure to corticosteroids in animals.[30, 31] Studies have shown decrease in lung cell size, cell number and lung weight and water following exposure to glucocorticoids. Significant decrease in brain weight and brain DNA content was observed by Howard following exposure of newborn mice to corticosteroids.[32] Decreased purposeful activity and increased nervousness in a group of newborn rats and mice exposed to cortisol was also demonstrated. Schapiro observed decreased brain cholesterol and delayed cortical dendritic branching in mature animals treated in the neonatal period with cortisol.[33] Treatment of newborn animals with steroids has also been reported to result in significant impairment of the immunologic responsiveness of these animals. However, study of the sequelae of early steroid administration to the newborn human infant has failed to reveal an effect on immune competence.[7]

Other significant toxic effects following maternal glucocorticoid therapy in animals include increased numbers of macerated and stillborn fetuses, decreased placental growth, increased placental senescence and impaired maternal-to-fetal glucose transfer.[7] Again, it should be emphasized that these experiments involve much larger doses of steroids than those used in humans.

In perhaps more significant studies, wherein primate monkeys were exposed to betamethasone in utero, DeLemos demonstrated a significant reduction in brain weight, total brain DNA and a reduction in newborn renal function.[34] Differences between the control and treated group with respect to brain weight, head circumference and DNA markedly narrowed by six months of postnatal age, suggesting the possibility of catch-up growth in these animals. Lung weight and lung DNA content were also reduced in the treated group. Significant differences in these pulmonary parameters, as well as a significantly lower overall fetal or neonatal weight of the treated animals, persisted at the follow-up neonatal examination at six months. Another more recent study also reported significant decreases in newborn weight and specific organ size following antepartum maternal administration of glucocorticoids to monkeys.[35] Smith reported that the growth of mixed fetal lung cell cultures was stimulated at 20 days' gestational age, but the overall growth of lung tissue was inhibited at the 28- to 30-day interval by exposure to cortisol.[12]

At this time, however, there is no good evidence to indicate unfavorable side effects or toxicity resulting from fetal or neonatal short-term exposure to glucocorticoids.[7] Clearly, more detailed studies and particularly long-term follow-up of the progeny of mothers treated in utero and in the neonatal period with steroids are needed before absolute statements regarding risks can be made. Nevertheless, the following considerations should be balanced against evidence of perinatal steroid toxicity suggested by previously described animal studies:

1. Comprehensive evaluation of newborns exposed to glucocorticoids in utero have failed to show any major adverse effect. Liggins[1] found no difference in IQ among 4-year-old children exposed to betamethasone in utero when compared with a control group. These workers also found no significant evidence of fetal growth retardation or increase in fetal or neonatal infection rates following antepartum administration of glucocorticoids.

2. Killam[3] reported normal growth rates for offspring from pregnancies in which the mother was treated with either betamethasone or hydrocortisone. He reported that head size,

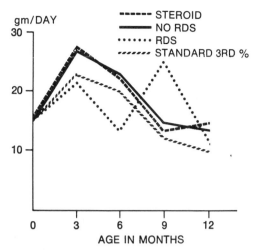

Figure 5. Effect of prenatal steroid treatment on rate of weight gain of preterm infants. (From Killam, A. P.: *In* Moore, T. D. (ed.): Lung Maturation and the Prevention of Hyaline Membrane Disease. Report of the Seventieth Ross Conference on Pediatric Research, Columbus, Ohio, Ross Laboratories, 1976, p. 113.)

weight and length were unaffected in the first year compared to a nontreated control group (Fig. 5). He also identified no other adverse effects in these newborns.

3. Ballard[36] reported that 12 to 24 mg of betamethasone, given to the mother 24 to 48 hours prior to delivery, resulted in maternal and cord blood plasma glucocorticoid activity within the physiologic stress range. That is, betamethasone plus the decreased amount of endogenous cortisol (total glucocorticoid activity in maternal or fetal plasma or both) was only approximately two to three times normal or in the range found in stress reactions (Fig. 6). This study also demonstrated that betamethasone was excreted in two days by mother and fetus (Fig. 7). Although fetal and neonatal endogenous cortisol suppression lasted at least three days, a postnatal increase in endogenous corticoids in response to stress was not suppressed by prenatal betamethasone exposure. On the basis of these observations, Ballard stated that prenatal glucocorticoid therapy for 48 hours is not associated with adverse effect in the human fetus. In addition, Ballard and his co-workers observed no differences in the ability to take feedings or to regain birth weight, in the incidence of late acidosis, unsuspected sepsis, patent ductus arteriosus or bilirubin levels in newborns exposed to betamethasone in utero compared with control groups. Head growth and IgM values were also within normal limits for this

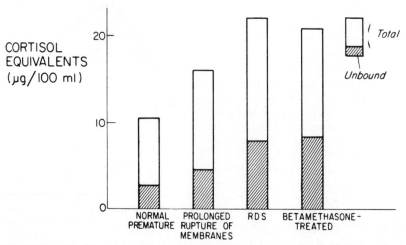

Figure 6. Total and unbound glucocorticoid activity in the premature infant. Normal values are mean levels in 14 infants without complications. Values for treated infants represent mean values 1 to 10 hours after the second dose of betamethasone. (From Ballard, P. L.: *In* Moore, T. D. (ed.): Lung Maturation and the Prevention of Hyaline Membrane Disease. Report of the Seventieth Ross Conference on Pediatric Research, Columbus, Ohio, Ross Laboratories, 1976, p. 87.)

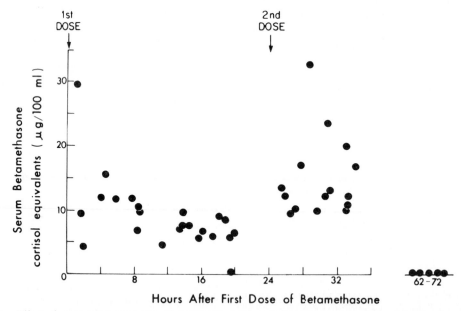

Figure 7. Effect of maternal treatment with betamethasone on betamethasone cord blood levels of premature infants. (From Ballard, P. L.: *In* Moore, T. D. (ed.): Lung Maturation and the Prevention of Hyaline Membrane Disease. Report of the Seventieth Ross Conference on Pediatric Research, Columbus, Ohio, Ross Laboratories, 1978, p. 86.)

group. Such preliminary findings support the concept that although significant toxicity may be the result in animal pregnancies following the antenatal administration of very large doses of glucocorticoids, no adverse consequences follow the use of smaller, therapeutically effective quantities of these agents during pregnancy.

Clinical Effectiveness of Antepartum Maternal Steroid Administration in Preventing Newborn Respiratory Distress Syndrome

The classic study demonstrating the effectiveness of maternal betamethasone administration in preventing newborn respiratory distress syndrome was reported by Liggins and Howie.[37] The most recent update of this well-controlled double-blind evaluation involved over 800 premature infants delivered between 1969 and 1974 and demonstrated that maternal betamethasone administration, particularly from 30 to 32 weeks of gestational age, achieved a striking reduction in respiratory distress in the neonate.[1] Other investigators have also reported clinical trials of betamethasone or other steroids administered to the mother prior to premature delivery that reduced the incidence of respiratory distress syndrome in the newborn.[2, 3, 4, 5, 6, 38] These studies either involved much smaller numbers of patients, or were not appropriate double-blind investigations.

In the Liggins study,[1] 443 mothers were treated with betamethasone prior to delivery of their premature infants and compared with 441 control mothers of the same gestational age and weight, according to a double-blind protocol. The standard maternal therapy in-

cluded 6 mg betamethasone phosphate and 6 mg betamethasone acetate administered intramuscularly upon entry into the study and 24 hours later. The control group received an identical injection with a small amount of cortisone acetate (6 mg) that resulted in no measurable increase in maternal glucocorticoid levels. Delivery was delayed if possible for 48 to 72 hours after the first injection. Improved perinatal survival was observed in the betamethasone-treated group, most likely owing to the lowering of the incidence of respiratory distress syndrome. The perinatal mortality (Table 1) in the control group was 15.9 per cent as opposed to 9.5 per cent in the treated group (p value <.01). Incidence of respiratory distress syndrome (Table 2) was reduced from 15.6 per cent in the control group to 10.0 per cent in the treatment group (p value <.02). However, if delivery occurred before 24 hours or was delayed for more than 7 days after initial maternal steroid administration, it appeared that no demonstrable benefit resulted. Therefore, with narrowing of the treatment group to those infants delivered within the time span for therapeutic effectiveness (Table 3), a striking reduction in perinatal mortality from 22.6 to 8.6 per cent was noted. Looking at the incidence of respiratory distress in this same group (Table 4), one is even more impressed by an overall decrease in respiratory distress from 23.7 to 8.8 per cent and a more striking reduction in respiratory distress in the 30- to 32-week gestational age category. This study concluded that significant benefit from this therapy was only demonstrable before 34 weeks' gestational age.

Other important findings included no significant hazard to fetus or mother resulting from ruptured membranes when exposed to this steroid therapy and no relationship between improved neonatal outcome and the use of uterine inhibitors, ethanol or salbuti-

TABLE 1.   INFANT SURVIVAL IN UNPLANNED PREMATURE LABOR (ALL INFANTS)

FETAL OUTCOME	BETAMETHASONE		CONTROL		p
	No.	%	No.	%	
Fetal deaths	12	2.7	19	4.3	NS
Early neonatal deaths	30	6.8	51	11.6	.02
Perinatal deaths	42	9.5	70	15.9	<.01
Survived 7 days	401	90.5	371	84.1	
All infants	443	100.0	441	100.0	

From Liggins, G. C.: *In* Lung Maturation and the Prevention of Hyaline Membrane Disease. Report of the 70th Ross Conference on Pediatric Research, Columbus, Ohio, Ross Laboratories, 1976, p. 98.

TABLE 2.   RDS Related to Entry-Delivery Interval (Liveborn Infants of Unplanned Deliveries)

Entry-Delivery Interval	Betamethasone			Control			
	No.	*RD*	*%RD*	*No.*	*RD*	*%RD*	*p*
Under 24 hr	77	19	24.7	82	25	30.5	NS
1 and under 7 days	182	16	8.8	156	37	23.7	0.001
7 days or more	172	8	4.7	184	4	2.2	NS
All infants	431	43	10.0	422	66	15.6	0.02

From Liggins, G. C.: *In* Lung Maturation and the Prevention of Hyaline Membrane Disease. Report of the 70th Ross Conference on Pediatric Research, Columbus, Ohio, Ross Laboratories, 1976, p. 98.

mol. The latter finding clearly contradicts several smaller and less well-controlled studies indicating reduction in respiratory distress syndrome following maternal antenatal treatment with a beta-adrenergic compound or ethanol.[40, 41]

On the basis of this large and impressive clinical trial, the following suggestions regarding therapy were advanced: (1) It seems advisable to attempt to forestall delivery for at least 24 hours and preferably 48 hours following the initial dose of betamethasone, by the use of an active inhibitory agent such as isoxsuprine. (2) It would seem advisable to avoid maternal glucocorticoid therapy in a pregnancy beyond 34 weeks without evidence by amniocentesis of pulmonary immaturity. (3) There may be a case for treatment if delivery has not occurred within 7 days following initial betamethasone administration. (4) According to Liggins' experience there seems to be a hazard to the neonate resulting from maternal betamethasone administration to the hypertensive mother. Table 5 shows a statistically significant increase in fetal death in the treated hypertensive group.

In several other less well-controlled studies similar results were reported, wherein maternal antenatal steroid treatment reduced newborn respiratory distress syndrome. Most of these studies involved much smaller treatment groups, ranging between 25 and 121 mothers. Nevertheless, a statistically significant reduction in respiratory distress in the newborn and some reduction in perinatal mortality were demonstrated, although mortality statistics were less impressive. A variety of steroids were used in these studies: betamethasone,[2-6] dexamethasone,[5, 38] and hydrocortisone[3] were reported to reduce neonatal respiratory distress syndrome, while methyl prednisolone[6] had no apparent effect on fetal lung maturity. Another recent study has demonstrated an increase in amniotic fluid L/S ratio following maternal intravenous hydrocortisone therapy.[42] Much larger maternal doses of hydrocortisone (1 to 4 g/24 hours), compared to betamethasone or dexamethasone (12 mg/24 hours), were required for therapeutic effectiveness corresponding to relative fetal lung–binding affinities for these compounds (Table 6). However, maternal intravenous hydrocortisone therapy lowered maternal serum unconjugated estriol levels by 60 per cent of pretreatment levels within an hour—or much more rapidly than decreases following intramuscular betamethasone administration. Differences in placental permeability to these agents[43] also parallel these findings. Betamethasone appears to cross the placenta more

TABLE 3.   Outcome of Infants of Unplanned Deliveries
24 Hours to 7 Days After Entry to Trial

Fetal Outcome	Betamethasone		Control		
	No.	*%*	*No.*	*%*	*p*
Fetal deaths	4	2.1	8	4.9	NS
Early neonatal deaths	12	6.5	29	17.7	0.002
Perinatal deaths	16	8.6	37	22.6	0.001
Survived 7 days	170	91.4	129	77.4	
All infants	186	100.0	164	100.0	

From Liggins, G. C.: *In* Lung Maturation and the Prevention of Hyaline Membrane Disease. Report of the 70th Ross Conference on Pediatric Research, Columbus, Ohio, Ross Laboratories, 1976, p. 99.

TABLE 4. RDS Related to Gestational Age, in Liveborn Infants of Unplanned Deliveries 24 Hours to 7 Days After Entry to Trial

Gestational Age at Delivery	Betamethasone			Control			
	No.	RD	%RD	No.	RD	%RD	p
Under 30 wk	36	10	27.8	26	15	57.7	.04
30 and under 32 wk	23	2	8.7	25	14	56.0	.001
32 and under 34 wk	50	0	0.0	31	4	12.9	.04
34 wk or more	73	4	5.5	74	4	5.4	NS
All infants	182	16	8.8	156	37	23.7	.001

From Liggins, G. C.: *In* Lung Maturation and the Prevention of Hyaline Membrane Disease. Report of the 70th Ross Conference on Pediatric Research, Columbus, Ohio, Ross Laboratories, 1976, p. 99.

readily than cortisol, while prednisolone crosses in very small amounts, possibly explaining its lack of clinical benefit.

Conclusions

Following these promising preliminary results, obstetricians in many centers have either completely or partially adopted a procedure whereby some mothers are given glucocorticoids, most commonly betamethasone, prior to the delivery of a premature infant at risk for respiratory distress syndrome. Others have continued to take a very cautious approach, maintaining that clear evidence of safety with antepartum maternal corticoid administration has not yet been established. Furthermore, some physicians still seek better proof of the clinical effectiveness of this technique. Clinicians of this persuasion are often heard to say, "I would like to see one more well-controlled double-blind study confirming the evidence before we adopt this method." In work previously cited, the effectiveness of maternal steroid administration seems very clear in reducing respiratory distress syn-

drome in the newborn; however, relatively high RDS rates in the control groups lead to some skepticism. In addition, the results in terms of reduction in neonatal mortality are less convincing (although still statistically significant in Liggins' work).

In weighing the pros and cons of this regimen, one must also consider the following facts: Even though only one well-controlled study exists to support antenatal maternal steroid administration, many less precisely controlled but still impressive clinical trials are being done that indicate the effectiveness of this procedure. At this point, to my knowledge, there is not one group of established clinical investigators reporting negative results or lack of effectiveness of this therapy in preventing newborn respiratory distress syndrome. Furthermore, it seems reasonable to say that only the most skeptical would doubt the clinical effectiveness of this agent in reducing respiratory distress, although the evidence is less clear as to ability in lowering neonatal mortality.

At this time, there is no clearly documented adverse effect of this agent on the mother or the newborn that would contraindicate its use.

TABLE 5. Fetal Outcome in Planned Delivery for Severe Hypertension-Edema-Proteinuria Syndromes

Fetal Outcome	Betamethasone		Control		
	No.	%	No.	%	p
Fetal deaths	12	25.6	3	7.0	.04
Early neonatal deaths	3	6.3	4	9.3	NS
Perinatal deaths	15	31.9	7	16.3	NS
Survived 7 days	32	68.1	36	83.7	
All infants	47	100.0	43	100.0	
RDS/Livebirths	4/35 (11.4%)		12/40 (30.0%)		NS

From Liggins, G. C.: *In* Lung Maturation and the Prevention of Hyaline Membrane Disease. Report of the 70th Ross Conference on Pediatric Research, Columbus, Ohio, Ross Laboratories, 1976, p. 99.

To be sure, with maternal steroid administration in pregnancy, one has to consider the possibility of an increased risk of infection in the mother and newborn, but this has yet to be demonstrated even after widespread experience. The clinician should be aware in employing this procedure in the diabetic pregnancy that insulin requirements will significantly increase[39] and hyperglycemic ketoacidosis may result (Fig. 8). It is also well to remember that in the study by Liggins[1] an increased fetal loss was reported in hypertensive pregnancies exposed to this regimen. Clearly, extra caution and consideration of the risk-to-benefit ratio should be exercised before using these agents in the hypertensive pregnancy.

Finally, the major hazard of maternal glucocorticoid administration in pregnancy remains the unknown possible long-term effects on the neonate from in utero exposure to such a potent hormone. The recent disastrous experience with diethylstilbestrol perhaps exaggerates our fears in this respect. Nevertheless, the large experience of Liggins, including neurologic and intellectual evaluation of a small

TABLE 6. RELATIVE AFFINITY OF VARIOUS STEROIDS FOR RECEPTORS IN THE CELLS OF HUMAN FETAL LUNG

STEROID	RELATIVE AFFINITY
Cortisol	100
6α-Methylprednisolone	1190
Fluocinolone Acetonide	1350
Dexamethasone	710
Betamethasone	540
Fluorometholone	400
9α-Fluorocortisol	350
Prednisolone	220
Triamcinolone Acetonide	190
Corticosterone	85
Estradiol	5
Testosterone	2
Estriol	<1
Androstenedione	<1

Mean values determined from dose-response competition experiments for each steroid using cytosol prepared from lungs of human fetuses of 16 to 20 weeks' gestation incubated with 13 nM ^{3}H-dexamethasone for 28 to 32 hr at 2° C.

From Liggins, G. C.: *In* Lung Maturation and the Prevention of Hyaline Membrane Disease. Report of the 70th Ross Conference on Pediatric Research, Columbus, Ohio, Ross Laboratories, 1976, p. 89.

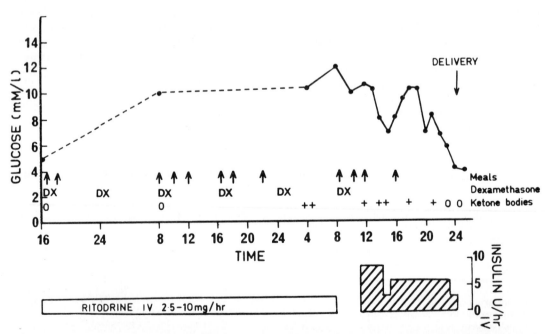

Figure 8. Plasma glucose concentration, urine ketones, diet and drug therapy in a chemical diabetic patient in premature labour. (DX indicates dexamethasone therapy.) (From Borberg, C., Gillmer, G. D. G., Beard, R. W. and Oakley, N. W.: Metabolic effects of beta-sympathomimetic drugs and beta-methasone in normal and diabetic pregnancy. Br. J. Obstet. Gynaecol. 85:184, 1978.)

group of children at 4 years of age, as well as careful evaluation of a larger number of offspring from 1 to 3 years of age, has failed at this point to show any evidence of adverse effects on growth and development of any organ system in these children. Furthermore, previous experience involving pregnancies in which the mother was treated throughout the gestation with significant quantities of steroids for autoimmune disease or other maternal problems and/or in which the newborn was treated in the neonatal period with steroids, has failed to reveal significant late adverse sequelae.[7] However, long-term results following dosages similar to those used to prevent respiratory distress syndrome are not clearly available so that ultimate and absolute proof of the safety of these agents awaits long-term follow-up of the offspring of the current therapeutic trials.

REFERENCES

1. Liggins, G.: Prenatal glucocorticoid treatment: prevention of respiratory distress. *In* Lung Maturation and the Prevention of Hyaline Membrane Disease. Report of the 70th Ross Conference on Pediatric Research, Columbus, Ross Laboratories, 1976, p. 97.
2. Kennedy, J. L.: Prenatal glucocorticoid treatment: prevention of respiratory distress syndrome. *In* Lung Maturation and the Prevention of Hyaline Membrane Disease. Report of the 70th Ross Conference on Pediatric Research, Columbus, Ross Laboratories, 1976, p. 105.
3. Killam, A. P.: Prenatal glucocorticoid treatment: effect on surviving infants. *In* Lung Maturation and the Prevention of Hyaline Membrane Disease. Report of the 70th Ross Conference on Pediatric Research, Columbus, Ross Laboratories, 1976, p. 110.
4. Stocker, J.: Prenatal glucocorticoid treatment: Reduction in neonatal deaths. *In* Lung Maturation and the Prevention of Hyaline Membrane Disease. Report of the 70th Ross Conference on Pediatric Research, Columbus, Ross Laboratories, 1976, p. 115.
5. Caspi, E., Schreyer, P., Weinraub, Z., Reif, R., Levi, I. and Mundel, G.: Prevention of the respiratory distress syndrome in premature infants by antepartum glucocorticoid therapy. Br. J. Obstet. Gynaecol. 83:187, 1976.
6. Block, M., Kling, O. R. and Crosby, W. M.: Antenatal glucocorticoid therapy for the prevention of respiratory distress syndrome in the premature infant. Obstet. Gynecol. 50:186, 1977.
7. Taeusch, H. W.: Glucocorticoid prophylaxis for respiratory distress syndrome: a review of potential toxicity. J. Pediatr. 87:617, 1975.
8. Schlesinger, M. and Mark, R.: Wasting disease induced in young mice by cortisol acetate. Administration Science 143:965, 1964.
9. Schapiro, S.: Neonatal cortisol administration: effect on growth, the adrenal gland and pituitary-adrenal response to stress. Proc. Soc. Exp. Biol. Med. 120:771, 1965.
10. Carson, S., Taeusch, H. W., Jr. and Avery, M.: Inhibition of lung cell division after hydrocortisone injection into fetal rabbits. J. Appl. Physiol. 34:660, 1973.
11. Kotas, R., Mims, L. and Hart, L.: Reversible inhibition of lung cell number after glucocorticoid injection. Pediatrics 53:358, 1974.
12. Smith, B.: Glucocorticoid effect on lung cell cultures. *In* Lung Maturation and the Prevention of Hyaline Membrane Disease. Report of the 70th Ross Conference on Pediatric Research, Columbus, Ross Laboratories, 1976, p. 60.
13. Howard, E.: Reduction in size and total DNA of cerebrum and cerebellum in adult mice after corticosterone treatment in infancy. Exp. Neurol. 22:191, 1968.
14. Fitzhardinge, P., Eisen, A., Lejtenyi, C., Metrakos, K. and Ramsay, M.: Sequelae of early steroid administration to the newborn infant. Pediatrics 53:877, 1974.
15. Baden, M., Bauer, C., Colle, E., Klein, G., Taeusch, H. W. and Stern, L.: Controlled trial of hydrocortisone therapy in infants with respiratory distress syndrome. Pediatrics 50:526, 1972.
16. Gluck, L. and Kulovich, M. V.: Lecithin/Sphingomyelin ratios in amniotic fluid in normal and abnormal pregnancy. Am. J. Obstet. Gynecol. 115:539, 1973.
17. Tulchinsky, D.: Amniotic fluid cortisol, lung maturation indicator. *In* Lung Maturation and the Prevention of Hyaline Membrane Disease. Report of the 70th Ross Conference on Pediatric Research. Columbus, Ross Laboratories, 1976, p. 80.
18. Chernik, V.: Glucocorticoid inhibition: delayed lung maturation. *In* Lung Maturation and the Prevention of Hyaline Membrane Disease. Report of the 70th Ross Conference on Pediatric Research, Columbus, Ross Laboratories, 1976, p. 67.
19. Robert, M. F., Bator, A. T. and Taeusch, H. W.: Pulmonary pressure-volume relationship after corticotropin and saline injections in fetal rabbits. Pediatr. Res. 9:760, 1975.
20. Sundell, H., Triantos, A., Relier, J. P. et al.: Prevention of hyaline disease with ACTH infusion in fetal lambs. Pediatr. Res. 7:407, 1973.
21. Fredrick, J. N. and Butler, N. R.: Hyaline membrane disease. Lancet 2:678, 1972.
22. Migeon, C. J., Prystowsky, H., Grumbach, M. M. and Byron, M. C.: Placental passage of 17-hydroxy corticosteroids: comparison of the levels in maternal and fetal plasma and effect of ACTH and hydrocortisone administration. J. Clin. Invest. 35:488, 1956.
23. Murphy, B. E. P.: Does the human fetal adrenal play a role in parturition? Am. J. Obstet. Gynecol. 115:52, 1973.
24. Barrett, C. T.: Cyclic AMP accelerator in lung maturation. *In* Lung Maturation and the Prevention of Hyaline Membrane Disease. Report of the 70th Ross Conference on Pediatric Research, Columbus, Ross Laboratories, 1976, p. 41.
25. Gilden, C., Sevanian, A., Tierney, D. V., Kaplan, S. A. and Barrett, C. T.: Regulation of fetal lung phosphatidyl choline synthesis by cortisol: role of glycogen and glucose. Pediatr. Res. 11:845, 1977.

26. Ferrell, P. M.: Enzymes: regulators of surfactant synthesis. *In* Lung Maturation and the Prevention of Hyaline Membrane Disease. Report of the 70th Ross Conference on Pediatric Research, Columbus, Ross Laboratories, 1976, p. 28.

27. Hallman, M. M., Kulovich, M. V., Kirkpatrick, R. G., Sugarman, G. and Gluck, L.: Phosphatidylinositol (PI) and phosphatidylglycerol (PG) in amniotic fluid: indices of lung maturity. Am. J. Obstet. Gynecol. 125:613, 1976.

28. Platzker, A. C. G., Kitterman, J. A., Mescher, E. J., Clements, J. A. and Tooley, W. H.: Surfactant in the lung and tracheal fluid of the fetal lamb and acceleration of its appearance by dexamethasone. Pediatrics 56:554, 1975.

29. Greengard, O.: Enzymic differentiation in mammalian tissues. *In* Campbell, P. N. and Dickens, F. (eds.): Essays in Biochemistry. Vol. 7, p. 159, 1971.

30. Carson, S., Taeusch, H. W., Jr. and Avery, M.: Inhibition of lung cell division after hydrocortisone injection into fetal rabbits. J. Appl. Physiol. 34:660, 1973.

31. Kotas, R., Mims, L. and Hart, L.: Reversible inhibition of lung cell number after glucocorticoid injection. Pediatrics 53:358, 1974.

32. Howard, E.: Reduction in size and total DNA of cerebrum and cerebellum in adult mice after corticosterone treatment in infancy. Exp. Neurol. 22:191, 1968.

33. Schapiro, S.: Some physiological, biochemical and behavioral consequences of neonatal hormone administration: cortisol and thyroxine. Gen. Comp. Endocrinol. 10:214, 1968.

34. DeLemos, R. A.: Glucocorticoid effect: organ development in monkeys. *In* Lung Maturation and the Prevention of Hyaline Membrane Disease. Report of the 70th Ross Conference on Pediatric Research. Columbus, Ross Laboratories, 1976, p. 77.

35. Johnson, J. W. C., Mitzner, W., London, W. T.,

Palmer, A. E. and Scott, R. E.: Betamethasone and fetal lung: evidence for major connective tissue changes. (Abstract.) Soc. Gyn. Research, p. 94, 1978.

36. Ballard, P. A.: Prenatal glucocorticoid treatment: Maternal and infant blood cortisol levels. *In* Lung Maturation and the Prevention of Hyaline Membrane Disease. Report of the 70th Ross Conference on Pediatric Research, Columbus, Ross Laboratories, 1976, pg. 85.

37. Liggins, G. C. and Howie, R. N.: A controlled trial of antepartum glucocorticoid treatment for prevention of the respiratory distress syndrome in premature infants. Pediatrics 50:515, 1972.

38. Thornfeldt, R. E., Franklin, R. W., Pickering, N. A., Thornfeldt, C. R. and Amell, G.: The effect of glucocorticoids on the maturation of premature lung membranes. Am. J. Obstet. Gynecol. 131:143, 1978.

39. Borberg, C., Gillmer, G. D. G., Beard, R. W. and Oakley, N. W.: Metabolic effects of beta-sympathomimetic drugs and betamethasone in normal and diabetic pregnancy. Br. J. Obstet. Gynaecol. 85:184, 1978.

40. Barrada, I. M., Vernig, N. L., Edwards, L. E. and Hakanson, E. Y.: Maternal intravenous ethanol in the prevention of respiratory distress syndrome. Am. J. Obstet. Gynecol. 129:25, 1977.

41. Kero, P., Hirvonen, T. and Välimäki, I.: Prenatal and postnatal isoxsuprine and respiratory distress syndrome. Lancet 2:198, 1973.

42. Zuspan, F. P., Cordero, L. and Semchyshyn, S.: Effects of hydrocortisone on lecithin-sphingomyelin ratio. Am. J. Obstet. Gynecol. 128:571, 1977.

43. Ballard, P. L., Granberg, P. and Ballard, R. A.: Glucocorticoid levels in maternal and cord serum after prenatal betamethasone therapy to prevent respiratory distress syndrome. J. Clin. Invest. 56:1548, 1975.

Editorial Comment

The authors in this chapter have raised the appropriate questions for controversy concerning the respiratory distress syndrome and whether it can be altered by the administration of glucocorticoids. As one might expect, all new modalities of therapy have a certain degree of polarization for enthusiasm or rejection and this topic is no exception. There tends to be a tone of acceptance of glucocorticoids for this use by most of the authors; however, physicians in some centers in this country feel that a more essential ingredient in the survival of the small baby is excellence in neonatal care, especially in the delivery room and for the first hour of life. It's too bad that the proponents and opponents can't get together and do randomized studies in each of their institutions on the use of glucocorticoids, but this now may never be done.

It was hoped that an answer to this question could be found in a double-blind multicenter study conducted under the auspices of the NICHD. The code for the study was broken in 1980 and the report published in *The American Journal of*

Obstetrics and Gynecology did not answer the question. The study did not control for variables that effect changes in fetal lung surfactant. The only positive finding in the report was that if the fetus was black and female, glucocorticoids would be helpful. A follow-up of these infants is essential if pertinent questions are yet to be answered. A survey of the world literature, utilizing "controlled studies," reveals that the neonatal mortality is 6.5 per cent for the treated and 29.1 per cent for the untreated with a neonatal incidence of RDS of 11 per cent for the treated and 30 per cent for the untreated. This literature survey was no better or worse than the multicenter double-blind study at answering pertinent questions.

The problem of fetal evaluation is that as time goes on better methods become available for caring for the small neonate and this variable is difficult to equate in any study. If the studies that have thus far been done are appropriate, then a logical and implied conclusion is that the administration of steroids results in a reduction in the incidence of respiratory distress syndrome in fetuses that have attained 28 to 32 weeks of gestation. There do not seem to be any problems of short-term effects on the offspring; however, the long-term effects are yet unknown even though a follow-up for seven years for those treated with betamethasone has been done and all children are normal. There are studies in animals in which extremely large pharmacologic doses have been administered that have produced adverse effect on growth and development. Great caution is needed in trying to extrapolate animal data to human medicine. There have been enough humans that have been treated— someone needs to institute the long-term follow-up.

The mechanism of action of glucocorticoids, regardless of the type used, deals with the induction of a local enzyme reaction with the type II pneumocyte to increase production of lecithin. We know that betamethasone does not increase the L/S ratio but hydrocortisone does in 80 per cent of the cases studied by serial amniocentesis. The explanation of how betamethasone works without altering the L/S ratio is still not known, since this glucocorticoid also reduces the incidence of RDS. It should be underscored that the optimal glucocorticoid agent, the dose and the mode of administration and long-term results are not known at this time.

6
The Management of Breech Presentations

Alternative Points of View

by Franklin C. Hugenberger

by Joseph V. Collea and Edward J. Quilligan

by James A. O'Leary and William W. Pasley

Editorial Comment

External Cephalic Version in Management of Breech Presentation

Franklin C. Hugenberger, M.D.

Columbus, Ohio

I am sure that every obstetrician will agree that breech presentation is an extra hazard to the pregnant woman and her baby. The first consideration is the possibility of prevention. If all breech presentations could be converted to cephalic presentations it would be a great boon to obstetrician, patient and baby.

With the trend in recent years to perform cesarean section to deliver infants presenting by the breech, it seems appropriate to try to stimulate interest in the ancient art of external cephalic version. This entails converting the breech presentation to a cephalic presentation as described in all the textbooks of obstetrics. Those of us who favor the procedure feel that it has not received the widespread use that it deserves. If external cephalic version can be done, many breech babies can be safely delivered as cephalic presentations.

External version may be attempted any time in the last 10 weeks of pregnancy. It may be easy, or quite difficult or impossible, especially in the presence of oligohydramnios. With hydramnics the turning is usually easy, but the breech presentation may be found again at the next examination. If this occurs, the version can be repeated. I have never used pads to prevent recurrence of the breech presentation. I have performed external version at term in early labor, but this is not to be expected usually.

For external version to be successful, diagnosis is naturally important. The patient must be examined: as the height of the fundus is checked, the hard round head is felt in the epigantrum and then the soft breech is felt at the pelvic brim. If there is doubt, vaginal examination may reveal the breech instead of the head at the inlet; then the procedure of external version is attempted. Sometimes if the technique is not successful early, it may be successful in a couple of weeks when the fetus is larger.

The technique in external version is relatively simple: the breech, if entering the pelvic brim, is displaced upward and then gently pushed to one side, probably preferably toward the infant's back, and at the same time the head in the fundus is gently pushed toward the opposite side, toward the fetal abdomen. If the fetus does not readily turn, the direction of turning may be reversed, the buttocks being pushed toward the abdomen and the head toward the back. I do not believe that one direction is better than the other; the important thing is to turn the fetus in the direction in which it can be turned. As the turning proceeds a little pressure is put on the buttocks, then on the head, then on the buttocks, until the fetus has transversed the 180-degree angle. Before the version is started the fetal heart rate should be checked and checked again when the turning is complete. If difficulty is encountered as the version proceeds slowly, the fetal heart rate is checked repeatedly. If the rate becomes alarmingly slow, as I have encountered a few times in 44 years, the version is quickly reversed. The fetal heart rate has always returned to normal and the version is repeated at the next prenatal visit, possibly in the opposite direction.

Anesthesia has never been used in external version in my practice; gentleness is essential, and nothing is done that is painful. The danger of placental separation may be theoretical, but I have never encountered the actual event. Cord entanglement is possible and is the reason for careful checking of the fetal heart rate. In my experience true knots in the cord have never been seen following version.

When I worked in an obstetric outpatient department with residents I tried to assist them to do external versions on the primigravida, but not on multiparas who had large pelves. If we are leaning toward cesarean section for all breeches I would urge attempting version on all breech presentations late in pregnancy, as I personally do in my private practice. The only exception is a breech pres-

entation in a patient who has had a previous cesarean section, for there is little advantage to having a cephalic presentation at cesarean section.

When should external version be done? I like to do it as soon as I discover the head in the fundus and the breech at the pelvic brim. Some early versions might be unnecessary as the fetus might change its presenting position spontaneously a few weeks later.

And what if the turned fetus is again presenting as a breech at the next prenatal visit? The external version is repeated. The patient is advised not to get down on her hands and knees as it allows the baby to fall away from the pelvic brim.

Unfortunately it is not possible to perform external cephalic version on all patients with breech presentations. Oligohydramnios is an obstacle, because there must be sufficient amniotic fluid for the fetus to turn in.

Despite our best efforts at external cephalic version there will be patients entering the hospital in active labor with the breech presenting. Some fetuses will have turned from cephalic to breech since the last examination; the procedure will not have been possible in others.

If careful physical examination, x-ray and ultrasonographic examination show any suggestion of disproportion, cesarean section should be elected. If the outlook is favorable and the obstetrician is trained in management of breech delivery, labor may be allowed to proceed. If at any time progress stops, cesarean section may be done.

Some obstetricians suggest that *all* breech presentations should be delivered by cesarean section. In this era of consumerism when it is suggested that the patient be told of alternatives and given an option, should this apply to the patient with a breech presentation? What of the young woman who wants to have a large family, has a good pelvis, a normal-sized fetus and would prefer to risk an attempt at vaginal delivery? Should she be forced to have abdominal delivery that might limit the size of her family? What if the uterus ruptures during a subsequent pregnancy with loss of uterus and infant, and possibly the mother's life? Do we have statistics showing that cesarean section for breech yields normal babies and a safe outcome for mothers in 100 per cent of cases?

With the growth of interest in home delivery, even without any trained attendant, it is apparent there is a trend "back to nature." It is also apparent we obstetricians must make every effort to make delivery at a hospital more attractive.

During the first two thirds of pregnancy we now feel at liberty to destroy the fetus at the mother's wish, but when some magic date arrives we must use every possible means, at whatever cost, to prevent a death. The patient may be forced to leave her family and friends to go to a distant special center for delivery. If the patient objects to this type of management, can we blame her? I have patients with four, six, eight children whose first baby was safely delivered through the vagina with the breech presenting. If a cesarean section had been done as a routine breech in the primi-

gravida, these women would not have had the families they wanted.

As for the malpractice fear, this is of our own doing.

We are sometimes too quick to criticize someone else's management of a case if the result is not good. Should not the liberal use of cesarean section for breech presentation be considered experimental until it has been proved ultimately to be the safer procedure for mothers and babies?

In checking my experience of several thousand deliveries the incidence of breech presentation has been about 1.8 per cent. I believe that this is about 50 per cent or less of the average; I think that this makes external cephalic version a worthwhile alternative.

The Management of Breech Presentation

Joseph V. Collea, M.D.

Georgetown University School of Medicine

Edward J. Quilligan, M.D.

University of California, Irvine

Successful management of breech labor and delivery has been a continual obstetric challenge. Until relatively recently, obstetricians, committed to vaginal delivery for most breech presentations, studied diligently to perfect "every movement imparted by the hands to the fetal body"[1] during breech delivery. Despite training and concerned care, however, breech perinatal morbidity and mortality rates remained considerably higher than those of comparable cephalic presentations. Hall and Kohl[2] in 1956, reporting on 1011 term breech infants, documented a perinatal mortality rate that was 5 times that of over 37,000 term cephalic presentations. Morgan and Kane,[3] in a computerized analysis of 404,847 deliveries including 16,327 breech births, reported a breech perinatal mortality rate of 30.1 compared with only 8.4 for the entire study population. In Copenhagen, Fischer-Rasmussen

and Trolle,[4] in a study of 9793 term singleton births including 431 breech deliveries, again confirmed the significantly increased breech perinatal mortality rate. When they corrected their data for perinatal deaths unrelated to fetal presentation, the reduced figures continued to show a term breech perinatal mortality rate approximately 5 times that of cephalic presentations. The authors noted that the major obstetric factors contributing to breech perinatal mortality were arrest of the aftercoming head, prolapse of the umbilical cord and prolonged labor, and concluded: "the advisability of wide indications for elective cesarean section in breech presentation is emphasized."

Analysis of breech statistics yields four principal causes of this increased breech perinatal mortality:

1. Low birth weight,
2. Congenital malformations,

3. Birth anoxia, or
4. Birth injury.

Low birth weight, defined as less than 2500 grams, is the most significant contributor to neonatal mortality today.[5] While occurrence of low birth weight infants in the general obstetric population is reported between 7 to 10 per cent, the incidence of low birth weight infants in breech presentation exceeds 30 per cent.[2, 3] During labor, the breech fetus presents to the maternal pelvis in succession the increasingly larger intertrochanteric, transthoracic and biparietal diameters. As the low birth weight breech fetus may easily deliver its body through a partially dilated cervix, entrapment of the larger fetal head may result. In addition, standard obstetric maneuvers to extract a low birth weight fetus even during a normal delivery process may result in significant fetal injury.[6]

Risks in Breech Presentation

Congenital malformations, such as congenital hip dislocation, hydrocephalus, anencephaly and meningomyelocele, occur more commonly in breech than in cephalic presentations and contribute significantly to breech perinatal morbidity and mortality.[7] Brenner[8] and his coworkers reported an incidence of 6.3 per cent congenital anomalies in 1016 singleton breech deliveries compared with an incidence of only 2.4 per cent congenital malformations in 29,343 singleton cephalic presentations. Retrospective analysis of infants born with chromosomal abnormalities and neuromuscular or structural anomalies yields convincing evidence that fetal malformations contribute to the incidence of breech presentation by physically preventing the fetus from actively assuming the cephalic presentation in late gestation.[7]

Birth anoxia may occur as a result of umbilical cord prolapse during labor or umbilical cord compression during prolonged breech extraction. The reported incidences of umbilical cord prolapse in the various types of breech presentation are listed in Table 1. It is apparent that the incidence of cord prolapse in frank breech presentation approaches the rate of 0.5 per cent found in cephalic presentations. Footling breech presentation, however, is associated with a rate that consistently exceeds 10 per cent, while complete breech presentation is associated with a rate of prolapse that approaches 5 per cent.

Umbilical cord compression resulting in birth anoxia is often seen in prolonged and difficult breech extractions. One factor contributing to difficult breech extraction is the arrest of the aftercoming head. Fischer-Rasmussen and Trolle[4] reported the occurrence of 27 cases of arrest of the aftercoming head during 319 term deliveries, for an incidence of 87.8 in 1000 breech deliveries. In comparison, they found only 12 cases of shoulder dystocia in 8723 term cephalic deliveries for an incidence of only 1.5 in 1000.

The breech fetus delivered vaginally is also at significant risk for birth injury. Gold,[14] in 1953, reported the incidence of birth injury in breech presentation as 17.5 in 1000 live births compared with 14.4 in 1000 for mid forceps, 1.3 in 1000 for low forceps and 0.21 in 1000 for spontaneous cephalic deliveries. Holland,[15] in 1922, described the mechanisms of tentorial tears and intracranial hemorrhage associated with vaginal breech delivery, while Caterini[16] and Bhagwanani[17] reported significant central nervous system damage and neonatal death associated with vaginal delivery of breech fetuses with deflexed heads in utero. Brachial palsy, the injury incurred by Emperor Wilhelm II of Germany at his breech birth in 1859,[18] occurs much more commonly

TABLE 1. Breech Presentation: Incidence of Cord Prolapse

Study	Overall Incidence (Percentage)	Type of Breech (Percentage)		
		Frank	Footling	Complete
Moore and Steptoe, 1943[9]	4.7	0.9	10.9	4.4
Kian, 1963[10]	4.6	1.3	13.1	2.3
Hall et al., 1965[11]	3.7	1.2	10.3	5.3
Morley, 1967[12]	4.1	0.0	15.0	5.1
Johnson, 1970[13]			18.0	

in breech than in cephalic presentations. Tan[19] reported the incidence of brachial palsy in breech presentation as 24.5 in 1000 breech deliveries compared to only 0.14 in 1000 cephalic deliveries and concluded from his data that difficult delivery of the aftercoming head was the most common cause of brachial palsy.

Management Methods

The increased incidence of umbilical cord prolapse, birth anoxia and birth injury led Wright[20] in 1959 to advocate cesarean section as the route of delivery for all viable breech presentations. At that time, however, while many investigators agreed that cesarean section avoided the increased risks to the fetus encountered in vaginal delivery, they believed that the maternal risks of cesarean section outweighed the fetal benefit. Obstetricians continued to utilize other methods such as external cephalic version, x-ray pelvimetry and Piper forceps to decrease breech perinatal morbidity and mortality.

External cephalic version performed by an experienced clinician during the early third trimester of pregnancy can significantly reduce the incidence of breech presentation at term.[20-22] Unfortunately, reported complications of the procedure, such as premature labor, premature rupture of the membranes, abruptio placenta, rupture of the uterus and fetal death secondary to umbilical cord entanglement, have curtailed enthusiasm to the point where few obstetricians perform this procedure. Consequently, external cephalic version is taught to only a small percentage of the obstetric residents in training today.[23] Recently, however, a report of external cephalic version under tocolysis has generated some interest in this procedure as a means of decreasing the rate of cesarean section for breech delivery.[23a]

The use of x-ray pelvimetry in the management of breech presentation is controversial. Several investigators[24-27] have reported the inability of pelvimetry to select patients who will have difficulty in labor or at delivery. In addition, Rovinsky[28] has reported no improvement in breech fetal outcome, and Kauppila[29] has shown no reduction in the incidence of difficult breech deliveries with the use of x-ray pelvimetry. Nevertheless, attempted vaginal breech delivery through a contracted maternal pelvis is associated with significant perinatal mortality and should be avoided.[30] Obstetricians who anticipate performing a vaginal breech delivery should obtain x-ray pelvimetry to rule out the possibility of an inadequate maternal pelvis.

Piper forceps have been used since 1929 by obstetricians for better control of delivery of the aftercoming head. Moore and Steptoe[9] reported that the use of Piper forceps in breech delivery reduced the incidence of breech neonatal mortality in infants with birth weights over 2500 grams. More recently, Milner[31] reported in the British literature that use of Piper forceps was associated with significantly reduced mortality rates in 1000- to 3000-g neonates.

Although external cephalic version, x-ray pelvimetry and Piper forceps are employed with the aim of improving breech perinatal outcome, many investigators argue that only cesarean section consistently avoids the risks—umbilical cord prolapse, birth injury and birth anoxia—that contribute so heavily to the perinatal morbidity and mortality. In their large series of over 16,000 breech deliveries, Morgan and Kane[3] reported that when primigravidas without obstetric complications were delivered at term by cesarean section, their perinatal mortality was zero. Likewise, other reports involving breech infants demonstrate that whenever cesarean section is performed in the management of patients with breech presentation, the perinatal mortality rate approaches zero.[4, 8, 29, 30, 32]

Favorable statistics in the breech situation by cesarean section have led to its ever-increasing use in management of breech presentation today. However, maternal morbidity and mortality from cesarean section have precluded the *absolute* recommendation of cesarean section in the management of all viable breech presentations. Furthermore, cesarean section cannot avoid or erase the perinatal losses related to low birth weight and congenital malformations. Consequently, appropriate management of patients with breech presentation must involve the careful selection of patients who require cesarean section from those who may be offered a trial of labor and vaginal delivery with a minimum of fetal and maternal risk.

At Women's Hospital, Los Angeles County-University of Southern California Medical Center, concern for the fetal risks during breech vaginal delivery has caused a steady increase in the breech cesarean section rate. During 1970, the overall cesarean section rate was 9.3 per cent, but 31.7 per cent of singleton breech infants were delivered by cesarean section. A retrospective analysis[33] of 375 patients with singleton breech presentations delivered during 1974 revealed a cesarean section rate of 67.6 per cent, while the overall rate for the hospital obstetric population remained at 9.3 per cent. Despite the increased rate of cesarean section for breech presentation in 1974, the breech perinatal mortality rate of 96 in 1000 deliveries (15 stillbirths and 21 neonatal deaths) was almost 5 times higher than the rate of 21 in 1000 recorded for the institution that year.

Analysis of the 21 breech neonatal deaths revealed that 6 were caused by congenital malformations incompatible with life, and 6 occurred in infants with birth weights less than 1000 grams. When neonatal deaths associated with congenital malformations were excluded, no death occurred in infants with birth weights greater than 1850 grams, regardless of their route of delivery. In addition, analysis of 5-minute Apgar scores demonstrated no significant difference in immediate outcome between infants delivered vaginally and by cesarean section. This study suggested that, given a high rate of cesarean section, properly selected breech infants can be vaginally delivered with immediate outcomes comparable to those in infants delivered by cesarean section.

Prospective Study

From these data, a prospective study[34] was designed to test the premise that selected breech infants could be safely delivered by the vaginal route. The outline of this study is presented in Figure 1. Patients with singleton frank breech presentation (confirmed by abdominal x-ray) at 36 or more weeks of gestation, with estimated fetal weight between 2500 grams and 3800 grams, were selected for study. Frank breech presentation was chosen because of its low incidence of umbilical cord prolapse. Excluded were (1) elderly primigravid patients in advanced labor (8 cm or more cervical dilatation), (2) patients with ob-

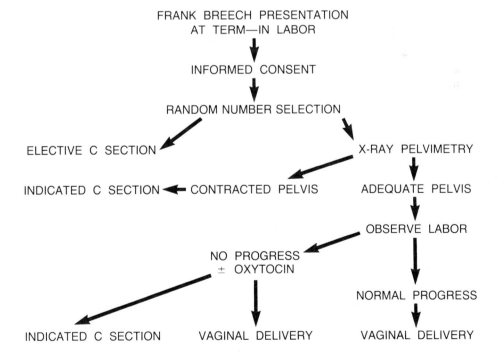

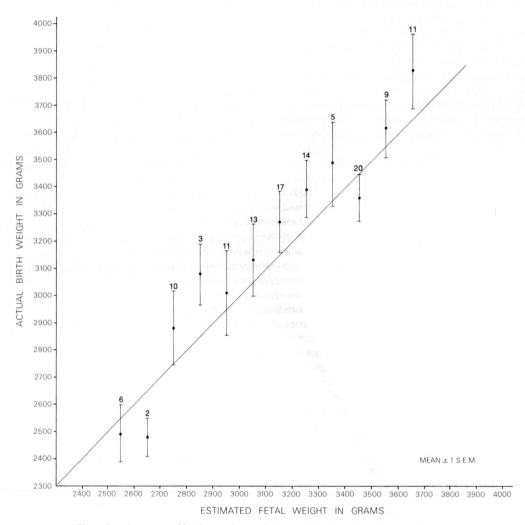

Figure 2. Accuracy of birth weight prediction in 121 frank breech presentations.

TABLE 2. FRANK BREECH PRESENTATION: PROSPECTIVE MANAGEMENT AND ESTIMATION
OF FETAL WEIGHT

PROTOCOL SELECTION	No.	ACTUAL BIRTH WEIGHT	ESTIMATED FETAL WEIGHT	
			Ave. Error (g)	*Error (g/kg)*
Vaginal	6	<2500 g	391.2	168.8
Vaginal	6	>3800 g	801.4	202.1
Cesarean	2	<2500 g	487.5	207.4
Cesarean	13	>3800 g	654.6	159.3
Total	27		609.2	172.4

stetric indications for cesarean section, (3) patients with abnormal abdominal x-ray findings such as hyperextension of the fetal head or fetal skeletal malformations, (4) patients with class B to F diabetes mellitus (White's classification) and (5) patients with a history of difficult or traumatic delivery.

Estimation of the fetal weight was obtained by performing Leopold's maneuvers[35] and compared favorably with the actual birth weight as demonstrated in Figure 2. Of the 127 patients who consented to the study, 70 were randomized to the vaginal delivery group and 57 to the cesarean section group. One hundred patients delivered infants with birth weights between 2500 g and 3800 g. As shown in Table 2, 27 patients delivered infants outside of the study's birth weight criteria. The average error of estimated fetal weight from actual birth weight are the error in grams per kilogram of actual birth weight are also recorded.

Fifty-five of the 57 patients selected for elective cesarean section were delivered according to protocol. Two delivered vaginally before surgery could be performed. In the vaginal group of 70 patients, 35 women had one or more contracted measurements on x-ray pelvimetry. Thirty-two of these patients were delivered by cesarean section, but 3 multiparous patients progressed rapidly in labor and were delivered vaginally before cesarean section could be performed. Of the 35 women with adequate pelvimetry, 30 delivered vaginally and 5 required cesarean section—4 for failure to progress in labor and 1 for acute fetal distress.

Although no perinatal deaths occurred in either the cesarean section group or the vaginal delivery group, two infants delivered vaginally sustained brachial plexus injuries, while no birth injury occurred in the cesarean section group. Patients in the cesarean section group, however, had significant maternal mor-

bidity when compared with patients who delivered vaginally.

Patients admitted to Women's Hospital in labor with term frank breech presentation are managed according to the study protocol. Patients at term with complete, incomplete and footling breech presentations are delivered by cesarean section to avoid the increased incidence of umbilical cord prolapse. All patients in labor with premature or low birth weight breech presentations and an estimated fetal weight between 1000 g and 2499 g are delivered by cesarean section to avoid the risks of birth trauma and entrapment of the aftercoming head.

Prior to the delivery of any patient with breech presentation, an abdominal x-ray is obtained to confirm the type of breech presentation and to determine the presence of structural anomalies in the fetus, such as anencephaly, hydrocephaly or spina bifida. In the event that an anencephalic or otherwise grossly deformed fetus is detected, cesarean section is averted and vaginal delivery is allowed.

Although the use of oxytocin is considered controversial by some investigators, the drug is employed for augmentation of labor in patients selected to deliver vaginally. Oxytocin is administered only in dilute solution by a continuous intravenous infusion method and is utilized to produce uterine contractions similar in frequency, duration and intensity to those seen in normal spontaneous labor. Whenever oxytocin is utilized, its effects on uterine activity should be monitored by an intra-amniotic catheter, which continuously records intrauterine pressure. Fetal well-being should also be monitored by a continuous recording of the fetal heart rate.

Vaginal delivery of the fetus in breech presentation is preferably accomplished by the assisted breech extraction technique. Total breech extraction is associated with increased rates of birth trauma and should be performed only in extreme circumstances when fetal survival is in jeopardy and the capability to perform cesarean section is not immediately available. Finally, for better traction on and control of the aftercoming head, Piper forceps should be applied.

The preferred method of pain relief for breech vaginal delivery is a continuous lumbar epidural anesthetic. This method allows for adequate pain relief during labor, a calm, stationary patient on the delivery table and a relaxed maternal perineum for the delivery. An alternate method of pain relief at delivery is a pudendal block anesthetic for delivery of the fetal body and a general anesthetic for application of the Piper forceps and delivery of the aftercoming head.

Maternal parity is not and should not be a deciding factor in the management of patients with breech presentation. Two studies[3, 36] have conclusively shown that breech perinatal morbidity and mortality rates in primigravid women are identical to those in multiparous women.

It is apparent from the retrospective report and from the prospective study that cesarean section plays an important role in the management of patients with breech presentation at Women's Hospital. Although we are aware of the maternal hazards associated with cesarean section, we believe that, where recommended, the benefits to the fetus of cesarean section justify the operative risks to the mother. Until the prospective study proves otherwise, cesarean section for all viable breech presentations is not recommended. In cases of advanced breech labor, for instance, more harm may come to both mother and fetus by a hastily performed and difficult cesarean section than by allowing for a controlled vaginal delivery. Proper selection of patients for cesarean section as well as vaginal delivery will ultimately result in improved maternal and infant outcome.

REFERENCES

1. DeLee, J. B.: Yearbook of Obstetrics and Gynecology. Year Book Medical Publishers, Inc., Chicago, 1939.
2. Hall, J. E. and Kohl, S. G.: Breech presentation. Am. J. Obstet. Gynecol. 72:977, 1956.
3. Morgan, H. S. and Kane, S. H.: An analysis of 16,327 breech births, J.A.M.A. 187:108, 1964.
4. Fischer-Rasmussen, W. and Trolle, D.: Abdominal versus vaginal delivery in breech presentation. Acta Obstet. Gynecol. Scand. 46:69, 1967.
5. Pritchard, J. A. and MacDonald, P. C.: Williams Obstetrics, 15th ed. Appleton-Century-Crofts, New York, 1976.
6. Alexopoulos, K. A.: The importance of breech delivery in the pathogenesis of brain damage. Clin. Pediatr. 12:248, 1973.
7. Braun, F. H. T., Jones, K. L. and Smith, D. W.: Breech presentation as an indicator of fetal abnormality. J. Pediatr. 86:419, 1975.
8. Brenner, W. E., Bruce, R. D. and Hendricks, C. H.: The characteristics and perils of breech presentation. Am. J. Obstet. Gynecol. 118:700, 1974.
9. Moore, W. T. and Steptoe, P. P.: The experience of the Johns Hopkins Hospital with breech presentation. South. Med. J. 36:295, 1943.
10. Kian, L. S.: Breech presentation. Am. J. Obstet. Gynecol. 86:1050, 1963.
11. Hall, J. E., Kohl, S. G., O'Brien, F. and Ginsberg, M.: Breech presentation at term. Am. J. Obstet. Gynecol. 91:665, 1965.
12. Morley, G. W.: Breech presentation—A 15-year review. Obstet. Gynecol. 30:745, 1967.
13. Johnson, C. E.: Breech presentation at term. Am. J. Obstet. Gynecol. 106:865, 1970.
14. Gold, E. M., Clyman, M. J., Wallace, H. M. and Rich, H.: Obstetric factors in birth injuries. Obstet. Gynecol. 1:43, 1953.
15. Holland, E.: Cranial stress in the fetus during labor and on the effects of excessive stress on the intracranial contents; with an analysis of 81 cases of torn tentorium cerebelli and subdural cerebral hemorrhage. J. Obstet. Gynaecol. Br. Commonwealth 29:549, 1922.
16. Caterini, H., Langer, A., Sana, J. C., Devanesan, M. and Pelosi, M. A.: Fetal risk in hyperextension of the fetal head in breech presentation. Am. J. Obstet. Gynecol. 123:632, 1975.
17. Bhagwanani, S. G., Price, H. V., Laurence, K. M. and Ginz, B.: Risks and prevention of cervical cord injury in the management of breech presentation with hyperextension of the fetal head. Am. J. Obstet. Gynecol. 115:1159, 1973.
18. Marx, R.: The birth of an emperor. Surg. Gynecol. Obstet. 89:366, 1949.
19. Tan, K. L.: Brachial palsy. J. Obstet. Gynaecol. Br. Commonwealth 80:60, 1973.
20. Wright, R. C.: Reduction of perinatal mortality and morbidity in breech delivery through routine use of cesarean section. Obstet. Gynecol. 14:758, 1959.
21. MacArthur, J. L.: Reduction of the hazards of breech presentation by external cephalic version. Am. J. Obstet. Gynecol. 88:302, 1964.
22. Bock, J. E.: The influence of prophylactic external cephalic version on the incidence of breech delivery. Acta Obstet. Gynecol. Scand. 48:215, 1969.
23. Ranney, B.: The gentle art of external cephalic version. Am. J. Obstet. Gynecol. 116:239, 1973.
23a. Saling, E. and Müller-Holve, W.: External cephalic versions under tocolysis. J. Perinatol. Med. 3:115, 1975.
24. Schifrin, B. S.: The case against pelvimetry. Contemp. Ob-Gyn. 4:77, 1974.
25. Russell, J. G. B. and Richards, B.: A review of pelvimetry data. Br. J. Radiol. 44:780, 1971.
26. Zatuchni, G. I. and Andros, G. J.: Prognostic index for vaginal delivery in breech presentation at term. Am. J. Obstet. Gynecol. 98:854, 1967.

27. Harris, J. M. and Nessim, J. A.: To do or not to do a cesarean section. J.A.M.A. 169:570, 1959.
28. Rovinsky, J. J., Miller, J. A. and Kaplan, S.: Management of breech presentation at term. Am. J. Obstet. Gynecol. 115:497, 1973.
29. Kauppila, O.: The perinatal mortality in breech deliveries and observations on affecting factors. Acta Obstet. Gynecol. Scand. (Suppl. 39) 1975.
30. Beischer, N. A.: Pelvic contraction in breech presentation. J. Obstet. Gynaecol. Br. Commonwealth 73:421, 1966.
31. Milner, R. D. G.: Neonatal mortality of breech deliveries with and without forceps to the aftercoming head. Br. J. Obstet. Gynaecol. 82:783, 1975.
32. Todd, W. D. and Steer, C. M.: Term breech: Review of 1006 term breech deliveries. Obstet. Gynecol. 22:583, 1963.

33. Collea, J. V., Weghorst, G. R. and Paul, R. H.: Singleton breech presentation—one year's experience. *In* Mandouzzato, G. P. and Keller, P. G. (eds.): Contributions to Gynecology and Obstetrics, Vol. 3, The Fetus at Risk, Basel, S. Karger A. G., 1977.
34. Collea, J. V., Rabin, S. C., Weghorst, G. R. and Quilligan, E. J.: The randomized management of term frank breech presentation: vaginal delivery vs. cesarean section. Am. J. Obstet. Gynecol. 131:186, 1978.
35. Leopold and Sporlin: Conduct of normal births through external examination alone. Arch. Gynaekol. 45:337, 1894.
36. Minogue, M.: Vaginal breech delivery in multiparae. J. Irish Med. Assoc. 67:117, 1974.

Once a Breech, Always a Cesarean Section?

James A. O'Leary, M.D.

University of Buffalo School of Medicine

William W. Pasley, M.D.

University of South Alabama Medical Center

In prior years the test of a good obstetrician was the manner in which he performed a breech delivery. At the present time a more valid test might be the manner in which the clinician evaluates and conducts the breech labor. Breech presentation challenges the clinician with many unique problems and difficult decisions. It should be emphasized that the art of modern obstetrics lies not in manual skills or clinical showmanship but rather in the ability to anticipate problems and prevent any and all injury to the mother and infant. It is our firm belief that there is still a place for the vaginal delivery of a breech. Statements such as "once a breech, always a cesarean," or "if in doubt, cut it out," are questionable at best.

Prognosis

Prognostically significant in the breech presentation is the condition of the cervix—consistency and dilatation—as well as the station of the presenting part. The prognosis for the breech is further affected by a twofold increase in fetopelvic disproportion, premature rupture of the membranes, dysfunctional labor and a threefold increase in macrosomia.[10] Antepartum and intrapartum deaths, neonatal deaths and low Apgar scores are much more common with this presentation.[4] The neonatal morbidity can be as high as 15.8 per cent, while the permanent and serious morbidity will be 7.2 per cent.[1] Also encountered on a more frequent basis are lower IQ scores.[9] A study of over 1000 children followed through the ninth grade showed that 24.5 per cent of those in breech presentation repeated grades, as opposed to 8.3 per cent in the control group.[15] Lower arithmetic scores, a need for remedial measures and a higher incidence of speech disorders and visual and auditory defects are encountered in breech presentation children.[8, 15]

The concern of a less-than-ideal offspring after a breech delivery is disturbing and clearly indicates that the overall prognosis for the breech is not good. There has been a 75 per cent increase in the number of cesarean sections for breech deliveries and a 35 per cent decrease in neonatal deaths in a larger city in this country.[12] Some investigators have emphasized the routine use of cesarean section in reducing the perinatal mortality and morbidity associated with the breech presentation.[24] We believe that the routine use of cesarean section is unjustified. It is our opinion that with careful evaluation of the patient it is possible to identify which infant in breech presentation can be delivered vaginally without increased risk to the mother or infant,[17] and which infant will require abdominal delivery.

Evaluation

Major concerns in the evaluation of the *term* breech should be the pelvis and the type of labor. Vaginal delivery should be attempted only in a well-formed gynecoid pelvis of average to large size. The transverse diameter of the inlet should be 17 cm and the anterior-posterior diameter of the inlet should be 11 cm as minimum measurements. In addition, the sacrum should be hollow and the subpubic arch normal. The interspinous diameter needs to measure 10 cm. The presence of a smaller or ill-formed pelvis is an indication for cesarean section.

Using these inlet criteria one can expect a perinatal mortality of 0.5 per cent in the term breech.[22] Even in the presence of adequate measurements and a normal pelvis the cesarean section rate will be 25 per cent. When the pelvic measurements are smaller and structure of the pelvic inlet is abnormal, 45 per cent of patients can be delivered vaginally, but the perinatal mortality will be 6 per cent.[22]

To adequately evaluate the pelvis, routine

TABLE 1. BREECH SCORE

	0	1	2
Parity	0	1	2
No. weeks	39 +	>37–39	37
Weight	8 + lbs	7–8	<7
Previous breech	0	1	2
Dilatation	2	3	4
Station	−3	−2	−1

x-ray pelvimetry is mandatory, as well as a flat plate of the abdomen to rule out hydrocephaly and hyperextension of the fetal head. Even with the most accurate measurements of the pelvis it is only possible to estimate fetal size by clinical examination. If possible, an ultrasonic measurement of the biparietal diameter should be obtained. A biparietal diameter greater than 9.5 cm should be an indication for cesarean section, if the ultrasonography is known to be reliable.

The Zatuchni-Andros Breech Score[3] should be utilized (Table 1). The score is weighed against the factors of first pregnancy and largeness in the infant, and this seems proper. The prognostic value of the score is greatest in low scores (0 to 4). A high score is of less value and is no guarantee of a normal labor and an easy delivery—and certainly is never a substitute for critical clinical judgment. All patients with low breech scores should undergo cesarean section.

The clinical assessment of the fetal size and type of breech is prognostically most important. All infants in excess of 3500 g and all footling breeches should be delivered by cesarean section.

The infant in breech presentation should be carefully scrutinized for any abnormality of labor, especially the rate of descent. This is best accomplished by constructing a Friedman labor curve and by keeping in mind that the infant in breech presentation usually starts at a higher station but should have a normal or rapid rate of descent.[10] Any abnormality in either the curve of descent or dilatation is an indication for cesarean section and not stimulation with oxytocin. The use of oxytocin in the presence of dysfunctional labor is associated with a perinatal mortality of 29.3 per cent, as opposed to 14.5 per cent with no labor augmentation.[22] Dysfunctional labor patterns are an ominous development, cannot be

TABLE 2. CESAREAN SECTION INDICATIONS

Excessive maternal obesity*
Excessive weight gain without edema*
Nongynecoid pelvis
Firm or rigid cervix
Prolonged rupture of membranes
Premature rupture of membranes
Dysfunctional labor
Footling breech
Prematurity
First pregnancy
Uncooperativeness in patient
Relative infertility
Uterine myomas
Post-term pregnancy*
Toxemia*
Diabetes*
Hyperextension of fetal head
High station
Poor obstetric history
Large infant
Request for sterilization*
Fetal distress
Abruptio placentae
Poor breech score

*Relative indications

easily remedied and represent an indication for abdominal delivery. Artificial rupture of the membranes is contraindicated. This philosophy is based on the fact that prolapse of the cord is increased from 3.1 per cent to 4.7 per cent with premature rupture of the membranes.[22]

Fetal distress is a relatively frequent complication of breech labors and usually is indicated by a pattern of variable decelerations of fetal heart rate. Therefore, every breech labor should have careful electronic monitoring of the fetal heart rate.

Indications for cesarean section should be liberal (Table 2). A careful search should be conducted to rule out actual or anticipated problems. A poor obstetric history is very revealing, but a normal obstetric history is never a reliable indication of pelvic size or structure, since many factors are involved.

Utilizing these criteria and indications, we have had excellent results. In a series of 150 breeches we have not had a single mortality. There was one instance of a low Apgar score, in which a birth injury was involved, following a total breech extraction for fetal distress. Our cesarean section rate was 65 per cent in the primigravida and 40 per cent in the multigravida.[17]

Analgesia and Anesthesia

Heavy sedation is clearly contraindicated; however, the patient can be sedated in the usual manner. Since alterations in the fetal heart rate are common, drugs that will change the baseline variability should not be used. In addition, scopolamine is contraindicated because its adverse effects can make the patient uncooperative. Patient cooperation is a most important factor.

A qualified anesthesiologist experienced in dealing with breech presentation is essential to a good outcome. As a rule, regional anesthesia is contraindicated because with it the patient is unable to bear down and the uterus will not be well relaxed for manipulations. It is our preference to use pudendal block and nitrous oxide analgesia for delivery of the baby to the level of the umbilicus, rapidly followed by general anesthesia for the remainder of the delivery, unless it is imminent.

The Delivery

Since spontaneous and assisted vaginal breech deliveries carry very little risk, they are much preferred over the dangerous total breech extraction. Complications and injuries to the fetus have been reported to be as high as 40 per cent with the latter procedure.[11] In breech extraction the presenting part has not reached the pelvic floor, and the cervix is usually not fully dilated. The procedure consists of extracting the entire infant from the birth canal. This is potentially very traumatic and usually a difficult maneuver. In most hands, it is associated with a significant increase in fetal injuries, morbidity and mortality. In such situations abdominal delivery is clearly preferable.

The spontaneous breech delivery is an infrequent event and should not be confused with an unattended delivery. In most circumstances an assisted delivery is preferable. An important factor in the vaginal breech delivery is the presence of an experienced and skilled assistant, since the presence of a second assistant is highly desirable.

The patient should be taken to the delivery room when the presenting part is distending the perineum. All patients should be catheterized and a generous episiotomy made. The patient can then be assisted in delivering the infant to the umbilicus. At this point there usually is traction on the cord; it should be advanced a few inches. The infant should be grasped so that the thumbs are on the sacrum and the fingers over the lower abdomen and pelvis. Traction should be directed downward at an angle of about 45 degrees, and the mother urged to bear down. No attempt should be made to deliver the arms until the scapulae are seen. The operator's hands should continue traction, and yet the grasp must remain on the pelvis. If the hands are advanced up the infant's body, the kidneys, spleen, liver and adrenals can be injured. If the shoulders do not deliver spontaneously, the infant is rotated slightly; and with the operator using one finger, the posterior shoulder is delivered. At times it may be easier to deliver the anterior shoulder first; or after delivering the posterior arm, the infant can be rotated 180 degrees and the opposite arm can be delivered over the perineum. Should the posterior arm not enter the hollow of the sacrum, two fingers placed on the humerus can bring the arm across the chest.

The head may be delivered with forceps or by the Mauriceau-Smellie-Veit maneuver, with or without the Wigand-Martin maneuver. The latter two techniques frequently result in last-minute uncontrolled popping of the head through the introitus, whereas the forceps delivery is more controlled and physiologic. A 20-year study of 1423 liveborn breech infants compared forceps and nonforceps deliveries and clearly demonstrated a lower mortality with forceps.[14] The application of forceps has two consequences. First, traction is applied to the skull and not to the shoulders, neck and mouth, all of which may be damaged by the aforementioned maneuvers. Second, the Piper forceps protect against decompression injury that may occur with crowning—especially in the premature breech.

Since the head is usually tightly applied to the maternal soft tissue, it is important for the operator to insert fingers into the vagina to protect the mother. In view of the shape of the shank the forceps should be inserted with the shank and handle below the horizontal. The obstetrician may have to be on one knee as the assistant supports the infant and keeps the cord out of the way. The right (superior) blade is inserted first so that the handles do not have to be crossed. The blades are locked and downward traction continued as the head

is delivered in flexion, and finally the handles of the forceps are raised upward.

It is important to emphasize that gentleness at this stage is most important—more so than timing. If necessary the nose and oropharynx can be cleared of secretions with a bulb syringe. It is easy to err by applying the forceps when the head is not well down in the pelvis and flexed. In these situations, a high forceps delivery is being attempted. During the delivery, gentle suprapubic pressure will aid in flexion of the head, if necessary. Excessive fundal pressure may cause deflexion.

Approximately one third of all infants in breech presentation will be premature, and the proper management of the premature breech can be an enigma. A most difficult decision is the correct fetal weight at which to perform a routine cesarean section. Until more statistics are available it is difficult to recommend a lower limit of gestational age or fetal size below which routine cesarean section should not be considered. In our experience that limit currently lies between 1000 and 1200 grams.

The cervix is the main problem with a premature breech. If a vaginal delivery is to be attempted, the delivery room should be equipped to perform Dührssen's incisions.

Summary

Evaluation of a breech presentation is a significant challenge to the obstetrician. It is the physician's obligation to bring to bear all available information and aids so that as normal labor and delivery as possible are ensured. It must be emphasized that there is no one single technique that will guarantee a safe vaginal delivery. A poor breech score is a helpful tool and a clear indication for cesarean section, while a good score is no guarantee of a normal labor and delivery. In regard to x-ray pelvimetry, abnormal morphology and small measurements are indications for abdominal delivery, while a normal pelvis may still produce a poor result unless all parameters are carefully studied.

The occurrence of a dysfunctional labor is always disconcerting, whether it is an abnormality of dilatation or descent. The association of a dysfunctional labor with a breech presentation is ominous. The use of an oxytocic in such circumstances is hazardous to the fetus and should be avoided.

There still is a place for the vaginal delivery of a term frank breech infant of average size. By utilizing the breech score and x-ray pelvimetry as described, closely scrutinizing the Friedman labor curve, avoiding oxytocics, employing the aforementioned indications for cesarean section and electronic fetal monitoring, it is possible to identify those infants that can be safely delivered by the vaginal route.

It should be emphasized that no protocol is a substitute for good clinical judgment. All such protocols are guidelines and cannot serve as a crutch or as a cookbook approach to obstetric management. All factors must be considered, such as the presence of diabetes, hypertension, uterine myomas and especially the personal experience of the obstetrician. The individual who rarely delivers a breech by the vaginal route may cause an additional hazard to the mother and/or the infant, and therefore may be an indication for cesarean section.

REFERENCES

1. Alexopoulos, K. A.: The importance of breech delivery in the pathogenesis of brain damage. Clin. Pediatr. 12:248, 1973.
2. Bird, C. C. and McElin, T. W.: 500 consecutive term breech deliveries. Obstet. Gynecol. 35:45, 1970.
3. Bird, C. C. and McElin, T. W.: A six-year prospective study of term breech deliveries utilizing the Zatuchni-Andros prognostic scoring index. Am. J. Gynecol. 121:551, 1975.
4. Brenner, W. E., Bruce, R. D. and Hendricks, C. H.: The characteristics and perils of breech presentations. Am. J. Obstet. Gynecol. 118:700, 1974.
5. Chez, R. A., Lovinsky, J. J., Weingold, A. B. and Andros, G. J.: Management of breech presentations. Contemporary Ob-Gyn. 10:118, 1977.
6. Cruikshank, D. P., and Pitkin, R. M.: Delivery of the premature breech. Obstet. Gynecol. 50:367, 1977.
7. Douglas, R. G. and Stromme, W. B.: Operative Obstetrics, 3rd ed. New York, Appleton-Century-Crofts, 1976.
8. Fiann, S.: Fetal mortality and morbidity following breech delivery. Acta Obstet. Gynecol. Scand. (Suppl.) 56, 1976.
9. Friedman, E. A., Schtleben, M. R. and Bresky, P. A.: Dysfunctional labor: XI. Long-term effects on infant. Am. J. Obstet. Gynecol. 127:779, 1977.
10. Friedman, E. A.: Labor Clinical Evaluation and Management. New York, Appleton-Century-Crofts, 1967.
11. Johnson, C. E.: Breech presentation at term. Am. J. Obstet. Gynecol. 106:865, 1970.
12. Lesinski, J.: High risk pregnancy. Obstet. Gynecol. 46:599, 1975.
13. Lyons, E. R. and Papsis, F. R.: Cesarean section in the management of breech presentation. Am. J. Obstet. Gynecol. 130:558, 1978.
14. Milner, R. T. G.: Neonatal mortality of breech deliveries with and without forceps to the aftercoming head. Br. J. Obstet. Gynecol. 82:783, 1975.
15. Muller, P. F., Campbell, H. E., Graham, W. E. et al.: Perinatal factors and their relationship to mental retardation and other parameters of development. Am. J. Obstet. Gynecol. 109:1205, 1971.
16. Neilson, D. R.: Management of the large breech infant. Am. J. Obstet. Gynecol. 107:345, 1970.
17. O'Leary, J. A.: Criteria for the management of the term breech: a preliminary report. Obstet. Gynecol. 53:341, 1979.
18. O'Leary, J. A.: Abnormal presentations. *In* Aladjem, S. (ed.): Obstetrical Practice. St. Louis, C. V. Mosby Co., 1980.
19. Pritchard, J. A. and McDonald, P. C.: Williams Obstetrics, 15th ed. New York, Appleton-Century-Crofts, 1974.
20. Rovinsky, J. J., Miller, J. A. and Kaplan, S.: Management of breech presentations at term. Am. J. Obstet. Gynecol. 115:497, 1973.
21. Smith, R. S. and Aldham, R. R.: Breech delivery. Obstet. Gynecol. 36:151, 1970.
22. Todd, W. D. and Steer, C. M.: Term breech: review of 1006 term breech deliveries. Obstet. Gynecol. 22:583, 1963.
23. Wheeler, T. and Greene, K.: Fetal heart rate monitoring during breech labor. Br. J. Obstet. Gynecol. 82:208, 1975.
24. Wright, R. C.: Reduction of perinatal mortality and morbidity in breech delivery through routine use of cesarean section. Obstet. Gynecol. 14:758, 1959.

Editorial Comment

There has been a gradual change in our thinking over the past decade in how best to manage the patient with a breech presentation. This change has occurred when clinical investigators identified that the outcome for the newborn from breech delivery differs from that of vertex delivery and that breech delivery may result in permanent damage to the baby. Two additional influences include the expectation of patients for a perfect result as well as a change in the medical-legal climate in this country. The practicing obstetrician who was trained more than 15 years ago will continue to selectively deliver the breech baby vaginally; however, those practicing obstetricians trained during the past 5 years will, in general, perform cesarean sections on most breech presentations, since their manual dexterity experience and thinking differ from that of others.

A controversy immediately emerges in residency training programs, since most residents want the challenge of a breech vaginal delivery. It is considered one of the more difficult to perform and offers an opportunity for clinical showmanship. This controversy that confronts the young obstetrician presents problems not only for the singleton in breech presentation but also for the second twin that is a breech. Should the delivery be by the vaginal or abdominal route? It is obvious that if we have obstetricians currently in practice who do not have expertise in breech delivery, then the second twin may indeed have a possibility of higher morbidity. Some centers in the country now encourage a cesarean section for the second twin if it is breech presentation. I never thought the time would come when a second twin would be considered for a cesarean section, but that time has now arrived in the 1980s. Cesarean section may be appropriate if the obstetrician feels uncomfortable in doing a vaginal breech delivery.

The challenge to the modern-day obstetrician should be to anticipate problems and prevent injuries or death in both mother and infant. In order to achieve this goal, care in each case must be highly individualized and no overall rule holds true. The difficulty we now face is that the well-trained obstetrician-gynecologist, no matter how clever and competent, will occasionally have a bad result from a breech delivered vaginally. This can be a major hazard for the infant and certainly opens the door for medical-legal implications if these babies are afflicted or cannot function to expected capacity. Since even the best obstetrician sometimes has a bad result, is this acceptable?

The authors of this chapter on breech delivery have posed specific issues for the breech presentation but have not promoted cesarean section for all breech presentations. They have identified the neonatal morbidity in the breech as approaching 15 per cent and stated that serious morbidity may be as high as 7 per cent. The morbidity in the offspring is underlined by the fact that one fourth (25 per cent) of all children who were breech deliveries must repeat grades in school as contrasted by one twelfth (8 per cent) of children with vertex deliveries. The central nervous system is the most vulnerable in the breech.

There are specific criteria that should be fulfilled for both the mother and fetus before the management method is decided for a breech delivery. Said another way, there are certain criteria that dictate a cesarean section, some of which are: a large breech baby (more than 3800 g), a small baby (under 1500 g), an incomplete breech, an unflexed fetal head and lack of obstetrician experience in breech deliveries. Some authors have pointed to the Zatuchni-Andros breech scoring index as an aid in helping them determine those patients who should be considered for a cesarean section. This scoring index is based upon parity, weeks of gestation, estimated fetal weight, dilatation and station and whether or not the patient has delivered a previous breech. It tends to have a weighted value for the primigravida toward a cesarean section even though the literature shows no difference between the primigravida and the multigravida patient for breech delivery complications. There is lower newborn morbidity if Piper forceps are used for the aftercoming head.

Breech presentation is more common in the low birth weight baby (30 per cent) and at most in 8 per cent of the total obstetric population. It has been generally accepted that the small baby (under 1500 g) usually benefits by cesarean section, which leaves 70 per cent of the breeches to cope with. From this remaining group another 25 per cent of infants in breech would most likely be delivered by cesarean section because of macrosomia or relative cephalopelvic disproportion. This leaves a remaining 40 per cent for whom management decisions need to be made. Out of this group 6 per cent will have congenital anomalies and some of these will be diagnosed antepartum and no cesarean section will be done. Thinking in the early 1980s is that a decision must be made in approximately 30 per cent of breeches, as decisions in the rest are being made for us on the basis of various other problems and situations in which the choice is obvious, such as a 4 per cent incidence of cord prolapse in the footling breech. Today most obstetricians agree there are specific criteria that must be fulfilled before vaginal delivery of a breech can be achieved, but this decision is not as ominous as it seems since it needs to be made in only one third of all breeches. If all breeches were delivered by cesarean section, the cesarean section rate would increase by only 2 per cent.

It should be underscored that if the individual is to do a breech delivery, one of the most essential prerequisites for that individual is expertise. If we diminish the total number of breech deliveries available for our residency training programs, then how are we going to adequately train obstetricians for the future? As of now a cesarean section cannot always be done instantly in every hospital in this country, and this underscores the need for adequate training for all obstetricians.

It is necessary that at least two skilled individuals be in the delivery room for the breech delivery and that one of them should know how to resuscitate the baby. Maximum cooperation of the patient is necessary if a pudendal block is used, but a qualified anesthesiologist should be present to administer "crash" halothane anesthesia in case of a trapped head or shoulders. Piper forceps should be used to protect the head, and the breech will be delivered without undue stress over a generous episiotomy.

Major tragedies are prevented by anticipation of problems and situations at the actual time of the delivery of the shoulders and head. There may be undue tugging and pulling, nuchal arms may be present, fetal distress may become manifest by cord compression and use of anesthesia may be less than desirable; hence, situations are often compounded. It is possible that excessive pressure can cause trauma to the spinal cord by overzealous rotation and traction to delivery of the shoulders and head. Cord trauma apparently is more common than we realize. The reason it has not been identified extensively is that most pathologists doing the morbid pathology do not dissect the cord critically in the breech delivery to look for contusion, separation and transection.

If the head and shoulders are trapped, deep halothane anesthesia should be first tried and if it fails, consider pushing the baby back into the vagina and uterus to relieve pressure, then do an immediate cesarean section. I personally did not think that this was possible, but at one of the perinatal seminar meetings, an individual in the audience stated that he had done this twice.

The controversy of management in the breech still remains as one of the greatest in obstetrics today, but we believe that this is a discussion that is gradually diminishing as fewer and fewer obstetricians deliver breeches vaginally or are competent to do so. Indeed, it is a dilemma as well as a controversy.

7

Identification and Management of Intrauterine Growth Retardation and the Post-Term Pregnancy

Alternative Points of View

by Leon I. Mann and David A. Baker
by James E. Thomasson and Harlan R. Giles
by Helmuth Vorherr and Robert H. Messer
by John A. Widness and William Oh

Editorial Comment

Identification and Management of Intrauterine Growth Retardation and the Postdate Pregnancy

Leon I. Mann, M.D.
University of Vermont College of Medicine

David A. Baker, M.D.
State University of New York at Stony Brook

Approximately 15 per cent of all pregnancies will be associated with the two problems of intrauterine growth retardation (IUGR) and post-term pregnancy. The incidence of IUGR, or smallness for gestational age, as it is more appropriately termed clinically, is 3 to 4 per cent.[1-3] When objective evaluation for gestational age by clinical and neurologic examination of all low birth weight neonates is conducted, and the neonate is properly classified from weight–gestational age curves, between 25 and 50 per cent will be determined to be small for gestational age (SGA) (less than tenth percentile, term or preterm) rather than average for gestational age (AGA) (tenth to ninetieth percentile, prior to term). In contrast to the AGA neonate, who is premature in terms of organ function—specifically the lung surfactant system—the SGA neonate is generally mature. The AGA neonate is most commonly the product of a gestation complicated by premature rupture of membranes or preterm labor and is primarily at risk during the neonatal period for hyaline membrane disease and the respiratory distress syndrome. The pregnancy complicated by IUGR is primarily at risk during the antepartum and intrapartum periods for fetal death because fetal oxygenation and substrate availability may be compromised irreversibly. Low birth weight in both AGA and SGA infants is associated with 70 to 80 per cent of all perinatal deaths.[4] IUGR has been reported to account for 15 to 20 per cent of total perinatal mortality and approximately one third of fetal mortality.

The postdate condition is reported to occur in 10 to 12 per cent of pregnancies.[5] "Postdatism" has been defined as the pregnancy that exceeds 294 days or 42 weeks from the first day of the last menstrual period. Eighty per cent of births will occur two weeks before or after the expected date of confinement, which leaves a 10 per cent chance of prior-to-term or postdate delivery. Because of frequent menstrual or ovulatory irregularities, many pregnancies calculated as postdate are in fact at term. Of those pregnancies that are truly postdate, some 20 to 40 per cent will result in the birth of a postmature neonate. It is the postmature fetus that is at increased risk of death due to impaired oxygenation and substrate availability. The prenatal mortality rate has been reported to increase some threefold to fivefold beyond 42 weeks, depending upon the parity and associated maternal complications.

Review of referral practices to the Maternal-Fetal Medicine Service within our perinatal regional program revealed that one third of referrals were for either the suspected diagnosis of IUGR or post-term pregnancy. One quarter to one third of our perinatal deaths during the past few years have been associated with one or another of the complications of IUGR and post-term pregnancy. It is obvious that the pregnancy complicated by either of these problems requires consultation with and supervision of a properly trained and experienced specialist in maternal-fetal medicine who functions within a perinatal center in which adequate facilities, personnel and equipment are available for proper diagnostic evaluation and management.

Pathophysiology

Pregnancies complicated by IUGR and the post-term syndrome have in common a similar pathophysiologic explanation. In both, substrate availability and uptake by the fetus is compromised so that continued fetal growth and eventually sustenance is in jeopardy. The mechanism by which substrate availability is impaired is different in the two conditions as is the time period of insult.

The IUGR fetus is most commonly affected by prolonged chronic nutritive deprivation due to inadequate uterine blood flow (hypertensive cardiovascular disease) or inadequate basic substrates, glucose, amino acids and fatty acids (malnutrition). IUGR is infrequently (3 to 5 per cent) associated with chronic infections (TORCH) that interfere with adequate placental transport. In the late stages of chronic nutritive deprivation, or in the more severe acute complications that develop late in pregnancy, the respiratory function of the placenta may be additionally compromised and fetal oxygenation jeopardized. The product of such a pregnancy is usually well developed but undergrown for its gestational age (low birth weight and small for gestational age) and is at increased risk for perinatal hypoxia at delivery because of further compromise of fetal oxygenation by the intermittent interruption of placental blood flow caused by labor contractions. Concern for the postdate pregnancy and the postmature neonate that may result from such a pregnancy involves the placenta that has outlived its ability to provide adequate substrate for fetal growth and sustenance. While maternal nutrition and uterine blood flow may be adequate, the nutritive and respiratory functions of the placenta are compromised. The postmature neonate appears, therefore, well developed and fully grown but wasted and potentially hypoxic and acidotic from events surrounding the perinatal period. Interference with placental transport in the postdate pregnancy has a shorter time frame than the more chronic IUGR problem. Proper identification and management of both of these situations requires an understanding and appreciation of these basic pathophysiologic observations.

Identification

With regular menstrual cycles prior to conception, accuracy of last menstrual period, uterine size–date consistency during antenatal visits, and proper dating of fetal milestones, such as quickening and audibility of heart tones, identification of the postdate pregnancy is not difficult. Upon completion of the 42nd week (294 days), the pregnancy is considered post-term. Often, however, the last menstrual period is in doubt, particularly when the patient presents for the first visit late in the pregnancy. When such a situation arises, or a discrepancy in size and date exists, serial ultrasonographic determination of biparietal diameter, measurement of abdominal circumference ratios and calculation of fetal weight[6] should be done. Twenty to 40 per cent of postdate pregnancies are, in fact, not post-term but are considered so because proper evaluation of fetal growth and maturation was not obtained. It is rarely necessary to perform amniocentesis for analysis of amniotic fluid for fetal lung maturation studies in postdate gestations (see later discussion).

In contrast to the ease of identification of the postdate pregnancy, the pregnancy complicated by IUGR is most difficult to identify. In our large series of 154 SGA neonates delivered of 148 pregnancies over a period of 3 years only one third were identified antenatally.[3] The key to identification seems to rest with an improved awareness on the part of obstetricians that the problem exists and that they should consider IUGR in size-date discrepancies. Of importance toward improved identification is a careful screening at the first antepartum visit for historical and previous obstetric information that may place the patient at risk for IUGR. These factors include a history of hypertensive cardiovascular disease of pregnancy, chronic medical problems such as diabetes and renal disease, previous delivery of a low birth weight or SGA infant or obstetric wastage, a history of smoking, alcohol or drug addiction and others.[3] Development of any of these medical problems during the pregnancy must be carefully evaluated. The female who is underweight or poorly nourished or both must be followed closely for adequate weight gain and properly counseled as to protein supplementation during her pregnancy. Size-date discrepancies and failure to document continued uterine growth or an increase in estimated fetal weight over a 2- to 4-week period should alert the obstetrician to the possibility of IUGR. Careful evaluation for IUGR should be carried out by serial ultrasonographic diameter/abdominal circumference ratios and calculated fetal weight. When charts were reviewed as to size-date discrepancies, nearly 50 per cent showed a failure of uterine growth over an interval of 1 to 4 months.[3]

Confirmation of Diagnosis

Confirmation of the diagnosis of post-term pregnancy can be obtained by serial ultrasonographic biparietal diameter, abdominal circumference ratios and fetal weight calculations. A decrease in the weekly increment of the growth of biparietal diameter occurs toward term so that the accuracy of these measurements in dating the gestation at this time depends on serial measurements. The variability of total uterine volume is also greatest at term. Single determinations would therefore be difficult to differentiate during the 40th to the 44th week of gestation. Wider discrepancies of size-date relationships are easier to solve by these ultrasonographic techniques.

Serial ultrasonographic biparietal diameter measurements are essential for the confirmation and proper diagnosis of IUGR. Two curves have been reported and consist of an early (low profile) and a late (late flattening) onset pattern.[3, 7] In the early pattern, the biparietal diameter measurement is consistently below two standard deviations from the normal for the stated gestational age and may later in pregnancy show a further increase in this discrepancy. Nutritional deprivation, chronic infection or genetic problems should be considered in such a situation. The late pattern reveals a biparietal diameter measurement consistent with gestational age up until 32 to 36 weeks of gestation, when the discrepancy between the abnormal biparietal diameter and the normal begins to exceed two standard deviations. The weight of the neonate will be less than the 10th percentile (low birth weight, small for gestational age), but its head circumference may be in the 20th to 60th percentile. This brain-sparing pattern of late onset IUGR is most found in association with maternal hypertensive cardiovascular disease. It has been explained by a redistribution of the fetal cardiac output in favor of the brain in response to chronic fetal hypoxia.[8] A single biparietal diameter measurement can be misleading and serial ultrasonographic studies are mandatory. If the patient is first seen or the diagnosis of IUGR is entertained late in pregnancy, a single biparietal diameter measurement may be incorrectly thought to represent a normal measurement at an earlier gestational age. A repeat biparietal diameter by ultrasonography should be obtained in this situation and an amniocentesis performed in order to obtain an analysis of amniotic fluid for fetal lung maturation. Serial 24-hour urinary collections for estriol determinations can be helpful in confirming the diagnosis of IUGR. Quite commonly, these values will be low, reflecting a smaller fetal placental-endocrine unit. This obviously limits their ability to interpret fetal condition. Newer laboratory tests such as qualitative amniotic fluid determinations have been suggested for detection of the IUGR pregnancy.[9]

Management

Once the diagnosis of a postdate pregnancy is confirmed, the goal of management is to deliver the patient at the most propitious moment. Ideally, this should involve the spontaneous onset of labor with a fetus in good condition and delivery by the vaginal route. Meddlesome obstetrics should be minimized in this situation. The postdate pregnancy may be continued and the onset of spontaneous labor expected up to the 44th week as long as the condition of the fetus has been properly evaluated and no evidence of stress determined. Associated medical or obstetric complications of a chronic nature, whether stable or not, or the onset of new complications such as toxemia are an indication for delivery prior to completion of the 42nd week. This may require induction of labor with delivery vaginally or by cesarean section.

The key to management rests with serial evaluation of fetal condition. Fetal condition can be evaluated by means of serial fetal activity–oxytocin challenge tests (FA–OCT; nonstress or stress monitoring) (see Chapter 1).[10, 11] Six to 10 fetal movements per 20 minutes with greater than 50 per cent associated with a fetal reactive tachycardia or a negative OCT have been reported[12] to represent results consistent with a stable fetal condition in greater than 95 per cent of cases. Any deviations from these normal results should lead the obstetrician to consider delivery within 24 to 48 hours. If amnioscopy can be performed, the presence of meconium-stained fluid would also represent an indication for induction of labor within 24 hours. A fall in serial 24-hour urinary estriol levels of greater than 40 per cent to an absolute value of less than 12 mg similarly represents an indication for delivery.

Induction of labor should be planned over a period of 2 to 4 days and should involve 6 hours a day of pitocin infusion beginning with a dilute solution. Continuous external fetal heart rate–uterine contraction monitoring (FHR–UC) must be performed simultaneously. Any observed ominous deceleration patterns should be followed by cesarean section if scalp blood pH testing cannot be performed. Under such induction circumstances the patient is maintained well hydrated and well rested, and artificial rupture of membranes is used as a last means of induction or when adequate effacement and dilatation and descent have occurred. Hyperstimulation, tachysystole and tetany must be avoided under such circumstances. Delivery in most of the patients considered postdate can be accomplished vaginally.

Once the suspicion of IUGR has been confirmed by serial ultrasonographic biparietal diameter determination and evidence of fetal lung maturity obtained by amniocentesis and surfactant evaluation, management involves the proper timing of delivery. A review of our collected cases indicated a significantly higher fetal death rate than neonatal death rate in this condition. All but one of seven fetal deaths occurred in pregnancies beyond 37 weeks.[3] Our protocol, therefore, is to initiate labor if necessary by the 38th week when the diagnosis of IUGR is confirmed and fetal lung maturity evident. If the associated maternal complications such as hypertensive cardiovascular disease are unstable, delivery may be necessary before 38 weeks and, on occasion, prior to evidence of fetal lung maturity. Often acceleration of fetal lung maturity and acceleration of brain function occur in the chronically distressed IUGR fetus.[13] Amniocentesis for evaluation of fetal lung maturity, therefore, may be performed in certain cases beginning at the 32nd to 34th week. Serial FA–OCTs must be performed at intervals determined by the stability of the clinical situation. These tests should be performed not less than twice weekly under any circumstance. Serial estriol determinations are often low-normal or low but can be of help if a decrease of 40 per cent or greater is documented. Other reported tests, such as of human placental lactogen, do not add more information than those described and are not used routinely in our Maternal-Fetal Medicine Service. Regardless of the stability of the associated maternal clinical condition and of fetal condition, the possibility of additional complications that may arise insidiously or acutely has led us to recommend delivery not later than the 38th week of pregnancy. As most of these patients will be in the period between the 36th to 38th week of pregnancy, a pitocin induction over two to four days with constant fetal monitoring and the aforementioned precautions is mandatory. Failed induction, evidence of fetal distress and other problems result in a cesarean section rate of approximately 25 per cent with this management protocol for IUGR.

Delivery

Delivery in both the postdate pregnancy and the pregnancy complicated with IUGR should be within a facility equipped with modern intrapartum monitoring equipment, including FHR–UC monitors and fetal scalp blood pH capability. In both situations there is increased risk for ominous decelerations that require scalp blood pH determinations for discrimination.[14, 15] The Perinatal Center Level 3 or in some instances Level 2 hospitals within a regional perinatal program are best able to handle these problems. Neonatologists should be alerted and in attendance at the delivery so that adequate preparation for immediate resuscitation and care of the newborn is available. Meconium detected during the intrapartum period should be extracted at birth by immediate intubation and suction of the pharynx to avoid aspiration and potential meconium pneumonitis. The newborn should be taken immediately to the neonatal intensive care unit under conditions that avoid any exposure to cold. Infants with either condition, but particularly the IUGR neonate, are at risk for hypoglycemia due to inadequate glycogen reserve within the liver parenchyma. Serial blood glucose determinations must be carefully monitored during the first 24 hours. Other newborn complications have been presented and reviewed previously.[3]

Conclusion

Following objective clinical and neurologic evaluation of the newborn, it is not uncommon to find that the fetus was in fact not postdate and postmature or small for gestational age. It is our opinion that it is better to be overly suspicious and cautious in the management of these two obstetric problems and err on the side of overdiagnosing than to underdiagnose with a resultant increase in fetal and perinatal mortality. With proper identification and management of the pregnancy that is post-term or complicated with IUGR, perinatal mortality ir it should not differ significantly from that in a low-risk obstetric population.

REFERENCES

1. Mann, L. I., Tejani, N. A., and Weiss, R. R.: Antenatal diagnosis and management of the small for gestational age fetus. Am. J. Obstet. Gynecol. 120:995, 1974.
2. Tejani, N. A., Mann, L. I., and Weiss, R. R.: Antenatal diagnosis and management of the small for gestational age fetus. Obstet. Gynecol. 47:31, 1976.
3. Tajani, N. A., and Mann, L. I.: Diagnosis and management of the small for gestational age fetus. Clin. Obstet. Gynecol. 20:943, 1977.
4. Mann, O. I., Baker, D. A., and Gallant, J. A.: The problem of low birth weight. Contemp. Ob/Gyn 8:141, 1981.
5. Vorherr, H.: Placental insufficiency in relation to postterm pregnancy and fetal postmaturity. Am. J. Obstet. Gynecol. 123:67, 1975.
6. Ott, W. J.: Clinical application of fetal weight determination by real-time U/S measurements. Obstet. Gynecol. 57:758, 1981.
7. Campbell, S.: The assessment of fetal development by diagnostic ultrasound. Clin. Perinatol. 1:507, 1974.
8. Mann, L. I.: Effect of hypoxia on fetal cephalic blood flow, cephalic metabolism and the EEG. Exp. Neurol. 29:336, 1970.
9. Manning, F. A., Hill, L. M. and Platt, L. D.: Qualitative amniotic fluid volume determination by ultrasound: Antepartum detection of IUGR. Am. J. Obstet. Gynecol. 139:254, 1981.
10. Bhakthavathsalan, A., Mann, L. I., Tejani, N. A. et al.: Correlation of the oxytocin challenge test with perinatal outcome. Obstet. Gynecol. 48:552, 1976.
11. Freeman, R. K., Garite, T. J., Modanlou, H., Dorchester, W., Rommal, C. and Devaney, M.: Postdate pregnancy: utilization of contraction stress testing for primary fetal surveillance. Am. J. Obstet. Gynecol. 140:128, 1981
12. Rouchard, F., Schifrin, B., Goupil, F. et al.: Nonstressed fetal heart rate monitoring in the antepartum period. Am. J. Obstet. Gynecol. 126:699, 1976.
13. Gould, J. B., Block, L. and Kulovich, M. V.: The relationship between accelerated pulmonary maturity and accelerated neurological maturity in certain chronically stressed pregnancies. Am. J. Obstet. Gynecol. 127:181, 1977.
14. Tejani, N. A., Mann, L. I., Bhakthavathsalan, A. et al.: Correlation of fetal heart rate-uterine contraction patterns with fetal scalp blood pH. Obstet. Gynecol. 46:392, 1975.
15. Tejani, N. A., Mann, L. I., Bhakthavathsalan, A. et al.: Correlation of fetal heart rate patterns and fetal pH with neonatal outcome. Obstet. Gynecol. 48:460, 1976.

Identification and Management of Intrauterine Growth Retardation

James E. Thomasson, M.D.
Harlan R. Giles, M.D.
University of Arizona Health Sciences Center

As a result of an early report concerning undergrown term infants by McBurney[1] and large retrospective studies by Lubchenco[2] and Gruenwald,[3] the attention of obstetricians and neonatologists has turned away from a total emphasis on *quantity* of intrauterine fetal existence and toward the *quality* of this existence. The once widely accepted assignment of gestational age based on arbitrary weight criteria has been largely abandoned and replaced by a resurgence of emphasis on early clinical evalution, ultrasonographic cephalometry and clinical and neurologic evaluation of the newborn.[4]

A closer look at the low birth weight infant—less than 2500 g—using the gestational age as calculated independently reveals two distinct populations. The first has a decrease in the quantity of intrauterine life, or true prematurity. For the second population, the quality of intrauterine life is suboptimal; it is this group of fetally deprived infants that are said to represent intrauterine growth retardation (IUGR).

Application of the intrauterine growth curves established by Lubchenco or Gruenwald allows diagnosis of IUGR at any gestational age to be made easily by the neonatologist. Unfortunately, diagnosis after delivery of the infant does little to reduce the high perinatal morbidity and mortality associated with this entity. Prenatal diagnosis based strictly on fundal height, estimated fetal weight and menstrual history has failed to recognize IUGR in 40 to 90 per cent of affected pregnancies.

Two types of growth retardation were originally proposed by Gruenwald[3] and have been amplified by numerous other investigators.[5-7] In one group of IUGR infants, the reduction in growth is primarily in terms of weight; crown-rump or overall infant lengths approach normal and the infant appears "wasted." These infants characteristically exhibit rapid postnatal weight gain and usually follow the normal infant and childhood growth pattern. It is presumed that the poor fetal nutrition in these infants developed late in gestation and that they possess a normal complement of nutritionally deprived cells. These infants have been described as having a low ponderal index (the ratio of birth weight in grams times 100 divided by crown-heel length in centimeters).[8]

The second type of IUGR infant has been described as being "short for dates."[6] Here, the total body growth of the infant is retarded. This appears to begin earlier in gestation and to be associated with an overall reduction in cellular number in many organs.[9] Eventual growth and development tends to remain in the same low percentiles exhibited at birth.[6]

Etiology

Intrauterine growth–retarded infants (using the criteria of Gruenwald) include 2 to 3 per cent of all newborns. Although the cause of this disorder is not completely understood, it does appear to be associated with chronic fetal malnutrition, hypoxia or both. In spite of the lack of definite cause-and-effect relationship, certain clinical states have shown an association with growth retardation. Unfortunately, a large percentage of intrauterine growth–retarded progeny are the result of an otherwise normal pregnancy.

Use of the ponderal index and the definition of short for gestational age infants does little to clarify the etiology of the disorder, as both types of IUGR can be seen in different patients with the same underlying pregnancy risk factors. This may mean that the disorder is similar but the timing—early versus late in gestation—is different.

The single most important reason for development of IUGR is fetal malnutrition. This can result from chronic maternal vascular disease as seen in chronic maternal hypertension, pregnancy-induced hypertension and diabetes mellitus. It is also seen with cyanotic heart disease, collagen vascular disease, severe maternal anemia and sickling disorders. In all of these conditions, the presumed mechanism is via reduced maternal blood flow to the placental bed. A concomitant increase in antepartum fetal death and intrapartum distress is seen in association with reduction of uterine perfusion in these maternal complications. Animal experiments have documented "runting" in preparations with compromised uterine circulations.[10]

Genetic factors may also be related to retardation of fetal growth in a relatively small number of cases. Growth retardation frequently coexists with trisomies of chromosomes 13 to 15, 18 or 21. Chromosomal analysis has occasionally been used[11] via amniocentesis in the third trimester to exclude chromosomal aberration in the clinically retarded fetus. Other presumably inherited developmental defects such as phocomelia and anencephaly may be the explanation for subnormal fetal growth. A higher percentage of short for gestational age infants is predictably found in this group of patients.

The degree of growth retardation associated with intrauterine infections such as rubella, herpes simplex, toxoplasmosis, syphilis and cytomegalic inclusion disease varies both with the etiologic agent and the duration of intrauterine infection. Infections during the period of organogenesis have the highest rate of morbidity and mortality as well as growth retardation.

External influences are difficult to evaluate as they relate to the fetal environment. Certain situations such as high altitude of residence,[12] maternal smoking[6, 13] and poor maternal nutrition as measured by weight gain[14] have all been associated with poor fetal growth, although isolation of such variables for analysis of causation is obviously impossible

Drugs taken by the mother have also been implicated. Immunosuppressive agents produce IUGR in animals[15] and presumably also in humans. The fetal alcohol syndrome has been well characterized over the past 2 to 3 years and it is associated with IUGR in over 95 per cent of cases reported.

Diagnosis

Most retrospective studies in which the neonatologist diagnoses IUGR show that the diagnosis was not clinically suspected by the obstetrician in 40 to 90 per cent of cases. This fact suggests the necessity for either a much higher index of suspicion (with use of clinical tools or laboratory and diagnostic tests or both for examination of growth) if the pick-up rate is to be increased.

The index of suspicion can be raised by a thorough history and physical examination, knowledge of the etiologic factors associated with IUGR and routine emphasis on clinical evaluation of gestational age at each prenatal visit.

A history of hypertension, diabetes, collagen vascular disease, maternal smoking or alcohol abuse would place the fetus at an increased risk of growth retardation. A past obstetric history revealing pregnancy complications, or a specific history of a previous infant with IUGR, can be very helpful in predicting fetal growth in the present gestation.

Establishment of gestational age is of paramount importance. This should be accomplished as early as possible in the pregnancy. The date of the last menstrual period should be determined with precision, and possible confounding factors such as recent use of oral contraceptives, history of anovulatory episodes or others should be considered. First trimester clinical examination and auscultation of the fetal heart (first with Doppler technique at 9 to 12 menstrual weeks and then by fetascope at 18 to 22 menstrual weeks) can help to identify those pregnancies with size-date discrepancies.

While the estimation of gestational age by fundal height can be fraught with error, a general rule we have used successfully is that "the fundal height in centimeters above the symphysis pubis is equal to gestational age in weeks between 18 and 28 weeks' gestation." This is particularly helpful if the patient is consistently evaluated by the same examiner. If gestational age and clinical size discrepancy develop during the course of prenatal care and the size lags more than three weeks behind expected growth, IUGR is suspected.

In those patients who have shown early size-date discrepancy of suboptimal uterine growth, the use of ultrasonography has been of increasing benefit for diagnosis. The early use of ultrasonographic biparietal diameter[16] has, with regional modification, become the standard for evaluation of gestational age by ultrasonography. Two evaluations between 22 and 28 weeks of menstrual age are the most reliable for assignment of gestational age by this technique.

With the increasing resolution capability of ultrasonic diagnostic equipment, this modality has become considerably more important in the evaluation of fetal growth. In a more or less temporal sequence, serial biparietal diameters,[16] abdominal circumference,[17, 18] cephalic circumference[19, 20] and, more recently, brain weight and ratio of brain weight to body weight have all been used to monitor intrauterine fetal growth. While the optimal measurement is not universally agreed upon, it is obvious that serial examinations are necessary for the diagnosis of growth retardation. Although this would appear to greatly simplify the problem, one nagging question persists: Which patients should receive the chosen ultrasonographic examination? One could, as recommended by Scheer,[21] obtain a scan on every obstetric patient, or one could scan only those patients with clinically suspected IUGR. The latter approach has, however, historically involved underestimation of the true incidence of IUGR. It has been our policy to liberally use ultrasonographic fetal evaluation for those patients who are historically or clinically at high risk for IUGR. In addition, for those patients who do not maintain normal clinical growth or who have size-date discrepancies, serial ultrasonography is performed.

Management

Once the diagnosis of suspected IUGR is made, we believe that this pregnancy is best followed by a single clinician, preferably in a perinatal center specializing in the high-risk patient. Consultation is frequently required with neonatologists, anesthesiologists, internists, cytogeneticists and virology laboratories. The patient is usually followed with weekly clinic visits and ultrasonography every two to four weeks to assess growth.

Evaluation in the remainder of the prenatal course is directed toward deciding the optimal time for delivery of this compromised infant. The balance between continuation of a pregnancy with documented fetal compromise and delivery of an immature infant is one requiring the utmost in individualization. Correction of the underlying maternal condition is rarely possible except in the case of nutritional deficiencies.

The capability for surveillance of the fetus in utero has expanded markedly over the past ten years. The fact that current literature continues to document efforts to improve current modalities and to suggest newer techniques points out the lack of agreement on a single test to follow the distressed or potentially distressed fetus. Most perinatologists would agree to the necessity of combining the various tests to assess the degree of compromise and plan delivery of an infant as soon as maturity can be documented or strong evidence for increasing distress is found.

Determination of urinary estriol levels has for years been the major test used for assessment of the fetus in utero. This test continues to have application, especially in the case of suspected IUGR. In our institution, however, we have replaced evaluation of urinary estriol levels with radioimmunoassay of unconjugated estriol for the purpose of surveillance of fetal metabolic status. A drop of 40 per cent from serial values obtained twice or thrice weekly is considered significant, but, because falsely low estriol levels occur frequently, an *immature* infant is never delivered for falling estriol level alone. Human placental lactogen has been used successfully by Spellacy[22] and others to predict the status of the fetus in utero. The 25 per cent false negativity and 50 per cent false positivity[23] requires, as with estriol, that this not become the sole means of monitoring these at-risk pregnancies.

Clinical experience by Hon and colleagues at the University of Southern California with fetal monitoring and the oxytocin challenge test (OCT) has made this the most commonly used test for evaluation of fetal status. Numerous other authors have confirmed the USC data and added refinements to the technique. This test, according to Freeman,[24] measures the respiratory reserve of the placenta. Although false-positive results have been reported in 25 to 40 per cent of patients, negative results have been highly reassuring if obtained weekly. False-negative results have been reported in less than 1 per cent of pregnancies in which the OCT was used as the sole criterion for intervention in high-risk pregnancies.[25]

Unstressed or baseline fetal monitoring has been investigated by several authors.[26-30] All of these authors suggest with high reliability that a fetus who shows good heart rate variability and accelerations with fetal movement will have a negative OCT and tolerate labor well. These nonstress tests may eventually become sufficiently predictive to eliminate the necessity for the OCT when the fetus is "reactive." We are currently combining the NST and the OCT and agree with published data that fetal reactivity on NST is rarely associated with either labor distress or an abnormal OCT.

A graphic approach to the delivery of a fetus with IUGR is depicted in Figure 1. With either falling estriol levels (more than 40 per cent decrease from previous values) or a positive OCT, amniocentesis is performed to document fetal maturity. Creatinine, uric acid ΔOD_{450}, and lecithin/sphingomyelin (L/S) ratio are obtained. Of primary importance is the L/S ratio. We currently use the method originally described by Gluck[31] without modification and agree with his contention that alteration of technique may require alteration in interpretation of results.[32] Avoidance of intrapartum asphyxia is of great importance in elimination of respiratory distress syndrome (RDS) in the neonate, even with mature L/S ratios.[32] We have had little experience with the foam stability, or "shake test," although others have reported good clinical correlation using this technique. Regardless of the test used, the IUGR infant generally exhibits precocious maturation of the L/S ratio presumably secondary to intrauterine stress.

In at least one case report,[11] amniocentesis has been used to obtain a karyotype of the infant with IUGR. Viral studies are probably also indicated at the same time, primarily for purposes of predicting the necessity for neonatal isolation.

Several long-term follow-up studies on IUGR infants have shown a high incidence of learning disabilities in these children.[33-35] This appears to occur even in those children with normal IQs by standard testing.[35] Learning disability has been found in 20 to 35 per cent of IUGR infants. Intrapartum compromise was not well controlled for in these series, but their findings suggest that allowing the fetus to remain in the intrauterine environment past the point of fetal lung maturity may be unwise.

The decision for delivery in the growth-retarded infant is based on the parameters listed in Figure 1. In addition, even in the patient who shows evidence of fetal growth retardation and normal OCT and estriol surveillance, amniocentesis is performed between 36 and 38 weeks and delivery effected with documentation of fetal lung maturity by an L/S ratio greater than 2.0. The method of delivery must be highly individualized. Vaginal delivery is attempted in those patients in whom labor can be easily initiated utilizing

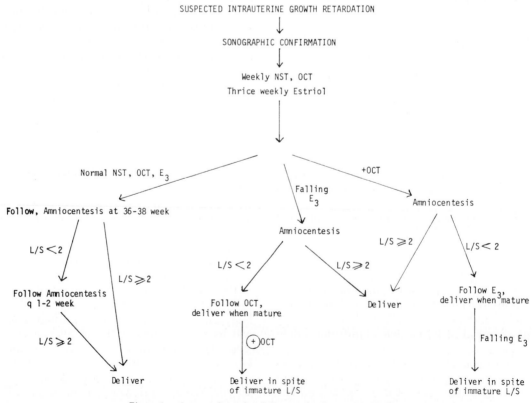

Figure 1. Approach to the delivery of a fetus with IUGR.

intravenous infusion of oxytocin. Intensive intrapartum fetal monitoring is mandatory via continuous techniques, since these infants have a high incidence of intrapartum asphyxia as evidenced by the increased frequency of ominous deceleration patterns and fetal acidosis.[36, 37] Fetal scalp pH measurements are used liberally as indicated.

If induction of labor is not easily accomplished, or if there is intrapartum evidence of acute fetal distress, operative intervention is rapidly undertaken. Regardless of the mode of delivery chosen, neonatologists should be present in the delivery suite. Aspiration of the oropharynx and nasopharynx prior to the delivery of the fetal body using a DeLee suction apparatus is strongly recommended for those infants with meconium-stained amniotic fluid.[36] The potential acute neonatal problems of asphyxia, hypoglycemia, hypocalcemia and meconium aspiration mandates the availability of a neonatal ICU nursery for these babies.

Summary

Management of intrauterine growth retardation requires knowledge of etiologic mechanisms, meticulous prenatal care, close fetal surveillance and atraumatic delivery to obtain the best possible outcome. This is best accomplished in a perinatal center with facilities for intensive obstetrical *and* neonatal care.

REFERENCES

1. McBurney, R. D.: The undernourished full term infant. West. J. Surg. Obstet. Gynecol. 55:363, 1947.
2. Lubchenco. L. O., Hansman, C., Dressler, M. and Boyd, E.: Intrauterine growth as estimated from live-born birth-weight data at 24 to 42 weeks of gestation. Pediatrics 32:793, 1963.
3. Gruenwald, P.: Growth of the human fetus. Am. J. Obstet. Gynecol. 94:1112, 1966.
4. Dubowitz, L. M. S., Dubowitz, V. and Goldberg, C.: Clinical assessment of gestational age in the newborn infant. J. Pediatr. 77:1, 1970.
5. Miller, H. D. and Hassanein, K.: Diagnosis of impaired fetal growth in newborn infants. Pediatrics 48:511, 1971.
6. Miller, H. C., Hassanein, K. and Hensleigh, P. A.: Fetal growth retardation in relation to maternal smoking and weight gain in pregnancy. Am. J. Obstet. Gynecol. 125:55, 1976.
7. Holmes, G. E., Miller, H. C., Hassanein, K., Lansky, S. B. and Goggin, J. E.: Postnatal somatic growth in infants with atypical fetal growth patterns. Am. J. Dis. Child. 131:1078, 1977.
8. Rohrer, F.: Der Index der Korperfulle als Mass des Ernahrungszustandes. Munch. Med. Wochenschr. 68:580, 1921.
9. Naeye, R. L.: Malnutrition. Arch. Pathol. 79:284, 1965.
10. Creasy, R. K., Barrett, C. T., de Swiet, M., Kahanpaa, K. V. and Rudolph, A. M.: Experimental intrauterine growth retardation in the sheep. Am. J. Obstet. Gynecol. 112:566, 1972.
11. Golbus, M. S., Hall, B. D. and Creasy, R. K.: Prenatal diagnosis of congenital anomalies in an intrauterine growth retarded fetus. Hum. Genet. 32:349, 1976.
12. McCullough, R. E., Reeves, J. T. and Liljegren, R. L.: Fetal growth retardation and increased infant mortality at high altitude. Arch. Environ. Health 32:36, 1977.
13. Kullander, S. and Kallen, B. A.: A prospective study of smoking and pregnancy. Acta Obstet. Gynecol. Scand. 50:83, 1971.
14. Niswander, K. R., Singer, J., Westphal, M. and Weiss, W.: Weight gain during pregnancy and prepregnancy weight. Association with birth weight term gestation. Obstet. Gynecol. 33:482, 1969.
15. Scott, J. R.: Fetal growth retardation associated with maternal administration of immunosuppressive drugs. Am. J. Obstet. Gynecol. 128:668, 1977.
16. Campbell, S., and Jurjak, A.: Comparison between urinary estrogen assay and serial ultrasonic cephalometry in assessment of fetal growth retardation. Br. Med. J. 4:336, 1972.
17. Campbell, S. and Wilkin, D.: Ultrasonic measurement of fetal abdomen circumference in the estimation of fetal weight. Br. J. Obstet. Gynecol. 82:689, 1975.
18. Higginbottom, J., Slater, J., Porter, G. and Whitfield, C. R.: Estimation of fetal weight from ultrasonic measurement of trunk circumference. Br. J. Obstet. Gynecol. 82:698, 1975.
19. Levi, S. and Erbsman, F.: Antenatal fetal growth from the nineteenth week. Am. J. Obstet. Gynecol. 121:262, 1975.
20. Campbell, S. and Thoms, A.: Ultrasound measurement of the fetal head to abdomen circumference ratio in the assessment of growth retardation. Br. J. Obstet. Gynecol. 84:165, 1977.
21. Scheer, K.: Sonography as a routine obstetrical diagnostic procedure. J. Clin. Ultrasound 5:101, 1976.
22. Spellacy, W. N., Teoh, E. S., Buhi, W. C., Birk, S. A. and McCreary, S. A.: Value of human chorionic somatomammotropin in managing high-risk pregnancies. Am. J. Obstet. Gynecol. 109:588, 1971.
23. Hensleigh, P. A., Cheatum, S. G. and Spellacy, W. N.: Oxytocin and human placental lactogen for prediction of intrauterine growth retardation. Am. J. Obstet. Gynecol. 129:675, 1977.
24. Freeman, R. K.: The use of the oxytocin challenge test for antepartum clinical evaluation of uteroplacental respiratory function. Am. J. Obstet. Gynecol. 121:481, 1975.
25. Egley, C. C. and Suzuki, K.: Intrauterine fetal demise after negative oxytocin challenge tests. Obstet. Gynecol. 50(Suppl.):54, 1977.
26. Lee, C. Y., DiLoreto, P. C. and O'Lane, J. M.: Study of fetal heart rate acceleration patterns. Obstet. Gynecol. 45:142, 1975.
27. Rochard, F. et al.: Nonstressed fetal heart rate monitoring in the antepartum period. Am. J. Obstet. Gynecol. 125:699, 1976.
28. Trierweiler, M. W., Freeman, R. K. and James, J.:

Baseline fetal heart rate characteristics as indicator of fetal status during the antepartum period. Am. J. Obstet. Gynecol. 125:618, 1976.

29. Tushuizen, P. B., Stoot, J. E. and Ubachs, J. M.: Clinical experience in nonstressed antepartum cardiotocography. Am. J. Obstet. Gynecol. 128:507, 1977.

30. Visser, G. H. A. and Huisjes, H. J.: Diagnostic value of the unstressed antepartum cardiotocogram. Br. J. Obstet. Gynecol. 84:321, 1977.

31. Gluck, L., Kulovich, M. V., Borer, R. C., Jr., Brenner, P. H., Anderson, G. G. and Spellacy, W. N.: Diagnosis of the respiratory distress syndrome by amniocentesis. Am. J. Obstet. Gynecol. 109:440, 1971.

32. Gluck, L., Kulovich, M. V., Borer, R. C., Jr. and Keidel, W. N.: The interpretation and significance of the lecithin/sphingomyelin ratio in amniotic fluid. Am. J. Obstet. Gynecol. 120:142, 1974.

33. Francis-Williams, J. and Davies, P. A.: Very low birth weight and later intelligence. Dev. Med. Child Neurol. 16:709, 1974.

34. Fancourt, R., Campbell, S., Harvey, D. and Norman, A. P.: Follow-up study of small-for-dates babies. Br. Med. J. 1:1435, 1976.

35. Fitzhardinge, P. M. and Steven, E. M.: The small for date infant. I. Neurological and intellectual séquelae. Pediatrics 50:50, 1972.

36. Modanlus, H., Yeatt, S-Y. and Hon, E. H.: Fetal and neonatal acid-base balance in normal and high-risk 'pregnancies. Obstet. Gynecol. 43:347, 1974.

37. Odendaal, H.: Fetal heart rate patterns in patients with intrauterine growth retardation. Obstet. Gynecol. 48:187, 1976.

38. Carson, B. S., Losey, R. W., Bowes, W. A., Jr. and Simmons, M. A.: Combined obstetric and pediatric approach to prevent meconium aspiration syndrome. Am. J. Obstet. Gynecol. 126:712, 1976.

Identification and Management of the Post-term Pregnancy — Postmaturity

Helmuth Vorherr, M.D.

Robert H. Messer, M.D.

University of New Mexico School of Medicine

Post-term pregnancy and potential development of fetal postmaturity are considered by most obstetricians to be realities. Perinatal losses due to respiratory and nutritive placental insufficiency in post-term fetuses are higher than in term pregnancies. A better understanding of the pathophysiology of post-term fetoplacental insufficiency and the identification of postmaturity may contribute to more successful management of post-term pregnancy with reduction of fetal and neonatal mortality and morbidity.

In view of this article's subject, it seems appropriate to quote Shakespeare (as already cited by Clifford in 1957[8]):

"And so, from hour to hour, we ripe and ripe, And then, from hour to hour, we rot and rot; And thereby hangs a tale."

Placental Aging

Full placental development, final thickness and specific functioning are achieved around the fifth month of gestation. Thereafter, until birth, signs of gradual placental aging are observed (Table 1). These are compensated for by increase in the number of trophoblastic villi and surface area of vaculosyncytial membranes to maintain adequate fetal oxygen and nutrient supply.

After the 36th week placental transport processes gradually decline and placental and fetal growth rate is reduced (Fig. 1), leveling off until the 42nd week; thereafter the birth weight decreases slightly. Amniotic fluid vol-

TABLE 1.   PLACENTAL AGING PROCESSES

Increase in thickness of basal membrane of chorionic epithelium, decrease in diameter of villi

Decrease in villous epithelium (disappearance of cytotrophoblastic cells), excess formation of syncytial knots

Progressive reduction in length of villi

Increase in free amino acids and in RNA, decrease in protein content

Increase in density of villous stroma (disappearance of most Hofbauer cells, sclerosis), decrease in capillaries and enhanced appearance of avascular villi, compensatory villous growth in peripheral parts of placenta

Increase in intervillous thrombosis and infarction

Increase in foci of fibrosis

Increase in cyst formation and excess of calcification

Increase in degenerative changes of decidual vessels (fibrinoid degeneration of intima)

From Vorherr, H.: Placental insufficiency in relation to post-term pregnancy and fetal postmaturity. Am. J. Obstet. Gynecol. 123:67, 1975.

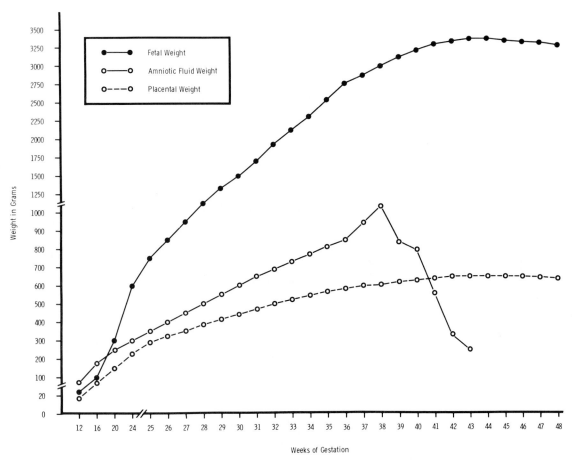

Figure 1. Average weights of fetus, placenta and amniotic fluid throughout human gestation. From the 16th week on, the fetus grows more rapidly than the placenta and the respective weight curves dissociate. Amniotic fluid correlates to placental weight until the 36th week; thereafter amniotic fluid volume declines rapidly. After the first half of gestation, the fetoplacental weight ratio is 2 to 3:1, increasing to a ratio of about 6:1 at term and remaining so during prolonged pregnancy. The standard deviation for fetal weight during the last trimester of gestation is ± 500 to 600 g. For placental weight and amniotic fluid volume, large variations (300 to 600 g) of single values are observed. The volume of amniotic fluid becomes greatly reduced post-term and only a few milliliters may be found after the 43rd week of gestation. (From Vorherr, H.: Placental insufficiency in relation to post-term pregnancy and fetal postmaturity. Am. J. Obstet. Gynecol. 123:67, 1975.)

ume decreases rapidly from the 38th week on (Fig. 1), and oligohydramnios is usually a sign of insufficient placental function. From the 35th week on, intervillous blood flow decreases and villous necrosis and fibrinoid deposition increase.[21] Placentas in post-term pregnancies show more villous necrosis and fibrinoid deposition than term placentas.[38]

Placental Insufficiency and Pathology

The rate of uteroplacental blood flow and the placental uptake of oxygen and nutrients are major determinants of placental and fetal growth. In 5 to 12 per cent of all pregnancies insufficient placental function is observed, and decreased uteroplacental circulation (toxemia, diabetes mellitus, multiple pregnancy) accounts for half of the cases causing chronic fetal hypoxia and growth retardation, or intrauterine asphyxia (hypoxia and acidosis) and fetal death. Placental pathology is connected with 20 to 40 per cent of all perinatal fetal deaths (Fig. 2).

At this time no specific treatment is known to prevent or alleviate placental insufficiency. In recent years an attempt has been made to treat placental insufficiency by increasing the uteroplacental flow in patients with toxemia through long-term infusion of the β_2-agonist agent ritodrine.[23]

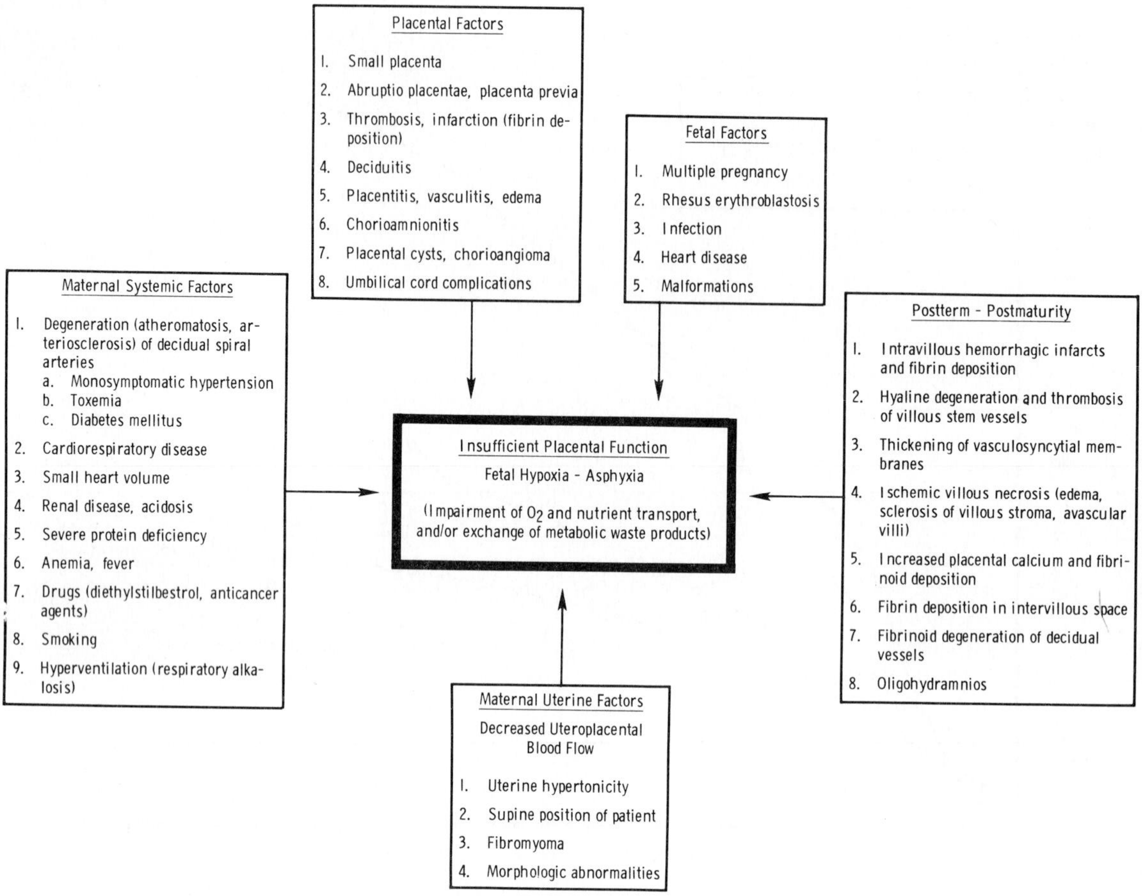

Placental Factors

1. Small placenta
2. Abruptio placentae, placenta previa
3. Thrombosis, infarction (fibrin deposition)
4. Deciduitis
5. Placentitis, vasculitis, edema
6. Chorioamnionitis
7. Placental cysts, chorioangioma
8. Umbilical cord complications

Fetal Factors

1. Multiple pregnancy
2. Rhesus erythroblastosis
3. Infection
4. Heart disease
5. Malformations

Maternal Systemic Factors

1. Degeneration (atheromatosis, arteriosclerosis) of decidual spiral arteries
   a. Monosymptomatic hypertension
   b. Toxemia
   c. Diabetes mellitus
2. Cardiorespiratory disease
3. Small heart volume
4. Renal disease, acidosis
5. Severe protein deficiency
6. Anemia, fever
7. Drugs (diethylstilbestrol, anticancer agents)
8. Smoking
9. Hyperventilation (respiratory alkalosis)

Insufficient Placental Function

Fetal Hypoxia - Asphyxia

(Impairment of O_2 and nutrient transport, and/or exchange of metabolic waste products)

Postterm - Postmaturity

1. Intravillous hemorrhagic infarcts and fibrin deposition
2. Hyaline degeneration and thrombosis of villous stem vessels
3. Thickening of vasculosyncytial membranes
4. Ischemic villous necrosis (edema, sclerosis of villous stroma, avascular villi)
5. Increased placental calcium and fibrinoid deposition
6. Fibrin deposition in intervillous space
7. Fibrinoid degeneration of decidual vessels
8. Oligohydramnios

Maternal Uterine Factors

Decreased Uteroplacental Blood Flow

1. Uterine hypertonicity
2. Supine position of patient
3. Fibromyoma
4. Morphologic abnormalities

Figure 2. Maternal and fetal factors in relation to placental insufficiency. (From Vorherr.[41])

Post-term Gestation in Relation to Placental Insufficiency, Fetal Distress and Postmaturity

POST-TERM GESTATION

Pregnancy is considered post term when it exceeds 294 days, calculated from the first day of the last menstrual period. The normal duration of gestation is 280 days from the first day of the last menstrual period, or 266 days following ovulation. The post-term state occurs in approximately 10 per cent of all pregnancies. It has been suggested that more than half of all diagnosed "post-term" pregnancies are actually term gestations;[32] the margin of error for estimates of post-term pregnancy by present diagnostic techniques is plus or minus 2 to 3 weeks.[13] In the absence of placental insufficiency, 70 to 80 per cent of fetuses carried beyond term do well, and large infants (4000 g and above) in good condition are born

2 to 3 times more often than in term pregnancies.[41] Increased fetal weight is always accompanied by higher placental weight, both in term and post-term pregnancies; in one newborn infant of 7500 g an excess of placental weight of 1770 g was observed.[12] The large size of some post-term fetuses does not ensure a better prognosis; even in large fetuses oxygen and nutrient supply may suddenly become decompensated.[11] Also, fetal weight does not always correlate with maturity, as for instance in pregnancies complicated by diabetes mellitus.

POST-TERM FETAL DISTRESS, POSTMATURITY AND PERINATAL MORTALITY

The post-term fetal growth curve flattens out because the placenta can no longer fulfill the demands of the growing conceptus; this results in a steadily increasing proportion of postmature fetuses with lower weight.[34]

The longer that gestation extends beyond term the greater is the likelihood for development of placental insufficiency, fetal growth retardation and fetal hypoxia-anoxia, i.e., fetal postmaturity. In approximately 35 per cent of post-term pregnancies fetal distress may be diagnosed, requiring delivery by cesarean section.[31] Most authors agree that in post-term pregnancies perinatal mortality is increased.

Pathophysiology of Fetal Post-term Postmaturity

PLACENTAL INSUFFICIENCY AND FETAL HYPOXIA

Fetus and placenta cease to grow at 42 to 43 weeks of gestation (Fig. 1) and their weights may even decrease, indicating insufficient fetoplacental function.

Placental insufficiency leading to the postmaturity syndrome (Tables 2 and 3) has to be considered as an imbalance between placental capacity and fetal nutritive and respiratory demands. Acute and extensive placental disturbances can cause fetal death due to hypoxia-

TABLE 2.   POSTMATURITY: PLACENTAL INSUFFICIENCY AND FETAL DISTRESS

CHRONIC PLACENTAL INSUFFICIENCY (EXTENDING OVER WEEKS):
 Predominantly nutritive insufficiency
 Urinary estriol on lower limit of norm (10 to 12 mg per 24 hours or less)
 Meconium release slight if any
 Wasting of subcutaneous tissues, growth retardation, dehydration, atrophy of thymus
 Oligohydramnios
 Disproportionate growth and maturation of brain
 Rarely: changes in fetal heart rate pattern

ACUTE AND SUBACUTE PLACENTAL INSUFFICIENCY (EXTENDING OVER A FEW HOURS OR DAYS):
 Predominantly respiratory insufficiency
 Decrease of urinary estriol to critical levels (5 mg per 24 hours or less)
 Aspiration of amniotic fluid
 Meconium release and staining of fetal skin and membranes
 Wasting of subcutaneous tissues (only when superimposed on chronic insufficiency)
 Necrosis or hemorrhage into adrenal glands or both
 Parenchymal damage of brain, myocardium and liver
 Pathologic fetal heart rate patterns due to fetal hypoxia and metabolic acidosis

Adapted from Vorherr, H.: Placental insufficiency in relation to post-term pregnancy and fetal postmaturity. Am. J. Obstet. Gynecol. 123:67, 1975.

TABLE 3.   CLINICAL PARAMETERS OF FETAL POSTMATURITY SYNDROME

Incidence of fetal postmaturity: ~2–4%

Perinatal mortality: 15–35% (~1 out of 4 postmature fetuses)

Distribution of perinatal mortality
 Before onset of labor: 9–30%
 During labor: 45–93%
 All intrauterine deaths: ~75%
 All birth: 7–25% (respiratory distress; brain, heart, liver, adrenal damage)

Postnatal morbidity: 16–46% (respiratory distress, mainly)

Amniotic fluid changes
 Volume: reduced to 250 ml or below (normal term values: 800 ml)
 Fat cells: increase of orange-staining fat cells over 50% (normal term values: 10–50%)

Vaginal smear: appearance of parabasal cells (normal term values: 0/85–95/5–15)

Fetal heart rate pattern: prolonged deceleration in cases of severe fetal asphyxia

Lowered urinary estriol excretion: 30% excrete less than 12 mg of estriol per 24 hours into the urine (normal term values: 15–25 mg per 24 hours)

Myometrium
 Persistent quiescence ("progesterone block")
 During labor: sluggish performance (uterine inertia)

Umbilical venous cord blood
 Decreased oxygen saturation: below 40% (normal term values: 55–70%); oxygen content below 8 vol % (normal term value: 12 vol %)
 Hemoglobin concentration increased: 16.8–20.5 g per dl (normal term values: 15–18.6 g per dl)

From Vorherr, H.: Placental insufficiency in relation to post-term pregnancy and fetal postmaturity. Am. J. Obstet. Gynecol. 123:67, 1975.

anoxia, whereas chronic and less pronounced morphologic and functional restrictions may lead to chronic hypoxia and to fetal malnutrition, i.e., fetal postmaturity (dysmaturity). In acute placental insufficiency fetal size is normal but in subacute, or more so in chronic placental insufficiency, retarded fetal growth is observed as well as a certain degree of hypoxia.[20] However, nutritive placental insufficiency (retarded fetal growth) is not always associated with respiratory placental insufficiency (fetal hypoxia).[22] In the condition of fetal hypoxia, placental diffusion-reserve capacity may become operative, increasing oxygen diffusion by 50 per cent (Fig. 3).[43] With exhaustion of placental reserve capacity the fetus cannot grow because brain, heart, liver and kidneys are incapable of functioning adequately; here fetal asphyxia and death are imminent (Fig. 4).

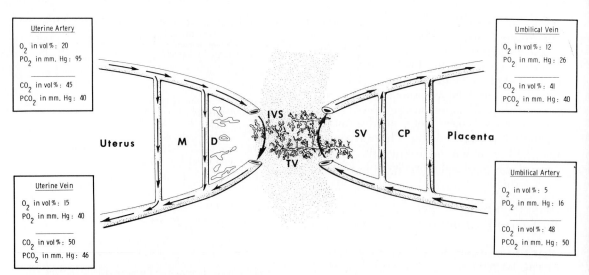

Figure 3. Uteroplacental-fetal circulation, blood gas content and arteriovenous shunting pathways. Near term, uteroplacental blood flow amounts to 500 to 600 ml per minute, intervillous blood flow to 400 to 500 ml per minute, and fetoplacental circulation to 300 to 400 ml per minute. The uterine arteriovenous oxygen difference is 5 to 7 volume per cent. The oxygen saturation of venous umbilical cord blood is 60 per cent, and that of arterial cord blood is about 40 per cent. It is thought that about 50 per cent of arterial blood does not participate in intervillous O_2-CO_2 exchange because it is shunted away with half on the maternal and half on the fetal side. A 40 per cent oxygen saturation of venous umbilical cord blood is the minimum required for adequate fetal oxygenation; the fetus needs 20 to 25 ml of O_2 per minute. Because approximately 300 to 350 ml of uteroplacental blood flow per minute can provide this amount of necessary oxygen to the fetus and in view of the existing higher uteroplacental blood flow (500 to 600 ml per minute), a certain uteroplacental–fetal reserve capacity (respiratory, nutritive, endocrine) must be assumed. When placental aging and degeneration lead to placental insufficiency and inadequate fetal oxygenation, a compensatory placental diffusion capacity for O_2 and for uptake of nutrients becomes operative by diminution of blood shunting on maternal and fetal side. Such shunt-reversal may provide a 50 per cent or more reserve capacity to cover fetal needs. When maternal myometrial-decidual and fetal chorionic plate-villous stem shunt-reversal mechanisms are not adequately functioning or the reserves become exhausted, fetal hypoxia and growth retardation may occur. (Symbols: M = myometrium; D = decidua; IVS = intervillous space; TV = terminal villi; SV = stem villi; CP = chorionic plate.) (From Vorherr.[41])

PLACENTAL INSUFFICIENCY: LESIONS, DYSFUNCTION AND FETAL FACTOR(S)

Post-term placental insufficiency is correlated with abnormal placental morphology (Table 4) and diminished placental hormone production (estriol, human placental lactogen). Although placental lesions are associated with a 10 times greater perinatal mortality rate,[2] it seems that fetal distress may also be due to placental dysfunction on a biochemical level without noticeable placental lesions.

Usually, development of postmaturity is related to placental factors (lesions, biochemical dysfunction). However, it also seems possible that in post-term pregnancy a fetal factor or factors, which participate in the regulation of placental function or fetal growth or both, functions abnormally, leading to postmaturity. At present nothing is known about the nature of such a factor or factors.

Identification of Post-term Placental Insufficiency and Fetal Postmaturity

Present clinical and biochemical methods (Table 5) do not permit reliable diagnosis of early placental insufficiency. This early insufficiency involves (1) failure to transport nutrients to the fetus and exchange of fetal metabolic waste products and (2) decline in fetal arterial and venous oxygen saturation.

MECONIUM STAINING OF AMNIOTIC FLUID

Release of meconium into amniotic fluid by the fetus in vertex presentation is still a valid, although rather insensitive, indicator of placental insufficiency and fetal hypoxia. A single hypoxic insult may cause meconium release

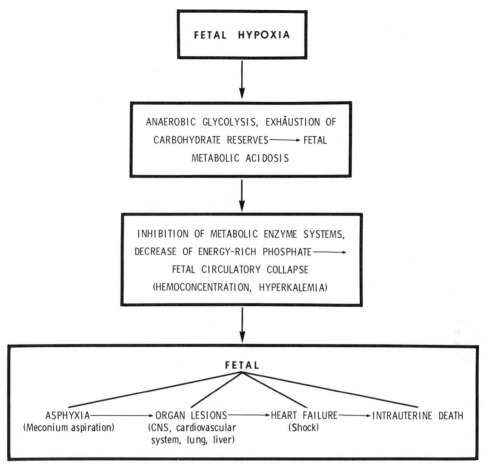

Figure 4. Fetal hypoxia and sequelae of metabolic acidosis. (From Vorherr.[41])

TABLE 4. MORPHOLOGY OF THE POST-TERM PLACENTA

COMPONENTS	EARLY POST-TERM PLACENTA (42–43 WEEKS GESTATION)	LATE POST-TERM PLACENTA (BEYOND 43 WEEKS GESTATION)
Placenta	Increased thickness and blood content; moderate increase in incidence of infarction, fibrin deposition and calcification	Decrease in placental thickness and blood content; pronounced increase in foci of infarction, fibrin deposition and calcification
Intervillous Space	Similar intervillous space volume as in term pregnancies	Diminution of intervillous space volume due to intervillous thrombosis and fibrin deposition
Villi	Overdifferentiation, i.e., diffuse hemangioma-like capillarization; increase in regenerative efforts; hyperplasia of cytotrophoblastic cells	Absence of villous regenerative efforts; stromal edema; hypovascularity, avascularity; villous fibrosis and shrinkage
Syncytium	Decreased syncytial sprouting; membrane thickening	Syncytial edema; increased syncytial thickening, vacuolization and degeneration
Syncytial knots	Increased knot formation	Greatly increased knot formation
Vessels of stem and anchoring villi	Moderate arterial narrowing and venous dilation	Arterial thrombosis; vascular hyalinization and obliteration
Vessels of resorptive villi	Sinusoidal dilation and increased blood content	Reduction in sinusoidal villous capillaries, vascular collapse and degeneration

From Vorherr, H.: Placental insufficiency in relation to post-term pregnancy and fetal postmaturity. Am. J. Obstet. Gynecol. 123:67, 1975.

TABLE 5. DIAGNOSIS OF POST-TERM PLACENTAL INSUFFICIENCY

Clinical examination (uterine size, abdominal circumference, maternal weight)*

Measurement of estriol*

Vaginal cytology‡

Fetal cephalometry and determination of intrauterine volume by ultrasound*

Amnioscopy,* amniocentesis* and amniotic fluid analysis (amount, color and constituents)*

Fetal EKG‡

Continuous recording of fetal heart rate (electrocardiography, phonocardiography)*

Recording of fetal heart rate and:
  Intravenous oxytocin challenge test (estimation of oxygen reserve of placenta and fetus)*
  Atropine and isoxsuprine test‡
  Physical exercise test†

Measurement of heat-stable alkaline phosphatase, oxytocinase, diamine oxidase‡

Measurement of uteroplacental circulation by radioisotopes (^{24}Na)†

Measurement of alpha fetoprotein‡ and serum enzymes‡

Amniography,‡ fetoscopy‡

Fetal scalp blood sampling during labor (P_{CO_2}, P_{O_2}, pH)*

Amniotomy during labor*

---

*Valuable.
†Theoretically valuable, no routine application.
‡Value not established.
Adapted from Vorherr, H.: Placental insufficiency in relation to post-term pregnancy and fetal postmaturity. Am. J. Obstet. Gynecol. 123:67, 1975.

into the amniotic fluid with subsequent fetal recovery. Therefore, the mere presence of meconium staining does not equate well with fetal distress. Meconium passage into amniotic fluid occurs when the oxygen saturation in the umbilical vein blood drops to 30 per cent; that is, half its normal value. Thick clumps of dark meconium indicate more severe fetal hypoxia than light greenish–tinted amniotic fluid.

CHANGES OF AMNIOTIC FLUID VOLUME AND CONSTITUENTS

In post-term patients scanty forewaters may be observed by amnioscopy. Reduction of the volume of amniotic forewater is accompanied by a perinatal mortality rate of 2 per cent and a 10 per cent incidence of low Apgar score. Amniotic fluid sodium, chlorine, glucose and osmolality diminish after 42 weeks of gesta-

tion; potassium remains constant and creatinine and urea concentrations increase.[41]

In cases of prolonged gestation more than 50 per cent of orange-staining fat cells are observed in the amniotic fluid, whereas values for term pregnancy range between 10 and 50 per cent.[13]

VAGINAL CYTODIAGNOSIS

Disappearance of intermediate cells and appearance of parabasal cells have been described as typical for post-term pregnancies with placental (hormonal) insufficiency. However, the vaginal smear does not appear to be a good indicator for the diagnosis of prolonged gestation and placental insufficiency because cell types vary greatly, and progressive (shift to superficial cells) as well as regressive smear types (shift to intermediate and parabasal cells) have been reported.[1]

ESTRIOL AND HUMAN PLACENTAL LACTOGEN (HPL)

Estriol still plays a dominant role in the assessment of fetoplacental function, even though great variations of single values are observed, with 10 to 50 per cent of endangered fetuses missed.[41] The diagnostic value of determinations of plasma estriol and urinary estriol seems equal.[44] Because of the great day-to-day variation of estriol values, only constantly low values are indicative of fetal danger. A precipitate decrease of urinary estriol values by 50 per cent or more is usually indicative of placental insufficiency and fetal hypoxia. When plasma levels of unconjugated estriol decline to below 4 ng per ml (normal: 12 ng per ml), insufficiency of the fetoplacental unit may be assumed. Similarly, when maternal 24-hour urinary estriol excretion is below 4 mg, fetal death is imminent. When estriol values were below 4 mg per 24 hours, in 65 per cent of cases fetal growth retardation was observed and the mortality rate was increased fivefold; conversely, in women with normal estriol values only 8 per cent fetal growth retardation existed.[22] Fetuses rarely die when 24-hour estriol excretion is above 5 mg. Nevertheless, estriol values below 8 to 12 mg, or a drop by 50 per cent of previous values, is a signal for termination of pregnancy. Approximately 30 per cent of patients with postmature fetuses excrete less than 12 mg of estriol per 24 hours into the urine;[13] fall in estriol values is due to impaired fetal adrenal and placental steroid metabolism. Increase in plasma estriol concentration or decrease in urinary estriol excretion may also occur as a consequence of impaired renal function (pre-eclampsia, diabetes mellitus). Moreover, in some cases low urinary estriol excretion may be the consequence of maternal treatment with prednisone and ampicillin or may be due to placental sulfatase deficiency; in these conditions delivery may not be indicated.

Serum measurements of HPL have been performed as adjunct to other tests for placental insufficiency.[6] With HPL plasma levels above 5 μg per ml, the risk of fetal distress or neonatal asphyxia is thought to be less than 10 per cent; HPL levels below 4 μg per ml may involve fetal complications in 71 per cent of pregnancies. On the other hand, it was found that in only 1 out of 12 instances of fetoplacental dysfunction were HPL values below 3 μg per ml. Whereas some investigators consider HPL valuable for the diagnosis of placental insufficiency and postmaturity, others deny such claims because no consistent HPL patterns in fetal dysmaturity, fetal heart rate abnormalities and post-term pregnancies could be traced.[33] According to Hobbins and co-workers,[16] HPL measurement is not very helpful in the diagnosis of intrauterine growth retardation.

So far, all the other placental hormone or enzyme tests have failed to fulfill expectations because normal values scatter over a wide range. Moreover, placental endocrine-metabolic activity (hormone and enzyme production) cannot be directly related to placental respiratory and nutrient transport functions.[2] Impaired production of placental HPL or estriol does not necessarily indicate that placental transport of nutrients and oxygen is decreased to a similar extent; as mentioned before, nutritive and respiratory placental functions are not necessarily affected simultaneously.

FETAL HEART RATE, OXYTOCIN CHALLENGE TEST AND FETAL BIPARIETAL DIAMETER AS DIAGNOSTIC TOOLS

Continuous recording of fetal heart rate pattern has become important in the observation of fetal well-being; however, this test also has pitfalls. Irregularities in fetal heart rate pattern may appear only in conditions of progressed placental insufficiency when the fetus is already asphyctic. On the other hand, in 50 per cent of cases of fetuses with abnormal heart rate, no hypoxia or acidosis exists. Accordingly, fetal heart rate patterns are best used as a screening system for fetal difficulty rather than as an absolute measure of distress. Only pH and P_{O_2} measurements in fetal scalp blood during labor can determine the extent of fetal danger.

Latent placental respiratory insufficiency may become overt and thus may be diagnosed by oxytocin challenge test (OCT). In response to uterine contractions, the placentofetal oxygen reserves become more compromised and provoke pathologic fetal heart rate patterns (persistent tachycardia, loss in beat-to-beat variation, variable deceleration, late or prolonged deceleration); especially prolonged deceleration has been related to placental insufficiency. In 10 to 15 per cent of pregnancies at high risk for placental insufficiency a positive OCT is observed. A positive OCT allows prediction of fetal distress with a 50 to 70 per cent validity; 30 to 50 per cent of OCTs are false positive. Conversely, in some cases in which OCT is negative, fetal distress develops during labor.[41]

Measurement of fetal biparietal diameter has proved valuable for determination of size and diagnosis of postmaturity. During normal fetal growth the biparietal diameter increases 1.6 mm per week on the average between weeks 31 and 37 and 0.7 to 1 mm between weeks 38 and 41.[39] In postmature fetuses the diameter shows arrest of growth or even regression. Serial values with an increase of less than 0.45 mm per week indicate fetal dysmaturity. With serial biparietal diameter measurements, fetal dysmaturity could be predicted in 90 per cent of cases as compared with a 70 per cent prediction rate with serial urinary estrogen estimations.[39] These favorable figures are not confirmed by Kubli and co-workers,[22] who stated that the diagnostic value of biparietal diameter for prediction of fetal growth retardation is limited (only 55 per cent correct predictions) (see later discussion).

COMPARISON OF TESTS. With four tests for evaluation of nutritive and respiratory placental function, a "correct" prediction of respiratory placental insufficiency of 59, 41, 40, and 46 per cent of cases was possible when the following served as test indices: meconium release into amniotic fluid, fetal biparietal diameter, fetal heart rate pattern during oxytocin-induced uterine contractility, and 24-hour urinary estriol excretion. The corresponding values for "correct" prediction of fetal growth retardation were 24, 55, 33, and 33 per cent.[22] According to Kubli and co-workers,[22] the best tests for placental nutritive function are estriol and biparietal diameter measurements, and for placental respiratory function, OCT and aminoscopy (amniocentesis). Not only is the predictive value of various tests limited, they often do not correlate. The diagnostic value of estriol for the management of post-term pregnancy has been doubted and the OCT has been held unsatisfactory to identify the compromised fetus. Unfortunately, no better tests are available.

Considering the procedures available for the identification of intrauterine growth retardation (see Table 5), it appears important that a thorough menstrual history be established, time of first quickening and audible heart action recorded, and periodic clinical examinations carried out in combination with appropriate tests for evaluation of fetoplacental function. Estimates of fetal weight by abdominal palpation are almost as accurate as measurement of biparietal diameter; they vary by plus or minus 500 and 400 g, respectively.[3] In evaluating fundal height and descent, decreasing body weight and abdominal circumference together with appropriate clinical and laboratory tests a prediction of fetal postmaturity seems possible in 70 to 80 per cent of pregnancies. Despite thorough clinical and laboratory surveillance, it may happen that a pregnant woman who showed no placental insufficiency and fetal distress during examination will return to the clinic a day or two later because she misses fetal movements. Also, sudden death of a postmature fetus due to acute placental insufficiency and fetal anoxia may occur during labor without warning by heart rate changes.[29]

Management of Post-term Pregnancy

Because most post-term fetuses (70 to 80 per cent) are delivered in good health, little concern has been voiced in regard to active management in cases of prolonged gestation. Post-term pregnancy and moderate placental insufficiency seldom result in fetal death.[5]

According to recent reports on a relatively small number of post-term pregnancies, no difference in perinatal mortality was observed compared with term pregnancies (0.3 to 0.4 per cent).[14, 36] In contrast, post-term pregnancies have been associated with a threefold to fourfold increase in perinatal mortality by several authors.[41] More recently, a perinatal mortality rate between 1 and 1.5 per cent and a fetal distress rate of 38 per cent have been reported for post-term pregnancies.[31] In cases with intrauterine growth retardation, the perinatal mortality rate may be increased fivefold to eightfold.[7]

Pregnancy should not be allowed to extend beyond term in women with an obstetric history of diabetes mellitus, toxemia, small-for-dates fetus or fetal erythroblastosis. About 20 to 30 per cent of post-term fetuses are potentially endangered because of postmaturity, and approximately 1 out of 4 postmature fetuses will die.[41] Reported incidence rates of postmaturity and perinatal mortality depend on whether post-term pregnancy is managed more aggressively or conservatively. At the present time the two styles of management are difficult to assess, even though it is conceivable that aggressive management involving routine induction of labor with oxytocin or amniotomy or both, and, if unsuccessful, delivery by cesarean section, can lower post-term perinatal mortality to term values. On the other hand it should be remembered that through cesarean section maternal mortality is increased as compared with vaginal delivery. Overall maternal mortality is 0.01 to 0.02 per cent, while cesarean section mortality ranges from 0.1 to 0.2 per cent. Moreover, postoperative morbidity is observed in 25 to 50 per cent of patients after cesarean section.

In view of these problems, neither routine induction of labor nor conservative watchful waiting can be advocated as a general rule for the management in the post-term pregnancy; each case necessitates individual assessment (Tables 5 and 6).

Post-term pregnancies are usually managed conservatively, that is, by semiweekly checks of fetal heart rate, estriol, HPL and amnioscopy. If amnioscopy is not possible, amniocentesis is indicated. Especially in "post-term" pregnancies with an unreliable gestational dating history, amniocentesis is helpful and amniotic fluid creatinine values of more than or equal to 2.5 mg per cent point to post-term pregnancy; also, measurement of biparietal diameter is helpful. For cases in which the fetal weight is estimated to be less than 2500 g, pregnancy should be allowed to continue

TABLE 6.　MANAGEMENT OF POST-TERM
PREGNANCY

BEFORE LABOR

Unfavorable cervix: biweekly estriol, fetal heart rate
(nonstress test, when negative OCT), amnioscopy
(amniocentesis)

Favorable cervix: induction of labor

Termination of pregnancy: intrauterine fetal growth
retardation, fetal distress

DURING LABOR

Monitoring of mother (uterine activity) and fetus
(heart rate, amniotic fluid, scalp blood)

Lateral positioning, especially in case of hypoactive
labor or fetal heart rate irregularities or both

Oxygen breathing in case of fetal distress

Avoidance of sedatives, analgesics, spinal block, inhalation anesthetics

Delivery by low forceps or by vacuum extraction in
case of fetal distress

Cesarean section in case of serious fetal bradycardia
and decrease of scalp blood pH below 7.2

Delay clamping of umbilical cord for additional fetal
blood supply

Observation of newborn for signs of dehydration, hypoglycemia, hypovolemia, acidosis, cerebral hypoxia, lung complications, adrenocortical insufficiency

as long as estriol values rise or remain stable
within normalcy, and as long as other test
parameters indicate adequate fetoplacental
function. A negative OCT, normal estriol values, adequately increasing biparietal diameter
values and clear amniotic forewaters indicate
that the pregnancy may be allowed to continue
for another half week or week before labor is
induced or retesting is done.

According to Saling,[30] post-term perinatal
deaths could be reduced by 40 per cent by
use of amnioscopy, but Henry[15] considered
amnioscopy not as satisfactory for the management of prolonged pregnancy. Nevertheless,
meconium staining of amniotic fluid or lack of
forewaters points to placental insufficiency and
fetal distress.

In post-term pregnancies with a favorable
cervix (Bishop score) and in the absence of
contraindications, induction of labor can save
fetuses that might be lost due to placental
insufficiency if pregnancy is allowed to continue.[24, 37] Because tests for fetal distress are
rather crude, efforts to promote cervical ripening and the onset of labor, such as membrane stripping or oxytocin infusion, seem
worthwhile. It is uncertain whether post-term

pregnancy in patients such as older primigravidous or gravidous women with a history of
abortion, stillbirth or dystocia requires more
aggressive measures for termination of gestation. Certainly, a post-term pregnancy with
the fetus in breech position should have delivery by cesarean section. Of the perinatal
losses, 50 per cent of term fetuses as well as
of post-term fetuses die before the onset of
labor; intrapartum deaths are thought to be
rare.[36] However, according to other reports
most post-term fetal deaths (see Table 3) occur
during labor and delivery because of further
reduction of fetoplacental oxygen reserve during uterine contractility.[41] Cefalo[7] reported
that a major cause of death of the growth-
retarded fetus is distress before and during
labor.

Induction of Labor in the Post-term Pregnancy

Approximately 40 per cent of women in
post-term pregnancy enter labor spontaneously and about 60 per cent require induction of labor or cesarean section.[14] Because in
approximately 70 per cent the cervix is unfavorable,[35, 42] induction of labor fails in a large
proportion. In 27 per cent of post-term pregnancies in which labor was induced, cesarean
section was required, compared with an incidence of 7 per cent in term patients.[26]
Whereas some authors reported an increase
in the rate of cesarean sections in post-term
pregnancies, two- to fourfold, others reported
cesarean section rates similar to term pregnancies.[41] Recently, Schneider and co-workers[31]
reported a cesarean section rate between 26
and 39 per cent for post-term pregnancies. In
the post-term pregnancy labor is tolerated
poorly,[35] and especially in post-term primigravidas labor is usually protracted; uterine
inertia has occurred twice as frequently in
post-term as in term pregnancies.[18, 32] However, it seems that only post-term fetuses with
compromised fetoplacental function tolerate
the stress of labor poorly; in post-term pregnancies with normal placental function labor
will not be different from that in term pregnancies.

Induction of labor in post-term pregnancies
requires continuous recording of fetal heart
rate and uterine activity because persistent
fetal tachycardia is the most common early
sign of hypoxia.[4] By positioning the woman on

her side (preferably left side) optimal utero-placental blood flow is ensured and uterine contractions become more intense but less frequent. Administration of a 5 per cent dextrose solution, 2 ml per minute, to prevent maternal dehydration and ketoacidosis represents a routine adjunctive measure. In addition, administration of oxygen by mask may alleviate fetal hypoxia as indicated by normalization of fetal heart rate irregularities.

Fetal Assessment During Labor

Development of fetal heart rate irregularities, scalp blood acidosis early in labor or meconium release during spontaneous or induced labor requires immediate attention. The fetal heart rate pattern is influenced by supine hypotension, sedatives, analgesics, paracervical and peridural block, head compression, umbilical cord compression and maternal acidosis.[4] Therefore, an abnormal rate is not necessarily due to primary placental insufficiency. On the basis of vaginal examination (station of presenting part, degree of cervix dilation) and course and estimated duration of labor, spontaneous delivery, forceps delivery or delivery by cesarean section must be decided on. Operative deliveries are usually performed in response to fetal asphyxia and uterine inertia. When fetal distress during labor can be alleviated by maternal lateral positioning and oxygen breathing and progress of labor are adequate, vaginal delivery may be anticipated. Recording of fetal heart rate, amnioscopy and fetal scalp blood sampling during labor allow prediction of fetal distress in 85 per cent of cases;[27] meconium release into amniotic fluid and irregularities of heart rate indicate distress in 44 to 69 per cent of fetuses.[9] Accordingly, despite meconium release and some irregularities of fetal heart rate, vaginal delivery within a few hours may be attempted as long as fetal scalp blood pH values do not drop below 7.20, indicating serious fetal acidosis and imminent death.[28] A cesarean section may be avoided by sampling of fetal scalp blood.[30] Uncontrollable severe variable and late decelerations require cesarean section.[7]

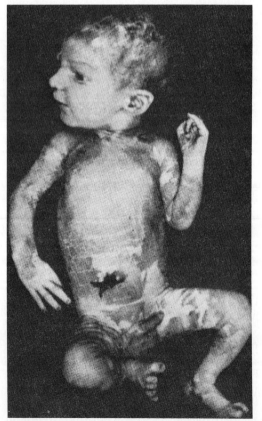

Figure 5. Fetoplacental dysfunction syndrome: postmaturity. This postmature male infant was delivered on day 308 of gestation by cesarean section after induction of labor had been complicated by fetal distress. Amniotic fluid, umbilical cord, fetal membranes and placenta were meconium-stained. The postmature newborn was long and very thin, appearing like a "wizened little old man." Skin and nails were intensely brown; large parts of the newborn's yellowish skin were desquamated. Despite the rather pronounced changes, this postmature baby survived. (From Clifford, S. H.: Postmaturity. Adv. Pediatr. 9:13, 1957.)

The Postmature Newborn

The postmaturity syndrome is clinically recognized in the newborn by (1) failure of growth (intrauterine inanition); (2) dehydration; (3) development of dry, cracked and wrinkled skin by reduction of subcutaneous fat depots; (4) long, thin arms and legs; (5) advanced hardness of the skull; (6) absence of vernix caseosa and lanugo hair; (7) skin maceration in flexion folds and external genital area; and (8) brownish-green or yellowish discoloration of skin, umbilical cord and membranes.[40] In the absence of vernix the fetal skin loses its protection, the normal red skin color disappears and skin maceration develops.[8] In postmature infants the body length is increased in relation to weight; such newborns are alert and look almost apprehensive (Fig. 5).[8, 13] Three different stages of the fetal postmaturity syndrome have been described.[8]

Stage 1 (Chronic Placental Insufficiency). Clinical signs include skin defects (maceration, loss of vernix), long nails, full scalp hair, malnutrition, long and thin body, older alert look, and usually no meconium staining. It seems that in Stage 1 the nutritional insufficiency is predominant over respiratory insufficiency of the placenta. Prognosis is for a normal course after delivery — in one out of three infants slight respiratory distress but no deaths.

Stage 2 (Acute Placental Insufficiency). If Stage 2 follows Stage 1 all the changes of Stage 1 are observed. Due to further reduction of placental respiratory function resulting in acute hypoxia (oxygen saturation in umbilical vein less than 30 per cent), meconium is released into the amniotic fluid. The bile of meconium stains skin, amniotic membranes and umbilical cord green. It is also possible that a normal post-term fetus will develop acute respiratory problems and in this case the symptoms of Stage 1 are missing. In 2 out of 3 infants respiratory distress is present at birth (aspiration of meconium-filled amniotic fluid, 50 per cent mortality rate); 1 out of 3 infants has brain damage and the overall mortality rate is 35 per cent.

Stage 3 (Subacute Placental Insufficiency). This is the state after survival of Stage 2; there is bright yellow staining of skin and nails with conversion of the green bile stain of meconium to yellow and yellowish-greenish-brownish staining of placental membranes, umbilical cord and placenta. The mor-tality rate is 15 per cent, mainly due to respiratory distress and brain damage.

Complications in the Postmature Newborn

Because of the danger of development of respiratory distress following meconium aspiration, a thorough suction and rinsing of nostrils, pharynx and trachea with physiological saline is important. Postmature infants may suffer from hypothermia, dehydration, hypovolemia, lung complications and symptoms of cerebral hypoxia and metabolic acidosis.[19, 25] Such newborns require special pediatric attention. Besides fluid and electrolyte therapy, sodium bicarbonate, glucose and antibiotics may become necessary.

Insufficient adrenocortical function may also endanger the postmature neonate. In post-term calves with an addisonian-like syndrome, glucose-cortisol infusions have proved to be lifesaving.[17] In postmature infants a tendency exists to develop hypoglycemia (decreased adrenocortical and hepatic function). Nevertheless, once delivered alive, postmature infants have a good chance to survive with proper care.[10]

Conclusion

As pregnancy extends beyond term, incidence of placental insufficiency, fetal postmaturity (dysmaturity), and perinatal mortality increase as a consequence of reduced nutritive and respiratory placental function. Postmaturity is correlated with increased incidence of placental lesions, fetal hypoxia and intrauterine growth retardation.

Early diagnosis of fetal postmaturity is difficult because currently applied test methods allow recognition only when placental insufficiency is far progressed. Conversely, an abnormal test or tests are not necessarily accompanied by fetal distress. Because induction of labor can save fetuses that might be lost due to placental insufficiency if pregnancy is allowed to continue, membrane stripping and oxytocin infusion for cervical ripening and induction of labor should be considered. Also in post-term pregnancies complicated by diabetes mellitus, toxemia or with small-for-dates fetus, pregnancy should be terminated. Pregnancy may be allowed to continue under close supervision in cases of uncertainty of duration of gestation or when the fetus is less than 2500 g and placentofetal function tests are normal.

As long as fetal scalp blood sampling during labor does not show dangerous fetal acidosis, despite abnormal fetal heart rate pattern and meconium release, vaginal delivery may be attempted when deemed possible within a few hours. Because during bearing-down efforts placentofetal respiratory reserves in post-term pregnancies may become further compromised, delivery by forceps or vacuum extraction may be considered. After delivery the umbilical cord should not be clamped immediately in order to allow for approximately 30 seconds' increased fetal blood supply and to counteract fetal hypovolemia. Dysmature newborn infants require special care by the neonatologist.

REFERENCES

1. Abdul-Karim, R.: Fetal physiology — A review. Obstet. Gynecol. Surv. 23:713, 1968.
2. Aladjem, S.: Fetal assessment through biopsy of the human placenta. *In* Pecile, A., and Finzi, C. (eds.): The Foeto-Placental Unit. Proceedings of an International Symposium held in Milan, Italy, Sept. 4–6, 1968. Amsterdam, Excerpta Medica Foundation, 1969, pp. 392–402.
3. Battaglia, F. C.: Intrauterine growth retardation. Am. J. Obstet. Gynecol. 106:1103, 1970.
4. Beard, R. W.: The detection of fetal asphyxia in labor. Obstet. Gynecol. Surv. 29:598, 1974.
5. Beischer, N. A. and Brown, J. B.: Current status of estrogen assays in obstetrics and gynecology. Part 2: Estrogen assays in late pregnancy. Obstet. Gynecol. Surv. 27:303, 1972.
6. Biggs, J. S. G.: Fetal assessment in late pregnancy: a current review. Aust. N.Z. J. Obstet. Gynaecol. 13:202, 1973.
7. Cefalo, R. C.: The hazards of labor and delivery for the intrauterine-growth-retarded fetus. J. Reprod. Med. 21:300, 1978.
8. Clifford, S. H.: Postmaturity. Adv. Pediatr. 9:13, 1957.
9. FitzGerald, T. B. and McFarlane, C. N.: Foetal distress and intrapartum foetal death. Br. Med. J. 2:358, 1955.
10. Gruenwald, P.: Chronic fetal distress and placental insufficiency. Biol. Neonate 5:215, 1963.
11. Gruenwald, P.: The fetus in prolonged pregnancy. Am. J. Obstet. Gynecol. 89.503, 1964.
12. Grünberger, V.: Relation zwischen Plazentagewicht und Geburtsgewicht von frühreifen, reifen und übertragenen Neugeborenen. Zentralbl. Gynaekol. 87:1367, 1965.
13. Harbert, G. M., Jr.: Evaluation of fetal maturity. Clin. Obstet. Gynecol. 16:171, 1973.
14. Hauth, J. C., Goodman, M. T., Gilstrap, L. C., III and Gilstrap, J. E. R.: Post-term pregnancy. I. Obstet. Gynecol. 56:467, 1980.
15. Henry, G. R.: Controlled trial of surgical induction of labour and amnioscopy in the management of prolonged pregnancy. J. Obstet. Gynaecol. Br. Commonwealth 76:795, 1969.
16. Hobbins, J. C., Berkowitz, R. L. and Grannum, P. A. T.: Diagnosis and antepartum management of intrauterine growth retardation. J. Reprod. Med. 21:319, 1978.
17. Holm, L. W: Prolonged pregnancy. Adv. Vet. Sci. 11:159, 1967.
18. Holtorff, J. and Schmidt, H.: Die verlängerte Schwangerschaft und ihr Einfluss auf das Schicksal des Kindes. Zentralbl. Gynaekol. 88:441, 1966.
19. Hosemann, H.: Schwangerschaftsdauer und Reifemerkmale des Neugeborenen. Arch. Gynaekol. 176:636, 1949.
20. Jenkins, D. M., Farquhar, J. B. and Oakey, R. E.: Urinary estrogen excretion in prolonged pregnancies. Obstet. Gynecol. 37:442, 1971.
21. Krantz, K. E. and Kubli, F.: Pathologie. *In* Käser, O., Friedberg, V., Ober, K. G., Thomsen, K. and Zander, J. (eds.): Gynäkologie und Geburtshilfe, Vol. 2. Stuttgart, Georg Thieme Verlag, 1967, pp. 52-76.
22. Kubli, F. W., Kaeser, O. and Hinselmann, M.: Diagnostic management of chronic placental insufficiency. *In* Pecile, A. and Finzi, C. (eds.) The Foeto-Placental Unit. Proceedings of an International Symposium held in Milan, Italy, Sept. 4–6, 1968. Amsterdam, Excerpta Medica Foundation, 1969, pp. 323-339.
23. Leodolter, S.: Neue Gesichtspunkte zur Erfassung und Behandlung der Plazentainsuffizienz. Wien. Klin. Wochenschr. 89(Supplementumm 70):3, 1977.
24. McClure Browne, J. C.: Postmaturity. Am. J. Obstet. Gynecol. 85:573, 1963.
25. McKay, R. J., Jr. and Smith, C. A.: Postmaturity and placental dysfunction. *In* Nelson, W. E. (ed.): Textbook of Pediatrics, 8th ed. Philadelphia, W. B. Saunders Co., 1964, pp. 358-359.
26. Martins, C. De Paula, Marques, A. M. Da Silva and Andreucci, D.: Guidelines for induction of labor in prolonged pregnancy. Obstet. Gynecol. 34:830, 1969.
27. Merger, R., Santarelli, J., Duval, Cl. and Lemoine, J.-P.: Fetale Herzfrequenz, ph-Wert des fetalen Kapillarblutes und Lebensfrische des Neugeborenen. Gynaekol. Rundsch. 11:177, 1971.
28. Mueller-Heubach, E. and Adamsons, K.: Surveillance of the fetus during the intrapartum period. Mt. Sinai J. Med. N.Y. 38:427, 1971.
29. Perkins, R. P.: Sudden fetal death in labor. The significance of antecedent monitoring characteristics and clinical circumstances. J. Reprod. Med. 25:309, 1978.
30. Saling, E.: Amnioscopy and foetal blood sampling: observations on foetal acidosis. Arch. Dis. Child 41:472, 1966.
31. Schneider, J. M., Olson, R. W. and Curet, L. B.: Screening for fetal and neonatal risk in the postdate pregnancy. Am. J. Obstet. Gynecol. 131:473, 1978.
32. Schüssling, G. and Radzuweit, H.: Zur Übertragung in der Schwangerschaft. Zentralbl. Gynaekol. 90:1705, 1968.
33. Seppälä, M. and Ruoslahti, E.: Serum concentration of human placental lactogenic hormone (HPL) in pregnancy complication. Acta Obstet. Gynecol. Scand. 49:143, 1970.
34. Sjöstedt, S., Engleson, G. and Rooth, G.: Dysmaturity. Arch. Dis. Child. 33:123, 1958.

35. Strand, A.: Prolonged pregnancy. Acta Obstet. Gynecol. Scand. 35:76, 1956.
36. Stubblefield, P. G. and Berek, J. S.: Perinatal mortality in term and post-term births. Obstet. Gynecol. 56:676, 1980.
37. Theobald, G. W.: The choice between death from postmaturity or prolapsed cord and life from induction of labour. Lancet 1:59, 1959.
38. Thliveris, J. A. and Baskett, T. F.: Fine structure of the human placenta in prolonged pregnancy. Preliminary report. Gynecol. Obstet. Invest. 9:40, 1978.
39. Varma, T. R.: A comparison of serial cephalometry and maternal urinary oestrogen excretion in assessing fetal prognosis. Aust. N.Z. J. Obstet. Gynaecol. 13:191, 1973.

40. Vorherr, H.: Disorders of uterine functions during pregnancy, labor, and puerperium. *In* Assali, N. S. (ed.): Pathophysiology of Gestation, Vol. 1. New York, Academic Press, 1972, pp. 145-268.
41. Vorherr, H.: Placental insufficiency in relation to post-term pregnancy and fetal postmaturity. Am. J. Obstet. Gynecol. 123:67, 1975.
42. Walker, J.: Prolonged pregnancy syndrome. Am. J. Obstet. Gynecol. 76:1231, 1958.
43. Wulf, H.: Störungen der intrauterinen Atmung. Arch. Gynaekol. 198:40, 1963.
44. Ylikorkala, O., Haapalahti, J. and Jouppila, P.: Comparison between serum estriol and urinary estrogens as indices of fetoplacental function. Arch. Gynaekol. 221:179, 1976.

Intrauterine Growth Retardation: The Current Approach to Perinatal Diagnosis and Management

John A. Widness, M.D.

William Oh, M.D.

Brown University Program in Medicine

For years the phenomenon of intrauterine growth retardation (IUGR) has been discussed under various terms including placental dysfunction, placental insufficiency, dysmaturity and so forth. The use of many variations in terminology to signify this condition strongly suggests its multifactorial etiology and pathogenesis. Since its recognition there has been broad interest on the part of obstetricians, pediatricians and pathologists in studying its many facets. This interest is derived from the fact that these growth-retarded infants of low birth weight and the pregnancies from which they arise constituted a unique high-risk group with its own individual set of problems in contrast with those low birth weight infants whose growth has been appropriate for their gestational age (AGA infants). The intrauterine growth–retarded infants have tenfold greater perinatal mortality than their full-term AGA counterparts owing primarily to an increased number of stillbirths and neonatal deaths often related to birth asphyxia.[1] Furthermore, the neonatal morbidities for these two low birth weight groups are different, with the IUGR group more often afflicted by the problems of meconium aspiration, hypoxia-induced seizures and renal insufficiency, polycythemia and hyperviscosity, hypocalcemia, and hypoglycemia.

In the early 1960s, Gruenwald[2] suggested that IUGR can be caused by one of three types of factors: fetal, placental or maternal. With primary fetal etiology there is adequate maternal and placental blood flow and nutrition, but for various reasons the fetus fails to grow because of abnormalities affecting it such as chromosomal defects, major congenital anomalies and intrauterine infections. This group accounts for approximately 10 per cent of all cases of IUGR.[3] In contrast, when placental or maternal causes are responsible for IUGR, reduced placental blood flow with its attendant decrease in oxygen and substrate transfer to the fetus are the primary mechanisms for fetal growth failure.

Although in many instances it may not be possible to separate the maternal from the placental causes, placental factors probably play a relatively small role in the overall incidence of IUGR. However, pathologic placental lesions such as extensive infarcts, large chorioangiomas or large areas of placental separation could lead to fetal runting. Maternal factors such as preeclampsia, drug addiction, chronic hypertensive disease, undernutrition and heavy smoking are believed to be the most common causes of IUGR. Furthermore, from the standpoint of fetal and neonatal morbidities, there are no distinct differences between those IUGR fetuses whose condition has maternal or placental causes, since the endpoint of both is placental insufficiency, either relative or absolute. In contrast, IUGR due to fetal factors manifests perinatal morbidities different from growth retardation caused by placental or maternal factors.

In a prospective study of risk factors during pregnancy by Hobel et al.,[3, 4] it was observed that 69 (4.8 per cent) of 1435 pregnancies had evidence of IUGR as indicated by clinical signs of wasting in the neonate and birth weight below the tenth percentile of the Colorado Intrauterine Growth Curve.[5] Using a predetermined set of criteria (Table 1), the IUGR infants were classified as to causal factors: maternal-placental and fetal. As shown in Table 2, only 47 of the 69 infants (68 per cent) demonstrated distinct evidence for classification into the maternal-placental factor category (87 per cent of those classified) or the fetal (13 per cent of those classified), while the remaining 22 infants (32 per cent) were growth retarded but did not have readily identifiable causes for the growth retardation. The latter phenomenon suggests the multiple and/or as yet unknown causes of IUGR or, alternatively, the incomplete nature of the present criteria for classifications.

One interesting finding in the study was the

TABLE 1. CRITERIA FOR CLASSIFICATION OF INTRAUTERINE GROWTH RETARDATION BY CAUSAL FACTORS

I. Maternal-placental
  A. Historical data
    1. Previous history of small-for-date infant
    2. Previous history of stillbirth or neonatal death
    3. Grand multiparity ($\geq$ 6 previous pregnancies)
    4. Maternal age ($\geq$36 or $\leq$15 years)
    5. Heavy smoking ($\geq$1 pack cigarettes/day)
    6. Drug addiction
    7. Anemia (hemoglobin $\leq$10 g/dl)
  B. Pregnancy events
    1. Preeclampsia or toxemia
    2. Chronic hypertension
    3. Urinary tract infection
    4. Multiple pregnancy
    5. First trimester vaginal bleeding
    6. Uterine anomalies
II. Fetal
    1. Congenital malformation of major organs
    2. Chromosomal anomalies
    3. First trimester infections (e.g., rubella)
    4. Cord IgM level $\geq$35 mg/dl

TABLE 2. PERINATAL MORBIDITIES OF VARIOUS TYPES OF INTRAUTERINE GROWTH RETARDATION

VARIETIES	NUMBER AND PERCENTAGE	FETAL DISTRESS DURING LABOR*	NEONATAL MORBIDITIES
Maternal-placental	41 (59)	10	18†
Fetal	6 (9)	0	6‡
Unclassified	22 (32)	3	4†
Total	69	13 (19)	28 (41)

*Based on one or more of the following: abnormal fetal heart rate pattern, meconium-stained amniotic fluid, persistent fetal bradycardia and Apgar score $\leq$4 at 1 minute.

†Asphyxia neonatorum, hypoglycemia, hypocalcemia and meconium aspiration syndrome.

‡Congenital heart disease, major gastrointestinal tract anomalies and congenital rubella syndrome.

clear difference in the type of perinatal morbidity observed between the two known varieties of IUGR. The maternal-placental causal variety of IUGR was associated with the occurrence of fetal distress during labor in 10 of the 41 cases (24 per cent), while none occurred in the fetal variety (Table 2). Also, the neonatal morbidities were different between the two groups. Meconium aspiration syndrome, neonatal hypoglycemia and hypocalcemia were observed in the maternal-placental variety while none of the infants in the fetal group had any of these complications. However, in this latter group there was a worse prognosis, since their neonatal morbidities were related to congenital defects, chromosomal anomalies and sequelae of congenital infections, all of which lead to potentially serious developmental problems.

In recent years, there have been studies striving to delineate a rational approach for the optimal management of these pregnancies and their offspring during the perinatal period. A variety of definitional approaches, theoretical models and technological changes during this same period have resulted in a number of controversial questions. They are addressed here as follows:

1. What is the definition of intrauterine growth retardation?

2. How can the prenatal diagnosis of IUGR best be made?

3. When should delivery be attempted?

One of the first lessons that the student of IUGR learns is that there is no clear, concise, universally accepted definition. Since IUGR babies had originally been lumped together with all low birth weight newborns despite the fact that they comprise only a third of that larger group, many of the definitions deal exclusively with the variables of birth weight and gestational age. Some authors have preferred to include only those infants whose weights are less than two standard deviations from the mean, while others have selected those less than the tenth percentile. In evaluating and comparing any studies, special care must be taken to consider those variables known to influence birth weight, e.g. altitude, socioeconomic status, sex, race and so forth. Many investigators use the intrauterine growth charts taken from Denver, Colorado, selecting the lowest tenth percentile as the cutoff for IUGR. If a population under study is selected from a middle class, sea level environment and the Denver tenth percentile criteria is used, then the infants under study will be a more severely affected group because they will be closer to the group below the third percentile for that population.

Recently, some investigators have come to think that while the birth weight for gestational age concept was helpful, a more detailed subclassification of IUGR was needed. This need grew out of follow-up data[6, 7] for these infants as well as a desire to better understand the diversity of etiologies for this syndrome.

Since brain growth and body length are often "spared" relative to body weight when IUGR is secondary to an insufficient nutrient supply, infants who are growth retarded for weight may not necessarily be growth retarded for length or head circumference. These IUGR infants with a low ponderal index (ratio of birth weight to body length or head circumference) demonstrate better catch-up growth during the first year of life than do those IUGR infants with a normal ponderal index.[8]

How well these two subclassifications of IUGR newborns will do in neurologic and psychologic follow-up when compared with each other and when matched with controls for birth weight, gestational age and date of birth remains to be determined. There is agreement, however, that as a whole, infants with IUGR do less well than matched siblings in areas of motor and school performance despite similar IQ scores.[9] Whether or not ponderal index subclassifications (or other subclassification) will better identify the infants at high and low risk for late neuropsychologic problems also remains to be seen. Nonetheless, the work of Winick and colleagues[10] in the area of brain growth and development in the rat model provides a theoretic basis for a

better outcome for those IUGR infants with a low ponderal index. These authors pointed out that somatic growth consists of two processes: (1) growth of cell number (hyperplasia), which is measured by unit weight (or protein) of tissue divided by DNA content, and (2) growth of cell size (hypertrophy), which is measured by tissue weight (or protein content) divided by DNA content. Hyperplasia takes place in the early phase of growth and is subsequently joined and then supplanted by hypertrophy. In the presence of undernutrition, the developing rat brain favors hyperplasia over hypertrophy in addition to favoring brain growth over growth of other body tissues.

How Can Intrauterine Diagnosis of IUGR Best Be Made?

Difficulty in making the in utero diagnosis of IUGR continues to be one of the chief obstacles in effectively reducing the associated high incidence of late fetal deaths. Since 10 to 20 per cent of all pregnancies are associated with inaccurate dating on the basis of menstrual history, the problem of making accurate diagnosis of IUGR at times centers on uncertainty in precisely dating the pregnancy. Under these circumstances, a serial ultrasonographic assessment of biparietal diameter (BPD) during the second trimester of pregnancy may be useful in estimating the gestational age. BPDs done between 16 to 26 weeks' gestation are usually within 1 week of true gestational age, since at this time the range of normal values is much narrower and the slope of the mean much steeper than later in pregnancy, when the discrepancy is not uncommonly 2 to 3 weeks.[11]

For an estimation of fetal growth, obstetricians often rely on the physical palpation of the gravid uterus for an estimation of fetal body size and hence gestational age. However, it is well recognized that even with the most experienced clinician, the error in fetal size assessment by physical examination is often large. Successive measurements of uterine fundal height by the same observer does afford some improvement in the assessment of fetal growth over that by multiple examiners. Nonetheless, in one report from Queen Charlotte's Hospital in London, only 29 per cent (33 of 115) of IUGR newborns were identified antenatally using this method.[11] In addition, to examiner variability, difficulty with this method of IUGR identification arises from variations in maternal abdominal size, maternal abdominal fat, amniotic fluid and fetal position. Therefore, improved methods of intrauterine diagnosis of IUGR have been sought.

Maternal hormonal assays have been suggested for prenatal identification of IUGR. These assays (e.g., estriol, human placental lactogen) are believed to be based on assessment of markers of placental function, but they have been generally disappointing in their specificity and sensitivity.[12] The obstetrician would do considerably better if he were to direct his attention to those women whose history places them at high risk for IUGR. These include women with a history of previous infants with IUGR, preeclampsia, severe chronic medical conditions (hypertension, cardiac or pulmonary disease), heavy smoking, drug addiction or grand multiparity (Table 1). An estimated 70 per cent of IUGR pregnancies can be identified by utilizing this screening procedure along with physical examination.[13]

Once the diagnosis of IUGR is suspected, ultrasonographic assessment of fetal biparietal diameter (BPD) after 18 to 20 weeks' gestation can be used as a tool to assist in the diagnosis of IUGR. Two general patterns of fetal head growth with IUGR have been described: low profile and late flattening.[11] The former is one in which head growth is retarded throughout the entire gestation and at a lower level paralleling the norm. This pattern is usually seen with primary fetal types of IUGR but may also represent a chronic form of fetal malnutrition. These fetuses usually have a low incidence of late fetal deaths, good Apgar scores and manifest no brain "sparing" with head circumference and length retarded to the same degree as weight. Moreover, postnatal persistence of this pattern of poor growth, despite adequate postnatal caloric intake, is further evidence for a primary fetal growth abnormality rather than malnutrition.

The late flattening ultrasonographic pattern of IUGR tends to be more common than the low profile, since this is often a result of maternal-placental causes. It is typified by biparietal growth that has followed the normal growth pattern until the third trimester of pregnancy, when it begins to fall off. This pattern is often witnessed in hypertensive pregnancies with the fetus being more prone to late antepartum death and intrapartum fetal distress with its resultant poor Apgar scores

and associated neonatal morbidities. These infants often demonstrate brain sparing as evidenced by head circumferences that are large relative to weights.

The determination of IUGR by serial BPD values alone suffers from a lack of specificity, since only two thirds of those pregnancies with IUGR patterns actually result in IUGR infants.[11] Recently, however, two additional ultrasonographic maneuvers have been utilized to increase accuracy of IUGR diagnosis. In one, the ratio of head circumference to abdominal circumference is determined and compared to normal values.[14] Since in IUGR secondary to maternal-placental causes, brain (head) growth occurs at the expense of visceral organs (in particular, the liver), a ratio favoring head over abdominal circumference relative to a gestational norm is found. This technique offers the additional advantage of being useful late in pregnancy even if no previous ultrasonographic BPD measurements are available for comparison.[15]

The second ultrasonographic technique that has been used to increase the specificity of diagnosing IUGR has been the estimation of total intrauterine volume (TIUV).[16] As the term implies, TIUV represents the sum of the uterine contents: fetus, placenta and amniotic fluid. Since decreased fetal mass is usually associated with decreased placental size and amniotic fluid volume, and since the TIUV is more easily estimated (it assumes the inner uterine cavity to be ellipsoid) than the complex geometry of the fetus, it has been shown to provide a good approximation of fetal weight. A recent study based on the same premise has found that a qualitative estimate of amniotic fluid volume may be helpful in selecting cases that manifest IUGR.[17] Since fetal renal and pulmonary blood flow are decreased in maternal-placental forms of IUGR because of fetal hypoxemia, the contribution that these organs make to amniotic fluid volume may be reduced. Pregnancies in which at least one pocket of amniotic fluid measures greater than 1 cm have a lower likelihood of involving IUGR.

Because of the dynamic nature of growth itself, both these ultrasonographic methods are entirely dependent on an accurate determination of gestational age. Additional confirmation of these promising techniques must be obtained from other investigators before they can be unconditionally recommended in all clinical settings.

When Should Delivery Be Attempted?

Perhaps the most controversial and yet most important issue involving IUGR centers on the optimal timing of delivery. Many clinicians monitor fetal status with weekly oxytocin challenge tests (OCT)[18, 19] or biweekly nonstress testing (NST)[20] or both, especially when a late flattening IUGR pattern is present. In the face of a normal OCT or NST, however, the timing or need for fetal pulmonary maturational indices is more controversial. If the lung maturity indices (lecithin/sphingomyelin [L/S] ratio[21] or foam stability test[22]) demonstrate fetal lung immaturity (L/S ratio less than 2.0 or negative foam stability test), consideration of maternal and fetal well-being along with conservative watchful waiting for fetal lung maturation would be the appropriate approach.

As shown in Table 3, a management plan (preferably with maternal hospitalization) can be outlined as follows. If, during the course of monitoring, the maternal and fetal conditions are stable and the fetal lung maturity is attained, delivery may be considered once the gestation is beyond 37 weeks. If lung maturity is not attained, the assessment of fetal well-being should be continued with biweekly serum or urinary estriol testing, weekly OCTs or alternatively biweekly NSTs, and clinical assessment of fetal activity by instructing the mother to count fetal movements between a specific time interval of the day. A significant reduction in "kick count" is strong evidence suggestive of fetal compromise and should be given serious clinical consideration. During this period, fetal lung maturity should be assessed at weekly intervals. When lung maturity is achieved, the decision to terminate pregnancy is relatively easier to make irrespective of the maternal and fetal clinical status, since the most significant risk for neonatal morbidity (respiratory distress syndrome) is virtually eliminated.

The problem becomes more difficult in the presence of a deteriorating maternal or fetal condition or both and fetal lung immaturity. In these instances, individual clinical judgment must be applied in considering the possibilities of delaying delivery (for 24 hours or longer) or treating the mother with a glucocorticoid or both in an effort to pharmacologically accelerate the fetal lung maturation. In the presence of hypertensive complications, particularly those with proteinuria (more than 5 g/day), maternal glucocorticoid administration should probably not be carried out because there is evidence that this maneuver may have an adverse effect on perinatal outcome.[23]

If the amniotic fluid analyses demonstrate fetal lung maturity in a preterm pregnancy, it has been questioned whether or not it is better for the fetus to remain in utero or be delivered prematurely. On this subject there are few data. On a theoretical basis, however, if the fetus is unable to grow because of nutritional deprivation secondary to placental or maternal factors, it is conceivable that growth may be accelerated ex utero by early delivery followed by adequate postnatal nutrition.

A recent study by Vohr et al.[24] may shed some light on this question. These investigators compared a group of 21 preterm (equal to or less than 37 weeks) IUGR newborns whose birth weights were less than 1500 g with a group of AGA newborns of similar birth weights, sex and socioeconomic status. These groups were followed for two years and evaluated for growth parameters as well as intellectual and neurologic outcomes. Head circumference was comparable for both groups at the end of the study (twenty-fifth percen-

TABLE 3. MANAGEMENT PLAN FOR PREGNANCY
COMPLICATED BY INTRAUTERINE GROWTH RETARDATION

PARAMETERS	STATUS AND MANAGEMENT			
Maternal and fetal conditions		Stable		Deteriorating
Fetal lung maturity	Mature	Immature	Mature	Immature
Delivery	Yes	No	Yes	Delay for <24 hours if clinically safe
Subsequent management plan	—	Continue monitoring of fetal well being; weekly assessment of fetal lung maturity; delivery when lung is mature	—	Consider maternal glucocorticoid treatment if no proteinuria ⩾5 g/day; then deliver

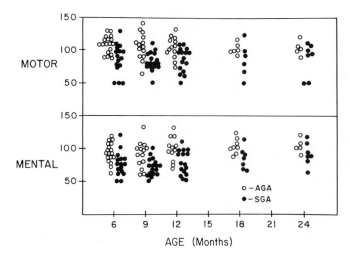

Figure 1. Scattergram of Bayley developmental score in preterm very low birth weight study infants. The difference in mean motor and mental score during the first 18 months of age are significant (p <.05). The discrepancies in the number of motor and mental observations at 18 and 24 months are due to a lack of patient's cooperation during the test. The small number at 2 years is due to patients' young age at the time of the follow-up report (From Vohr et al.[24]).

tile); similarly, the neurologic assessment as well as the Bayley scores showed no differences (Table 4 and Fig. 1). Hence, the poor outcome reported by some observers for term IUGR infants[9] may be modified for the preterm IUGR newborn who survives the perinatal period and who has the benefits of modern neonatal intensive care. It should be pointed out, however, that the neonatal mortality of the IUGR and AGA infants from which these infants were selected were 40 and 45 per cent, respectively. Clearly, additional perinatal and longer term follow-up experience needs to be collected and evaluated before an answer can be given to the question of when is the best time to deliver the IUGR fetus.

TABLE 4. FOLLOW-UP DATA ON PRETERM INTRAUTERINE GROWTH–RETARDED (IUGR) AND APPROPRIATE FOR GESTATIONAL AGE (AGA) INFANTS*

		IUGR	AGA
Number of infants		21	20
Gestational age (wks)		33.4 ± 2.2†	29.3 ± 0.7
Birth weight (g)		1220 ± 185	1195 ± 190
Total perinatal risk score‡		119 ± 48	119 ± 27
Neurological findings at 1 and 2 years	Normal	14 (7)	16 (7)
	Suspect	2 (0)	2 (0)
	Abnormal	1 (1)	1 (2)

*Adopted from the data of Vohr et al.[24]
†M ± SEM, p <.05
§The small number is due to the fact that some subjects were too young at the time for follow-up study.

Summary

1. The difficulties involved in a precise definition of IUGR are discussed in reference to a diversity of proposed pathogeneses. Studies of IUGR must be evaluated in light of the exact conditions of the study and with consideration given to the known variables affecting fetal growth.

2. Deficiencies in the clinician's ability to diagnose IUGR exist despite clinical, biochemical and ultrasonographic modes of evaluation. The screening of maternal past medical and obstetric histories, attention to the development of hypertension in pregnancy and evaluation of serial measurements of fundal growth should alert the physician to the possibility of IUGR. These women should be evaluated by serial ultrasonographic techniques.

3. The timing of delivery in the IUGR pregnancy without evidence of impending fetal death remains controversial and must be individualized.

REFERENCES

1. Usher, R. H.: Clinical implications of perinatal mortality statistics. Clin. Obstet. Gynecol. 14:885, 1971.
2. Gruenwald, P.: Chronic fetal distress and placental insufficiency. Biol. Neonate 5:215, 1963.
3. Hobel, C. J. and Oh, W.: Unpublished data.
4. Hobel, C. J., Hyvarien, M. A., Okada, D. M. and Oh, W.: Prenatal and intrapartum high risk screening. I. Prediction of the high risk neonate. Am. J. Obstet. Gynecol. 117:1, 1973.

5. Lubchenco, L. O., Hansman, C., Dressler, M. and Boyd, E.: Intrauterine growth as estimated from liveborn birth weight data at 24 to 42 weeks' gestation. Pediatrics 32:793, 1963.

6. Lubchenco, L. O.: The High Risk Infant. W. B. Saunders Co., Philadelphia, 1976, pp. 181–201.

7. Babson, S. G., Behrman, R. E. and Lessel, R.: Fetal growth: liveborn birth weights for gestational age of white middle-class infants. Pediatrics 45:937, 1970.

8. Holmes, G. E., Miller, H. C., Khatab, H., Lansky, S. B. and Goggin, J. E.: Postnatal somatic growth in infants with atypical fetal growth patterns. Am. J. Dis. Child. 131:1078, 1977.

9. Fitzhardinge, P. M. and Steven, E. M.: The small-for-date infant. II. Neurological and intellectual sequelae. Pediatrics 50:50, 1972.

10. Winick, M.: Cellular growth during early malnutrition. Pediatrics 47:969, 1971.

11. Campbell, S.: Fetal growth. Clin. Obstet. Gynecol. 1:41, 1974.

12. Tulchinsky, D.: Endocrine evaluation in the diagnosis of intrauterine growth retardation. Clin. Obstet. Gynecol. 20:969, 1977.

13. Mann, L. I., Tejani, N. A. and Weiss, R. F.: Antenatal diagnosis and management of the small-for-gestational age fetus. Am. J. Obstet. Gynecol. 120:995, 1974.

14. Campbell, S. and Thomas, A.: Ultrasonic measurement of the fetal head to abdomen circumference ratio in the assessment of head growth. Br. J. Obstet. Gynaecol. 84:165, 1977.

15. Crane, J. P. and Kopta, M. M.: Prediction of intrauterine growth retardation via ultrasonically measured head/abdominal circumference ratios. Obstet. Gynecol. 54:597, 1979.

16. Gohari, P., Berkowitz, R. L. and Hobbins, J. C.: Prediction of intrauterine growth retardation by determination of total intrauterine volume. Am. J. Obstet. Gynecol. 127:255, 1977.

17. Manning, F. A., Hill, L. M. and Platt, L. D.: Qualitative amniotic fluid volume determination by ultrasound: antepartum detection of intrauterine growth retardation. Am. J. Obstet. Gynecol. 139:254, 1981.

18. Freeman, R. K.: The use of oxytocin challenge test for antepartum clinical evaluation of uteroplacental respiratory function. Am. J. Obstet. Gynecol. 121:481, 1975.

19. Odendaal, H. J.: The fetal and labor outcome of 102 positive contraction stress tests. Obstet. Gynecol. 54:591, 1979.

20. Flynn, A. M., Kelly, J. and O'Connor, M.: Unstressed antepartum cardiotocography in the management of the fetus suspected of growth retardation. Br. J. Obstet. Gynaecol. 86:106, 1979.

21. Gluck, L., Kulovich, M. C., Borer, R. C., Jr., Brenner, P. H., Anderson, G. G. and Spellacy, W. N: Diagnosis of the respiratory distress syndrome by amniocentesis. Am. J. Obstet. Gynecol. 109:440, 1971.

22. Clements, J. A., Platzker, A. C. G., Tierney, D. et al.: Assessment of the risk of the respiratory distress syndrome by a rapid test for surfactant in amniotic fluid. N. Engl. J. Med. 286:1077, 1972.

23. Liggins, G. C. and Howie, R. N.: A controlled trial of antepartum glucocorticoid treatment for prevention of the respiratory distress syndrome in premature infants. Pediatrics 50:515, 1972.

24. Vohr, B. R., Oh, W., Rosenfeld, A. G. and Cowett, R. M.: The preterm small-for-gestational age infant: a two-year follow-up. Am. J. Obstet. Gynecol. 133:425, 1979.

Editorial Comment

It may first appear that the topics of intrauterine growth retardation and post-term pregnancy are divergent; however, the underlying pathophysiologic mechanisms may be similar. During the past decade greater emphasis has been placed on assuring the patient and her obstetrician of the well-being of the fetus. One of the most bothersome conditions, especially for the woman with her first full-term pregnancy, is that of "postdatism;" it underscores the necessity of accurate early documentation of expected delivery dates. The contributors to this chapter have identified this condition as more common than is usually appreciated and have discussed how it should be managed.

The post-term state (longer than 294 days) is observed in 10 to 20 per cent of pregnancies and intrauterine growth retardation in 4 per cent of pregnancies.

Depending on the type of patient population, intrauterine growth retardation may be as high as 10 per cent. A significant point is the fact that the problem in 25 to 35 per cent of referrals to a tertiary care center for definitive evaluation and care may well be caused by a combination of intrauterine growth retardation and post-term pregnancy. The question to consider is: What should be done? Even more importantly, 35 per cent of perinatal mortality is contributed to by these two conditions—hence the importance of understanding what this means to the fetus and the newborn.

It is often said, with tongue in cheek, that we are here because of the quality of the placenta and the lack of central nervous system defects due to hypoxia during fetal life. Problems that pertain to placentas are reflected in the syndrome of intrauterine growth retardation that results in offspring with classifications such as low birth weight (LBW), small for gestational age (SGA), and average for gestational age (AGA). These terms are used for comparison or for classifying weights with charts devised by Lubchenko, Gruenwald, and Hendricks.

The quality of the offspring is the bottom line, since some investigators feel that 25 per cent of children who had significant intrauterine growth retardation will show some central nervous system defect manifested by a decrease in growth and development as well as a lower IQ. Others now believe that with modern aggressive neonatal intensive care methods, along with the scientific skills of obstetricians identifying problems and employing good antenatal surveillance, this type of defect should occur only infrequently. Let us hope it is the latter opinion that holds true and not the former.

When the retrospectroscope is used, if congenital anomalies and fetal infections can be ruled out, the culprit in problems of fetal growth and well-being is usually the placenta. The degree of placental aging and the amount of placental reserve afford safety margins for the fetus. Meconium is an insensitive indicator of chronic hypoxia, but its presence in amniotic fluid is not considered a sign of a normal healthy fetus. Its effect can best be equated by the amount present and fetal behavior in this situation.

The key to the problem of understanding both intrauterine growth retardation and the post-term pregnancy is establishment of the true length of gestation. We have found that clinical evaluation should not be disregarded when a number of parameters are used together and they all agree. A pelvic examination before 12 weeks of gestation should establish the exact size of the uterus. An early ultrasonogram and a record of 20 weeks of fetal heart tones is correlated to a fundal height measurement from the symphysis that 28 cm equals 28 weeks' gestation. Along with appropriate quickening, this provides a collage of clinical data from which a determination can be made as to whether or not the pregnancy is post-term, affected by IUGR, or both. Do not be misled by a spurious result. One of the most useful clinical tools to confirm IUGR is a decreasing amount of amniotic fluid as seen by serial ultrasonography. The biochemical parameter of urinary estriol or estriol-creatinine ratio is useful in firming up the diagnosis but is not diagnostic. Biweekly biophysical monitoring such as the nonstress test or the oxytocin challenge test should reassure the clinician that the fetus still has placental reserve and good health. Sooner or later an aggressive decision must be made for delivery of the baby when pulmonary maturity is present.

Intrauterine growth retardation is often associated with maternal conditions such as hypertension, chronic renal disease and so forth. When this is the situation there seems to be a decrease in the amount of Wharton's jelly in the umbilical cord and easier vessel compression. These can produce a higher incidence of intrapartum fetal distress since there is usually diminished amniotic fluid.

The dilemma of the post-term pregnancy can be overcome by knowing when the patient is at 42 weeks of gestation. The time of worry about this is early in pregnancy—appropriate observations should be documented so that at term these can be reviewed. Once the patient reaches 42 weeks' gestation, appropriate biophysical (NST, OCT) and biochemical (estriol) testing should begin. Many obstetricians avoid the problem of post-term pregnancy by not letting the patient go beyond 42 to 43 weeks of gestation.

There also seems to be a decrease in Wharton's jelly in the umbilical cord in a postdate pregnancy. This, combined with the oligohydramnios that is commonly present in the postdate pregnancy and with meconium in the amniotic fluid, is an ominous indicator of chronic fetal distress. The cesarean section rate in both the IUGR and the postdate situation will be at least twice that expected in a normal population.

8
Deep Vein Thrombophlebitis During Pregnancy

Alternative Points of View

by Umberto VillaSanta and Juan L. Granados

by Jack W. Pearson and Lillie-Mae Padilla

Editorial Comment

Deep Vein Thrombophlebitis During Pregnancy

Umberto VillaSanta, M.D.
University of Maryland School of Medicine

Juan L. Granados, M.D.
University of West Virginia School of Medicine

Deep venous thrombosis, although rarely seen in the antepartum period of gestation, is a source of anxiety for the obstetrician who is often unable to confirm his diagnostic impression and must confront a patient with the unsolved therapeutic dilemma of anticoagulant use during pregnancy.

The incidence of antepartum deep venous thrombosis varies between 0.3 and 0.5 per 1000 pregnancies.[1-3] This rate is similar to the one reported for nonpregnant females[2] and is three to eight times lower than the rate found among patients in the puerperium.[1-3]

Pathogenesis

Venous stasis of the lower extremities is one of the physiologic changes of pregnancy. Increased vein distensibility[4] and a decreased velocity of the venous blood, due at least in part to the mechanical obstruction to venous return by the gravid uterus,[5] are responsible for this change.

Pregnancy is associated with a notable increase in fibrinogen and factors VII, VIII, IX, and X[6] and a reduction in plasma factor XIII (fibrin-stabilizing factor) concentration.[7]

It is interesting that, in spite of these mechanical and biochemical changes, increased risk of deep venous thrombosis seems to be confined only to the postpartum period.

Diagnosis

The most common symptoms and signs of deep venous thrombophlebitis are muscular pain, tenderness and swelling of the leg and a positive Homans' sign (pain in the calf following passive dorsiflexion of the toe), or Lowenberg test (pain in the calf or thigh associated with the rapid inflation of a blood pressure cuff to 180 mm Hg pressure) or positive results of both the sign and test.

Unfortunately, these signs and symptoms are not specific. Some of them occur in normal pregnancies. Haeger, using phlebography, was able to confirm the clinical suspicion of deep venous thrombosis in only 55 per cent of the patients he tested. The remaining 45 per cent experienced signs and symptoms attributed to venous obstruction with the same frequency but had a completely normal venous system by venography.[8]

Several diagnostic methods are available to the physician trying to prove the suspicion of deep venous thrombosis.

Doppler ultrasound is the most popular among the noninvasive methods. The technique is based on the fact that manual compression of the leg produces a pulse wave that propagates in the deep veins and is detected readily by a Doppler ultrasound detector. This wave is the manifestation of an increased flow, and will be either diminished or absent in case of thrombosis. The Doppler examination agreed with phlebography in 75.9 per cent of the limbs containing venous thrombosis in a large study conducted by Sigel.[9] This method is unable to detect clots, however, if the tributary veins only are affected and when patent collateral veins are present. False-positive results may be found in uncomplicated pregnancies in which venous outflow from the lower extremities is restricted to a degree similar to that found with mild venous thrombosis. We are not familiar with this technique, but others have used it as the main diagnostic tool for the detection of venous thrombosis during pregnancy, or as a screening procedure (especially in conjunction with impedance plethysmography) of patients at risk for venous obstruction by thrombi. No adverse effects to the fetus have yet been reported by the use of the ultrasound technique.

Impedance plethysmography shares many of the limitations of the Doppler ultrasound, especially the inability to detect minor venous obstructions and the high rate of false-positive results. This technique is more sensitive in detecting thigh deep venous thrombosis than the Doppler ultrasound, but it has demonstrated significantly less ability to detect popliteal and calf venous thrombosis.[10] The method is also noninvasive and harmless to the fetus.

Fibrinogen, labeled ^{125}I, is a useful procedure for the diagnosis of venous thrombosis of the lower extremities. Unfortunately, this technique loses sensitivity in the upper thigh and pelvis due to the relatively poor penetration of the ^{125}I and the background radioactivity produced by the femoral artery and bladder.[11] Its use during pregnancy is not recommended because the isotopic iodine crosses the placenta and concentrates in the fetal thyroid.

Phlebography is the reference standard in the diagnosis of deep venous thrombosis, being capable of detecting the vast majority of clinically significant venous thrombi. Its drawback is the exposure of the fetus to radiation. However, the actual dose received by the unborn child, although it varies with a number of factors, is less than with pelvimetry. Care should be taken to properly shield the uterus when the procedure is performed.

In conclusion, the diagnosis of deep venous thrombosis during pregnancy is complicated by the specificity of each of the signs and symptoms of the disease and by the unreliability or hazards to the fetus of the various diagnostic techniques.

At present, the decision to treat is most often based on the clinical impression. In selected cases, phlebography should be used after carefully weighing, with the patient, the risk of radiation to the fetus against the problems associated with prolonged anticoagulant therapy.

Complications

The most severe complication of deep venous thrombosis is pulmonary embolism. One of us (VillaSanta)[12] reported a 15.9 per cent incidence of embolization among patients with antepartum deep venous thrombosis who were not treated with anticoagulants. The maternal mortality of this untreated group was 12.8 per cent. In contrast, in the group treated with anticoagulants, the embolization rate was 5.2 per cent and the maternal mortality, 0.7 per cent.

Dyspnea is the most characteristic sign of pulmonary embolism; however, the most constant one is tachypnea. Small emboli, lodged into the secondary or tertiary branches of the pulmonary artery, may produce infarction, which is associated with pleural signs. Pleuritic pain, cough, splinted respirations, hemoptysis, and a friction rub may ensue. Obstruction of the primary branches of the pulmonary artery or multiple emboli produce symptoms of massive embolism. In these cases, signs of right ventricular failure, such as jugular venous distension, enlarged liver, left parasternal heave and fixed splitting of the second pulmonic sound, are present. Auscultation of the heart during normal pregnancy may reveal "functional" systolic murmurs or an increased P_2. These auscultatory changes, if they are new, will only be suggestive of pulmonary embolism.

The following laboratory aids are useful in confirming the diagnosis of pulmonary embolism:

1. Arterial blood gases. With a few exceptions, the arterial PaO_2 is less than 80 mm Hg when the patient is breathing room air.

2. EKG. Tachycardia is the most common abnormality. Nonspecific inversion of the T wave is found in about half of the patients. Shift of the axis to the right may be present in patients with massive embolism.

3. Chest x-ray. An infiltrate may be seen. Areas of increased radiolucency, elevation of the diaphragm and pleural effusion are some of the other radiologic findings.

4. Liver function tests. In cases in which pulmonary embolism is complicated by congestive heart failure, an elevated LDH and bilirubin with a normal SGOT is characteristically present.

5. Hematologic studies. Leukocytosis and an elevated erythrocyte sedimentation rate may be found. Fibrin split products are always present, and although sometimes detectable in uncomplicated pregnancies, their absence practically excludes the diagnosis of embolism.[13]

6. Lung scan. This is probably the most reliable test to prove or rule out pulmonary embolism. If a lung scan is needed, it is important to use technetium instead of iodine and to shield the uterus.

7. Angiography. If vena caval ligation is contemplated, angiography provides the only reliable means of distinguishing between embolization by a new clot and fragmentation of an old one.[14]

Management

Anticoagulant therapy is the main treatment of deep venous thrombosis with or without embolism.

Before the use of anticoagulants during pregnancy is discussed, it is useful to review some of the adjuvant therapies helpful for the symptomatic relief of the patient.

DEEP VENOUS THROMBOSIS

Trendelenburg position of patients immobilized in bed is helpful to promote venous circulation and to decrease edema of the affected extremity. Simple elevation of the leg and thigh may, by impeding femoral flow, produce the opposite effect.[15] The patient should be instructed to perform flexion and extension exercises of both legs on a regular basis. Early ambulation should be encouraged as soon as the symptoms subside and the temperature has come down to normal for at least 24 hours. Application of moist heat to the affected area can be beneficial. If analgesic drugs are required, those that affect platelet function, such as aspirin, should not be used. Elastic stockings designed to provide a decreasing pressure gradient from ankle to thigh and improve venous flow have replaced frequently inadequate elastic bandages.

PULMONARY EMBOLISM

In addition to these measures, if the source of the embolism is in the lower extremities, oxygen, with the goal of maintaining a PaO_2 above 70 mm Hg, is essential to prevent maternal and fetal hypoxia. Narcotics (morphine or meperidine) will relieve pain and decrease anxiety. Stool softeners to avoid straining at defecation may be helpful. Treat shock, if present, with vasopressor drugs such as isoproterenol by drip (2 to 4 mg in 500 ml of 5% dextrose in water), adjusting the rate of infusion to maintain the systolic pressure at about 90 mm Hg. In cardiac failure, digoxin may be needed. Antibiotics are only indicated in suspected cases of septic embolism.

The Use of Anticoagulants
During Pregnancy

At the present time, three major types of anticoagulants are available: agents that inhibit fibrin formation (heparin and coumarin derivatives); agents that alter platelet physiology (aspirin and dextran); and finally, those that facilitate fibrinolysis (streptokinase and urokinase).

We will discuss only the first two, since they are by far the most effective and widely used anticoagulants in the United States. The fibrinolytic agents are not yet commercially available.

Heparin is a mucoitin polysulfuric acid produced by the mast cells of Ehrlich or heparinocytes. Due to its high molecular weight, it does not cross the placental barrier.[16] With a co-factor, which is a plasma alpha-globulin known as antithrombin III, heparin forms a complex that has a powerful antithrombin action, thus preventing the formation of fibrin from fibrinogen. Heparin effects can be neutralized by a very slow intravenous injection (in 1 to 3 minutes) of 1 to 1.5 mg of protamine sulfate per 100 U of administered heparin. No more than 50 mg of protamine sulfate should be used in any 10-minute period. (Protamine alone may cause bleeding if given in excessive amounts.)

Complications of heparin therapy include hemorrhage,[17, 18] osteoporosis (if more than 15,000 U per day are given for more than 6 months),[19] and some other rare effects such as pain at the injection site, allergic reactions, alopecia and thrombocytopenia.[17]

A number of clotting studies can be used to monitor heparin therapy. The initial Lee-White clotting time has been replaced by the more sensitive and accurate partial thromboplastin times (PTT, aPTT, WBPTT).[20, 21] In order to achieve an effective anticoagulation, we aim to maintain the PTT of 2.5 to 3 times the control value.

Treatment is started with a loading dose of 5000 U for deep venous thrombosis and 10,000 to 15,000 U for pulmonary embolism, administered intravenously. This initial dose is followed by a continuous intravenous infusion of 400 U/kg/24 hr, which is maintained for 10 days or until the symptoms disappear. At this time, subcutaneous heparin or oral coumarin may be used for long-term anticoagulation. If it is decided to use subcutaneous heparin, the patient is instructed in the self-administration of 150 to 200 U/kg every 12 hours. The patient is kept on anticoagulant therapy for six weeks after an acute episode of thrombophlebitis and for six months following pulmonary embolization. If the patient is on coumarin derivatives, conversion to heparin is accomplished at 36 weeks of gestation. Heparin is discontinued at the onset of spontaneous labor or prior to elective induction of labor. Patients who had a recent pulmonary embolism or a recent thrombosis of the iliac or femoral vein receive intrapartum continuous intravenous heparin at a dose to keep their PTT at 1.5 to 2 times the control value. Six hours postpartum, heparin can be restarted in those patients in whom it was discontinued and given in full dose (PTT, 2.5 to 3 times control) to those who received it during labor and delivery.

Heparin prophylaxis is indicated in patients with a history of thrombophlebitis or pulmonary embolism and in patients at high risk for thrombophlebitis. Henderson et al. found that 10 per cent of the patients who had pulmonary embolism during pregnancy had a previous history of this condition.[22] Prophylaxis is achieved by administering 5000 U of heparin subcutaneously in early labor and every 12 hours thereafter until the patient is fully ambulatory.

Coumarin derivatives reduce the production of prothrombin factor VII, factor IX and factor X by inhibiting the actions of vitamin K. Vitamin K is a co-factor in the synthesis of these four essential clotting factors. Coumarin derivatives, due to their small molecular weight, cross the placenta and are excreted in breast milk.[23] Their use during the first trimester of pregnancy may result in multiple congenital anomalies of the newborn. Shaul and Hall, in a recent review of the literature, reported 14 cases of the so-called vitamin K antagonists embriopathy in newborns whose mothers received coumarin during the first 8 weeks of pregnancy.[24] Sodium warfarin and phenindione (a vitamin K antagonist related to warfarin) were the drugs implicated. The most typical defects included nasal hypoplasia, stippled epiphyses, ophthalmologic abnormalities, intrauterine growth retardation and developmental delay. Recently, two reports have indicated that warfarin may cause birth defects in newborns whose mothers receive the drug only during the second and third trimesters of pregnancy.[25, 26] Although the characteristic nasal hypoplasia and stippled epiphyses were not present, mental retardation, ophthalmologic abnormalities and generalized central nervous system anomalies were found. In addition, the use of coumarin derivatives during the second and third trimester may result in fetal death due to placental and fetal hemorrhage. In 1965, VillaSanta[12] reported a 15.7 per cent fetal loss due to hemorrhagic complications when mothers received oral anticoagulants,[3] and recently, Laros reported a fetal mortality of 11.7 per cent among the same type of patients[27] and Tejani,[28] a 30 per cent fetal wastage in a group of patients with cardiac valve prosthesis.

In view of the teratogenicity and fetal hemorrhagic complications associated with the use of coumarin derivatives, we consider them to be contraindicated during pregnancy. However, a number of patients may find it difficult, if not impossible, to inject themselves with heparin or may be allergic to the drug. In these cases, after informing them of the potential risk associated with the use of coumarin, we recommend the following therapeutic guidelines:

1. Heparin should be used during the acute phase of the disease and the first trimester of pregnancy.

2. When sodium warfarin is used during the second and third trimester of gestation, the prothrombin time should be kept between 1.5 to 2 times the control value. Initially, the patient is given 10 to 15 mg daily, by mouth, until the therapeutic prothrombin time mentioned previously is achieved. A maintenance dose of 2 to 10 mg a day with prothrombin times repeated once or twice a week is used thereafter.

3. At 36 weeks of gestation, if the patient is still in need of anticoagulant therapy, warfarin is discontinued and heparin restarted. This is done to avoid the possibility of neonatal bleeding and based on the fact that the effects of coumarin derivatives on the fetus may last for up to 14 days after the drug is discontinued.[29] If preterm labor occurs, warfarin anticoagulation can be reversed by using vitamin K and fresh frozen plasma.

4. Warfarin therapy is reinstituted soon after delivery, and heparin is discontinued on the seventh day postpartum. Mothers are not allowed to breast feed their infants.

Dextran, widely used as a plasma expander, has been shown to reduce clot formation in injured femoral vessels from 95 to only 10 per cent.[30] Because of its high molecular weight, it does not cross the placenta.[31] Its use in pregnancy was first proposed by VillaSanta,[12] and several reports of its efficacy have followed.[32, 33] Dextran is effective if used in early stages of thrombophlebitis, but its action is much less satisfactory if this condition has been present for more than 48 hours. The empiric formula is $(C_6H_{10}O_5)n$, and the average molecular weight is about 75,000. For the average patient, weighing between 110 and 130 pounds, therapeutic treatment consists of 500 ml of a 6 per cent solution administered as a slow intravenous drip for 3 consecutive days. The PTT is slightly increased after dextran infusion, but only 5 times the therapeutic dose will prolong bleeding time to dangerous levels,[30] so that repeated tests for coagulation control are not necessary. So far, no adverse effects on pregnancy have been reported and no cases of thrombophlebitis treated with dextran have been found to progress to embolization.

Rarely, when anticoagulants are contraindicated or have failed, surgical interruption of the vena cava and both ovarian veins may be necessary to save the mother's life. This operation is compatible with fetal life.[34] Finally, in patients with massive embolization of the main pulmonary artery demonstrated by angiography and persistent cardiac failure, pulmonary embolectomy may have to be performed.[14] In these cases, although fetal survivals have been reported,[35] the main concern is the maternal outcome.

REFERENCES

1. Aaro, L. A. and Juergens, J. L.: Thrombophlebitis associated with pregnancy. Am. J. Obstet. Gynecol. 109:1128, 1971.
2. Drill, A.: Oral contraceptives and thromboembolic disease. J.A.M.A. 219:583, 1972.
3. VillaSanta, U.: Therapy in antepartum thrombophlebitis. Obstet. Gynecol. 26:534, 1965.
4. McCausland, A. M., Hyman, C., Winsor, T. et al.: Venous distensibility during pregnancy. Am. J. Obstet. Gynecol. 81:472, 1961.
5. Wright, H. P., Osborn, S. B. and Edmonds, D. G.: Changes in the rate of flow of venous blood in the leg during pregnancy measured with radioactive sodium. Surg. Gynecolog. Obstet. 90:481, 1950.
6. Todd, M. E., Thompson, J. H., Bowie, E. J. W. et al.: Changes in blood coagulation during pregnancy. Mayo Clin. Proc. 40:370, 1965.
7. Coopland, A., Alkjaersig, N. and Fletcher, A. P.:

Reduction in plasma factor XIII (fibrin stabilizing factor) conceptration during pregnancy. J. Lab. Clin. Med. 73:144, 1969.

8. Haeger, K.: Problems of acute deep venous thrombosis. Angiology 20:219, 1969.

9. Sigel, B., Robert, W. R., Popky, G. L. and Ipsen, J.: Diagnosis of lower limb venous thrombosis by Doppler ultrasound technique. Arch. Surg. 104:174, 1972.

10. Richards, K. L., Armstrong, J. D. and Tikoff, G. et al.: Non-invasive diagnosis of deep venous thrombosis. Arch. Intern. Med. 136:1091, 1976.

11. Kakkar, V. V.: The diagnosis of deep venous thrombosis using the ^{125}I-fibrinogen test. Arch. Surg. 104:152, 1972.

12. VillaSanta, U.: Thromboembolic disease in pregnancy. Am. J. Obstet. Gynecol. 93:142, 1965.

13. Gurewich, V., Hume, M. and Patrick, M.: The laboratory diagnosis of venous thromboembolic disease by measurement of fibrinogen/fibrin degradation products and fibrin monomer. Chest 64:585, 1973.

14. Sasahara, A. A.: Therapy for pulmonary embolism. J.A.M.A. 229:1795, 1974.

15. Burns, W. T.: Thromboembolic disease in obstetrics and gynecology. The value of early diagnosis and adequate treatment. Am. J. Obstet. Gynecol. 71:260, 1956.

16. Finnerty, J. J. and MacKay, B. R.: Antepartum thrombophlebitis and pulmonary embolism: Report of a case and review of the literature. Obstet. Gynecol. 19:405, 1962.

17. Gervin, A. S.: Complications of heparin therapy. Surg. Gynecol. Obstet. 140:789, 1975.

18. Basu, D., Gallus, A., Hirch, J. et al.: A prospective study of the value of monitoring heparin treatment with the activated partial thromboplastin time. N. Engl. J. Med. 287:324, 1972.

19. Griffith, G. C., Nichols, G., Asher, J. D. et al.: Heparin osteoporosis. J.A.M.A. 193:185, 1965.

20. Estes, J. W.: Kinetics of the anticoagulant effect of heparin. J.A.M.A. 212:1492, 1970.

21. Godal, H. C.: Heparin assay methods for the control of in vivo heparin effects. Thromb. Diath. Haemorrh. 33:77, 1974.

22. Henderson, S. R., Curtis, J. L. and Creasman, W. T.: Antepartum pulmonary embolism. Am. J. Obstet. Gynecol. 112:476, 1972.

23. Deykin, D.: Warfarin therapy. N. Engl. J. Med. 283:691, 1970.

24. Shaul, W. L. and Hall, J. G.: Multiple congenital anomalies associated with oral anticoagulants. Am. J. Obstet. Gynecol. 127:191, 1977.

25. Sherman, S. and Hall, B. D.: Warfarin and fetal abnormality. Lancet 1:692, 1976.

26. Larson, M. and Reid, M.: Warfarin and fetal abnormality. Lancet 1:1356, 1976.

27. Laros, R. K., Jr.: Anticoagulants: indications and use. Contemp. Obstet. Gynecol. 5:67, 1975.

28. Tejani, N.: Anticoagulant therapy with cardiac valve prosthesis during pregnancy. Obstet. Gynecol. 42:785, 1973.

29. Pridmore, B. R., Murray, K. H. and MacAllen, P. M.: The management of anticoagulant therapy during and after pregnancy. Br. J. Obstet. Gynaecol. 82:740, 1975.

30. Bryant, M. F., Bloom, W. L. and Brewer, S. S., Jr.: Use of dextran in preventing thrombosis of small arteries following surgical trauma. J. Med. Assoc. Georgia 50:580, 1961.

31. Falk, V., Forkman, B. and Arfors, K. E.: The permeability of the (human) placenta to dextrans. Acta Obstet. Gynecol. Scand. 46:414, 1967.

32. Husni, E. A., Pena, L. I. and Lehnert, A. E.: Thrombophlebitis in pregnancy. Am. J. Obstet. Gynecol. 97:901, 1967.

33. Wallach, R. C.: Dextran therapy for pregnancy-associated deep thrombophlebitis. Am. J. Obstet. Gynecol. 112:613, 1972.

34. Collins, C. G.: Suppurative pelvic thrombophlebitis. A study of 202 cases in which the disease was treated by ligation of the vena cava and ovarian vein. Am. J. Obstet. Gynecol. 108:681, 1970.

35. Evans, G. L., Dalen, J. E. and Dexter, L.: Pulmonary embolism during pregnancy. J.A.M.A. 206:320, 19768.

Preferable Management of Complications of the Venous System in Pregnancy: An Update

Jack W. Pearson, M.D.

Lillie-Mae Padilla, M.D.

Indiana University School of Medicine

Complications or compromise of the venous system associated with pregnancy are frequently seen in the obstetrician's office. Problems that present range from a patient's complaint of pain, swelling and cosmetic disfiguration to the more serious and even life-threatening problems associated with thrombophlebitis and thromboembolism. Close attention must be paid, at the time of the patient's initial visit, to any past history of thrombophlebitis or embolization that may have occurred either in prior pregnancies or while the patient was taking oral contraceptives. Patients with such histories are followed in our high-risk clinic. Although individual clinicians' anxiety levels vary, as do criteria for seriousness of the observed disease process, the impression gained is that the incidence of venous complications in pregnant women ranges from 5 to 33 per cent. Parity, age, degree of symptoms considered significant, and the amount of time the physician spends with the patient during a routine prenatal visit contribute to the number of problems recognized. The purpose of this article is to point out and attempt to place in proper perspective the significance of these complications and to present a method of management in each situation. Our primary purpose will be to discuss the efficacy of medical management in the vast majority of these patients. There will be no attempt to discuss in any depth the pathogenesis of venous disease or predisposing factors in pregnancy, as this has been done well in many other texts and articles.

Varicose Veins in Pregnancy

Among the most frequent and aggravating problems for the patient are those related to varicose veins that develop in pregnancy. The patient's complaints are primarily those of cosmetic disfiguration, leg pain and swelling that occur as the pregnancy progresses. The problem is obviously self-limited and we consider conservative management to be optimal in these circumstances. We recommend daily rest periods with the legs elevated and emphasize that the patient lie on her side rather than supine to further facilitate venous return from the lower extremities. Angiographic studies have shown the detrimental effect of the supine position on venous return in the pregnant patient. In the more severe cases we also prescribe full leg support, usually with prescription panty support hose.* According to Nabatoff and Pincus,[40] 20 per cent of patients with varicose veins in the lower extremities in pregnancy will demonstrate associated

---

*Jobst Institute, Inc., P. O. Box 653, Toledo, Ohio 43601.

vulvar varicosities. In most cases we have found that support of the perineal area can be obtained by use of panty support hose. Severe edema that compromises the patient in spite of the elastic hose is one of the exceptions to our usual rule of not using diuretics in pregnancy. Dyazide is prescribed every other day for this patient.

Several articles have been published, particularly from European countries, advocating a surgical attack on varices in pregnancy, using the same indications as for nonpregnant patients. The majority of American physicians and surgeons believe that any consideration of surgical correction of the varices appearing in or aggravated by pregnancy should be postponed from six weeks to three months after parturition. The preponderance of literature indicates that both injection techniques and surgical techniques, including the so-called radical surgical approach, have less optimal results in pregnant than in nonpregnant patients. In view of the fact that conservative measures are so effective and the temporal nature of pregnancy so certain, there should be little question that the conservative approach is by far the best. However, it goes without saying that these patients are at significant risk in terms of developing more serious complications and close attention must be paid to persisting or recurrent symptoms that might indicate a change in clinical status.

In our practice over the past 11 years all patients with varices have been considered for prophylactic administration of 500 ml of low molecular weight dextran during labor and on each of the first three postpartum days. This has been done to prevent the occurrence of puerperal thrombophlebitis. During this time 7220 patients were delivered at the William Beaumont General Hospital (WBGH), 6569 patients at the R. E. Thomason General Hospital (RETGH) (1970 to 1973) and 25,701 patients at the Indiana University Medical Center (IUMC) (1974 to 1980). The incidence of postpartum thrombophlebitis in patients so treated was negligible and there was no instance of pulmonary embolus in these cases. We believe that administration of low molecular weight dextran has little risk. Obvious precautions must be taken in those cases of severe cardiovascular disease in which the blood volume expansion inherent in the dextran administration can cause cardiac decompensation.

Superficial Thrombophlebitis

If the patient develops symptoms and findings of superficial phlebitis either antepartum or postpartum, our approach and management remains the same. In all cases we first rule out deep thrombophlebitis using techniques to be described. After this is done, bed rest is prescribed and the patient is advised to lie on either side but not on her back. The foot of the bed is elevated and local heat, elastic bandages and bed exercises are prescribed. The patient is ambulated as soon as she no longer experiences leg pain. In addition, she is given 500 ml of dextran daily for 3 days. We have been impressed by the fact that in the vast majority of cases the patient's symptoms disappear within 12 to 24 hours after therapy is instituted. The patient is discharged to the high-risk clinic in 3 to 5 days from the time of initiation of therapy. We do not use anticoagulation therapy in these cases and believe that surgery is certainly contraindicated.

Deep Thrombophlebitis

Perhaps the most significant problem in considering deep thrombophlebitis during pregnancy is the importance of an accurate diagnosis and the difficulty of obtaining one. Although accuracy of clinical diagnosis is higher when the process has extended to the inguinal area, more than 50 per cent of *postoperative* nonpregnant patients with phlebographic or isotopic evidence of venous thrombosis have no signs or symptoms of the disorder, and nearly half of patients thought to have deep vein thrombophlebitis may have a normal venous system by venography. Moreover, up to 50 per cent of fatal emboli in these patients arise from clinically unsuspected thrombi.

In contrast to the series reported by Henderson et al., suggesting that this is also the case in the pregnant patient, all our cases have been clinically evident and we have seen embolization in pregnancy without apparent phlebitis in only one case. We have seen no instance of bilateral antepartum deep phlebitis and the overwhelming majority of cases have involved the left leg. In addition, most of our patients have been nulligravid or of low parity. All have been diagnosed by methods to be outlined.

The pregnant patient who has varices or has a significant history of venous complications in a previous pregnancy or while taking oral contraceptives should be made aware of the following symptoms: unilateral or bilateral extremity swelling, acute leg pain, chest pain, chronic cough or hemoptysis. She is instructed to seek medical care at the earliest possible moment if these symptoms develop.

The incidence of deep phlebitis has been variously reported to be between 0.018 and 0.52 per cent in the antepartum period, and between 0.1 and 1.0 per cent in the puerperium. Although thrombophlebitis can occur at any stage of gestation, it appears to increase in frequency as pregnancy advances. After delivery, deep phlebitis is most frequently seen within the first three postpartum days but may occur up to four weeks after delivery. As noted in Table 1, our experience in El Paso with antepartum disease reflected an incidence of 0.073 per cent. At Indiana University Medical Center over the past 8 years we have encountered an incidence of approximately 0.095 per cent. The IUMC data actually represent the years 1975 to 1977, and the rate has been essentially stable since that time. It may be a bit skewed, reflecting the effect of referral cases.

TABLE 1.   INCIDENCE OF DEEP THROMBOPHLEBITIS

No. DELIVERIES	No. CASES OF DEEP THROMBO- PHLEBITIS	INCIDENCE OF ANTEPARTUM DEEP THROMBO- PHLEBITIS	MATERNAL MORTALITY	EMBOLIZA- TION	FETAL DEATH
13,500 (literature review)	7	0.52/1000	0	1*	0
13,789 (WBGH and RETGH)	10	0.73/1000	0	0	1
8371 (IUMC)	8	0.95/1000	0	1*	0

*Episodes occurred when heparin treatment was discontinued and phlebitis recurred.

Methods we routinely use to diagnose deep thrombophlebitis in pregnancy are as follows:

1. Physical examination, with particular emphasis on observation and documentation of any areas of redness or cord formation in the peripheral venous system, and also auscultation of the lungs.

2. Careful documentation in the patient's chart of comparable leg measurements taken 6 cm above and below the patella on each leg.

3. The Lowenberg blood pressure cuff test is utilized bilaterally and any difference noted in the pressure necessary to produce pain in each leg.

4. We use the technique of Doppler assessment of the venous system, placing the transducer over or cephalad to the apparent area of involvement and noting presence or absence of increased venous flow when pressure is applied over the muscle mass of the calf.

Venography is the most specific laboratory evaluation but is invasive, expensive, subject to difficulty of interpretation, exposes the fetus to some radiation even with shielding and can *induce* phlebitis in 3 to 5 per cent of patients. Because of our success with noninvasive methods, we have resorted to venography only when clinical evaluation and other methods were equivocal for symptomatic patients early in pregnancy in whom a diagnosis would necessitate a long period of treatment. Radioactive iodine–labeled fibrinogen scans have not been used because of the danger of hepatitis and because of the possibility of free isotope reaching the fetus. We have had no experience with technetium colloid scans of the extremities. Similarly, we have no experience with plethysmography, although this technique has been reported by several investigators to offer comparable usefulness to Doppler evaluation.

The Doppler technique is most useful with unilateral disease because blood flow in both femoral veins may be retarded late in pregnancy without thrombus formation. Furthermore, major venous obstruction must be present to allow unequivocal detection. Doppler evaluation has been shown by several authors to have a high correlation with venographic studies. The accuracy of this technique is further improved if ileofemoral disease is present. Since we find that deep thrombophlebitis in pregnancy is almost always unilateral and because Doppler equipment is readily available to the obstetrician, we have found this technique of primary value in assessing suspected deep thrombophlebitis.

TREATMENT REGIMEN

Upon establishing the diagnosis of deep thrombophlebitis our policy is to treat the patient with anticoagulation throughout the remainder of the pregnancy. Our technique is as follows:

The patient is admitted to the hospital and an intravenous catheter of the pediatric disposable type* is utilized with an adapter.† Over the first 24 hours sodium heparin is administered intravenously every 4 hours to establish a coagulation time between 2 and 3 times control levels when measured one half hour before the administration of the next injection. Over the next 24 to 48 hours, the patient is educated in the technique of self-administration of intravenous heparin, and from that point on she administers the heparin to herself through the indwelling catheter, with usual dosage of between 10,000 and 12,000 units every 6 hours. This is continued throughout the remainder of the pregnancy (Fig. 1). The patient is ambulated as soon as she is relatively asymptomatic, and when she is fully ambulatory she is discharged from the hospital. She maintains her therapy with weekly visits to the high-risk obstetric clinic until delivery. We have found that the indwelling catheter technique is satisfactory and that the catheters need to be replaced at intervals of two weeks to three months. We believe that the self-administration of heparin is quite safe and is analogous to the case of diabetic patients, who traditionally have administered insulin to themselves and treated their own disease with medical supervision and guidance.

We have personal experience with over 40 cases and know of at least 16 others in which the technique has been utilized. Seven of these were reported by Gurll and associates and the other nine disclosed in personal communication with the physicians involved. There has been one fetal death. Of all patients (now over 25) treated at IUMC, there was only one incident of infection occurring at the catheter site.

We are aware of no instances of recurrence of the disease process during the pregnancy when therapy has been continuous, and there have been no reports of embolization while

---

*Endo Laboratories, Inc., 1000 Stewart Ave., Garden City, N.Y. 11530

†Deseret Pharmaceutical Co., Inc., 9450 S. State St., Sandy, Utah 84070

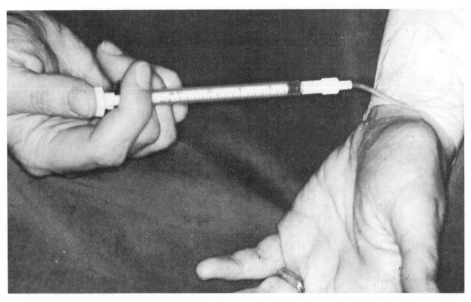

Figure 1. Demonstration of technique in which the patient administers heparin with indwelling catheter in place.

this regimen is followed. The anticoagulation is continued throughout pregnancy and discontinued 4 to 8 hours prior to delivery. Heparin is resumed approximately 4 hours after delivery and continued for the first 24 to 48 hours of the puerperium. Treatment with a coumarin derivative is begun on the first or second postpartum day and continued for 6 weeks.

We believe strongly that this type of long-term therapy is indicated because it has been reported that 24 per cent of patients with antenatal deep thrombophlebitis will develop pulmonary emboli if their condition is not treated, with an associated death rate of 15 to 18 per cent. The incidence of embolization is decreased to 4.5 per cent in those patients who are receiving anticoagulants, and the death rate drops to 0.7 per cent. Of the patients treated at IUMC three discontinued self-administration of heparin upon leaving the hospital and were readmitted with recurrent thrombophlebitis, one with a pulmonary embolus. One of these patients, who had left the hospital against medical advice, was then switched to Coumadin until just prior to delivery. She had one subsequent episode of hematemesis after taking the wrong dose of Coumadin. The patient with cellulitis at the catheter site, whose medication was changed to Coumadin, had a subsequent episode of epistaxis. She had had hematemesis after administering herself the wrong dose of heparin

in a prior pregnancy. Two additional patients each had an episode of hematemesis while on outpatient heparin, one because she was administering the wrong dose. In only one case did a patient bleed to the point of needing transfusion and all were maintained on continued anticoagulation.

We have had no maternal mortality in association with this regimen, and there have been only two instances in which there has been significant maternal morbidity. In the first case (at RETGH), a massive retroperitoneal hematoma developed secondary to trauma in a 300-pound patient in the early third trimester of pregnancy. The mother did well but the attendant maternal hypovolemia caused fetal hypoxia and death. In the second instance (IUMC), the patient suffered a hematoma of the anterior abdominal wall and left broad ligament after moving furniture. She was delivered by cesarean section because of subsequent premature labor and a breech presentation. Both mother and infant did well.

There have been no significant bleeding complications in labor or the puerperium. In two instances in which lochia was somewhat increased, anticoagulation therapy was continued and bleeding was controlled with the administration of methergine. A literature review and our partial personal experience with cases in which intravenous heparin therapy was used from the time of diagnosis until delivery are summarized in Table 1.

We recognize that anticoagulation with coumarin derivatives has been advocated in several publications, but we have also noted significant fetal loss in association with this regimen from both fetal and neonatal bleeding as well as from associated maternal complications. A high incidence of abortion and some documentation of teratogenesis associated with Coumadin treatment have strengthened our belief that heparin therapy is the preferred approach to management. Fogarty and co-workers have recommended thrombectomy as an optimal means of management, particularly in cases of deep iliofemoral thrombophlebitis. In view of the fact that recurrence of thrombosis is not uncommon after this procedure, the only circumstances in which we think that surgery (e.g., vena caval ligation) might be indicated are those in which recurrent embolism complicates the disease process in spite of optimal anticoagulant therapy.

Pelvic Thrombophlebitis

Puerperal pelvic or ovarian thrombophlebitis is a serious complication and an extremely difficult diagnosis to establish. We believe that any puerpera in whom fever and pelvic tenderness indicate the presence of endometritis and parametritis that do not resolve within 48 to 72 hours after the initiation of systemic antibiotic therapy should be considered to have pelvic phlebitis, whether or not the diagnosis is apparent on pelvic or abdominal examination. In these circumstances, the patient is treated with intravenous heparin therapy, which is continued from 5 to 10 days, with conversion to Coumadin therapy. This in turn is continued on an empiric basis for 6 weeks. If resolution of the fever and pelvic complaints is not apparent 48 to 72 hours after initiation of the heparin therapy, one must consider the possibility of adnexal abscess or other surgical complications of the puerperium, and laparotomy is indicated.

Thromboembolic Disease

Diagnosis of pulmonary emboli in any patient requires firm documentation before or during the institution of a therapeutic approach. The patient's symptoms are significant and close attention should be paid to any complaints or findings of tachypnea, dyspnea, chest pain (especially pleuritic in nature), apprehension, chronic cough, tachycardia or hemoptysis, even in the absence of apparent thrombophlebitis in the extremities or pelvis. The usual diagnostic measures of enzyme studies, EKG, auscultation and x-ray assessment of the chest should be performed. Pulmonary angiographic studies should be obtained to confirm the diagnosis in order to effectively document the condition of these patients prior to treatment. Lung scanning techniques utilizing radioactive substances have been shown to be inaccurate. This is particularly true in the pregnant or postpartum patient.

We believe that the first line of defense and management is anticoagulation, and until the patient's course in the hospital is well established, we rely entirely upon intravenous heparinization in an attempt to control the disease process and prevent further emboli. Coumadin is not to be utilized in this phase of treatment. If repeat embolization occurs despite adequate anticoagulation, a surgical approach may be necessary. In this case, the anticoagulation achieved by heparin is readily reversed, whereas that obtained with coumarin derivatives presents definite hazards to the patient in the operating room. We further think that the coumarin derivatives are a poor second choice to heparin as an immediate and early agent of anticoagulation in these patients because of their delayed action and questionable value in preventing repeat embolization. In view of the fact that embolization has not occurred in antepartum patients with deep thrombophlebitis who were treated as described, we have found no need for surgical intervention in the pregnant patient.

History of Embolism Involving Birth Control Pills

There is a last group of pregnant patients who present with a history of embolization, vascular accident or both while previously taking birth control pills. To date, we do not know if these patients are analogous to those who have had phlebitis or thromboembolism in a prior pregnancy and therefore we have not placed them on the heparin regimen. We have empirically advised 600 mg of aspirin twice a day throughout the pregnancy. We have seen six patients in this category and none have evidenced vascular problems during pregnancy. None of the newborn have been clinically abnormal in any way nor evidenced a bleeding diathesis.

The following selected bibliography of pertinent articles has been of value in preparing this article and is recommended to the interested reader.

REFERENCES

1. Aaro, L. A. and Juergens, J. L.: Thrombophlebitis associated with pregnancy. Am. J. Obstet. Gynecol. 109:1128, 1971.
2. Abbott, A., Sibert, J. R. and Weaver, J. B.: Chondrodysplasia punctata and maternal warfarin treatment. Br. Med. J. 2:1639, 1977.
3. Alger, L. S. and Laros, R. K.: Thromboembolic disease and pregnancy. J.C.E. Obstet. Gynecol. 20:13, 1978.
4. Barner, H. B., William, V. L., Kaiser, C. C. and Hanlon, C. R.: Thrombectomy for iliofemoral venous thrombosis. J.A.M.A. 208:2442, 1969.
5. Bates, M. M.: Venous thromboembolic disease and ABO blood type. Lancet 1:239, 1971.
6. Beller, F. K.: Thromboembolic disease in pregnancy. Clin. Obstet. Gynecol. 11:290, 1968.
7. Bettmann, M. A. and Paulin, S.: Leg phlebography: the incidence, nature and modification of undesirable side effects. Radiology 122:101, 1977.
8. Bonnar, J. and Walsh, J.: Prevention of thrombosis after pelvic surgery by British Dextran 70. Lancet 1:615, 1972.
9. Brown, T. K. and Munsick, R. A.: Puerperal ovarian vein thrombophlebitis: a syndrome. Am. J. Obstet. Gynecol. 109:263, 1971.
10. Burstein, R., Alkjaersig, M. and Fletcher, A.: Thromboembolism during pregnancy and the postpartum state. J. Lab. Clin. Med. 78:838, 1971.
11. Byrne, J. J.: Thrombophlebitis in pregnancy. Clin. Obstet. Gynecol. 13:305, 1970.
12. Clagett, G. P. and Salzman, E. W.: Prevention of venous thromboembolism. Prog. Cardiovasc. Dis. 17:345, 1975.
13. Coon, W. W.: Epidemiology of venous thromboembolism. Ann. Surg. 186:149, 1977.
14. Crane, C., Hartsuck, J., Birtch, A., Couch, N. P., Zollinger, R., Matloff, J., Dalen, J. and Dexter, L.: The management of major pulmonary embolism. Surg. Gynecol. Obstet. 128:27, 1969.
15. Dale, W. A. and Lewis, M. R.: Heparin control of venous thromboembolism. Arch. Surg. 101:744, 1970.
16. Dodson, M. G., Mobin-Uddin, K. and O'Leary, J. A.: Intracaval umbrella-filter for prevention of recurrent pulmonary embolism. South. Med. J. 64:1017, 1971.
17. Duncan, I. D., Coyle, M. G. and Walker, J.: Management and treatment of 34 cases of antepartum thromboembolism. J. Obstet. Gynaec. Br. Commonwealth 78:904, 1971.
18. Evans, D. S. and Cockett, F. B.: Diagnosis of deep-vein thrombosis with an ultrasonic doppler technique. Br. Med. J. 2:802, 1969.
19. Flanigan, D. P., Goodreau, J. J., Burnham, S. J., Bergan, J. J. and Yao, J. S. T.: Vascular-laboratory diagnosis of clinically suspected acute deep-vein thrombosis. Lancet 1:331, 1978.
20. Flessa, H. C., Glueck, H. I. and Dritschilo, A.: Thromboembolic disorders in pregnancy: pathophysiology, diagnosis and treatment, with emphasis on heparin. Clin. Obstet. Gynecol. 17:195, 1974.
21. Fogarty, T. J., Wood, J. A., Krippaehne, W. S. and Dennis, D. L.: Management of iliofemoral venous thrombosis in the antepartum state. Surg. Gynecol. Obstet. 128:546, 1969.
22. Fogarty, T. J. and Hallin, R. W.: Temporary caval occlusion during venous thrombectomy. Surg. Gynecol. Obstet. 122:1269, 1966.
23. Gurll, N., Helfand, Z., Salzman, E. F. and Silen, W.: Peripheral venous thrombophlebitis during pregnancy. Am. J. Surg. 121:449, 1971.
24. Haeger, K.: The treatment of varicose veins in pregnancy by radical operation or conservatively. Acta Obstet. Gynecol. Scand. 47:223, 1968.
25. Henderson, S. R., Lund, C. J. and Creasman, W. T.: Antepartum pulmonary embolism. Am. J. Obstet. Gynecol. 112:476, 1972.
26. Hill, W. C. and Pearson, J. W.: Outpatient intravenous heparin therapy for antepartum iliofemoral thrombophlebitis. Obstet. Gynecol. 37:785, 1971.
27. Hirsh, J., Cade, J. F. and O'Sullivan, E. F.: Clinical experience with anticoagulant therapy during pregnancy. Br. Med. J. 1:270, 1970.
28. Hirsh, J., Cade, J. F. and Gallus, A. S.: Anticoagulants in pregnancy: a review of indications and complications. Am. Heart J. 83:301, 1971.
29. Howie, P. W.: Thromboembolism. Clin. Obstet. Gynaecol. 4:397, 1977.
30. Hull, R., Hirsh, J., Sackett, D. L., Powers, P., Turpie, A. G. G. and Walker, J.: Combined use of leg scanning and impedance plethysmography in suspected venous thrombosis. N. Engl. J. Med. 296:1497, 1977.
31. Hull, R., Hirsh, J., Sackett, D. L. and Stoddart, G.: Cost effectiveness of clinical diagnosis, venography, and non-invasive testing in patients with symptomatic deep vein thrombosis. N. Engl. J. Med. 304:1561, 1981.
32. Hushni, E. A., Leopoldo, I. P. and Lenhert, A. E.: Thrombophlebitis in pregnancy. Am. J. Obstet. Gynecol. 97:901, 1967.
33. Ikard, R. W., Ueland, K. and Folse, R.: Lower limb venous dynamics in pregnant women. Surg. Gynecol. Obstet. 132:483, 1971.
34. Jick, H., Westerholm, B., Vessey, M. P. et al.: Venous thromboembolism and ABO blood type. Lancet 1:539, 1969.
35. Juergens, J. L.: Venous thromboembolism. Cardiovasc. Clin. 3:233, 1971.
36. Marcus, A. J.: Aspirin and thromboembolism—a possible dilemma. N. Engl. J. Med. 297:1284, 1977.
37. Mavor, G. E. and Galloway, J. M. D.: Iliofemoral venous thrombosis. Br. J. Surg. 56:45, 11969.
38. Moncrief, J. A., Darin, J. C., Canizdro, P. C. et al.: Use of dextran to prevent arterial and venous thrombosis. Ann. Surg. 148:553, 1963.
39. Mueller, M. J. and Lebherz, T. B.: Antepartum thrombophlebitis. Obstet. Gynecol. 34:874, 1969.
40. Nabatoff, R. A. and Pincus, J. A.: Management of varicose veins during pregnancy. Obstet. Gynecol. 36:928, 1970.
41. Olwin, J. H. and Koppel, J. L.: Anticoagulant therapy during pregnancy. Obstet. Gynecol. 34:847, 1969.
42. Ramsay, D. M.: Thromboembolism in pregnancy. Obstet. Gynecol. 45:129, 1975.

43. Richards, K. L., Armstrong, J. D., Jr., Gerasim, T., Hershgold, E. J., Jeffery, L. B. and Rampton, J. B.: Noninvasive diagnosis of deep venous thrombosis. Arch. Intern. Med. 136:1091, 1976.

44. Robin, E. D.: Overdiagnosis and overtreatment of pulmonary embolism: The emperor may have no clothes. Ann. Intern. Med. 87:775–781, 1977.

45. Ross, M., Norwicki, J. and Rangarajan, N. S.: Asymptomatic pulmonary embolism during pregnancy. Obstet. Gynecol. 37:131, 1971.

46. Shaul, W. L. and Hall, J. G.: Multiple congenital anomalies associated with oral anticoagulants. Am. J. Obstet. Gynecol. 127:191, 1977.

47. Sher, M. H.: Management of antepartum thrombophlebitis. Am. Surg. 37:587, 1971.

48. Standness, D. E., Jr., Ward, K., Krugmire, R., Jr.: The present status of acute deep venous thrombosis. Surg. Gynecol. Obstet. 145:433, 1977.

49. Talbot, S., Ryrie, D., Wakley, E. J. and Langman, J. J. S.: ABO blood groups and venous thromboembolic disease. Lancet 1:1257, 1970.

50. Turnbull, A. C., Daniel, D. G. and McCarry, J. M.: Antenatal and postnatal thromboembolism. Practitioner 206:727, 1971.

51. VillaSanta, U.: Thromboembolic disease in pregnancy. Am. J. Obstet. Gynecol. 93:142, 1965.

52. Wallach, R. C.: Dextran therapy for pregnancy-associated deep thrombophlebitis. Am. J. Obstet. Gynecol. 112:613, 1971.

53. Weekes, L. R. and Duekmedjian, A. G.: Thromboembolic disease in pregnancy. Am. J. Obstet. Gynecol. 107:649, 1970.

54. Wessler, S.: Medical management of venous thrombosis. Ann. Rev. Med. 27:313, 1976.

55. Thromboembolic disease in obstetrics and gynaecology. Med. J. Aust. 2:1283, 1969.

56. Antenatal thromboembolism. Br. Med. J. 1:249, 1970.

Editorial Comment

Deep vein thrombophlebitis in pregnancy and the puerperium is infrequently seen but is associated with high morbidity and potential mortality. The authors of articles in this chapter agree that an accurate diagnosis is difficult to make, especially in pregnancy, when invasive diagnostic techniques are contraindicated. They are equally in agreement that it is of utmost importance that the diagnosis be made and proper treatment instituted.

It is apparent that because of the high fetal losses associated with coumarin derivative therapy and the embryopathy (apparently in all trimesters) associated with coumarin therapy such agents are contraindicated in pregnancy. The use of coumarin derivatives should therefore be restricted to the very rare management situation when anticoagulation is necessary and heparin therapy is just not possible.

The problem patient is the one who has deep vein thrombophlebitis in the first trimester and who is adequately treated with hospitalization and intravenous heparin therapy for ten days. The physician's dilemma then begins as to whether she should be started on oral coumarin derivatives or be given intermittent intravenous heparin or self-administered subcutaneous heparin. Most would agree that coumarin derivatives should not be given until after 18 weeks of gestation and only then under special considerations. We have found that self-administered subcutaneous heparin is satisfactory and affords the patient ambulatory therapy. The minimum dose is 5000 U every 12 hours for prophylaxis, but for a person who has had deep vein thrombophlebitis, at least 6000 to 7000 U of heparin are needed 3 times a day. The innovation of using an indwelling venous catheter for self-administration of heparin, as advocated by Pearson and Padilla, is an excellent one. It allows the patient to be ambulatory and out of the hospital, and is apparently associated with few complications and very little inconvenience. The heparin infusion prevents clotting in the catheter that would otherwise lead to potential infection at the catheter site.

It is unclear to us whether the presence of varicose veins is associated with a higher incidence of deep vein thrombophlebitis, but in any event it would do no harm to look a little harder at patients who do have varicosities. Such patients would then join those who had a history of previous thromboembolism or phlebitis in the high-risk category, whether or not such had been associated with use of oral contraceptives. The role of subcutaneous minidose heparin (5000 U twice a day) as a means of prevention should also be considered in the high-risk group of patients. (This group also includes women with morbid obesity, past history of pulmonary embolism and so forth.) The true value of minidose heparin in obstetrics has yet to be determined by randomized studies.

9
Idiopathic Thrombocytopenic Purpura in Pregnancy

Alternative Points of View

by Joseph J. Kryc and James J. Corrigan, Jr.
by Robert A. Knuppel and Heidi McNaney

Editorial Comment

The Preferred Management of Idiopathic Thrombocytopenic Purpura in Pregnancy

Joseph J. Kryc, M.D.
Ohio State University School of Medicine

James J. Corrigan, Jr., M.D.
University of Arizona Health Sciences Center

General Features of Idiopathic Thrombocytopenic Purpura

The entity called idiopathic thrombocytopenic purpura (ITP) has been known since 1735. In 1765, Arand reported the first case of pregnancy associated with ITP, and 100 years later the first reported case of ITP in a newborn was noted by Dohrn.[1] It was not until the 1940s that the distinction between primary and secondary thrombocytopenia was made. ITP is defined as thrombocytopenia of unknown etiology characterized by a reduced platelet count, the presence of mild to moderate bleeding, normal to increased numbers of megakaryocytes in the bone marrow, increased platelet destruction, and the absence of disease states that are known to produce thrombocytopenia.[2] ITP, therefore, is a diagnosis made by exclusion.

The two clinically recognized varieties of ITP are acute and chronic.[3, 3a] The acute form generally occurs in children and is self-limiting. The chronic form is predominantly seen in adults and persists for years. At least four fifths of all cases of ITP in adults are of the chronic variety. ITP is more common in females than in males, the ratio being 3–4 to 1. Although chronic ITP can occur in all age groups, it is more commonly seen in the second and third decades.

Since this also coincides with the childbearing age, it is not surprising that ITP is encountered in pregnancy. Current data suggest that chronic ITP is an autoimmune disease, and it has been called autoimmune thrombocytopenia by some investigators. Depending upon the methods used, platelet antibodies can be detected in well over 50 per cent of the patients with chronic ITP.[3, 3a, 3b] The clinical presentation of patients with chronic ITP consists of a fluctuating course as noted by hemorrhagic episodes lasting weeks to months. This can be interrupted by periods of apparent remission with no active bleeding. Spontaneous complete remissions are very rare. Frequently, the clinical course appears quite benign despite the low platelet count. With appropriate therapy, complete or partial remission can be achieved in over 90 per cent of the chronic cases.[3a, 4] The mortality rate in adults with chronic ITP ranges from 2.5 to 5.4 per cent, but with modern therapy it is probably closer to 2 per cent.[3, 3a, 4–6] In the pediatric age group the overall mortality for acute and chronic ITP ranges from 0.6 to 1.2 per cent, or around 1 per cent of the cases.[7–9] In most cases, death is due to intracranial bleeding episodes.

General Features of Maternal ITP

The clinical manifestations of the pregnant and the nonpregnant patient are the same in that bleeding is of the purpuric variety.[3a, 9a, 9b] In acute ITP the onset is sudden, whereas in the chronic cases it tends to be insidious. In chronic cases, there is often a long history of mild bleeding, characterized by easy bruising in the absence of trauma, frequent episodes of epistaxis or prolonged menses or all of these. In addition, bleeding from mucous membranes following trauma (tooth extractions, minor operations) may be the first symptom of the thrombocytopenic condition.

During pregnancy, chronic cases may be detected for the first time, acute cases may appear for the first time or relapses of chronic cases may occur. Although some investigators have suggested that ITP worsens or is aggravated during pregnancy, this is difficult to assess because of the known variable course of the illness. In addition, the presumed deterioration does not tend to recur in all pregnancies in the same patient.[1, 10, 11] The prognosis for this condition during pregnancy is excellent; there has not been a maternal death reported as caused by ITP since 1965, and with modern obstetric care supplemented by appropriate medical management, morbidity has also declined (Table 1).[11]

It is known that ITP does not cause sterility; however, very few studies have been undertaken to study its influence on fertility. In one investigation a high rate of spontaneous abor-

TABLE 1. MATERNAL ITP: MATERNAL AND FETAL MORTALITY SINCE 1954

AUTHOR	YEAR	PERCENTAGE MATERNAL MORTALITY	PERCENTAGE FETAL MORTALITY
Peterson and Larson[18]	1954	2.1	15.1
Mendel and Sparkman[14]	1957	1.6	19
Tancer[1]	1960	5.5	16.5
Goodhue and Evans[15]	1963	5.6	5.7
Heys[12]	1966	0	17
Laros and Sweet[11]	1975	0	21

tions (33 per cent) was noted in such patients, compared with the random rate of 8 to 15 per cent.[10] However, other studies have noted spontaneous abortions occurring with a frequency of 5.7 to 7 per cent.[12]

Except for splenectomy, no treatment was available before the 1950s. Early studies suggested that the patients with the highest risk of mortality were those who had not had a splenectomy prior to pregnancy or who required this operation during pregnancy[1, 12–15] (Table 2). Splenectomy during pregnancy is difficult because of technical problems and problems in controlling hemostasis at the operative site. Thus the attendant fetal mortality in these patients is equally high (approaching 25 to 30 per cent in some studies), being secondary to maternal death, premature labor, spontaneous abortions and the effects of anesthesia as well as the neonatal thrombocytopenia.

Bleeding at the time of delivery was studied by many investigators; little evidence was produced to suggest a high incidence of postpartum hemorrhage. This is understandable because the mechanism for controlling uterine bleeding is contraction of the uterus after expulsion of the fetus and placenta. Of greater concern is the possibility of vaginal or perineal lacerations that could result in uncontrolled bleeding.[10–13]

During the 1950s the efficacy of steroids in the therapy of ITP was assessed in a number of studies of nonpregnant patients. However, the value of this mode of therapy had not been established in pregnancy and, in addition, the possible fetal side effects were unknown. In 1966, Heys reported on 16 females with 21 pregnancies associated with ITP.[12] As noted in Table 2, the risk of ITP in pregnancy seemed to be minimal in patients who had previously undergone splenectomy. The danger, however, seemed to be considerable if splenectomy had not been performed. In this

TABLE 2. MATERNAL ITP: MATERNAL MORTALITY AND RELATIONSHIP TO SPLENECTOMY

AUTHOR	SPLENECTOMY	TOTAL NUMBER OF PREGNANCIES	MATERNAL (NUMBER)	MORTALITY (PERCENTAGE)
Peterson and Larson, 1954[18]	Before pregnancy	27	0	0
	During pregnancy	13	1	7.6
	None	26	0	0
Mendel and Sparkman, 1957[14]	Before pregnancy	31	0	0
	During pregnancy	22	1	4.5
	None	31	0	0
Tancer, 1960[1]	Before pregnancy	34	0	0
	During pregnancy	12	1	8.3
	None	27	3	11
Laros and Sweet, 1975[11]	Before pregnancy	4	0	0
	During pregnancy	2	0	0
	None	5	0	0

particular series, 12 patients did not have a prior splenectomy and in many the symptoms were quite severe. Steroid therapy resulted in full symptomatic remission in approximately the same number of patients for both acute and chronic duration ITP. However, the total number of patients studied was small. The morbidity of 14 per cent in this series, as estimated by postpartum hemorrhage, was no greater than that for other obstetric situations.

The efficacy of platelet transfusions made an impact on therapy during the 1960s and has been successful in halting acute bleeding episodes and in preparing patients for surgery. Chronic usage of platelets, however, has not been found to affect the course of ITP favorably and may indeed result in a more rapid disappearance of platelets from the systemic circulation by stimulating antibody production. At the present time, ITP seems to have a minimal effect on the course of pregnancy if the patient is managed properly both medically and surgically.

Effect of Maternal ITP on the Infant

The overall fetal mortality (see Table 1) in this condition ranges between 13 and 25 per cent.[9, 11, 16] Since the pioneering work of Harrington et al in 1953, numerous reports have shown that the majority of women with chronic ITP have a material that crosses the placenta and can affect the infant's platelet count.[17] The data strongly indicate that this is gamma globulin.[3b, 17, 17a] Results of a number of studies have shown that in mothers with demonstrable thrombocytopenia, with or without prior splenectomy, 75 to 80 per cent of the infants have thrombocytopenia. Involvement is reduced to 27 to 40 per cent if the maternal platelet count is normal[14, 18, 19] (Table 3). In addition, the infant mortality rate is quite high in those with thrombocytopenia, as is discussed later.

Management of the Nonpregnant Patient with ITP

Corticosteroids are used as the initial management of patients with ITP. Sixty to 80 per cent of patients will achieve some improvement in the platelet count, but persistent remissions occur in only 10 to 15 per cent.[4, 20] In those patients who are steroid unresponsive or in whom steroids cannot maintain a remission without dependence upon the drug, splenectomy is the next usual form of management. Response to this procedure has been excellent, with a 70 to 80 per cent remission rate. For patients who are acutely bleeding, with or without the presence of the spleen, platelet transfusions have been quite beneficial in controlling the bleeding. Plasmapheresis, although an interesting approach to the problem, has not been studied adequately to determine its effectiveness. In the nonpregnant patient with ongoing symptomatic thrombocytopenia, despite usage of steroids and splenectomy, immunosuppressive therapy has been employed and varying results obtained.[4, 21, 22]

Management of the Pregnant Patient with ITP

Management of the pregnant patient with ITP consists of steroids, splenectomy and platelet transfusions.[11, 19, 23-26a] In general, the dosages of corticosteroids used have been similar to those in the nonpregnant adult patient with ITP. In addition, the response rate in the pregnant patient appears to be the same as in the nonpregnant patient. No studies have been done, however, to evaluate whether the dose response relationship is different in pregnancy due to higher transcortin levels. This may mean that increased dosages are required. Splenectomy has been performed for the usual indications; that is, steroid unresponsiveness, steroid side effects (especially diabetes mellitus) and bleeding into the vital areas such as the central nervous system. Earlier data suggested that splenectomy during pregnancy was associated with a significant risk in both mother and fetus. This increased risk was in part secondary to an inability to achieve adequate surgical hemostasis, a problem that is now overcome by the availability of platelet transfusions. Because splenectomy becomes technically more difficult as pregnancy advances and the uterus enlarges, it should be performed prior to the third trimester whenever possible.

Although present-day techniques make surgery during pregnancy safer, there are still important risks to consider: anesthetic effects on the embryo, the possibility of spontaneous abortion and the possibility of premature labor. Previous studies have shown that although maternal morbidity is markedly improved with splenectomy, fetal morbidity and mortality are not (Table 3). Although a variety of cytotoxic agents have been used safely in the second and third trimester of pregnant women with acute leukemia,[27] to our knowledge these have not been employed as a method of management of the pregnant woman with ITP. Plasmapheresis also has not been reported to have been attempted during pregnancy.

Effect of Maternal ITP on the Fetus

Current data would suggest that corticosteroids and splenectomy are the treatments of choice in controlling the manifestation of ITP in the mother. With these modalities, it has been found that maternal mortality is zero and morbidity is considerably less than in those women who have not been treated with corticosteroids or splenectomy.[11] What continues to be a problem is the unacceptably high fetal mortality rate associated with ITP during pregnancy. Steroids, splenectomy, or a combination of these treatment modalities have had no effect on improving perinatal mortality or decreasing the incidence in severity of neonatal purpura. The most significant factor in determining fetal involvement at the time of delivery is the activity of ITP in the mother at that same time. Territo and associates showed that 79 per cent of newborns had thrombocytopenia when the maternal platelet counts were less than 100,000 at delivery, and 27 per cent of the infants demonstrated thrombocytopenia when the maternal platelet counts were above 100,000.[19] However, these data could not be confirmed by Noriega-Guerra et al.[27a] The risk seems to be higher in the woman with active disease as demonstrated by the platelet count, but there is also considerable

TABLE 3. MATERNAL ITP: RELATIONSHIP OF MATERNAL SPLENECTOMY AND FETAL INVOLVEMENT

AUTHOR	SPLENECTOMY	TOTAL NO.	INFANTS INVOLVED	
			No.	*Percentage*
Peterson and Larson[18]	Before pregnancy	31	27	87.1
	None	20	14	70
	Totals	51	41	82.3
Mendel and Sparkman[14]	Before pregnancy	40	31	77.5
	None	25	16	64
	Totals	65	47	72.3
Tancer[1]	Before pregnancy	34	26	76
	None	27	19	70
	Totals	61	45	73

TABLE 4. RELATIONSHIP OF MATERNAL PLATELET COUNT AND FETAL INVOLVEMENT IN MATERNAL ITP

AUTHOR	MATERNAL PLATELET COUNT AT DELIVERY	TOTAL NO.	INFANTS INVOLVED No.	INFANTS INVOLVED Percentage
Peterson and Larson[18]	>100,000	11	5	45.5
1954	<100,000	39	29	74.4
	Total	50	34	68.0
Mendel and Sparkman[14]	>100,000	15	6	40.0
1957	<100,000	41	30	73.0
	Total	56	36	64.3
Territo et al.[19]	>100,000	22	6	27.0
1973	<100,000	63	50	79.0
	Total	85	56	66.0
Scott et al.[29a]	>100,000	8	4	50.0
1980	<100,000	4	2	50.0
	Total	12	6	50.0

risk in the woman who has a normal platelet count. Thus, the hematologic status of the mother may or may not be a useful predictor of fetal involvement (Table 4).

Management of Labor and Delivery of the Pregnant Patient with ITP: The Cesarean Section Controversy

Serious consideration has to be given to the method of delivery in the pregnant patient with ITP. It is clear that there is no uniform opinion on this issue. Initially, cesarean section was recommended for obstetric indications only, with complete disregard for the fetus. Since the overwhelming cause of neonatal death in this condition is central nervous system bleeding, trauma to the fetal head plays a significant role. An elective cesarean section would be the most nontraumatic delivery for the fetus.[16, 21–23] With realization that fetal involvement is greater when the mother has thrombocytopenia, cesarean section has gained increased popularity as a method of delivery for these patients. In addition, it avoids the risk of hemorrhage in the mother secondary to the expulsive forces, as the most frequent type of bleeding following vaginal delivery has been associated with maternal lacerations and not uterine bleeding.

Cesarean section, however, could expose the mother to the increased risk of hemorrhage secondary to the surgical procedure. Although these are controlled incisions, bleeding may be just as difficult to halt as would bleeding from vaginal lacerations. The di-

lemma of whether cesarean section should be done or vaginal delivery allowed is difficult if not impossible to resolve. Fetal involvement is as high as 80 per cent in mothers with demonstrable thrombocytopenia (platelet counts less than 100,000); therefore, the attendant maternal morbidity secondary to cesarean section may be acceptable. However, it may not be as acceptable in mothers with normal platelet counts. Fetal involvement in these patients is only 30 to 40 per cent, so 60 per cent of these mothers would be subjected to unnecessary risks. Since the overall neonatal-perinatal mortality figure for infants born to mothers with ITP is still on the order of 13 to 25 per cent, as compared with the overall neonatal mortality of 1.2 per cent and the overall perinatal mortality rate of 1.8 per cent, it clearly indicates that something has to be done differently to try to identify the fetus at risk and avoid exposing the mother to the risks of unnecessary cesarean section.

Recently, fetal scalp sampling was utilized to try to identify the fetus at risk at the time of delivery.[29, 29a] Platelet counts of less than 50,000 in fetal scalp samples were interpreted as indicating fetal involvement, and recommendations were that these infants should be delivered by cesarean section.

The studies in this review have focused on perinatal and neonatal mortality. There are, however, instances of infants who have had active bleeding in the neonatal period and who survived with subsequent neurologic damage.[30] It is suggested that long-term studies be done on these infants no matter what the mode of delivery.

Recommended Management

Maternal ITP should be managed first by corticosteroids. If the hemorrhagic manifestations cannot be controlled or if significant side effects appear with the steroid therapy, splenectomy can be done relatively safely during pregnancy. In addition, platelet transfusions can be utilized for transient control of hemorrhagic manifestations. Immunosuppressive agents are not recommended at this time. As was appreciated, the most useful prognosticator of fetal involvement appears to be the activity of ITP in the mother as determined by the platelet count. Since perinatal mortality occurs in 13 to 25 per cent of the cases with modern therapy and the incidence of fetal involvement varies between 40 to 80 per cent, dependent upon the maternal platelet counts, we would like to propose the scheme shown in Table 5 for the management of these patients at labor and delivery.

MOTHERS IN LABOR WITH PLATELET COUNTS OF GREATER THAN 100,000

Fetal thrombocytopenia in this group of patients varies and is as high as 40 per cent. It would be highly advantageous to differentiate those infants who are involved from those who are not. A recent communication by Ayromlooi suggests that fetal scalp samples be performed during labor and fetal platelet counts obtained.[29, 29a] If involvement is confirmed, management of labor and delivery could be based on these values. In the mother with a normal platelet count and a fetus with a normal platelet count, the likelihood of fetal involvement is negligible. Vaginal delivery may, therefore, be safely contemplated and cesarean section performed for routine obstetric indications. However, if the fetal platelet count is low, intracranial hemorrhage is a strong possibility in this group, and procedures to obviate this should be considered.

TABLE 5.   RECOMMENDED MANAGEMENT OF LABOR AND DELIVERY

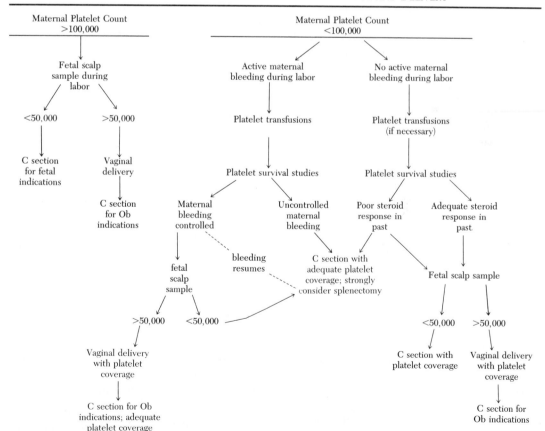

Cesarean section would therefore be recommended to ensure minimal fetal trauma at the time of delivery.

MOTHERS WITH THROMBOCYTOPENIA IN LABOR

Mothers who present in labor with thrombocytopenia and active bleeding should be considered medical and surgical emergencies. Platelet transfusions should be utilized liberally to abate bleeding, and if time permits platelet survival studies should be performed as suggested by Angiulo et al.[26] If adequate maternal hemostasis is achieved and can be maintained during labor, fetal scalp samples can be obtained to detect fetal involvement, because fetal thrombocytopenia occurs in 60 to 80 per cent of the patients. Therefore, the method of delivery can be appropriately selected on the basis of maternal hemostasis and fetal involvement. If hemostasis is adequate and fetal platelet counts are normal, vaginal delivery may be contemplated with liberal use of cesarean section in situations in which maternal pelvic trauma may be expected.

If maternal hemostasis cannot be adequately achieved or if platelet counts remain markedly low despite the use of platelet transfusions or if fetal involvement is strongly suspected, cesarean section with or without concomitant splenectomy, as described by Jones et al., is suggested.[23]

Mothers who present in labor with thrombocytopenia but without active bleeding have the potential for major hemorrhage during delivery. Factors other than bleeding may help determine an appropriate plan of management. Platelet transfusions could be utilized to assess adequate hemostasis, and if time permits, platelet survival studies may be useful. In addition, the patient's past response to steroid therapy may be used as an indicator of the responsiveness of her disease. If the patient has had an adequate trial of steroids in the past with poor response, the method of delivery can be approached from the standpoint of the activity of maternal disease at the time of labor, with consideration being given to cesarean section with possible splenectomy. Alternative management would be to opt for cesarean section on the basis of fetal involvement. For patients who have had a good response to steroids in the past, the method of delivery can be based on fetal involvement with adequate platelet coverage.

REFERENCES

1. Tancer, M. L.: Idiopathic thrombocytopenia purpura and pregnancy. Am. J. Obstet. Gynecol. 79:148, 1960.
2. Wintrobe, M. M.: Clinical Hematology, 7th ed. Philadelphia, Lea and Febiger, 1974, pp. 1075–1089.
3. Mueller-Eckhardt, C.: Idiopathic thrombocytopenia purpura (ITP): Clinical and immunologic considerations. Semin. Thromb. Hemostas. 3:125, 1977.
3a. McMillan, R.: Chronic idiopathic thrombocytopenic purpura. N. Engl. J. Med. 304:1135, 1981.
3b. Karpatkin, M., Siskind, G. W. and Karpatkin, S.: The platelet factor 3 immunoinjury technique reevaluated. Development of a rapid test for antiplatelet antibody. Detection in various clinical disorders, including immunologic drug-induced and neonatal thrombocytopenia. J. Lab. Clin. Med. 89:400, 1977.
4. Lacey, J. V. and Penner, J. A.: Management of idiopathic thrombocytopenic purpura in the adult. Semin. Thromb. Hemostas. 3:160, 1977.
5. Watson-Williams, E. J., Macpherson, A. I. S. and Davidson, S. The treatment of idiopathic thrombocytopenic purpura. A review of 93 cases. Lancet 2:221, 1959.
6. Carpenter, A. F., Wintrobe, M. M., Fuller, E. A., Haut, A. and Cartwright, G. E.: Treatment of idiopathic thrombocytopenic purpura. J.A.M.A. 171:1911, 1959.
7. Komrower, G. M. and Watson, G. H.: Prognosis in idiopathic thrombocytopenic purpura of childhood. Arch. Dis. Child. 29:502, 1954.
8. McClure, P. D.: Idiopathic thrombocytopenic purpura in children: diagnosis and management. Pediatrics 55:68, 1975.
9. Lusher, J. M. and Iyer, R.: Idiopathic thrombocytopenic purpura in children. Semin. Thromb. Hemostas. 3:175, 1977.
9a. Goldsweig, H. and Chediak, J.: Quantitative and qualitative platelet disorders that complicate pregnancy. J. Reprod. Med. 19:205, 1977.
9b. Perkins, R. P.: Thrombocytopenia in obstetric syndromes. A review. Obstet. Gynecol. Sur. 34:101, 1979.
10. Schenker, J. G. and Polishuk, W. Z.: Idiopathic thrombocytopenia in pregnancy. Gynaecologia 165:271, 1968.
11. Laros, R. K. and Sweek, R. L.: Management of idiopathic thrombocytopenic purpura during pregnancy. Am. J. Obstet. Gynecol. 122:182, 1975.
12. Heys, R. F.: Child bearing and idiopathic thrombocytopenic purpura. J. Obstet. Gynaecol. Br. Commonwealth 73:205, 1966.
13. Heys, R. F.: Steroid therapy for idiopathic thrombocytopenic purpura during pregnancy. Obstet. Gynecol. 28:532, 1966.
14. Mendel, E. B. and Sparkman, R.: Idiopathic thrombocytopenic purpura in pregnancy. J. Int. Coll. Surg. 28:156, 1957.
15. Goodhue, P. A. and Evans, T. S.: Idiopathic thrombocytopenic purpura in pregnancy. Ob-Gyn Sur. 18:671, 1962.
16. Pochedly, C.: Thrombocytopenic purpura of the newborn. Ob-Gyn Sur. 26:63, 1971.
17. Harrington, W. J., Sprague, C. C., Minnich, V. et al.: Immunologic mechanisms of idiopathic and neonatal thrombocytopenic purpura. Ann. Intern. Med. 39:433, 1953.

17a. Kernoff, L. M., Malan, E. and Gunston, K.: Neonatal thrombocytopenia complicating idiopathic thrombocytopenic purpura in pregnancy: evidence for transplacental passage of antiplatelet antibody. Ann. Intern. Med. 90:55, 1979.

18. Peterson, O. and Larson, P.: Thrombocytopenic purpura in pregnancy. Obstet. Gynecol. 4:454, 1954.

19. Territo, M., Finklestein, J., Oh, W. et al.: Management of autoimmune thrombocytopenia in pregnancy and in the neonate. Obstet. Gynecol. 41:579, 1973.

20. Ahn, Y. S. and Harrington, W. J.: Treatment of idiopathic thrombocytopenic purpura. Ann. Rev. Med. 28:299, 1977.

21. Bouroncle, B. A. and Doan, C. A.: Refractory idiopathic thrombocytopenic purpura treated with azathioprine. N. Engl. J. Med. 275:630, 2966.

22. Ahn, Y. S., Harrington, W. J., Seelman, R. C. and Eytel, C. S.: Vincristine therapy of idiopathic and secondary thrombocytopenias. N. Engl. J. Med. 291:376, 1974.

23. Jones, W. R., Storey, B., Norton, G. and Neische, F. W.: Pregnancy complicated by acute idiopathic thrombocytopenic purpura. A report of two patients treated by simultaneous C-section and splenectomy. J. Obstet. Gynaecol. Br. Commonwealth 81:330, 1974.

24. Murray, J. and Harris, R. E.: The management of the pregnant patient with idiopathic thrombocytopenic purpura. Am. J. Obstet. Gynecol. 126:499, 1976.

25. Jones, R. W., Asher, M. I., Rutherford, C. J. and Munro, H. M.: Autoimmune (idiopathic) thrombocytopenia in pregnancy and the newborn. Br. J. Obstet. Gynaecol. 84:679, 1977.

26. Angiulo, J. P., Temple, J. T., Corrigan, J. J., Jr. and Galindo, J. H.: Management of cesarean section in a patient with idiopathic thrombocytopenia purpura. Anesthesiology 46:145, 1977.

26a. Carloss, H. W., McMillan, R. and Crosby, W. H.: Management of pregnancy in women with immune thrombocytopenic purpura. J.A.M.A. 244:2756, 1980.

27. Durie, B. G. M. and Giles, H.R.: Successful treatment of acute leukemia during pregnancy. Arch. Intern. Med. 137:90, 1977.

27a. Noriega-Guerra, L., Aviles-Miranda, A., Alvarez de la Cadena, O. et al.: Pregnancy in patients with autoimmune thrombocytopenic purpura. Am. J. Obstet. Gynecol. 133:439, 1979.

28. Levine, P. R.: Idiopathic thrombocytopenia, diabetes mellitus and pregnancy. Obstet. Gynecol. 48:1 (suppl) 315, 1976.

29. Ayromlooi, J.: A new approach to the management of immunologic thrombocytopenia in pregnancy. Am. J. Obstet. Gynecol. 130:235, 1978.

29a. Scott, J. R., Cruikshank, D. P., Kochenour, N. K., Pitkin, R. M. and Warenski, J. C.: Fetal platelet counts in the obstetric management of immunologic thrombocytopenic purpura. Am. J. Obstet. Gynecol. 136:495, 1980.

30. Matoth, Y., Zaizov, R. and Frankel, J. J.: Minimal cerebral dysfunction in children with chronic thrombocytopenia. Pediatrics 47:698, 1971.

Idiopathic Thrombocytopenic Purpura and Pregnancy

Robert A. Knuppel, M.D., M.P.H.

Heidi McNaney, M.D.

University of South Florida College of Medicine

We re-evaluated idiopathic thrombocytopenic purpura (ITP) during pregnancy by reviewing the literature since 1939, with emphasis on the immunologic basis of the disorder and progressive improvement in maternal and fetal outcomes. Overall improvement in maternal and fetal morbidity and mortality reflects advances in treatment of all patients with ITP. Only one maternal death has been reported since 1951. The reasons for reduced maternal mortality rates of ITP, including use of corticosteroids and splenectomy, are discussed, along with current treatment. Although some investigators recommend primary elective cesarean section in ITP patients, the efficacy of cesarean section as opposed to vaginal delivery is still under debate. Fetal scalp blood sampling early in the course of labor has facilitated identification of the thrombocytopenic fetus. How successful this technique will be in community hospitals remains to be demonstrated.

A comprehensive review of the literature will serve as a resource from which to evaluate new frontiers in ITP. Future noninvasive technologic advances will more exactly predict which fetus and newborn may or may not suffer from thrombocytopenic sequelae (hemorrhage, petechiae) if vaginal delivery is allowed.

Definition

Idiopathic (immunologic) thrombocytopenic purpura (ITP) is a term applied to a clinical picture of thrombocytopenia of unknown etiology, which is characterized by a reduced platelet count, the presence of normal or increased megakaryocytes in the bone marrow and increased platelet destruction. ITP is an autoimmune disease in which the patient produces antibodies against his or her own platelets. Affected platelets are then recognized and destroyed by the spleen and other components of the reticuloendothelial system.

Historical Background

In 1735 a German physician, Paul Gottlieb Werlhof, described for the first time a purpural disease in two young girls.[1] Thirty years later, Arand described the first case of purpura in pregnancy.[2] No further reports appeared until 1867, when Barnes[3] and Byrne[4] each reported a case of purpura in pregnancy. Barnes' case, which was most likely a secondary purpura, resulted in premature labor with neonatal and maternal death. This condition was reflected in the ominous prognoses in all subsequent reports for the next 75 years.

Many advances were made in the understanding of ITP after 1842, when Donne first described blood platelets. Later, Brohn and Krause in 1883 and Denys in 1887 independently discovered the pathogenetic role of thrombocytopenia in the clinical state of purpura. These advances made possible differentiation among various forms of purpura. Nevertheless, for the next century, obstetricians continued to classify all cases of purpura associated with pregnancy as a single group.

Frank in 1915 was the first investigator to suggest that the production of platelets by megakaryocytes became arrested by a factor produced by the spleen.[5] The following year Kaznelson observed the beneficial effect of splenectomy in a patient with ITP and postulated that the thrombocytopenia was due to an increased rate of platelet destruction by the spleen.

By 1923, Mosher had found 40 cases of purpura in pregnancy.[6] He concluded that the maternal mortality rate was nearly 100 per cent from postpartum hemorrhage and that the fetal mortality rate was 50 per cent. Two years later, Rushmore reported 48 cases with a maternal mortality rate of 58 per cent and a fetal mortality rate of 64 per cent.[7] Neither author made any attempt to distinguish among the various types of purpura. Not until years later did investigators recognize that in a case of purpura in pregnancy the prognosis depends largely upon whether the purpura is idiopathic or secondary. Desaussure and Townsend[8] in 1935, Polowe[9] in 1944, Patterson[10] in 1945 and Rosenvasser and Ramazzi[11] in 1956 continued to quote Rushmore's mortality rates and implied that they were applicable to ITP in pregnancy.

The first attempt to evaluate the recorded results of pregnancy associated with true ITP was made by Burnett and Klass[12] in 1943. They concluded that this combination was not necessarily fatal. Robson and Davidson in 1950 suggested that the mortality in pregnant women with ITP was no higher than that which could be expected from ITP alone; however, fetal mortality was 15 per cent.[13] In the same year Epstein and colleagues reported a maternal mortality rate of 8.7 per cent in 39 cases of ITP and a fetal mortality of 26 per cent; they observed thrombocytopenia in some of the neonates.[14] In a series of brilliant investigations from 1951 to 1953, Harrington and co-workers showed by in vivo infusions of blood or plasma from patients with ITP to volunteer recipients that a thrombocytopenic factor, which was able to damage circulating platelets, was present.[15, 16] They also noted that this factor could be transmitted through the placenta and that mothers with the disease bore babies with short-lived thrombocytopenic purpura. In 1957 Mendel and Sparkman reported 84 pregnancies in 65 mothers with a maternal mortality rate of 1.6 per cent and a fetal mortality rate of 1.9 per cent.[17] Slaughter and associates reviewed cases of ITP in pregnancy with special reference to splenectomy.[18] They concluded that any infant born to a mother with ITP, whether or not splenectomy had been performed, could have thrombocytopenia.

Clinical Picture

DIAGNOSTIC CRITERIA

The prognosis and therapy, especially in pregnant patients, depend on an accurate hematologic diagnosis. The following criteria have generally been followed in making the diagnosis: (1) thrombocytopenia less than 100,000 per cu mm, (2) normal to increased megakaryocyte mass, (3) absence of identified sources of platelet destruction, (4) absence of splenomegaly, (5) normal coagulation studies, (6) history excluding drug ingestion, exposure to noxious substances, recent infections or family history of bleeding, and (7) demonstration of an antiplatelet antibody.[5, 19] This last criterion is usually unrealistic because techniques are generally unavailable.

These diagnostic criteria can usually be determined at the initial evaluation that includes a complete history, physical examination and appropriate laboratory studies. Careful attention to the history will rule out many secondary forms, as will negative serologic studies such as an antinuclear antibody (ANA) assay, antiDNA assay and systemic lupus erythematosus (LE) prep.

Signs and Symptoms

There are two distinct varieties of ITP, the acute and the chronic.[1, 20–22] The acute ITP usually occurs in children, 85 per cent of whom are under 8 but over 1 year of age, with equal numbers of males and females affected.[23] It is self-limited to a few weeks or months. About two thirds of these patients give a clear history of an antecedent infection occurring a week or two before the onset of purpura. The infection is acute, febrile, non-bacterial and probably viral. Sometimes it is associated with an exanthematous state such as rubella, rubeola or chickenpox. Onset of purpura is generally sudden, and mild fever, headache and backache, or nausea may be present. Acute ITP in pregnancy is rare and usually self-limiting. Most patients show a spontaneous cure in a period of weeks. Unless this form of ITP presents in late pregnancy, it represents little risk to the mother or fetus unless associated with a teratogenic viral illness. Supportive care is all that is needed. When acute ITP occurs in late pregnancy, it is handled in the same way as the chronic form. In general, fewer than 10 per cent of cases of this form of ITP will progress to the chronic, self-perpetuating type. Further research may very well prove that acute ITP is not a true idiopathic thrombocytopenic purpura.

The chronic form of ITP is found primarily in young adults. Females are affected more frequently than males in a ratio of 34:1.[23] In these women the incidence is greatest in the second and third decades of life. The calcu-

lated morbidity is 4.5 males and 7.5 females with ITP per 100,000 persons per year;[24] overall mortality ranges from 4.4 to 6.8 per cent in the nonpregnant patient, depending on the series.[1, 20] The designation of chronic usually refers to the truly idiopathic variety with characteristics of an insidious onset, a long history of easy bruising and prolonged menses, relatively mild bleeding manifestations, a lowering of the platelet count, and a platelet survival indicating increased platelet destruction with no significant anemia, leukopenia or splenomegaly. Hemorrhagic manifestations are of the purpural type, predominantly dermal and mucosal. Spontaneous bleeding into the skin is primarily in the form of petechiae. Menorrhagia and metrorrhagia are common and may be the only manifestations of the disease. They may be the reason for the nonpregnant patient's first visit to a gynecologist. The most serious and life-threatening complications of ITP are intracranial hemorrhages, which have an overall frequency of about 1 per cent.[1]

Chronic ITP is a self-perpetuating disorder that may last for many years. Complete cure probably never occurs spontaneously.[20] The clinical course fluctuates with hemorrhagic episodes of a few weeks' duration, then it is interrupted by symptomless intervals. Hemorrhagic manifestations are generally related to the degree of thrombocytopenia. Although the cessation of bleeding may be associated with an increased number of platelets, the thrombocytopenia of various degrees persists. With appropriate therapy a complete or partial remission can be obtained in greater than 90 per cent of the chronic cases.

Laboratory Findings

The number of circulating platelets is reduced to levels between 20,000 to 80,000 per cu mm. Platelet size and morphology are often abnormal. Large and giant forms (megathrombocytes), small platelets and bizarre shapes may be seen on peripheral smear. The megathrombocytes are associated with destruction and accelerated thrombocytopoiesis with release of these immature forms. Red blood cells, hemoglobin, total leukocyte count and differential are often normal except for changes resulting from severe blood loss. In these cases a slight anemia with or without iron deficiency may develop, especially in the menstruating or pregnant female.

Alterations of bone marrow are normally

restricted to megakaryocytes. They are plentiful in number and increased in size. Immature forms increase, and the presence of cytoplasmic and nuclear degeneratives, vascularization, lack of granular development and deficient platelet budding is noted. Eosinophilia frequently occurs in the acute form. Defects in hemostasis are solely attributable to a reduced platelet count, but the correlation is variable. The bleeding time may be less than expected for the platelet count from 10,000 to 80,000 per microliter due to the increased hemostatic competence of the young platelets. Clot retraction in vitro is diminished. Coagulation tests are normal. Platelets have decreased thromboelasticity on thromboelastograms. Decreased adhesion, release of platelet Factor III and aggregation may be seen.

An informative and almost indispensable method in the evaluation of ITP patients is the measurement of platelet survival and sequestration sites.[20] In ITP a variable but rapid removal of radioactively labeled autologous or compatible isologous platelets from the circulation occurs. In contrast to the normal life span of 7 to 10 days, the platelet life span is shortened to a few hours or days in ITP.[25] Major sequestration is in the spleen and liver.[26] In normal persons, as well as in ITP patients, the spleen is the only exchangeable platelet pool and acts as a reservoir containing about 30 per cent of the total platelet mass.

Simple and unanimously approved immunohematologic tests for the detection of platelet autoantibodies are not available. Kelton et al. in 1980 noted that a number of methods had been developed to measure platelet-associated IgG (PAIgG).[27] Their studies support the fact that the antiglobulin consumption directly quantitates IgG on the platelet and is sensitive and specific. When they compared the results of the two PAIgG assays in immune and nonimmune thrombocytopenia and nonthrombocytopenic controls, the antiglobulin consumption assay was clearly superior, with overall sensitivity and specificity rates of 94 and 95 per cent, respectively. Although these new assays remain removed from clinical practice, their import may be felt in future years. At present, they have been utilized satisfactorily in the prenatal diagnosis and distinction between maternal platelet–associated IgG and serum platelet–bindable IgG in neonatal thrombocytopenia due to passive immunization.[28]

Pathogenesis

HUMORAL ANTIPLATELET FACTOR

The idea that a hormone-like substance may be one of the etiologic factors in ITP was supported by Liebling[29] in 1926, Davidson[30] in 1937, Epstein[14] in 1950 and Robson[13] in 1950. They reported that mothers with this disease frequently delivered babies with transient purpura. These researchers suggested transplacental transmission of a thrombocytopenic factor occurring independently of the presence or absence of a spleen. ITP has been referred to as an autoimmune disorder principally since Harrington's studies starting in 1951.[15, 16] Harrington also thought that neonatal thrombocytopenia developed as a result of transmission across the placenta of maternal autoagglutinins for platelets.[16, 31, 32]

The platelet-depressing factor in the plasma of patients with typical ITP has these characteristics: it is present in the 7S gamma globulin fraction (IgG), it is absorbed by normal human platelets, it affects autologous as well as homologous platelets (regardless of platelet antigenic type) and it is species-specific.[33] It remains present after splenectomy. The factor produces increased platelet destruction and most likely some depression of megakaryocyte function by binding to their antigenic sites, which explains the absence of a compensatory increase in platelet production in the presence of the increase in megakaryocyte mass.[21]

Although some studies have shown that the antiplatelet factor can be demonstrated in only 60 to 80 per cent of patients with ITP,[1, 21] the sensitivity of present techniques is probably inadequate. Platelet autoantibodies in serum may not be demonstrated satisfactorily in vitro, whereas in vivo studies have given clearcut results proving that an antiplatelet factor is present and has the characteristics of an antibody. Independent of the clinical picture, the antibody in the circulation may be different in various patients and can be low because of the great avidity of the platelets; it is tissue-fixed and noncirculating.[21]

Role of the Spleen

The importance of the spleen in the pathogenesis of ITP has been recognized since 1916, when Kaznelson first suggested that the spleen acts as a sieve to remove platelets from the circulation. Sprague and Harrington[32, 34] have given the most convincing demonstration that, with similar antibody concentrations, the spleen serves an important role in removing sensitized antibody-coated platelets. This is the main function of the spleen in ITP and accounts for the therapeutic effect of splenectomy. After splenectomy, the antiplatelet factor is still present despite apparent clinical remission. Shulman[33] demonstrated that platelets moderately sensitized by antibodies are removed in the spleen, whereas highly sensitized platelets are removed primarily in the liver. Thus the protection afforded by splenectomy works in conjunction with smaller antibody concentrations, but higher concentrations lead to destruction even in the absence of the spleen. The latter fact may also explain the relapse in patients after splenectomy. Recent reports have also implicated the spleen as an important site of platelet autoantibody production of ITP.[21]

Thrombopoiesis

The role of thrombopoiesis in ITP has been debated for years. It has definitely been established that platelet turnover is significantly increased in ITP. The turnover is mediated by a feedback mechanism through the peripheral platelet count. Although megakaryocyte hyperplasia is frequently seen on bone marrow examination, it often cannot compensate for platelet destruction and is ineffective. This hyperplasia may be influenced by direct megakaryocyte inhibition by platelet autoantibodies, since platelets and megakaryocytes share common antigenic sites.[21] Direct evidence for this hypothesis is still lacking.

Treatment

In general, the existence of a platelet count of 30,000 per cu mm is sufficient to prohibit serious bleeding in ITP and a count of 50,000 per cu mm is sufficient to ensure safety.[34, 35] Regardless of the causes, bleeding at any level will be enhanced by trauma, fever, infection, increase in metabolic rate from any etiology, azotemia or the administration of any agent that decreases platelet production or alters platelet function (alcohol, aspirin). Avoidance and rapid correction of these problems are important.

PLATELET TRANSFUSIONS

Platelet transfusions are generally ineffective and should be reserved for an attempt to stop hemorrhage. On the average, a single pint of donor blood contains 1×10^{11} platelets. During processing, however, unavoidable losses occur so that platelet concentrate contains 0.5 to 0.7×10^{11} platelets. Newer methods of collection (plateletpheresis) using the Latham blood processor* allow for a significant harvest of platelets. An average of 2.6×10^{11} platelets are collected from a single donor by use of the Haemonetics 30. Further viability of platelets and their function may be influenced by: (1) the anticoagulant solution used, (2) bad composition, (3) mixing, (4) storage temperature and (5) starting platelet concentration.[36] Interestingly, disagreement regarding storage time and temperature for platelet concentrates continues. The storage characteristics of whole blood may reduce the functional capabilities of the platelets even if the unit is less than 72 hours old. Some recent studies indicated that storage at room temperature of 30 to 50 cc of plasma with gentle agitation results in good preservation of functional platelets. Although platelets, when used for ITP patients, should be infused as soon as possible after they have been collected, the majority of collected platelets remain viable after 48 to 72 hours of storage, depending upon preservation procedures.

ADRENOCORTICOSTEROIDS

Steroids were first demonstrated to be effective in the treatment of ITP in 1950 by Bonnin.[38] Adrenocorticotropin (ACTH) and cortisone were then used, but prednisone is now the steroid of choice. The initial benefits of steroids on platelet levels probably represent handicaps imposed upon the reticuloendothelial macrophages, although a decrease in autoantibody production also occurs with more protracted therapy. Sprague and Harrington also proposed that steroids decrease capillary fragility independent of their effect on platelet counts and may also promote bone marrow production of platelets.[37, 39]

When a patient with ITP is initially seen, steroids are generally used after the diagnostic

---

*Model 30, Haemonetics Corp., Natick, Mass.

work has been completed. The major aims of steroid therapy are to obtain immediate control of bleeding and to keep the patient in good health until remission occurs either spontaneously or with splenectomy. Only occasionally will a complete remission be obtained following discontinuance of steroids (10 to 15 per cent). For initial therapy in patients who have clinical bleeding, doses of 1 to 1½ mg per kg of prednisone per day are used.[39] Therapy should be continued for two to three weeks. If the platelet count does not exceed a level of 50,000 per cu mm, splenectomy is indicated. If greater improvement takes place, the dosage of steroids should be decreased progressively to a maintenance dose or the lowest dose compatible with adequate platelet counts that can be maintained safely (e.g., 0.25 mg per kg a day). If relapse occurs, steroids should be increased and splenectomy considered. Steroids may again be indicated after failure of splenectomy to raise platelet counts. Steroids are also indicated in patients in whom splenectomy is contraindicated. Steroid therapy is generally not satisfactory for long-range management and its use is regarded as adjunctive in most patients.

SPLENECTOMY

Splenectomy is the treatment of choice in the nonpregnant patient when surgery is not otherwise contraindicated. Although the percentage of remissions from splenectomy varies in different centers, the general result is still similar to that obtained by Harrington[16] in 1953: namely, a sustained remission will occur in about 70 per cent of the patients after splenectomy. A small fraction (10 to 20 per cent) will respond temporarily for several weeks. The platelet count six weeks after surgery is a good indicator of response since later relapse is infrequent.[37]

The risks from splenectomy in the nonpregnant patient are small; mortality is generally less than 1 per cent. Therefore, splenectomy affords a prompt and lasting clinical cure in most patients with ITP, and presents acceptably low risk in pregnant patients.

IMMUNOSUPPRESSANTS

Since 1960,[40] a variety of nonsteroidal immunosuppressant agents have been used in the treatment of ITP refractory to steroids and splenectomy. In general, these agents handicap multiple aspects of the immune response, including macrophage function. Patients may require prolonged periods of treatment, weeks to months, before an effect is seen. The more frequently employed agents are azathioprine, cyclophosphamide and the vinca alkaloids.

Azathioprine[41] is used in dosages of 1.2 to 2.4 mg per kg (50 to 250 mg per day), and a minimum of 3 months and up to 2 years of therapy is required before the platelet count is stabilized. Steroids are used concomitantly. The most common side effects are leukopenia, alopecia, ulcerations of the mucous membranes and diarrhea.

Cyclophosphamide is used in dosages of 50 to 200 mg per day or intermittently 300 to 600 mg per m², intravenously or orally, over a 4-hour period every 2 to 3 weeks.[42] Improvement in the platelet count may be evident in 2 to 4 weeks, but longer periods of treatment are usually needed. Side effects are severe leukopenia, alopecia and hemorrhagic cystitis. The overall response rate to azathioprine or cyclophosphamide or both in splenectomy failure ranges from 25 to 66 per cent. Cyclophosphamide seems to be more effective than azathioprine, but its potential side effects are more serious.

The vinca alkaloids, vincristine and vinblastine, were recently introduced in the treatment of ITP.[43] In contrast to most immunosuppressants that cause thrombocytopenia, these agents induce thrombocytosis in animals and man. Vincristine is used in dosages of 0.025 mg per kg; vinblastine in dosages of 0.125 mg per kg. Injections are repeated every 7 to 10 days. A rise in platelets is usually observed within 5 to 7 days after injection. This early response is an advantage over cyclophosphamide and azathioprine. If there is no response after three injections, benefit is unlikely and side effects are increased. Once remission occurs, no maintenance is used. Therapy is usually well tolerated. Transient malaise, jaw pain and fever may be observed shortly after injections of vincristine. Various neuropathies, seen more commonly in older people, are troublesome and are reversible after discontinuation of treatment. Neutropenia is the major side effect of vinblastine. The use of vinca alkaloids after steroids and splenectomy failure has induced partial to complete remission in 69 per cent of cases.

Immunosuppressants should not be used as the primary modality of treatment because of more potential risks associated with their prolonged use. Potential teratogenicity discourages their use in women of childbearing age.

The ability to define and monitor the effects of any therapy is limited by the failure to develop clinical assays to measure the circulating antibody.

ITP in Pregnancy

There are numerous reports in the modern (since 1960) literature regarding the problem of ITP in pregnancy.[44–82] Some authors describe the management of a few patients, some review the literature,[2, 5, 52, 57, 59] some make proposals of policies to be followed on the basis of a few personal cases[45, 50, 51, 52] and still others seem to decide the success or failure of management on magic figures derived from laboratory reports. Very few present experience with a group of pregnancies in which the value of an overall multidisciplinary intensive management is stressed.[52–54]

Tancer searched the literature from 1924 to 1957, and accepted the cases of 53 women as having had a reasonably accurate diagnosis of ITP made either before or during pregnancy.[2] He also reported 5 new cases for a total of 58 patients with 72 deliveries and 73 fetuses. The maternal mortality rate was 5.5 per cent. Of the four deaths, two were from cerebral hemorrhage in the first trimester; one occurred after a splenectomy in the sixth month, and one came after postpartum splenectomy. The fetal mortality rate was 12.9 per cent. Three fetuses died in utero in the immediate postsplenectomy period, three died of neonatal purpura including one tentorial tear after low forceps delivery, one died of atelectasis after cesarean section and one died of prematurity. Of the remaining 54 patients, 26 delivered without prior splenectomy, 34 after prior splenectomy and 12 had splenectomy performed during pregnancy. Four mothers received ACTH or cortisone and none of their infnts displayed neonatal purpura.

Tancer concluded that maternal mortality was equivalent to mortality among nonpregnant patients with ITP and that pregnancy was not contraindicated. He did not recommend splenectomy in the pregnant patient, and warned that neonatal purpura might occur with ITP despite previous splenectomy or the absence of antepartum purpura or thrombocytopenia in the mother.

Goodhue and Evans in 1962 again reviewed the literature and reported a new case of ITP in pregnancy.[5] The investigators were impressed by the lack of uniformity in the use of the term ITP and thought that a number of cases accepted by many authors, including Tancer, used varying criteria for diagnosis. Many cases were accepted before the era of bone marrow study and had been carried on by succeeding workers under the term ITP. Goodhue and Evans attempted more strictly to separate primary cases of ITP from those that may well have been secondary. They separated cases from 1939 to 1963 into proved (satisfying all diagnostic criteria presented earlier) and probable (usually lacking bone marrow evaluation) cases. More than half of Tancer's cases fell into Goodhue and Evans' "probable" category. Goodhue and Evans' outcomes of mother and infant were based only on cases classified as proved. These included 37 pregnancies in 36 mothers with proved ITP. The maternal morbidity rate in this group was 5.6 per cent. The two maternal deaths were (1) from cerebral hemorrhage at 14 weeks of pregnancy and (2) in the postoperative period after splenectomy at the sixth month of gestation. Of the remaining 35 viable pregnancies, there was one neonatal death because of prematurity and one stillbirth occurred in a mother treated with splenectomy at 6 months of gestation, resulting in a perinatal mortality rate of 5.7 per cent. Postpartum hemorrhage occurred in 13.5 per cent of the cases. All of these cases were in patients with low platelet counts at delivery. Purpura in the newborn of mothers with ITP appeared mild. In this series, 12 infants had purpura or thrombocytopenia or both, for an involvement rate of 34.3 per cent. There were no deaths among these infants. The incidence was lowest in mothers treated only with steroids; moderate in those treated with splenectomy during gestation, no treatment or splenectomy and steroid therapy; and highest in mothers with splenectomies performed prior to the pregnancy.

Only 21 of the mothers who accounted for the 37 pregnancies had a platelet count reported during delivery. Five had normal platelet counts and delivered normal infants. Sixteen of the women with low platelet counts delivered 8 infants with purpura and 8 without. Of the mothers, 16 had splenectomies during gestation (with 1 death), 6 had previous splenectomy and 15 had spleens intact during pregnancy. Ten patients were treated with steroids. No conclusions concerning the cure rate with various types of therapy were made because of the small number of cases. Goodhue and Evans, however, recommended steroid therapy and indicated that treatment with splenectomy should be reserved for those patients whose disease was not controlled clinically by any other modality.

Heys in a 1966 study evaluated steroid therapy in ITP during pregnancy by a review of previously published case histories from 1953 to 1966 in conjunction with three new cases.[47] Again there were overlaps with cases already presented by Tancer and Goodhue and Evans, but most of Heys' patients fell in a "proved" category. His study presented 21 pregnancies in 19 mothers in whom confirmed ITP was treated by steroid therapy. Heys reported no maternal deaths. In 12 of the pregnancies splenectomy had not been previously performed. Complete hematologic or symptomatic remission or both types for the duration of the pregnancy was achieved in 30 per cent of patients with active purpura. Significant symptomatic improvement occurred in another 25 per cent. Treatment failed in the remaining 45 per cent. A high incidence of severe toxemia was found, as was one case of postpartum psychosis. Of the 21 pregnancies, 2 ended in stillbirths, the result of cranial hemorrhage. One neonatal death was also due to severe hemorrhagic thrombocytopenia. In all, 9 infants (43 per cent) showed clinical evidence of purpura; 2 had asymptomatic low platelet counts of less than 100,000. Steroid therapy during pregnancy did not significantly improve perinatal mortality or the incidence of neonatal ITP.

Again in 1966, Heys presented a second article on ITP and pregnancy.[54] Rather than analyzing isolated pregnancies or small groups collected from literature, he reported a retrospective study of all pregnancies occurring in a group of women affected by the disease in one 5-year period (1959 to 1964). Forty-four pregnancies occurred in 21 women; 38 in women who had previous splenectomy; 1 woman had antepartum splenectomy, and there were 5 complete pregnancies without splenectomy. There were no maternal deaths, but maternal morbidity (especially postpartum hemorrhage) increased among mothers who had intact spleens. The spontaneous abortion rate was only 7 per cent of all pregnancies in this series. The perinatal mortality rate was 17 per cent. There were 6 stillbirths: 1 associated with a bleeding placenta previa, 1 the result of an abruptio placenta, 1 due to asphyxia and 3 due to intracranial hemorrhage.

Purpuric manifestations (thrombocytopenia or purpura or both) occurred in 9 cases of the 29 liveborn infants (35 per cent); 3 in women who had had their spleens removed previously and were symptomatically and hematologically free from disease. The actual incidence of involvement may well have been higher— many normal-appearing infants had not had a platelet count done. Heys concluded that platelet counts should be done on all infants and mothers with ITP, even when in remission. He also recommended forceps delivery to minimize the danger of maternal hemorrhage due to expulsive efforts of labor.

Territo et al. in 1973 reviewed 80 previously reported cases from 1946 to 1972 and 5 new cases of ITP during pregnancy.[48] Again there was an overlap of previous reviews. Except for Heys' views on forceps delivery, previous authors had extended much attention to the influence on neonatal outcome from the severity of maternal disease, prior to splenectomy, and steroid therapy without regard to the method of delivery.

Territo found that children born to mothers who had platelet counts of greater than 100,000 per cu mm at delivery had a 27 per cent incidence of thrombocytopenia, whereas children born to mothers with platelets of less than 100,000 per cu mm had a 79 per cent incidence of thrombocytopenia. Before this time, infants of ITP mothers were primarily delivered vaginally. Cesarean section had been avoided except for strict obstetric criteria because excessive bleeding from surgery was feared. In her review of the 16 reported cases in which cesarean section was performed, plus her own 4 cases, Territo found only 3 instances in which excessive bleeding had occurred and these were controlled with blood transfusions. In no case was there a death. She believed that because cesarean section can avoid the risk of cerebral hemorrhage in the mother from expulsive efforts of labor, it may be the procedure of choice in selected patients with platelet counts less than 100,000 per cu mm with prolonged labor or in any patient with platelet count greater than 100,000 per cu mm with prolonged labor or fetal distress.

These views on cesarean section were supported by the work of Jones et al. in 1974.[46] Jones concluded that maternal morbidity and mortality were rare as a result of advances in the treatment of ITP in nonpregnant individuals and that the significant risk of neonatal complications was not the major factor in obstetric management. He described two patients with acute ITP presenting in late pregnancy. In both there was little or no response to steroids; therefore, elective cesarean section and splenectomy were performed. Both infants had marked thrombocytopenia. Whole blood and platelet transfusions adequately restored hemostasis during surgery. The uncomplicated postoperative course run by both mothers and their infants attested to the success of the therapeutic approach used.

Another review of the literature by Laros and Sweet, which appeared in 1975, included literature cases from 1969 to 1974 and five of their own pregnant patients with ITP.[44] No maternal deaths occurred in this series of 14 pregnancies; however, significant maternal symptomatology occurred relative to the ITP. Steroids were used in 8 pregnancies — 4 women had previous splenectomy and 2 had splenectomy performed during pregnancy. Platelet transfusions were used in 5 mothers. The perinatal mortality rate was 21 per cent: 1 fetal death in utero occurred at 7 months (of unknown cause) and 1 at 37½ weeks secondary to cerebral and pulmonary hemorrhages. One infant delivered by cesarean section because of maternal cardiopulmonary disease died on the third day of life as a result of cerebral hemorrhage. Fifty per cent of the infants had normal platelet counts, 25 per cent had asymptomatic thrombocytopenia, and 25 per cent had purpura and thrombocytopenia.

Laros and Sweet recommended steroids as the first treatment of choice but recommended splenectomy during pregnancy if platelet response was unsatisfactory. They were of the opinion that the high mortality rate associated with splenectomy in the past was related to inadequate surgical hemostasis. Laros and Sweet also indicated that no hard data were available to support Territo's recommendations to perform cesarean section prophylactically in cases in which the maternal platelet count at term is less than 100,000 per cu mm, especially since the only neonatal death in their series occurred in an infant delivered by cesarean section. As a better way of treating the fetus in utero, they proposed finding a steroid that would cross the placenta better than prednisone. Since betamethasone crosses the placenta considerably more effectively than prednisone, it would be logical to use this drug during the last weeks of pregnancy in an attempt to treat the fetus. There are no hard data, however, to support this approach.

Murray and Harris in 1976 discussed the problem of ITP in pregnancy, especially with regard to the controversy over the method of delivery.[45] They presented two personally managed patients and addressed themselves to the problem of persistently high perinatal mortality rates in patients with ITP in pregnancy by delivering both of their patients by cesarean section. The first patient, who had new onset of ITP during pregnancy, had a good response to steroid therapy and normal platelet counts at delivery. She delivered a thrombocytopenic infant. The second patient, who had had previous onset of ITP at age 11, had had a splenectomy at that time. She was asymptomatic with good platelet counts during her pregnancy and also delivered a thrombocytopenic infant. In commenting on Territo's work, Murray and Harris agreed that cesarean section was best for mothers with platelet counts up to 100,000 per cu mm, since they had a 79 per cent chance of delivering a thrombocytopenic infant. They went a step further, however, and indicated that the incidence of 29 per cent neonatal purpura in the group with platelets greater than 100,000 per cu mm was not acceptable, and that these patients should also be delivered by cesarean section.

Levine et al. also shared Territo's views, and presented a case of ITP, complicated by diabetes mellitus, in pregnancy.[50] Their patient presented with new onset of ITP during pregnancy and had a platelet count of 32,000 per cu mm at the time of delivery. The patient subsequently underwent primary cesarean section and splenectomy. Her infant was born with an initial cord blood platelet count of 5,000 per cu mm. After exchange and platelet transfusions the infant did well on 10 days of prednisone. The authors were of the opinion that cerebral damage to the neonate was avoided because of the cesarean section, and they supported the view that this procedure is indicated in all women whose platelet count is less than 100,000 per cu mm at the time of delivery. They concluded that splenectomy at the time of cesarean section should be seriously considered in new-onset ITP.

In the following year (1977), another patient with ITP during pregnancy was managed by cesarean section. Anguilo et al. presented a patient in whom ITP had been diagnosed at 39 weeks of gestation.[51] During the first five hospital days, the platelet counts ranged from 3000 to 16,000 per cu mm and a cesarean section was planned for the sixth day. Before the operation the patient's response to a platelet challenge was determined. Six platelet concentrates produced a 19,000 per cu mm increase in the platelet count. On the basis of this result, Anguilo estimated that 18 platelet concentrates would acutely increase the platelet count by 58,000 per cu mm. (A count of 60,000 to 70,000 per cu mm is recommended to provide normal hemostatic mechanisms.)[34] The procedure was tolerated well by both mother and infant. The initial platelet count in the infant was 112,000 per cu mm.

The following year, Jones et al. presented a personal series of pregnancies in 29 women with ITP.[55] They reported no increased incidence of obstetric complications, no maternal deaths, and no problems following spontaneous vaginal delivery (88 per cent) or low forceps delivery (12 per cent). No cesarean sections were performed. There were eight spontaneous abortions but no perinatal deaths. One infant, however, developed a cerebral hemorrhage at 60 hours of life and now has moderate psychomotor retardation. After studying serial platelet counts, Jones and colleagues found that the time of maximum risk to the infant is not at birth but two to four days later, when the lowest platelet counts are found. A detailed study of the 20 most recently treated liveborn infants (1972 to 1976) was presented. Five mothers with intact spleens received no treatment; six received steroid therapy. Eight women had had previous splenectomy, and one had a splenectomy during gestation. Four of these women also received steroid therapy. Ten (50 per cent) of the infants had thrombocytopenia of less than 100,000 per cu mm, and four had symptoms that included intracerebral bleeding with psychomotor retardation. The lack of perinatal mortality in Jones' series is encouraging but hard to explain in light of both earlier and later studies.

O'Reilly and Taber were the next investigators to approach the subject of ITP in pregnancy (1977).[49] They reported cases of six new patients, one of whom delivered triplets (a first). In addition, they reviewed all the "verified" literature cases for a total of 84 women with 129 pregnancies. These included the cases of Goodhue and Evans, Heys, Territo, Jones, Laros and Sweet and Murray and Harris. Previous recommendations for elective cesarean section in all mothers with platelet counts of less than 100,000 per cu mm at delivery were not supported by O'Reilly and Taber's data. It is of interest that the patient carrying triplets developed a new onset of ITP during her 36th week of pregnancy. An initial platelet count was 15,000 per cu mm. The patient was treated with a daily dose of prednisone of 60 mg orally. The subsequent weekly platelet counts were 8000, 14,000 and 4000 per cu mm. Elective splenectomy with cesarean section was recommended at this time but was refused. During the mother's 40th gestational week, membranes ruptured and spontaneous labor commenced. Female triplets were delivered vaginally. Maternal platelet count at delivery was 4000 per cu mm. The triplets had platelet counts of 48,000, 32,000 and 59,000 per cu mm, respectively. The platelet counts remained depressed in all three infants for three weeks. By the fourth week the platelet counts began to rise, and one month after delivery all three infants had counts over 200,000 per cu mm.

In O'Reilly's review, the maternal mortality rate was 4 per cent, with the last maternal death reported in 1951. Fetal mortality rate for the entire series was 18 per cent. Of the mothers with intact spleen, the rate was 15 per cent, and 20 per cent for those who had had their spleens removed. The overall incidence of neonatal thrombocytopenia or purpura or both was 44 per cent. When the maternal platelet count at delivery was greater than 100,000 per cu mm, the incidence of hemorrhagic neonatal deaths was the same for the two groups. The presence or absence of the maternal spleen had little effect on fetal outcome. Of the 88 pregnancies in which the mothers had prior splenectomy before delivery, 43 per cent of the fetuses developed purpura or thrombocytopenia or both. Of the 45 pregnancies in which maternal spleen was present, 41 per cent of the infants developed purpura or thrombocytopenia or both. The causes of the 24 fetal deaths were as follows: spontaneous abortion 6; stillbirth 13 (6 with marked hemorrhage, 5 intracranially); neonatal hemorrhage 3; nonhemorrhagic unrelated deaths, 2. Cesarean section was performed in 12 per cent (13) of the live births. Simultaneous cesarean section and splenectomy was performed in six of these patients. A high incidence (26 per cent) of postpartum maternal hemorrhage was found overall.

Ayromlooi[52] in 1978 stressed that the intrapartum diagnosis of fetal thrombocytopenia is an important tool for the management of ITP in pregnancy and proposed for the first time fetal scalp blood sampling as a method of evaluation. Fetal scalp sampling in two patients with ITP was performed early in labor. Both fetal platelet counts were greater than

100,000 per cu mm and both patients were allowed to deliver vaginally without complications. Neither infant developed neonatal thrombocytopenia. Ayromlooi stated that not all pregnant patients should be delivered by cesarean section because more than one third of infants delivered vaginally are perfectly normal. With this approach, it is hoped that intracranial hemorrhage and perinatal mortality can be prevented without unnecessary cesarean sections.

A more recent report from Noriega-Guerra et al.[56] (1979) analyzes the evolution and treatment of 21 pregnancies in 18 patients with ITP and stresses the value of multidisciplinary, intensive management in a large group of pregnancies.[56] Unfortunately, scalp sampling was not used as a diagnostic tool. In these patients ITP was diagnosed from 3 months to 31 years before the pregnancy (16 patients), and prenatal control was achieved in the remaining 5 during pregnancy by frequent monitoring in a high-risk obstetric unit, where recording of platelet counts and serial urinary estriols was carried out. Steroid control of the disease was initiated in 4 of the patients during the first trimester, in 11 during the second and in 6 during the third. Genetic malformations, an increase in the frequency of toxemia, and postpartum psychosis, all mentioned in the literature as being caused by the use of steroids, were not observed. Eighteen women received hydrocortisone intravenously throughout labor and delivery.

One maternal death occurred as a result of incomplete hemostatic control. In week 38, the patient developed hypertension, followed shortly by pulmonary hemorrhage, pneumonia, heart failure and acute fetal distress. Prompt cesarean section was performed. Death occurred during the second postoperative day after pulmonary and cerebral hemorrhage. One fetal death occurred in a patient with a history of toxemia, diabetes mellitus, transfusional hepatitis and meconium in the amniotic fluid. The fetus was found to have an edematous hemorrhagic nuchal umbilicus at the time of death at 36 weeks. Delivery was vaginal in 18 cases (3 with low forceps) and by cesarean section in 3 cases for obstetric indications only. Seven infants had no problems, 9 (43 per cent) had thrombocytopenia (4 asymptomatic), and 3 had petechiae with normal counts.

Serial estriol studies were carried out in ten gestations. All patients had low estriol values but those who did not receive high-dose steroids had low values that showed no increase, obviously because of suppression of the fetal adrenal gland. Oxytocinase values were also in the lower part of the normal curve and apparently were not influenced by steroids.

In this series no incidence of intracranial hemorrhage took place. Only 33 per cent of infants born to mothers with platelet counts of less than 100,000 per cu mm at the time of delivery showed evidence of purpura. On this basis, the authors disagreed with Territo and others that cesarean section was indicated in mothers with platelet counts less than 100,000 per cu mm at the time of delivery. They were of the opinion that the procedure was indicated only for purely obstetric reasons in these patients.

Kernoff et al. in 1979 took a completely different and still somewhat experimental approach to the identification of the thrombocytopenic fetus antenatally by identifying the presence of antiplatelet antibodies in the mother.[53] Before this study, the platelet antibody had never appeared in either the serum or attached to the platelets of both affected mother and child. A sensitive antiglobulin consumption assay that is capable of measuring nanogram amounts of platelet-bound IgG had recently been reported and was used in study. In the series of three patients, the first mother had active disease with a platelet count of 75,000 per cu mm at the time of delivery and 17.1 ng IgG/10^6 platelets at delivery (control levels 3.3 to 10.0 ng IgG/10^6). She delivered by cesarean section an infant with a cord platelet count of 98,000 per cu mm and 26.4 ng IgG/10^6 platelets. Over the next 12 weeks, this newborn's platelet count rose to 401,000 and platelet antibody fell to 2.9 ng IgG/10^6 platelets.

The two remaining patients had ITP remission with normal platelet counts and antibody levels during pregnancy and delivery. Neither infant had thrombocytopenia. Unfortunately, the rarity of the condition denied Kernoff and co-workers an opportunity to make observations on the outcome of pregnancies in women who have normal platelet counts and an increased antiplatelet antibody level. A review by Perkins[80] of thrombocytopenia in obstetrics appeared in 1979. In this paper, he discussed the subject of ITP briefly. Perkins had also found it helpful in a few cases to attempt to measure platelet counts in the fetus directly by scalp blood sampling during early labor. He stressed, however, the risk of inducing hemorrhage from the scalp in a severely thrombocytopenic infant. Such hemorrhaging can be overcome by prolonged pressure to the scalp wound. Perkins presented one illustrative case of a patient with a platelet count of 80,000 per cu mm at the time of delivery. At 6 mm of cervical dilation, the infant underwent fetal scalp sampling that revealed a platelet count of 52,000 per cu mm. Cesarean section was performed. Both mother and infant had an unremarkable postpartum course.

A recent report on the subject of ITP in pregnancy seems to provide a rational basis for obstetric management to date. In this study, Scott and colleagues employed the technique of platelet counts on fetal scalp blood obtained before or early in the course of labor in 12 patients with ITP.[81] A count of 50,000 per cu mm was used to define fetal thrombocytopenia. Three thrombocytopenic fetuses were delivered by cesarean section. A trial of labor was permitted in the other nine cases in which fetal scalp platelets exceeded 50,000 per cu mm. The outcome was good in all cases, except for petechiae. Therefore, Scott recommended that, in pregnancy complicated by ITP, amniotomy should be done as soon as conditions permit fetal blood sampling, either at the time of labor induction or early in the course of labor.[81] If platelet counts obtained are greater than 50,000 per cu mm, vaginal delivery should be anticipated, whereas fetuses with lower counts should be delivered by cesarean section as soon as possible. This approach, although considerably more specific than a decision based solely on the maternal platelet count, requires further evaluation.

Summary

The number of reported proved ITP cases probably does not reflect the true incidence of ITP as a complication of pregnancy. Only three maternal deaths have been reported and only one since 1951. More maternal deaths may remain unreported because authors are more likely to report their successes than their failures. Maternal mortality rates have, however, been significantly reduced. This improvement is a result of several factors, including (1) better diagnostic criteria, (2) steroid therapy, (3) the reduced surgical risk of splenectomy during pregnancy and (4) the availability of platelets for transfusion. The favorable data for maternal mortality suggest that conception should not be prohibited in patients with known ITP. Perinatal mortality in this review is 9.1 per cent; before 1960 the rate was 12.9 per cent; from 1969 to 1980 the rate was 8.6 per cent.

The overall incidence of infants with thrombocytopenia (platelet count less than 50,000 per cu mm) or purpura or both, including hemorrhagic stillborn fetuses, was 42.4 per cent. The incidence of thrombocytopenia in liveborn infants born to mothers with maternal platelet counts of less than 100,000 per cu mm at delivery was 53.9 per cent. The incidence of thrombocytopenia in infants born to mothers with platelet counts greater than 100,000 per cu mm was 23 per cent. The absence of a spleen made little difference in the group with maternal platelets of less than 100,000 per cu mm at delivery; 52 per cent were thrombocytopenic infants of mothers without spleens; 55 per cent were thrombocytopenic infants of those with spleens intact and 50 per cent were thrombocytopenic infants whose mothers' spleen status was not reported. This condition was not valid for mothers with platelet counts of greater than 100,000 per cu mm at delivery. The incidence of thrombocytopenic infants among mothers without a spleen was 32 per cent, whereas it was only 7 per cent among mothers with intact spleens. This finding is consistent with the fact that after splenectomy, even with normal maternal platelet counts, the antiplatelet antibody is still being produced and is available for transplacental transfer to the fetus.

These data compiled from a review of the literature support other reviews that do not bear out the reliability of maternal platelet counts at the time of delivery for predicting thrombocytopenia in the fetus. If the incidence of thrombocytopenia in infants born to mothers with platelet counts of less than 100,000 per cu mm at delivery was 53.9 per cent, cesarean sections performed for this reason would have been unnecessary in 46.1 per cent of the patients. Moreover, vaginal delivery would have posed an increased risk for 23 per cent of infants born to mothers with platelet counts of greater than 100,000 per cu mm at time of delivery.

The incidence of ITP is approximately three to four times greater in females than males. Because its onset occurs most frequently before the age of 30, pregnancy and ITP do occasionally coexist. When faced with this situation the obstetrician has a dual concern— the welfare of both mother and fetus—and must tailor management of the case to obtain optimal results for both. This situation is further complicated by multiple gestation.

The effect of pregnancy on the clinical course of ITP is variable. Untreated, the symptoms associated with ITP tend to worsen during pregnancy, despite an increase of free cortisol. If remission has been achieved by prior splenectomy, steroid therapy or cytotoxic immunosuppressants, the majority of women will not have relapse during pregnancy. The risk of exacerbation of active disease is 30 to 40 per cent. In the treatment of active ITP, either new-onset or recurrent exacerbation, the first modality to be employed should be corticosteroids, as it is in nonpregnant patients. If a satisfactory response is obtained (50,000 to 100,000 per cu mm), patients may be maintained on a low-dose regimen until after delivery. These patients may be at increased risk for toxemia of pregnancy and postpartum psychosis, and any other side effects of steroid therapy that the nonpregnant patient may develop. The possibility of teratogenicity must always be considered.

If the response to steroids is unsatisfactory, splenectomy should be performed. The use of platelet transfusions (especially HLA matched) should overcome any problems with surgical hemostasis. This procedure is best performed in the first and second trimesters; as the uterus further enlarges, splenectomy becomes technically more difficult. If it cannot be performed by the second trimester, splenectomy should be postponed until after delivery or done in conjunction with cesarean section. Splenectomy does impose increased risk to the fetus and may result in fetal death in utero or in spontaneous abortion.

The use of cytotoxic immunosuppressive drugs in pregnancy is still experimental because of their possible teratogenic effects. They are not recommended during the first trimester. No adequate data are available on their use at any time during pregnancy.

The administration of platelets is indicated only in severe cases of hemorrhage or as immediate preparation for surgery.

The rates of spontaneous abortion reported in the recent series reviewed range from 7 to 23 per cent. A higher incidence of postpartum hemorrhage has been observed, especially in patients with low platelet counts. Since bleeding from the placental site is initially controlled mechanically by myometrial contraction and retraction, the occurrence of postpartum hemorrhage may reflect bleeding

due to trauma to the cervix and other maternal soft tissues and to episiotomy sites. Obviously, lacerations and trauma should be avoided whenever possible. The bleeding sites may require the use of platelet packs for hemostasis. Meticulous repair is essential to avoid the formation of hematoma.

Maternal ITP is associated with a 10 to 15 per cent perinatal mortality rate; most intrauterine or neonatal deaths are caused by cerebral hemorrhage. The thrombocytopenia in the newborn is a self-limited disease, which results from the transplacental transfer of maternal antiplatelet antibodies. Since the child does not produce any of the antibodies, the duration of the disease will depend on the level and rate at which maternal antibodies are cleared from the baby's circulation. The clinical neonatal disease often becomes worse after delivery and the platelet count often does not reach a nadir until the fourth to sixth day.[49] The thrombocytopenia may not be evident on physical examination. Frequently, however, generalized petechiae and frank bleeding are seen. Early platelet counts should be determined on all babies of affected mothers. Many patients do not require special treatment. The main justification for active therapeutic measures is to prevent or treat the serious life-threatening hemorrhage. Platelet transfusions can be given in a dose of 10 ml per kg. These should be freshly prepared. In an effort to decrease the length of the thrombocytopenic phase in the child by removing maternal antibodies, exchange transfusions may be considered. However, the benefit of this procedure has not been proved. Steroids (1 mg per kg prednisone) have been used, but their influence on the course of the disease is doubtful. Splenectomy has even been performed in serious cases, but is not recommended.

In a review of the literature, several schools of thought on the management of labor emerge: in one vaginal delivery is preferred; in one a decision is made on the basis of the maternal platelet count at the time of delivery, and in one cesarean section is favored, regardless of maternal platelet counts, especially in postsplenectomy mothers in whom circulating antiplatelet antibodies can be high in the presence of a normal platelet count. The basis for the use of cesarean section is the greater risk in labor of cranial trauma, which is especially dangerous to newborns who may develop transient neonatal thrombocytopenia.

Newer guidelines for the obstetric management of the gravid woman with ITP propose identifying fetuses that are truly thrombocytopenic and delivering vaginally the infants who are not thrombocytopenic. This identification can be accomplished by platelet counts via fetal scalp blood sampling before or early in the course of labor. Only about 0.1 cc of fetal blood is needed for the count. If the count is low (less than 50,000 per cu mm), abdominal delivery as soon as possible is the method of choice. If the count is higher, vaginal delivery may be allowed to progress.

Conclusions

The improvement in maternal and fetal morbidity and mortality resulting from idiopathic thrombocytopenic purpura during pregnancy has largely been a reflection of advances in therapy of ITP in all patients. Maternal morbidity and mortality are now rare, but the significant risk of neonatal complications is still a major factor in perinatal management. This risk stems from the transplacental transfer of maternal antiplatelet autoantibodies, which may cause reduction in the fetal or neonatal platelet counts. The literature supports a poor correlation between maternal and fetal platelet counts.

This problem has created a controversy over the use of elective cesarean section to avoid the trauma of labor and its resultant complications (particularly cerebral hemorrhage) in the thrombocytopenic fetus or newborn. There has not been enough experience to learn if elective cesarean section will significantly reduce the fetal and neonatal morbidity and mortality without increasing maternal morbidity and mortality. A more specific approach is the identification of the thrombocytopenic infant through fetal scalp sampling. This procedure should allow development of a more selective use of cesarean section and allow the fetus with an adequate platelet count to be delivered vaginally. However, it requires rupture of the membranes, a cervix 3 cm dilated, appropriate collecting and transport equipment and personnel experienced in fetal scalp sampling.

Ideally, all pregnant patients suffering from ITP should be managed by medical personnel with experience in selecting the thrombocytopenic fetus. If this is not realistically feasible, a cesarean section should be performed. The hazard of surgery is justified when compared with the risk of vaginal delivery to the thrombocytopenic fetus. Platelets should be transfused immediately prior to surgery if the mother is thrombocytopenic. Platelet concentrates can be prepared from random units of anticoagulated whole blood. Each unit of concentrate contains at least 5.5×10^{10} platelets, as well as lymphocytes and a few red blood cells, suspended in plasma to a final volume of 30 to 50 ml. The transfusion of one unit of platelet concentrate will usually raise the platelet count to 9000 to 10,000 per microliter per m^2 of body surface, the usual dose being between 6 and 8 units. An alternative method of obtaining adequate numbers of donor platelets is harvesting them from a single donor (plateletpheresis) by using a cell separator, which allows the collection of an average of 2.6×10^{11} platelets per donation. This method has the advantage of a small risk of post-transfusion hepatitis as well as of platelet alloimmunization.

One of the main problems remaining is that there is no way to predict the number of platelets that have to be transfused to arrest a bleeding episode. Similarly, when preparing the patient for surgery, there are no accurate tests that make it possible to foretell the number of units that will be necessary to achieve previously set levels. Furthermore, in states in which there is a high turnover rate such as ITP, we cannot predict how long these levels will be maintained. Therefore, the transfusion of platelets just one hour before surgery has been proposed by several authors. An additional consideration is the possibility of $Rh_o(D)$ sensitization when an $Rh_o(D)$ negative woman receives platelet concentrates from $Rh_o(D)$ positive donors (especially when a large number of units is transfused as in ITP), since platelet concentrates contain small amounts of red blood cells as "contaminants." This problem can be overcome by practicing Rh immunoprophylaxis with Rh immune globulin.

Platelets must be available for all women who are thrombocytopenic, because obstetric factors may dictate surgical intervention.

It must be remembered that even with the scalp sample technique or with cesarean section, the physician should not expect that all these babies will be normal, because fetal bleeding has been documented prior to the onset of labor.

Future advances may obviate the need for

invasive fetal studies. New research methods for defining mothers with platelet-associated IgG present at the time of delivery may select appropriate candidates for cesarean section. Furthermore, the effect of steroid administration to all mothers with ITP, regardless of previous splenectomy or platelet count, appears to reduce reticuloendothelial removal of the fetal platelets.[82] Plasma exchange may prove to be clinically useful to accelerate clearance of antiplatelet antibodies in patients suffering anamnestic immune phenomena without recurring antigenic stimulation. The rarity of ITP has restricted research; however, double-blind longitudinal studies are indicated while sound clinical judgment and experience prevail.

REFERENCES

1. Mueller-Eckhardt, C.: Idiopathic thrombocytopenic purpura: clinical and immunologic considerations. Semin. Thromb. Hemostas. 3:125, 1977.
2. Tancer, L.: Idiopathic thrombocytopenic purpura and pregnancy. Am. J. Obstet. Gynecol. 79:148, 1960.
3. Barnes, R.: A case of fever in a pregnant woman marked by extensive purpura effusion in the skin. Br. Med. J. 2:375, 1867.
4. Byrne, J.: Case of purpura hemorrhagica preceding and following labor. Br. Med. J. 2:383, 1867.
5. Goodhue, P. and Evans, T.: Idiopathic thrombocytopenic purpura in pregnancy. Obstet. Gynecol. Surv. 18:671, 1962.
6. Moeher, G.: The complication of purpura with gestation. Surg. Gynecol. Obstet. 36:502, 1923.
7. Rushmore, S.: Purpura complicating pregnancy. Am. J. Obstet. Gynecol. 10:553, 1925.
8. DeSaussure, H. and Townsend, E.: Purpura hemorrhagic in pregnancy. Am. J. Obstet. Gynecol. 29:597, 1935.
9. Polowe, D.: Splenectomy in pregnancy complicated by thrombocytopenic purpura hemorrhagicum. J.A.M.A. 124:771, 1944.
10. Patterson, W.: Thrombocytopenic purpura in pregnancy and the newborn. J.A.M.A. 130:700, 1946.
11. Rosenvasser, E. and Ramazzi, P.: Hemopatia trombopenia y embarazo. Rev. Esp. Obstet. Ginecol. 15:17, 1956.
12. Burnett, C. and Klass, I.: A review of the problem of purpura during pregnancy. J. Obstet. Gynaecol. Br. Commonwealth 50:393, 1943.
13. Robson, J. and Walker, G.: Congenital and neonatal thrombocytopenic purpura. Arch. Dis. Child. 26:175, 1951.
14. Epstein, R. et al.: Congenital thrombocytopenic purpura; purpura haemorrhagica in pregnancy and the newborn. Am. J. Med. 9:44, 1950.
15. Harrington, W. et al.: Demonstration of a thrombocytopenic factor in the blood of patients with idiopathic thrombocytopenic purpura. J. Clin. Invest. 30:646, 1951.
16. Harrington, W. et al.: Immunologic mechanisms in idiopathic and neonatal thrombocytopenic purpura. Ann. Intern. Med. 38:433, 1953.
17. Mendel, E. and Sparkman, R.: Idiopathic thrombocytopenic purpura in pregnancy. J. Int. Coll. Surg. 28:156, 1957.
18. Slaughter, D. et al.: Splenectomy and cesarean section in pregnancy, complicated by acute thrombocytopenic purpura. Arch. Surg. 63:132, 1951.
19. Lacey, J. V. and Penner, J. A.: Management of idiopathic thrombocytopenic purpura in the adult. Semin. Thromb. Hemostas. 3:160, 1977.
20. Baldini, M.: Idiopathic thrombocytopenic purpura, Part I. N. Engl. J. Med. 274:1245, 1977.
21. Baldini, M.: Idiopathic thrombocytopenic purpura, Part II. N. Engl. J. Med. 274:1301, 1977.
22. Baldini, M.: Idiopathic thrombocytopenic purpura, Part III. N. Engl. J. Med. 274:1360, 1977.
23. Doan, C. et al.: Idiopathic and secondary thrombocytopenic purpura. Ann. Int. Med. 53:861, 1960.
24. Miescher, P. A. and Muller-Eberhard, H. J. (eds.): Textbook of Immunopathology, Vol. II. New York, Grune and Stratton, 1969.
25. Najean, Y. et al.: Survival of radiochromium-labeled platelets in thrombocytopenias. Blood 22:718, 1963.
26. Aster, R. and Jandl, J.: Platelet sequestration in man. J. Clin. Invest. 43:843, 1964.
27. Kelton, J., Giles, A., Neame, P., Powers, P. and Hirsch, J.: Comparison of two direct assays for platelet-associated IgG (PAIgG) in assessment of immune and nonimmune thrombocytopenia. Blood 55:424, 1980.
28. Kelton, J. et al.: Neonatal thrombocytopenia due to passive immunization. N. Engl. J. Med. 25:1401, 1980.
29. Liebling, P.: Purpura hemorrhagica in pregnancy. Am. J. Obstet. Gynecol. 11:847, 1926.
30. Davidson, L.: Congenital thrombocytopenia. Am. J. Dis. Child. 54:1324, 1937.
31. Lozner, E.: Differential diagnosis, pathogenesis and treatment of the thrombocytopenic purpuras. Am. J. Med. 14:459, 1953.
32. Harrington, W. et al.: The autoimmune thrombocytopenias. Prog. Hematol. 1:166, 1956.
33. Shulman, R. et al.: Similarities between known antiplatelet antibodies and factors responsible for thrombocytopenia in idiopathic purpura. Ann. N.Y. Acad. Sci. 124:499, 1965.
34. Sprague, C.: Use of fluorescent antibody technique in detection of platelet antibodies in blood platelets. Boston, Little, Brown & Co., 1961.
35. Shulman, N. et al.: Role of reticuloendothelial system in pathogenesis of idiopathic thrombocytopenic purpura. Trans. Assoc. Am. Physicians 78:374, 1965.
36. Huestis, D. et al.: Practical Blood Transfusion. Boston, Little, Brown & Co., 1976.
37. Sprague, C. et al.: Platelet transfusions and the pathogenesis of idiopathic thrombocytopenic purpura. J.A.M.A. 150:1193, 1952.
38. Bonnin, J.: Management of thrombocytopenic states with particular reference to platelet thromboplastic function. Br. J. Haematol. 7:250, 1961.
39. Ahn, Y. S. and Harrington, W. J.: Treatment of idiopathic thrombocytopenic purpura. Ann. Rev. Med. 28:299, 1977.
40. Damishek, W. and Schwartz, R.: Treatment of certain autoimmune diseases with antimetabolites: a preliminary report. Trans. Assoc. Am. Physicians 73:113,1960.
41. Bouroncle, B.A. and Doan, C. A.: Refractory idi-

opathic thrombocytopenic purpura treated with Imuran. N. Engl. J. Med. 275:630, 1966.

42. Laros, R. K. and Penner, J.: Refractory thrombocytopenic purpura treated successfully with cyclophosphamide. J.A.M.A. 215:445, 1971.

43. Aisenberg, A. and Wilkes, B.: Studies on the suppression of immune responses by the periwinkle alkaloids vincristine and vinblastine. J. Clin. Invest. 43:2394, 1964.

44. Laros, R. K. and Sweet, R. L.: Management of idiopathic thrombocytopenic purpura during pregnancy. Am. J. Obstet. Gynecol. 122:182, 1975.

45. Murray, J. and Harris, R.: Management of the pregnant patient with ITP. Am. J. Obstet. Gynecol. 126:449, 1976.

46. Jones, W. R., Storey, B., Norton, G. and Neische, F. W., Jr.: Pregnancy complicated by acute idiopathic thrombocytopenic purpura. J. Obstet. Gynaecol. Br. Commonwealth. 81:330, 1974.

47. Heys, R.: Steroid therapy for idiopathic thrombocytopenic purpura during pregnancy. Obstet. Gynecol. 28:532, 1966.

48. Territo, M., Finklestein, J., and Oh, W. et al.: Management of autoimmune thrombocytopenia in pregnancy and in the neonate. Obstet. Gynecol. 41:579,1973.

49. O'Reilly, R. and Taber, B.: Immunologic thrombocytopenic purpura and pregnancy. Obstet. Gynecol. 51:590, 1977.

50. Levine, P. et al.: Idiopathic thrombocytopenic purpura, diabetes mellitus and pregnancy. Obstet. Gynecol. (Suppl.) 48:31, 1976.

51. Anguilo, J. et al.: Management of cesarean section in a patient with idiopathic thrombocytopenic purpura. Anesthesiology. 46:145, 1977.

52. Ayromlooi, J.: A new approach to the management of idiopathic thrombocytopenic purpura in pregnancy. Am. J. Obstet. Gynecol. 130:235, 1978.

53. Kernoff, L. M., Malan, E. and Gunston, K.: Neonatal thrombocytopenia complicating autoimmune thrombocytopenia in pregnancy. Ann. Intern. Med. 90:55, 1979.

54. Heys, R.: Childbearing and idiopathic thrombocytopenic purpura. J. Obstet. Gynaecol. Br. Commonwealth 73:205, 1966.

55. Jones, R. et al.: Idiopathic thrombocytopenic purpura in pregnancy and the newborn. Br. J. Obstet. Gynaecol. 84:679, 1977.

56. Noriega-Guerra, L., Aviles-Miranda, A., Alvarez de la Cadena, O. et al.: Pregnancy in patients with autoimmune thrombocytopenic purpura. Am. J. Obstet. Gynecol. 133:439, 1979.

57. Bernstein, P. et al.: The problem of idiopathic purpura in pregnancy and the neonatal period. Am. J. Obstet. Gynecol. 38:323, 1939.

58. Limarzi, L.: Thrombocytopenia of the newborn. Med. Clin. North Am. 28:153, 1944.

59. Barnes, A. and Doan, C.: Splenectomy in pregnancy. Am. J. Obstet. Gynecol. 55:864, 1948.

60. Arrowsmith, W. et al.: Simultaneous cesarean section and splenectomy in idiopathic thrombocytopenic purpura. J. Lab. Clin. Med. 34:1580, 1949.

61. Peterson, O. and Larson, P.: Idiopathic thrombocy-

topenic purpura in pregnancy. Obstet. Gynecol. 4:454, 1954.

62. Coopersmith, B.: Two cases of thrombocytopenia during pregnancy treated with splenectomy. Am. J. Obstet. Gynecol. 69:450, 1955.

63. Newmark, F.: Thrombocytopenic purpura in pregnancy. J.A.M.A. 158:646, 1955.

64. Poulhes, J. et al.: Splenectomy in pregnancy complicated by thrombocytopenic purpura. J.A.M.A. 124:771, 1944.

65. Vandenbrouche, J. and Verstraete, M.: Thrombocytopenia due to platelet agglutinins in the newborn. Lancet 268:593,1955.

66. Schoen, E. et al.: Neonatal thrombocytopenic purpura. Pediatrics 17:72, 1956.

67. Kaye, B. and Dufault, F.: Idiopathic thrombocytopenic purpura with pregnancy. Obstet. Gynecol. 9:228, 1957.

68. Salzberg, M. and Koren, Z.: Pregnancy associated with thrombocytopenic purpura and eclampsia. Am. J. Obstet. Gynecol. 76:1275, 1958.

69. Hershman, A. and Matthews, J.: Idiopathic thrombocytopenic purpura in pregnancy: review and case report. J. Am. Osteopath. Assn. 59:302, 1959.

70. Hoadley, W.: Pregnancy complication: idiopathic thrombocytopenic purpura treated with steroids and splenectomy. Mo. Med. 56:544, 1959.

71. Marks, R. and Wegryn, S.: Idiopathic thrombocytopenic purpura in pregnancy. Am. J. Obstet. Gynecol. 77:895,1959.

72. Rogers, T.: Thrombocytopenia in pregnancy following splenectomy. Am. J. Obstet. Gynecol. 78:806, 1959.

73. Watson, P.: Pregnancy with idiopathic thrombocytopenic purpura. J. Obstet. Gynaecol. Br. Commonwealth 66:124, 1959.

74. Peretti, F.: Pregnancy with the Werlhof type of thrombocytopenic hemorrhagic syndrome. Minerva Anestesiol. 2:661, 1960.

75. Zilliacies, H. and Kallio, H.: Idiopathic thrombocytopenic purpura with pregnancy. J. Obstet. Gynaecol. Br. Commonwealth 69:472, 1962.

76. Glodt, H.: Idiopathic thrombocytopenic purpura with pregnancy. Obstet. Gynecol. 23:132, 1964

77. Lambeth, S.: Idiopathic thrombocytopenic purpura with pregnancy with follow-up. Am. J. Obstet. Gynecol. 89:839, 1964.

78. Glick, L. and Weiser, N.: Thrombocytopenic purpura in pregnancy. J.A.M.A. 147:44, 1951.

79. Oski, F. and Naiman, J.: Hematologic Problems of the Newborn. Philadelphia, W. B. Saunders Co., 1972.

80. Perkins, R.: Thrombocytopenia in obstetric syndromes: a review. Obstet. Gynecol. Surv. 34:101, 1979.

81. Scott, J. et al.: Fetal platelet counts in the obstetric management of immunologic thrombocytopenic purpura. Am. J. Obstet. Gynecol. 136:495, 1980.

82. Karpatkin, M., Porges, R. and Karpatkin, S.: Platelet counts in infants of women with autoimmune thrombocytopenia. N. Engl. J. Med. 305:936, 1981.

Editorial Comment

Idiopathic thrombocytopenia during pregnancy, fortunately, is a very uncommon disease. Each tertiary care center sees between 6 to 16 such cases per year. If it is assumed that different physicians manage these patients and that it would take a number of years for any individual physician to have treated a respectable number of patients with ITP, it is no wonder that there has been disagreement about what should be done. If we assume that an obstetrician is in a tertiary care center that handles sick obstetric patients, and furthermore, if we assume that somewhere between 5 to 20 per cent of the babies will die whose mothers have this disease, it would take 18 months for one death to occur at that center. Statistically, it would be unusual for the same obstetrician to manage all the center's patients over a period of three years; hence, there will be no firm and fixed guidelines as to what should be done. It's nice to talk about the problem when you see the patient in the antepartum period and evaluate whether or not the mother has positive antibodies, which occur in chronic cases approximately 50 per cent of the time. Do these antibodies then cross the placenta and affect the fetus, who also then will have ITP? Can we tell if the fetus is affected during the antepartum period? The authors of this chapter answer, "No." Our rock and a hard place becomes even firmer when we realize that during the past 15 years there have been no reported maternal deaths from ITP. (I am sure they have occurred, but they have not been reported in the literature to our knowledge.) The problem then is not maternal safety but fetal safety. Will a cesarean section on a patient not in labor prevent damage to the fetus? This is the root of the controversy.

The authors have had good experience in this area and have done a thorough job of looking at the literature. It is interesting in this controversy that they do not necessarily agree, nor do they generally disagree, and they get down to the management of the individual patient. They identify the fact that valuable weapons in the treatment of the patient who has ITP are corticosteroids, splenectomy and platelet transfusions. There has been some recent information leading to the conclusion that platelet transfusion should be withheld if at all possible until after the delivery of the baby, but as yet this theory has not permeated our literature. Knuppel and McNaney stress that if the mother has thrombocytopenia a platelet transfusion is in order prior to surgery.

Interestingly, the authors point out that approximately 80 per cent of infants have ITP whose mothers have platelet counts of less than 100,000. Not 80 per cent of these babies die; the mortality rate is somewhere between 5 to 20 per cent. The real point of controversy is whether the patient should have cesarean section or vaginal delivery. The opinion of Knuppel is that most patients should be delivered by cesarean section, for the simple reason that it is impossible to differentiate in a reasonable manner what the problems are for the fetus. Kryc and Corrigan take a somewhat different point of view, looking at the individual patient and dividing the patients according to whether the mother who is in labor has a platelet count of greater than 100,000 and has no signs of disrupted homeostasis. They would state, knowing full well that when the mother has more than 100,000 platelets, 40 per cent of the babies may have ITP. As labor progresses, they would recommend that scalp blood sampling be done, and as long as the fetus does not have ITP, vaginal delivery should be permitted.

The mother who goes into labor with ITP and a platelet count of less than

100,000 should be declared a medical and surgical emergency. Kryc and Corrigan recommend platelet transfusion and, more importantly, platelet survival studies. The fetal scalp blood sample can be taken, and most likely there will be a problem of ITP in the fetus. If this is true, they recommend in the event of maternal hemostasis and fetal involvement that a cesarean section be done.

The final answer is yet to come, except to state that unless you have sophisticated diagnostic weapons at your disposal, and if you think that the mother with a clotting disorder can survive a cesarean section, it may be best to do cesarean section for fetal indications. If the mother does not have good homeostasis and you don't have the facilities, then it's best that you try to refer the patient to an institution that has sophisticated blood banking and excellence in clinical pathology in the area of hematology. It takes a concerted effort on the part of many people to treat the critically ill pregnant patient who has ITP if you are going to end up with a live mother and a live baby, both of whom will do okay. You will probably never be criticized for doing a cesarean section for fetal indications in these patients if in doubt, unless the mother develops a serious complication and death follows. The problems that pertain to the patient with ITP are sometimes misleading in that we assume that the magic number for the platelet count is around 100,000. The patient could have 200,000 platelets, and if they were not normal, they would not afford any more hemostasis than otherwise; hence, it is important that other profiles be used to indicate the problem. The answers are far from complete, and there does continue to be disagreement about whether or not the patient should have vaginal or abdominal delivery in ITP.

10
Preferred Management of Gestational Trophoblastic Neoplasms

Alternative Points of View

by Donald P. Goldstein and Ross S. Berkowitz
by Charles B. Hammond and Thomas N. Suciu

Editorial Comment

Preferred Management of Gestational Trophoblastic Disease

Donald P. Goldstein, M.D.
Ross S. Berkowitz, M.D.
Harvard Medical School

In 1956, Li, Hertz and Spencer inaugurated a new era in the management of gestational trophoblastic disease (GTD) when they reported complete regression of metastatic choriocarcinoma in three women treated with methotrexate.[1] During the succeeding two decades, our knowledge of the natural history and pathophysiology of GTD has advanced considerably, and with it a gratifying improvement in treatment has ensued.

Advances in the therapy of GTD have been made in several inter-related areas. First, the development of a specific and sensitive radioimmunoassay for human chorionic gonadotropin (hCG) has facilitated effective diagnosis, treatment and follow-up of patients with all types of trophoblastic tumors. In fact, the sequential measurement of hCG now serves as the sole criterion for the administration of chemotherapy. Second, because of the increased understanding of the natural history of GTD, a new therapeutic classification has been developed at the New England Trophoblastic Center (NETDC), that provides for greater individualization of therapy. Third, study of the morphologic variations in patients with GTD has elucidated various features that are of prognostic importance. Fourth, while several chemotherapy regimens have achieved excellent results, one has emerged in which reduced toxicity is combined with optimal therapeutic outcome.

This article will review in detail these major advances and outline an optimal program for the evaluation and management of this disease.

313

The Measurement of Human Chorionic Gonadotropin

One of the most important advances in oncology has been the recognition that serum proteins may serve as cell markers in the detection and management of malignancy. The cytotrophoblastic and syncytiotrophoblastic cells that constitute the functional elements of all trophoblastic tumors invariably secrete hCG. Serial determination of hCG has become an invaluable tool in the detection of viable trophoblastic tumor cells, in monitoring the effectiveness of chemotherapy and in ensuring that remission is sustained upon completion of chemotherapy.[2]

Measurement of hCG has become progressively more sensitive and specific with the development of improved assay methods. The determination of hCG was initially performed by biologic assays such as the Klinefelter mouse uterine weight assay, which did not discriminate between follicle-stimulating hormone (FSH), luteinizing hormone (LH) and thyroid-stimulating hormone (TSH).[3]

HCG, like the other glycoprotein hormones (FSH, LH, TSH), consists of two polypeptide chains (alpha and beta) attached to a carbohydrate moiety. The alpha chain of hCG is immunologically indistinguishable from alpha chains of other glycopeptide hormones. Because hCG and LH share indistinguishable alpha chains, there is substantial cross-reactivity between hCG and LH in several biological and immunologic assays. The beta chain of each of the four glycopeptide hormones is biochemically unique and confers biologic and immunologic specificity. In 1972, Vaitukaitis and co-workers reported the development of a highly specific and sensitive radioimmunoassay for hCG based upon the immunologic properties of the beta subunit structure.[4] The present beta subunit radioimmunoassay has a sensitivity of 10 mIU per ml and is specific for hCG, thereby permitting accurate measurement of hCG without interference from other glycopeptide hormones, particularly LH (Fig. 1). Recently a radioreceptor assay* has become commercially available and is more rapidly performed and less costly than the BSU method.[5] Regrettably, this assay is not specific for hCG and has a sensitivity of only 200 mIU per ml, limiting its usefulness for the measurement of low levels of hCG that overlap with endogenous levels of LH. The beta sub-

*Biocept 6, Wampole Laboratories, Stamford, Conn.

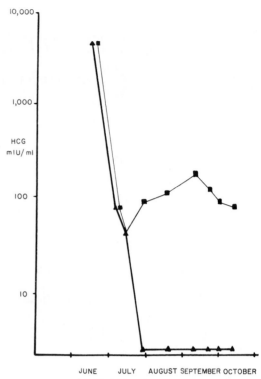

Figure 1. Graph illustrating the serum hCG regression curves following treatment in a 14-year-old female with nongestational choriocarcinoma of the ovary as performed by the specific beta subunit (—▲—) and the nonspecific hLH radioimmunoassays (—■—). Note that hCG levels are undetectable by the beta subunit assay despite the presence of postcastration levels of hLH following total removal of tumor by total abdominal hysterectomy and bilateral salpingo-oophorectomy.

unit radioimmunoassay appears to be the optimal test for patients with GTD because it permits more accurate diagnosis.

The Role of Histology

Hertig and Sheldon assessed the histologic features of 200 hydatidiform moles and assigned them to six categories that correlated with the clinical outcome.[6] Since this initial study, few additional insights have been gained regarding the prognostic importance of the morphology of GTD.

Histopathologic variations of GTD have recently been restudied in detail to evaluate possible correlations among morphology, biologic behavior and response to chemotherapy.[7] Fifty-seven patients with GTD treated between 1965 and 1975 were selected at random from the records of the NETDC. Favorable response to chemotherapy was associated with

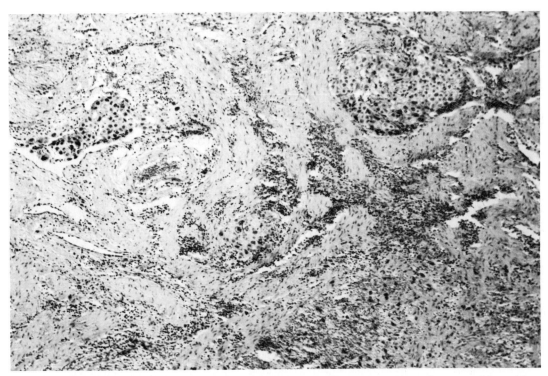

Figure 2. Photomicrograph showing the typical morphologic pattern seen in patients who respond favorably to single-agent chemotherapy. Note the fibrinoid layer at the host-tumor interface. (H & E, 10×)

degree of maturation of the trophoblastic cells, the presence of a plexiform pattern of trophoblastic growth, and the deposition of a fibrinoid layer at the interface between trophoblastic and host tissues (Fig. 2). Trophoblastic tumors with marked mitotic activity, nuclear atypia and compact growth of cytotrophoblast were noted to require more intensive chemotherapy to achieve sustained remission (Fig. 3). The absence of fibrinoid and lymphocytic infiltration at the tumor-host interface was also associated with relative resistance to chemotherapy. In six of seven cases studied at autopsy, there was a striking absence of fibrinoid material and lymphocytic infiltration in the host tissues and marked depletion of lymphocytes in the patients' lymph nodes and spleen. The final outcome in these patients may have been influenced by their inability to sustain a vigorous immunologic response to their tumors as manifested by the deficiency of the lymphocytic and plasma cell infiltration. Improved understanding of the histopathologic features of GTD further enables the clinician to anticipate which patients are more likely to require primary intensive chemotherapy.

Classification

GTD has been traditionally divided into three histopathologic types—hydatidiform mole, invasive mole and choriocarcinoma. This morphologic classification is currently of limited utility because precise pathologic diagnoses of metastatic foci are frequently unavailable and most patients are treated with chemotherapy regardless of histology. Hertz, Lewis and Lipsett introduced a clinically oriented staging system in 1961 based primarily on the presence or absence of metastatic disease.[3] Hammond and Parker modified the Hertz classification system because of the observation that certain factors placed some patients with metastatic disease at higher risk.[8] Criteria for high-risk metastatic disease included metastases to brain or liver or both, an hCG titer greater than 100,000 milliIU per ml, and a duration of disease longer than four months.

A new therapeutic classification has been in use for the past eight years at the NETDC that incorporates concepts from both the older morphologic system and the clinical staging of Hertz et al. and Hammond and Parker (Fig.

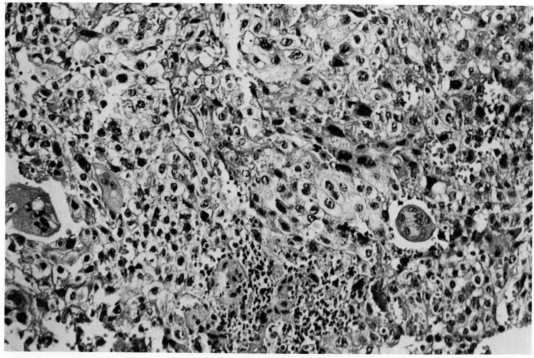

Figure 3. Photomicrograph showing the typical morphologic pattern seen in patients who respond poorly to single-agent chemotherapy. Note the marked trophoblastic activity, nuclear atypia, and compact growth of cytotrophoblast. (H&E, 10×)

4). The importance of this classification system rests in its ability to provide for greater individualization of treatment.

Revised Staging Classification and Preferred Management

CLASS I. MOLAR PREGNANCY

The accumulated experience in management of molar pregnancy at the NETDC has recently been reviewed in order to clarify the factors that predispose to proliferative complications. The most important prognostic elements encountered are: hCG titer greater than 100,000 mIU per ml, uterus larger than dates (usually more than 16 weeks' size), ovaries larger than 6 cm, other factors such as maternal age more than 40, toxemia, hyperthyroidism, coagulopathy, trophoblastic embolization and the history of a previous molar pregnancy or other type of trophoblastic tumor. Patients with these high-risk factors developed nonmetastatic and metastatic proliferative compli-

cations at a rate of 19 and 7 per cent, respectively, whereas patients without these factors developed nonmetastatic and metastatic proliferative sequelae at a rate of 4 and 0.2 per cent, respectively (Table 1). It therefore seems prudent to divide patients with molar pregnancy either into categories of low-risk disease (IA) or high-risk disease (IB).

CLASS II. LOW-RISK NONMETASTATIC GTD

Patients with low-risk nonmetastatic GTD (Class II), following evacuation of an hydatidiform mole, usually have persistently elevated hCG levels, uterine subinvolution and persistent vaginal bleeding. Clinical symptoms are related to the presence of a small amount of residual molar tissue in the endometrial cavity. Criteria for the diagnosis of Class II GTD include the following: hCG level less than 5000 mIU per ml, uterine cavity less than 11 cm in depth, ovaries less than 6 cm in diameter, and pathology restricted to Grades I to IV hydatidiform mole.

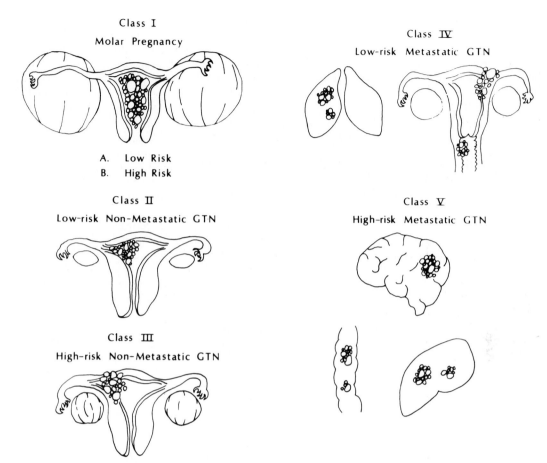

Figure 4. Schematic summary of therapeutic classification of gestational trophoblastic neoplasms utilized at the New England Trophoblastic Disease Center.

CLASS III. HIGH-RISK NONMETASTATIC GTD

Following evacuation of an hydatidiform mole, patients with high-risk nonmetastatic GTD (Class III) usually experience ovarian cysts, vaginal bleeding, uterine subinvolution and persistently elevated hCG titers. Clinical symptoms are secondary to invasive islands of viable trophoblastic tissue in the myometrium. The presence of deep myometrial invasion may be confirmed by clinical examination, curettage or pelvic arteriography or both. The diagnosis of Class III GTD is guided by the following criteria: hCG titer more than 5000 mIU per ml, uterine cavity more than 11 cm in depth, ovaries more than 6 cm in diameter, and pathology that includes all grades of hydatidiform mole or choriocarcinoma.

TABLE 1.   PROLIFERATIVE TROPHOBLASTIC COMPLICATION RATE FOLLOWING EVACUATION OF MOLAR PREGNANCY (JULY 1, 1965–JUNE 30, 1978)

	NO. AND PERCENTAGE OF PATIENTS	
OUTCOME*	*Low Risk*	*High Risk*
Normal involution	323/337 (96)	360/486 (74)
Proliferative trophoblastic sequelae		
Nonmetastatic	13/337 (4)	94/486 (19)
Metastatic	1/337 (0.2)	32/486 (7)
Totals	337/823 (41)	486/823 (59)

*Evacuation only; no chemotherapy administered.

CLASS IV. LOW-RISK METASTATIC GTD

In low-risk metastatic GTD (Class IV), metastases involve the lungs, vagina, pelvis or other organs excluding the liver, brain and bowel. The hCG titer is less than 100,000 mIU per ml and the duration of disease is less than four months from the termination of the antecedent pregnancy or the onset of symptoms. The histologic diagnosis in Class IV GTD may be either hydatidiform mole or choriocarcinoma, although hydatidiform mole predominates.

CLASS V. HIGH-RISK METASTATIC GTD

Patients with high-risk metastatic GTD (Class V) have the following characteristics: metastases involving the brain, liver or bowel, or all these organs, hCG titer greater than 100,000 mIU per ml, and duration of disease longer than four months from the termination of the preceding pregnancy or the onset of symptoms. Many patients with Class V disease have had prolonged symptoms after a term pregnancy before the diagnosis of GTD was considered. All patients with Class V GTD have been found to have choriocarcinoma. The most common cause of death in Class V disease has been spontaneous hemorrhage from cerebral or hepatic metastases.

Selection of Chemotherapeutic Agents

Excellent remission rates have been achieved in the treatment of nonmetastatic and metastatic GTD with several different chemotherapeutic regimens (Table 2). Both nonmetastatic GTD (Classes II and III) and low-risk metastatic GTD (Class IV) can be adequately treated with either actinomycin D or methotrexate with comparable results. The optimal goal of treatment is to reduce systemic toxicity while maximizing therapeutic response. The introduction of methotrexate with citrovorum factor rescue as primary treatment of Classes II to IV disease is an important step toward achieving that goal.

Methotrexate exerts its antineoplastic effect by inhibiting nucleic acid synthesis. The drug combines with dihydrofolate reductase, thereby inhibiting the formation of tetrahydrofolic acid. Tetrahydrofolic acid, or citrovorum factor, is vital in the transfer of single-carbon fragments, which are essential to synthesis of nucleic acids. With administration of citrovorum factor, the metabolic block induced by methotrexate may be neutralized and systemic toxicity may be reduced. It is tempting to theorize that escalating the dosage of methotrexate in combination with citrovorum factor rescue will improve results, since the intracellular concentration of methotrexate would be increased, enhancing its tumoricidal effects.

During the past four years, methotrexate with citrovorum factor has been utilized in the management of Classes II to IV GTD according to the protocols outlined in Table 3. Use of this regimen has achieved sustained remission of nonmetastatic and metastatic GTD in 98 and 100 per cent of patients, respectively. Treatment with methotrexate and citrovorum factor used with hCG monitoring has also reduced the number of courses of chemotherapy required to induce complete remission in comparison to methotrexate without citrovorum factor or actinomycin D.[10-13]

Between September 1974 and June 1978, 51 patients with nonmetastatic GTD were treated with either 4 mg per kg or 6 mg per kg methotrexate with citrovorum factor rescue to determine if the higher dosage could further reduce the number of courses of chemotherapy required to induce remission. Thirty-six of 41 patients (88 per cent) treated with 4 mg per kg methotrexate in 4 divided doses with citrovorum factor rescue achieved complete remission with only one course of chemotherapy. Increasing the initial dose of methotrexate to 6 mg per kg in 10 patients did not reduce the need for subsequent courses of chemotherapy but did increase associated morbidity. The incidence of hepatic or hematologic toxicity or both due to 4 mg per kg and 6 per kg methotrexate with citrovorum factor rescue was 2.5 and 30 per cent, respectively. Treatment of GTD with 4 mg per kg methotrexate in 4 divided doses with citrovorum factor rescue achieved excellent therapeutic results with virtually no marrow or hepatic toxicity.

Another study was undertaken to determine if treatment with methotrexate and citrovorum factor resulted in a significant reduction in toxicity. Seventy-five patients from the files of the NETDC who were treated with either methotrexate and citrovorum factor, metho-

TABLE 2. Published Results of Treatment of GTD

Author/Year	Remission Agents	No. Patients	Percentage Remission
Nonmetastatic disease			
Hammond, 1967	Mtx	38	93
Hammond, 1970	Mtx/act D	29	90
Brewer, 1971	Mtx/act D/triple therapy	80	100
NETDC, 1975	Act D	31	94
NETDC, 1978	Mtx-CF	51	98
Metastatic Disease			
Hertz, 1961	Mtx, vinblastine	63	47
Ross, 1965	Mtx, act D	50	74
Hammond, 1970	Mtx, act D	29	72
Brewer, 1971	Mtx/act D/triple therapy	71	86
NETDC, 1975	Act D	39	67
NETDC, 1978	Mtx-CF	8	100

trexate alone or actinomycin D were selected at random to assess their comparative marrow, hepatic and epithelial toxicities. The criteria for hepatic, hematologic and epithelial toxicity were as follows: (1) hepatocellular dysfunction as reflected in SGOT level more than 50 units, (2) platelet count less than 100,000 per cu mm, (3) a total white count less than 2500 per cu mm, (4) a total polymorphonuclear leukocyte count less than 1500 per cu mm, (5) generalized rash, (6) marked thinning and loss of scalp hair, and (7) marked mouth ulcerations with dysphagia. While methotrexate and citrovorum factor was associated with only a 4 per cent incidence of hepatic or hematologic toxicity or both, methotrexate alone and actinomycin D incurred a 48 per cent incidence of hepatic or marrow toxicity or both (Table 4). Whereas methotrexate and citrovorum factor and methotrexate alone were associated with no generalized rash or marked alopecia, actinomycin D induced a generalized rash or marked alopecia in 24 and 52 per cent, respectively. Methotrexate and citrovorum factor and methotrexate alone caused marked stomatitis in only 16 and 20 per cent of the patients, respectively, while actinomycin D induced marked stomatitis in 40 per cent.

It appears that methotrexate with citrovorum factor rescue is the least toxic and most effective single-agent chemotherapy regimen in the management of GTD. This regimen not only reduces the number of courses of chemotherapy required to induce remission but also minimizes associated morbidity. In the absence of pre-existing liver disease, methotrexate with citrovorum factor rescue should be the primary chemotherapeutic agent in the management of GTD, except in molar pregnancy and Class V patients. This regimen fulfills the goal of maximizing therapeutic outcome while limiting associated morbidity.

TABLE 3. Methotrexate-Citrovorum Factor Rescue Protocol

Day	Time	Therapy
1	8 am	CBC, platelet count, SGOT
	4 pm	Mtx, 1.0 mg/kg, IM
2	4 pm	CF, 0.1 mg/kg, IM
3	8 am	CBC, platelet count, SGOT
	4 pm	Mtx, 1.0 mg/kg, IM
4	4 pm	CF, 0.1 mg/kg, IM
5	8 am	CBC, platelet count, SGOT
	4 pm	Mtx, 1.0 mg/kg, IM
6	4 pm	CF, 0.1 mg/kg, IM
7	8 am	CBC, platelet count, SGOT
	4 pm	Mtx, 1.0 mg/kg, IM
8	4 pm	CF, 0.1 mg/kg, IM

Follow-up: CBC, platelet count, SGOT: 3× weekly for 2 weeks and PRN. hCG: weekly.

Subsequent course(s): With response: retreat at same dose. Without response: add 0.5 mg to initial dose; if no response, switch agent.

TABLE 4. Comparative Hepatic and Hematologic Toxicity of Chemotherapy in GTD

Drug	No. Patients	Hepatic Toxicity	Myelosuppression and/or Hepatic Toxicity
Mtx-CF	25	0	1 (4%)
Mtx	25	5 (20%)	12 (48%)
Act D	25	0	12 (48%)

However, if a patient proves to be resistant to it, actinomycin D should be used.

HCG Monitoring and Chemotherapy

CLASS I. MOLAR PREGNANCY

Whether or not prophylactic chemotherapy is administered, all patients with molar pregnancy must be followed closely with weekly hCG titers until the hCG level is less than 10 mIU per ml for 3 consecutive weeks. The hCG titer should then be monitored monthly for 6 consecutive months and during this interval effective contraception utilized. If the hCG titer rises or plateaus for more than 2 consecutive weeks, the patient must be readmitted for metastatic evaluation, repeat curettage and chemotherapy treatment (Fig. 5). After 6 months of normal hCG titers, the patient may discontinue contraception and become pregnant if she desires. The patient should be reassured that subsequent pregnancies in general are not more prone to increased complications, although there is a slightly increased risk of repeat molar pregnancy and spontaneous abortion. Furthermore, patients treated with chemotherapy for GTD have no increased risk of obstetric complications or congenital malformations in later pregnancies. Because of the risk of recurrent GTD, it seems prudent to pathologically evaluate all subsequent placentas from later pregnancies.

CLASSES II TO V. GTD

After each course of chemotherapy, serum hCG levels are measured weekly and serve as the sole basis for determining the need for further treatment. Further chemotherapy is withheld as long as the hCG titer is falling serially. A second course of treatment is administered if the hCG level plateaus for more than 2 consecutive weeks or becomes elevated. If the serum hCG titer is less than 10 mIU per ml for 3 consecutive weeks, the patient is then followed with monthly hCG levels for at least 6 months. The required interval of hCG follow-up is determined by the patient's class of GTD.

We have recently evaluated the rate of fall

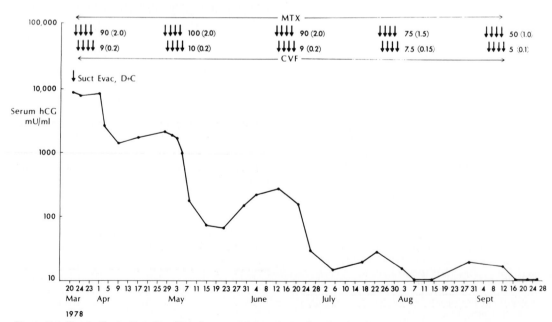

Figure 5. Graph illustrating the clinical curve of a patient who developed proliferative trophoblastic sequelae following evacuation of molar pregnancy. The serum hCG titer dropped sharply following suction curettage, then plateaued before rising. This pattern indicates proliferation of residual trophoblastic tissue requiring chemotherapy.

TABLE 5. HUMAN CHORIONIC GONADOTROPIN RESPONSE FOLLOWING INITIAL COURSE OF METHOTREXATE–CITROVORUM FACTOR AND CLINICAL OUTCOME

		NO. PATIENTS	NO. IN COMPLETE REMISSION
No. days for hCG titer to fall 1 log	> 18	3	0
	< 18	38	33 (87%)

TABLE 6. RESULTS OF PROPHYLACTIC CHEMOTHERAPY IN MOLAR PREGNANCY (JULY 1, 1965–JUNE 30, 1978)

	NO. PATIENTS (%)			
OUTCOME	Evac. and Chemotherapy*		Evac. Only†	
Normal involution	229	(96)	683	(83)
Proliferative trophoblastic sequelae				
Nonmetastatic	10	(4)‡	107	(13)
Metastatic	0		33	(4)
Totals	239	(100)	823	(100)

*Suction evacuation (or hysterectomy) with prophylactic act D.

†Suction evacuation (or hysterectomy only) *no* act D.

‡Required only 1 course of single agent chemotherapy for remission.

of the hCG titer following the initial course of chemotherapy as a predictor of therapeutic response. The number of days for the hCG level to fall 1 log after chemotherapy was recorded in 41 patients with nonmetastatic GTD. Table 5 compares the rate of fall of the hCG titer after the initial course of chemotherapy to the ensuing therapeutic outcome. Subsequent chemotherapy was needed in only 5 of 38 patients (13 per cent) in whom a 1-log fall in hCG titer occurred in less than 18 days. In contrast, all 3 patients in whom hCG levels took longer than 18 days to fall 1 log required additional chemotherapy to achieve remission. Therefore, if the hCG titer does not decline by 1 log at 18 days after chemotherapy, another course of treatment should be instituted. Chemotherapy may therefore be administered before remaining viable neoplastic cells have the opportunity to fully recover from previous cytotoxic injury.

If a second course of methotrexate and citrovorum factor is required, the dose of methotrexate is unaltered if the patient's response to the first treatment was adequate. Adequate response is defined as a 1-log fall in hCG titer following a course of chemotherapy. When the response to the first treatment was inadequate, the methotrexate dosage is escalated by an increment of 2 mg per kg in four divided doses. If the response to 2 consecutive courses of methotrexate and citrovorum factor is inadequate, the patient is considered to be resistant to methotrexate, and actinomycin D is substituted.

Treatment

CLASS I. MOLAR PREGNANCY

Effective management of molar pregnancy requires a thorough suction evacuation of the molar tissue and careful follow-up of serial hCG titers. A chest x-ray should be obtained prior to therapy and repeated in four weeks.

Weekly hCG measurements will differentiate those patients who develop proliferative trophoblastic sequelae from those whose course after evacuation is benign. Approximately 83 per cent of patients with molar pregnancy will have complete spontaneous regression of serum hCG activity within 12 to 14 weeks following evacuation. Proliferative trophoblastic complications ensue in 17 per cent of patients with molar pregnancy, with 4 per cent developing metastatic involvement.

At the NETDC, utilization of actinomycin D prophylactically in patients with molar pregnancy has led to a significant reduction in the incidence of proliferative trophoblastic sequelae (Table 6). No patient treated with prophylactic chemotherapy developed metastatic involvement and only 4 per cent experienced nonmetastatic proliferative complications. Actinomycin D was selected for prophylactic treatment because methotrexate was found to have prohibitive hepatic toxicity when used in pregnant women.[9] Currently, prophylactic chemotherapy with actinomycin D is reserved for high-risk molar pregnancy (Class IB). The protocol for the use of prophylactic actinomycin D is summarized in Table 7.

CLASS II. LOW-RISK NONMETASTATIC GTD

Class II GTD may be successfully and comparably managed with either single agent chemotherapy or hysterectomy (Table 8).[10, 11] If the patient desires to conserve reproductive potential, primary treatment should consist of chemotherapy. If hysterectomy is planned, adjunctive single-agent chemotherapy should

TABLE 7. ACTINOMYCIN D PROTOCOL

DAY	TIME	THERAPY
1	8 AM	CBC, platelet count, SGOT
	7 PM	Compazine, 10 mg, IM
	8 PM	Act D, 12 µg/kg, stat IV
2	8 AM	CBC, platelet count
	7 PM	Compazine, 10 mg, IM
	8 PM	Act D, 12 µg/kg, stat IV
3	8 AM	CBC, platelet count, SGOT
	7 PM	Compazine, 10 mg, IM
	8 PM	Act D, 12 µg/kg, stat IV
4	8 AM	CBC, platelet count
	7 PM	Compazine, 10 mg, IM
	8 PM	Act D, 12 µg/kg, stat IV
5	8 AM	CBC, platelet count, SGOT
	7 PM	Compazine, 10 mg, IM
	8 PM	Act D, 12 µg/kg, stat IV

Follow-up: CBC, platelet count: 3× weekly for 2 weeks, and PRN. hCG: weekly.

Subsequent course(s): With response: retreat at same dose. Without response: add 3 µg/kg to initial dose, if no response, switch agent.

still be employed. Adjunctive chemotherapy is not associated with increased postoperative morbidity when meticulous surgical technique is employed. Regardless of the treatment regimen, hCG titers should be monitored weekly until they are normal for three consecutive weeks, and then measured monthly for six consecutive months. After six months of normal hCG titers, patients with Class II GTD may become pregnant.

CLASS III. HIGH-RISK NONMETASTATIC GTD

Patients with Class III GTD may achieve complete sustained remission with either single-agent chemotherapy or hysterectomy (Table 9).[12] If hysterectomy is performed, adjunc-

TABLE 8. TREATMENT RESULTS IN LOW-RISK NONMETASTATIC GTD AT NETDC (JULY 1, 1965– JUNE 30, 1978)

REMISSION THERAPY	REMISSION/NO. PATIENTS (% REMISSIONS)	
1° Mtx*	26/26	(100)
1° Act D	11/11	(100)
1° Hysterectomy†	3/3	(100)
Totals	40/40	(100)

*One course only.
†Adjunctive single-agent chemotherapy used prophylactically.

TABLE 9. TREATMENT RESULTS IN HIGH-RISK NONMETASTATIC GTD AT NETDC (JULY 1, 1965– JUNE 30, 1978)

REMISSION THERAPY	REMISSION/NO. PATIENTS (% REMISSIONS)	
1° Mtx	66/83	(80)
1° Act D	28/38	(74)
Sequential Mtx/Act D	27/27	(100)
1° Hysterectomy*	14/14	(100)
Totals	135/135	(100)

*Adjunctive single-agent chemotherapy used prophylactically.

tive single-agent chemotherapy should still be administered. If the patient wants to retain reproductive function, chemotherapy should be the primary treatment modality. Serum hCG titers must be monitored weekly until they are normal for three consecutive weeks regardless of the treatment regimen. The hCG level should then be measured monthly for six consecutive months and then bimonthly for another six months. After 12 months of normal hCG titers, patients with Class III GTD may then become pregnant. The interval of hCG follow-up is longer in Class III GTD because of the greater biological virulence of this type.

CLASS IV. LOW-RISK METASTATIC GTD

Class IV GTD should be initially managed with single-agent chemotherapy. Methotrexate with citrovorum factor is the treatment of choice unless there is pre-existing hepatic disease. If the tumor is resistant to this therapy, actinomycin D should be promptly substituted.[13] When there is inadequate response to single-agent chemotherapy, combination chemotherapy with methotrexate and citrovorum factor, actinomycin D and cyclophosphamide should be instituted (Table 10). Hysterectomy is indicated in metastatic GTD only for reasons such as uterine hemorrhage, sepsis, the presence of large bulky tumor, or other specific problems. During the past 13 years, 76 patients with Class IV GTD have been managed with this outlined therapeutic regimen and all have achieved complete sustained remission (Table 11).

The hCG titer must be measured weekly until the level is less than 10 mIU per ml for 3 consecutive weeks. The hCG titer is then monitored monthly for 6 consecutive months and bimonthly for an additional 6 months.

TABLE 10.   TRIPLE-AGENT CHEMOTHERAPY
PROTOCOL

DAY	TIME	THERAPY
1	8 AM	CBC, platelet count, SGOT
	7 PM	Compazine, 10 mg, IM
	8 PM	Mtx, 1.0 mg/kg, IM
		Act D, 12 μg/kg, stat IV
		Cyclophosphamide, 3 mg/kg, stat IV
2	8 AM	CBC, platelet count
	7 PM	Compazine, 10 mg, IM
	8 PM	CF, 0.1 mg/kg, IM
		Act D, 12 μg/kg, stat IV
		Cyclophosphamide, 3 mg/kg, stat IV
3	8 AM	CBC, platelet count, SGOT
	7 PM	Compazine, 10 mg, IM
	8 PM	Mtx, 1.0 mg/kg, IM
		Act D, 12 μg/kg, stat IV
		Cyclophosphamide, 3 mg/kg, stat IV
4	8 AM	CBC, platelet count
	7 PM	Compazine, 10 mg, IM
	8 PM	CF, 0.1 mg/kg, IM
		Act D, 12 μg/kg, stat IV
		Cyclophosphamide, 3 mg/kg, stat IV
5	8 AM	CBC, platelet count, SGOT
	7 PM	Compazine, 10 mg, IM
	8 PM	Mtx, 1.0 mg/kg, IM
		Act D, 12 μg/kg, stat IV
		Cyclophosphamide, 3 mg/kg, stat IV
6	8 PM	CF, 0.1 mg/kg, IM
7	8 AM	CBC, platelet count, SGOT
	8 PM	Mtx, 1.0 mg/kg, IM
8	8 PM	CF, 0.1 mg/kg, IM

Follow-up: CBC, platelet count, SGOT: 3× weekly for 2 weeks, and PRN. hCG: weekly.

Subsequent course(s): With response: retreat at same dose. Without response:

↑ MTX to 1.5 mg/kg
↑ CF to 0.15 mg/kg
↑ Act D to 15 μg/kg
If no response, switch agent.

After 12 months of normal hCG titers, the patient may discontinue contraception and become pregnant, but hCG titers should be obtained every 6 months for 5 years.

CLASS V.   HIGH-RISK METASTATIC GTD

The optimal management of Class V GTD requires the selective utilization of combination chemotherapy, radiotherapy and surgical treatment. Primary combination chemotherapy includes the use of methotrexate and citrovorum factor, actinomycin D and cyclo-

TABLE 11.   TREATMENT RESULTS IN LOW-RISK
METASTATIC GTD AT NETDC (JULY 1, 1965–
JUNE 30, 1978)

REMISSION	REMISSION/NO. PATIENTS (% REMISSION)	
1° Mtx	24/35	(69)
1° Act D	19/35	(54)
Sequential Mtx or Act D	21/27	(78)
2° Triple TX	4/4	(100)
2° ITMA	2/2	(100)
Totals	76/76	(100)

phosphamide as outlined in Table 10. If brain metastases are present, the risk of death from intracerebral hemorrhage is considerable. Whole-head irradiation should therefore be immediately employed (3000 rads over 10 to 15 days) if cerebral metastases are documented or even strongly suspected on the basis of computerized tomography scan or elevated cerebral spinal fluid hCG levels. Adjunctive radiation therapy may also be utilized in the management of hepatic metastases. If a hepatic metastasis ruptures and precipitates intraperitoneal bleeding, the bleeding must be controlled by surgical intervention. Bowel metastases should be locally resected when diagnosed by stool guaiac tests and localized by roentgenographic study of the intestinal tract. Hysterectomy is more commonly indicated in Class V disease because of increased frequency of associated serious uterine infection or hemorrhage. During the past 4 years, the described therapeutic program has achieved complete sustained remission in 8 of 11 patients with high-risk metastatic GTD (Table 12). Duration and frequency of hCG monitoring in Class V GTD is the same as described for Class IV disease.

Immunotherapy of GTD

Half of the genetic material of the trophoblast cell is of paternal or foreign origin. The

TABLE 12.   TREATMENT RESULTS IN HIGH-RISK
METASTATIC GTD AT NETDC (JULY 1, 1965–
JUNE 30, 1978)

REMISSION	REMISSION/NO. PATIENTS (% REMISSION)	
< 1975 1° single agent 2° multiple agents	6/20	(30)
> 1975 1° multiple agents	8/11	(72)
Totals	14/31	(45)

*X-ray therapy and surgery utilized when indicated.

gestational trophoblastic tumor may therefore be appropriately viewed as a foreign graft or allograft. HLA or transplantation antigens and blood group antigens have been demonstrated to be expressed on the cellular membranes of trophoblast cells.[14-15] Furthermore, hCG and its beta subunit is also represented on the trophoblastic cellular membrane in a continuous and dense manner.[16] The unique sensitivity of GTD to chemotherapy has been attributed to immunologic rejection of the malignant allograft. Because GTD should possess a full complement of paternal antigens, this malignant allograft should elicit a viable and vigorous immunologic reaction.

Certain clinical observations have indicated that regression of GTD may be associated with allograft rejection. The prognosis of patients with choriocarcinoma has been related to the intensity of lymphocytic infiltration at the host-tumor interface. When the lymphocytic reaction was marked, the clinical outcome was more favorable. Metastatic choriocarcinoma has been reported to spontaneously regress after removal of the primary tumor. Host immunologic defenses may be able to cope with metastatic foci after the bulk of the primary tumor is excised. Patients with metastatic choriocarcinoma have also achieved prolonged sustained remission after immunization therapy with paternal antigens.[17]

As our understanding of the immunologic response to GTD expands, immunotherapy may play an important role in the management of this disease.

REFERENCES

1. Li, M. C., Hertz, R. and Spencer, D. B.: Effect of methotrexate therapy upon choriocarcinoma and chorioadenomas. Proc. Soc. Exp. Biol. Med. 93:361, 1956.
2. Goldstein, D. P.: Chorionic gonadotropin. Cancer 38:453, 1976.
3. Hertz, R., Lewis, J. Jr. and Lipsett, M. B.: Five years' experience with the chemotherapy of meta-static choriocarcinoma and related trophoblastic tumors in women. Am. J. Obstet. Gynecol. 82:631, 1961.
4. Vaitukaitis, J. L., Braunstein, G. D. and Ross, G. T.: A radioimmunoassay which specifically measures human chorionic gonadotropin in the presence of human luteinizing hormone. Am. J. Obstet. Gynecol. 113:751, 1972.
5. Saxena, B. B. and Hasan, S. H.: Radioreceptor assay of human chorionic gonadotropin—detection of early pregnancy. Science 184:793, 1974.
6. Hertig, A. J. and Sheldon, W. H.: Hydatidiform mole: a pathologicoclinical correlation. Am. J. Obstet. Gynecol. 53:1, 1947.
7. Deligdisch, L., Driscoll, S. G. and Goldstein, D P.: Gestational trophoblastic neoplasms: morphologic correlates of therapeutic response. Am. J. Obstet. Gynecol. 130:801, 1978.
8. Hammond, C. B. and Parker, R. T.: Diagnosis and treatment of trophoblastic disease. A report from the Southeastern Regional Center. Obstet. Gynecol. 35:132, 1970.
9. Goldstein, D. P.: The prevention of gestational trophoblastic disease by the use of actinomycin D in patients with molar pregnancy. Obstet. Gynecol. 43:475, 1974.
10. Goldstein, D. P., Saracco, P., Osathanondh, R. et al.: Methotrexate with citrovorum factor rescue for gestational trophoblastic neoplasms. Obstet. Gynecol. 51:93, 1978.
11. Goldstein, D. P., Goldstein, P. R., Bottomley, P. et al.: Methotrexate with citrovorum factor rescue for nonmetastatic gestational trophoblastic neoplasms. Obstet. Gynecol. 48:321, 1976.
12. Hammond, C. B., Hertz, R., Ross, G. T. et al.: Primary chemotherapy for nonmetastatic gestational trophoblastic neoplasms. Am. J. Obstet. Gynecol. 98:71, 1967.
13. Osathanondh, R., Goldstein, D. P., and Pastorfide, G. B.: Actinomycin D as the primary agent for gestational trophoblastic disease. Cancer 36:863, 1975.
14. Loke, Y. W. and Ballard, A. C.: Blood group A antigens on human trophoblast cells. Nature 245:329, 1973.
15. Loke, Y. W., Joysey, V. C. and Borland, R.: HL-A antigens on human trophoblast cells. Nature 232:403, 1971.
16. Naughton, M. A., Merrill, D. A., McManus, L. M. et al.: Localization of the beta chain of human chorionic gonadotropin on human tumor cells and placental cells. Cancer Res. 35:1887, 1975.
17. Cinander, B., Hayley, M. A., Rider, W. D. et al.: Immunotherapy of a patient with choriocarcinoma. Can. Med. Assoc. J. 84:306, 1961.

Preferable Management of Gestational Trophoblastic Disease

Charles B. Hammond, M.D.

Duke University Medical Center

Thomas N. Suciu, M. D.

University of Arizona Health Sciences Center

Prior to the introduction of chemotherapy, the survival rate for patients with gestational trophoblastic neoplasms, choriocarcinoma and related tumors was unusually poor.[1, 2] However, in 1956, a patient with metastatic choriocarcinoma was successfully treated chemotherapeutically and a new era in tumor therapy began.[3] Many reports followed in rapid succession, including a 10-year study by Hertz and co-workers in Bethesda, who investigated the effects of various chemotherapeutic agents upon nearly 200 patients with these malignancies.[4-6] From all these studies came several conclusions: First, a significant number of these patients can be cured with chemotherapy; second, early disease is more often limited in amount and is associated with higher cure rates and less therapy; third, the toxic side effects of chemotherapeutic agents are predictable and rarely fatal if the person administering them is experienced with their use and both clinical and laboratory expertise are available; finally, less than adequate therapy often results in the subsequent development of resistant disease.[7]

Equal in importance to aggressive therapy of patients with gestational trophoblastic neoplasms (GTN) is the availability of a laboratory in which the human chorionic gonadotropin (hCG) levels may be accurately measured. This hormone is produced in essentially all patients with these tumors.[8] Through precise measurement of the amount of hCG present, one can accurately follow the progress of therapy, document remission and maintain follow-up. Precise and sensitive assays, including radioimmunoassay which specifically detects hCG or which measure well into the normal pituitary gonadotropin ranges, are necessary if tragic consequences are to be avoided.

In the past several years, treatment centers have been developed to treat and investigate patients with GTN. This article will attempt to review our concept of adequate therapy for patients with both benign and malignant trophoblastic disease, and to discuss several newer treatment methodologies.

Benign Trophoblastic Disease

By benign trophoblastic disease, we mean primary hydatidiform mole, a gestation that usually lacks an intact fetus and is characterized by cystic swelling of the chorionic villi. The histopathologic criteria of hydatidiform mole are edema of the villous stroma, loss of the vascular pattern and varying degrees of trophoblastic proliferation. The frequency of mole has marked geographic variation, and best estimates of incidence in the United States are 1:1000 to 2000 pregnancies. Approximately 50 per cent of patients with metastatic gestational trophoblastic neoplasms, and 75 per cent of GTN patients without metastases, initially had molar pregnancies.

DIAGNOSIS

Hydatidiform mole is often diagnosed relatively late because, in the early stages of gestation, there are few characteristics to distinguish it from normal pregnancy. We have recently reviewed 347 patients with molar pregnancy[9] and noted several findings: Uterine bleeding is the single outstanding characteristic (89 per cent) and varies from spotting to profuse hemorrhage. Anemia is a common finding. Early molar abortion may occur, but if not, the uterus may enlarge disproportionately to what would be expected for the gestational duration. At the time of evacuation, 46 per cent had a uterus larger than expected size, 16 per cent had an expected-sized uterus, and 38 per cent had a uterus *smaller* than that anticipated. Massive enlargement of the ovaries may occur with in situ hydatidiform mole, owing to the effect of the greatly elevated levels of hCG (15 per cent). Toxemia of pregnancy was noted in 12 per cent of these 350 patients, a problem not usually seen until considerably later in normal pregnancy. Hyperemesis gravidarum was a frequent finding (14 per cent) in this group, and 2 per cent had thyrotoxicosis due to the increased level of thyroid-stimulating hormone (hCT) from the molar tissue.

Diagnosis of hydatidiform mole varies from quite easy to very difficult.(A large percentage of the patients were seen to have molar vesicles extruding through the cervix when vaginal examination was done for bleeding.) If the uterus is enlarged to adequate size, other useful findings include palpation of fetal parts or movement, detection of fetal heart tones and x-ray visualization of a fetal skeleton. Positive evidence is reliable, because the coexistence of a fetus with a mole is quite unusual. Negative findings may be misleading. The most useful diagnostic test is pelvic ultrasound, which usually provides quite accurate results. Amniography, using transabsominal instillation of a radiopaque dye, is probably the most accurate test, as a classic "honeycomb" pattern is produced by the dye around the dilated vesicles. Tests for hCG in these patients usually show significant elevations over those seen in normal pregnancy, and they do not decline to lower levels as normally occurs after 80 to 90 days of nonmolar pregnancy. It must be remembered, however, that no single value for hCG is diagnostic for hydatidiform mole. Assays for a variety of other hormonal substances have been of little use to facilitate the diagnosis of molar pregnancy for the individual patient.

MANAGEMENT

The mortality rate in primary hydatidiform mole can be quite low with aggressive management. Initial therapy should be aimed at correction of anemia, management of other superimposed medical problems (cardiovascular, infection, metabolic) and uterine evacuation. Data now exist to suggest that the method of evacuation may influence the incidence of postevacuation malignancy (dilation and curettage 19 per cent; hysterotomy 36 per cent; hysterectomy 2 per cent), but these data are trends only.[7] In general, a 10 to 20 per cent secondary malignancy rate is anticipated after uterine evacuation only. We utilize the status of the patient with regard to labor, bleeding, uterine size, age, parity and the patient's wishes regarding further reproduction to assist in this choice. It has been suggested that oxytoxin alone or vaginal prostaglandin E stimulation of labor may increase the incidence of major blood loss, infection and trophoblastic pulmonary embolization; and even with this, dilation and curettage is usually needed.[10, 11] Hysterotomy is likewise often associated with greater blood loss, greater postoperative morbidity and the usual need for repeat cesarean section in later pregnancies. For these reasons, we rarely evacuate the uterus by any of these techniques. Primary evacuation should be by suction if further childbearing is desired, and we have evacuated uteri as large as those at 28 weeks gestational size using this approach. If no further pregnancies are wished, abdominal hysterectomy with mole in situ is utilized as the primary evacuative technique.

Several studies have demonstrated that there is a 10 to 20 per cent chance that patients with hydatidiform mole will later develop malignant trophoblastic disease.[12, 13] The initial histopathology is of little aid in predicting which particular patients will develop malignancies.[14] Classical findings such as prompt uterine involution, regression of cystic ovarian enlargement and cessation of bleeding are all favorable clinical signs, but a definitive follow-up of the patient after evacuation of hydatidiform mole is made with hCG assays to detect residual or proliferating trophoblastic malignancy. For such follow-ups, the assay must be sufficiently sensitive and specific to measure levels of hCG well into normal pituitary gonadotropin ranges. Radioimmunoassays for hCG, either intact molecule or β-subunit type ("hCG-specific") are required for these levels of sensitivity. Pregnancy tests are of use only when positive.[15] We suggest that hCG assays be performed at one- to two-week intervals after the evacuation of the mole. Delfs has well shown that secretion of hCG persisting six to eight weeks after molar evacuation is associated with a significant likelihood that malignant trophoblastic disease is present or will develop.[12] If the hCG titer fails to decline, rises or plateaus after evacuation, or if metastases are noted, we suggest that systemic therapy be instituted. If the hCG titer falls to nonmeasurable levels, follow-up is instituted with hCG assays at one- to two-month intervals for one year. We have not found that repeated curettage was of assistance in follow-up or management of these patients.

PROPHYLACTIC CHEMOTHERAPY

Several authors have reported a reduction in the incidence of postmolar trophoblastic malignancy if patients received systemic chemotherapy at the time of evacuation of the mole.[10, 16, 17] To date, however, studies have been small and conducted by experts in the use of chemotherapeutic agents, and even in these the malignant sequelae of hydatidiform mole have not been totally eradicated. In fact, Ratnam and co-authors have reported that, although the incidence of postmolar trophoblastic malignancy appears to be reduced by prophylactic chemotherapy, mortality rate may be increased overall because of toxic complication and the development of resistant disease.[18] We have seen several patients who received such "prophylactic therapy" administered by community physicians not familiar with these potent agents, and the subsequent toxicity was severe. Unfortunately, several deaths have occurred. It will be shown later in this article that the 10 to 20 per cent of patients who develop malignant disease after molar pregnancy can be readily identified and that such early diagnosis can be equated with a cure rate of essentially 100 per cent with appropriate therapy.[19] Additionally, the long-term genetic and carcinogenic consequences of exposing a large population of patients to prophylactic chemotherapy are as yet unknown. For these reasons, we have not recommended prophylactic chemotherapy for all patients with hydatidiform mole. This is not to condemn a needed experimental approach by qualified investigators; instead, it is an effort to reduce unnecessary morbidity and mortality for most of these patients.

Malignant Trophoblastic Disease

The spectrum of disease in the category of GTN includes malignancies under the pathologic terms of hydatidiform mole (after initial evacuation), invasive mole (chorioadenoma destruens) and choriocarcinoma. All are preceded by some type of pregnancy, although

TABLE 1. PATIENT CATEGORIZATION

1. Nonmetastatic trophoblastic disease–hCG elevated, disease confined to the uterus (negative staging studies).
2. Metastatic trophoblastic disease (good prognosis)–hCG elevated, metastases present but not to brain or liver, none of the poor prognostic findings present.
3. Metastatic trophoblastic disease (poor prognosis)–hCG elevated and greater than 40,000 mIU/ml at start of therapy, metastases to brain or liver, duration of symptoms of malignancy greater than 4 months, trophoblastic malignancy after term gestation, or significant unsuccessful chemotherapy prior to referral.

over 50 per cent initially were molar gestations.

Once the decision has been reached that a patient has malignant trophoblastic disease (by pathologic analysis or in the follow-up after molar pregnancy, or curettage or biopsy), we determine the hCG level and stage the patient for metastatic disease. A thorough history and physical, chest x-ray, computerized tomography or isotopic liver and brain scans, electroencephalogram, intravenous pyelogram, and complete hematologic and chemical evaluations are utilized in this process. On occasion dilation and curettage, pelvic ultrasound, tomography or arteriography may be indicated. After these studies, we categorize the patient according to the system in Table 1. Further comments regarding this categorization and its influence upon therapy will follow.

NONMETASTATIC TROPHOBLASTIC DISEASE

Nonmetastatic GTN, or disease confined to the uterus without evidence of distant metastases, will be seen with greater frequency if the examiners' index of suspicion is high. In approximately 75 per cent of patients the diagnosis will be achieved during follow-up of individuals who have had molar pregnancy, and in the remainder diagnosis will follow other types of pregnancy. In both situations, abnormal gestational tissue may be discovered on curettage and gonadotropins will be elevated. It is important when possible to diagnose histopathologically one of the various categories of trophoblastic disease. Patients are then best followed by monitoring gonadotropin titers. Metastatic staging studies, as just outlined, should be carried out. The patient and physicians should then come to a

TABLE 2. METHOD OF SINGLE AGENT CHEMOTHERAPY

1. Repetitive 5-day courses: methotrexate, 15 to 25 mg intramuscularly qd or actinomycin D to 13 µg/kg body weight intravenously qd
   a. Consider hysterectomy during first course of chemotherapy if further reproduction is not desired.
   b. Minimum interval between courses: 7 days
   c. Maximum interval between courses: 14 days (unless laboratory values are too low)
   d. Consider oral contraception for pituitary suppression
2. Continue repetitive 5-day courses of the *same* drug until:
   a. If hCG titer drops to normal pituitary range, then cease therapy
   b. If hCG titer "plateaus" and is elevated
   c. If hCG titer rises by tenfold
   d. If new metastases appear
3. Monitor oncolytic effect by *weekly* hCG titers, chest x-rays and pelvic examinations
4. Treatment is terminated when hCG titer is within *normal pituitary ranges;* 3 consecutive normal weekly hCG titers are necessary to diagnose remission
5. Treatment safety factor (done daily during therapy regimen, less frequently between course)—do not start, continue or resume a dose of medication if:
   a. White blood count is less than 3000/mm
   b. Polymorphonuclear leukocytes number less than 1500/mm
   c. Platelets number less than 100,000/mm
   d. Significant elevations of BUN, SGOT, or SGPT occur
6. Follow-up:
   a. hCG titers monthly for 6 months, bimonthly for 6 months, then every 6 months thereafter
   b. Physical, pelvic exams, chest x-rays, blood survey every 3 months for 1 year, every 6 months thereafter
   c. No pregnancy for 1 year

decision for or against further reproduction, as the choice will influence management. If the reproductive potential is to be preserved, the patient is begun on single-agent methotrexate or actinomycin D as outlined in Table 2. Therapy is continued with repetitive courses of either agent, utilizing the response of the hCG titer as the primary index of oncolytic effectiveness. Treatment is maintained in this fashion until the hCG titer is reduced to nonmeasurable levels. If the hCG titer fails to decline, if it rises or if metastases (other than cerebral or hepatic) appear, the other drug is tried.

Recently, Bagshawe[20] and Goldstein and colleagues[21] have published their experiences in the therapy of patients with a regimen of higher-dose methotrexate alternating with folinic acid (eight days alternating) and reported excellent results with dramatic reduction in toxicity. We have recently begun to use this approach with similar success for patients with nonmetastatic disease. However, we have elected to give therapy in repetitive courses until remission is achieved rather than to withhold further courses as long as the hCG titer continues to decline, because of the potential for producing resistant disease through less aggressive therapy.

If the patient with nonmetastatic GTN does not desire further pregnancies, we suggest that the uterus be removed by total abdominal hysterectomy on the third day of the initial five-day course of chemotherapy. Lewis and others have reported no increase in postsurgical morbidity among patients who received these agents and who underwent a variety of surgical procedures.[22] Repetitive courses of chemotherapy must be continued in the postoperative period as if surgery had not been performed. If treatment is not continued in the postsurgical period, a tumor that has either been disseminated during the procedure or that was present but unidentified at the time of surgery may be given the opportunity to expand.

A small percentage of patients with nonmetastatic GTN will fail to achieve remission with systemic chemotherapy. Pelvic arteriography may demonstrate a focus of trophoblastic disease deep in the myometrium, and resistant disease is manifested by persistent elevation of the hCG titer despite repetitive systemic chemotherapy. In these patients, one can consider either arterial infusional chemotherapy in a last attempt to preserve the uterus or hysterectomy during chemotherapy. Caution should be exercised when interpreting pelvic arteriography on patients who have received chemotherapy because a false-positive rate of as high as 20 per cent has been reported in this clinical setting.[23] As a rule, we do not believe that multiple-agent chemotherapy with its higher toxicity is warranted unless hysterectomy has been unsuccessfully attempted.

It is now anticipated that essentially all patients with nonmetastatic GTN can be cured. In 1966, the Bethesda group reported that 98 per cent of a series of 58 patients achieved cure with the methods outlined previously.[6] In 1978, Hammond and associates reported cures in all of a group of 112 patients[24] (Table 3). In both of these series, nearly 90 per cent of patients who desired to preserve reproductive capacity were able to do so. In neither series were there any toxic

TABLE 3. GESTATIONAL TROPHOBLASTIC NEOPLASIA NONMETASTATIC DISEASE
(DUKE THERAPY 1966–1975)

TYPE OF THERAPY	PRIMARY THERAPY	PRIMARY RX CURE	SECONDARY THERAPY	SECONDARY RX CURE
Single agent (Mtx/act D)	91	84	X	X
Pelvic arterial infusion	1	0	2	2
Elective initial hysterectomy*	15	15	X	X
Indicated initial hysterectomy*	5	5	X	X
Delayed hysterectomy* (resistance)	X	X	6	6
Totals	112	104	8	8

*Whenever hysterectomy was done patients continued to receive single agent chemotherapy (Mtx/Act D) after surgery until no hCG detected. 112/112 (100%) patients cured. 86/97 (89%) patients who desired preservation of uterus had this.

deaths owing to therapy, nor have there been any recurrences up to the time of this report. Ross and others have reported normally successful reproduction rates in this group.[6]

METASTATIC TROPHOBLASTIC DISEASE

Patients with GTN in whom metastases are present beyond the uterus are classified as having "good" or "poor" prognosis. This categorization is based on data from the Bethesda study, which demonstrated that a successful outcome to chemotherapy was greatly influenced by the duration of disease, the height of the initial pretreatment hCG titer and the presence or absence of either cerebral or hepatic metastases. Patients who were diagnosed promptly, even with metastases beyond the uterus other than cerebral and hepatic and who had note of the other signs and findings giving a poor prognosis, could expect a 90 per cent cure rate with chemotherapy. For the patients who had these "poor prognosis" signs and findings, the survival rate was less than 30 per cent.[4, 5] Thus, if a patient has metastatic GTN and a pretreatment hCG titer in excess of 100,000 mIU per 24-hour urine sample or 40,000 mIU/ml by serum radioimmunoassay, or cerebral or hepatic metastases, or a duration of symptoms attributable to the disease for longer than four months, it is believed that she has "poor prognosis metastatic disease." Recently we have added two additional "poor

prognostic" findings: the patient with metastatic disease developing after term gestation[25] and the patient who has received significant unsuccessful chemotherapy prior to referral to our institution.[19]

GOOD-PROGNOSIS METASTATIC DISEASE

Patients with good-prognosis metastatic GTN are treated in similar fashion to those with nonmetastatic disease (see Table 2). We continue to utilize methotrexate as our initial drug in patients if they have received recent blood transfusions, and if renal and hepatic function is normal. Despite the fact that actinomycin D has seemed to be somewhat less toxic than methotrexate, one must recall that approximately half of these patients will ultimately require treatment with both agents, owing to development of resistance to one of the drugs. We have chosen to utilize methotrexate initially but change to actinomycin D in the event that serum hepatitis develops. To date we have not treated any of these patients with the Bagshawe-Goldstein regimen of alternating methotrexate and folinic acid (see nonmetastatic disease section). Despite the apparent superiority of this regimen over traditional single-agent therapy, because of reduction in toxicity, we do not believe that it has been adequately tested to date.

After institution of treatment, repetitive five-day courses of chemotherapy are continued, and the patient's progress is monitored by weekly hCG assays. Treatment is changed to the other drug if a patient's assays fail to show a significant decline through two courses of chemotherapy. It appears that peripheral metastases in patients with good-prognosis GTN are usually even more sensitive to these drugs than is deep-seated myometrial disease. Experimental data are accumulating that hysterectomy done during the first course of therapy may influence the outcome for patients who do not desire further pregnancies and in whom there is either curettage evidence or arteriographic signs of uterine disease. It must be stressed that this technique remains in experimental stages, and that a few cases of apparent dissemination of disease have been reported by Bagshawe,[36] even when operating under cover of chemotherapy. This, however, has not been our experience if continued aggressive chemotherapy is utilized in the postoperative interval. If a patient desires to preserve her reproductive potential or if local uterine disease cannot be identified, systemic chemotherapy alone is continued. If resistance to both agents develops, delayed hysterectomy with chemotherapy or arterial infusional chemotherapy with the uterus in situ may be indicated. In any of these situations in which surgery is performed, repetitive courses of the drugs are continued postoperatively until the hCG titer falls into the normal pituitary gonadotropin range. Hysterectomy must be approached with extreme caution if there is evidence of extrauterine pelvic extension of tumor. Hemorrhage may be severe during such a procedure. If all of these approaches fail, then one can consider multiple-agent chemotherapy, as well as adjunctive radiotherapy. Table 4 shows our results with these forms of therapy for patients with "good-prognosis GTN."

POOR-PROGNOSIS METASTATIC DISEASE

Earlier in this section the findings in patients with metastatic GTN that mark poor prognosis were listed. Since the prognosis for such patients has remained so poor with conventional single-agent chemotherapy, we have recently completed a study in which more vigorous initial therapy was carried out. We now suggest that these patients be initially treated with high-dose combination chemotherapy consisting of methotrexate (15 mg intramuscularly), actinomycin D (10 μg per kg body weight intravenously), and chlorambucil (8 mg orally), all given daily for 5 days per course. The safety criteria listed in Table 2 are used, except the between-course interval is increased to a minimum of 12 days. After two or three courses of this combination therapy, treatment may be diverted to single-agent actinomycin D in standard fashion. If cerebral or hepatic metastases are present, the patient is begun on 2000 rads whole liver or 3000 rads whole brain irradiation simultaneous with the start of chemotherapy. Weekly monitoring with hCG assay is utilized. Toxic results from this approach are a major hazard, and this radical form of therapy should be undertaken only by an experienced physician with considerable laboratory and therapeutic support available. Extreme caution must be

TABLE 4. GESTATIONAL TROPHOBLASTIC NEOPLASIA: GOOD PROGNOSIS, METASTATIC (DUKE THERAPY 1966–1975)

TYPE OF THERAPY	PRIMARY THERAPY	PRIMARY RX CURE	SECONDARY THERAPY	SECONDARY RX CURE
Single agent (Mtx/act D)	49	41	X	X
Pelvic arterial infusion	X	X	3	3
Indicated 1° hysterectomy*	2	2	X	X
Delayed hysterectomy* (resistance)	X	X	5	5
Totals	51	43	8	8

*Whenever hysterectomy was done, patients continued to receive single agent chemotherapy (Mtx/act D) after surgery until no hCG detected. 51/51 (100%) patients cured. 44/51 (86%) patients who desired preservation of uterus had this.

TABLE 5. GESTATIONAL TROPHOBLASTIC
NEOPLASIA: POOR PROGNOSIS—METASTATIC
(DUKE THERAPY 1966–1975)

I. 1966–1968, 7 patients *initially* treated with single
agent Mtx/act D, and *secondarily* treated with combination chemotherapy: Cure, 1 (14%); died, 6 (3
toxicity, 3 disease).
II. 1968–1975, 40 patients initially treated with combination chemotherapy: Cure, 31 (78%); died, 9 (3
toxicity, 6 disease).

used when the patient has impaired renal or
hepatic function. Results from our studies
comparing conventional therapy with more
vigorous triple therapy are shown in Table 5.
Finally, we have had considerable experience
with other combinations of chemotherapy for
patients with disease resistant to single agent
or triple therapy. Most promising seems to be
a modification of Bagshawe's "chamoma"
regimen[27] (Table 6) which utilizes seven drugs
during a nine-day treatment interval. At our
center, remission has been achieved in the

TABLE 6. MULTIAGENT CHEMOTHERAPY REGI-
MEN FOR RESISTANT GESTATIONAL TROPHOBLASTIC
DISEASE

Day 1	0700 hrs	Hydroxyurea 500 mg PO
	1900 hrs	Hydroxyurea 500 mg PO
Day 2	0700 hrs	Hydroxyurea 500 mg PO
	1900 hrs	Hydroxyurea 500 mg PO
		Actinomycin D 0.2 mg IV
Day 3	0700 hrs	Vincristine 1 mg/M² IV
	1900 hrs	Methotrexate 100 mg/M² IV push
		Methotrexate 200 mg/M² IV over 12 hrs
		Actinomycin D 0.2 mg IV
Day 4	1900 hrs	Actinomycin D 0.2 mg IV
		Cytoxan 500 mg/M² IV
		Folinic acid 14 mg IM
Day 5	0100 hrs	Folinic acid 14 mg IM
	0700 hrs	Folinic acid 14 mg IM
	1300 hrs	Folinic acid 14 mg IM
	1900 hrs	Folinic acid 14 mg IM
		Actinomycin D 0.5 mg IV
Day 6	0100 hrs	Folinic acid 14 mg IM
	1900 hrs	Actinomycin D 0.5 mg IV
Day 7	No treatment	
Day 8	No treatment	
Day 9		Melphalan 6 mg/M²
		Adriamycin 30 mg/M²

first five of six patients with resistant "poor
prognosis" disease with this protocol.[28]

Comment

Regardless of the therapy utilized, treatment of malignant trophoblastic disease is
continued until the hCG titer has returned to
normal by an assay sensitive enough to measure well into normal pituitary gonadotropin
ranges. Pregnancy tests are of use only when
positive; then full-range assays must be utilized. Early and accurate diagnosis can be
achieved with frequent and repeated use of
such sensitive and precise hCG assays. High
remission rates and successful therapy are
dependent upon the use of such assays. We
also have utilized pituitary gonadotropin
suppression via oral contraceptives in all patients who do not have contraindications to
these agents. This allows a more accurate
determination of remission by hCG assays,
which also react with pituitary LH.[19] Recent
studies have shown that the beta subunit hCG
radioimmunoassay is a more specific and reliable technique for sensitive hCG monitoring.[29]

Stone and co-workers have noted the fact
that a patient placed on oral contraceptives
after evacuation of hydatidiform mole and before remission has been documented has a
greater likelihood of developing secondary malignancy.[30] Our impression has not supported
this observation, and we have studies currently underway to evaluate this factor. However, because an intercurrent pregnancy is
such a major problem for these patients, we
have continued to utilize these agents unless
there are other, more traditional contraindications to their use.

Systemic single-agent chemotherapy with
methotrexate or actinomycin D remains the
primary treatment modality for patients with
gestational trophoblastic disease. The clinical
identification of these patients as to the presence or absence of metastases and the subdi-
viding of the group with metastases into
"good" and "poor" prognosis patients are major aids in determining the initial method of
therapy most likely to achieve remission with
the least toxic hazard. Arterial infusion chemotherapy and hysterectomy in conjunction
with chemotherapy are now being studied,
and both certainly seem to warrant further
use. The newer regimen of alternating methotrexate and folinic acid seems likely to continue the excellent results obtained with the

standard single-agent therapy but with a major reduction of toxicity for the patient with limited disease. Initial therapy of the poor-prognosis patient with combination chemotherapy—with and without cerebral or hepatic irradiation—seems to improve the salvage rate markedly, while such therapy administered after resistant disease has developed offers little in the way of improving mortality rates. The recurring point these data seem to emphasize is that the type of initial therapy must be tailored to the individual patient.

Hysterectomy performed during the first course of chemotherapy in patients who have clinical evidence of uterine disease and who do not desire further reproduction has been associated with high cure rates and less need for chemotherapy. Arterial infusion of chemotherapeutic drugs may provide an alternative to hysterectomy for selected patients. The role of prophylactic chemotherapy before and after evacuation of a hydatidiform mole seems promising, but we believe that the toxic hazard outweighs the possible reduction in malignant persistence. All of these treatment methodologies require further investigation before widespread clinical use is acceptable.

Treatment centralization of patients with gestational trophoblastic neoplasms has resulted in a marked reduction in morbidity and mortality.[31] Further, centralization has allowed a limited number of physicians to gain a vast amount of expertise in treating these patients while promoting the development of more individualized treatment protocols based upon the extent and prognosis of disease. It seems mandatory to use this experience combined with highly individualized and intensive therapy for the patient who develops resistant disease. Protocols such as the modified Bagshawe multiagent regimen may offer improved therapy.

In the future, it seems likely that development of other agents and regimens will occur to further increase remission rates for patients with malignant trophoblastic disease. It is anticipated that such agents and techniques will also be associated with reduced toxicity, which remains a most desirable goal. The demand for more rapid, more easily available and less expensive hCG assays remains. Despite the possibility that all these improvements will be made in the future, it now appears that malignant trophoblastic disease is amenable to nearly complete control with the therapeutic modalities currently available.

REFERENCES

1. Brewer, J. I., Rinehart, J. J. and Dunbar, R.: Choriocarcinoma. Am. J. Obstet. Gynecol. 81:574, 1961.
2. Greene, R. R.: Chorioadenoma destruens. Ann. NY Acad. Sci. 80:143, 1959.
3. Li, M. C., Hertz, R. and Spencer, D. B.: Effects of methotrexate therapy upon choriocarcinoma and chorioadenoma destruens. Proc. Soc. Exp. Biol. Med. 93:361, 1956.
4. Hertz, R., Lewis, J. L., Jr. and Lipsett, M. G.: Five years' experience with the chemotherapy of metastatic choriocarcinoma and related trophoblastic tumors in women. Am. J. Obstet. Gynecol. 82:631, 1961.
5. Ross, G. T., Goldstein, D. P., Hertz, R., Lipsett, M. B. and Odell, W. D.: Sequential use of methotrexate and actinomycin D in the treatment of metastatic choriocarcinoma and related trophoblastic diseases in women. Am. J. Obstet. Gynecol. 93:223, 1965.
6. Hammond, C. B., Hertz, R., Ross, G. T., Lipsett, M. B. and Odell, W. D.: Primary chemotherapy for nonmetastatic gestational trophoblastic neoplasms. Am. J. Obstet. Gynecol. 98:71, 1967.
7. Lewis, J. L., Jr.,: Chemotherapy for metastatic gestational trophoblastic neoplasms. Clin. Obstet. Gynecol. 10:330, 1967.
8. Odell, W. D., Hertz, R., Lipsett, M. B., Ross, G. T. and Hammond, C. B.: Endocrine aspects of trophoblastic neoplasms. Clin. Obstet. Gynecol. 10:290, 1967.
9. Curry, S. L., Hammond, C. B., Tyrey, L., Creasman, W. T., and Parker, R. T.: Hydatidiform mole: diagnosis, management and long-term follow-up of 347 patients. Obstet. Gynecol. 45:1, 1975.
10. Goldstein, D. P.: Prevention of gestational trophoblastic disease by use of Actinomycin D in molar pregnancies. J. Obstet. Gynecol. 43:475, 1974.
11. Attwood, H. D. and Park, W. W.: Embolism to the lungs by trophoblast. J. Obstet. Gynaecol. Br. Commonwealth 68:611, 1961.
12. Delfs, E.: Quantitative chorionic gonadotropin; prognostic value in hydatidiform mole and chorionepithelioma. Obstet. Gynecol. 9:1, 1957.
13. Brewer, J. I., Smith, R. T. and Pratt, G. B..: Choriocarcinoma. Am. J. Obstet. Gynecol. 85:841, 1962.
14. Hammond, C. B. and Parker, R. T.: Diagnosis and treatment of trophoblastic disease. Obstet. Gynecol. 35:132, 1970.
15. Hammond, C. B., Hertz, R., Ross, G. T., Lipsett, M. B. and Odell, W. B.: Diagnostic problems of choriocarcinoma and related trophoblastic neoplasms. Obstet. Gynecol. 29:224, 1967.
16. Holland, J. F., Hreshchylshyn, M. M. and Glidewell, O.: Controlled clinical trials of methotrexate in the treatment and prophylaxis of trophoblastic neoplasia. Abstracts, 10th International Cancer Congress, Houston, May 1970. Detroit, Medical Arts Publishing, 1970.
17. Goldstein, D. P. and Reid, D. E.: Recent developments in the management of molar pregnancy. Clin. Obstet. Gynecol. 10:313, 1967.
18. Ratnam, S. S., Teoh, E. S. and Dawood, M. Y.: Methotrexate for prophylaxis of choriocarcinoma. Am. J. Obstet. Gynecol. 111:1021, 1971.

19. Hammond, C. B., Borchert, L. G., Tyrey, L., Creasman, W. T. and Parker, R. T.: Treatment of metastatic trophoblastic disease: good and poor prognosis. Am. J. Obstet. Gynecol. 115:451, 1973.

20. Bagshawe, K. D.: Choriocarcinoma: The Clinical Biology of the Trophoblast and its Tumors. London, Edward Arnold, 1968.

21. Goldstein, D. P., Saracco, P., Osathamondh, R., Goldstein, P. R., Marean, A. R. and Bernstein, M. R.: Methotrexate with citrovorum factor rescue for gestational trophoblastic neoplasms. Obstet. Gynecol. 51:93,1978.

22. Lewis, J. L., Jr., Gore, H., Hertig, A. T. and Goss, D. A.: Treatment of trophoblastic neoplasms. With rationale for the use of adjunctive chemotherapy at the time of indicated operation. Am. J. Obstet. Gynecol. 96:710, 1966.

23. Boronow, R. C.: Pelvic arteriography after chemotherapy of malignant trophoblastic disease – a cause for caution. Obstet. Gynecol. 36:675, 1970.

24. Hammond, C. B., Schmidt, H. J. and Parker, R. T.: Gestational trophoblastic disease. *In* McGowan, L. (ed.): Gynecologic Oncology. New York, Appleton-Century-Crofts, 1978, pp. 287.

25. Miller, J. M., Surwit, E. A. and Hammond, C. B.: Choriocarcinoma following term pregnancy. Obstet. Gynecol. 53:207, 1978.

26. Bagshawe, K. D.: Choriocarcinoma. Baltimore, Williams and Wilkins Co., 1969.

27. Bagshawe, K. D.: Treatment of trophoblastic tumors. Ann. Acad. Med. (GB) 5:273, 1976.

28. Surwit, E. A., Hammond, C. B., Suciu, T. N. and Schmidt, H. J.: A new combination chemotherapy for resistant gestational trophoblastic disease. Gynecol. Obstet. 8:110, 1979.

29. Vaitukaitis, J. L., Braunstein, G. B. and Ross, G. T.: A radioimmunoassay which specifically measures human chorionic gonadotropin in the presence of human luteinizing hormone. Am. J. Obstet. Gynecol. 113:751,1972.

30. Stone, J., Dent, J., Kardana, A. and Bagshawe, K. D.: Relationship of oral contraception to development of trophoblastic tumor after evacuation of hydatidiform mole. Br. J. Obstet. Gynecol. 83:913, 1976.

31. Brewer, J. I., Eckman, T. R., Dolkart, R. E., Toruk, E. E. and Webster, A.: Gestational trophoblastic disease—a comparative study of the results of therapy in patients with invasive mole and with choriocarcinoma. Am. J. Obstet. Gynecol. 109:335, 1971.

Editorial Comment

It is clear that the proper chemotherapeutic management of gestational trophoblastic disease is one of the major advances in treatment of cancer and represents the first medical cure of a malignancy. Such therapy in correct amounts and over the proper time span has converted a uniformly fatal disease to one that is curable near the 100 per cent level. Therapy has changed from surgical to medical. It is equally clear that the chemotherapeutic agents of choice in this disease are associated with toxicity and the potential for both morbidity and mortality. For this reason, all patients who receive chemotherapy for gestational trophoblastic disease should be treated by a gynecologic oncologist in a center that has all clinical and laboratory facilities for monitoring. The medical oncologist deals with this disease so rarely that he should consult the gynecologic oncologist regarding appropriate management. Inadequately treated patients may convert from a good prognosis to a poor prognosis category by the development of resistant disease. Hence, the initial diagnosis and proper management are of utmost importance.

The authors of these two articles are in charge of two of the four regional trophoblastic treatment centers in the United States and accordingly have acquired great experience and expertise in management of this disease. Such experience and the salutary outcomes that it provides emphasize that such diseases should be treated in a center in which the disease is treated many times a year rather than occasionally.

There is no controversy in diagnosis, diagnostic methods and classification of trophoblastic disease. The only point of divergence is the thought expressed by the Duke group that there is no role for prophylactic actinomycin in molar pregnancies and the belief of the Boston group that this drug will prevent the 10 to 20 per cent of molar pregnancies that would develop into malignant trophoblastic disease from doing so. It is certainly fair to say that if prophylactic treatment is used it should be given only in centers with experience in monitoring its toxicity and that prophylactic treatment is probably not indicated in benign trophoblastic disease (hydatidiform mole).

It is of great importance that routine pregnancy tests not be used alone to follow molar pregnancies after evacuation. It must be remembered that routine pregnancy tests are helpful only so long as they are positive (down to hCG levels of 60 to 800 mIU per ml). There is a range (200 to 800 mIU per ml) in which the radio receptor assay (Biocept G) is useful, but likewise when it becomes negative a beta subunit h(LC)CG assay is required and must be followed to the point that it is negative ($<$ mIU per ml). The beta subunit assay now provides the clinician with a tool to monitor low levels of the hCG marker in this disease.

11

Genetic Counseling in Obstetrics and Gynecology

Alternative Points of View

by Joe Leigh Simpson
by Morton A. Stenchever and
David A. Luthy
by Arthur C. Christakos

Editorial Comment

Genital Ambiguity

Joe Leigh Simpson
Northwestern University

Birth of an infant with genital ambiguity requires that the correct diagnosis and the proper sex for rearing be determined in rapid, systematic fashion. Parents must also be helped to cope with both their own emotional reactions and with those of inquisitive relatives and peers.

Immediate Management

Immediate management of the infant with genital ambiguity (Fig. 1) requires attention to both medical and psychological factors. If a competent group of gynecologists, urologists, pediatricians, psychiatrists, geneticists and endocrinologists is not available, it is best to refer the patient to a center having such a team.

Both cytogenetic and endocrine studies should be initiated. To determine the genetic sex, one should rely upon lymphocyte cultures, not solely upon analysis of buccal epithelial cells (buccal smear), for the presence or absence of X-chromatin or Y-chromatin. To exclude the syndromes of adrenal hyperplasia, the most common cause of genital ambiguity, serum sodium, serum potassium, serum 17α-hydroxyprogesterone, and the urinary excretion of 17-ketosteroids, pregnanetriol and possibly tetrahydrodeoxycortisol should be determined. Proper urine collection in infants requires that they be placed in metabolic beds designed to guarantee complete collection.

During the 72 to 96 hours required for these tests, the emotional status of the parents must be considered. The preferable approach is to avoid any public indication that a special situation exists: that is, the physician should attach no unusual significance to the occurrence of genital ambiguity. Inform the parents that their child has a "birth defect" involving the external genitalia, just as another birth defect might involve the heart. Counsel that the child can expect normal psychosexual development, regardless of the sex of rearing chosen.

Some parents may be poorly equipped to cope with peer pressures. If so, it might be preferable to advise them to withhold infor-

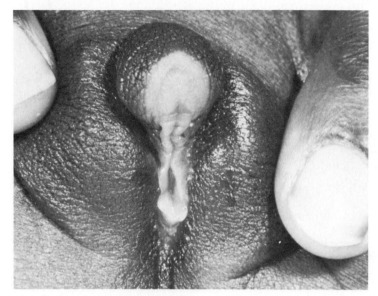

Figure 1. External genitalia of an infant with 45,X/46,X,dup(Yq) mosaicism. The phallus is larger than expected for a clitoris but less than that expected for a penis. Incomplete labioscrotal fusion is present. (From Morillo-Cucci, G. and German, J.: Abnormal Y chromosomes and monosomy 45,X: a concept derived from the study of three patients. Birth Defects 7:210, 1971.)

mation concerning the sex of the infant from relatives; certainly birth announcements should be deferred. If relatives live a long distance away, they could even be told that labor was "false." If legally possible, the first name should be withheld from the birth certificate until the sex of rearing is chosen. Alternatively, names suitable for either a boy or girl might be chosen: Chris, Courtney, Frances, Jean, Hilary, Lee, Leigh, Leslie, Pat. Occasionally, formal psychiatric consultation is necessary.

Physical Examination

Although a careful physical examination should be performed on every infant with genital ambiguity, diagnosis of a specific disorder cannot usually be made by physical examination alone. Nonetheless, some important generalizations are applicable. Assessment of potential penile function should be completed prior to arriving at the specific diagnosis.

That the external genitalia are rarely sufficiently distinctive to diagnose a particular disorder is not surprising because early in embryogenesis both male and female embryos have identical external genitalia. The genital tubercle and the genital folds can differentiate as follows: (1) the normal manner for embryos of a given sex, (2) incomplete masculinization of male embryos or (3) unexpected virilization of female embryos. At birth, the normal penis

is usually 3 to 4 cm long and about 1 cm wide. The size of the phallus is less helpful diagnostically than the location of the urethral opening. In normal males, the urethral orifice is located at the tip of the glans penis. In incomplete virilization, which presumably results from either decreased synthesis of fetal androgens or phallic unresponsiveness to androgens, the urethral orifice is located on the proximal glans penis, the shaft of the penis or the perineum. Sometimes the physician can distinguish an underdeveloped penis from an overdeveloped clitoris by inspecting the frenulum on the ventral surface of the phallus. In normal males, there is only a single midline frenulum; in normal females, there are two frenula, each lateral to the midline. Thus, a female with clitoral hypertrophy has two paramedian frenula, whereas a male with hypospadias has either a single midline frenulum or several irregularly spaced fibrous bands (chordee) that extend between the perineum and the penile shaft. A very large clitoris associated with normal urethral placement suggests exposure to androgens or progestins after genital differentiation (first trimester).

Fusion of the labioscrotal folds results in formation of the scrotum and obliteration of the potential vagina. This process occurs in a posteroanterior direction, the fusion site represented by the scrotal raphe. The processes that cause a hypoplastic penis also cause incomplete fusion of the labioscrotal folds. Likewise, the processes that cause clitoral hypertrophy cause unexpected fusion of the labioscrotal folds. If partial fusion occurs, the fused portion will be posterior.

If müllerian derivatives (fallopian tubes, uterus, upper vagina) are present in an infant with genital ambiguity, that infant has either female pseudohermaphroditism, true hermaphroditism or a cytogenetic form of male pseudohermaphroditism. A genetic form of male pseudohermaphroditism is unlikely to be associated with müllerian development. Frequently, a uterus can be palpated during the rectal examination; however, cystoscopic studies, roentgenographic studies (vaginogram) or an examination with anesthesia may be necessary to verify presence or absence of a uterus.

The composition of a gonad can sometimes be deduced by location, consistency or surrounding organs. First, a gonad located in the labial or inguinal regions almost invariably contains testicular tissue. In fact, in true hermaphroditism, the greater the amount of testicular tissue, the greater the probability of gonadal descent. Second, a testis is not only softer than an ovary or a streak gonad but also more often is surrounded by blood vessels that impart a reddish appearance. By contrast, an ovary is white, convoluted and of fibrous consistency. If different portions of a single gonad differ in consistency, one should consider presence of either an ovotestis or a testis or streak gonad that has undergone neoplastic transformation. If a well-differentiated fallopian tube is absent on only one side, the gonad on that side is probably a testis or ovotestis.

The presence of somatic anomalies comprising the Turner stigmata suggests that the associated genital ambiguity is caused by 45,X/46,XY mosaicism because the Turner stigmata (see Simpson[1]) presumably reflect the coexistence of 45,X cells. Similarly, increased areolar and scrotal pigmentation may result from increased levels of ACTH, a hormone with melanocyte-stimulating properties.

Classification of Common Disorders Causing Genital Ambiguity

Although there are several ways to delineate disorders of sexual differentiation,[1-3] it seems clinically preferable to place an affected individual initially into one of several broad categories that can be recognized readily on the basis of chromosomal complement and gonadal

TABLE 1. CLASSIFICATION OF DISORDERS OF SEXUAL DIFFERENTIATION

1. Male pseudohermaphroditism*
2. Female pseudohermaphroditism*
3. True hermaphroditism*
4. Gonadal dysgenesis (bilateral)
5. Polysomy for the X or Y chromosome
6. Hypogonadism associated with normal external genitalia and normal chromosomal complements
7. Anomalies limited to wolffian or müllerian derivatives

*Categories usually associated with genital ambiguity. Tables 1–3 are modified from Simpson, J. L.: Diagnosis and management of the infant with genital ambiguity. Am. J. Obstet. Gynecol. 128:137, 1977.

status. These categories include gonadal dysgenesis, true hermaphroditism, female pseudohermaphroditism, male pseudohermaphroditism, sex-reversed (46,XX) males, anomalies limited to müllerian or wolffian derivatives, and forms of hypogonadotropic hypogonadism occurring in individuals with normal external genitalia and normal chromosomal complements[1] (Table 1). Within each category, the various disorders are probably best delineated on the basis of their etiology: chromosomal abnormalities, recessive or dominant genes or teratogenic factors. The most common disorders associated with genital ambiguity are summarized in the following paragraphs.

Female Pseudohermaphroditism

Individuals with female pseudohermaphroditism are genetic females (46,XX) in whom genital development is not that expected for normal females (Table 2). Individuals with true hermaphroditism may also have a 46,XX com-

TABLE 2. COMMON FORMS OF FEMALE PSEUDOHERMAPHRODITISM

Genetic etology
  Syndromes of adrenal hyperplasia
    21-Hydroxylase deficiency
    11β-Hydroxylase deficiency
    3β-ol-Dehydrogenase deficiency
  Nonadrenal genetic forms associated with somatic anomalies
Teratogenic etiology
  Maternal ingestion of progestins or androgens
  Androgen-producing neoplasia
Uncertain etiology
  Exstrophy of bladder
  Exstrophy of cloaca
  Sirenomelia

plement, but they are best considered separately. Most subjects with female pseudohermaphroditism have adrenal hyperplasia, although nonadrenal female pseudohermaphroditism has been reported.

SYNDROMES OF ADRENAL HYPERPLASIA

In adrenal hyperplasia, an enzyme deficiency leads to decreased production of cortisol by the adrenal cortex.[1, 4] The syndromes of adrenal hyperplasia are the most common cause of genital ambiguity. Diminished glucocorticoid production leads to decreased negative feedback inhibition of adrenocorticotropic hormone (ACTH) by cortisol. Thus, ACTH secretion increases. In addition, alternate biosynthetic pathways are utilized (Fig. 2), and excessive synthesis of androgens occurs. Excessive androgens during embryogenesis virilize androgen-dependent organs, thereby causing genital ambiguity in females (female pseudohermaphroditism). Müllerian derivatives and ovaries develop as expected for females. Several forms of adrenal hyperplasia cause genital ambiguity: deficiencies of 21-hydroxylase, 11β-hydroxylase and 3β-ol-dehydrogenase. Each is inherited in autosomal recessive fashion.

21-HYDROXYLASE DEFICIENCY. Two forms of 21-hydroxylase deficiency exist, one form with and one form without sodium wasting.

In both forms, excess synthesis of androgens causes genital virilization. In the mild form, ACTH compensation apparently produces normal amounts of cortisol; thus, neither sodium wasting nor adrenal insufficiency occurs. In the severe form sodium wasting occurs, but it can be corrected by the administration of cortisol. Early diagnosis is imperative, since uncorrected hyponatremia and hyperkalemia may lead to death because of electrolyte imbalance. Males with 21-hydroxylase deficiency have normal external genitalia; however, the disorder can sometimes be diagnosed at birth on the basis of scrotal and areolar hyperpigmentation. If salt wasting is not present, diagnosis in males may not be made until pubic hair growth or increased statural growth occurs around 2 years of age. Plasma 17α-hydroxyprogesterone and urinary excretion of pregnanetriol are increased. Linkage of HLA to the 21-hydroxylase locus permits antenatal diagnosis and heterozygote detection.[5]

11β-HYDROXYLASE DEFICIENCY. Deficiency of 11β-hydroxylase results in increased secretion of deoxycortisol and deoxycorticosterone, steroids that promote salt retention. Hypervolemia and concomitant hypertension may be present. 11β-hydroxylase deficiency may or may not be associated with salt retention. Virilization of external genitalia occurs, as in 21-hydroxylase deficiency. Urinary tetrahydrodeoxycortisol is increased.

3β-OL-DEHYDROGENASE DEFICIENCY. In this disorder the major androgen produced is

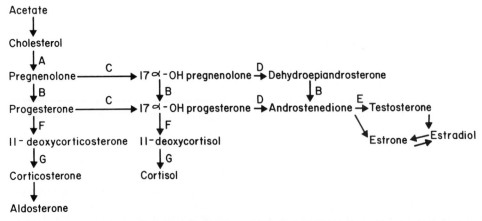

Figure 2. Summary of important adrenal and gonadal biosynthetic pathways. Letters designate enzymes required to complete the appropriate conversions. A: 20α-hydroxylase, 22α-hydroxylase, and 20,22-desmolase (adrenal lipoid hyperplasia); B: 3β-ol-dehydrogenase; C: 17α-hydroxylase; D: 17,20-desmolase; E: 17-ketosteroid reductase; F: 21-hydroxylase; G: 11β-hydroxylase. (From Simpson, J. L.: Disorders of Sexual Differentiation: Etiology and Clinic Delineation. New York, Academic Press, 1976.)

dehydroepiandrosterone (DHEA). Although DHEA is a relatively weak androgen, females with 3β-ol-dehydrogenase are virilized. However, virilization is often less pronounced than in 21- or 11β-hydroxylase deficiencies. Males deficient for 3β-ol-dehydrogenase have underdeveloped external genitalia and incomplete scrotal fusion (male pseudohermaphroditism). 3β-ol-dehydrogenase deficiency is associated with severe sodium loss. Many patients survive only a few days, but the disorder has also been detected in older children. Urinary pregnenetriol is increased.

17α-HYDROXYLASE DEFICIENCY. Females with 17α-hydroxylase deficiency cannot synthesize adequate amounts of either androgens or estrogens. They do not have genital ambiguity, but they may consult a gynecologist because of primary amenorrhea. 46,XX patients have infantile, yet well-differentiated female external genitalias, ovaries, uterus and vagina. Hypertension may be present as result of increased synthesis of mineralocorticoids, particularly corticosterone.[1, 6]

OTHER FORMS OF FEMALE PSEUDOHERMAPHRODITISM

Other causes of female pseudohermaphroditism include (1) genetically determined nonadrenal forms that are associated with multiple somatic anomalies,[1] (2) maternal ingestion of testosterone or certain synthetic progestins during the sixth to twelfth weeks of embryonic development (see Simpson[1] for discussion of specific hormones), (3) an androgen-producing tumor in pregnancy, and (4) exstrophy of the bladder, exstrophy of the cloaca, and sirenomelia, all of which produce an abnormal perineal appearance that may cause confusion concerning sex assignment.[1]

Male Pseudohermaphroditism

Individuals with male pseudohermaphroditism have a Y chromosome, but their internal or external genitalia develop incompletely (Table 3). This broad definition includes persons in whom the phenotype may be predominantly male, predominantly female or ambiguous. The gynecologist is usually concerned only with those male pseudohermaphrodites whose genitalia are female or ambiguous.

TABLE 3. COMMON FORMS OF MALE PSEUDOHERMAPHRODITISM CAUSING GENITAL AMBIGUITY

Cytogenic etiology (45,X/46,XY)
Genetic etiology
  Disorders with multiple malformation patterns
  Disorders with an enzyme deficiency in testosterone biosynthesis
    Deficiency prior to the synthesis of pregnenolone (adrenal lipoid hyperplasia)
    Deficiency of 3β-ol-dehydrogenase
    Deficiency of 17α-hydroxylase
    Deficiency of 17,20-ketosteroid reductase
    Deficiency of 5α-reductase (pseudovaginal perineoscrotal hypospadias phenotype)
  Incomplete androgen insensitivity and Reifenstein syndrome
  Pseudovaginal perineoscrotal hypospadias and 5α-reductase deficiency
  Agonadia
  Leydig cell agenesis

CYTOGENETIC FORMS

The presence in a single individual of both 45,X and 46,XY cells usually results in an abnormal phenotype. Although 45,X/46,XY mosaicism is associated with a spectrum of phenotypes, these individuals may be grouped into one of three clinical categories[1]: (1) individuals with ambiguous external genitalia, in whom the gonads usually consist of one streak gonad and one dysgenetic testis (mixed gonadal dysgenesis), (2) individuals of female phenotype, who have sexual infantilism and bilateral streak gonads and in whom short stature and other features of the Turner stigmata[1] may exist, and (3) individuals of predominantly male appearance, who have bilateral testes and in whom the external genitalia are unmistakably male but rarely completely normal.

Individuals in the first and second categories usually show müllerian development (uterus and fallopian tubes). By contrast, individuals with a genetic (mendelian) form of male pseudohermaphroditism (see later discussion) usually have no uterus. Therefore, the presence of a uterus in an individual with ambiguous external genitalia and testes suggests 45,X/46,XY mosaicism. Finally, about 15 per cent of 45,X/46,XY individuals have a gonadoblastoma or dysgerminoma.[7] Thus, extirpation of gonads of patients with female or ambiguous external genitalia who have a uterus and a 46,XY cell line is obligatory.

GENETIC (MENDELIAN) FORMS

Male pseudohermaphroditism may be genetic (mendelian) in etiology (Table 3). Genetic forms characterized by either predominantly male external genitalia (e.g., penile hypospadias or persistence of müllerian derivatives in otherwise normal males) or predominantly female external genitalia (e.g., XY gonadal dysgenesis or complete testicular feminization) are not immediately relevant to this discussion, and likewise multiple malformation syndromes associated with genital ambiguity may be excluded. All are discussed elsewhere.[1] Other genetic forms are summarized in the following paragraphs. Their most important common diagnostic feature is absence of a uterus.

ERRORS IN TESTOSTERONE BIOSYNTHESIS. Errors in testicular biosynthesis include adrenal lipoid hyperplasia, 3β-ol-dehydrogenase deficiency, 17α-hydroxylase deficiency, 17,20-desmolase deficiency, and 17-ketosteroid reductase deficiency (Fig. 2). In each disorder, plasma testosterone and urinary excretion of 17α-ketosteroids are usually decreased. Differentiation between these various types requires direct enzyme studies or assays of appropriate androgen precursors. 17,20-desmolase and 17-ketosteroid reductase deficiencies have been reported only in males; thus, these two disorders could be either X-linked recessive or male-limited autosomal recessive. The other deficiencies are probably inherited in autosomal recessive fashion,[1, 2] and of these 17α-hydroxlase is probably most common in males.[8]

It is important to identify individuals with these forms of male pseudohermaphroditism because life-threatening electrolyte imbalances may occur. In both adrenal lipoid hyperplasia and 3β-ol-dehydrogenase deficiency, males show both genital ambiguity and severe salt wasting. Males with 17α-hydroxylase deficiency have both genital ambiguity and hypertension, the latter resulting from increased synthesis of mineralocorticoids. Individuals with 17,20-desmolase deficiency and 17-ketosteroid reductase deficiency have genital ambiguity but no electrolyte imbalance. Deficiency of 5α-reductase, the enzyme that converts testosterone to dihydrotestosterone, is discussed in conjunction with pseudovaginal perineoscrotal hypospadias.

INCOMPLETE ANDROGEN INSENSITIVITY AND REIFENSTEIN SYNDROME. In *complete androgen insensitivity*, 46,XY individuals fail to virilize because of androgen insensitivity that usually, but not always,[9] results from an abnormality involving the androgen cytosol receptor.[10] Affected patients have normal female external genitalia, no müllerian derivatives, and a blindly ending vaginal pouch contributed solely by invagination of the urogenital sinus. Breast development occurs at puberty, but little if any pubic or axillary hair develops. Complete androgen insensitivity is an X-linked recessive disorder.

In *incomplete androgen insensitivity*, inherited in the same fashion as complete testicular feminization, the external genitalia are ambiguous (clitoral hypertrophy and labioscrotal fusion); however, breast development occurs at puberty.[1, 10] Pubic and axillary hair are present.[1] In incomplete androgen insensitivity, plasma testosterone levels are also normal for males, and administration of testosterone does not increase nitrogen retention. Despite their similar modes of inheritance, complete androgen insensitivity and incomplete androgen insensitivity are definitely distinct conditions because in a given kindred all affected individuals have either the complete form or the incomplete form.

The appellation *Reifenstein syndrome*[11] was traditionally applied to individuals with (1) phallic development that is abnormal yet more masculine than in incomplete testicular feminization (i.e., affected patients have hypospadias but the external genitalia are unmistakably male), and (2) small scrotal testes, as a result of which gonadotropin levels are elevated. Individuals with the Reifenstein syndrome develop gynecomastia but not impressive breast development. Androgen sensitivity has traditionally been considered intact.

Incomplete androgen insensitivity and Reifenstein syndrome were thus considered separate traits, characterized by androgen insensitivity and androgen sensitivity, respectively. However, later data suggest that the two may merely reflect varied expression of a single mutant allele.[12, 13] On the other hand, the situation may not be quite so simple.[13, 14]

I have observed cases of androgen-insensitive individuals who have normal female external genitalia except for posterior labioscrotal fusion. Wilson and McDonald[10] designate this condition "incomplete testicular feminization."[10] I do not favor such designation, because for many years "incomplete testicular feminization" and incomplete androgen insensitivity have been used interchangeably.

PSEUDOVAGINAL PERINEOSCROTAL HYPO-

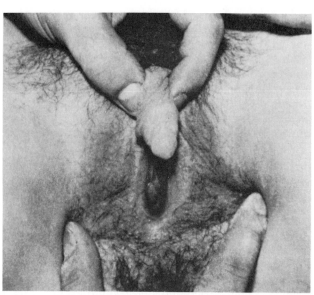

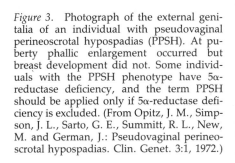

Figure 3. Photograph of the external genitalia of an individual with pseudovaginal perineoscrotal hypospadias (PPSH). At puberty phallic enlargement occurred but breast development did not. Some individuals with the PPSH phenotype have 5α-reductase deficiency, and the term PPSH should be applied only if 5α-reductase deficiency is excluded. (From Opitz, J. M., Simpson, J. L., Sarto, G. E., Summitt, R. L., New, M. and German, J.: Pseudovaginal perineoscrotal hypospadias. Clin. Genet. 3:1, 1972.)

SPADIAS (PPSH) AND 5α-REDUCTASE DEFICIENCY. PPSH is a descriptive title applied to 46,XY individuals who undergo normal puberal virilization despite genital ambiguity.[15, 16] In PPSH, the phallus is hypoplastic and a prominent ventral groove is often present (Fig. 3). Labioscrotal fusion is common. The vagina ends blindly, and no müllerian derivatives are present. At puberty virilization occurs, as evidenced by beard growth, voice deepening and development of a masculine habitus. Breast development does not occur. The testes of affected patients secrete normal amounts of testosterone, respond normally to feedback inhibition and may show spermatogenesis.[13, 15, 16]

Some individuals with the PPSH phenotype are deficient in 5α-reductase, the enzyme that converts testosterone to dihydrotestosterone.[17-19] Dihydrotestosterone is responsible for genital virilization during embryogenesis, but testosterone alone appears to be responsible for puberal virilization. If an individual were deficient in 5α-reductase, one would thus predict the occurrence of a PPSH-like phenotype. If all individuals with the PPSH phenotype were deficient in 5α-reductase, one could delete the appellation "PPSH" in lieu of the specific enzyme defect. However, clinical and presumably genetic heterogeneity exists among patients with the PPSH phenotype. Thus, the appellation PPSH retains nosologic usefulness; however, in the future we can hope that the molecular etiology of all forms of male pseudohermaphroditism will be elucidated, permitting abandonment of unwieldly terms such as PPSH.[20]

The combination of PPSH and 5α-reductase deficiency differs clinically from incomplete testicular feminization in that puberal virilization occurs only in the former. Thus, breast development occurs in incomplete testicular feminization but not in PPSH. Before puberty, it is difficult clinically to distinguish PPSH from incomplete testicular feminization, unless other family members are affected. However, administration of testosterone[21] produces phallic enlargement in infants with PPSH but not in those with incomplete testicular feminization, and cultured genital fibroblasts show abnormalities in androgen receptors in the latter.[22]

AGONADIA. In this disorder neither gonads nor internal ducts are present. The external genitalia resemble those of a female more than those of a male. The vagina is absent and labioscrotal fusion is present.[13, 23, 24] A small penis-like structure is usually the only identifiable external genital structure. Neither wolffian nor müllerian structures are consistently present. Somatic anomalies may be present.

Because both genital and gonadal development are deficient, pathogenesis must involve a developmental defect of the entire reproductive system—gonads, internal ducts and external genitalia. Absence of gonadal tissue alone would be expected to produce not agonadia but the XY gonadal dysgenesis phenotype (streak gonads, female external genitalia and a normal uterus), because normal müllerian development and normal female external genital development occur despite absence of gonadal tissue.

OTHER FORMS. Other genetic forms of male pseudohermaphroditism may exist. For example, in at least three families, one sib was reported to have XY gonadal dysgenesis, whereas another sib had genital ambiguity and müllerian development. Such families are difficult to classify.[1] One possible explanation is that 45,X/46,XY mosaicism is present—that is, a gene causing mosaicism is present. Another possible explanation is that the gene causing XY gonadal dysgenesis is capable of varied expression, occasionally producing an incompletely expressed form of XY gonadal dysgenesis in which limited testicular development occurs. (See German et al.[25] for further speculation.)

In addition, male pseudohermaphroditism may result from Leydig cell agenesis.[26]

True Hermaphroditism

True hermaphrodites have both ovarian and testicular tissue. They may have a separate ovary and a separate testis or, more often, one or more ovotestes. Most true hermaphrodites have a 46,XX complement, although a few are 46,XY or 46,XX/46,XY.[27-29] In the present context it will suffice to generalize about the phenotype of all true hermaphroditism, irrespective of the chromosomal complement. However, there is evidence for both clinical and etiologic heterogeneity.[28]

About two thirds of true hermaphrodites are reared as male. The external genitalia are usually either frankly ambiguous or predominantly male, but occasionally a vagina and a well-differentiated uterus are present. Gonadal tissue may be located in the ovarian region, the inguinal region or the labioscrotal region.[27-29] The greater the proportion of testicular tissue in an ovotestis, the greater the likelihood of gonadal descent.[27] In 80 per cent of ovotestes, the testicular and ovarian components are juxtaposed end-to-end.[27] Thus, most ovotestes can be detected by inspection or possibly by palpation because testicular tissue is softer and more vascular than ovarian tissue. A testis or ovotestis is more likely to be present on the left. Spermatozoa are rarely present in the testes or ovotestes of true hermaphrodites, but oocytes are usually present. Neoplasia may arise in the gonads of true hermaphrodites, but apparently less frequently than in XY gonadal dysgenesis or 45,X/46,XY mosaicism.[28] Testicular neoplasia is most common, but gonadoblastomas have also been reported.

Some cases result from chimerism, the presence of both 46,XX and 46,XY cells in a single individual (46,XX/46,XY). However, experimental production of XX/XY mouse chimeras usually does not result in true hermaphroditism, and most 46,XX/46,XY humans are not true hermaphrodites.

46,XX true hermaphroditism is almost certainly heterogeneous in etiology.[28] A few individuals doubtless have undetected chimerism, but for phenotypic reasons as well as genetic ones, undetected chimerism probably cannot be the explanation for all cases of 46,XX true hermaphroditism. The presence of testicular tissue in 46,XX individuals is perplexing, because male determinants are believed to be located in the Y chromosome. Possible explanations for the occurrence of testicular differentiation in individuals who apparently lack a Y chromosome are (1) translocation of the testicular determinant(s) from the Y to an X chromosome, (2) translocation of the testicular determinant(s) from the Y to an autosome, (3) undetected mosaicism or chimerism (i.e., 46,XX/46,XY) and (4) sex-reversal genes. Consistent with the first two hypotheses are (1) existence of families in which anomalous distributions of the X-linked antigen Xg have occurred,[1] and (2) detection of H-Y antigen in 46,XX true hermaphrodites.[30]

Differential Diagnosis

After the genetic and endocrine data just discussed become available, the physician can usually determine the proper diagnosis. Differential diagnosis is conveniently approached on the basis of chromosomal complement.

If a 46,XX/46,XY complement is detected in an infant with genital ambiguity, that infant probably has true hermaphroditism. However, a 46,XX/46,XY complement is not always associated with true hermaphroditism, nor do most true hermaphrodites have a 46,XX/46,XY complement.

If an infant with genital ambiguity has a 46,XX complement, she probably has female pseudohermaphroditism. (However, 46,XX true hermaphroditism occurs.) If endocrine studies are abnormal, adrenal hyperplasia is present. The most common forms of female pseudohermaphroditism are the syndromes of adrenal hyperplasia, particularly 21-hydroxylase deficiency and 11β-hydroxylase deficiency. The former is present if serum 17α-OH progesterone or urinary pregnanetriol are elevated, whereas the latter is present if urinary tetrahydrodeoxycortisol is elevated. In 3β-ol-dehydrogenase, other hormone abnormalities exist.[4] If a 46,XX infant with genital ambiguity has normal endocrine function, one should suspect either a nonadrenal genetic form of female pseudohermaphroditism or a teratogenic form of female pseudohermaphroditism (Table 2). 46,XX true hermaphroditism is usually not detected until surgical exploration, although the diagnosis should be suspected if (1) a gonad shows areas of different consistencies, suggesting an ovotestis; (2) the cervical canal either is obliterated or shows squamous metaplasia; or (3) other family members have true hermaphroditism or sex reversal.

If an infant with genital ambiguity has a 46,XY chromosomal complement, he probably has a form of male pseudohermaphroditism; however, a few 46,XY true hermaphrodites have been reported. If a uterus is present in a male pseudohermaphrodite, 45,X/46,XY mosaicism exists. Well-developed müllerian derivatives are usually not present in genetic forms of male pseudohermaphroditism associated with genital ambiguity. It is important to detect 45,X/46,XY mosaicism because 15 to 20 per cent of such patients develop gonadoblastomas or dysgerminomas; thus, gonadal extirpation should be offered. Incidentally, detection of H-Y antigen does not indicate the presence of testes, because nonmosaic 45,X individuals show H-Y, albeit low levels.[31] The latter indicates that the structural locus for H-Y is not on the Y.[31, 32]

If no uterus is present, a genetic form of male pseudohermaphroditism exists (Table 3). If testosterone is deficient, an enzyme deficiency probably exists. However, the specific enzyme deficiency must be deduced on the basis of elevations or deficiencies of specific testosterone precursors. In practice, it is often difficult to confirm a defect in testosterone biosynthesis in a neonate, because testosterone levels in normal neonates are relatively low and hence subject to laboratory variations. Some endocrinologists prefer to administer gonadotropin and observe androgen response. If traditional endocrine studies are normal in a male pseudohermaphrodite without a

uterus, other genetic forms (Table 3) must be considered. The choice usually lies between incomplete testicular feminization/the Reifenstein syndrome or PPSH/5α-reductase deficiency. In the androgen insensitivity conditions—incomplete testicular feminization and Reifenstein syndrome—patients usually fail to show nitrogen retention following testosterone administration. Their labial fibroblasts also show androgen receptor abnormalities, and testosterone cream fails to produce clitoral enlargement. In PPSH and 5α-reductase deficiency, postnatal androgen sensitivity is intact. Specific confirmation of 5α-reductase deficiency requires measurement of the conversion of testosterone to dihydrotestosterone.

Management Following Specific Diagnosis

The sex of rearing appropriate for a child with genital ambiguity may not necessarily agree with the genetic sex because one must consider not only the disorder itself but the status of the external genitalia. Ideally a child should be raised according to its genetic sex, i.e., female if a female pseudohermaphrodite and male if a male pseudohermaphrodite.

Female pseudohermaphrodites should nearly always be raised female. If an infant has female pseudohermaphroditism as a result of adrenal hyperplasia, administration of cortisol and possibly also mineralocorticoids is necessary. The clitoris should be reduced surgically, and any labioscrotal fusion corrected. Genital surgery is usually performed at 2 to 4 years of age. Individuals with adrenal hyperplasia may require increased dosage of mineralocorticoids during operation; however, surgery need not necessarily be deferred until the adrenal status is absolutely stable. Cortisol must be administered throughout childhood and possibly adult life, although requirements per unit of mass may decrease. Paradoxically, mineralocorticoids sometimes may not be required immediately after birth, yet required later in life. Nonadrenal female pseudohermaphroditism requires surgery but not hormone administration.

If an individual has male pseudohermaphroditism or true hermaphroditism, a decision must be made on whether genital reconstruction can produce a phallus capable of normal male function and whether androgen sensitivity exists. This decision is best made by a team of physicians: obstetrician-gynecologists, pediatricians, urologists, geneticists and endocrinologists. If an infant's capacity to function as a male is in doubt, it should be raised as female, irrespective of genetic sex. If a female gender role is chosen, the external genitalia must naturally be reconstructed along female lines and the testes must be extirpated. Depending upon the specific condition, male pseudohermaphrodites raised as male may be infertile and may require hormones as adults; however, sexual orientation will be normal if the parents show no ambivalence concerning the chosen sex of rearing. A male role is especially preferable if a male infant has an enzyme error preventing biosynthesis of testosterone, because in such disorders testicular architecture is usually normal. In addition, males with PPSH and 5α-reductase deficiency have virilization at puberty and may even show spermatogenesis.[8] It thus seems unwise to raise all infants with genital ambiguity as female, as some investigators have proposed. On the other hand, any male pseudohermaphrodite whose external genitalia are too poorly developed to permit construction of a functional penis should be raised as female. In addition, androgen insensitivity must be excluded by assays for cytosol androgen receptors. Some investigators administer topical testosterone to exclude androgen insensitivity and possibly to facilitate genital reconstruction. However, testosterone administration is not without potential hazard and should be used cautiously.

If individuals with true hermaphroditism are raised as male, ovarian tissue should be removed to preclude puberal feminization. Similarly, a hysterectomy should be performed. Even if the sex of rearing is male, intra-abdominal testes should probably be extirpated. If true hermaphrodites are raised as females, testicular tissue should be extirpated to prevent inappropriate virilization.

There is no scientific evidence that any specific surgical technique for genital, ductal or gonadal surgery is uniquely advantageous. Jones and Scott,[3] among other investigators, describe useful procedures.

REFERENCES

1. Simpson, J. L.: Disorders of Sexual Differentiation: Etiology and Clinical Delineation. New York, Academic Press, 1976.
2. Wilson, J. D. and Goldstein, J. D.: Classification of hereditary disorders of sexual development. Birth Defects 11(4):1, 1975.
3. Jones, H. W., Jr. and Scott, W. M.: Hermaphroditism, Genital Anomalies, and Related Endocrine Disorders, 2nd ed. Baltimore, Williams and Wilkins, 1971.
4. New, M. I. and Levine, L. S.: Congenital adrenal hyperplasia. Adv. Genet. 4:251, 1973.
5. Levine, L. S., Zachmann, M., New, M. I. et al.: Genetic mapping of the 21-hydroxylase deficiency gene within the HLA linkage group. N. Engl. J. Med. 299:911, 1978.
6. De Lange, W. E., Lappöhn, R. E., Sluiter, W. J. and Doorenbos, H.: Primäre amenorrhoe und hypokaliämie infolge 17alpha-hydroxylase-mangels. Dtsch. Med. Wochenschr. 102:1024, 1977.
7. Simpson, J. L. and Photopulos, G.: The relationship of neoplasia to disorders of abnormal sexual differentiation. Birth Defects 12(1):15, 1976.
8. Jones, H. W., Jr., Lee, P. A., Rock, J. A., Archer, D. F. and Migeon, C. J.: A genetic male patient with 17α-hydroxylase deficiency. Obstet. Gynecol. 59:254, 1982.
9. Amrhein, J. A., Meyer, W. J., III, Jones, H. W., Jr. and Migeon, C. J.: Androgen insensitivity in man. Evidence for genetic heterogeneity. Proc. Natl. Acad. Sci. USA 73:891, 1976.
10. Wilson, J. D. and McDonald, P. C.: Male pseudohermaphroditism due to androgen resistance: testicular feminization and related syndromes. *In* Stanbury, J. B., Wyngaarden, J. B. and Frederickson, D. S. (eds.): The Metabolic Basis of Inherited Disease, 4th ed.: New York, McGraw-Hill, 1978, p. 894.
11. Bowen, P., Lee, C. S. N., Migeon, C. J. et al.: Hereditary male pseudohermaphroditism with hypogonadism, hypospadias, and gynecomastia (Reifenstein's syndrome). Ann. Intern. Med. 62:252, 1965.
12. Amrhein, J. A., Klingensmith, C. J., Walsh, P. C., McKusick, V. A. and Migeon, C. J.: Partial androgen insensitivity. The Reifenstein syndrome revisited. N. Engl. J. Med. 297:350, 1977.
13. Simpson, J. L.: Male pseudohermaphroditism. Genetics and clinical delineation. Hum. Genet. 44:1, 1978.
14. Simpson, J. L. and Summitt, R. L.: Androgen insensitivity syndrome, incomplete. *In* Bergmsa, D. (ed.): Birth Defects: Atlas and Compendium, 2nd ed. White Plains, National Foundation, 1979, p. 80.
15. Simpson, J. L., New, M. I., Peterson, R. E. and German, J.: Pseudovaginal perineoscrotal hypospadias (PPSH) in sibs. Birth Defects 7(6):140, 1971.
16. Opitz, J. M., Simpson, J. L., Sarto, G. E., Summitt, R. L., New, M. and German, J.: Pseudovaginal perineoscrotal hypospadias. Clin. Genet. 3:1, 1972.
17. Imperato-McGinley, J., Guerrero, L., Gautier, T. and Peterson, R. E.: Steroid 5α-reductase deficiency in man: an inherited form of male pseudohermaphroditism. Science 186:1213, 1974.
18. Walsh, P. C., Madden, J. D., Harrod, M. J., Goldstein, J. L., McDonald, P. C. and Wilson, J. D.: Familial incomplete male pseudohermaphroditism, type 2. N. Engl. J. Med. 291:944, 1974.
19. Peterson, R. E., Imperato-McGinley, J., Gautier, R. and Sturia, E.: Male pseudohermaphroditism due to steroid 5α-reductase deficiency. Am. J. Med. 62:170, 1977.

20. Simpson, J. L. and Summitt, R. L.: Pseudovaginal perineoscrotal hypospadias. *In* Bergsma, D. (ed.): Birth Defects: Atlas and Compendium, 2nd ed. 1979, p. 893.

21. Smith, D. W. and Jones, K. L.: Testosterone in the early management of the ambiguous genitalia in the XY individual. Birth Defects 11(4):143, 1975.

22. Pinsky, L., Kaufman, M., Straisfeld, C., Zilahi, B. and Hall, C. St.-G.: 5α-reductase activity of genital and nongenital skin fibroblasts from patients with 5α-reductase deficiency, androgen insensitivity, or unknown forms of male pseudohermaphroditism. Am. J. Med. Genet. 1:407, 1976.

23. Sarto, G. E., and Optiz, J. M.: The XY gonadal agenesis syndrome. J. Med. Genet. 10:288, 1973.

24. Coulam, C. B.: Testicular regression syndrome. Obstet. Gynecol. 53:45, 1979.

25. German, J., Simpson, J. L., Chaganti, R. S. K., Summitt, R. L., Reid, L. B. and Merkatz, I. R.: Genetically determined sex determination in man. Science 202:53, 1978.

26. Brown, D. M., Markland, C. and Dehner, L. P.: Leydig cell agenesis: a cause of male pseudohermaphroditism. J. Clin. Endocrinol. Metab. 46:1, 1978.

27. VanNiekerk, W. A.: True Hermaphroditism. Hagerstown, Harper and Row, 1978.

28. Simpson, J. L.: True hermaphroditism. Genetic and etiologic aspects. Birth Defects 14(6C):9, 1978.

29. Van Neikerk, W. A. and Retief, A. E.: The gonads of human true hermaphrodites. Hum. Genet. 58:117, 1981.

30. Wachtel, S. S., Koo, G. C., Breg, W. R. et al.: Serologic detection of a Y-linked gene in XX males and XX true hermaphrodites. N. Engl. J. Med. 295:750, 1976.

31. Wolf, U., Fraccaro, M., Mayerová, A., Hecht, T., Zuffardi, O. and Hameister, H.: Turner syndrome patients are H-Y positive. Hum. Genet. 54:149, 1980.

32. Wolf, U.: Genetic aspects of H-Y antigen. Hum. Genet. 58:25, 1981.

33. Morillo-Cucci, G. and German, J.: Abnormal Y chromosomes and monosony 45,X: a concept derived from the study of three patients. Birth Defects 7(6):210, 1971.

34. Simpson, J. L.: Diagnosis and management of the infant with genital ambiguity. Am. J. Obstet. Gynecol. 128:137, 1977.

Genetic Counseling: Who, What, When, Where and How

Morton A. Stenchever

David A. Luthy

University of Washington College of Medicine

The role of consultant, as well as primary health care provider, gives the obstetrician a unique opportunity to provide genetic counseling to individuals who might benefit from such service. The effect of a genetic condition on ability to reproduce, the risk of passing a given condition to offspring, the effect of poor pregnancy outcome on future pregnancies and the possibilities of antenatal detection in genetic high-risk pregnancies are areas of increasing interest to health care consumers. The physician can no longer dismiss such questions but must either provide adequate counseling or access to such counseling.

Obstetricians and gynecologists are frequently the primary physicians for female patients, in addition to providing specialized health care. This role places added responsibility for the recognition and assessment of patients who might benefit from genetic counseling (Table 1). A family history should be a part of every new gynecologic and obstetric evaluation. Data recorded in pedigree fashion (Fig. 1) provide maximal information quickly and allow hereditary patterns to be recognized more easily. In addition, a few simple questions such as: "Are there any birth defects in the family? Is there any mental retardation in the family? Is there anything in the family that you think might be hereditary?" provide a quick and efficient screen for genetic problems. Specific areas can then be dealt with in more detail and the appropriate referral made. Pediatricians have frequently functioned in the capacity of screening and referral of genetic disorders. However, it is clearly incumbent upon those who care for pregnant women to assume this responsibility.

Who Should Provide Genetic Counseling

Genetic counseling may be provided by any well-trained individual—obstetrician, family practitioner, pediatrician, geneticist or genetic associate (paramedical person specially trained in genetic disorders and counseling tech-

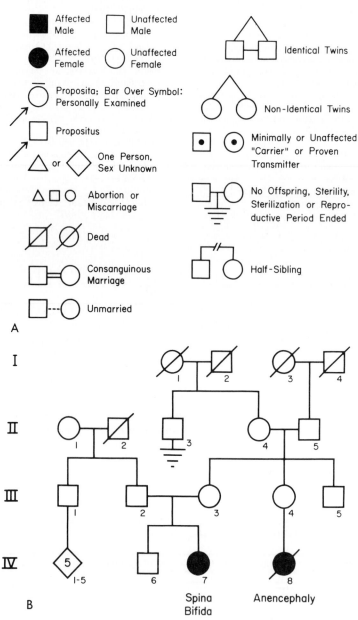

Figure 1. A, pedigree symbols and B, sample pedigree of family with neural tube defect.

TABLE 1. CONDITIONS IN WHICH GENETIC
COUNSELING MAY BE BENEFICIAL

1. Family history of any inheritable or potentially inheritable disorder
2. Pregnancy at risk for disorder amenable to antenatal detection
3. Repeated reproductive failure
4. Rhesus isoimmunization
5. Amenorrhea and infertility

niques). The counselor should have enough experience to handle the problems in question and be sensitive to the patient's needs and anxieties. Difficult problems are usually best handled by a skilled geneticist.

In order to provide effective counseling, an accurate diagnosis must be established. This may be difficult with scattered or deceased family members. However, without an accurate diagnosis all counseling is based on an unstable foundation. The counselor must know the mode of inheritance and the family history in order to estimate risk of occurrence and recurrence and to assess other family members who might be at risk. The counselor should know the natural history of the disease and its possible variations and must also be cognizant of methods of antenatal detection and reproduction options possible for the patient.

When, Where and How

In general, questions should be handled at the time they arise. Frequently, counseling situations can be anticipated by the physician—as in the case of the pregnant woman over 35—and brought to the attention of the patient, thus avoiding last-minute scheduling. Couples benefit from immediate counseling because their questions are answered and many fears allayed and they have time to reach a rational decision—in the case of the woman over 35, regarding amniocentesis.

Two exceptions to the rule on immediate counseling include infants with multiple anomalies and stillborn fetuses. In such cases it is wise to wait three to four months until appropriate studies have been performed. In addition, parents will have time to cope with the initial trauma and will be more receptive to counseling. Decisions regretted later about future reproduction or sterilization may be avoided in this manner.

Counseling is best given in a quiet room with the patient and her husband present. All distractions should be eliminated. The importance of the couple as a unit in genetic counseling, especially with respect to reproduction, cannot be overemphasized, as decisions based on counseling affect both individuals. Information is best disseminated in simple, straightforward language. Repetition is necessary and the facts should be repeated, perhaps with change in context, as often as needed to transmit the desired information. Counseling should be nondirective, and the goal should be to impart enough information to the couple to allow them to make rational decisions concerning their problem.

Who Should Receive Genetic Counseling and What Should be Discussed

When genetic counseling is done, the calculations of recurrence or occurrence risk is usually the center of focus. In many cases, an assessment of risk is all that is required, such as a pregnant woman inquiring about a birth defect within her family. However, one must be careful to avoid offhand advice if the facts are not clear; the implications could be enormous.

Complete counseling should provide the patient with much more than a risk figure. It is important at the outset to ascertain what the patient knows and what he or she wishes to know. Counseling can then be directed toward that end. In addition to risk, the natural history of the disease involved should be discussed along with anticipated problems. Variability in onset or expression of the disease should be thoroughly discussed, as should methods of treatment.

Reproductive risks are often of foremost concern, and reproductive options should be thoroughly explained, including antenatal detection, contraception, sterilization, adoption or artificial insemination when appropriate. Methods of carrier detection should be discussed when applicable.

Comprehensive counseling of families with complicated genetic disorders such as Huntington's chorea is usually best handled by a genetics clinic staffed by geneticists and adequate ancillary personnel, including social service workers, in conjunction with the referring physician. The situation of reproduction and its implications in such cases, in addition to day-to-day problems and questions, may be more easily handled in this manner.

Antenatal Diagnosis

The obstetrician will be confronted with questions regarding antenatal diagnosis more often than with any other topic in genetic counseling. The field of antenatal diagnosis has literally exploded with technologic advances and capabilities in recent years, and the disorders detectable prenatally are increasing daily (Table 2). Most antenatal detection centers on assays or tissue culture performed on amniotic fluid cells. Thus, it is imperative to discuss methods of amniocentesis, risks of the procedure and reliability of the assay or culture in question with the couple, in addition to the genetic risk.

Mid-trimester amniocentesis is a simple outpatient procedure ideally performed at 15 to 17 weeks of gestation. Large collaborative studies in both the United States and Canada were undertaken in the early 1970s to assess the safety and accuracy of mid-trimester amniocentesis for genetic purposes. In the United States study 1040 women undergoing mid-trimester amniocentesis were matched as closely as possible to a similar number of controls. An overall accuracy of 99.4 per cent was reported. The rate of spontaneous abortion and fetal death (3.4 per cent) was not statistically different between the two groups. Growth and developmental testing performed

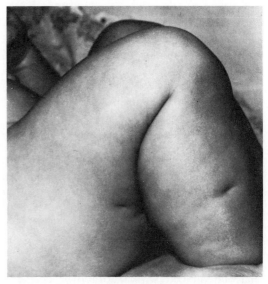

Figure 2. Residual skin depression secondary to fetal puncture during mid-trimester amniocentesis.

on the infants after one year revealed no difference between the two groups. Similar results were reported in the Canadian study.

Although the immediate complication rate was approximately 2 per cent in the United States study (vaginal bleeding or leakage of amniotic fluid), most centers are now reporting a much lower rate. Fetal puncture has been recognized as an infrequent potential complication, usually not of serious consequence (Fig. 2).

TYPES OF DISORDERS

CYTOGENETIC INDICATIONS. Fetal chromosome analysis is an accurate and reliable procedure when performed in an experienced facility—the accuracy being in excess of 99 per cent in most major centers. Because of the small number of cells in amniotic fluid, two to four weeks in tissue culture are necessary before analysis. Cell growth in tissue culture occurs in over 90 per cent of cases at most centers.

Advanced maternal age is the most common indication for antenatal diagnosis. The relationship between advanced maternal age and Down's syndrome has been recognized since the 1930s. Most centers consider advanced maternal age to be 35 years or more at the time of delivery. Of the women over 35 years of age tested in the United States collaborative study, 2.0 per cent had fetuses with chromo-

---

TABLE 2. PRENATAL DIAGNOSIS IN GENETIC
COUNSELING

COMMONLY ACCEPTED INDICATIONS
  Maternal age ≥ 35 years
  Previous child with autosomal trisomy
  Balanced translocation carrier
  Sex determination in X-linked disorders
  Family history of previous child with neural
    tube defect
  Inborn errors of metabolism detectable prenatally

NEWER APPLICATIONS
  Risk for structural defects in the fetus detectable by
    direct or indirect fetal visualization: anencephaly,
    hydrocephaly, renal agenesis, Ellis-van Creveld,
    TAR
  Gene studies on amniotic fluid cells: pregnancy at risk
    for homozygous α-thalassemia
  Fetal blood sampling: hemoglobinopathies

somal abnormalities. Despite the safety of amniocentesis and accuracy of fetal chromosome analysis, only a small percentage of women 35 years of age or older seek antenatal diagnosis.

A balanced translocation in one of the parents represents a high risk for producing chromosomally abnormal offspring. The risk in such cases depends on the chromosomes involved and the location of the translocation. Figure 3 demonstrates the R-banded karyotype of a woman with a balanced reciprocal translocation involving the long arm of chromosomes 13 and 17. The karyotype was performed because of a history of repeated reproductive failure including spontaneous abortions and malformed offspring. The patient underwent anmiocentesis in each of her three subsequent pregnancies, resulting respectively in the birth of a normal male, the elective abortion of a trisomy 13 fetus, and the birth of a male with the same translocation as his mother.

Other indications for cytogenetic evaluation of the fetus would include a previous child with a chromosomal abnormality (trisomy 21, trisomy 18, trisomy 13). The recurrence risk for trisomy 21 is approximately 1 per cent. Although the recurrence risk for trisomy 18 and trisomy 13 is low, couples so affected may be at increased risk for trisomy 21 and therefore amniocentesis is warranted. In addition, couples who have been through the experience of a child with a chromosomal abnormality frequently seek antenatal diagnosis even in cases in which the risk is low.

Sex determination can be used in pregnancies at risk for X-linked disorders. Since only males are affected in such cases, a couple can choose to continue gestation of female fetuses only. A full karyotype should be performed to most accurately determine sex. Affected and unaffected male fetuses can now be distinguished in several X-linked conditions, and active research is being directed toward distinguishing affected from unaffected males in classic hemophilia and Duchenne muscular dystrophy.

NEURAL TUBE DEFECTS. Open neural tube defects including anencephaly and spina bifida can be detected prenatally through elevated levels of amniotic fluid alpha-fetoprotein (AFP) when sampling is done at 16 to 20 weeks of gestation. Women who have previously borne a child with either anencephaly or spina bifida have a 2 to 5 per cent recurrence risk (one half for anencephaly; one half for spina bifida) with each subsequent pregnancy. Sisters of these women may be at a 1 per cent risk for such offspring. AFP is a fetospecific protein that is present in fetal serum and amniotic fluid, with concentrations in fetal serum approximately 150 times that of amniotic fluid. Amniotic fluid AFP elevations due to open

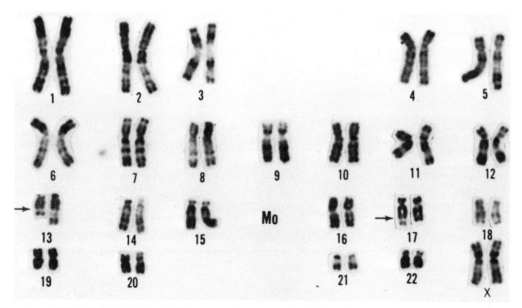

Figure 3. 46,XX,t(13q;17q). R-banded karyotype demonstrating balanced reciprocal translocation involving the long arms of chromosomes 13 and 17. The patient's condition was ascertained through a history of repetitive reproductive failure including spontaneous abortions and malformed liveborn infants.

neural tube defects are thought to occur by transudation of AFP across the exposed defect. Although AFP is a nonspecific indicator of neural tube defects, and other conditions may be associated with elevated levels of AFP, the AFP assay has proved invaluable in monitoring high-risk pregnancies. In the future, ultrasonography will be used more frequently to detect neural tube defects, and in many centers most cases of anencephaly are now detected by this method.

INBORN ERRORS OF METABOLISM. Inborn errors of metabolism that result from enzyme deficiencies should be amenable to prenatal diagnosis if the deficiency can be demonstrated in cultured fibroblasts. Tay-Sachs disease, which can be detected prenatally, is especially frequent among Ashkenazic Jews, and is caused by a deficiency in the enzyme hexosaminidase A. The enzyme deficiency results in the accumulation of sphingolipid due to the block in its degradative pathway, and this is responsible for the progressive neurologic deterioration. The enzyme can be demonstrated to be deficient in cultured amniotic fluid cells in fetuses affected with Tay-Sachs. Effective heterozygote screening exists, and couples at risk may be screened prior to pregnancy. Biochemical assays on cultured amniotic fluid cells are highly complex and frequently require four to six weeks to complete. Therefore early referral is mandatory. In the future microassays performed on fetal blood obtained by fetoscopy may be available for the diagnosis of certain biochemical defects.

FETAL VISUALIZATION

Many genetic disorders are without recognizable biochemical or chromosomal abnormalities. Prenatal diagnosis may be feasible in some cases by visualizing structural defects in the fetus. Indirect fetal visualization using ultrasonography may be useful in evaluating fetuses at risk for anencephaly (Fig. 4), hydrocephaly, omphalocoele, congenital heart disease, renal agenesis or polycystic kidneys. Fetal radiography can be used to determine the presence or absence of fetal radii in the autosomal recessive disorder of thrombocytopenia with absent radii, thus correctly differentiating affected from nonaffected fetuses (Fig. 5).

Direct fetal visualization using a small 1.7 mm endoscope has found limited application in detecting fetal structural abnormalities. Fetoscopy has been used to confirm the diagnosis of spina bifida and to make the diagnosis of Ellis-van Creveld syndrome. At present, the major role for fetoscopy resides in fetal blood sampling.

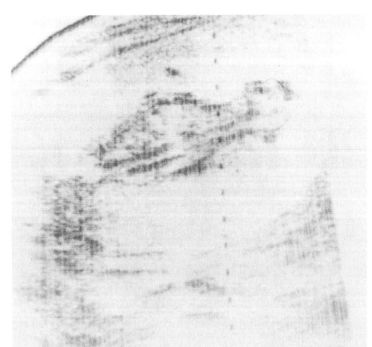

Figure 4. Anencephalic fetus at 16 weeks' gestation. Diagnosis made by ultrasound.

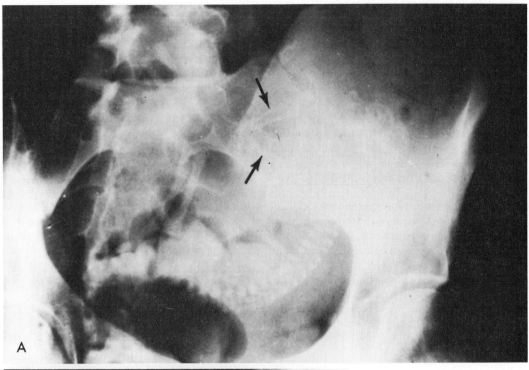

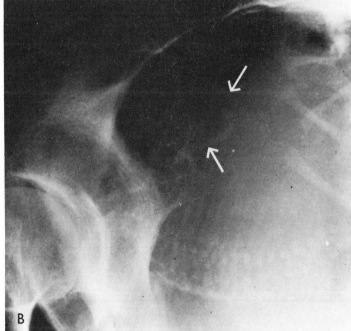

Figure 5. Fetal radiographs at 19 weeks' gestation in two pregnancies at risk for TAR syndrome. *A,* Humerus, ulna, and radius demonstrated (arrows) indicating unaffected fetus. *B,* Humerus, rudimentary ulna (arrows), and absent radius indicating an affected fetus.

FETAL BLOOD SAMPLING

With small quantities of fetal blood obtained by fetoscopically directed aspiration, the prenatal detection of hemoglobinopathies is possible. Although discussion of the methods used are beyond the scope of this article, sickle cell disease and the thalassemias may be detected using fetal blood. Future applications of fetal blood sampling may allow detection of affected males at risk for factor VIII deficiency or Duchenne muscular dystrophy in addition to biochemical abnormalities. More experience is needed to assess the safety of fetoscopy and the accuracy of microassays for biochemical abnormalities. Spontaneous fetal loss following fetoscopy appears to range from 5 to 10 per cent.

The most elegant advances in prenatal diagnosis have been the use of DNA hybridization and restriction endonuclease mapping of DNA from amniotic fluid cells for the prenatal diagnosis of alpha-thalassemia. Using this method, homozygous alpha-thalassemia can be detected by using DNA from amniotic fluid cells obtained at amniocentesis without the requirement of fetal blood. Similar applications have recently been repeated in sickle cell disease.

Repeated Reproductive Failure

Couples with repeated reproductive failure frequently seek genetic counseling because they have serious doubts about future reproduction. Such couples may have a history of habitual abortion, abortion of offspring with congenital malformations, or abortions interspersed with normal pregnancies. A history of three spontaneous abortions or any combination of abortions and stillborn or malformed infants warrants evaluation. Of the factors suspected in reproductive failure only uterine anomalies and cytogenetic abnormalities have definitely been identified as playing a causative role.

Early cytogenetic evaluation of both members of the couple with full-banded karyotypes is warranted, because cytogenetic abnormalities may result not only in repeated abortion but also liveborn infants with anomalies. The frequency of chromosomal abnormalities, most frequently balanced translocations (see Fig. 3) among couples with repetitive abortion is 5 to 10 per cent. When there is an additional history of a stillborn or malformed infant the frequency of chromosomal abnormalities is 15 to 25 per cent (see Table 3).

Couples with reproductive failure benefit greatly from counseling and evaluation. Couples with cytogenetic abnormalities may elect prenatal diagnosis or other reproductive options. If no abnormalities are found, the couple is often reassured by negative findings.

STILLBIRTHS OR INFANTS WITH ANOMALIES

When a stillborn infant or infant with anomalies is delivered, the parents are usually distraught and have feelings of guilt. Direct, gentle reassurance and prompt evaluation of the infant should be undertaken. However, any definitive counseling should await the outcome of evaluation and should be deferred until the couple has adjusted to the initial trauma of the event.

In the case of stillbirths, questions invariably arise in future pregnancies, and there are usually only sketchy records to use as reference. Complete reports of autopsy, karyotyping, pictures and x-rays of stillborn fetuses will

TABLE 3. Frequency of Chromosomal Abnormalities Among Couples with Repeated Reproductive Failure

Author	Reference	Percentage Abortions	Percentage Abortions and Stillborn Infants or Infants with Anomalies
Kim et al.	N. Engl. J. Med. 293:844, 1975		25
Schmidt et al.	J.A.M.A. 236:369, 1976	9.1	11.8
Byrd et al.	Fertil. Steril. 28:246, 1977	6.8	27.3
Stenchever et al.	Am. J. Obstet. Gynecol. 127:143, 1977	31.2	16.7

provide information for future counseling. The cause in approximately 50 per cent of stillborn infants with anomalies may be genetic.

Rh Disease

Rh isoimmunization remains a problem occasionally encountered by the obstretrician despite the use of Rh immune globulin. Couples who have had an Rh-sensitized pregnancy frequently seek counseling concerning risks of future pregnancies.

The genetics and mechanics of Rh sensitization should be reviewed. The major blood group and most probable genotype of each member of the couple should be reviewed with them as well as past pregnancy history and the implications of these findings on future pregnancies. Potential risks of future pregnancies should be discussed, as should amniocentesis, the techniques, hazards and outcome of intrauterine fetal transfusion, and risks of fetal death and prematurity.

Reproductive options including adoption, artificial insemination and sterilization should be discussed. When a couple has received this information they can more easily make decisions about future reproduction.

Amenorrhea and Infertility

With many of the disorders discovered during the evaluation of primary amenorrhea, the patient will benefit from sensitive counseling.

Chromosomal abnormalities enter the differential diagnosis of several gynecologic disorders, and whenever chromosomal analysis is considered, full-banded karyotyping should be performed. When a chromosomal abnormality is discovered, patients may benefit from sessions with a skilled geneticist.

A karyotype is indicated in the evaluation of primary amenorrhea, and chromosomal abnormalities may be found in 25 to 30 per cent of these patients. The most frequent abnormalities include 45,X, 45,X mosaicism and 46XY. Patients with secondary amenorrhea may occasionally warrant chromsomal evaluation, particularly if the condition is associated with elevated serum FSH and low serum estradiol. X-chromosome abnormalities may be found in a small percentage of these patients.

Occasionally during the course of an infertility evaluation, a severely oligospermic or azospermic male will be encountered. Chromosomal abnormalities can be found in 5 to 10 per cent of these cases, with 47,XXY and 47,XXY mosaicism being the most common abnormalities.

Once the diagnosis is established, it should be discussed with the patient in simple terms. Disorders such as Turner's syndrome, testicular feminization, and Klinefelter's syndrome have major reproductive implications. Proposed management, both medical and surgical, should be discussed. A strong emphasis should be placed on the positive aspects of each condition. As in all counseling, repetition and simple explanations are the most useful and satisfying to the patient.

Conclusions

The obstetrician-gynecologist is in a unique position to provide genetic counseling for a variety of conditions that have reproductive implications. Some of these conditions have been outlined. Successful counseling depends on an interested and informed counselor who is attentive to the desires of the patient. Information should be given in a nondirective manner and in sufficient depth to allow the patient to make rational decisions about the future.

REFERENCES

1. Bowman, J. W.: Management of Rh-isoimmunization. Obstet. Gynecol. 52:1, 1978.
2. Lowe, C. V., Alexander, D., Bryla, D. and Seigel, D.: The Safety and Accuracy of Mid-trimester Amniocentesis. The NICHD Amniocentesis Registry, DHEW Publication No. (NIH) 78–190.
3. Milunsky, A.: The Prenatal Diagnosis of Hereditary Disorders. Springfield, Charles C Thomas, 1973.
4. Milunsky, A.: The Prevention of Genetic Disease and Mental Retardation. Philadelphia, W. B. Saunders, 1975.
5. Murphy, E. A. and Chase, G. A.: Principles of Genetic Counseling. Chicago, Year Book Publishers, 1975.
6. Poland, B. J. and Lowry, R. B.: The use of spontaneous abortuses and stillbirths in genetic counselling. Am. J. Obstet. Gynecol. 118:332, 1974.
7. Simpson, N. E., Dallaire, L., Miller, J. R. et al.: Prenatal diagnosis of genetic disease in Canada: Report of a collaborative study. Can. Med. Assoc. J. 115:739, 1976.
8. Stenchever, M. A., Parks, K. J., Daines, T. L. et al.: Cytogenetics of habitual abortion and other reproductive wastage. Am. J. Obstet. Gynecol. 127:143, 1977.

Antenatal Diagnosis of Chromosomal Abnormalities

Arthur C. Christakos, M.D., F.A.C.O.G.

Duke University School of Medicine

Until recent years, antenatal diagnosis of genetic disease or any other fetal condition would have been an educated guess, at best. With Bevis' invasion of the amniotic cavity in the early 1950s, more accurate assessment of the fetal condition could be made.[1] Since that time, additional invasive and noninvasive techniques of fetal study have been developed.

Physical and chemical studies of amniotic fluid and of amniotic fluid cells as well as acoustical studies of intrauterine contents have allowed obstetricians to detect prenatally some 60 or more genetically determined diseases. More conditions are being detected yearly by application of various techniques of study. Most medical centers are unprepared to perform extensive studies; therefore, requests for specific tests should be made of those centers having expertise in detecting specific conditions.

The obstetrician has become one of the professionals to whom families turn for advice regarding genetic disease. Primarily, most requests for genetic counseling involve inquiries about risk figures for future progeny. Secondarily, requests are made for prognostic forecasts for the affected family members. We obstetricians may not be prepared to impart such information for a specific condition, but we should be familiar with patterns of inheritance so that intelligent answers may be given for the primary question. Furthermore, those of us trained in prenatal care and family planning should be prepared to help a family follow the course of action that seems appropriate *to them* in view of the risks they face and their family goals.

Whenever we encounter a particular genetic condition that is not familiar to us, we should seek consultation with those professionals who have expertise. Above all, we should do no harm by giving families unrealistic hope or unwarranted discouragement for the prognosis on their affected members and for recurrence risks.

Genetic counseling is that process of communication dealing with the human problems associated with the occurrence or the risk of occurrence of genetic disorder. Clark Fraser[2] listed several components of the process of genetic counseling as helping the family:

1. To comprehend the medical facts, including the diagnosis, the probable cause and the available management.

2. To appreciate the contribution of heredity to the disorder and the risk of recurrence in specific relatives.

3. To understand the options for dealing with the risks of recurrence.

4. To choose the course of action that seems appropriate *to them* in view of risks and family goals and act in accordance with that decision.

5. To make the best possible adjustment to the disorder and to the affected family member, and to the risk of recurrence of that disorder if a decision is made to take the risk.

Before engaging in genetic counseling, one must make an accurate diagnosis. This involves, among other things, the taking of a detailed family history or the development of a pedigree. Other prerequisites for an accurate diagnosis include a thorough physical examination, pertinent laboratory studies and extensive review of the literature and pertinent medical records. If these steps have been followed and the family then seeks advice from the obstetrician, more authoritative counsel can be given.

In this presentation I will outline the magnitude of the problem of chromosomal disorders and how antenatal karyotypic analysis may help in solving some of the worrisome dilemmas encountered by at-risk populations.

Historical Perspective

Within the past 20 years, the study of human chromosomes has developed from a process of squashing metaphase figures to one of developing by automation karyotypes of differentially stained chromosomes. What was once a process of incubating bone marrow for a few hours is now a sophisticated technique of culturing viable cells obtained from any site, including the previously sacrosanct amniotic sac.

That humans have 23 pairs of chromosomes was established by Tjio and Levan in 1956.[3] The first clinical entity associated with abnormal chromosomes was described by Lejeune in three mongol children in 1959.[4] Since then an entirely new literature has developed in human cytogenetics.

Magnitude of the Problem

Chromosomal disorders have been found to be associated with sterility, reduced fertility, fetal or infant death or congenital malformations or both. It is estimated that in the United States 175,000 spontaneous abortions of fetuses having a chromosomal disorder occur yearly. Additionally, 15,000 infants with chromosomal abnormalities are born in the United States each year. If one surveys the neonatal population in the United States for chromosomal abnormalities, an incidence of 0.59 per cent is found.[5] If the population under consideration is composed of full-term low birth weight infants, the incidence jumps to 2.2 per cent[6] and if the population includes all perinatal deaths as well, the incidence is 5.8 per cent.[7, 8] Stated differently, if all fetal wastage and congenitally defective neonates are considered, chromosomal abnormalities are present in about 36 per cent of all conceptions.

If maternal age at the time of delivery is considered, there is a definite positive correlation between increasing incidence of chromosomally abnormal conceptions and increasing maternal age. This is especially true for Down's syndrome[9] and to a lesser degree for other chromosomal abnormalities.[10, 11] Increasing paternal age does not seem to be so positively correlated.[12] Some investigators, however, have suggested that markedly advanced paternal age may be positively correlated.[13-16] Once a child with trisomy 21 is born to a woman, the risk for recurrence is at least 1 to 2 per cent, irrespective of maternal age.[17, 18] Recurrence risks for other chromosomal abnormalities are not as well established.

Translocation carrier parents run a much greater risk of having abnormal offspring. Even though these conditions are relatively rare, their existence has such an impact on families that the known presence of a translocation carrier state is sufficient grounds for prenatal chromosome studies.

Compared with chromosomal disorders per se, X-linked recessive traits probably do not have the same statistical significance. However, whenever an X-linked recessive trait that threatens life and health exists in a sibship, the 50 per cent risk to all male offspring should be considered. Presently only a small number of X-linked recessive conditions can be accurately diagnosed in utero. Therefore, karyotypic analysis to determine the sex of the fetus has been the only means of identifying the potentially affected fetus.

Indications for Antenatal Chromosome Studies

There are essentially four indications for antenatal karyotypic analysis. The practicing obstetrician will be privileged to care for pregnant women from these various categories not infrequently. If there is a facility available to perform chromosome studies, patients identified as "at-risk" should be informed of the risks involved and offered antenatal karyotypic analysis. The category representing the largest segment of the gravid population with an indication for antenatal chromosome studies is the group with increasing parental age, especially increasing maternal age.

As mentioned, increasing maternal age has been positively correlated with aneuploidies in the offspring. Antenatal karyotypic analysis is recommended for pregnant woman 35 years of age or older. Some investigators in the field of cytogenetics also advise pregnant woman whose mates are 55 years of age or older to undergo antenatal chromosome studies.[19] Paternal age of 55 years is admittedly arbitrarily chosen because of a lack of evidence defining a specific paternal age beyond which an indisputable increased risk for chromosomal abnormalities exists for the offspring.[20-22]

The proportion of pregnant women 35 years of age or older varies in different geographic areas of this country. There are sufficient numbers in North Carolina, a state with a population of about 5.5 million with about 80,000 deliveries yearly, so that about 1500 antenatal karyotypic analyses are done. Four laboratories located in different regions of the state perform the bulk of these studies. It is estimated on the basis of 4 per cent of mothers 35 and over that there may be another 1000 to 1500 "at-risk" patients who are not served. Cytogenetic abnormalities are diagnosed in about 3 per cent of the fetuses of these older women. Forty-five potentially abnormal newborns are identified through these efforts, while another 30 to 45 are missed because antenatal karyotyping is not done in the other at-risk patients. Golbus and his co-workers at the University of California Medical Center, San Francisco, reported 2.4 per cent incidence of chromosomal abnormalities in over 2000 pregnancies tested because of advanced maternal age.[23]

The relationship between advanced maternal age and chromosomal aneuploidies among the conceptuses was well illustrated by Tsuji and Nakano[24] in a karyotypic study of fetal material obtained from induced abortions in older women. These abortions were performed for nonmedical reasons. For the 35- to 39-year-old group, an incidence of 1.6 per cent chromosomal anomalies was found. The incidence increased to 6.0 per cent for the 40- to 44-year-old group while the 45- to 49-year-old group, admittedly small in numbers, demonstrated an incidence of 25 per cent. The overall incidence of chromosomal aberrations in all patients 35 years and older was 5.1 per cent.

The second indication for antenatal chromosome studies is a previous child with chromosomal abnormality. Following the birth of one child with an autosomal trisomy or sex chromosomal aneuploidy, the likelihood that subsequent progeny will have some kind of chromosomal aneuploidy is increased. Indeed, the occurrence of a chromosomal aneuploidy in a previous conceptus, whether surviving gestation or resulting in early abortion, is definitely associated with an increased risk of abnormal karyotypes in subsequent conceptuses. The recurrence risk for trisomy 21 (Down's syndrome) is 1 to 2 per cent, irrespective of parental age, assuming that parental karyotypes are normal.[25] It is conceivable that a predisposition to nondisjunction in some individuals is responsible for recurrent aneuploidies. The true etiology for this phenomenon is not yet known. This increased risk is present irrespective of parental ages or chromosomal constitutions.

Parental chromosomal abnormalities such as balanced translocations and inversions are a third indication for fetal karyotyping. Such aberrations are rare but should be suspected when repeated fetal wastage occurs or when an abnormal baby is born with an unbalanced translocation. Approximately 2 to 3 per cent of newborns with Down's syndrome have translocations involving the No. 21 chromo-

some. It appears that about one fourth of translocations are inherited from carrier parents, while the remainder arise de novo.[26] Paternal translocation carriers are responsible for a smaller proportion of the inherited translocation Down's syndrome babies than are the maternal translocation carriers.[27] Most translocation Down's syndrome babies have translocations between a No. 14 chromosome and a No. 21. Rare occurrences of translocation between both Nos. 21 can likewise result in Down's syndrome. A carrier parent for such a translocation can produce only two kinds of gametes, namely (1) unbalanced t21/21 or (2) nullisomic gametes. These gametes result in only two types of zygotes: unbalanced translocation Down's syndrome or lethal monosomic conceptuses.

Chromosomal inversions may also produce unbalanced gametes and zygotes. Carriers for translocations and inversions may experience repeated fetal wastage through early spontaneous abortion and premature delivery of abnormal progeny or stillbirths as a result of these unbalanced zygotes.

A fourth category of patient recommended for antenatal (fetal) karyotyping is the known carrier for a debilitating or lethal X-linked trait such as Duchenne muscular dystrophy or hemophilia. For those X-linked traits in which biochemical methods are already well developed and applicable for the fetus, the karyotypic identification of a male can lead to identification of the affected fetus and of the fetus free of disease. For those X-linked traits for which no antenatal techniques of identification have yet been developed, the antenatal karyotype can identify only the male fetus.

All concerned parties are aware that theoretically 50 per cent of male fetuses are free of the disease in question. Such information is used by parents of affected progeny in planning future reproduction according to the dictates of their previous experience, their conscience and their emotions. The pros and cons of directive counseling can be debated in other places. It is my practice to present information in an objective way to parents so that they may make their own decision regarding continuation or interruption of pregnancy. Furthermore, determination of fetal sex under these circumstances should not be denied because of announced parental decision not to abort regardless of karyotypic results. The satisfaction and reassurance afforded by a female karyotype are undeniable. In

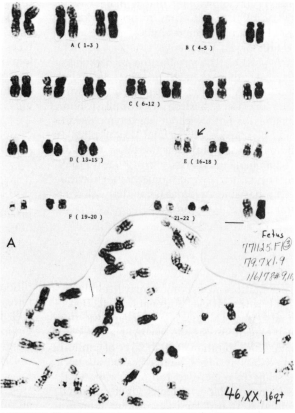

Figure 1. A, Large No. 16 in fetus. *B,* Large No. 16 in father.

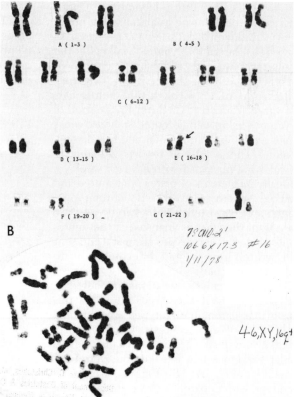

addition, foreknowledge that a male will be born can offer couples time to prepare for the possibility of an affected child.

A fifth or miscellaneous category for fetal karyotyping can be proposed which includes situations other than those just discussed. Couples with a history of repeated fetal wastage or previous children with multisystemic anomalies or both without karyotypic studies should be considered for fetal karyotyping. In addition, those couples who report exposure to hallucinogenic drugs during early pregnancy or within several months of fertilization may be possible candidates for discussion regarding fetal karyotyping.

Amniocentesis and Karyotyping

The amniocentesis procedure itself is described in the article "Antenatal Detection of Neural Tube Defects," which follows this. Sterile plastic disposable syringes are recommended for aspiration of 20 to 25 cc of amniotic fluid. (Glass syringes tend to cause amniotic fluid cells to adhere to the side walls while plastic avoids this problem.) Once obtained, the fluid is transported at ambient temperature to a tissue culture laboratory. Under sterile conditions, using a laminar flow hood, as many individual cultures are prepared as allowed by the sample volume, following the simple technique described by Gray and co-workers at the State University of New York at Buffalo in 1971.[28] Growth time before harvest varies from 16 to 32 days. Preparation of karyotypes using well-accepted standard techniques and stains requires an additional week or more. This results in reports available to the referring physician within 3 to 5 weeks.

Ideally 20 metaphase plates are counted and analyzed microscopically. If chromosome counts are consistent, four karyotypes are made from the 20 cells analyzed at the microscope. Copies of karyotypes are made and sent with written reports and interpretations to referring physicians.

Occasionally minor variations are noted in analyzing the fetal karyotypes. It is for this reason that parental karyotypes are obtained at the time of amniocentesis. Comparison of parental and fetal chromosomes may reveal similar variations that are not considered abnormalities (Fig. 1A, 1B). Figure 1A is a fetal karyotype with apparent extra material on the long arm of a No. 16 chromosome. Figure 1B

represents the karyotype of the phenotypically normal father demonstrating an identical unusually long No. 16 chromosome. In addition, balanced translocations in the fetus may be found in one or the other parent. It is reassuring to translocation carriers to realize that fetuses with such abnormal chromosome findings can be as "normal" as their parents.

Conclusion

Fetal karyotypic analyses offer couples at risk of chromosomal abnormalities in their progeny the opportunity to identify cytogenetically abnormal fetuses sufficiently early in pregnancy to allow relatively safe induced abortion if they, in their informed deliberations, decide to interrupt pregnancy. In addition, the couple with a known abnormal fetus who decides against induced abortion will have time before delivery to prepare emotionally and otherwise for the abnormal offspring.

Determination of sex in those fetuses at risk for severe X-linked disease can at least reassure in the case of the female fetus and offer an opportunity to make a difficult decision in the case of the male fetus. If the condition is one that can be detected by biochemical or other methods once a male fetus has been identified, the parents can be given even more information with which a more meaningful decision can be made.

REFERENCES

1. Bevis, D. C. A.: The antenatal prediction of hemolytic disease of the newborn. Lancet 1:395, 1952.
2. Fraser, F. C.: Genetic counseling. Am. J. Hum. Genet. 36:636, 1974.
3. Tjio, J. H. and Levan, A.: The chromosome number of man. Hereditas 42:1, 1956.
4. Lejeune, J., Gautier, M. and Turpin, R.: Étude des chromosomes somatiques de neuf enfants mongoliens. Compt. Rend. Acad. Sci. 248:1721, 1959.
5. Golbus, M. S.: The antenatal detection of genetic disorders. Obstet. Gynecol. 48:496, 1976.
6. Chen, A. and Falek, A.: Chromosome aberrations in full-term low birth weight neonates. Humangenetik 21:13, 1974.
7. Machin, G.: Chromosome abnormality and perinatal death. Lancet 1:549, 1974.
8. Sutherland, G., Bauld, R. and Bain, A.: Chromosome abnormality and perinatal death. (Letter) Lancet 1:752, 1976.
9. Mitchell, A.: J. Ment. Sci. 98:174 (1876) quoted in Richards, B. W.: Mongols and their mothers. Br. J. Psychiat. 122:1, 1973.

10. Smith, D. W., Patau, K. and Therman, E.: Autosomal trisomy syndromes. Lancet 2:211, 1961.
11. Smith, D. W.: Autosomal abnormalities. Am. J. Obstet. Gynecol. 90:1055, 1964.
12. Penrose, L. S.: The relative effects of paternal and maternal age in mongolism. J. Genet. 27:219, 1933.
13. Mikkelson, M., Halberg, A. and Paulson, H.: Maternal and paternal origin of extra chromosome in trisomy 21. Hum. Genet. 32:17, 1976.
14. Wagenbichler, P., Killian, W., Rett, A. and Schnedl, W.: Origin of the extra chromosome no. 21 in Down's syndrome. Hum. Genet. 32:13, 1976.
15. Hansson, A. and Mikkelson, M.: The origin of the extra chromosome 21 in Down's syndrome. Studies of fluorescent variants and satellite association in 26 informative families. Cytogenet. Cell Genet. 20:194, 1978.
16. Matsunaga, E., Akisa, T., Hidetsune, O. and Ki Kuchi, Y.: Reexamination of paternal age effect in Down's syndrome. Hum. Genet. 40:259, 1978.
17. Milunsky, A.: The Prenatal Diagnosis of Hereditary Diseases. Springfield, Charles C Thomas, 1973.
18. Mikkelson, M. and Stene, J.: Genetic counselling in Down's syndrome. Hum. Hered. 20:457, 1970.
19. Buchanan, P.: Personal communication, 1980.
20. Erickson, J. D.: Paternal age and Down's syndrome. Am. J. Hum. Genet. 31:489, 1979.
21. Stene, J. and Stene, E.: Statistical methods for detecting a moderate paternal age effect on incidence when a strong maternal one is present. Ann. Hum. Genet. 40:343, 1977.
22. Stene, J. and Stene, E.: Paternal age effect in Down's syndrome. Ann. Hum. Genet. 40:299, 1977.
23. Golbus, M. S. et al.: Prenatal genetic diagnosis in 3000 amniocenteses. N. Engl. J. Med. 300:157, 1979.
24. Tsuji, K. and Nakano, R.: Chromosome studies in embryos from induced abortions in pregnant women age 35 and over. Obstet. Gynecol. 52:542, 1978.
25. Mikkelson, M.: Down's syndrome: current state of cytogenetic research. Hum. Genet. 12:1, 1971.
26. Wright, S. W. et al.: Frequency of trisomy and translocation in Down's syndrome. J. Pediatr. 70:420, 1967.
27. Nadler, H. L.: Prenatal diagnosis of genetic defects. Adv. Pediatr. 22:1, 1976.
28. Gray, C., Davidson, R. G. and Cohen, M. M.: A simplified technique for the culture of amniotic fluid cells. J. Pediatr. 79:119, 1971.

Antenatal Diagnosis of Neural Tube Defects

Arthur C. Christakos, M.D., F.A.C.O.G.

Duke University School of Medicine

In the United States each year there are about 8000 children born with neural tube defects. The projected cost of lifetime care for one infant surviving with a significant opening in the neural tube has been estimated at between $100,000 and $250,000. The mental anguish of parents and other family members cannot be measured. Nor can the physical and emotional impact on the affected individuals themselves be appreciated by society.

During the past 20 years relatively safe techniques of interrupting pregnancy during the second trimester have been perfected and accepted by the medical and legal professions and by many societies and jurisdictions. Accurate diagnosis of neural tube defects early enough in the second trimester can allow for pregnancy interruption—if that is the desire of the parents—thereby avoiding financial, physical and emotional burdens on society and family.

The material in this presentation consists of some definitions of neural tube defects and some discussion of incidence and recurrence risk figures. In addition, a brief historical account of the development of practical and accurate methods of antenatal detection of neural tube defects is given, followed by a discussion of their application in the clinical setting.

Definitions

The most common forms of open neural tube defects or myelodysplastic diseases are anencephaly and spina bifida cystica. The former is characterized by absence of the cranial vault associated with amorphous brain substance. Survival for more than a few hours after birth is rare. Spina bifida cystica, in contrast to anencephaly, is compatible with postnatal survival, although with differing degrees of impaired quality of survival. Sacular protrusions from the spinal canal through midline spinal defects characterize this type of

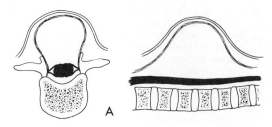

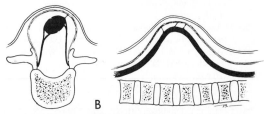

Figure 1. A, Meningocele; *B*, myelomeningocele.

TABLE 1. INCIDENCE RATES FOR NEURAL TUBAL DEFECTS	
GEOGRAPHIC AREA	PER THOUSAND BIRTHS
Northern Ireland	7.2
Wales	5.8
Scotland	5.6
Republic of Ireland	4.8
England	4.0
United States	1 to 3 (East>West)

neural tube defect. If the sac contains meninges *without* neural elements, it is characterized as a *meningocele* (Fig. 1A). More common than the meningocele is the *myelomeningocele* (or *myelocele*), which contains neural elements in addition to meninges (Fig. 1B). This type is frequently associated with hydrocephaly. Other variations of greater or lesser degree may occur throughout the central nervous system, including *encephalocele* (defects in the skull with protrusion) and *spina bifida occulta*, characterized by bony defects without protrusion of meninges or neural elements.

Incidence and Recurrence Risks

Globally a marked variation in incidence has been reported, suggesting environmental as well as genetic factors etiologically. The highest rates are seen in Britain and Ireland, while the lowest rates are found in Africa, Asia and South America. Intermediate incidence figures are seen in continental Europe, North America and Israel. There are marked differences in incidence rates between the eastern and western coasts of the United States with three times the number of cases in the east as in the west (Table 1).[1]

These defects are second in incidence only to heart anomalies at birth and, like cardiac defects, are considered multifactorial or polygenic in origin. Rarely, recurrence of affected

siblings is seen, suggesting either autosomal recessive or X-linked inheritance.[2]

Recurrence risks in a sibship are similar to those for other polygenic diseases and are empirically stated, as seen in Table 2.[1] Unfortunately, 90 per cent of all neural tube defects occur without a previous history in a family or in a sibship. In recent years, Milunsky and Alpert have suggested that there may very well be a positive correlation between advancing maternal age and increased incidence of neural tube defects.[3]

History of Development of Antenatal Diagnostic Techniques

In the late 1960s, reports of measurable bilirubin in amniotic fluids of anencephalics raised the possibility of reliable antenatal diagnosis of these myelodysplastic disorders.[4, 5] When bilirubin was found in amniotic fluid of anencephalics near term, it was thought that leakage or transudate of fetal blood components may occur directly from serum or indirectly via cerebrospinal fluid. Bilirubin is not considered a very specific indicator because it can originate in either maternal or fetal circulation. Because of its relatively low molecular weight (585), rapid turnover is a distinct probability. Brock and Sutcliffe[6] recognized alpha fetoprotein (AFP) as a more specific indicator of neural tube defects because of its more specific fetal origin. Having a molecular weight of 64,000, it is a glycoprotein with alpha-1-electronphoretic mobility. Embryologically synthesized by the yolk sac, it is

TABLE 2. RECURRENCE RISKS FOR NEURAL TUBAL DEFECTS		
One child affected	1:20	(5%)
Two previously affected	1:10	(10%)
Three previously affected	1:5	(21%)
Either parent affected	1:30	(3%)
Parent and child affected	—	(13%)

produced later by the fetal liver and gastrointestinal tract. AFP first appears in fetal serum at about four to six weeks, increasing in concentration until the thirteenth gestational week, after which it declines steadily toward term, reaching low adult levels of less than 10 nanograms per ml early in the neonatal period. Peak concentrations in fetal serum at 13 weeks may attain levels as high as 4 mg per ml.

In adults elevated serum AFP levels have been recorded in association with hepatitis, cirrhosis and primary and metastatic malignancies of the liver. Testicular and ovarian teratocarcinomas and gastric and pancreatic carcinomas have also been associated with elevated serum AFP levels.

There is a marked concentration gradient for AFP between fetal serum and amniotic fluid at 150 to 200:1 with an even greater concentration gradient between fetal serum and maternal serum in the order of 10,000:1. It is no wonder then that even small fetal-maternal transfusions that occur during amniocentesis or during abortion could grossly affect maternal serum levels of AFP.

When studied prior to the end of the second trimester, neural tube defects have been associated with grossly elevated AFP levels in amniotic fluid. The optimal stage of gestation for AFP determinations on amniotic fluid is at 15 to 16 weeks on the basis of the first day of the last normal menstrual period. There is an adequate volume of fluid available for safe and successful amniocentesis at that time. In addition, concentrations of AFP are still sufficiently high to be measured accurately. Furthermore, interruption of pregnancy is easier and safer prior to 20 weeks in the event that a significant defect is considered present and the parents choose induced abortion.

Fetal conditions other than neural tube defects may also be associated with elevated amniotic fluid AFP. Some such conditions have been reported are severe Rh isoimmunization, fetal maceration, twin pregnancy, XO sex chromosome constitution[7] and fetal cystic hygroma.[8, 9] Still other fetal conditions include omphalocele and gastroschisis,[10] esophageal atresia[11] and congenital nephrosis.[12] Because of the high concentration gradient between fetal serum and amniotic fluid, contamination with fetal blood can also give false-positive results.

Falsely negative AFP levels in amniotic fluid (i.e., normal values) in the presence of neural tube defects may be due to small lesions or to lesions covered by full-thickness skin, restricting leakage of fetal serum or cerebrospinal fluid into amniotic fluid. It has been estimated that these conditions are present in about 4 per cent of infants surviving severe neurologic defects.[13]

If no AFP is detected in the fluid sample, the possibility that the sample is maternal urine should be considered. In addition, renal agenesis of the fetus could be responsible for undetectable AFP levels in amniotic fluid.

There have been other amniotic fluid parameters investigated for their potential as diagnostic tools in the early detection of neural tube defects. As mentioned earlier, bilirubin has been elevated in association with these conditions. Certain amino acids and a beta trace protein (B-TP) have likewise been measured at high levels in amniotic fluid in association with neural tube defects. Reproducibility of results has been extremely poor, precluding practical use of these parameters.

Smith et al.[14] from Oxford and Stockholm reported from a preliminary study that acetylcholinesterase (AChE) levels are increased in amniotic fluids of fetuses with open neural tube defects. They studied samples from 77 pregnancies previously subjected to AFP testing, including 5 misclassified by the AFP test; that is, 4 were false positive and one was false negative. Fifty-six were true negatives and 16 were true positives. This study revealed a close association between elevated AChE levels and anencephaly and open spina bifida. There was not a strong relationship between AChE level and period of gestation. The authors believe that a very large survey would be needed to determine whether the amniotic fluid AChE test alone is a better test than amniotic fluid AFP in the early diagnosis of neural tube defects.

Fetal macrophage counts in amniotic fluid have revealed a high proportion in comparison with other cellular constituents in amniotic fluids of fetuses with myelodysplastic lesions. Again, the use of this parameter is precluded because the specificity of macrophage counting in amniotic fluid would appear to be less than that of AFP determination.

Maternal serum AFP levels have been found to be elevated in third trimester fetal distress and intrauterine fetal death. Because of this, the potential of serum AFP in detecting neural tube defects has been investigated. Maternal serum concentrations of AFP steadily increase as pregnancy progresses in contrast to amniotic fluid concentrations, which diminish after 13 weeks. Normal adult nonpregnant serum AFP levels rarely exceed 10 ng per ml. At 14 weeks, levels reach about 30 ng per ml, rising to about 50 ng per ml at 18 weeks and 90 ng per ml at 22 weeks. Wide variations occur when maximum concentrations occur between 32 and 35 weeks.

Some investigators suggest that grossly deviating levels of AFP in maternal serum may be helpful in early detection of neural tube defects, but the use of this method is not yet practical in most hospitals. When such abnormal levels are found, they should be confirmed by amniotic fluid AFP measurements and by ultrasonographic studies (see later discussion). When maternal serum AFP determinations are within normal range, it is conceivable that 80 per cent of neural tube defects can be ruled out. Some false negatives can and do occur.

A variety of physical methods have been developed for antenatal study to detect fetal structural defects. Those currently available include radiography, amniography, fetoscopy and ultrasonography. Because of the hazards of ionizing irradiation when radiographic techniques are employed, radiography and amniography can be essentially ruled out for practical application. The risk of abortion inherent in fetoscopy likewise precludes practical utilization of this method. Ultrasonography, on the other hand, can be quite helpful. Until recently the chief disadvantage of this modality has been the relatively poor degree of resolution achieved with very expensive and complex equipment. Modern sonographic equipment now offers much better resolution (to about 1 to 2 cm) as well as real-time scanning properties.

Normal growth curves of fetal biparietal diameter have been plotted so that deviations from normal can be determined. It is conceivable that by comparing biparietal and transthoracic diameters at any point during gestation, hydrocephaly and microcephaly can be suspected when these differences are found to exceed or fall short by 1 cm, respectively. Cystic dilatation of the fetal cerebral ventricles may also suggest hydrocephaly.

By 14 weeks anencephaly can readily be diagnosed when sonographic absence of skull echoes is demonstrated. Indeed, such findings make AFP studies on amniotic fluid unnecessary.

Practical Application of These Modalities

For all practical purposes, the combined use of amniotic fluid AFP and ultrasonographic studies should identify essentially 95 per cent of all significant open neural tube defects. Until such time as amniotic fluid measurements of acetylcholinesterase have been shown to be more reliable and better than AFP studies in the early detection of neural tube defects, AChE studies cannot be expected to be readily available and to replace AFP and ultrasonography. Maternal serum AFP studies could conceivably serve as useful screening in those populations with high incidence figures, such as in the United Kingdom.

Clinical Application of Diagnostic Techniques

The typical patient for whom the clinician should consider ultrasonographic and amniotic fluid AFP studies to rule out neural tube defects during mid trimester will give a history of having had a child with a spina bifida cystica (myelocele). Because of the recurrence risk of about 5 per cent that each subsequent child may have a similar abnormality or anencephaly, these studies should be recommended. They should be performed at about 15 to 16 weeks' gestation. Fetal skull and spinal development will have progressed to the point that ultrasonographic evidence of structural defects may be detectable.

AFP levels in amniotic fluid over 2 log standard deviations above the mean at any specific gestation were found by Milford-Ward to be associated with open neural tube defects in 95 per cent.[15] Each laboratory should establish its own standards for each stage of gestation. Generally speaking, AFP levels after 20 weeks' gestation are less reliable. It is mandatory that gestational age be as accurately determined as possible for proper interpretation. Miscalculation of gestational age may be one of the most common causes of error in interpretation of AFP. Another common cause of error is fetal blood contamination of amniotic fluid. Use of ultrasonography prior to amniocentesis can help in avoiding errors in calculating gestational age. In addition, placental localization via ultrasonography may assist the operator in avoiding the placenta during amniocentesis, thereby reducing the risk of fetal blood contamination.

During the past 20 years or longer, neurosurgical approaches to neural tube defects have resulted in larger numbers of affected individuals surviving childhood and entering reproductive years. Not infrequently, patients with such histories require counseling if they are pregnant or are planning pregnancy. The risk of neural tube defects in the progeny of such individuals is about 3 per cent (see Table 2). This risk is sufficiently high to warrant studies to rule out these defects during early mid trimester.

It stands to reason that patients undergoing amniocentesis for chromosome or other studies would also have amniotic fluid AFP tests performed. Most antenatal chromosome studies are done because of advanced maternal age (35 years or older), which may also play a role in the etiology of neural tube defects. Furthermore, it follows that AFP testing would be employed on available fluid obtained during mid trimester for whatever purpose from patients living in localities considered "endemic" for neural tube defects, such as in Northern Ireland, Wales, Scotland and the Republic of Ireland.

A fourth category of patients considered candidates for amniotic fluid AFP tests to detect neural tube defects are those with previous offspring with hydrocephaly. Cohen and his co-workers of the Hadassah-Hebrew University reported a 1.6 per cent frequency of anencephaly or spina bifida among sibs of children with hydrocephaly.[16] This frequency represents a twofold to eightfold increase in population frequencies at large. Because a risk figure of 1 per cent is usually considered adequate to suggest prenatal diagnosis by amniocentesis, the 1.6 per cent risk indicates that amniotic fluid AFP tests should be made in mothers of hydrocephalic children.

Regardless of the indication for AFP testing, the pregnant patient for study should be managed with the objective of subjecting the mother and fetus to as little risk as possible. Based on the first day of the last menstrual period, clinical evaluation of uterine size and ultrasonographic biparietal diameters, amniocentesis is planned for the gestational period between 15 and 17 weeks. Ideally, real-time ultrasonographic studies done in the same room as the amniocentesis, without moving the patient, helps avoid puncturing the fetus and affords the operator with the best view to avoid penetrating the placenta. If this luxury is not available, ultrasonographic studies for estimation of fetal age and localization of the placenta just prior to amniocentesis serves much the same purpose as these real-time studies.

With the patient lying comfortably in the supine position, the abdomen is prepared with multiple layers of Betadine (povidone-iodine) solution and then draped as a sterile field. Indeed, the patient is informed beforehand that the procedure is regarded in the same way as is a minor operative procedure and an operative permit is obtained based on the form developed by Schwarz and Mennuti for the American College of Obstetricians and Gynecologists (Fig. 2).

The best site for amniocentesis as demonstrated by ultrasonography is identified. One per cent xylocaine (Lidocaine) solution is injected into the skin with a 26-gauge needle to form a wheal. A 20-gauge needle measuring 1½ inches is used to infiltrate the depths of the abdominal wall, especially the level of the parietal peritoneum, which is essentially the only pain-sensitive area other than skin. A 20-gauge spinal needle with obturator in place is then thrust fairly abruptly through the abdominal wall and myometrium. The operator experiences a popping sensation as the amniotic cavity is entered reminiscent of the sensation of lumbar puncture or paracentesis for ascites. This abrupt technique is used in order to avoid tenting the chorioamnion as the needle point traverses those membranes. The experience with this technique has been good in obtaining fluid readily. Fetal injury by the needle has been virtually nonexistent, with one report of dimpling on the buttock of one fetus in a limited experience with approximately 450 amniocenteses in the clinic under my supervision.

Short sterile plastic connector tubing is attached to the hub of the needle after removal of the obturator, and the flow of fluid is noted. A syringe is then connected to the other end of the connector tubing for slow but steady aspiration of approximately 6 ml fluid for AFP testing. If other studies are to be done, syringes are changed without disturbing the needle. Occasionally there is an impediment to flow that is usually corrected by rotating the needle gently. Rarely is it necessary to reintroduce the obturator or to attempt amniocentesis in another site. There are times when blood appears in the initial portion of the aspirate. This clears with a slightly deeper placement of the needle as a rule. If blood clots occlude the needle, it is best to attempt amniocentesis in another site or on another day.

Slow but steady aspiration of fluid is recommended for best results. If fluid is aspirated too rapidly, it is conceivable that the uterine

INFORMED CONSENT AND RELEASE

I, _____request that an amniocentesis be performed for the purpose of prenatal diagnosis.

I consent to the use of ultrasound examination prior to amniocentesis as an aid to determine location of the placenta (afterbirth) and placement of the needle.

I understand that 20 to 25 cc of amniotic fluid will be removed from my uterus by a needle puncture through my abdomen.

I understand that the major risk of the procedure is less than a 1 per cent chance of spontaneous abortion.

I understand that the successful completion of the test is not guaranteed as it is dependent upon satisfactory growth of cells. I also understand that the accuracy of the test is dependent upon the growth of fetal cell rather than maternal cells (cells from the mother). I understand that the chance of this problem occurring is also less than 1 per cent.

The test is being performed for the purpose of detecting _____
_____in my unborn child.

It is my desire that a test also be attempted on the same cells to determine if there is anything unusual about the chromosomes of my unborn child. I understand that any finding will be explained to me. (Initials) _____

It is my desire that a test be performed to determine the level of alpha fetoprotein in the amniotic fluid with the understanding that this may detect the presence of certain other birth defects as "neural closure defects." I understand that any finding other than normal will be explained to me. (Initials) _____

I realize that this test will only identify the conditions named above and does not guarantee a normal, healthy baby.

I understand that after completion of the diagnostic tests, some of the sample may be saved for research purposes.

Signature: _____

Witness: _____Date: _____

Revised 5/76

Figure 2. Form for informed consent and release developed by Schwarz and Mennuti. Used by permission of the American College of Obstetricians and Gynecologists.

wall could contract sufficiently to dislodge the placenta, resulting in abortion. This is thought to have been the cause of the only abortion attributed to amniocentesis in the series of approximately 450 studies in my experience.

The risk for spontaneous abortion resulting from amniocentesis has been reported as between 0.1 and 1.0 per cent.[17, 18] I quote the risk of 1 in 250 to my patients.

For my peace of mind, a Doppler instrument is used to auscultate fetal heart tones before and after the procedure. The patient and her husband are also reassured by hearing their fetus' heartbeat. As soon as possible, fluid is centrifuged and the clear supernatant is submitted to laboratory for AFP testing. If fluid cannot be processed within 24 hours, it is frozen in a standard freezer at 0 degrees C until it can be processed. The cell button is saved for fetal hemoglobin assay, especially if AFP level is elevated. It is clear how contamination of amniotic fluid with fetal blood could significantly alter AFP concentrations, since the concentration gradient between fetal' serum and amniotic fluid is 150 to 200 to 1.

It is also clinically important to be aware of fetal blood contamination, especially in Rh-negative women. If blood does contaminate the fluid, it is certainly possible that a feto-maternal transfusion has occurred. Whenever this happens, it is recommended that Rho(D) immune globulin (RhoGAM) be administered to the mother to prevent Rh antibody production by her reticuloendothelial system. Once the mother's immune system is challenged by the Rh antigen, repeated challenges during pregnancy provoke larger quantities of Rh antibody production resulting in fetal erythroblastosis. Passive immunization by 300 μg RhoGAM should prevent the initial challenge to the maternal reticuloendothelial system without significantly affecting fetal red blood cells.

Some mention of those conditions other than fetal neural tube defects that are associated with elevated amniotic fluid AFP has already been made. With this in mind, some workers in the field recommend that amniocentesis for AFP testing be done on all patients with a history of a previous infant with congenital nephrosis or with gastrointestinal or abdominal wall defects. Some workers even recommend amniocentesis if there is a history of these conditions or of neural tube defects in close relatives.[19]

This discussion concludes with the recounting of two patients' problems, their evaluation and management as examples of fetal structural defects detected in mid trimester. One involved a neural tube defect while in the other a condition confused with a neural tube defect occurred.

CASE REPORTS

Case 1. In conjunction with my colleagues Morgan, Haney, and Phillips, I reported the case of a 26-year-old gravida 4, para 3–1–1, whose third pregnancy had produced a premature stillborn female with an encephalocele and a cystic hygroma. Because of the increased risk of recurring neural tube defect, amniocentesis for AFP testing was performed at 16 weeks after preliminary ultrasonography revealed a large cystic structure extending from the fetal vertex to the upper thoracic spine (Fig. 3). The mass appeared symmetrical and located directly posterior to the fetal skull, cervical spine and upper thoracic spine. Amniography confirmed the characteristics of the mass (Fig. 4). Even though no bony defect was demonstrable, the size of the mass coupled with the previous history and an AFP level in the amniotic fluid of 22.9 µg per ml (14.8 to 23.0, normal range at 16 weeks) led to the interpretation of recurring encephalocele or cervical spina bifida. The patient and her husband were offered interruption of pregnancy via hypertonic saline injection, which they accepted.

At delivery the fetus demonstrated a large cystic structure precisely as described by ultrasonography and amniography. Postmortem fetal x-rays failed to reveal a spinal or true skull defect (Fig. 5). Microscopic sections of the mass were consistent with classical findings of a cystic hygroma (Fig. 6).

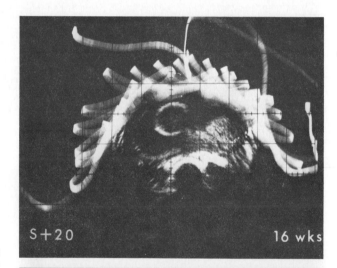

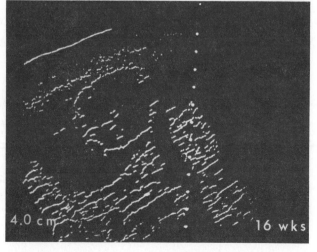

Figure 3. Ultrasonography of large cystic structure extending from fetal vertex to upper thoracic spine.

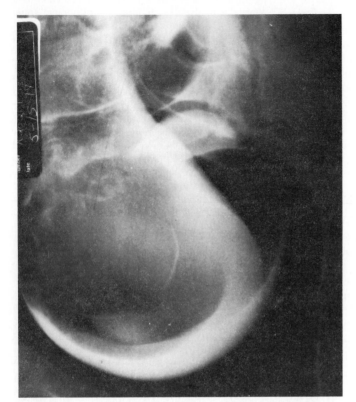

Figure 4. Amniography of mass.

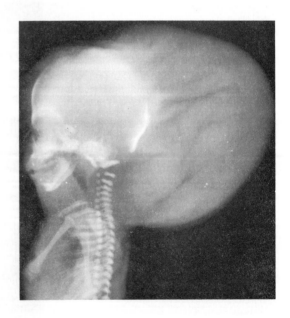

Figure 5. Postmortem fetal skull x-ray that showed no spinal or true skull defect.

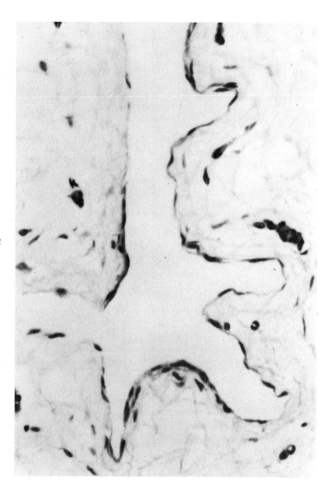

Figure 6. Microscopic characteristics of cystic hygroma.

Given the same set of circumstances, even without a grossly elevated amniotic fluid AFP, it is anticipated that identical management would be offered.

Case 2. This 36-year-old woman underwent amniocentesis at 16 weeks after ultrasonography for antenatal karyotypic analysis. Fetal skull echoes were absent and fetal age was estimated on the basis of poor transthoracic measurements ranging from 33 to 40 mm (Fig. 7). Amniotic fluid AFP was measured at 295 μg per ml, a level approximately 20 log standard deviations above the mean for 16 weeks' gestation.

The findings were explained to the couple, who asked for and received interruption of pregnancy via hypertonic saline injection. Anencephaly was confirmed at the time of abortion. Karyotypic analysis was normal on the amniotic fluid cell cultures.

These two patients illustrate the procedures used in evaluation of pregnancy at risk for neural tube defects. Furthermore, these cases illustrate examples of true positive findings and false positive findings.

Conclusion

The practical application of amniotic fluid AFP testing in conjunction with careful ultrasonographic studies is accepted as the most accurate technique in midtrimester detection of neural tubal defects. This approach is recommended for all patients at risk, including those with previous history of neural tube defects in themselves or in their offspring, those with previous history of hydrocephaly in their offspring, and those having amniocentesis done in mid trimester for any other reason. Additionally, the combined use of ultrasonography and amniotic fluid AFP testing is recommended for all patients with previous offspring having gastroschisis, esophageal atresia or congenital nephrosis.

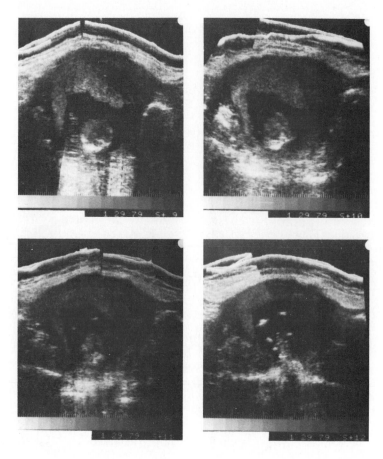

Figure 7. Estimation of fetal age by ultrasonography.

REFERENCES

1. Brock, D. J. H.: The prenatal diagnosis of neural tube defects. Ob-Gyn Surv. 31:32, 1976.
2. Christakos, A. C. and Simpson, J. L.: Anencephaly in three siblings. Obstet. Gynecol. 33:267, 1969.
3. Milunsky, A. and Alpert, E.: Antenatal diagnosis, alpha-fetoprotein and the FDA. N. Engl. J. Med. 295:168, 1976.
4. Cassady, G. and Cailliteau, J.: The amniotic fluid in anencephaly. Am. J. Obstet. Gynecol. 97:395, 1967.
5. Lee, T. J. and Wei, P. Y.: Spectrophotometric analyses of amniotic fluid in anencephalic pregnancies. Am. J. Obstet. Gynecol. 107:917, 1970.
6. Brock, D. J. H. and Sutcliffe, R. G.: Alpha-fetoprotein in the antenatal diagnosis of anencephaly and spina bifida. Lancet 2:197, 1972.
7. Hunter, A., Hammerton, J. L., Baskett, T. and Lyons, E.: Raised amniotic fluid alpha-fetoprotein in Turner syndrome. Lancet 1:598, 1976.
8. Seller, J. J., Creasy, M. R. and Alberman, E. D.: Alpha-fetoprotein levels in amniotic fluids from spontaneous abortions. Br. Med. J. 1:524, 1974.
9. Morgan, C. L., Haney, A. F., Christakos, A. C. and Phillips, J.: Antenatal detection of fetal structural defects with ultrasound. J. Clin. Ultrasound 3:287, 1975.
10. Seppälä, M., Karjalainen, O., Rapola, J. et al.: Maternal alpha-fetoprotein and fetal exomphalos. Lancet 1:303, 1976.
11. Seppälä, M. and Lindgren, J.: Alpha-fetoprotein in normal and abnormal gestation. *In* Peeters, H. (ed.): Protides of Biological Fluids, 24th Colloquium. Oxford, Pergamon Press, 1976.
12. Seppälä, M., Rapola, J., Huttunen, N. et al.: Congenital nephrotic syndrome: prenatal diagnosis and genetic counseling by estimation of amniotic fluid and maternal serum alpha-fetoprotein. Lancet 2:123, 1976.
13. Laurence, K. M.: Effect of early surgery for spina bifida cystica on survival and quality of life. Lancet 1:301, 1974.
14. Smith, A. D., Wold, N. J., Cuckle, H. S., Stirrat, G. M., Bobrow, M. and Lagerkrantz, H.: Amniotic fluid acetylcholinesterase as a possible diagnostic test for neural tube defects in early pregnancy. Lancet 1:685, 1979.
15. Milford-Ward, A.: The clinical relevance of alpha-fetoprotein in maternal serum in pregnancy. *In* Peeters, H. (ed.): Protides of Biological Fluids, 24th Colloquium. Oxford, Pergamon Press, 1976.
16. Cohen, T., Stern, E. and Rosenmann, A.: Sib risk of neural tube defect: is prenatal diagnosis indicated

in pregnancies following birth of a hydrocephalic child? J. Med. Genet. 16:14, 1979.

17. Lowe, C. U., Alexander, D., Bryla, D. and Seigel, D.: The safety and accuracy of mid-trimester amniocentesis. The NICHD Amniocentesis Registry. U.S. Dept. of HEW Public Health Service, Publication No. (NIH) 78–190, 1978.

18. Chayen, S. (ed.): An assessment of the hazards of amniocentesis. Report to the Medical Research Council by their working party on amniocentesis. Br. J. Obstet. Gynecol. 85: (Suppl) 2:1, 1978.

19. Johnson, A. M. et al.: Amniotic fluid alpha-fetoprotein levels in antenatal diagnosis of neural tube defects. N.C. Med. J. 39:98, 1978.

Editorial Comment

These articles are related and yet unrelated for a controversy chapter. The article on prenatal detection of chromosomal abnormalities indicates in its content that the author has never seen a case in which the antenatal diagnosis of sex and the diagnosis of sex at birth proved to be different. I thought this could not occur until three years ago. I performed an amniocentesis on a physician because of advanced age, who was a physician's wife, and lo and behold, the antenatal results showed a normal female karyotype, but at the time of birth the child was a boy. When I saw the mother the next time two years later for her next pregnancy, she said, "I thought you would like to know that the normal girl you predicted by antenatal diagnosis had a penis." It's obvious that what grew out of the sample was maternal cells, undoubtedly from a needle track, perhaps from either the uterus or the abdominal wall. Because of this I no longer tell people that we're absolutely positive as to sex, as there are exceptions that we all want to forget about. We think this problem has now been solved by the use of a small Whitaker No. 23 gauge needle with a stylet. It is now necessary to aspirate amniotic fluid instead of having free flow with the larger needle that we used at that time.

One item of omission in these chapters is the fact that somewhere up to 4 per cent of offspring will have some form of congenital anomaly; hence, on antenatal diagnosis it would always seem wise to emphasize to the patient precisely what antenatal diagnosis does predict and following that statement to say that there are other anomalies that cannot be identified by conventional methods of karyotyping, amniotic fluid analysis and ultrasound. Everybody knows this, but it should be underscored that it is an important point to make to the patient on each genetic consultation.

The finding of ambiguous genitalia in a child is often devastating for the parents, but, interestingly, the anomaly may go unnoticed unless careful examination is done. It is most important not to make snap decisions, but to work the problem up in a scientific manner and also give the parents much support. Culturing the lymphocytes of a newborn baby does not take too long and it determines whether or not the child is an XY, XX, or mosaic; this would be the first important item to know for counseling. If there is a great deal of compulsion to name the baby, the excellent suggestion was made by Simpson for the parents to choose a name that could either be for a boy or a girl, such as Chris, Frances, Lee, Hilary. A statement once made was that if in doubt raise the child as a girl as it is easier to cope with such problems in women, but that's not good enough at the present time. We now have sophisticated ways to find out precisely the gender identity.

Articles in this chapter are welcome additions to controversies, but the disputed matter actually does not rest with the articles themselves. The problem is, "Is it a boy or a girl?" or "Is the baby normal or is it abnormal?" There are no overriding, sweeping generalizations that can be made about counseling except to remember that statistics are great to lean on, but when it comes to the individual patient, either the patient has the problem or does not have it—0 to 100 per cent. That is the stark reality we face each time we counsel a patient. The one thing we all know is the more we look, the more we find. If we ignore the patient's problem, sweeping statements can be made that there really are few difficulties and such identifications and scientific work-up really aren't necessary. That no longer is a controversy, as we now have available tools to give precise definitions to the parents.

Once the precise definitions are given, the hard work begins, and that is to counsel the family on what is best for their individual situation at the time. I happen to believe that it's necessary for physicians to help patients solve problems, but I'm not implying by saying this that the physician makes the decision on what a patient should do. However, patients, even with the best objective knowledge, have to have some help. It's best to present the objective data to the patient about the particular problem and not expect or insist on them making a decision at that time. It takes time for them to digest the facts and address their problem; there are many personal ramifications for each patient.

The next visit should include an additional review of the problem. Then the physician should try to learn whether the patient needs any other facts in helping arrive at the proper conclusion. Judgments on these very deep personal, moral and emotional problems take time, and there is no shortcut for this. It is part of the physician's responsibility and obligation to help the family arrive at what they feel is an equitable and sound decision for them at that time and then support the decision. I think you'll find that if counseling is done in this manner, patients will be forever grateful to you, no matter how major the problem seems.

Some physicians feel they do not want to become this emotionally involved in a particular issue with the patient and ask for guidance and help from other professionals. These other professionals maybe do not understand the problem as well as they should, and often erroneous information is given. If physicians are unable to cope with these problems themselves, then it would be my suggestion that they not become involved in caring for these patients but refer them for specialized consultations. The complaint that we frequently hear occurs when the patient is referred to an important consultant and the consultant always seems to be too busy to sit down and take the time necessary for human counseling. The secret in handling these problems, if you do not do it yourself, is to choose a wise, concerned consultant who knows how to hold a patient's hand, look her in the eye, and tell her things that nobody really wants to hear, and understand how she feels about it. These people are hard to come by, but they are there. The question is, are you going to be the one or are you going to try to find one?

12
Second Trimester Abortion

Alternative Points of View

by William E. Brenner
by David A. Grimes and Carl W. Tyler, Jr.

Editorial Comment

The Appropriate Use of Prostaglandins in Induction of Labor and Interruption of Pregnancy

William E. Brenner, M.D.

Chapel Hill, North Carolina

To use prostaglandins appropriately, the physician must be aware of their general chemistry, physiologic role, pharmacologic properties and appropriate uses. With this information he can appropriately use prostaglandins and understand the complications of their use as well as the benefits.

Chemistry

Prostaglandins are synthesized from arachidonic acid and rapidly metabolized to inactive substances in most tissues. Essentially, all tissues studied have the capability of converting arachidonic acid to prostaglandin E_2 or prostaglandin $F_{2\alpha}$ or both. They are catabolized in most tissues. The effects of exogenously administered prostaglandins are short, because about 90 per cent of prostaglandin E_2 and $F_{2\alpha}$ are metabolized in one circulation through the lungs.[1] Constant or repeated systemic administration is necessary to accomplish effects. However, reactions from systemic dosages are usually rapidly alleviated because of the rapid metabolism.

Physiology

Natural prostaglandins apparently play an important role in the normal physiology and pathophysiology of the fetus and the mother. In physiologic and pathologic conditions, prostaglandins probably act at a local level rather than acting through systemic circulation. Prostaglandins act as local regulators by (1) contracting smooth muscle, (2) altering exocrine and endocrine gland excretion and (3) affecting neurologic conduction through altering the release of substances such as epinephrine, norenephrine and acetycholine[2] (Fig. 1).

The physiologic actions are unknown for three reasons: the effects of prostaglandins are local, the concentrations at the local sites are unknown and all of the circumstances of the "local climate" are unknown. Since most of our hypotheses are derived from measurements of systemic levels of prostaglandins in physiologic and pathologic conditions and the observations of effects of infusing pharmacologic doses, they are probably incorrect. However, prostaglandins appear pertinent to autoregulation and pathophysiology.[2]

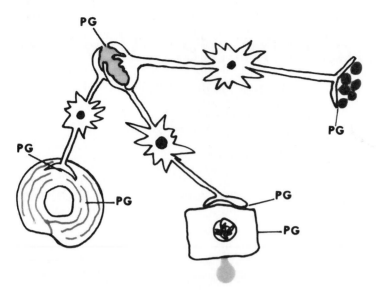

Figure 1. Actions of prostaglandins.

Natural prostaglandins may express themselves in normal physiology and pathophysiology by an absence or decrease in production, excessive production, production of inappropriate proportions of different types and inadequate metabolism. Although it is thought that prostaglandins play an important role in all physiologic and pathophysiologic circumstances in obstetrics, there is no adequate information to justify this speculation. Specifically, there is a small amount of information suggesting that prostaglandins play a role in the fetus for maintaining blood flow in the umbilical vessels and the ductus arteriosus and maintaining uterine blood flow. Interference with the production of prostaglandins may be important in the genesis of preeclampsia. Initiation and maintenance of labor, especially as it relates to uterine contractions and cervical dilatation, may be important effects of endogenous prostaglandins.

We in obstetrics and gynecology have been able to exploit only two capacities of prostaglandins: their capacity to induce delivery at every stage of gestation, and their capacity to induce cervical dilatation. These reactions may not be distinct from each other. Since prostaglandins ordinarily produce their effects at a local level and in most organ systems, pharmacologic administration of significant systemic levels ordinarily results in many undesirable effects as well as the desired effect. Fortunately, since prostaglandins are rapidly metabolized to inactive substances, the side effects resolve rapidly once the drug is discontinued. However, to accomplish effects

through systemic administration, a relatively high administration rate has to be maintained to counteract the rapid metabolism rate.

How prostaglandins affect delivery at any time of pregnancy is unknown. An important aspect is prostaglandins' oxytoxic property, and their ability to initiate and maintain uterine contractions can be explained by the hypothesis illustrated in Figure 2.

Prostaglandin E_2 and prostaglandin $F_{2\alpha}$ increase the intracellular free calcium concentration of the myometrial cell by freeing calcium from the reticulum. This results in myometrial contraction. Myometrial contraction results in conversion of inactive phospholipase from stable lysosomes into active phospholipase A_2. Phospholipase A_2 acting on the fetal membrane converts an esterified "inactive" arachidonic acid to free arachidonic acid. Free arachidonic acid is converted to prostaglandin E_2 and $F_{2\alpha}$ in the decidua.[3] In this manner, a continuing cycle of uterine contractility occurs that is compatible with labor.

Pharmacology

The property of prostaglandin to induce delivery at any stage of gestation is more than one of merely inducing contractility. Although prostaglandins are effective oxytoxic agents and are exceedingly effective in inducing uterine contractions at all stages of gestation, similar types of uterine contractility can be produced with extremely high doses of oxytocin. Yet oxytocin rarely causes delivery in spite of

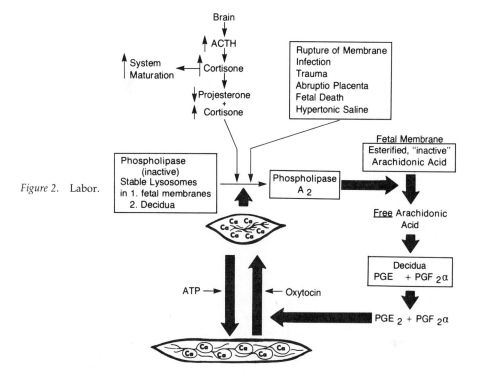

Figure 2. Labor.

high myometrial contractility over several days' duration, except in the term patient. In contrast, prostaglandins cause delivery in a short period of time, indicating that they possess important properties that make them effective abortifacients and dilators of the cervix, in addition to their ability to cause uterine contractility.[4]

Induction of Labor

Although prostaglandins are as effective as oxytocin for inducing labor, the incidence of hypercontractility with prostaglandins may result in increased morbidity. In the doses necessary to induce at term, prostaglandins are well tolerated orally; this is more convenient than oxytocin administration. Buccal oxytocin is often not effective and constant intravenous infusions are inconvenient. However, hypercontractility may occur more frequently with prostaglandins.[5]

For *elective induction* of term labor in patients in whom the cervix is partially dilated, well effaced and has a total Bishop's score greater than 7, the only benefit of using prostaglandin rather than oxytocin is that it can be given orally (Fig. 3). In the study illustrated in Figure 3, over 80 per cent of patients

delivered, independent of whether oxytocin or prostaglandin was used.

The disadvantage of oral prostaglandin is that hypercontractility may be more common than with the use of continuous intravenous infusion of oxytocin.[5] Ordinarily, the hyper-

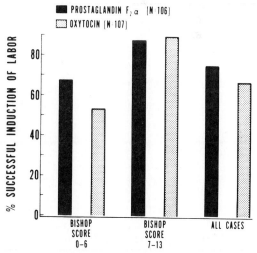

Figure 3. Comparison between intravenous prostaglandin $F_{2\alpha}$ and oxytocin for the induction of labor at term (N = 213). (From Spellacy, W. N. et al.: Prostaglandin $F_{2\alpha}$ and Oxytocin for Term Labor Induction. *In* The Prostaglandins. Clinical Applications in Human Reproduction. Symposia Specialists, Inc., Post Office Box 610397, Miami, Florida 33161.

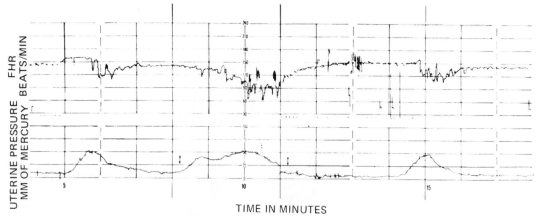

Figure 4. Reversible hypercontractility with prostaglandins. Illustration of hypertonicity that occurred on PGF_2 causing prolonged contraction and that resulted in temporary fetal bradycardia. Reduction in dose rate immediately corrected the situation. (From Vakhariya, V. R. and Sherman, A. I.: Prostaglandin $F_{2\alpha}$ for induction of labor. Am. J. Obstet. Gynecol. 113:219, 1972.)

contractility occurs shortly after the initiation of prostaglandin infusion and disappears rapidly when it is discontinued, and the fetal heart rate pattern returns to one that is not associated with fetal distress, as in Figure 4.[6]

However, on occasion hypercontractility may continue even after the prostaglandin is discontinued, even when administered by intravenous infusion. Fetal distress may continue until fetal death occurs, as illustrated in Figure 5.[5]

In summary, for the elective induction of labor, it does not appear appropriate to use prostaglandin rather than oxytocin even

though it is more convenient to administer. It has a rate of effectiveness that is similar to intravenous oxytocin, and hypercontractility may be more common with its use. However, as experience increases, this opinion may change.

INDICATED INDUCTION OF LABOR

Prostaglandins may be slightly more effective than oxytocin for inducing labor and delivery in patients for *nonelective* "indicated" reasons. Ordinarily, these patients have an

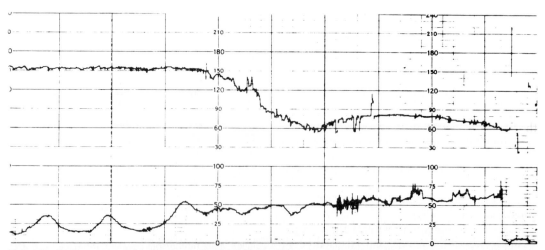

Figure 5. Hypercontractility with prostaglandins. Fetal monitor tracing demonstrating uterine hypertonicity and fetal bradycardia during a prostaglandin $F_{2\alpha}$ induction of labor. The upper line denotes the fetal heart rate in beats per min. and the lower line represents amniotic fluid pressure in mm Hg. The infusion (rate 20 μg/min of $PGF_{2\alpha}$) had been discontinued prior to this segment of the tracing. (From Spellacy, W. N. et al.: Prostaglandin $F_{2\alpha}$ and oxytocin for term labor induction. In Southern, E. M. (ed.): The Prostaglandins. Mt. Kisco, N.Y., Futura Pub. Co., 1972, p. 111.)

"unripe" cervix with a Bishop's score of 6 or less. Although there was not a statistically significant difference in the study results depicted in Figure 3,[5] larger series may eventually demonstrate that prostaglandins are more effective than oxytocin in these patients. However, hypercontractility may be especially dangerous in these patients because they are usually having induction for medical conditions and they have a compromised fetus. Prostaglandins have also been used to "ripen" the cervix before induction by either oxytocin or prostaglandin. No conclusive benefits have been demonstrated for this approach. In summary, there are no data to indicate that it is appropriate for the obstetrician to use prostaglandins for nonelective induction of labor. However, it may eventually be demonstrated that prostaglandins are slightly more effective than oxytocin in these patients. If this happens, the risk-to-benefit ratio of utilizing prostaglandins rather than oxytocin for the small proportion of patients who will deliver with prostaglandins, but not deliver with oxytocin, or for use in patients to "ripen" the cervix prior to oxytocin induction must be evaluated against the increased risk of hypercontractility.

INDUCTION WHEN A DEAD FETUS IS ANTICIPATED

The use of prostaglandins is most appropriate for inducing delivery after the first trimester when a dead fetus is anticipated. Prostaglandins are useful for managing patients with:

1. Death in utero
2. Severe congenital abnormalities
3. Severe maternal disease incompatible with childbirth
4. Large molar pregnancies
5. Premature rupture of the membranes in the previable period
6. Need for therapeutic abortion

The only methods approved by the Food and Drug Administration are (1) intra-amniotic administration of prostaglandin $F_{2\alpha}$ for the termination of gestation in the second trimester; (2) prostaglandin E_2 in vaginal suppositories (20 mg) for these indications: termination of pregnancy from the twelfth week of gestation through the second trimester, termination of missed abortion or intrauterine fetal death to the twenty-eighth week of gestation, and termination of nonmetastatic gestational trophoblastic disease (benign hydatidiform mole);

and (3) intramuscular administration of 15-Me prostaglandin $F_{2\alpha}$ for induction of abortion. However, I will discuss my impressions based upon limited trials, since it is anticipated that some analogues may be available in the future.

Several routes and rates of prostaglandin administration are practicable. Oral administration is unsatisfactory because of the high incidence of vomiting and diarrhea with the levels necessary to cause induction in patients before term. Intra-amniotic, extra-amniotic and vaginal administration of prostaglandin $F_{2\alpha}$ and prostaglandin E_2 is practicable, as is intramuscular and vaginal administration of analogues.

Induction of Abortion

INTRA-AMNIOTIC ADMINISTRATION

Intra-amniotic administration of prostaglandin $F_{2\alpha}$ is appropriate for induction of midtrimester abortion after 16 weeks' gestation and is approved by the Food and Drug Administration. Dilatation and surgical evacuation are ordinarily the preferred methods before 16 weeks' gestation because of effectiveness, rapid action and relatively low morbidity.[7]

Intra-amniotic administration is appropriately accomplished by one of two methods. In both, sterile technique is used. One technique consists of insertion of an 18 thin wall-spinal type needle and of a flexible catheter into the amniotic fluid, through which serial doses of prostaglandin may be administered without repeated amniocentesis. The other technique consists of insertion of a 22-gauge spinal needle to perform the amniocentesis for drug administration, and removal of the needle. Repeat amniocentesis is necessary if more doses are to be administered—this is advantageous in about 20 per cent of patients. With both techniques, the drug is administered in the same manner. A small test dose of 5 mg is administered slowly, followed by 35 mg administered slowly about 5 minutes later if there are no adverse effects from the test dose.[8]

Intra-amniotic administration of prostaglandin $F_{2\alpha}$ is more effective than other unaugmented methods and is as effective as other augmented medical methods for inducing midtrimester abortion (Fig. 6).

As compared with other commonly used medical methods (hypertonic saline, hyper-

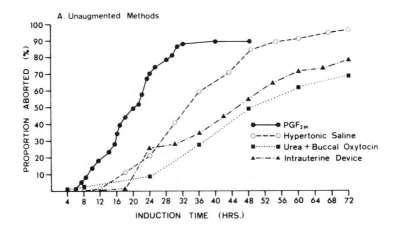

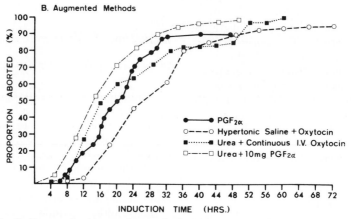

Figure 6. Prostaglandin $F_{2\alpha}$ vs. other intrauterine methods. (1) Intrauterine devices–Karman coils, balsa, catheters–77 subjects.[9] (2) Urea with buccal oxytocin–50 subjects having induction with 80 g of intra-amniotic urea and a course of buccal oxytocin 24 hours later.[10] (3) Hypertonic saline–306 patients having induction with 200 ml of 20% saline.[7] (4) $PGF_{2\alpha}$–42 patients having induction with an initial intra-amniotic dose of 40 mg of $PGF_{2\alpha}$ with a 20 mg dose 24 hours later.[7] (5) Hypertonic saline plus continuous intravenous oxytocin–3943 patients treated with intra-amniotic administration of about 200 ml of 20% hypertonic saline and a continuous intravenous infusion of about 200 mu of oxytocin per minute.[7] (6) Urea plus continuous intravenous oxytocin–30 patients induced with 80 g of intra-amniotic urea and the continuous intravenous infusion of 138 or 276 mu of oxytocin per minute.[11] Urea plus $PGF_{2\alpha}$–150 patients induced with 80 g of urea and 10 mg of $PGF_{2\alpha}$ intra-amniotically with intravenous oxytocin 24 hours later.[12] (From Brenner, W. E. and Berger, G. S.: Risks, Benefits and Controversies in Fertility Control. In Sciara, J. J., Zatuchni, G. L., and Speidel, J. J. (eds.): Advances in Female Sterilization Techniques. Harper and Row, Hagerstown, Maryland. pp. 292–321, 1977.[8])

tonic saline augmented with prostaglandin $F_{2\alpha}$ and hypertonic urea augmented with prostaglandin $F_{2\alpha}$), the intra-amniotic administration of prostaglandin $F_{2\alpha}$ alone appears to have a similar degree of safety under controlled conditions (Table 1).

Comparing prostaglandin $F_{2\alpha}$ with hypertonic saline, disseminated intravascular coagulation and infection are less common, and blood transfusion and major operative intervention are necessary less often. Cervical injury, retained placenta and gastrointestinal side effects of nausea and vomiting are more common with prostaglandin $F_{2\alpha}$. Compared with the combination of urea plus intra-am-

niotic prostaglandin $F_{2\alpha}$, blood transfusion, cervical injury, retained placenta and side effects of nausea and vomiting and diarrhea are less common. Compared with the combination of saline plus prostaglandin $F_{2\alpha}$, blood transfusion is less frequently needed and coagulopathy is less common with the prostaglandin $F_{2\alpha}$ method.[15]

There are hypothetical reasons to believe that prostaglandins may be safer in patients with specific problems such as cardiac, renal, metabolic and clotting abnormalities. The infusion of prostaglandin $F_{2\alpha}$ in high doses that could be a result of inadvertent intravascular administration does not usually result in significant cardiovascular effects. Significant hematologic changes and coagulation and intravascular volume changes do not occur after prostaglandin administration as they do with hypertonic saline and hypertonic urea administration.[16] However, constriction of the bronchi occurs with high systemic doses of prostaglandin $F_{2\alpha}$. This is a rare, potentially serious complication of high systemic doses of prostaglandin $F_{2\alpha}$. The other complications of prostaglandin use (cervical injury, uterine rupture, retained placenta) appear to result from prostaglandin's oxytoxic property.[2]

Unfortunately, the safety of prostaglandin $F_{2\alpha}$ methods as they are used in clinical prac-

tice does not appear to be as reliable as it is in controlled studies (Table 2). Clinical practice safety depends upon at least (1) complications of the drug per se, (2) abortion process initiated, and (3) management by the physician. Prospective survey studies, which have many variables and biases, indicate that prostaglandin $F_{2\alpha}$ used in clinical practice, when augmented with oxytocin and given by several different methods, may be less safe than hypertonic saline and urea. Although complications appear to be more common with prostaglandin $F_{2\alpha}$ than with saline, the death rate is higher with saline.

The prostaglandin $F_{2\alpha}$ method alone or aug-

TABLE 1. COMPLICATION RATES OF MIDTRIMESTER INTRA-AMNIOTIC INSTILLATION ABORTION METHODS

COMPLICATION	SALINE* 20% (N = 314) (%)	$PGF_{2\alpha}$* (N = 328) (%)	UREA† + $PGF_{2\alpha}$ (N = 150) (%)	SALINE‡ + $PGF_{2\alpha}$ (N = 500) (%)
Death	0.0	0.0	0.0	0.0
Hemorrhage requiring transfusion	2.2	1.4	7.5	2.0
Consumptive coagulopathy	0.3	0.0	0.0	1.4
Cervical injury	1.0	1.4	4.0	0.0
Anesthesia	0.0	2.2	NR	0.0
Fever	15.6	8.5	NR	NR
Treated with antibiotics	8.3	6.1	NR	NR
Not treated with antibiotics	6.1	2.4	NR	NR
Pelvic infection	2.9	0.3	7.3	3.9
Convulsions	0.0	0.6	NR	0.0
Bronchospasm	0.0	1.0	NR	0.4
Other§	3.4	4.7	NR	NR
One or more major complications	4.8	5.0	NR	7.2
Major operative intervention	2.2	1.3	0.0	0.8
Side effects				
Vomiting	8.9	36.3		73
Diarrhea	5.7	15.6	70	45
Number of women with any side effect or complication	59.3*	55.8*	NR	73

*Unpublished data are from an International Fertility Research Program randomized study.[12]

†Burkman et al.: Am. J. Obstet. Gynecol. 126:328, 1976. Intravenous oxytocin was initiated in 24 hours if abortion had not occurred.[13]

‡Kerenyi, T. et al. Personal communication. Oxytocin was initiated when labor began.[14]

§Includes dizziness, pain, vaginal discharge or prolonged bleeding not diagnosed as hemorrhage, tachycardia, bradycardia and diaphoresis, or chills without fever.

NR = Not reported.

From Brenner, W. E.: Artificial abortion of early midtrimester pregnancy with commercially available prostaglandin. Program for Applied Research on Fertility Regulation, April 19, 1978.

TABLE 2. COMPLICATION RATES OF MID-TRIMESTER ABORTIONS BASED ON SURVEILLANCE STUDIES

COMPLICATIONS	UREA-PGF$_{2\alpha}$ (+ OXYTOCIN AFTER 24 HRS) (N = 150) [13]	SALINE-PGF$_{2\alpha}$ (+ OXYTOCIN AT ACTIVE LABOR) (N = 500)	SALINE W/O OXYTOCIN (N = 307) [14]	SALINE + OXYTOCIN (N = 3,945)	SALINE + OR W/O OXYTOCIN (N = 10,013)	PGF$_{2\alpha}$ MOST + OXYTOCIN (N = 1,241) [17,7,18,19]	D & E 13–20 WKS (N = 6,213)	D & E 13–15 WKS (N = 152) [20]	SALINE 16–18 WKS (N = 442) [18,21]	HYSTEROTOMY (N = 942)	HYSTERECTOMY (N = 813) [18,21]
Uterine perforation (%)	0.0	0.0	0.0	0.03	0.1	NR	0.3	0.0	0.0	NA	NA
Cervical injury (%)	4.0	0.0	0.0	0.1	0.6	NR	1.2	3.3	0.7	NA	NA
Hemorrhage[c] requiring transfusion (%)	7.5	2.0	0.3	0.7	1.9	5.8	0.2	0.7	0.9	1.7	2.6
Infection/fever (%)	7.3	3.9	4.2	6.0	7.4	13.3	2.4	3.3	7.9	38.6	47.2
Anesthesia-related[a] (%)	NA	NA	NA	NA	NA	NA	NR	2.0	0.0	0.7	2.7
"Retained products" (%)	46.7**	41.8	28.0*	41.4*	28.3	36.1	0.9	4.6	23.1	0.3	0.1
Women with one or more major complications[b]	NR	7.2	1.3	2.0	1.8	2.9	0.7	0.0	0.7	8.1	15.4

From Brenner.[7]
*Rate of placental retention 1 hr after fetal expulsion.
**Rate of placental retention 2 hrs after fetal expulsion.
[a]General anesthesia, [b]As defined by each author, [c]Blood loss >500 cc.

mented with hypertonic urea or saline is much safer than hysterotomy or hysterectomy in clinical practice (Table 3).[18, 21] Even when an intra-amniotic prostaglandin $F_{2\alpha}$ abortion is followed by laparoscopy or "minilap" sterilization, the morbidity is lower than with hysterotomy or hysterectomy. Hysterotomy and hysterectomy are rarely indicated and should be reserved for patients in whom the procedure is medically indicated because of complications or underlying pathology.

Use of cervical dilatation and surgical evacuation (D&E) in the 13- to 15-week period appears safer than postponing the abortion until 16 weeks' gestation and performing it with intra-amniotic methods[20] (Tables 2, 3). D&E also appears safer in the 13- to 20-week period in the hands of some obstetricians than intra-amniotic methods when performed by some investigators.[17] However, after 14 weeks' gestation, large Pratt dilators or intracervical laminaria tents and special forceps are necessary for safe evacuation.

The long-term effects of abortion by intra-amniotic methods are unknown. Cervical incompetency, prematurity and placenta previa are probably more common after midtrimester abortion than after term delivery or first trimester abortion. Whether these complications are more common after acute mechanical dilatation by either dilators or intracervical laminaria tents or by pharmacologic methods is unknown.

Under specific circumstances it appears appropriate to augment intra-amniotic prostaglandin $F_{2\alpha}$ with oxytoxics, hypertonic solutions or intracervical laminaria tents or all these.

Although higher rates of uterine injury and retained placenta probably occur when the potent oxytoxic prostaglandin is further augmented with oxytocin, it is appropriate to give intravenous oxytocin to obtain an adequate amount of uterine contractility when the dosage of intra-amniotic $F_{2\alpha}$ is no longer effective. For example, ordinarily insignificant levels of intra-amniotic prostaglandin $F_{2\alpha}$ are found six hours after administration and after the membranes have ruptured. Institution of intravenous oxytocin in these cases at levels to obtain adequate uterine contractility is warranted to prevent unnecessary delay in abortion, because such delay results in increased chance of infection.[7]

The advantages of augmenting intra-amniotic prostaglandin $F_{2\alpha}$ with hypertonic solutions are that smaller doses of prostaglandin may be used, and there are lower rates of fetuses born with signs of life. These potential advantages must be balanced against the increased risk of complications of using hypertonic solutions of saline, urea, alcohol or mannitol in deciding whether to augment prostaglandin with these solutions.

Insertion of intracervical laminaria appears to be an appropriate method of augmenting intra-amniotic prostaglandin $F_{2\alpha}$. Insertion of laminaria either in the afternoon before the next morning's injection[22] or concomitant with the prostaglandin $F_{2\alpha}$ injection[23] significantly shortens the time until abortion without apparently increasing the incidence of side effects and complications (Fig. 7). Although placement of intracervical laminaria may eventually be shown to decrease the incidence of cervical injury, it will not totally protect the cervix; cervical rupture has occurred with use of intracervical laminaria tents.

In summary, intra-amniotic administration of prostaglandin $F_{2\alpha}$ for termination of midtrimester pregnancy after 16 weeks' gestation is appropriate. It is more effective than other unaugmented methods and as effective as other augmented methods. When used appropriately, it is as safe as hypertonic saline and prostaglandin $F_{2\alpha}$ augmented with hypertonic urea or saline methods, and it is safer than major surgical methods. Although dilatation and evacuation with special equipment by some surgeons may be safer in patients with less than 20 weeks' gestation, prostaglandin $F_{2\alpha}$ may be safer for other practitioners.

VAGINAL ADMINISTRATION OF PROSTAGLANDIN E_2

Vaginal administration of prostaglandin E_2 for induction of abortion during the midtrimester after at least 14 weeks' gestation is appropriate under conditions in which intra-amniotic administration is not suitable. Prior to the 14 to 16-week period, dilatation and evacuation is ordinarily more satisfactory. In dosages effective enough to induce abortion, prostaglandin E_2 results in high rates of vomiting and diarrhea. Although the diarrhea can be attenuated to clinically acceptable rates with Lomotil, nausea and vomiting remain a significant problem even when prochlorperazine is administered. Absorption from the vagina is often unpredictable, especially after occurrence of rupture of the membranes or bleeding. Satisfactory rates of abortion oc-

TABLE 3. Rates of Indicators of Risk in Percent of Midtrimester Abortion Procedures Classified by Primary Procedure Based on Surveillance Studies

Indicators	Urea, PGF$_{2\alpha}$ + Oxytocin at 24 hrs (N = 150)	Saline, PGF$_{2\alpha}$ + Oxytocin at active labor (N = 500)	Saline w/o Oxytocin 16-24 wks (N = 307)	Saline + Oxytocin 16-24 wks (N = 3,945)	Saline +, w/o Oxytocin (N = 10,013)	PGF$_{2\alpha}$ Most + Oxytocin (N = 1,241)	D & E 13-20 wks (N = 6,213)	D & E 13-15 wks (N = 152)	Saline 16-18 wks (N = 442)	Hysterotomy (N = 942)	Hysterectomy (N = 813)
	(13)		(14)		(7,17,18,19)			(20)		(18,21)	(18,21)
Death* No./100,000	—	—	—	25.3	16.0	10.5	13.0	—	—	63	100
Major operative intervention (%)	0.0	0.8	0.0	0.1	0.1	0.6	0.2	0.7	0.0	NA	NA
Minor operative intervention (%)	NR	22.8	12.4	20.8	32.8	41.3	1.0	3.3	23.1	NA	NA
Hospital readmissions (%)	3.0	NR	0.3	0.5	1.4	2.9	1.16	3.9	1.8	NR	NR
Total complications (%)	NR	NR	9.8	11.7	27.2	NR	5.9 (13–16 wks.) 5.4 (17 + wks)	12.5	10.8	32.9	50.4
Median hospital days	NR	NR	2	2	2	NR	0.2	0.2	1.7	5	6

From Bremner.[7]

*Death rate = No. per 100,000 abortions, calculated only for denominations of 1000 or more. NR = Not reported; NA = Not applicable.

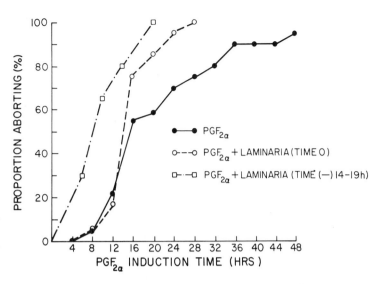

Figure 7. Cumulative abortion rate with laminaria-augmented intra-amniotic PGF$_{2\alpha}$ dose schedules. Eleven subjects received 40 mg of PGF$_{2\alpha}$ intra-amniotically 14 to 16 hours after placement of intracervical laminaria tents (PGF$_{2\alpha}$ + Laminaria [Time (−)14–19]).[22] Subjects[22] received intra-amniotic PGF$_{2\alpha}$ 25 mg initially with an identical dose at 6, 24, and 30 hours (PGF$_{2\alpha}$). Subjects[21] had intracervical laminaria tents placed immediately prior to the initiation of the same PGF$_{2\alpha}$ dose schedule (PGF$_{2\alpha}$ + Laminaria [Time 0]).[23] (From Brenner, W. E.: The current status of prostaglandins as abortifacients. Am. J. Obstet. Gynecol. 123:306–328, 1975.)

curred in *unaugmented* methods only when 20 mg prostaglandin E$_2$ suppositories were administered at a minimum of every 3 hours. With this dosage, 73 per cent of patients had vomiting, 45 per cent had diarrhea, and 63 per cent had transient oral temperature of greater than 100°F, all of which appeared drug-related; 64 per cent had incomplete abortion[2] (Fig. 8).

Because of the commonly occurring side effects, unpredictability of absorption and frequent need for intravenous oxytocin, vaginal administration is ordinarily appropriate only when intra-amniotic administration of prostaglandin F$_{2\alpha}$ or dilatation and evacuation is contraindicated.

INDUCTION AFTER FETAL DEATH IN UTERO

In contrast, use of vaginal suppositories is usually the preferred method to induce abortion in patients with death in utero after 16 weeks' gestation, when dilatation and evacuation is often difficult. Vaginal administration of prostaglandin E$_2$ suppositories every 4 hours is highly effective (Fig. 9).

Side effects are acceptable. The method is more convenient and probably safer than other methods of managing patients with death in utero, which are waiting for spontaneous labor, and abortion after constant intravenous infusion of oxytocin, intra-amniotic saline and intra-amniotic administration of prostaglandin F$_{2\alpha}$. Carrying a dead fetus until labor occurs may cause an emotional hardship and subclin-

ical coagulopathy and rarely a clinically significant coagulopathy. Constant intravenous infusion of high doses of oxytocin over several days is often necessary to induce abortion in these patients, resulting in immobilization, prolonged hospitalization and potential water intoxication from oxytocin mismanagement.

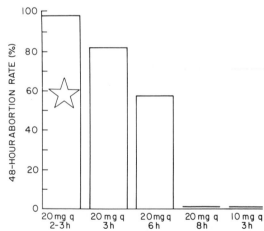

Figure 8. The efficacy of different PGE$_2$ vaginal suppository dose schedules. The proportion of 64 midtrimester subjects who aborted within 48 hours after induction was initiated with 20 mg PGE$_2$ vaginal suppositories administered every 2 to 3 hours. (Subjects who had rupture of the membranes received augmentation with intravenous oxytocin). Results are graphed from the data reported by Bolognese and Corson.[24] Twenty-nine first and second trimester subjects had induction with PGE$_2$ triglyceride suppositories without augmentation and the proportion of subjects aborting within 48 hours in each treatment group is graphed.[2] (From Brenner, W. E.: The current status of prostaglandins as abortifacients. Am. J. Obstet. Gynecol. 123:306–328, 1975.)

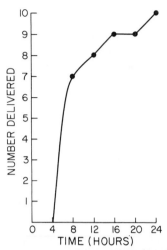

Figure 9. Cumulative delivery rates among 10 patients treated with $PGE_{2\alpha}$ vaginal suppositories for intrauterine fetal death. The number of subjects aborting by each time in hours after beginning the administration of a 20 mg PGE_2 vaginal suppository every 4 hours to 10 subjects with death in utero.[15] Program for Applied Research on Fertility Regulation, April 19, 1978.

Intra-amniotic administration of saline has a longer induction time than the prostaglandin E_2 method, and saline is more frequently rapidly absorbed intravascularly with a dead fetus than it is with a live fetus. The subclinical coagulopathy that ordinarily occurs with intra-amniotic saline may be more frequently clinically significant in patients with death in utero, especially if they already have a subclinical coagulopathy from the dead fetus. Similar problems probably occur with other hypertonic solutions such as urea and mannitol. Even though the intra-amniotic and extra-amniotic administration of prostaglandin $F_{2\alpha}$ and E_2 is highly effective, careful titration is necessary, since uterine response and systemic absorption are more variable than when the fetus is alive. Excessive prostaglandin cannot be removed and infection may be more common than with the vaginal method.

The obstetrician must be especially cautious inducing abortion in patients with death in utero in later pregnancy to ensure that the fetus is in a favorable presentation. Inducing abortion with the fetus in an unfavorable position such as transverse lie and overstimulation of contractility in grand multiparous women has resulted in uterine rupture.[25] Although prostaglandins per se do not result in disseminated intravascular coagulation, this condition may occur in patients with death in utero, especially during labor and delivery.

In summary, vaginal administration of prostaglandin E_2 for induction of abortion is ordinarily less effective, with higher incidences of side effects, and overall it is less satisfactory than intra-amniotic prostaglandin $F_{2\alpha}$ methods. However, it appears appropriate and, in fact, it is the method of choice for inducing abortion in patients with death in utero when the fetus is too large for satisfactory vaginal surgical evacuation.

EXTRA-AMNIOTIC ADMINISTRATION

Extra-amniotic administration of prostaglandins for abortion may be appropriate and useful when intra-amniotic and vaginal administration is not satisfactory. Either single doses of 15 (S)–15 methyl prostaglandin $F_{2\alpha}$ or multiple serial injections of prostaglandin $F_{2\alpha}$ or prostaglandin E_2 are not satisfactory unless they are augmented by the continuous intravenous infusion of oxytocin.[2] Generally, the method is inconvenient and confining, and many physicians report high rates of infection associated with this method. No method of extra-amniotic administration of prostaglandins is approved by the Food and Drug Administration.

INTRAMUSCULAR ADMINISTRATION

Serial intramuscular administration of the 15 (S) 15 methyl analogues of prostaglandin $F_{2\alpha}$ and prostaglandin E_2 is potentially appropriate when intra-amniotic administration is not suitable. With dose schedules that are clinically effective, relatively high rates of vomiting and diarrhea with the $F_{2\alpha}$ analogue[2] and fever with the E_2 analogue are common.[2] Serial intramuscular injections are inconvenient (Fig. 10).

Intramuscular administration may be especially useful in patients in whom the membranes have ruptured and in whom abortion fails after intra-amniotic administration when further intra-amniotic administration may not be possible and vaginal evacuation is not as safe. Under some circumstances, intramuscular administration may be a satisfactory primary induction method. Effective dosage of 15 (S) 15 methyl prostaglandin $F_{2\alpha}$ is 250 µg every 2 hours. The incidence of side effects (80 per cent vomiting, 30 per cent diarrhea, 10 per cent shivering), even when the patients

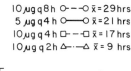

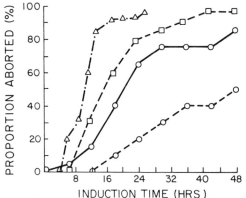

Figure 10. The cumulative abortion rates with different intramuscular 15 (S)–15 methyl prostaglandin E₂ methyl ester dose schedules. The cumulative proportion of 20 second trimester subjects in percentage aborting over the trial period in hours with 10 μg 15 (S)–15 methyl prostaglandin E₂ methyl ester [15 (S) ME PGE₂] administered intramuscularly every 2 hours is graphed from data reported by Ballard and Quilligan.[26] The 20 subjects treated with 5 μg every four hours have been previously reported. Twenty subjects had induction with 10 μg every 4 hours and 10 subjects had induction with 10 μg every 8 hours. ($\bar{x}$ = mean.[2]) (From Brenner, W. E.: The current status of prostaglandins as abortifacients. Am. J. Obstet. Gynecol. 123:306–328, 1975.)

are premedicated with prochlorperazine and Lomotil, limits its use as a primary abortifacient. The prostaglandin E₂ analogue has the additional disadvantage of causing fever.[2] Intramuscular administration of prostaglandin analogues has not been satisfactorily studied in terminating pregnancy in patients with death in utero.

In summary, intramuscular administration of 15 (S) 15 methyl prostaglandin F₂α may be appropriate for the management of patients when other methods have failed to terminate the pregnancy, and vaginal evacuation or intra-amniotic administration or both are not appropriate. Under special circumstances, it may be the primary agent for inducing abortion for patients with fetal death in utero.

Vaginal Prostaglandin for Induction of Cervical Dilatation Before Surgical Evacuation

Vaginal administration of prostaglandin F₂α suppositories is appropriate for inducing cervical dilatation prior to surgical evacuation. Vaginally administered prostaglandin F₂α is highly effective within a short period of time for inducing cervical dilatation in nulliparous women. Three hours after placement of a 50 mg prostaglandin F₂α suppository, 85 per cent of nulliparous women in the first trimester had sufficient dilatation with clinically acceptable side effects to evacuate the uterus without further dilatation.[23] Among patients needing further dilatation, the force necessary to accomplish that dilatation was less than among nontreated patients. If further studies confirm the preliminary trials, it may be appropriate for prostaglandin F₂α vaginal suppositories to be administered for inducing cervical dilatation prior to surgical evacuation. Although the long-range effects of pharmacologic dilatation of the cervix are unknown, they may be less than with mechanical dilatation, especially in second trimester pregnancies. Unfortunately, the retail cost of prostaglandin F₂α is too high for this method of cervical dilatation to be practical now.

Control of Postpartum Atony

Diluted prostaglandin F₂α by constant intravenous infusion or direct injection into the myometrium and intramuscular injection of 15 mL prostaglandin F₂α may be effective in treating postpartum atony when intravenous oxytocin and methyl ergonovine fail.

Future

It is anticipated that the following developments may make prostaglandins more practical and appropriate to use for more indications in the future:

1. More specific analogues
2. Better delivery systems
3. Better augmentation methods
4. More specific knowledge about the physiologic role of prostaglandins

Summary

The appropriate use of prostaglandins depends upon the physician's awareness of the chemistry of prostaglandins and their physiologic role and pharmacologic use. For induction of labor and abortion, only two capabilities of prostaglandins have been exploited: the induction of delivery at any stage of gestation and cervical dilatation. With these capabilities, prostaglandins are potentially useful for the following:

1. Postcoital contraception
2. Induction of abortion
3. Cervical dilatation prior to surgical abortion
4. Induction of abortion of a dead fetus
5. Induction when a fetus incapable of survival is expected
6. "Indicated" induction of labor
7. "Elective" induction of labor

However, because of the other properties of prostaglandins, side effects are common, especially when prostaglandins are used systemically.

For "indicated" and "elective" induction of labor, prostaglandins are as effective as intravenous oxytocin. However, hypercontractility may be more common with prostaglandin. Therefore, it does not appear appropriate to use prostaglandin for induction of labor because the only advantage appears to be the convenience of oral administration.

Intra-amniotic administration of prostaglandin for induction of second trimester abortion has effectiveness and complication rates similar to those for hypertonic saline. It is less safe than cervical dilatation and surgical evacuation when performed by experienced surgeons. Augmentation of intra-amniotic prostaglandin with intracervical laminaria tents and in special circumstances with continuous infusion with intravenous oxytocin or intra-amniotic hypertonic saline or urea appears appropriate.

Vaginal administration of prostaglandin E_2 is probably the method of choice in most cases of death in utero when surgical vaginal evacuation is unsatisfactory. Vaginal administration as the primary abortion method may be appropriate only in cases when D&E and intra-amniotic administration are not satisfactory. Intramuscular administration of analogues is appropriate in cases in which surgical evacuation and intra-amniotic administration and vaginal administration are unsatisfactory. If further study of prostaglandin $F_{2\alpha}$ and its analogues confirms the effectiveness of these prostaglandins in producing cervical dilatation, it will be appropriate to administer them to cause cervical dilatation before surgical evacuation if the cost of prostaglandins can be reduced enough. We can hope that more specific analogues, better delivery systems and

better knowledge of prostaglandins' physiologic role and pharmacologic properties will make prostaglandins and antiprostaglandins practical for many needs in obstetrics and gynecology.

REFERENCES

1. Von Euler, U. S.: *In* Ramwell, P. W. (ed.): The Prostaglandins, vol. 1. New York, Plenum Press, 1973.
2. Brenner, W. E.: The current status of prostaglandins as abortifacients. Am. J. Obstet. Gynecol. 123:306, 1975.
3. Pritchard, J. A. and MacDonald, P. C.: Williams Obstetrics. New York, Prentice-Hall, 1976.
4. Hendricks, C. H., Brenner, W. E., Ekbladh, L., Brotanek, V. and Fishburne, J. I.: Efficacy and tolerance of intravenous prostaglandins $F_{2\alpha}$ and E_2. Am. J. Obstet. Gynecol. 111:564, 1971.
5. Spellacy, W. N. and Gall, S. A.: Prostaglandin $F_{2\alpha}$ and oxytocin for term labor induction. *In* The Prostaglandins. Clinical Applications in Human Reproduction, Symposia Specialists, Inc., Post Office Box 610397, Miami, Florida 33161.
6. Vakhariya, V. R. and Sherman, A. I.: Prostaglandin $F_{2\alpha}$ for induction of labor. Am. J. Obstet. Gynecol. 113:212, 1972.
7. Brenner, W. E. and Berger, G. S.: Pharmacological methods of inducing midtrimester abortion: risks and benefits. Program for Applied Research on Fertility Regulation Workshop on Risks, Benefits and Controversies in Fertility Control, 1977.
8. Brenner, W. E.: Termination of second trimester pregnancy using prostaglandin $F_{2\alpha}$. ACOG Technical Bulletin, #27, April 1974.
9. Mullick, B., Brenner, W. E. and Berger, G.: Termination of pregnancy with intrauterine devices. A comparative study of coils, coils and balsa, and catheters. Am. J. Obstet. Gynecol. 116:305, 1973.
10. Greenhalf, J. O.: Termination of pregnancy during the midtrimester by intra-amniotic injection of urea. Br. J. Clin. Pract. 26:24, 1972.
11. Craft, I. and Musa, B.: Induction of midtrimester therapeutic abortion by intra-amniotic urea and intravenous oxytocin. Lancet 1:1058, 1971.
12. Unpublished data of International Fertility Research Program.
13. Burkman, R. T., Atienza, M. F., King, T. M. and Burnett, L. S.: Intraamniotic urea and prostaglandin $F_{2\alpha}$ for midtrimester abortion: a modified regimen. Am. J. Obstet. Gynecol. 126:328, 1976.
14. Kerenyi, T.: Personal communication.
15. Brenner, W. E.: Artificial abortion of early midtrimester pregnancy with commercially available prostaglandin. Program for Applied Research on Fertility Regulation, April 19, 1978.
16. Brenner, W. E., Fishburne, J. I., McMillan, C. W., Johnson, A. M. and Hendricks, C. H.: Coagulation changes during abortion induced by prostaglandin $F_{2\alpha}$. Am. J. Obstet. Gynecol. 117:1080, 1973.
17. Grimes, D. A., Schultz, K. F., Cates, W. and Tyler, C. W.: Midtrimester abortion by dilatation and

evacuation: a safe and practical alternative. N. Engl. J. Med. 296:1141, 1977.

18. Tietze, C. and Murstein, M. C.: Induced abortion: 1975 factbook. Rep. Pop./Fam. Plan. 14, p. 55, 1975.

19. Cates, W.: Prostaglandin may be "too safe" for abortions. J.A.M.A. 236:247, 1976.

20. Brenner, W. E. and Edelman, D. A.: Therapeutic abortion by dilatation and evacuation in the 13 to 15 weeks' gestation gravida versus intraamniotic saline instillation after 15 weeks' gestation. Contraception 10:171, 1974.

21. Tietze, C. and Lewit, S.: Joint program for the study of abortion (JPSA): early medical complications of legal abortion. Stud. Fam. Plan. 3:97, 1972.

22. Stubblefield, P. G., Naftolin, F., Frigoletto, F. D. and Ryan, K. J.: Pretreatment with laminaria tents before midtrimester abortion with intra-amniotic prostaglandin $F_{2\alpha}$. Am. J. Obstet. Gynecol. 118:284, 1974.

23. Brenner, W. E., Hendricks, C. H., Dingfelder, J. and Staurovsky, L.: Laminaria augmentation of intraamniotic prostaglandin $F_{2\alpha}$ for the induction of midtrimester abortion. Prostaglandins 3:879, 1973.

24. Bolognese, R. J. and Corson, S. L.: Prostaglandin E_2 vaginal suppository as an early second trimester abortifacient. Obstet. Gynecol. 43:104, 1974.

25. Schulman, H.: Personal communication.

26. Ballard, C. A. and Quilligan, E. J.: Midtrimester abortion with intramuscular injection of 15-methyl prostaglandin E_2. Contraception 9:523, 1974.

27. Brenner, W. E., Dingfelder, J. R., Staurovsky, L. G. and Hendricks, C. H.: Vaginally administered prostaglandin $F_{2\alpha}$ for cervical dilatation in nulliparas prior to suction curettage. Prostaglandins 4:819, 1973.

Controversies Concerning Midtrimester Dilatation and Evacuation Abortion

David A. Grimes, M.D.

Carl W. Tyler, Jr., M.D.

Centers for Disease Control

During the late 1970s, the emergence of dilatation and evacuation (D&E) as an acceptable method of midtrimester abortion created intense controversy in the United States. Several factors contribute to this: (1) midtrimester abortion is an area of gynecology with unique ethical, aesthetic and legal concerns; (2) the concept of D&E contradicted traditional gynecologic tenets; and (3) the technology spread primarily from private practice settings to academic centers, rather than the reverse.

First, midtrimester abortion involves difficult decisions concerning the competing rights and interests of the woman versus those of her fetus. Midtrimester abortion can be a distasteful experience for both the woman and her medical attendants. In addition, the legal limitations on midtrimester abortion vary from state to state. In this regard, nonmedical concerns may obscure or outweigh scientific evidence when methods of abortion are chosen.

Second, the concept of a 12-week ceiling for instrumental abortion had been espoused by gynecologic authorities for many years.[1] The finding that the risk of mortality for the pregnant woman increases continuously as the duration of pregnancy increases conflicted with this concept. Midtrimester D&E was a direct challenge to this concept.

Third, the dissemination of this new technology was centripetal. Traditionally, new technologies in obstetrics and gynecology are developed and tested in academic centers; the technologies then diffuse into nonacademic practice. Residency training programs rapidly incorporate new technologies into their curricula, and medical schools offer postgraduate courses for physicians already in practice. Recent examples include colposcopy, laparoscopy, electronic fetal monitoring and microsurgery. In the case of midtrimester D&E, however, most of the innovative changes began in private nonacademic centers. D&E was adopted by private practitioners in the United States, who, apparently fearful of criticism by their peers, practiced D&E discreetly. After publication in 1977 of two large studies[2, 3] that gave credibility to this procedure, numerous confirmative reports, summarized in a previous article,[4] followed in rapid succession. With the exception of a few academic medical centers,[5-7] midtrimester D&E is not widely taught to residents at the present time. Moreover, in contrast to other new technologies, formal continuing education courses in D&E are virtually nonexistent.

This article updates the ongoing controversy surrounding midtrimester D&E. After reviewing the incidence, advantages, and disadvantages of D&E, we will focus on some of the unresolved questions concerning this method of abortion.

Incidence

Unparalleled changes in abortion practice took place in the United States during the 1970s. Induced abortion, previously a clandestine and hazardous procedure, rapidly became the most frequently performed operation on adults in the United States—and one of the safest.[8] Similarly, D&E, once anathema, emerged in 1977 as the most frequently used method of abortion at 13 weeks or more of gestation.[4]

The use of D&E in current practice is inversely related to gestational age during the second trimester (Table 1). The principal impact of D&E has been in the 13- to 15-week interval. According to 1978 US data, this method accounted for 82 per cent of abortions at this stage of pregnancy, and accounted for 25 per cent of abortions at 16- to 20-weeks' gestation. Even at this later stage of pregnancy, D&E was used more often for abortions than intrauterine prostaglandin instillation. At gestational ages of 21 weeks or more, D&E was used for 13 per cent of abortions.[8]

TABLE 1. PERCENTAGE OF REPORTED LEGAL ABORTIONS AT ≥ 13 WEEKS' GESTATION, BY TYPE OF PROCEDURE, UNITED STATES,* 1978

		TYPE OF PROCEDURE				
WEEKS OF GESTATION	DILATATION AND EVACUATION	INTRAUTERINE SALINE INSTILLATION	INTRAUTERINE PROSTAGLANDIN INSTILLATION	HYSTEREOTOMY/ HYSTERECTOMY	OTHER	TOTAL
13–15	82.1	10.0	4.3	0.3	3.3	100.0
16–20	24.6	45.6	18.7	0.5	10.6	100.0
≥ 21	12.8	52.8	15.4	0.4	18.6	100.0

*Based on data from 32 states.
Source: Center for Disease Control: Abortion Surveillance 1978, issued November, 1980.

Advantages and Disadvantages

D&E for midtrimester abortion has a number of important advantages compared with alternative methods. First, there is compelling evidence that D&E is safer than either induction of labor or hysterotomy or hysterectomy.[4]

All comparative studies published to date have consistently found D&E to have lower morbidity rates than alternative techniques. We[4] previously summarized the findings of five prospective nonrandomized cohort studies (one single institution and four multicenter) and one randomized clinical trial. Since that study, two additional nonrandomized cohort studies have confirmed these findings. Cadesky and associates[9] in Toronto compared the results of 29 D&E abortions with 29 abortions by instillation of prostaglandin $F_{2\alpha}$ at 16 to 19 weeks' gestation. The Canadian group observed a significantly lower complication rate with D&E than with instillation (7 and 55 per cent), although the latter figure includes curettage required to remove the placenta. The

total hospital stay was one day shorter for the D&E group.

Stubblefield and associates[10] in Boston compared 406 D&E abortions at 13 to 18 weeks' gestation with 623 abortions by instillation of prostaglandin $F_{2\alpha}$ augmented by laminaria tents at 10 to 23 weeks' gestation. Ten complications (e.g., fever and endometritis) occurred significantly more often with prostaglandin $F_{2\alpha}$ abortions. The only complication that occurred more often with D&E was intraoperative hemorrhage. This appears to have had little clinical impact, since the prostaglandin group had significantly higher rates of postabortal hemorrhage, anemia after abortion and blood transfusion.

D&E also carries a significantly lower risk of death than alternative methods of abortion. Nationwide surveillance[8] of abortion deaths from 1972 to 1978 documented an overall death-to-case rate of 7.7 deaths per 100,000 D&E procedures, compared with 13.9 for saline instillation, and 9.0 for instillation of prostaglandin and other agents (Table 2). The

TABLE 2. DEATH-TO-CASE RATES BY TYPE OF ABORTION METHOD AND GESTATIONAL AGE, UNITED STATES, 1972–1978

TYPE OF METHOD AND GESTATIONAL AGE	NO. OF DEATHS	ESTIMATED NO. OF PROCEDURES	DEATH-TO-CASE RATE*	95% CONFIDENCE LIMITS
D&E (≥ 13 weeks)	18	234,257	7.7	5–12
13–15 weeks	10	177,239	5.6	3–10
≥ 16 weeks	8	57,018	14.0	6–28
Curettage (≤ 12 weeks)	53	5,385,199	1.0	0.7–1.3
Instillation (≥ 13 weeks)	50	405,893	12.3	9–16
Saline	38	273,035	13.9	10–19
Prostaglandin and other agents	12	132,858	9.0	5–16
Hysterotomy/hysterectomy	9	21,044	42.8	20–81

*Deaths per 100,000 procedures.

marked variation in rates for saline and pros- taglandin instillation at different gestational ages probably is a statistical artifact reflecting the relatively few deaths and abortions in- volved. The death-to-case rate for hysterotomy or hysterectomy is far higher than that for D&E at each gestational age. Thus, in terms of both morbidity and mortality, D&E appears to be the safest available method of midtrimes- ter abortion.

Not only is D&E a safer abortion procedure than instillation of abortifacients at comparable gestational ages, but D&E also has another benefit: its use has allowed a shifting of mid- trimester abortions to earlier stages of preg- nancy. Gestational age is the single most powerful determinant of the likelihood of com- plications or death from abortion; both mor- bidity and mortality rates increase progres- sively with advancing gestational age (Fig. 1).[11] Hence, delays of any kind increase the risks from abortion.

Traditional tenets of gynecology have inad- vertently increased the risks from abortion by introducing needless delays. Because it was widely held that there is no safe or practical method of abortion at 13 to 15 weeks' gestation (the "gray zone"), women who requested abor- tions during this interval were often delayed until 16 weeks' gestation for an instillation procedure.[1] This policy subjected women to an inherently less safe procedure at a less safe gestational age.

Adherence to the "gray zone" concept cre- ated a bimodal distribution of gestational age at the time of abortion in the United States (Fig. 2). The clustering of abortions around 16 weeks' gestation presumably represents women whose abortions were delayed from 13 to 15 weeks' gestation because of adherence to the "gray zone" concept. In contrast, the projected distribution of abortions without such delays reveals a smooth decline. Between 1975 and 1978, the actual distribution shifted toward the projected distribution, reflecting increasing use of D&E in the 13- to 15-week interval. Thus, the impact of D&E on the safety of abortion has been twofold: it has provided a safer method and it has helped to eliminate delays that themselves increase the risks from abortion.

Second, D&E costs less than alternative methods of midtrimester abortion. D&E pro- cedures are usually performed on an outpa- tient basis, obviating expensive hospital charges for overnight stays. The difference in price between D&E and instillation abortions

is as much as $275.[12] Since approximately 100,000 women undergo abortions at 13 weeks or more of gestation in the United States each year,[8] the economic impact of D&E is large on a nationwide scale.

Third, D&E is faster and more convenient for women and their physicians than other

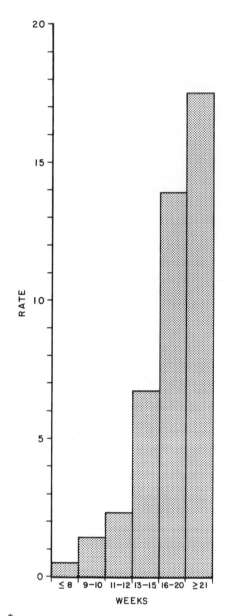

* DEATHS PER 100,000 LEGAL ABORTIONS
** MENSTRUAL WEEKS OF GESTATION

Figure 1. Death to case rate* for legal abortions, by weeks of gestation,** United States, 1972–1978. (Modi- fied from Cates, W., Jr., Schulz, K. F., Gold, J. and Tyler, C. W., Jr.: Complications of surgical evacuation procedures for abortions after 12 weeks' gestation. Pregnancy termination, procedures, safety, and new developments, 1979.)

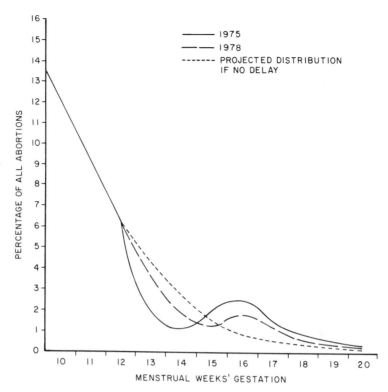

Figure 2. Change in distribution of abortions by gestational age, 1975 and 1978, and projected distribution if no delay. (Modified from Cates, W., Jr.: D & C after 12 weeks: safe or hazardous? Cont. Ob./Gyn. 13:23, 1979.)

methods. Women can be scheduled for abortion at specific times, rather than having to wait for an available hospital bed. Similarly, the duration of the abortion procedure can be predicted more accurately with the D&E method. With D&E the physician performs a brief operation; with instillation abortions the physician must be available to attend to problems encountered during a lengthy labor and delivery.

Fourth, D&E is less painful than available alternatives. With D&E anesthesia is routinely used; with instillation abortions women endure hours of labor, usually with analgesia rather than anesthesia to minimize pain. This has been termed a "maxi-labor followed by a mini-delivery."[13] In addition, D&E is less emotionally stressful for women.[14] Women are spared both labor and viewing the fetus. Kaltreider and associates[5] documented fewer adverse psychologic sequelae in women who had D&E abortions compared with those women who had instillation procedures.

Fifth, D&E can facilitate the management of septic spontaneous midtrimester abortions. Traditional means of evacuating the products of conception in this situation have been oxytocin administration, which may be slow or ineffective, and hysterotomy, which adds a major operation to the woman's medical prob-

lems. Facility with the D&E technique enables the physician to empty the uterus promptly and safely.[7] Early removal of the infected tissue hastens recovery.[15]

On the other hand, D&E has the disadvantage of being more emotionally stressful for the physician and operating room personnel than instillation abortions. In general, the stress felt by participants in midtrimester abortion is related to the extent of contact with the fetus; with D&E the physician's contact is direct and destructive. This may evoke strong emotional reactions during or after the abortion, including occasional disquieting dreams. Empathy for the woman undergoing D&E and peer support can reduce this stress to manageable levels.[5, 16]

Remaining Questions

A number of questions about D&E remain unanswered. First, what level of training or skill is required to perform D&E abortions safely? Although some have alleged that extraordinary expertise is necessary,[17] there are few data to support this assertion. The procedure is less difficult technically than vaginal hysterectomy, an operation all gynecologists learn to do. Residents at Boston Hospital for

Women have been taught to perform D&E procedures,[18] and morbidity rates have been low. It seems reasonable to conclude that D&E is an operation that can be taught and learned by most gynecologists. Experts usually advise those learning the technique to obtain appropriate supervision and then gradually to extend the gestational age range of their abortions. As noted before, formal learning experiences with D&E are scarce. To the extent that this situation persists, the claim that few physicians are adept at D&E may be a self-fulfilling prophecy.

Second, in what type of facility can D&E be safely performed? Most existing information about the safety of D&E has come from hospitals.[4] Nevertheless, reports[19-21] of D&E abortions performed in clinics have documented low morbidity rates. Nationwide mortality surveillance from 1972–1978[22] indicates that D&E abortions performed in nonhospital facilities had a death-to-case rate of 6.9 deaths per 100,000 procedures similar to the rate for those performed in hospitals (9.4 deaths per 100,000 procedures).

Should D&E abortions be limited to hospitals if these procedures can be performed with comparable safety and at lower cost in clinics? These morbidity and mortality data do not support regulations in some states that require all midtrimester abortions to be performed in hospitals. Recent judicial decisions have liberalized the upper gestational age limit at which D&E abortions can be done in nonhospital facilities in certain states. New Jersey, North Carolina, Louisiana and Missouri now allow D&E abortions through 16 weeks' gestation in nonhospital clinics. Other decisions in Ohio and Indiana, upheld by the U.S. Supreme Court, limit all midtrimester abortions to hospitals; 17 states currently have such restrictions.[22]

Third, what is the preferred type of anesthesia for D&E abortions? Good results have been described with paracervical[23] and intracervical[24] as well as general anesthesia,[5] and each technique has its proponents. Paracervical anesthesia, familiar to most gynecologists, is safe and effective. Intracervical blocks may use an anesthetic with a vasoconstrictor, such as epinephrine, which has been reported subjectively to diminish uterine bleeding during the evacuation. Whether using a vasoconstrictor decreases blood loss, however, has not been quantified. General anesthesia is more expensive to provide but offers both pain relief and amnesia for the operation.

Little is known of the comparative safety of these anesthesia techniques for D&E. Data from first trimester suction curettage, however, indicate that uterine hemorrhage, cervical injury and uterine perforation occur significantly more often when general anesthesia rather than local anesthesia is used.[26] Nationwide mortality surveillance has revealed that the risk of dying from suction curettage is twofold to fourfold greater when general anesthesia is used.[27] Whether these findings can be extrapolated to midtrimester abortion is not yet known.

Fourth, what is the optimal means of dilating the cervix to the diameters required for D&E? Two general approaches are used: acute mechanical dilatation or laminaria. The use of dilators has the advantage of brevity, and reported experience with this technique has been favorable both in the United States[2] and in Europe.[20, 21] Disadvantages include difficult dilatation in some instances, particularly with very young primigravidous women, and occasional cervical tears. Moreover, many physicians are concerned about the potential for damaging the integrity of the cervix with subsequent implications for future fertility.

Most gynecologists who perform D&E in the United States place laminaria tents in the cervix for varying intervals of time.[4] The duration of laminaria treatment ranges from a few hours to overnight. One physician[19] relies on sequential packings of laminaria over several days to achieve wide cervical dilatation. Use of laminaria facilitates dilatation for the operation but prolongs the abortion procedure for the woman. Even if overnight laminaria are used, hospital admission is not necessary.[13, 18, 24] On the other hand, some physicians[23] reserve laminaria use for selected women, on the basis of the dimensions and elasticity of the cervix. The risk-to-benefit ratio of acute dilatation versus laminaria treatment is unknown at present.

Fifth, should oxytocin be administered during the evacuation? Some physicians,[9] hoping to decrease uterine bleeding and provide a firm uterine wall, routinely give oxytocin intravenously. Others[13] intentionally avoid using oxytocin for fear of "trapping" the fetal calvarium. Again, data are lacking to evaluate this practice. With first trimester suction curettage abortions, concurrent oxytocin administration decreases blood loss when general anesthesia is used.[28] Whether this finding applies to midtrimester D&E is unknown.

Sixth, what instruments should be used to evacuate the uterus? Most D&E procedures rely on suction curettage, forceps extraction and sharp curettage. The available instruments have been reviewed in detail by Hern.[29] Little comparative information is available, however, concerning the choice of equipment. Stubblefield and associates[6] found in a randomized clinical trial that a 15.9 mm diameter suction cannula would effectively abort pregnancies up to 16 weeks' gestation. Avoiding the need for forceps extraction may make D&E less distasteful to physicians, which may in turn promote dissemination of the technique.

Seventh, what should the upper gestational age limit for D&E be? As fetal growth and ossification progress, evacuating the uterus may be more difficult, and complication rates may be higher. Most physicians performing D&E establish an upper limit based on personal skill and experience. The limits of some stop at 16 weeks' gestation,[9] while those of others extend as far as 24 weeks' gestation.[19, 30] In the largest prospective study[13] it was found that D&E is significantly safer than instillation abortions through 20 weeks' gestation; because of the relatively few D&E abortions performed at 21 weeks' gestation or longer, data on the comparative safety of abortion methods at this stage of pregnancy are insufficient. Neither morbidity nor mortality data available at present indicate what the upper limit for D&E should be.

Finally, are there adverse late effects of D&E? Most speculation is centered on the possibility of cervical trauma sustained during dilatation leading to adverse outcomes in subsequent pregnancies. Postulated problems include spontaneous abortion, cervical incompetence and premature birth. Follow-up data on the reproductive experience of women who have had D&E abortions is insufficient at present to substantiate or refute these concerns. Investigation of potential late sequelae of D&E should be a priority for future research.

Conclusion

The evolution of D&E has been surrounded by controversy. In spite of its skeptical reception by academia, D&E has become the most frequently performed method of abortion at 13 weeks' gestation or longer in the United States. Comparative morbidity studies and nationwide mortality surveillance indicate that D&E is safer than alternative methods through 16 weeks' and as safe as any other technique through 20 weeks' gestation. D&E also is less expensive, more convenient, more comfortable and more compassionate for the woman. On the other hand, D&E clearly requires more technical skill than instillation abortion, and D&E transfers much of the emotional burden of midtrimester abortion from the woman and nurse to the physician.

Although data about D&E are accumulating rapidly, a number of important questions remain unanswered. These include the level of operator training required, the safety of non-hospital D&E procedures, the choice of drugs and instruments, the upper gestational age limit for D&E and potential late sequelae. Further studies are needed to answer these questions.

Midtrimester abortion may well be the most difficult aspect of the most controversial medical and political issue confronting our society today. Hence, it is especially important that the decisions concerning midtrimester abortion methods be based on good science as well as on good intentions. As noted by Hern,[29] D&E "brings the physician into confrontation with the act of late abortion as no other method does. There is no other choice that requires more commitment on the part of the physician to freedom of reproductive choice for women. . . . Many tasks in medicine are difficult, and this is one of them."

REFERENCES

1. Grimes, D. A., and Cates, W., Jr.: Gestational age limit of 12 weeks for abortion by curettage. Am. J. Obstet. Gynecol. 132:207, 1978.
2. Hodari, A. A., Peralta, J., Quiroga, P. J. and Gerbi, E. B.: Dilatation and curettage for second trimester abortions. Am. J. Obstet. Gynecol. 127:850, 1977.
3. Grimes, D. A., Schulz, K. F., Cates, W., Jr. and Tyler, C. W., Jr.: Midtrimester abortion by dilatation and evacuation: a safe and practical alternative. N. Engl. J. Med. 296:1141, 1977.
4. Grimes, D. A. and Cates, W., Jr.: Midtrimester abortion by dilatation and evaluation. *In* Berger, G. S., Keith, L. and Brenner, W. E. (eds.): Second Trimester Abortion. Perspectives After a Decade of Experience. Boston, John Wright. PSG Inc., 1981.
5. Kaltreider, N. B., Goldsmith, S. and Margolis, A. J.: The impact of midtrimester abortion techniques on

patients and staff. Am. J. Obstet. Gynecol. 135:235, 1979.

6. Stubblefield, P. G., Albrecht, B. H., Koos, B. et al.: A randomized study of 12-mm and 15.9-mm cannulas in midtrimester abortion by laminaria and vacuum curettage. Fertil. Steril. 29:512, 1978.

7. Grimes, D. A. and Hulka, J. F.: Midtrimester abortion by dilatation and evacuation. South. Med. J. 73:448, 1980.

8. Centers for Disease Control: Abortion surveillance 1978, issued November 1980.

9. Cadesky, K. I., Ravinsky, E. and Lyons, E. R.: Dilation and evacuation: A preferred method of midtrimester abortion. Am. J. Obstet. Gynecol. 139:329, 1981.

10. Stubblefield, P. G., Kayman, D. J. and Osorio-Burns, L.: Midtrimester abortion by dilatation and evacuation and by laminaria and prostaglandin F_{2a}: Experience in a teaching hospital. Unpublished manuscript.

11. Cates, W., Jr., Schulz, K. F., Grimes, D. A. and Tyler, C. W., Jr.: The effect of delay and choice of method on the risk of abortion morbidity. Fam. Plann. Perspect. 9:266, 1977.

12. National Abortion Federation: 1979 Membership Directory. New York, National Abortion Federation, 1979.

13. Hanson, M. S.: D&E midtrimester abortion. Presented at 16th annual meeting, Association of Planned Parenthood Physicians, San Diego, California, October 25–27, 1977.

14. Rooks, J. B. and Cates, W., Jr.: Emotional impact of D&E versus instillation. Fam. Plann. Perspect. 9:276, 1977.

15. Grimes, D. A., Cates, W., Jr. and Selik, R. M.: Fatal septic abortion in the United States, 1975–1977. Obstet. Gynecol. 57:739, 1981.

16. Hern, W. M. and Corrigan, B.: What about us? Staff reactions to D&E. Adv. Plann. Parent. 15:3, 1980.

17. Flowers, C. E.: Discussion. Am. J. Obstet. Gynecol. 131:14, 1978.

18. Altman, A.: Stubblefield, P. G., Parker, K. et al.: Midtrimester abortion by laminaria and vacuum evacuation (L&E) on a teaching service: a review of 789 cases. Adv. Plann. Parent. 16:1, 1981.

19. Hern, W. M.: Outpatient second-trimester D&E abortion through 24 menstrual weeks' gestation. Adv. Plann. Parent. 16:7, 1981.

20. Van Den Berg, A. S.: Abortion procured in the second trimester of pregnancy. Medisch. Contact 29:1555, 1974.

21. van Lith, D. A. F., Beekhuizen, W. and van Schie, K. J.: Complications of aspirotomy (AT): A modified dilatation and curettage procedure for terminating early second-trimester pregnancies. *In* Zatuchni, G. I., Sciarra, J. J., Speidel, J. J. (eds.): Pregnancy Termination: Procedures, Safety, and New Developments. Hagerstown, Harper and Row, 1979.

22. Cates, W., Jr. and Grimes, D. A.: Deaths from second-trimester abortion by dilatation and evacuation: causes, prevention, facilities. Obstet. Gynecol. 58:401, 1981.

23. Peterson, W. F., Berry, F. N., Grace, M. R. et al.: Second trimester abortion by D&E: an analysis of 10,584 cases. Obstet. Gynecol. (in press).

24. Grimes, D. A., Hulka, J. F. and McCutchen, M. E.: Midtrimester abortion by dilatation and evacuation versus intra-amniotic instillation of prostaglandin F_{2a}: a randomized clinical trial. Am. J. Obstet. Gynecol. 137:785, 1980.

25. Finks, A. A.: Mid-trimester abortion. Lancet 1:263, 1973.

26. Grimes, D. A., Schulz, K. F., Cates, W., Jr. and Tyler, C. W., Jr.: Local versus general anesthesia: which is safer for performing suction curettage abortions? Am. J. Obstet. Gynecol. 135:1030, 1979.

27. Peterson, H. B., Grimes, D. A., Cates, W., Jr. and Rubin, G. L.: Comparative risk of death from induced abortion at ≤12 weeks' gestation performed with local versus general anesthesia. Am. J. Obstet. Gynecol. 141:763, 1981.

28. Lauersen, N. H. and Conrad, P.: Effect of oxytocic agents on blood loss during first trimester suction curettage. Obstet. Gynecol. 44:428, 1974.

29. Hern, W. M.: Midtrimester abortion. In Wynn, R. M. (ed.): Obstetrics and Gynecology Annual, vol. 10. New York, Appleton-Century-Crofts, 1981.

30. Hubacker, A. S.: Dilatation and extraction for late second-trimester abortion. Adv. Plann. Parent. 15:119, 1981.

Editorial Comment

This chapter is indeed a true controversy, since there are two points of view as to the best method of terminating midtrimester pregnancies. Brenner, who was one of the early and persistent investigators in the use of prostaglandins, outlines the area of use for prostaglandins, not only in second trimester pregnancies but also in induction of labor and for the dead fetus. He outlines the different routes of administration of prostaglandins, which include intra-amniotic instillation, vaginal suppositories and intramuscular therapy. Grimes and Tyler, who have been at the Centers for Disease Control in Atlanta for a number of years, were the first individuals to identify that dilatation and evacuation after 14 weeks of pregnancy was safer than intra-amniotic administration of uterotonic materials.

This chapter was written by the true experts in their fields, and interestingly, their conclusions are dissimilar. Brenner concedes that dilation and evacuation (D&E) is most likely preferable up to 16 weeks of gestation; however, after 16 weeks of gestation intra-amniotic prostaglandin is most likely the safest form of medication when all things are taken together by everyone doing pregnancy terminations. Importantly, it is pointed out that a 5 mg test dose must be given before intra-amniotic injection of the drug to rule out any allergic phenomenon, especially in those individuals with history of asthma; then the remaining 35 mg. of prostaglandin is injected. The problems involved in future childbearing—cervical incompetence, premature labor and placenta previa—are most common after second trimester abortions, but the true long-term effects are unknown. The discussion touches on use of intra-amniotic urea both with and without prostaglandins so that there is no life in the fetus. This obviates some of the emotional problems encountered by health care personnel who care for these patients.

Laminaria tents are used to induce cervical ripening and are usually inserted at the time the intra-amniotic medication is given. The laminaria tents reach their maximum absorption of local secretions and gradual dilatation of the cervix; this often coincides with the onset of contractions caused by the prostaglandins. The two seem to work in synergism. Brenner points out that vaginal prostaglandins are especially applicable for the patient who has an intrauterine fetal death but that they are of little use in promoting terminations of pregnancies of less than 16 weeks' gestation if the pregnancy is viable. An inordinate number of side effects are reported, such as vomiting, temperature elevation and diarrhea, and in one study 64 per cent had aborted incompletely. Vaginal prostaglandins, however, are useful if in the process of doing the intra-amniotic injection membranes are ruptured. Additionally, intramuscular prostaglandins with 15 (S) 15 methyl prostaglandin $F_{2\alpha}$ can be used if membranes are ruptured. There is now some suggestion that vaginal prostaglandins in the dose of 50 mg of $F_{2\alpha}$ may be used 3 hours prior to D&E to induce cervical dilatation; this may assist in the future but is still under investigation. Brenner correctly points out that prostaglandins are potentially useful for postcoital contraception, induction of abortion, cervical dilatation prior to surgical abortion, induction of a dead fetus, induction when a fetus incapable of survival is expected, indicated induction of labor, as well as elective induction of labor. The indicated and elective induction of labor with prostaglandins has never really caught on, since oxytocin seems to work so very well in a predictable fashion.

Grimes and Tyler point out the historical reason for the problem of acceptance of dilatation and evacuation as the safest mechanism of pregnancy termination up to 20 weeks of gestation. Most innovative medical programs are usually begun in an academic center with clinical investigation and are then transposed into private practice; however, dilatation and evacuation began in a reverse fashion, in private practice, and because of this, academic centers have not wholeheartedly accepted and endorsed it. One of the problems is the fact that few residents are trained in the evacuation of the uterus beyond 12 weeks of gestation. Some of the controversies that still exist have to do with the level of operator training needed, whether it is safe to do D&E in nonhospital environments, the drugs that could be used in conjunction with the D&E as well as the instrumentation and the late sequelae. These are questions that need to be answered.

Grimes and Tyler forget to mention that it was the CDC and the abortion surveillance group that promoted the termination of early pregnancies as the safest method five to eight years ago; this may account for the difficulty in accepting D&E as safest for second trimester abortions. The randomized trials that proved D&E as safest for abortions from 14 weeks to 20 weeks of gestation were somewhat loaded in that only individuals with very impeccable credentials and great skill in pregnancy termination were utilized for this study. It is not surprising that the results were good. This would be what you would expect for any surgical procedure if you chose the best people to do it; their patients should have the fewest complications. The real question, as Grimes and Tyler point out, is whether anybody can do this and end up with statistics as good as those that are already reported; i.e., a death rate from abortions of all kinds of 7.7 per 100,000, contrasted to 13.9 for second trimester saline abortions and 9.0 for prostaglandin abortions. The real controversy that they point out remains the level of skill needed to do the procedure; this skill must be identified in an appropriate manner. They aptly state that doing a second trimester abortion is easier than doing a vaginal hysterectomy, and everybody would agree with this. The formal learning experience available is very scarce and is really not advertized as something the physician should have before doing these. The question of anesthesia still has not been settled: whether or not a paracervical block or whether paracervical block and a short-acting analgesic can be used or whether it is necessary for a general anesthetic to be used. One of the concerns that we all have is dilatation of the cervix. If this is traumatic, will it cause pregnancy wastage in the future in the form of a torn internal os that will result in preterm labor?

There are many questions that need to be answered, and with time the answers will be useful to the obstetrician-gynecologist who is concerned with pregnancy terminations.

13
Optimal Management of the Rape Victim

Alternative Points of View

by Norman F. Gant, Johann H.
Duenhoelter and Daniel E. Scott
by Dorothy J. Hicks and Raphael S. Good

Editorial Comment

Optimal Treatment of the Rape Victim

Norman F. Gant, M.D.

Johann H. Duenhoelter, M.D.

Daniel E. Scott, M.D.

University of Texas Southwestern Medical School

In recent years, the crime of rape has become a matter of increasing public concern, particularly to women's groups, forensic scientists and physicians. Interestingly, these three diverse groups working co-operatively have significantly improved the quality and quantity of care provided for the victims of this age-old crime. Women's groups have worked to help the victim and to aid in the prosecution of the rapist. Forensic scientists have worked to improve laboratory methods that might be used to identify the offender. Physicians in general, and gynecologists specifically, have worked to provide dignified and compassionate care for the victim and to ensure that this care includes rapid medical examination, collection of evidence and administration of appropriate agents to prevent venereal disease and pregnancy.

The number of women and young girls who report the crime of sexual assault has increased markedly in the United States during recent years. In most large cities victims are referred to the emergency rooms of general hospitals where physicians are available who have special expertise in dealing with such matters and can provide the medical examination and treatment of the victim and also can ensure that evidence is properly collected. The availability of such experts in rural areas and smaller cities is less than uniform. Victims of sexual assault may, nonetheless, receive excellent care by family physicians and gynecologists who, even though they have not received special training in the areas of medicolegal gynecology and are not provided with appropriate forensic pathology support, now have available to them special "kits" that include necessary instructions and provide the appropriate containers to be used for the collection and preservation of specimens. However, all persons dealing with patients who present with the complaint of sexual assault must remember that the designation of "rape" is not made in a doctor's office or in an emergency room by physicians or nurses but

395

in the courtroom by a judge and jury. Therefore, the role of medical personnel and forensic scientists is of great importance: some offenders have pleaded guilty solely on the basis of an accurate and detailed record describing physical findings and other evidence collected during an initial examination. Thus, a court appearance and the psychologic trauma so often associated with it may be avoided if medical personnel provide adequate services.

In order to ensure that victims of sexual assault receive compassionate and professional care, it is important that all health care providers involved in caring for these women be trained medically and emotionally to meet these patients' needs. It is unfortunate but true that the victim may evoke sympathetic or hostile feelings or both among the personnel caring for her. Therefore, all personnel concerned with a patient who states that she has been sexually assaulted should be carefully screened and counseled regarding their own feelings, whether these feelings are hostile or sympathetic. All such medical personnel should understand that until proven otherwise in court the patient is a victim of a violent crime.

Optimal care of sexual assault victims requires a well-designed system to provide rapid identification of victims and their speedy transport to a medical facility and expert examination by sympathetic personnel. An optimal system frequently cannot be initiated or operated by a single group, such as the police force, child welfare officials, women's volunteer organizations, forensic scientists or physicians. On the other hand, if all these groups cooperate in the planning, design and implementation of such a program, the results for the community and the victims can be remarkable, as evidenced by the system in operation in Dallas County, Texas, since 1971.

This article will deal with identification of female victims of sexual assault, their medical examination and treatment, collection of evidence, and development of a cooperative effort between police, women's action groups, physicians, forensic scientists, child welfare authorities and prosecuting attorneys. Such a system has been designed and implemented by the Faculty of the Departments of Obstetrics and Gynecology, and Forensic Pathology at the University of Texas Southwestern Medical School. The medical system to be discussed has been tailored to the special resources and needs of a specific community, but many of the components to be described

are fundamental and are required to ensure a successful operation.

Identification of Victim

Most victims are identified by law enforcement officials to whom a sexual assault is reported or through counseling in a "rape crisis center" or other similar institution devoted to counseling and providing care for such women. Occasionally victims seek the care of a physician in an office or emergency room after trauma has occurred or to receive preventive treatment for venereal disease and pregnancy. If police officers have not been informed of an incident, the patient is counseled to inform them. In most instances the victims are interested in identification and prosecution of their assailant. If the patient wishes to file a criminal charge, a police officer is summoned and will file the case under a specific number, which subsequently serves as a unique identifying number during investigation and possible later prosecution.

If the victim of a sexual assault is not interested in a police investigation and does not want to press charges against the assailant, the physician cares for any physical injury and provides treatment to prevent venereal disease and unwanted pregnancy. These techniques will be described subsequently. There may be a variety of reasons for the victim not to press charges, although we counsel patients who are hesitant about the prosecution of the assailant that the results of the examination and the evaluation of the physical evidence may preclude a trial and may help ensure that a similar crime not be repeated against another woman.*

Admission and Registration

When a victim of sexual assault enters a physician's office or the emergency room of a hospital, attempts should be made to provide special privacy for the patient and to deal with her with the highest degree of discretion. All clerks, aides, nurses and physicians should be

---

*In some states evidence may be collected even when the victim does not wish to press charges because, should the victim decide later to press charges, this may be done within a time limitation such as two years.

instructed accordingly. Special codes have been suggested and their use may, under certain circumstances, prevent outsiders from becoming aware of the victim's presenting complaint. The victims should be considered primarily as patients who deserve compassion because they frequently have been subjected to threats on their lives and severe injury only minutes to hours before their admission. In many instances the emotional instability this causes is all too apparent, while in others, the psychological response may be characterized by withdrawal and indifference. There is no single immediate characteristic emotional response.

After a patient has been identified as a rape victim, she should receive immediate attention. A separate interviewing area or an examining room must provide privacy. A nurse or a physician should counsel her about the availability of medical care and the methods used to collect evidence, which may become important for the prosecution of the assailant. The victim is asked to sign appropriate consent forms that allow for examination and treatment as well as collection of evidence and release of relevant information to law enforcement and prosecuting authorities. The signature of the victim should be witnessed. If the victim is a minor, the consent of a parent, relative or guardian needs to be obtained, either directly, or if this is not possible, over the telephone in the presence of a witness. Specific informed consent procedures depend upon local and state laws that govern such authorizations of medical care. Before the physician obtains a history or performs the physical examination, it is advisable that he discuss the case with the investigating police officers, who may be able to direct the physician's attention to certain areas. In the presence of a nurse, the physician will ask the victim relevant questions and should record the data on a form specially designed for this purpose.[1]

History

Although a victim's statements to physicians frequently cannot be quoted in court because they are considered "hearsay," a careful history should be obtained for two reasons. First, unusual areas of injury may be revealed and sites for evidence collection thus identified. Second, the recorded history may help the physician later during a court appearance to recall details and circumstances of the event.

Preferably, the history is obtained in the presence of a female chaperon. Initially, some general information is obtained from the victim such as age, gravidity, parity and, if applicable, the date and outcome of her last pregnancy. The menstrual history is recorded in as much detail as possible. An analysis of this information later allows certain conclusions about the likelihood of a pregnancy resulting from a specific episode of sexual intercourse. The patient is asked if she might already be pregnant or if she has any symptoms of pregnancy. The use of contraceptive techniques is recorded. The date of the patient's last voluntary intercourse is noted and whether condoms were used or whether she cleansed the vagina with a douching solution. If the victim indicates that she was virginal before the sexual assault, this information needs to be recorded. Previous use of vaginal tampons is noted because this may influence the size and distensibility of the hymenal opening.

While these preliminary data are being obtained, victims usually begin to relate to the physician, who then may begin to focus on the history of the actual sexual assault. Did an abduction take place? Was the victim threatened with a weapon and, if so, what type of a weapon? Was a weapon actually used? Were any witnesses present and were they involved in the crime? Did she attempt to resist the assailant, possibly by scratching him or by causing any other injury? Was she subjected to vaginal intercourse or did fellatio, cunnilingus, anal intercourse or other sexual practices occur? The answers to the questions of whether the penis penetrated the vulva, intromission took place, orgasm occurred and the assailant wore a condom are of obvious importance during the search for spermatozoa and acid phosphatase. It is also important to record if the victim bathed or showered, defecated or urinated after the assault and prior to the examination.

The history is concluded with some general inquiries about recent illnesses and their treatment. If the patient has undergone a surgical procedure in the vaginal area, this is recorded. Use of any medications, alcohol or illegal drugs during the 24 hours preceding the alleged sexual assault is noted. The quantity, times of ingestion, injection or inhalation are recorded. Finally, the victim is asked if she has ever been sexually assaulted before and if this assault was brought to the attention of law enforcement officers.

Physical Examination

A physical examination of a victim of sexual assault should never be performed without a witness. Blood pressure, pulse and temperature are measured and recorded together with the victim's height and weight. A careful assessment of her general appearance follows, including the level of consciousness and orientation and the apparent influence of alcohol or drugs. The body surface is carefully inspected for bruises, fractures and lacerations and, if any are present, they should be described in detail and possibly photographed.

An examination of the mouth may reveal loose teeth, soft tissue trauma or other evidence of injury. The saliva may be bloody from injuries or it may contain acid phosphatase and spermatozoa, which can be detected with forensic methods.

Inspection of the pubic area may reveal foreign bodies such as leaves and small wood or dirt particles, which need to be secured. If the pubic hair is matted together this should be noted; bruises, abrasions and lacerations in the vulva and hymenal areas are carefully described and, occasionally, a sketch of the perineal area may be useful to record the location of injuries. Not infrequently, an attempt at anal intercourse, although unsuccessful, may result in bruising in the perineal area. Using an unlubricated speculum of appropriate size (the patient's own secretions should be used for lubrication), the vagina and cervix are searched for evidence of injury. The gross appearance of vaginal contents is described. After obtaining evidence, the process of which will be described later, bimanual, rectal and vaginal examinations are performed and the organs that can be palpated are described in a fashion similar to the usual gynecologic examination. Finally, any injuries of the extremities are recorded.

Collection of Evidence

During the trial of a suspected assailant, proper collection and evaluation of evidence is of utmost importance to attorneys for both the prosecution and the defense. Defendants may plead guilt singly on the basis of evidence collected in a physician's office and, in many instances, juries have become convinced that a suspect was guilty on the basis of this evidence.

Every specimen collected for medicolegal purposes in a physician's office or an emergency room needs to be labeled individually with the name of the victim, the name of the physician who obtained it, the name of the nurse who witnessed the collection, the date and time of collection, and a description of the anatomic location from which the specimen was obtained. At Parkland Memorial Hospital a kit is used containing the supplies necessary for collection and preservation of these specimens. The kit is supplied by the Southwestern Institute of Forensic Sciences and has been an invaluable aid. Similar kits are now commercially available and one has been developed by Simpson/Basye, Inc.* in cooperation with the American College of Obstetrics and Gynecology.

Clothing in the possession of the victim, which may contain foreign bodies, blood or seminal fluid stains, is submitted after appropriate identification. Two tubes of venous blood are collected: one specimen is submitted for a serologic test for syphilis and a second to the forensic laboratory for assessment of the victim's blood group and type. If there was a history of recent alcohol ingestion, a separate specimen is collected from which the blood alcohol level can be measured. If the patient relates that fellatio occurred and that it was accompanied by ejaculation, sputum is sampled with a cotton tip applicator and submitted in order to detect the presence of acid phosphatase, e.g., in a tube containing 1 ml normal saline. A second cotton swab is used to obtain another sputum sample that is then applied to a glass slide, preserved with a fixative and submitted for identification of spermatozoa.

If the victim has scratched the assailant, tissue from his skin may be found under her fingernails. To identify these skin particles, the victim's fingernails are clipped and the clippings collected.

If the pubic hair is matted, the matted areas are removed with scissors and submitted for detection of acid phosphatase and spermatozoa. Free hair can be found by combing the pubic area. This specimen is usually called "combings" and submitted separately from pubic hair removed from the victim with scissors and labeled "cuttings." In some instances, the assailant's hair can be differentiated microscopically from that of the victim. Any

---

*430 Ayre Street, Wilmington, DE 19804.

other loose hair on the victim should be collected and labeled similarly.

After the vagina has been inspected as just described, two specimens of vaginal fluid are collected with a swab and are then smeared on two glass slides, which are subsequently preserved with a fixative. In the forensic laboratory these specimens are stained appropriately for identification of spermatozoa. In some laboratories, semen typing can also be performed on these specimens, while other laboratories require specimens collected with a swab that are subsequently submitted in a dry test tube.

A so-called wet mount is prepared by collecting a drop of vaginal fluid from the posterior fornix with a dropper, mixing it with a drop of normal saline and applying it to a glass slide. If the vagina appears dry, 1 to 2 ml of saline is introduced into the vagina and gently mixed by several opening and closing motions of the speculum. This fluid is then used to prepare a wet mount. Care should be taken not to aspirate cervical mucus, because spermatozoa remain motile and detectable there for longer but less predictable time periods than in vaginal fluid. The wet mount can be inspected under a microscope for the presence or absence of motile or nonmotile spermatozoa. Material for the endocervix is removed with a cotton tip applicator and is plated out on Thayer-Martin medium for culture of gonococci.

If the victim reports rectal penetration, the respective samples are collected from the rectum.

If indicated, a urine pregnancy test should be done.

After all samples for forensic investigation are collected, they should be placed into a container, which is subsequently sealed and placed in a locked cabinet until the forensic laboratory assumes responsibility for the samples. These precautions are taken to ensure that the chain of evidence is preserved. In the Parkland Memorial Hospital Emergency Room a locked box, bolted in a refrigerator, is utilized for this purpose. All specimens are deposited into this container and only authorized persons from the forensic laboratory can unlock it and assume possession of the specimens. While the physician is responsible for proper collection, identification and safeguarding of the evidence—he may be questioned about the procedure in court—the forensic scientists must assume the responsibility for appropriate identification and processing in his laboratory.

Treatment

The medical treatment of victims of sexual assault has three objectives: repair of injury, prevention of pregnancy and prevention of venereal disease.

Repair of injury includes care that is routinely administered in the emergency trauma area: suture of lacerations, setting of fractures, surgical exploration of gunshot and stab wounds, and so forth. If genital lacerations are present, they may require exploration and repair under anesthesia in the operating room by an experienced gynecologic surgeon. In any case in which skin trauma has occurred, tetanus toxoid should be administered.

In every patient the possibility has to be considered that a pregnancy may be the result of the involuntary intercourse. Prevention of pregnancy is not necessary when the victim uses a reliable ongoing contraceptive technique, has been sterilized or has just begun her menstrual period. On the other hand, victims who are unsure about the date of their last normal menstrual period and are at risk to conceive from the involuntary intercourse are offered a prescription for postcoital contraceptive. Diethylstilbestrol, in a dose of 25 mg twice a day, as recommended by Kuchera,[2] has generally proved to be effective. When this regimen was administered to 1217 patients within 72 hours of sexual intercourse, not a single pregnancy was observed.[3] Patients are counseled that the next menstrual period usually occurs at the expected time, but not uncommonly the period may come earlier or later. In order to prevent nausea and vomiting, side effects that occur in about half the patients treated with diethylstilbestrol, an antiemetic in suppository form (e.g., TGAN 200 mg every 6 hours) is prescribed and should be administered prophylactically.

Each woman who has been sexually assaulted is at risk of contracting venereal disease and needs to be treated accordingly. The treatment recommended by the Centers for Disease Control consists of 4.8 million units of aqueous procaine penicillin in two intramuscular injections of 2.4 million units each in conjunction with 1 gram of Probenecid administered orally. Patients should be observed for approximately 30 minutes after the injection for signs of an allergic reaction. Patients who are allergic to penicillin should be treated with an intramuscular injection of 2 g of spectinomycin. The third treatment modality for patients who refuse parenteral medications is tetracycline, 1.5 g initially by mouth followed by 0.5 g orally 4 times a day for the next 4 days. In most patients these treatment regimens are adequate to eradicate incubating gonococci, but a subsequent examination should be scheduled for a repeat cervical culture and for a repeat serologic test to detect syphilis.

Subsequent Care

After collection of evidence and after appropriate therapy has been provided for the physical injury, the physician needs to decide if the victim requires psychological or psychiatric care, either immediately in the emergency room or subsequently in a clinic or private office. He may then prescribe a sedative to provide the patient with some rest.

In several cities, women's action groups have organized individual and group counseling that may begin immediately after identification of the assault victim and may continue through the trial and even after the trial. Some large city hospitals are staffed around the clock by such groups to provide support and counsel to assault victims as needed.

Subsequent medical care of these victims should include a second cervical culture for gonococci and a serologic test for syphilis, and, if indicated, pregnancy testing. An interval of four to six weeks after the sexual assault has been found useful because enough time has passed to allow for detection of syphilis and gonorrhea that may not have been eradicated by the prophylactic treatment. Additionally, most women can be expected to have a menstrual period by this time so that appropriate steps can be undertaken in those instances in which a bleeding episode has not occurred. It is the obligation of the physician who cares for the patient immediately after the assault to convince her of the importance of these subsequent visits and the potential consequences if she is not re-evaluated. Even under these circumstances the incidence of return for subsequent diagnosis and treatment has been disappointing.[4]

Alleged Sexual Abuse in Prepubertal Females

Prepubertal females are involved in approximately one third to one half of cases in which a sexual assault is alleged (personal observations). These girls present special problems for a variety of reasons. First, it is difficult to substantiate events that are frequently only suspected and only rarely witnessed. Second, the patients may be under duress not to discuss events surrounding the incident.

An atmosphere of trust must be created by the physician before he can even hope to obtain a reliable history from a child. This is even more important than in adults since these children often have been threatened by their assailants with reprisals if they discuss the event. Not infrequently, the assailant remains a threat to the victim after discharge from the physicians' care because the assailant may be a member of the victim's family. It may be impossible to alleviate the child's fear when another relative is present who, in the victim's mind, may try to protect the assailant.

When children are too young to report or recall an event, the persons who presume that sexual abuse occurred should relate their observations and suspicions. If a child is old enough to communicate, she should be interviewed separately from the parents. An interview with the child requires patience and special skills because all questions have to be phrased in terms that children will understand and even then these children frequently are hesitant to answer. It may help to relate the events of the suspected sexual assault to events in the life of the child that she clearly remembers. In most instances, the child will be able to identify the person involved in the alleged sexual activity.

Before an examination, the child should be prepared and her cooperation won. Previous trips to a physician's office or to a hospital emergency room may have been associated by this young patient with pain. Gentleness during the examination cannot be overemphasized. The force applied by two persons during the examination of an uncooperative child may be perceived by the child as greater trauma than the actual sexual assault.

The general physical examination of the young girl does not differ from that performed on the adult. The external genitalia and perineal area can be inspected easily if the patient places her heels together with the knees in a flexed position and allows her thighs to fall apart. Touching of the genitalia during this initial inspection is not necessary. Subsequently, the labia majora are separated gently to expose labia minora, clitoris, urethral orifice and vagina. The lower third of the vagina and some of the vaginal secretions can even be identified with this maneuver. Any injury, be it recent or old, is described in detail. A clean plastic medicine dropper can be gently passed through the hymenal opening to collect specimens for culture and microscopic examination. If no evidence of injury is found, a digital rectal exploration is needed to complete the examination.

In most cases a more detailed examination of the vagina and cervix is unnecessary. Injuries in children resulting from sexual assault are usually apparent during inspection of the external genitalia. If a penetrating injury has occurred in an area that is not accessible to examination without pain, general anesthesia in an operating room may be indicated in order to ensure exploration and surgical repair. Anesthesia is also indicated when foreign bodies that cannot be easily removed are found in the vagina, urethra, bladder or rectum. In cases of serious trauma, immediate care of injuries obviously takes precedence over the medicolegal examination. Evidence in these prepubertal girls is collected in similar fashion as in adult women. Vaginal secretions are examined for motile and nonmotile spermatozoa and acid phosphatase. Cultures for gonococci from the vaginal fluid should also be performed and blood for a serologic detection of syphilis should be obtained.

Several preventive treatment regimens have been recommended against venereal disease in young girls. Aqueous procaine penicillin (100,000 units/kg up to a maximum of 4.8 million units) in addition to Probenecid (25 mg/kg orally up to a maximum of 1 g) is the most frequently used regimen. For girls who are allergic to penicillin, spectinomycin hydrochloride intramuscularly (50 mg/kg, 2 g maximum) or tetracycline (25 mg/kg, 1.5 g maximum) in a single oral dose followed by 10 mg/kg (500 mg maximum) by mouth 4 times daily over a 4-day period offers protection in most instances.

Sexual assault is just one form of child abuse and the procedures for notifying the proper authorities, in most communities a local child welfare department, have to be carried out according to the organization of the services within the specific community.

The Physician as a Court Witness

In most instances cases of sexual assault are not brought to trial because either the alleged assailant is not apprehended, the case is unfounded or the assailant pleads guilty. However, if the case goes to trial, the examining physician often plays a critical role and needs to be knowledgeable about the legal consequences of examination and treatment of a victim as well as of the collection of evidence. Therefore, it must be remembered that any facet of the victim's time in the physician's office and her previous or subsequent care may be brought up in the trial.

While the physician should be the victim's advocate during her visit to his office, in court he has to be an objective witness. The prosecuting or defending attorney who calls the physician as a witness will attempt to qualify him as an expert by presenting to the court the course of his general medical education, specialization, experience in treating victims of sexual assault and his previous experience in court.

The physician should be prepared to use lay terms during his testimony. In most instances he is questioned about the circumstances under which he examined and cared for the victim. He is asked to describe the patient's emotional and physical condition. Additionally, he is often asked to describe injuries and if he detected motile or nonmotile spermatozoa. The physician is expected to know how long spermatozoa remain motile and detectable in the female reproductive tract under the circumstances in which the victim was first examined.[5] Although the physician rarely will be asked about the results and interpretation of the forensic examination, he should be prepared to answer questions about the collection of evidence and the safeguarding of specimens. The answers of the expert witness should be short and precise and, if the physician is unfamiliar with a topic, does not understand a question or does not know an answer, he should unhesitatingly so state.

TABLE 1. Convictions of Rape in 3 Texas Counties Between 1974 and 1977

| | County 1 | | County 2 | | Dallas County | |
	No.	Percentage†	No.	Percentage†	No.	Percentage†
Convicted						
Guilty plea	60	30.3	396	37.1	378	46.3
Not guilty plea	24	12.1	114	10.7	109	13.3
Total convictions	84	42.4	510	47.8	487	59.6
Total cases disposed*	198	100.0	1066	100.0	817	100.0
Convictions per 100,000 population	2.3		6.3		8.2	
Cases disposed per 100,000 population	6.3		13.1		13.8	

*Includes convictions, acquittals and dismissals.
†% of cases disposed.
From Texas Judicial Council Annual Reports 1975–1977, Austin, Texas.

Experience of the Dallas Center

An evaluation of the impact of rape examination centers on the number of rapes occurring and on the frequency of conviction is difficult. Many victims do not report the crime, police departments apprehend assailants in varying numbers and the success or failure of a prosecutor depends on factors too numerous to mention. Unfortunately, comparison of data from Dallas County before and after the opening of our center is impossible, because methods of data collection and reporting have changed during recent years. Nevertheless, some data obtained between 1974 and 1977 could be compiled from three urban Texas counties[6] (Table 1). In county 1 no coordinated system for examination of rape victims exists. In county 2 victims are seen by many physicians, at all levels of training, in a variety of hospitals; in Dallas all victims are attended by a single group of board-certified obstetrician-gynecologists within one hospital. Fewer convictions were made and fewer cases were disposed of per population unit in counties 2 and 3 than in Dallas County. If the premise is correct, that a similar number of rapes occur per population unit in all three counties, the success in Dallas has indeed been remarkable.

Many physicians consider examination and treatment of rape victims an ungratifying experience. However, it is a civic responsibility that needs to be fulfilled to make our society safer for women and to protect suspected assailants from unjust indictment, prosecution and conviction.

REFERENCES

1. McCubbin, J. H. and Scott, D. E.: Management of alleged sexual assault. Texas Medicine 69:59, 1973.
2. Kuchera, L. K.: Postcoital contraception with diethylstilbestrol. J.A.M.A. 218:562, 1971.
3. Kuchera, L. K.: Postcoital contraception with diethylstilbestrol—updated. Contraception 10:47, 1974.
4. Soules, M. R., Stewart, S. K., Brown, K. M. et al.: The spectrum of alleged rape. J. Reprod. Med. 20:33, 1978.
5. Soules, M. R., Pollard, A. A., Brown, K. M. et al.: The forensic laboratory evaluation of evidence in alleged rape. Am. J. Obstet. Gynecol. 130:142, 1978.
6. Texas Judicial Council Annual Reports 1975-1977, Austin, Texas.

Management of the Rape Victim

Dorothy J. Hicks, M.D.
Raphael S. Good, M.D.
University of Miami School of Medicine

Rape is the fastest growing crime in the United States according to the law enforcement authorities, and most authorities believe that at best only one in four rapes is reported. The Uniform Crime statistics show an almost 200 per cent increase in the number of rapes reported in 1960 and 1976. These figures do not include the numbers of sexual assaults on children, the homosexual rapes or the rape-murders. Law enforcement people estimate that in the United States, a rape occurs every two minutes. The crime is not reported because the victims are afraid of embarrassment and intimidated by the attitude of the public that the woman is to blame for the assault. Also, she may fear reprisal by her attacker. Forcible rape is a violent crime and is a form of sexual deviance. The object of the attacker is not sexual gratification as is understood by a normal male but is rather to humiliate and hurt the woman or to prove to himself that he is a virile male.

Some information about rapists may be helpful. The average rapist strikes once a week, sometimes more frequently, and the violence tends to increase with each attack. The crimes are planned in detail and each rapist has a distinct mode of operation. The study done by the Queens Bench Foundation of San Francisco showed that 82.2 per cent chose their victim because she "was available," 71.2 per cent because she "was defenseless," and less than 50 per cent because she "was sexy" or "attractive."[19] To the rapist, the female is an object and many cannot even describe the appearance of the victim once the attack is completed. Most series show that 50 per cent of rapes occur in the home of either the victim or the offender. In our series, the age of female patients ranged from 2 months to 91 years. Five per cent of our patients were male and 30 per cent of the patients were below the age of 15 years.

Sexual assault precipitates a crisis situation, and the victim of this crime needs empathy, not just sympathy, from all those who come in contact with her. Bard states that rape may be thought of as "the ultimate invasion of self (short of homicide)" and this fact may help people to understand just what rape does to the victim. The psychological trauma of the rape victim is far more serious than the physical abuse in most instances. In our series of 3562 patients seen since January 1974, only 15 per cent had physical injuries and less than 1 per cent were hospitalized, although two patients died as a result of the attack. All patients need medical care and psychological counseling at the time of the attack and should have adequate follow-up care if they are to survive this crisis without permanent damage.

The attitude, not the sex, of persons dealing with rape victims is extremely important. The first person who comes in contact with the patient may set the tone for the entire experience. These persons cannot be judgmental. The patient must be given the opportunity to realize that she is again in control of her life. It is important that she be given the right to make decisions as to what will be done to and for her. This privilege was denied her from the time the attack began until she was released.

It must be possible for the victim to receive medical treatment and counseling even though she chooses not to report the crime to law authorities. If the police are involved, they must be understanding and should take the victim to a treatment center as soon as possible after the attack. The patient should be encouraged to report the crime, and usually, when patients understand the psychology of the rapist and that sexual assault is a crime, they decide to report the incident even though they may not wish to prosecute.

Medical Aspects

The area to which rape victims are taken should be a quiet, peaceful place adjacent to but not a part of a full-service emergency room. It should be obvious, however, that if serious injury has occurred this is taken care of before the specific examinations are done; therefore, some patients will go directly into the trauma section.

Written informed consent forms properly signed and witnessed conforming to the hospitals protocols are mandatory. The consent should include the taking of photographs and the release of information to the authorities if the police are involved. State laws vary where minors are concerned. In some states, parental consent is necessary and in others it is not necessary for minors to receive care.

When the patient arrives at the treatment center, she should not be made to repeat the story of the attack over and over again. The physician should be the one to take the history from the patient. If the patient has volunteered the story to the nurse or a counselor, however, the physician should use that material as a basis and proceed from there. The history taken at the time of the medical examination should not be detailed. At this time, the patient is likely to be confused and the official statements taken later by the police are likely to differ in minor areas from the emergency room history. These discrepancies, even though minor, may jeopardize the case at prosecution. Rape is a legal term and as Braen states, "The physician should keep in mind that it is not his responsibility to determine whether the patient has been raped, but . . . to report his findings."

The chart should include the patient's name, address, birth date, marital status and, if any police are involved, their names and other identification.

The personal history should include the parity and gravidity of the patient, the date of the last menses and whether or not it was normal. The date of last voluntary intercourse is essential because the sperm found may be residual from that exposure. Whether or not the patient practices contraception is important.

If the patient has had hepatitis or venereal disease and whether or not it has been treated is important, both from the standpoint of the attack and also for the protection of the laboratory people who will be handling the specimens.

Whether or not the patient has douched, bathed, voided or defecated since the incident is useful information. Whether the patient changed clothes is part of the history.

The history of the assault should include its date, time and location. The number of assailants and whether or not they were known to the victim should be documented. Whether the attacker threatened the victim and had a weapon is important. The physician should find out if restraints were used and if so, any markings are left on the skin as evidence of this.

Particulars of the attack should include the following: the anatomic type of attack—oral, vaginal, rectal—and whether there was penetration and ejaculation. If a foreign body was inserted into any body cavity, this is recorded. Any visible injuries as a result of the attack should be documented.

The physical examination has a dual purpose: to locate injuries and to allow collection of specimens that can be used as evidence.

In the general part of the examination, the state of consciousness should be noted and any bruises, lacerations, fractures and so forth described in detail. Foreign material such as sand or grass should be collected and placed in a clean envelope. Particular attention should be paid to the hair and scalp, the breasts and back. A Wood's lamp may be used to locate seminal stains on the skin. The ultraviolet light causes semen to fluoresce and it is easily identifiable. Moistened cotton swabs will lift these stains. If there has been a struggle, scrapings should be taken from under the fingernails. If the nail has been broken, a part of the remaining nail should be clipped and the portion kept as a match for the broken piece if it is found.

Even if the patient denies fellatio or sodomy, swabs should be taken from the oral cavity and nasopharynx. The areas should be cultured for gonococci and the material plated immediately on Thayer-Martin medium. Any evidence of trauma or lubricating material in the perianal area should be noted. Swabs should be taken from the rectum and the rectum cultured for gonococci.

Most of the specific testing is done in the pelvic area. The patient is placed in the lithotomy position. The pubic hair is combed carefully and the comb and combings placed in a clean envelope. Some hairs should be trimmed and placed with the combings.

The vulvar area is examined carefully for evidence of trauma and semen. Any findings should be carefully described. Cotton swabs may be used to collect any foreign material or semen from the vulvar area. These are then placed in a clean envelope and sealed as the other specimens were.

The appearance of the hymen is important.

Any evidence of trauma should be documented and carefully described; including whether the hymen is intact. If lacerations are present, they should be described as either fresh or old. A Pederson speculum moistened only with water should be used to inspect the vaginal canal and cervix. The smaller speculum is helpful because there is seldom any natural lubrication since the prime emotion in rape is fear, and the use of jelly may affect the acid phosphatase test. Any fluid in the canal should be described. Swabs from the cervical area and near the introitus are taken. Air-dried smears are made from these swabs and the swabs and smears are sent to the laboratory. In our center we then inject 2 cc of sterile saline into the vagina and retrieve it with a pipet. This is the "vaginal aspirate." The fluid is injected into the fornices rather than at the cervix in an attempt to avoid the endocervical mucus.

After the forensic tests are done, the endocervical canal is cultured for gonococci and a pap test is done to provide a permanent record of sperm.

A bimanual pelvic examination is then performed to determine the presence of lacerations in the vault and the state of the pelvic organs. A rectovaginal examination should also be done.

The physician should examine the vaginal aspirate as soon as possible and note the presence or absence of sperm and whether or not they are motile. Anything unusual in the aspirate should be noted. If no sperm are found, the aspirate should be tested for the presence of acid phosphatase, an enzyme found in all body fluids but in high concentration only in seminal fluid.

A specimen of the patient's saliva is then obtained by asking the victim to chew a small piece of clean cloth. This is then used by the laboratory to check the secretor status of the victim, because 80 per cent of people secrete blood antigens in their body fluids. It is extremely important that no one but the victim touch this piece of cloth at any time.

Any clothes that may prove to be evidence are placed in a paper bag. Plastic should not be used because the moisture will cause an overgrowth of bacteria and mold and prevent accurate laboratory diagnosis.

Photographs that are indicated should be taken by a police photographer. If this is not feasible, the undeveloped film should be given to the police so that it is processed in their laboratory.

Each and every specimen collected as evidence must be carefully labeled with the patient's name, the date and time of the examination and identifying numbers. These must be signed by everyone who handles the specimens and ideally should be handed to the police after the examination is completed. Whenever custody of the specimens is transferred, a written receipt should be obtained. We have built this into our sexual battery form (Fig. 1). The specimens should be processed in a crime laboratory whenever possible so that the "chain of evidence" (the custody of evidence) is kept intact. A copy of the form should be given to the officer at the conclusion of the examination. Any break in the "chain of evidence" may jeopardize prosecution.

Medical treatment for the rape victim should consist of prophylaxis for venereal disease and pregnancy as well as tetanus when indicated. It is especially important to offer protection for venereal disease because many patients do not return for the follow-up examination four to six weeks after the attack. In our clinic we use the dosage regimen of the Centers for Disease Control: Probenecid 1 g by mouth and aqueous procaine penicillin G 4.8 million units intramuscularly. This will protect the patient from incubating syphilis as well as treat gonorrhea. If the patient is allergic to penicillin, we offer spectinomycin hydrocloride 2 g intramuscularly in a single injection. This will not protect a patient against syphilis. Tetracycline may be used: 1.5 g orally immediately, then 500 mg 4 times a day for 15 days.

Although the risk of rape related pregnancy is said to be about 1 per cent, few patients care to take that chance. In view of this, we offer them the "morning-after" pill: Diethylstilbestrol 25 mg twice a day for 5 consecutive days. This must be started within 72 hours of exposure to be effective. Because the side effects include nausea, we offer antiemetics to be taken before the DES. Because DES will damage a fetus, we withhold the medication if the patient is adamant in refusing menstrual extraction or abortion should pregnancy occur.

After the medical examination is completed, the patient receives formal counseling, although actually the counseling has begun from the time the patient enters our care.

Unless she refuses, arrangements are made for follow-up care for counseling for the patient and any significant others in her circle and for re-examination for venereal disease and pregnancy four to six weeks after the attack.

RAPE TREATMENT CENTER

JACKSON MEMORIAL HOSPITAL

UNIVERSITY OF MIAMI SCHOOL OF
MEDICINE

Address_____

Place of exam_____ Time_____

Birth date_____ Race____ M S W D SEP

Police dept._____ Case #_____

Officer_____

PERSONAL HISTORY

Para____ ____ ____ ____ Gr._____

LMP: Date_____Normal   Abnormal

Last coitus: Date_____Time_____

Contraception: Yes   No   Type:_____

Douche   Bath   Defecate   Void since assault

Venereal Disease: Yes   No   Type_____RX_____

Hepatitis: Yes   No   When_____RX_____

HISTORY OF ASSAULT
Date:_____ Time:_____

Location:_____

No. of assailants_____Race: B W L O UNK

Attacker: Known_____ Unk_____ Relative_____

Threats: Yes   No   Type_____

Restraints: Yes   No   Type_____

Weapon: Yes   No   Type_____

	Oral	Anal	Vaginal	Digital	For. Body
Type of sex:	___	___	___	___	___
Penetration:	___	___	___	___	___
Ejaculation:	___	___	___	___	___

Comments:_____

_____

GENERAL EXAM: (brusies, trauma, laceration
marks)

NO HISTORY

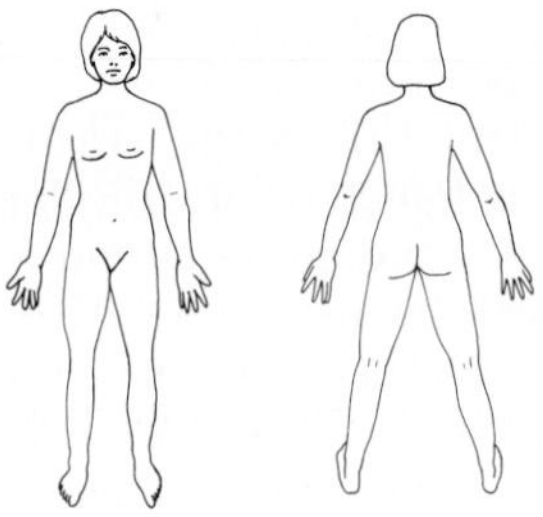

PELVIC EXAM: (include signs of trauma,
bleeding, foreign bodies)

Vulva_____

Hymen_____

Vagina_____

Cervix_____

Fundus_____

Adnexae_____

Rectal_____

_____

_____

_____

Figure 1.   Sexual battery form, Jackson Memorial Hospital, University of Miami School of Medicine, pages 1
and 2.

RAPE TREATMENT CENTER

JACKSON MEMORIAL HOSPITAL   UNIVERSITY OF MIAMI SCHOOL OF MEDICINE

Physician_____ Nurse_____ Counselor_____

TESTS

GC Culture: Oral   Anal   Cervical   Other_____

VDRL: Yes   No (5 cc venous blood—red top)

PAP Test: Yes   No

TREATMENT

VD Prophylaxis: Yes   No   Type_____
Pregnancy Prophylaxis: Yes No Type____

Tetanus: Yes   No   Other meds:_____

EVIDENTIAL SPECIMENS, TESTING AND RECEIPT

Results of preliminary tests: AP: Negative   Weak   Moderate   Strong

Sperm:: None   1–5   6–10   10+   Motile   Nonmotile

SPECIMENS OBTAINED;	GIVEN TO POLICE	OTHER TREATMENT
10 cc Venous blood (red top)_____	_____	X-ray_____
Fingernail scrapings_____	_____	Surg. consult_____
Pubic hair combings_____	_____	Psych. consult_____
Vaginal Smear_____	_____	Other: (Explain)_____
Vaginal Swab_____	_____	
Cervical Smear_____	_____	
Cervical Swab_____	_____	
Vaginal aspirate_____	_____	
Rectal Smear_____	_____	
Rectal Swab_____	_____	
Oral Smear_____	_____	
Oral Swab_____	_____	
Saliva specimen_____	_____	GIVEN TO POLICE

Clothing (number)_____   Type_____   Condition_____

Foreign bodies (number)_____   Type_____   Location_____

Other specimens_____   Photographs: Yes   No   Taken by_____

TOTAL NUMBER SPECIMENS   TOTAL TO POLICE

Receipt of Evidence: The above evidence has been received by me on (date)_____at

(Time)_____   (Officer's signature)_____

Physician's signature:_____

Witness signature_____

Psychological Aspects

The psychological reactions to rape can be conceptualized within the framework of general crisis theory. Rape represents a specific crisis with attendant intrapsychic and interpersonal aspects that determine emotional, behavioral and physical responses. Even though sexual assault has its idiosyncratic characteristics, an understanding of the process of adaptation to any hazardous event aids in appreciating responses to rape so that meaningful interventions can be initiated to bolster coping mechanisms and prevent extended periods of emotional, behavioral or physical invalidism.

A crisis can be defined as a stressful life event—a hazard that poses a threat—the threat may be real or imagined. The threat of bodily harm is frequently real when rape is the event but only fantasized when a natural disaster such as a hurricane or earthquake causes a panic reaction and fear of bodily harm in a person far removed from the disaster site; the psychological, physical and behavioral symptoms may be similar even though the event and threat are markedly different. Hazardous events not only result in threats to bodily integrity but also may include, though are not necessarily limited to, threats to self-esteem, to social or financial status, to instinctual needs related to dependency or control, and to significant interpersonal relationships.

Previous life experiences also affect the response to a hazardous event. One who might have been exposed to a similar event in the past and was able to deal effectively with resultant fears without serious sequelae is better able to cope with a similar situation. The successful resolution of the crisis confirms that one has the ability to deal with a similar event, which in turn tends to decrease the likelihood of disorganization and symptom formation. A stressful event tends to rekindle thoughts, feelings and fantasies associated with similar past events. If the victim recalls that she was able to successfully cope with the past event, it adds to her sense of confidence that she can cope with the current event—self-esteem increases and nonpathologic resolution is more apt to ensue.

The wider the range of coping mechanisms available to an individual exposed to stress the more likely is the individual to be able to deal with the crisis adaptively. The individual whose major defense following rape is denial may prejudice her future physical and emotional well-being. Due to her denial, she may delay seeking medical advice, thereby increasing the risk of pregnancy and infection. The inability to deal with painful feelings such as anger and guilt may lead to phobic behavior and to both psychological and physical symptoms.

The ability to effectively deal with losses is a very significant factor in the successful resolution of a crisis. This is particularly true for rape, since rape may represent not only one but numerous losses. Some of these include the loss of virginity, which may imply loss of status, loss of self-esteem related to the feeling of having been defiled, which may also be interpreted as a loss of cleanliness, and fear of loss of interpersonal relationships, which is frequently expressed by the rape victim as a fear that her sexual partner will reject her. These losses are interwoven because rejection by the sexual partner reinforces the sense of lowered self-esteem and worthlessness.

Losses account, in part, for the feelings of guilt and anger so frequently exhibited by individuals exposed to stressful events. The psychodynamics of the feelings of guilt and anger have been well delineated by numerous investigators. However, in rape victims, the intrapsychic determinants are reinforced by environmental factors. Many segments of our society continue to view the rape victim as being in some way responsible for the assault, and attitudes about her manner of dress, the nature of her walk, her previous sexual activity and so forth only tend to increase her sense of guilt. It is well documented that anger accompanies losses based on infantile developmental factors, which are probably never completely resolved by any individual. However, the sexual assault victim has a specific target for her anger—namely, her assailant. She can focus her anger on a specific individual who is actually responsible for her losses. The rape victim who is not able to effectively deal with this anger due to her feelings of guilt may direct it toward herself with resultant depression. Alternatively, she may displace her anger to other males, possibly producing strains in work, social and sexual relationships.

The social support system available to the rape victim is, as it is for any individual in crisis, a vital aspect in abetting coping responses. If the parents of a victim are able to openly deal with the event, this has positive aspects that aid coping. It implies to the victim that the assault is not shameful and can be freely discussed, thus reducing guilt. It gives the victim the opportunity to retell the details and thereby to re-establish a sense of mastery and control. It also gives the assault victim an opportunity to verbalize some of her feelings and to deal more effectively with painful affects. The parents, children, husband or male friend who creates an atmosphere of silence implying that the assault did not occur or that it has little meaning reinforces the assault victim's sense of shame and guilt and encourages suppression of anger.

Even though the events that lead to crisis are protean and variable and even though personality structure, previous life experiences, coping mechanisms, response to losses and availability of social support systems vary from individual to individual, nevertheless the disequilibrium resulting from the attack is manifested in clearly defined physical, psychological and behavioral reactions. Regardless of the strategies employed by the rape victim to deal with the attack itself, the ultimate response and readjustment can be divided into distinct phases.

An understanding of the sequential nature of the reactions permits planned, supportive interventions so essential for the prevention of long-term disability. Horowitz, who conducted extensive studies of individuals exposed to stressful events, describes five stages of the stress response syndrome: (1) the outcry or immediate emotional response to the actual event; (2) denial or emotional numbness as a defense; (3) intrusiveness of repetitive unbidden thoughts, frequently with nightmares; (4) working through, which may require specific counseling or even brief psychotherapy; and finally, (5) cognitive completion with attainment of emotional mastery in the context of one's current life.[14]

Others have specifically studied the stress response syndrome in assault victims. Burgess and Holmstrom analyzed the symptoms of 92 adult women who were victims of forcible rape and delineated an "acute phase" in which there is disorganization and a "long-term process" in which there is reorganization.[6] This schema is consistent with the syndrome described by Horowitz. In the study of the rape victims, the acute phase was characterized by impact reactions, somatic manifestations and emotional reactions.

The impact reaction occurred in the first few hours following the rape and was characterized by a wide variety of emotions ranging from shock exhibited by feelings of fear and anger, to disbelief with an outward, exaggerated calm.

The somatic reactions persisted for several weeks following the rape and included soreness from physical trauma, tension headaches and sleep disturbances. Gastrointestinal symptoms such as abdominal pain, anorexia and nausea were also present. Genitourinary disturbances were common; there were many complaints of vaginal discharge, vulvar itching and a burning sensation on urination.

Emotional reactions during the acute phase covered a wide spectrum. The victims expressed feelings of fear, humiliation, anger, guilt and desire for revenge. The fear of physical violence and death frequently persisted. These acute phase reactions led to a general disorganization, and only after several weeks did most victims begin the longer term process of reorganization. These investigators found that during this reorganization process, which frequently persisted for a few months, approximately 50 per cent of the patients raped in their homes changed their residence and many changed phone numbers; it seemed to be a mechanism for dealing with the fear of the return of the assailant. During this phase, victims gradually overcame the common fears of being indoors if the rape had occurred while they were sleeping in bed or of being outdoors if the attack had occurred outside the home. The fear of being anywhere alone was almost universally expressed. Many women developed sexual fears that required time for resolution. During this phase, victims frequently sought out family members and close friends for support.

The counseling program at the Rape Treatment Center of the University of Miami-Jackson Memorial Medical Complex is based on a crisis intervention model that is applicable to most individuals exposed to a hazardous event but tailored to the specific problems of victims of sexual assault. The counseling is not considered psychotherapy, nor does it replace psychotherapy. The symptomatology is considered to be the response of average, normal individuals to a hazardous event. It is assumed that these individuals will be able to mobilize adaptive coping mechanisms and that they had been functioning adequately prior to the rape.

The major goal of the counselor is to promote mastery; this is accomplished by support and the sustaining of hope. As a role model, the counselor expresses concern and confidence that the victim will be able to return to at least her former level of functioning. The counseling is issue-oriented and there is no perceived need to deal with developmental or environmental problems. The counselor encourages the victim to consider choices and come to her own decisions concerning solutions; the temptation to act for the client is rigorously avoided as it tends to increase dependency. However, the counselor recognizes and legitimatizes the individual's increased dependency needs and may use these needs to marshal family supports. Bolstering the network of family and close friends gives the victim a sense of support that increases self-esteem without interfering with decision-making and leads to the eventual achieving of mastery.

The verbalization of fears and the discussion of dreams and nightmares is encouraged. The patient is also encouraged to speak freely of her feelings toward her assailant as this is frequently linked to changed feelings toward significant males in her life.

In order to counsel effectively, it is necessary to have an understanding of the victim's life adjustment prior to the assault as well as a knowledge of the quality of the victim's object relations, ability to tolerate stress, adaptive resources and available social supports. This assessment can be made rapidly by ascertaining school or work history, current interpersonal relationships and how leisure time is spent. With this knowledge the counselor is better able to formulate the needs of the individual victim and can more effectively help the patient in her reorganization tasks. Finally, the continued availability of the counselor is emphasized. This reaffirms for the victim that someone is caring and concerned and that there is someone to whom she can freely communicate her fears, thoughts and feelings.

In summary, sexual assault presents a crisis for the victim that results in definable symptomatology. An appreciation of crisis theory and the stress response syndrome aids the clinician in planning interventions to enhance an early return to normal function and to prevent prolonged disability.

REFERENCES

1. Bard, M. and Ellison, K.: Crisis Intervention and Investigation of Forcible Rape. The Police Chief 41:68, 1974.
2. Boozer, D. G.: Personal communications, 1970-1978.
3. Bowlby, J.: Processes of mourning. Int. J. Psychoanal., 42:317, 1961.
4. Braen, G. R.: The Rape Examination. North Chicago, Abbott Laboratories, 1976.
5. Burgess, A. W. and Groth, A. N.: Address at Workshop for Victimology, Fresno, California, May 1976.
6. Burgess, A. W. and Holmstrom, L. L.: Rape trauma syndrome. Am. J. Psychiatr. 131:981, 1974.
7. Burgess, A. W. and Holmstrom, L. L.: Rape: Victims of Crisis. Robert J. Brady, Bowie, Md., 1974.
8. Caplan, G.: An Approach to Community Mental Health. New York, Grune & Stratton, 1961.
9. Freud, S.: Mourning and Melancholia, Standard ed., Vol. XIV. London, Hogarth Press, 1957.
10. Halpern, S., Hicks, D. J. and Crenshaw, T.: Rape: Helping the Victim. Oradel, N.J., Medical Economics Book Co., 1978.
11. Hicks, D. J.: Rape: Sexual Assault. Obstetrics & Gynecology Annual, 7:447, 1978.
12. Hicks, D. J.: Rape: A Crime of Violence. Contemporary Ob/Gyn, 11:67, 1978.
13. Hirschowitz, R. G.: Crisis theory: A formulation. Psychiat. Ann. 3:36, 1973.
14. Horowitz, M. J.: Stress Response Syndrome. New York, Jason Aronson, Inc., 1976.
15. Jacobson, G., Strickler, M. and Morley, W. E.: Generic and individual approaches to crisis intervention. Am. J. Public Health 58:339, 1968.
16. Lindemann, E.: Symptomatology and management of acute grief. Am. J. Psychiat. 101:141, 1944.
17. Morley, W. E., Messick, J. M. and Aquilera, D. C.: Crisis: paradigms of intervention. Journal of Psychiatric Nursing 5:537, 1967.
18. Planned Parenthood Memo: FDA approved DES for emergency use. February 13, 1975, p. 34.
19. Queen's Bench Foundation: Rape: Prevention and Resistance. San Francisco, 1976.
20. Sexual Assault Manual, Miami, Jackson Memorial Hospital, 1977.
21. Solomon, M.: After the Rape: A Report of Metro's Rape Awareness Program, Miami, Florida, 1974.
22. Sutherland, S. and Scherl, D. J.: Patterns of response among victims of rape. Am. J. Orthopsychiat. 40:503, 1970.
23. Tyhurst, J. G.: Individual reactions to community disaster: the habitual history of psychiatric phenomena. Am. J. Psychiat. 107:764, 1951.
24. Uniform Crime Reports: Crime in the United States. Federal Bureau of Investigation, Washington, DC, U.S. Government Printing Office, p. 37, 1975.

Editorial Comment

The information in this chapter on the rape victim underscores the changes in and growing sophistication of treatment that has taken place in this area over the past decade. The authors of these articles have made major contributions in establishing regional health planning for the assault victim in the Miami and the Dallas areas. There are more points of agreement than disagreement in these two articles; agreement would be expected since these come from the authors who have made major contributions in changing the management of the rape victim for their areas. Everyone agrees that women's groups, forensic scientists, physicians and law enforcement agencies, all working together, have improved the quality of health care for the rape victim. The rape victim now is treated like any other patient in a dignified approach to health care.

If we all agree that rape is one of the most villainous forms of body invasion, then our attention should be turned to the work of Dallas group. They have developed a systematic, scientific method in which the rape victim is taken to one location, Parkland Hospital, and seen by board-certified obstetricians-gynecologists. Interestingly, the percentage of convictions for rape was statistically greater there than in two other comparable Texas counties in which no such services were offered. I know of no other major city in the country that has accepted this civic responsibility of having all rape victims brought to one rape crisis center for care and having each person seen by a board-certified obstetrician-gynecologist. All too often an intern or first-year resident is sent to the emergency department to evaluate a rape victim, and this is probably inexcusable health care. I don't mean to imply that interns and first-year residents are not capable of doing some of the technical things that are necessary, but certainly the sophistication of a fully trained obstetrician-gynecologist is what a woman needs at this time of great crisis.

The controversy in the past has been about the dictum that a female gynecologist should see the rape victim, along with a female police officer. Disagreement with this has come from female gynecologists, who say that this certainly is not necessary, and this is underscored by the Miami group, who state that it is the attitude of the person that is important and not the sex. This is true for both police officers and physicians as well as other health care personnel.

Both groups have underscored the importance of having the victim sign a form that allows data collection and that a witness be present. It is important for the people seeing an alleged rape victim that documentation be made with appropriate witnesses to identify that specimens were taken from the patient and that these were placed in sealed containers as a group and then taken care of by appropriate people. A difference in methods is that the Miami group collects the information and gives it to the police, whereas the Dallas group collects the information and then gives it under lock and key to the forensic pathologist, who then establishes the laboratory evidence of rape and provides this information to the police.

Both groups agree that as far as the physician is concerned, there are three objectives for therapy: repair of the injury, prevention of pregnancy and prevention of venereal disease. The Miami authors go into great detail about the psychological support that is necessary and give us a good understanding of the attitude of the female who has been raped. They emphasize that rape is a legal term and that physicians should not decide if it did or did not occur but that they should determine the specific findings and report them accurately. One thing the Miami group does that the Dallas group does not do is that they ask the patient to chew a clean cloth to try to determine secretor antigens, and this cloth, untouched by anyone but the victim, is then put in an envelope for later analysis. They also emphasize that a photograph should be taken, if possible by police photographers rather than by others. The Miami group emphasizes that if the patient can't focus on rage and hostility of the assailant, then she ends up with psychological problems because she directs inward this hostility and rage, and this in turn creates a depressive reaction. The depressive reaction may or may not displace anger in relationships with other males, and this can cause a strain on relationships in all settings for the future. The friends of the victim who know of the attack, if they say nothing and act as though it never happened, make the patient have more guilt and shame than usual. It's interesting to note that 50 per cent of the victims change phone numbers and location of residence over the next two months, and this is felt to be due to fear, guilt and shame. There is a heavier psychic toll than most people realize, and there is no simple approach for each person because therapy must be highly individualized.

Both groups abide by the CDC guidelines for the prevention of venereal disease in that they use 4.8 million units of penicillin plus 1 gram of Probenecid. The idea is to eliminate incubating syphilis and to cure gonorrhea if present.

The risk of pregnancy for the rape victim is low. It's important to know whether the victim was protected by a contraceptive method at the time of the incident. If not, both groups agree in that they give diethylstilbestrol, 25 mg, twice a day for 5 days, to prevent conception. It was brought out by the Miami group that this has a potential of causing a damaged fetus; hence, if the victim refuses to have an abortion or a menstrual extraction if pregnant, they do not give the stilbestrol. Other groups in this country are now prescribing oral contraceptives, given three or four times a day for two or three days, which causes basically the same abnormal endometrial reaction with prevention of implantation, and obviates the problems of gastrointestinal symptoms from a large dose of stilbestrol estrogen. The results apparently are equally effective with both methods.

There is some mild disagreement on reporting the event of alleged rape, and each physician must understand the particular state laws; in some states an alleged attack must be reported to the police. However, if the victim does not wish to pursue charges, then nothing more is done. The important point is made that once the victim understands the problem, she often is quite amenable to discussing this with the police. The most important duty of the physician is to be an accurate recorder of facts and to try to prevent discrepancies in what is recorded at the time the patient is seen. This should involve an accurate, scientific approach to the problem. The Dallas group mentions that there are kits available that can be used for collection of specimens; however, they have their own particular kit made up by the forensic scientists. The Miami group does not use any kit form, but collects data on an individualized basis. One group says it's important to obtain the history in front of a chaperon and the other doesn't think that this is essential. The chaperon is used principally as a witness; however, by the time most of these incidents come to trial it is difficult to remember precisely what went on, and it would seem that this is not absolutely essential.

The end result of both groups is the same: the giving of adequate, expert scientific care to the rape victim. We would hope that all women are afforded similar care opportunities.

14

Management of Recurrent and Refractory Vaginitis

Alternative Points of View

by Raymond H. Kaufman, Ivor L. Safro and
Herman L. Gardner
by Marvin S. Amstey and Sangithan
Moodley

Editorial Comment

Management of Recurrent and Refractory Vaginitis

Raymond H. Kaufman, M.D.

Ivor L. Safro, M.D.

Herman L. Gardner, M.D.

Baylor College of Medicine

The increasing occurrence of venereally transmitted infection has presented the clinician with new problems in the management of vulvovaginal disease. Many of the problems related to persistent vaginal infections are also related to reinfection. Rarely are they a result of resistance of the causative organisms to therapy. These problems are so numerous that it would take a textbook to cover the subject thoroughly. This presentation will be limited to the more commonly encountered and more frustrating problems seen by the clinician.

The subjects discussed will be *Trichomonas vaginalis* vaginitis, *Gardnerella vaginalis* vaginitis, candidiasis, herpes genitalis, *Torulopsis* (Candida) *glabrata* vulvovaginitis and desquamative inflammatory vaginitis.

Before the refractory nature of vulvovaginitis can be established, the physician must first make the proper diagnosis. Too often,

women who have had bacteriologic cure continue to complain of symptoms and continue to be treated by the overzealous physician. Unless the diagnosis can be substantiated, specific therapy should be deferred. The individual with persistent or recurrent vaginitis poses a significant diagnostic and therapeutic problem. Many of these individuals have been treated repeatedly by many physicians, often for several years. Frequently, they are seen by a gynecologist only after many years of frustrating therapeutic experiences. In addition to the distress of ongoing disturbing symptoms, severe strain often has been placed upon the emotional stability of the patient as well as on her marital relationship. It is important that the gynecologist obtain an accurate history and perform a careful examination, utilizing appropriate laboratory tests to establish the correct diagnosis. Not infrequently, patients with successfully treated vaginitis will continue to have persistent symptoms and are repeatedly treated even in the absence of detectable infection. In addition, cultures often have been taken from the vagina and organisms identified that probably play no part in causing clinical vaginitis, but that are vigorously and unnecessarily treated. Careful physical examination and appropriate studies in the overwhelming majority of patients will establish the correct diagnosis and lead to effective therapy.

The most meaningful examination of a patient with a vaginal infection or discharge is made when the patient is experiencing symptoms, when she has not douched for at least two or three days and when she has not used a vaginal medication or a contraceptive cream or gel for at least five to seven days. Vaginal flora is changed by chemicals circulating in the vaginal pool. Almost any chemical agent that is instilled into the vagina shortly before examination distorts the clinical pattern and makes isolation of an infectious agent difficult, if not impossible. Some medications have a residual effect, lasting several days. The intensity of a patient's complaint of discharge often correlates poorly with objective findings. Some patients with no demonstrable abnormal vaginal secretions complain bitterly of discharge, whereas others with profuse discharge and repulsive odor deny its presence. Nevertheless, the complaint of discharge, especially when associated with irritative symptoms or malodor, is significant. The more fluid the discharge, the less likely it is to accumulate in the vagina in large volume, and therefore the complaint of profuse discharge by the patient may be justified even though it is not apparent to the physician.

Vulvar tissues should be carefully inspected for gross lesions, irritative signs such as erythema, edema and excoriation, and for the characteristics of the secretions that may have accumulated in the vestibule. The urethra is stripped, and the Bartholin's gland area is palpated. A dry, unlubricated, bivalve speculum is then inserted into the vagina and the cervix and vagina inspected for evidence of gross tissue disease and to determine the features of vaginal secretion. Inspection of secretion on the withdrawn speculum is also important. The volume, consistency, color and odor of the secretion are determined. The pH is assessed by using pH indicator paper. Some patients may have two or more causes for their discharge. For example, 25 per cent of patients with trichomoniasis also have *G. vaginalis* vaginitis. Both conditions are clear-cut examples of minor venereal diseases. Logic dictates and experience shows that patients with one venereal disease are more apt to acquire a second or even third sexually transmitted infection.

In establishing the cause of recurrent or persistent vaginitis, various laboratory determinations are of great value. No technique can be better than the technologist who performs the test. Unfortunately, medical technologists often are trained to run complex analytic equipment, but they often do not have the interest or background to make a reliable study of vaginal secretions. This, combined with the fact that the material presented for study is often improperly collected and transported, makes for an even worse situation.

Diagnostic Techniques

The physiologic saline wet mount is probably the most important laboratory method used to establish the differential diagnosis of vaginitis or discharge. It should be employed in the investigation of every symptomatic patient. Preparation of a saline wet mount requires only a few simple steps.

A small cotton-tipped applicator is dipped into fresh physiologic saline and a drop of the solution is transferred to a glass slide. Using the same cotton-tipped applicator, a small amount of vaginal secretion is mixed with the saline on the slide. This suspension is coverslipped and examined microscopically through both low-power and high-power objectives. Only when a delay in examining the slide is anticipated is it necessary to mix the vaginal material in a test tube of saline. Old saline can become contaminated with various microbes and cause confusion. Lactobacilli are easily visualized in the saline wet mount, and the three most common organisms that cause vaginitis can usually be readily identified by finding motile trichomonads, the "clue cells" of *G. vaginalis*, or the spores and filaments of Candida. *G. vaginalis*, being a surface parasite, does not provoke an outpouring of leukocytes, and for this reason never accounts for a truly purulent discharge. A large number of pus cells in vaginal secretions in patients with *G. vaginalis* vaginitis indicates an associated pathologic condition, such as cervicitis.

The KOH (10 to 20 per cent) wet mount is a highly accurate method of diagnosing candidiasis. It is prepared by using a small glass rod to place a droplet of the solution onto the slide. An excess of solution can make a smear too dilute and poses a danger to the microscope objectives. An applicator stick is used to transfer a small amount of the vaginal secretion to the slide and to mix the secretion with the KOH solution. The slide is then coverslipped and examined through the microscope through both high power and low power. Most of the cellular material on the slide dissolves immediately or becomes transparent, making detection of intact Candida particles easy. Candida is the only vaginal fungus with both spores and filaments. Spores in large numbers without associated filaments suggest *Torulopsis glabrata* infection.

Stained smears of vaginal secretions are only occasionally required for the differential diagnosis of vaginitis and discharge, because an accurate diagnosis can usually be made by correlating clinical findings with saline and KOH wet mount. The smear, however, is a reliable method of identifying candidal spores and filaments and the pores of *Torulopsis glabrata*, and at times may be of some value in identifying the organisms of *G. vaginalis*. It is useless in the diagnosis of trichomoniasis.

The Papanicolaou smear is sometimes of value in providing a clue as to the cause of a vaginitis. In our experience, however, the cervical-vaginal smear is not a reliable method for the differential diagnosis of vaginitis. Exceptions to this rule are the characteristic findings of giant cells and intranuclear inclusion bodies in patients with herpes genitalis. This is often the first clue to the presence of an asymptomatic viral infection.

Clinicians are prone to place too much confidence in microbiologic cultures. In most clinical laboratories, microbiology is not the precise science that some consider it to be. Cultures are only occasionally required in the differential diagnosis of vaginitis. In our practice, their use is primarily reserved for investigative protocols or to confirm gonorrhea, Chlamydia, or herpes genitalis. Vaginal bacterial cultures are rarely informative. Cultural isolation of a bacterium, even though it is the predominant vaginal agent isolated, does not always prove an etiologic relationship between that bacterium and the discharge of the vaginitis present. Clinicians must guard against always assigning etiologic significance to bacterial agents enumerated in the laboratory report. In fact, few clinical laboratories are geared to provide useful answers to gynecologists; most utilize only routine culture media.

For these procedures to be useful at all, there must be good communication between clinician and microbiologist. Since special media must be used to confirm or rule out most organisms causing specific infections, pertinent information about the patient's problem must be furnished by the clinician. Microbiologists should be provided with air-dried slides to assist them in giving useful answers. For example, Casman's blood agar medium with 5 per cent defibrinated rabbit blood has proved to be an excellent medium for culturing *G. vaginalis*. Candida species can be readily identified on Nickerson's medium, which is readily available and keeps well in storage. *Trichomonas vaginalis* can be cultured on simplified Trypticase serum of Kupferberg and Wittington-Feinburg medium. Using culture techniques to identify the three most common causes of vaginitis (Candida, *Trichomonas vaginalis*, *G. vaginalis*), however, is very rarely indicated, since careful examination of saline wet mount and KOH preparations almost always reveals the offending organism in the symptomatic patient. Culture techniques can be used, however, when the wet mount, and KOH preparations are consistently negative and the patient's symptoms persist. In most instances, however, in the absence of objective clinical findings, it will be rare to grow out one of the aforementioned organisms.

Determining the pH of vaginal secretion on the unlubricated withdrawn speculum is one of the most rapidly accomplished but one of the most informative tests available. A pH in the normal range (3.8 to 4.2) essentially eliminates the possibility of trichomoniasis and *G. vaginalis* vaginitis. In general, any patient with a white or slate-colored curdy vaginal secretion, without offensive odor and of normal volume, with a pH of 3.8 to 4.2, has a normal vaginal secretion and not a discharge. Lactobacilli or diphtheroids usually predominate in the flora of the normal vagina.

Once the diagnosis is specifically arrived at, appropriate therapy can more appropriately be instituted. However, each of the various vaginal infections does present specific problems relative to permanent cure. Several of the more difficult problems will now be discussed.

Trichomoniasis

Since the development and proof of the therapeutic value of systemically administered metronidazole (Flagyl), the management of trichomoniasis has become a simple matter. Correcting the problem is predicated on establishing an accurate diagnosis in the laboratory and understanding that this is a sexually transmitted disease. The limited value of topical medicaments to eradicate trichomonads from the host and the necessity of a systemic agent to reach inaccessible foci in the urinary tract of both sexes have long been recognized. Metronidazole is presently the only systemic agent with FDA approval in this country. Other effective systemic agents, including tinidazole, flunidazole and nimorazole, are being used in other countries, but none appears superior to metronidazole. Its success and safety have been confirmed by hundreds of investigators, and the opinion is essentially unanimous that it affords a cure rate approaching 100 per cent.

The current recommended schedule for treatment is 250 mg t.i.d. for 7 days. We recommend 500 mg every 12 hours for 5 days. Gardner's results in over 900 patients utilizing this regimen are comparable to any reported.[15] A single dose of 2 g of metronidazole has been extensively investigated and results thus far are encouraging. Fleury obtained a 95 per cent cure rate with a single 2-g dose.[12, 13] His criterion for cure, however, was based on a single post-treatment wet mount at 7 to 10 days. Csonka's results with the 2 g dose showed an 18 per cent failure rate at the end of 3 months, but his failure rate for the 7-day regimen was only 6 per cent.[6] Morton estimated his failure rate using a single 2 g dose at 20 per cent.[32]

Since the majority of men with infected sexual partners also harbor trichomonads, they are a continuous source of reinfection for the women; logic dictates, therefore, that these men should receive treatment simultaneously. We recommend this treatment without even attempting to isolate the organism from the male. In a study by Gardner and Dukes the reinfection rate in women was two and one half times higher in patients whose sexual partners had not been treated.[18] The dosage schedule for the male partner is identical to that for the woman.

Despite the almost 100 per cent effectiveness of oral metronidazole, occasional patients (probably less than 1 per cent) fail to respond to the drug. Whether this results from poor absorption, organismal resistance, or failure of a vaginal transudation has not been settled. Pretreatment with estrogens to stimulate the vagina has been suggested. Any advantage here would seem to be the effect of augmented vaginal transudation. In the patient who does not respond to standard therapy, the dosage should be increased to 500 mg t.i.d. for 10 days. In the individual with repeated recurrent episodes of trichomoniasis, suspicion should be aroused to the possibility of another sexual consort as the source of reinfection. This often is a delicate problem that requires frank and open discussion with the patient. Many individuals do not realize that their source of reinfection is from a sexual contact, and this must be explained to them.

Contraindications to metronidazole include blood dyscrasia, diseases of the central nervous system, and pregnancy (although no detrimental effect on either the mother or unborn child has been observed and no teratogenic influence on human beings has been reported). Thus, it sometimes is necessary to resort to topical agents to control this infection. Intravaginal medications, in our experience, usually provide only temporary relief of symptoms. Some of the topical agents still available include Tricofuron suppositories, which contain the trichomonacide furazolidone; AVC cream and Vagitrol cream, both of which contain allantoin and aminacrine; and Betadine vaginal gel, which contains povidone-iodine. Whatever the topical agent used, it should be continued for 15 days or longer, including the period of menstrual flow. No vaginal medicament will eradicate the organisms from Skene's gland and the urinary tract, and urethral instillations are largely ineffective in destroying organisms in the urethra.

PROPHYLAXIS

Douching with a strongly acid or medicated preparation soon after intercourse with an infected man probably affords considerable protection against trichomoniasis. The number of vaginal trichomonads would be reduced, and according to clinical and laboratory evidence, a large number of organisms is necessary to incite an infection.

EPIDEMIOLOGY

Epidemiologic measures have not received sufficient attention and investigation. Some of the same methods used to control other venereal diseases should perhaps be applied to trichomoniasis. Even with the availability of metronidazole, trichomoniasis will remain one of the most widespread of the current vaginal infections unless the sexual partner of each patient is treated, and unless appropriate community and educational control measures are applied. The management of trichomoniasis should be less formidable than that of other venereal diseases since it is considerably less contagious. In view of the fact that the disease affects the general health of the patient to a relatively mild degree, health authorities have little interest in community projects directed toward its eradication.

TRICHOMONIASIS IN MEN

Keutel[27] discovered Trichomonas in 79 per cent of the sexual partners of infected women. Watt and Jennison[39] noted the parasite in 60 per cent of the sexual partners of infected women, Bedoya et al.[3] in 78 per cent, and Block[4] in 61.5 per cent. We have recovered Trichomonas from the urethras of the majority of husbands of infected wives, generally without resorting to culturing techniques. Many failures to detect Trichomonas in men can be attributed to technical difficulties rather than to absence of infection.

Most men harboring Trichomonas are unaware of having infection; probably fewer than 20 per cent have signs or symptoms of the disease. Most often, any discharge is minimal; reportedly, however, in the rare patient it is abundant and purulent. Block found that 21 per cent of 91 patients either had discharge, dysuria, burning and irritation after coitus, or a combination of these manifestations. It is Keutel's opinion that more than 90 per cent of infected male patients have symptoms of prostatitis, and it can be assumed that the seminal vesicles are infected.[27] Further proof

of the fact that the male is often a carrier of this organism is the study of Catterall and Nicol, who demonstrated *T. vaginalis* in all female partners of 56 men with *T. vaginalis* urethritis.[5] It is imperative that urologists become more interested in trichomonal infection and give some recognition to its overall importance.

The diagnosis of trichomoniasis in men is much more difficult than in women because of the difficulty in isolating Trichomonas from the male urethra. Failure to demonstrate the organisms on one or two microscopic or even culture examinations is not proof that the man is not a carrier. The organism can usually be detected in a drop of secretion that has been removed from the urethra after the patient has not voided for several hours. The secretion is placed on a glass slide, firmly pressed with a coverslip and examined under high microscopic power. If the secretion is profusely purulent, dilution with physiologic saline may be necessary. The first ounce of an early morning voided specimen of urine is also a useful source of the organisms. The specimen must be thoroughly centrifuged and the sediment examined under the high-power objective. Some investigators find that the organisms are more easily isolated in prostatic secretion after massage. If Trichomonas cannot be identified by slide technique, cultures are necessary; however, we have observed many positive smears of material that failed to yield positive cultures. The reasons for emphasizing the occurrence of male infection is to stress again the importance of the male role as a source of constant reinfection of the female, and that treatment of the male partner is a necessary part of the overall therapy of this infection.

Gardnerella Vaginalis Vaginitis

Any woman whose ovarian activity is normal, and who has a gray, homogeneous, malodorous vaginal discharge with a pH of 5.0 to 5.5 but whose specimen yields no trichomonads, is likely to have *G. vaginalis* vaginitis. A wet smear preparation from the vagina of such a patient contains the "clue cells" of *G. vaginalis*. In the stained smear, the bacterial flora consists primarily of heavy fields of short gramnegative bacilli. Rarely is it necessary to utilize culture to confirm the diagnosis. When, however, this is done, the organism can be grown on Casman's blood agar base, adjusted to pH 5.5 before autoclaving and containing 5 per cent fresh defibrinated rabbit blood.

A problem in eradicating this infection is a lack of understanding that it is a sexually transmitted disease. *G. vaginalis* vaginitis is probably our most common venereal disease, and also one of the most contagious. In a study reported by Gardner and Dukes in 1959, the predominant organism in the urethras of 91 husbands of 101 infected wives was *G. vaginalis*.[19] In contrast, in the study of urethral cultures obtained from male medical students used as a control group, rarely was one found to harbor the organism. Pheifer et al. recovered *G. vaginalis* from 79 per cent of male sex partners of infected women.[35] Numerous other investigators have also reported a high recovery rate of *G. vaginalis* from the urethras of husbands of infected wives. Moreover, it has been repeatedly observed that the majority of successfully treated patients have recurrence of the disease if their consorts are not treated simultaneously and successfully with appropriate therapy.

A lasting cure for this infection is often difficult to accomplish because of the enormous problem of reinfection. The situation is easily compounded when third parties or multiple sex partners are involved. An insoluble therapeutic exercise can develop.

THERAPY METHODS

Topical agents such as intravaginal sulfonomides have been advocated for the management of this infection for many years. Unfortunately, the use of these medications is of minimal value in eradicating the infection. In our own experience utilizing various sulfa creams and tablets the infection was eradicated (as confirmed by cultures 10 and 30 days after completion of therapy) in less than 30 per cent of women treated. In all instances, the consorts were simultaneously treated with systemic antibacterial agents. In other studies, the use of intravaginal "sulfa" therapy proved to be of no more value than the use of the "base" substance in several of the utilized "sulfa" preparations.[36] Providone-iodine instilled twice daily for 10 to 14 days has also proved to be relatively unsuccessful.

In recent years, systemically administered antibiotics have been of some value. Ampicillin 500 mg administered every 6 hours for 5 days proved to be an effective systemic agent, but it appears that many resistant strains have since developed and, in our experience, therapy has been less than uniformly successful. Cephalexin 500 mg every 6 hours for 6 days is about as effective as ampicillin but probably has fewer side effects than the latter drug. Cephradine, administered 250 mg to 500 mg every 6 hours for 6 days, appears to give a better cure rate than the two previously mentioned agents, but here again its use is not uniformly successful. Unfortunately, the use of these antibiotics often precipitates vulvovaginal candidiasis, and if they are utilized, the concurrent use of a vaginal fungicide should be considered.

After the introduction of metronidazole, we observed that many patients with concomitant *G. vaginalis* vaginitis and trichomoniasis were cured of both infections when they and their consorts were treated with metronidazole. Smith and Dunkelberg found varying degrees of inhibition of *G. vaginalis* by metronidazole when used in in vitro experiments.[38] Pheifer et al. treated 81 patients with metronidazole utilizing 500 twice daily for 7 days.[35] They recorded immediate post-treatment negative cultures in 100 per cent of their patients. Fleury has obtained a 93.5 per cent cure rate for *G. vaginalis* using metronidazole. It would thus appear that this drug is the most efficacious therapeutic agent for the management of *G. vaginalis*. It cannot, however, be emphasized enough that all sexual partners must be treated at the same time as the patient or there will be a rapid recurrence of infection.

One of the most difficult problems the gynecologist has in treating patients with *G. vaginalis* is convincing the male partners that their treatment is necessary. Not uncommonly, the man visits his personal physician only to be told that without clinical evidence of the disease there is nothing to treat. A considerable body of evidence has been accrued supporting the fact that the male frequently is infected with this organism. De La Fuente and colleagues found *G. vaginalis* in the urethras of 37 of 44 men whose wives had *G. vaginalis* vaginitis.[8] Gardner and Dukes found that *G. vaginalis* was the predominant bacterial organism of the urethra in 91 of 101 men whose wives were infected.[9] Since these men were not examined for evidence of clinical disease, the effects of *G. vaginalis* were not determined; nevertheless, the failure of most of this group to report the symptoms of urethritis voluntarily might suggest that they suffered no such discomfort. Dunkelberg and Woolvin observed that *G. vaginalis* was the predominant organism in the urethral discharge of five males suspected of having gonorrhea yet whose specimens did not yield gonococci.[11] The microscopic and cultural findings were identical to those seen in *G. vaginalis* vaginitis. We suspect that the finding of *G. vaginalis* was coincidental. Hughes and Carpenter discovered an unidentified small gram-negative bacilli in some of the discharges of 216 male patients with urethritis, all of whom had received a clinical diagnosis of penicillin-resistant gonorrhea.[24] Dunkelberg and Woolvin suggested that many of these may have actually been cases of *G. vaginalis* urethritis.[11] In our opinion, *G. vaginalis* is rarely if ever a primary cause of symptomatic genitourinary infection in men, although it has been well established that many men with "nonspecific" urethritis harbor *G. vaginalis*.

Since the specimens of more than 90 per cent of men whose sexual partners are infected with *G. vaginalis* also yield the organism, these men constitute a continuous source of reinfection. For this reason, the male sexual partner must be treated simultaneously with the patient if reinfection is to be prevented. The reinfection rate in women whose sexual partners are not treated far exceeds the rate of those whose consorts are successfully treated. In fact, reinfection is predictable if the consort is not treated. Treatment schedules that have proved most successful in men are the same regimens using systemic agents as are used in the treatment of women.

Candidiasis

One of the most perplexing problems the gynecologist encounters is that of recurrent or persistent candidiasis. The patient with a sporadic infection poses no therapeutic problem, but the chronically recurrent disease is a true enigma to the physician. This perplexing situation is being encountered with increasing frequency by the practicing physician and may very well be related to the fact that candidiasis is probably being seen more frequently today, and compared with the other common varieties of vaginitis (Trichomonas and *G. vaginalis*) is also being seen relatively more often.

Gardner, 1944, detected clinical candidiasis in 2.8 per cent of the gynecologic patients seen in his private office practice.[17] In 1957, in a study of patients from the same practice, candidiasis was found in 4.3 per cent of nonpregnant patients. In 1965, Gardner noted that 5.9 per cent of 1000 consecutive gynecologic patients had clinical candidiasis.[16] Gardner also studied the relative frequency of the three most common pathogens recovered in gynecologic patients with vulvovaginitis in the same private office practice in 1956, 1966 and 1976 (Table 1).

The many predisposing and perpetuating factors inherent in chronically recurrent candidiasis make this infection an especially troublesome one. Factors purported to increase the incidence of this infection include pregnancy; variations in the menstrual cycle; use of oral contraceptives, antibiotics and corticosteroids; diabetes mellitus; nondiabetic glycosuria; diet; debilitation; and changes in immunologic competence.

PREGNANCY. Pregnancy is the most common predisposing factor, with the occurrence and severity of the infection increasing with the duration of gestation. Worldwide studies show that approximately one third of specimens of all pregnant women yield Candida on any particular day. After delivery and the rapid change in the endocrine milieu of the individual there is a radical change in vaginal metabolism, chemistry and cytology, and in most patients rapid disappearance of the clinical signs of candidiasis. Negative cultures are usually obtained in a few days, since the new vaginal environment is extremely unfavorable to the growth of species of Candida.

TABLE 1. RELATIVE FREQUENCY OF THE THREE COMMON VAGINITIDES IN NONPREGNANT PATIENTS IN 3 STUDIES A DECADE APART

	1956 (301 cases)	1966 (200 cases)	1976 (1000 cases)
Candidiasis	19.9%	47.5%	39.7%
Gardnerella vaginalis vaginitis	55.8	30.5	45.2
Trichomoniasis	40.5	45.0	15.1

MENSTRUAL CYCLE. The intensity of the clinical features of candidiasis tends to coincide with the hormonal pattern of the menstrual cycle. Because of the altered physiology just before menstruation, clinical manifestations are usually more severe at this time with some degree of relief being experienced during and after the menstrual flow. It is not at all uncommon in individuals with recurrent disease to note a relationship of exacerbation with menses.

ORAL CONTRACEPTIVES. There is no uniform agreement as to the relationship of combination birth control pills to the occurrence and resistance to treatment of vaginal candidiasis. Morris and Morris[31a] reported essentially the same recovery of Candida from users and nonusers, as have many other investigators. Oriel et al., in screening a large number of patients, found the overall incidence of "yeasts" is almost twice as great in those taking oral contraceptives. The most common consensus today is that while oral contraceptives do not increase the incidence of symptomatic candidiasis, their continued use sometimes makes successful therapy more difficult.

ANTIBIOTICS. Since the introduction of antibiotics, the incidence of candidiasis has risen to a degree parallel to their increased usage, whether they are administered systemically or topically. The broad-spectrum agents such as the tetracyclines are more likely to be associated in this respect than penicillin. One theory explaining this relationship is that candidal organisms multiply more rapidly because of the reduction of bacterial competition. Dukes and Tettenbaum demonstrated that mice injected intraperitoneally with *C. albicans* survived, but that when the same inoculum was mixed with tetracycline the mice died of candidal infection.[9] There is an increased colonization of the host by species of Candida after the administration of antibiotics. Loh and Baker reported an increase of 100 to 1000 times in the intestinal population of Candida in patients who were taking chlortetracycline and oxytetracycline.[29] These findings, along with those of many other investigators, indicate that the use of antibiotics increases the growth of Candida in the intestinal tract. Regardless of the precise mechanism involved, the incidence and severity of the disease are clearly related to the use of antibiotics.

CORTICOSTEROIDS. Adrenal steroids have an adverse effect on established candidal infections. In laboratory studies, the susceptibility of animals to candidal infection after administration of corticosteroids was increased, although the steroid agents seemed to have no effect on organisms grown in vitro. Corticosteroids applied topically to the vulvovaginal tissues do not seem to aggravate the disease, a fact worthy of note in the symptomatic treatment for severe candida infections. The full relationship of systemic corticosteroids to vaginal candidiasis has not yet been fully clarified.

DIABETES MELLITUS. Only a small percentage of patients with candidiasis observed by the gynecologist has sugar in the urine or abnormal glucose tolerance curves. This is not to say, however, that diabetes mellitus is not a potent predisposing factor, since a high percentage of diabetic patients will have obstinate candidiasis if treatment is neglected. What is termed *diabetic vulvovaginitis* is inseparably allied to the increased susceptibility of diabetic patients to candidiasis, this being related to increased concentrations of glucose in the tissue, blood and urine or possibly to the glycosuria alone. Thus, it is worthwhile to study glucose tolerance in individuals with persistent or recurrent candidiasis even though the likelihood of detecting diabetes in such patients is quite small.

HOST IMMUNITY. The role of host immunity in resisting Candida has received renewed emphasis recently. Although alterations of immune competence, especially changes in immunoglobulin levels and anti-Candida antibody titers, have been reported in patients with systemic candidiasis, comparable studies of vaginal candidiasis are relatively few. Mathur et al. found elevated serum titers of anti-Candida immunoglobulins of the secretory IgA and IgE types in patients with vaginal candidiasis.[30] Elevated levels of IgE in cervicalvaginal washings were also found. Absorption of Candida antigen showed these immunoglobulins to be antibodies predominantly specific for Candida.

The authors comment on the possible synergistic role of IgE and secretory IgA in the local immune response in the cervical-vaginal area. They speculate whether IgE plays a defensive role (the mode of action of which is as yet unknown) in concert with secretory IgA in the mucous membrane site. Moreover, in studies of atopic dermatitis, elevated IgE has been associated with alterations of leukocyte chemotaxis and cell-mediated responsiveness. Thus the presence of elevated IgE in patients with chronic vaginal candidiasis may represent a subtle defect in cell-mediated immunity—perhaps a decrease in suppressor T-cells, which normally oversee IgE production.

Other evidence of cell-mediated abnormalities in candidiasis may be culled from the results of immune profiling of patients with systemic candidiasis. These findings suggest the possibility of utilizing immune therapy in the individual with chronic or recurrent candidiasis. Palacios found that "resistant forms" of candidiasis are often found in patients with allergic states and multiple hypersensitivities.[34] He accomplished a high rate of improvement by "densensitizing" patients with injections of *Candida albicans* antigen. Kudelko has also reported limited success with *C. albicans* injections.[28]

MALE FACTOR. Men are more likely to be recipients than donors of candidiasis; nevertheless, men can harbor Candida organisms beneath the foreskin and on the genitocrural tissues and thus constitute a reservoir of infection for women. Gilpin reported that the ejaculate of husbands of women with recurrent disease often yields Candida species.[21] Isolating Candida from the male genitals is a simple matter, though their overall importance as a potential source of infection is unknown.

TREATMENT FOR CHRONICALLY RECURRENT CANDIDIASIS

The patient with sporadic infection poses no therapeutic problem, but the chronically recurrent disease is a true medical puzzle to the physician. In view of the several predisposing and perpetuating factors, chronically recurrent candidiasis is increasingly troublesome. Most cases are probably caused by autogenous reinfection. No uniformly successful approach to this vexing problem has been found. Obviously, not only must the vulvovaginal organisms be eradicated but every effort must be made to remove foci of infection and to correct all predisposing factors. Reassurance of the patient also becomes an important part of the treatment.

For the patient with chronically recurrent disease — the patient who has repeatedly used every medication available — we recommend from the following suggestions those that seem to best fit the needs for each particular patient.

1. Use a candidicidal agent continuously for a period of four to six weeks, rather than for the recommended one to two weeks.

2. Use intravaginal candidicide nightly for a few days before each menstrual period as a prophylactic measure, since recurrence is common just before menses.

3. Use intravaginal candidicide during and for several days after any course of antibiotic therapy.

4. Discontinue oral contraceptives. This appears to be beneficial in some instances.

5. Apply candidicidal cream to the preputial folds twice daily for seven to ten days. Organisms are sometimes harbored beneath the foreskin of the clitoris. The consort's penis should be likewise treated. He should also be examined for the presence of genitocrural cutaneous candidiasis.

Wearing protective sheaths can sometimes be helpful. For the patient who still develops new infections, we use one of the following two plans.

1. Allow the patient to use a vaginal candidicide ad lib whenever there is the slightest evidence of new irritation. Often the patient finds it necessary to use medication for only two to three days to abort a new infection.

2. The plan we most often resort to is the use of long-term prophylactic medication. After intensive treatment to eliminate vaginal Candida, the patient is instructed to insert one of the newer candidicides into the vagina every second, third or fourth night for an indefinite period, usually three to four months.

These two approaches perhaps appear to be an admission of defeat, but if the patient's infection is controlled and she remains asymptomatic, then they can be considered beneficial.

The use of an oral candidicidal agent such as nystatin, 500,000 units t.i.d. for 10 to 14 days, is allegedly valuable in reducing or eliminating intestinal colonization and thus reducing the reinfection rate. Its suggested benefit has not been demonstrated. Our own experience in a double-blind study following this treatment plan showed that the number of reinfections in the treated and control groups was essentially identical.

Since species of Candida are recoverable from the oral cavity in many adults, the factor of cunnilingus should be considered in every case of intractable candidiasis. When this is thought to be the source of reinfection, oral rinses using nystatin suspension are recommended.

The role of contaminated douche nozzles, bathtubs and wet bathing suits as sources of reinfection is probably unimportant. However, sterilization of the douche nozzle and the use of a shower instead of the tub would be simple undertakings.

In the patient whose disease persists in spite of strict adherence to the treatment protocol outlined, consideration can be given to immunotherapy utilizing a Candida vaccine, as reported by Kudelko.[28]

Recurrent Herpes Genitalis

Another of the frustrating problems the clinician deals with is related to the management and prevention of recurrent herpes genitalis. Unfortunately, despite the numerous proposed therapeutic regimens, no satisfactory treatment is currently available for genital herpes virus infection. Numerous approaches have been advocated including the use of BCG, Betadine solution, photoinactivation, topically applied ether, chloroform, 5 iodo-2-deoxyuridine (IDU), adenine arabinoside, and acyclovir. None of these approaches, however, has proved to be completely effective in treating either the primary or the recurrent infection. Initially, photoinactivation using neutral red or proflavine was thought to be of some benefit in shortening the duration of clinical infection and preventing recurrence. The more recent randomized double-blind studies of Myers et al.[33] and Kaufman et al.,[25] however, have demonstrated that these medications are no more efficacious than control nonactive dyes.

On the assumption that the viruses of smallpox and herpes are related immunologically, repeated inoculations with smallpox vaccine has been advocated for the prevention of herpes genitalis. The results of such treatments have been disputed repeatedly by numerous investigators, including Kern and Schiff.[26] The latter authors also conducted a well-controlled study to evaluate a specific vaccine prepared from inactive herpes virus. The results from the control material and vaccine were essentially identical. Vaccines prepared from heat-inactivated chorioallantoic membrane cultures of embryonic hen eggs consisting of Type I vaccine (Lupidon H) and

Type II vaccine (Lupidon G) were prepared by Hermal (Hermal-Chemie Kurt Hermann Laboratories of Hamburg). Reports on the use of this vaccine, like the results with so many therapeutic agents, were initially glowing, but to date we have not seen a well-conducted double-blind randomized study to suggest this therapy is of any greater benefit than .other methods currently available. Furthermore, considering the potential oncogenic effects of HSV Type II, there is some question regarding the safety of using the whole inactivated virus in a vaccine.

One obvious reason for the ineffectiveness of most therapies is the fact that between recurrences the virus is habored in a latent fashion in the sensory ganglion supplying the area affected. Thus, local treatment may eradicate or inactivate virus on the vulva or cervix but does not eradicate the latent virus still present in the nerve root ganglia. Acyclovir ointment 5 per cent has recently become available for the treatment of herpes genitalis. However, in non-immunocompromised patients, no evidence of clinical benefit has been demonstrated. Vidarabine therapy has been used for several systemic viral infections with some benefit, and more recently has been used to treat systemic infections of the newborn, with a degree of success. However, recent clinical trials by Goodman et al.[22] and by Adams et al.[2] have demonstrated its lack of efficacy when used topically to treat genital herpes virus infection.

Lacking a specific treatment, palliative measures become necessary. Symptomatic relief is often obtained by hot sitz baths, wet dressings, or various shake lotions. Wet dressings are quite difficult to use because of the necessity of almost constant application. Such dressings as Burow's solution diluted 1/20 parts in water or a saturated solution of boric acid afford some relief of symptoms. Various antibiotic ointments (Neosporin G) may expedite healing in some persons, presumably by preventing a secondary infection. Smith believes that topically applied corticosteroids relieve symptoms and hasten healing; however, the use of corticosteroids, even topically, in the presence of a viral infection should be cautioned against.[37] The application of various local anesthetic ointments such as lidocaine gel has been advocated, but it has been our experience that occasionally this can result in a severe contact dermatitis. Thus this approach is seldom recommended. Thymol 4 per cent (an antiviral agent) in chloroform has been reported to shorten the course of the acute infection. In our experience, it has somewhat enhanced lesion healing and decreased the duration of pain, but the drug has been of no benefit in preventing recurrent infection.

Recurrent herpes genitalis is extremely distressing to the patient, and every effort should be made to discover and control those factors that are responsible for recurrence. An understanding of the patient's emotional problems is helpful, as is the use of tranquilizers and sedatives at appropriate times. In some individuals, recurrence appears at the onset of menses or following sexual intercourse. In these individuals there is little that can be done to prevent recurrence except to offer assurance that in most instances, as time passes, the frequency of recurrence tends to decrease.

PREVENTION OF INFECTION

Genital herpes virus infection is sexually transmitted, and a question of great concern to the individual with recurrent infection is the likelihood of transmissibility of the infection to a sexual partner. During the acute infection, disease is transmitted to the consort by direct sexual contact in a large percentage of instances. Thus, it is wise to recommend abstinence from sexual contact during the period of active infection. Once the lesions are completely healed, the likelihood of transmitting the disease is extremely small. The probability of transmitting the infection in the absence of clinical disease, although remote, is still possible as indicated by the fact that the virus has been recovered from the cervix of asymptomatic women and from the urethra and prostate of asymptomatic men. If coitus is engaged in during the course of active infection, the use of a condom by the man may offer some degree of protection, although this certainly will not guarantee against transmission of infection to him from an infected female. Singh et al.[36a] have demonstrated the viricidal effects of various intravaginal contraceptive agents, and theoretically one might suggest their use if coitus is engaged in during an acute infection. Certainly, the male partner with active lesions should avoid any sexual contact with his female partner during pregnancy.

Torulopsis (Candida) Glabrata Vulvovaginitis

Since the early 1960s, new interest has been aroused in *T. glabrata*. The fungus has been discovered in many patients with mild vaginal pruritus and an increased discharge from which no other fungus or known vaginal pathogen could be isolated. Gardner found *T. glabrata* as the causative agent in 13 of 1000 consecutive cases of an infectious vulvovaginitis. Since the organism is usually commensal, its presence in even a larger number of asymptomatic patients is probable. Oriel et al.[33a] reported that only half of their patients whose specimens yielded the organism had symptoms. After analyzing and correlating all available reports, it seems that *T. glabrata* may be considered a weak pathogen that is capable of producing mild vulvovaginitis in susceptible patients. Actually, it is rather like Candida in that it is often in evidence without inciting clinical disease.

The reason for presenting a discussion of *T. glabrata* in this chapter is the infrequency with which the clinician makes this diagnosis. However, the disease certainly should be kept in mind when vulvovaginal mycosis is considered and the typical hyphae and spores of candidiasis are not found but numerous spores characteristic of *T. glabrata* are present in the wet mount preparation. It is also being discussed because of the extreme difficulty of eradicating this infection when symptomatic.

The most common clinical picture noted in a patient with this infection is an increase in vaginal secretion — its gross characteristics are only slightly different from those of normal secretions. No malodor is present, the color is white or slate, the consistency is slightly more curdy than normal, thrush patches do not form, and the acidity is usually about pH of 4.5 in contrast with pH 3.8 to 4.2 in normal subjects. Erythema, if present, is only slight. Discharge, mild itching and a burning sensation are manifestations most often mentioned by the patient.

The patient with mild irritative symptoms of vulvovaginitis who harbors none of the usual vaginal pathogens might be suspected of having *T. glabrata* infection. As a rule, a wet mount of secretions in physiologic saline when viewed under high-power magnification contains a tremendous number of spores similar to those of Candida, though much smaller and highly variable in size. No hyphae are present

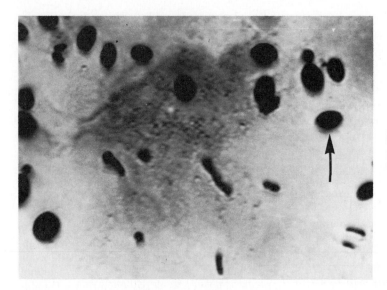

Figure 1. Torulopsis glabrata. Spores without the presence of hyphae are present (arrow). Wet mount × 700.

and pus cells are relatively few (Fig. 1). Vaginal secretions treated with 20 per cent potassium hydroxide as well as stained smears show numerous small spores but no hyphae. Wickerham reported that *T. glabrata* produces smooth colonies without hyphal tips on culture.[40] He also noted that the organisms cause gaseous fermentation of glucose and trehalose, and no other species of yeast is known to cause fermentation of these sugars. In his opinion, *T. glabrata* is readily differentiated from other fungi by its carbon assimilation reactions and by its ability to assimilate nitrate.

In our experience, *T. glabrata* infections respond poorly to the newer antifungal agents such as miconazole and chlortrimazole, which are so effective against candidal infections. We have found that 1 to 2 per cent aqueous gentian violet applied every 2 to 3 days for 10 to 12 days is the most dependable therapy available for this infection. Even after use of gentian violet, there is a high recurrence rate of clinical infection.

Desquamative Inflammatory Vaginitis

Fortunately, this condition is very infrequently seen, since it is such an enigma to both patient and physician. Desquamative inflammatory vaginitis displays some of the clinical and microscopic features of postmenopausal atrophic vaginitis, yet it develops in women with normal estrogen levels. Its peculiar distribution, persistence, poor response to treatment and tendency to recrudescence after treatment is discontinued are also striking features. In 1968, Gardner reported finding this vaginitis in only 8 of more than 3000 patients with vaginitis examined in private practice between 1952 and 1967.[14] From 1967 through 1976 he found an additional six cases. The clinical and microscopic features closely resembled those observed in six cases reported by Gray and Barnes in 1965.[23] Neither Gray and Barnes nor Gardner could detect a specific causative bacterium in this unusual vaginitis. An unidentified chronic viral infection has not been excluded as the primary cause; however, this possibility seems remote even though the cytologic and histologic studies of the vagina in two patients disclosed some inconclusive evidence of a viral infection. Theoretically, a dystrophic process involving vaginal metabolism is another etiologic possibility. No patients have displayed a dietary deficiency or obvious allergenic or primary irritant reaction. The pathogenesis of the atrophic status of the vaginal mucosa in this disease remains obscure. Gray and Barnes suggested that infection dissolves the superficial cells of the vagina or prevents their maturity.

CLINICAL APPEARANCE

The clinical features of this problem are characteristic. The mucosa of all or part of the upper half of the vagina, especially the op-

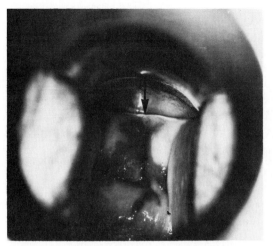

Figure 2. Sharply demarcated erythematous area is depicted by arrow.

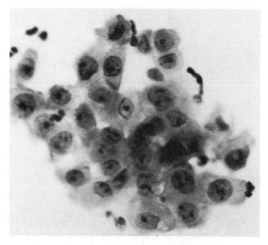

Figure 3. Vaginal smear from patient with desquamative inflammatory vaginitis demonstrating primarily parabasal cells.

posed surfaces of the posterior fornix and the ectocervix, is acutely inflamed. The margins of the affected areas are usually well delineated and at times they have a serpiginous configuration (Fig. 2).

Trauma to the lesions frequently leads to superficial ulceration and ecchymotic bleeding points and streaks. Some areas of epithelium may be covered by a gray pseudomembrane; this peals off when the vagina is wiped as though it had been parboiled, exposing the inflamed surfaces.

Most patients complain of a moderate to copious vaginal discharge, usually homogeneous and purulent, although it may be seromucoid or bloody. Malodor is not a feature. Mild burning and pruritus are reported by the majority of the patients and are the only irritative symptoms. The vaginal pH is diminished to 5.0 to 6.8. Gardner, in his 1968 report, reported minor stenosis secondary to scarring in the upper vagina in several patients.

CYTOLOGY AND HISTOPATHOLOGY

As in vaginal atrophy from estrogen deficiency, cytologic smears from the vaginal secretions of these affected patients exhibit a high percentage of basal and parabasal vaginal epithelial cells (Fig. 3) as well as many pus cells, and usually small numbers of intermediate and superficial cells. Relatively few bacteria are present and lactobacilli are essentially lacking. On biopsy, acute and chronic inflam-

matory reaction involve both mucosal and submucosal tissues. Some areas of the epithelium are thin and superficially ulcerated. Vacuolization of a few epithelial cells is sometimes observed (Fig. 4). Focal areas of stromal hemorrhage are commonly present.

A patient who has normal ovarian activity, persistent localized vaginitis (especially of the vaginal vault), and abnormal discharge containing a high percentage of immature epithelial cells and many pus cells not attributable to any known specific cause should perhaps be given a diagnosis of desquamative inflammatory vaginitis. Other diseases associated with unusual numbers of immature vaginal epithelial cells in women with normal estrogen levels include trichomoniasis, primary irritant vaginitis and occasionally certain bacterial infections.

TREATMENT

With or without treatment, the course of this disease is protracted. None of the lesions reported by Gardner healed spontaneously, and whether they healed completely with treatment is conjectural.

On the basis of the cytologic evidence of vaginal immaturity, several patients were repeatedly given estrogens, both intravaginally and orally. Little or no beneficial effect upon either the clinical or microscopic patterns of the disease was observed. Actually, this would be expected, since the usual prerequisite to the diagnosis of desquamative inflammatory

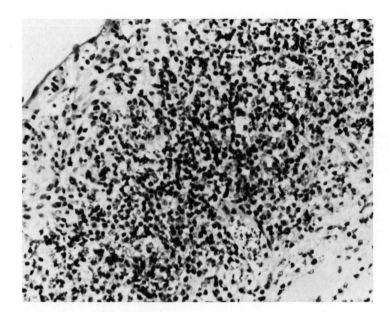

Figure 4. Desquamative inflammatory vaginitis. There is a very marked acute and chronic inflammatory infiltrate extending from the submucosa to the epithelium. Lining epithelium is thin and atrophic.

vaginitis is active ovarian function. The response to antibacterial agents administered systemically or locally is also discouraging. The use of intravaginal corticosteroid suppositories appears to be of some benefit in managing this condition. Response to therapy is slow, covering a period of months; and even after improvement or apparent cure, the vaginitis tends to recur. Nevertheless, intravaginal application of corticosteroid preparations thus far has proved to be the most effective treatment.

REFERENCES

1. Adam, E., Kaufman, R. H., Mirkovic, R. R. and Melnick, J. L: Persistence of virus shedding after herpes genitalis. Am. J. Obstet. Gynecol. 137:827, 1980.
2. Adams, H. G., Benson, E. A., Alexander, E. R., Bontver, L. A., Remington, M. A. and Holmes, K. K.: Genital herpetic infection in men and women: clinical course and effect of topical application of adenine arabinoside. J. Infect. Dis. 133A:151, 1976.
3. Bedoya, J. M., Rico, L. R. and Rios, G.: Trichomoniasis der Menschlichen Genitalien; venerarishce Erkrankung II, Geburtsch. Frauenheilk 18:994, 1958.
4. Block, E.: Occurrence of trichominis in sexual partners of women with trichomoniasis. Acta Obstet. Gynecol. Scand. 38:398, 1959.
5. Catterall, R. D. and Nicol, C. S.: Is trichomonal infestation a venereal disease? Br. Med. J. 1:1177, 1960.
6. Csonka, G. W.: Trichomonal vaginitis treated with one dose of metronidazole. Br. J. Venereol. Dis. 47:456, 1971.
7. Deardorff, S. L., Detura, F. A., Drylie, D. M.,

Centifano, Y. and Kaufman, H.: Association between herpes hominis type II and the male genitourinary tract. J. Urol. 112:126, 1974.
8. De La Fuente, F., Rico, L. R. and Soria, F.: Hemofilasis urogenital afeccion benerea? Rev. Esp. Ob. Ginec. 18:252, 1959.
9. Dukes, C. D. and Tettenbaum, I. S.: Studies on the potentiation of monilial and staphylococcal infections by tetracycline. New York, Antibiotics Annual Med. Encyclopedia, Inc., 1954–1955, p. 674.
10. Dunkelberg, W. E. and Bosman, R. I.: *Hemophilus vaginalis:* incidence among 431 specimens examined. Milit. Med. 126:920, 1961.
11. Dunkelberg, W. E. and Woolvin, S. S. C.: *Hemophilus vaginalis* relative to gonorrhea and male urethritis. Milit. Med. 128:1098, 1963.
12. Fleury, F. J.: Personal communication, 1978.
13. Fluery, F. J., Von Virgen, W. S., Prentice, R. I., Russell, J. G., Singleton, J. A. and Standard, J. V.: Single dose of two grams of metronidazole for *Trichomonas vaginalis* vaginitis. Am. J. Obstet. Gynecol. 128:320, 1977.
14. Gardner, H. L.: Desquamative inflammatory vaginitis: a newly defined entity. Am. J. Obstet. Gynecol. 102:1102, 1968.
15. Gardner, H. L.: Trichomoniasis. Obstet. Gynecol. 19:279, 1962.
16. Gardner, H. L.: Unpublished Data, 1965.
17. Gardner, H. L.: Vaginal thrush. Texas J. Med. 40:333, 1944.
18. Gardner, H. L. and Dukes, C. D.: Clinical and laboratory effects of metronidazole. Am. J. Obstet. Gynecol. 89:990, 1964.
19. Gardner, H. L. and Dukes, C. D.: *Hemophilus vaginalis* vaginitis. Ann. N.Y. Acad. Sci. 83:280, 1959.
20. Gardner, H. L., Dukes, C. D. and Dampier, T. K.: The prevalence of vaginitis. Am. J. Obstet. Gynecol. 73:1080, 1957.
21. Gilpin, C. A.: Resistant monilial vaginitis: the male aspect. Florida State Med. J. 54:337, 1967.
22. Goodman, E. L., Luby, J. P. and Johnson, M. T.: Prospective double-blind evaluation of topical ad-

enine arabinoside in male herpes progenitalis. Antimicrob. Agents Chemother. 8:693, 1975.

23. Gray, L. A. and Barnes, M. L.: Vaginitis in women — diagnosis and treatment. Am. J. Obstet. Gynecol. 92:125, 1965.

24. Hughes, R. B. and Carpenter, C. M.: Alleged penicillin-resistant gonorrhea. Am. J. Syph. Gonor. Ven. Dis. 32:265, 1948.

25. Kaufman, R. H., Adam, E., Mirkovic, R. R., Melnick, J. L. and Young, R. L.: Treatment of genital herpes simplex virus infection with photodynamic inactivation. Am. J. Obstet. Gynecol. 132:861, 1978.

26. Kern, A. B. and Schiff, B. L.: Vaccine therapy in recurrent herpes simplex. Arch. Derm. 89:844, 1964.

27. Keutel, H. J.: Trichomonadenerkrankung des Mannes. Verh. Deutsch. Ges. Urol. 7:159, 1959.

28. Kudelko, N.: Allergy in chronic monilial vaginitis. Ann. Allergy 29:266, 1971.

29. Loh, W. P. and Baker, E. E.: Fecal flora of man after oral administration of chlortetracycline or oxytetracycline. Arch. Intern. Med. 95:74, 1955.

30. Mathur, S., Goust, J. M., Horger, III, E. O. et al.: Immunoglobulin anti-Candida antibodies and candidiasis. Infect. Immunol. 18:257, 1977.

31. Mathur, S., Virella, G., Koistinen, J., Horger, III, E. O. et al.: Humoral immunity in vaginal candidiasis. Infect. Immunol. 15:287, 1977.

31a. Morris, C. H. and Morris, D. F.: Normal vaginal microbiology of women of childbearing age in relation to the use of oral contraceptives and vaginal tampons. J. Clin. Pathol. 20:636, 1967.

32. Morton, R. S.: Metronidazole in the single dose treatment of trichomoniasis in men and women. Br. J. Vener. Dis. 48:525, 1972.

33. Myers, M. G., Oxman, M. N., Clark, J. E. and Arndt, K. S.: Failure of neutral-red photodynamic inactivation in recurrent herpes simplex virus infections. N. Engl. J. Med. 293:945, 1975.

33a. Oriel, J. D. et al.: Genital yeast infections. Br. Med. J. 4:761, 1972.

34. Palacios, H. J.: Hypersensitivity as a cause of dermatologic and vaginal moniliasis resistant to topical therapy. Ann. Allergy 37:110, 1976.

35. Pheifer, T. A., Forsyth, P. S., Durfee, M. A. et al.: Nonspecific vaginitis: role of *Hemophilus vaginalis* and treatment with metronidazole. N. Engl. J. Med. 298:1429, 1978.

36. Schwartz, B.: Personal communication.

36a. Singh, B. Rostio, B., and Cutler, J. G.: Viricidal effect of certain chemical contraceptives on type 2 herpesvirus. Am. J. Obstet. Gynecol. 126:422, 1976.

37. Smith, E.: Management of herpes simplex infections of the skin. J.A.M.A. 235:1731, 1976.

38. Smith, R. F. and Dunkelberg, W. E., Jr.: Inhibition of *Corynebacterium vaginale* by metronidazole. Sex. Transm. Dis. 4:20, 1977.

39. Watt, L. and Jennison, R. F.: Incidence of *Trichomonas vaginalis* in marital partners. Br. J. Vener. Dis. 36:163, 1960.

40. Wickerham, L. J.: Apparent increase in frequency of infections involving *Torulopsis glabrata*. J.A.M.A. 165:47, 1957.

Recurrent and Refractory Vulvovaginitis

Marvin S. Amstey, M.D.
Sangithan Moodley, M.B., Ch.B., M.D.
University of Rochester School of Medicine and Dentistry

Alterations in the biologic characteristics of the vaginal environment induced by infectious and other agents are a significant cause of morbidity. The vaginal environment has been the subject of much research over the last decade, which indicates that the vagina is a dynamic structure rather than an inert copulatory channel connecting the lower genital tract to the upper.

The spectrum of infections involving the vagina has been undergoing a change that may be explained partially by recent sophistication in laboratory diagnosis and by changing behavioral patterns — for example, extensive use of various methods of contraception, changes in sexual behavior and use of various proprietary medications.

To the practicing physician the treatment of recurrent and refractory vulvovaginitis can prove to be an exercise in frustration, very often stemming from failure to follow basic principles. It is a condition the treatment of which frequently results in loss of patient confidence; in this group of patients will be found a large percentage who have already sought help from many physicians. It is important, therefore, to participate as an interested and caring physician rather than acting as a dispenser of antibiotics and vaginal creams.

Physioanatomic Considerations

Anatomically the vagina connects the lower to the upper genital tract. This is an important consideration, since upper genital problems frequently cause symptoms referable to the vagina or vulva. For example, a chronically infected cervix can be the cause of persistent vaginal discharge; if not managed properly, this may result in a significant percentage of treatment failures.

At childbirth the vagina of the neonate, due to stimulation from estrogens of maternal origin, is covered by a thick stratified squamous epithelium and has good vascularity. The vagina is initially sterile but soon becomes colonized by microorganisms, particularly lactobacillus. These organisms have long been considered the "guardian" organisms of the vagina in view of the fact that their presence often inhibits growth of other organisms. Vulvovaginitis in the neonate rarely, if ever, proves to be a problem.

Following withdrawal of estrogen stimulation of maternal origin the vagina and external genitalia atrophy. The epithelium becomes thinner and the vascularity decreases. The labial folds atrophy, and the introitus and urethra lose their protective covering from apposition of the labia in the midline. Because of these changes there is increased susceptibility of the genital tract to infections. Gonorrhea, for example, can prove to be a difficult vaginal infection to eradicate at this stage and may necessitate the use of exogenous estrogens to induce the maturation of the genital tract, which is associated with increased resistance to infection.

The menopausal vagina, with withdrawal of endogenous estrogens, may undergo atrophic changes and show an increased liability to infection. The use of topical or exogenous estrogen in these patients often leads to dramatic relief without use of antibiotic substances.

The proximity of the urethra and rectum to the vagina is another important consideration. The rectum, for example, may provide a reservoir of *C. albicans*, and if not eradicated, this organism could lead to chronic and refractory moniliasis. Urethral involvement by Trichomonas is a contributing factor for failure of topical therapy against vaginal trichomoniasis. Skene's glands, Bartholin's glands, infected nabothian follicles and the rectum are some important reservoirs of infection; these infections should be looked for and treated. The principle of looking for reservoirs of infection in the female's consort is important in the management of the patient with persistent disease.

Another important consideration is the nerve supply to the genital tract. The external genitalia have a somatic supply, while the vagina and upper genital tract have an autonomic supply. Pain, pruritus and dyspareunia are thus experienced from irritation of nerve fibers on the vulva. It behooves the physician to be thorough in his examination and evaluate the condition of the upper genital tract structures, which could harbor more serious pathology. Small vaginal carcinomas presenting with persistent vaginal discharge are known to have been missed by inadequate examination of the patient. The act of routinely prescribing vaginal creams over the phone is poor practice.

Microbiologic Characteristics

Several investigators within the last decade have attempted to study the normal flora of the vagina. A review of these studies reveals one pertinent fact: the marked variability of isolation of microorganism types by different workers. This is not surprising and can be explained by factors such as varying availability and sophistication of microbiologic techniques and marked differences in population types studied. The term "normal vaginal flora" should be defined as the flora of an asymptomatic female excluding *N. gonorrhoeae*, *T. pallidum* and Trichomonas. Some of the common isolates from the vagina of asymptomatic females are shown in Table 1.

The few differences reported appear to be in qualitative colonization among pregnant patients, users of oral contraceptives, and premenopausal and postmenopausal patients; there is a greater incidence of gram-negative aerobic bacilli other than *E. coli* in postmenopausal women.

In general any alteration in vaginal homeostasis may result in infectious morbidity. Physiologic alterations include factors such as changes in the hormonal milieu induced by cyclic ovarian function and age. Acquired alterations include the use of various types of contraceptive methods, and use of antibiotics, douches and tampons. The concept of infection being related to environmental influences has many examples in clinical practice: the susceptibility of pregnant patients to candidi-

TABLE 1. COMMON ORGANISMS WITHIN THE NORMAL ADULT VAGINA

AEROBIC AND FACULATATIVE ANAEROBIC	ANAEROBIC
S. epidermidis	Veillonella
Lactobacillus	Peptostreptococcus spp.
Streptococcus (many groups, but particularly B and D)	Peptococcus spp.
Gardnerella vaginalis	Bacteroides spp. (including fragilis)
S. aureus	Clostridia spp.
E. coli	(including
Klebsiella	perfringens)
Proteus spp.	Eubacterium spp.
Candida albicans	Torulopsis
Chlamydia trachomatis	Other fungi
Ureaplasma urealyticum	
Mycoplasma hominis	

asis; the frequent accompaniment of vaginal candidiasis with use of long-term antibiotic therapy; the leukorrhea associated with intrauterine contraceptive device (IUD) usage. Changing the vaginal environment also has been employed in therapeutic considerations: for example, attempts at altering vaginal pH and the use of natural yogurt to replace vaginal lactobacilli.

The concept of an abnormal environment induced physiologically or otherwise is important and may be the cause of many treatment failures if not investigated and treated appropriately. Antibiotics represent only a small part of the total therapeutic modality in that antibiotics reduce the load of microorganisms that enable local defense mechanisms to overcome infection. The discharge associated with IUD use, for example, rarely abates with antibiotic treatments but generally improves considerably after removal of the device.

Approach to the Patient with Chronic Vulvovaginitis

The general attitude of physicians toward vulvovaginitis over the years has been rather casual. The management of patients with vulvovaginitis does not involve a two-minute history and pelvic examination alone but a complete history, the pertinent physical examination and the intelligent use of laboratory methods.

The primary complaints of patients with vulvovaginitis include vaginal discharge, pain (from vulvitis and dyspareunia), vaginal odor, itching of vulva or vagina or both and occasionally vaginal bleeding. These questions should be answered: (1) Is it caused by an infectious agent? (2) Is it the result of a disturbed environment? (3) Is it the manifestation of a psychologic dysfunction?

The first important aspect with regard to an infectious agent is to distinguish whether it is transmitted venereally. One should inquire about the presence of symptoms in the male consort. Not infrequently recurrence and "chronicity" are secondary to reinfection from a "third partner." Unfortunately such information is usually not forthcoming until after repeated visits when the patient comes to trust and confide in her physician. Common causes of vaginitis are listed in Table 2 along with significant clinical characteristics. It is important to use laboratory aids in diagnosis since a large percentage of patients harbor multiple pathogens. In addition, many patients with infections caused by organisms listed in Table 2 may have any or none of these symptoms. Only the laboratory will diagnose them satisfactorily.

Conditions leading to chronicity or recurrence include factors such as incorrect diagnosis and treatment, presence of multiple organisms, failure to eradicate the reservoir of infection, drug resistance (rarely encountered for the common vaginal pathogens) and presence of an abnormal environment. One must also include factors such as failure to treat the male consort(s), iatrogenic influences upon the vaginal environment (douching, IUD usage) and the presence of other metabolic changes in the patient (diabetes mellitus, lymphomas).

One must obtain information from history-taking that can enable the identification of symptoms related to emotional stress. This

TABLE 2. COMMON VAGINAL INFECTIONS AND THEIR CLINICAL CHARACTERISTICS

ORGANISM	AMOUNT	CONSISTENCY	ODOR	COLOR
Trichomonas vaginalis	Profuse	Thin/Frothy	Foul + +	Green-Yellow
Candida albicans	Moderate	Curd-like	Musty	White
Gardnerella vaginalis	Profuse	Thick/Foamy	Foul + + +	Gray-White

information may be obtained during the second or third visit when it becomes apparent that no specific agent or problem with the vaginal environment can be found. The physician should keep the concept of vulvovaginitis as a symptom of emotional distress in the forefront. Appropriate historical data should be obtained early before the patient starts "doctor shopping" because the physician, frustrated by not finding the cause of the infection, has forgotten that chronic vulvovaginitis is a common psychosomatic illness.

It is important when scheduling a patient with vulvovaginitis to inform her not to douche or use any vaginal medication for at least one week and abstain from intercourse for a day or more prior to that visit. This enables the physician to determine the extent and nature of the symptoms. Patients with complaints of profuse discharge may be found on occasion to have little exudate visible because of watery discharges that drain easily. A fastidious female, obsessed by hygiene, may complain vehemently of a trivial discharge, whereas the patient with a profuse, malodorous discharge may be relatively asymptomatic. Patients' perceptions of their condition vary greatly; women with both types of perception need attention.

Several features from a general physical examination should be noted: general health, habits of cleanliness, nutritional status, condition of other mucous membranes (an allergic manifestation may be reflected by swelling of the mucous membranes throughout the body) and any general manifestations of systemic disease. Some information from "social history" may be useful. The pelvic examination should be complete.

Skene's glands and Bartholin's glands should be palpated. The cervix should be visualized and infected nabothian follicles sought. A particularly large ectropion is often the cause of a persistent mucoid vaginal discharge, which can be annoying. The urethra should be milked and note made of any discharge. The perianal area should be inspected for evidence of inflammation as might occur secondary to candidal infection from a large rectal reservoir following chronic antibiotic usage. In gonorrheal proctitis the rectum may be resistant to conventional antibiotic dosages, and recurrence of infection from this source is not uncommon. Rarely, chronic vaginitis may be secondary to a small rectovaginal fistula and should be considered in patients recently postpartum who had sustained injury during childbirth.

TABLE 3 illustrates some of the products of metabolism of both Gardnerella and anaerobic organisms. When both organisms are present, the new products such as putrescine, cadaverine and other amines have pungent and "putrid" odors that help in the diagnosis of the presence of Gardnerella infection.

TABLE 3. PRODUCTS OF GARDNERELLA VAGINALIS AND ANAEROBES

GARDNERELLA VAGINALIS	ANAEROBES	BOTH
Acetate	Acetate	Putrescine*
Pyruvic	Butyrate	Cadaverine*
Amino acids	Proprionate	Histamine*
	Succinate	Tyramine*
		Isobutylamine*

*Disappears after metronidazole therapy.

LABORATORY AIDS

These generally are simple procedures. The most important step involves microscopy of the vaginal exudate suspended in saline. A Gram stain usually does not add further to the diagnosis. Diagnostic features of common vaginal pathogens are summarized in Table 4. Although these organisms comprise the majority of infectious causes, this may not be true for recurrent and refractory cases of vulvovaginitis. Multiple infectious agents frequently coexist and each requires specific therapy. Other fungi, protozoa and viruses must be considered.

The Prepubertal Female

Vulvovaginitis is the commonest gynecologic problem encountered in the prepubertal female. Numerous reasons have been cited for this in the past, such as poor hygiene and frequent manipulation of the external genitalia from curiosity and masturbation. One of the most important factors contributing to this inflammation is the lack of estrogen stimulation of the tissues.

Common causative factors in this age group can be categorized as infectious and noninfectious.

TABLE 4. COMMON LABORATORY AIDS FOR DIAGNOSIS OF VAGINITIS

ORGANISM	LIGHT MICROSCOPY	MEDIUM FOR CULTURE
Gardnerella vaginalis	"Clue" cells (vaginal epithelial cells covered with microorganisms) Presence of many organisms on the slide	Casman's agar Dunkelberg medium
Trichomonas vaginalis	Many white blood cells on the smear Motile trichomonads Nonmotile trichomonads	Diamond's medium C.P.I.M. medium
Monilia	Pseudohyphae, budding yeasts	Sabouraud's medium Nickerson's medium

INFECTIOUS CAUSES

NONSPECIFIC INFECTIONS. This comprises about 80 per cent of vaginitis and is due to poor hygiene. Fecal staining of the vestibule follows improper cleansing of the rectum. As a consequence *E. coli* is the common organism isolated. Other organisms include *S. aureus*, the streptococci and Proteus species.

SPECIFIC INFECTIONS. These comprise the remaining 20 per cent of causes. Isolates in order of frequency include *Candida albicans*, Trichomonas, Neisseria, Gardnerella and Streptococcus. These organisms can be identified by either microscopy or culture technique.

RARER INFECTIOUS PROCESSES. These include cellulitis from skin abrasions and inflammation secondary to a urinary infection. *Enterobius vermicularis* (pinworms) may infect the vagina and produce inflammation.

NONINFECTIOUS CAUSES

FOREIGN BODIES. These objects lead to a nonspecific vaginitis with a malodorous discharge and vaginal spotting. They may be the most common cause of "nonspecific" vaginitis.

ALLERGIC MANIFESTATIONS. This may be part of the generalized allergic phenomenon or a local one secondary to the fabric in new underclothing, a laundry detergent, clothes softeners, powders, bath oils, bubble baths and the like.

EPITHELIAL DYSTROPHIES. This rarely may present a problem in childhood.

NEOPLASMS. Even rarer is the presence of benign and malignant tumors, which may present with a vaginal discharge. Vaginal adenosis is included in this group but usually does not produce a mucoid exudate until the glands are stimulated by endogenous estrogen.

Women of Childbearing Age

INFECTIOUS CAUSES

The three most common types of vaginitis have been discussed. Other infectious causes include recurrent *Herpes genitalis*, foreign body vaginitis (e.g., retained tampons), gonorrhea (in this disease vaginitis, per se, is rare), chronic infection of Bartholin's and Skene's glands and pyodermas of the vulvar skin. Recurrent infection from upper genital tract conditions (chronic cervicitis, endometritis) contribute a significant percentage to the morbidity.

Recurrent genital herpes viral infection is a special problem in that its pathogenesis is unknown. In contrast to reinfection, in which an organism is reintroduced to the vulva or vagina, this viral infection has a latent stage. Once the original herpetic infection has disappeared, the genetic material of the virus is still present in the host. The best guess today is that the virus (or its DNA) resides in the sacral ganglia. A number of events will trigger the production of new virus, which probably migrates down the efferent limbs of the nerves to the genitalia to become manifest as a recurrent herpetic lesion shedding large amounts of virus. Some of the "trigger events" include other pelvic infections, intercourse, menstrual periods, emotional disturbances, temperature changes and cyclic hormone therapy with birth control pills. Whenever an herpetic lesion is present, it is infectious to anyone coming into contact with the virus. The major difference between a primary genital herpesvirus infection and a recurrent infection is that the latter persists for fewer days with little or no systemic symptoms.

A multitude of studies have not been able to demonstrate any difference in humoral or cellular immune responses between patients who never develop recurrences and those with frequent genital herpesvirus recurrences. Therefore, at this point it is not possible to predict which patient will have recurrent infections. It is estimated that 30 to 50 per cent of patients will have occasional recurrences. Fortunately, only a fraction (perhaps 5 to 10 per cent) will have frequent recurrences triggered by factors mentioned.

NONINFECTIOUS CAUSES

Similar considerations exist for this group of causes as are listed for the premenarchal female. With the widespread use of contraceptives in this group of patients, and the common practice of douching and use of vaginal medications, allergic vulvovaginitis (or nonspecific inflammation) is an extremely common problem. Once the infectious causes for vulvovaginitis are excluded, allergic reactions and psychosomatic reactions are the most common causes of recurrent vulvovaginitis.

The Postmenopausal Female

INFECTIOUS CAUSES

In the sexually active postmenopausal female, consideration will still have to be given to venereally transmitted pathogens. As noted, infections in the postmenopausal female can result in serious morbidity due to atrophy of the genital structures following estrogen withdrawal. Most studies on asymptomatic patients reveal no differences in the vaginal flora between the postmenopausal female and other groups of patients. Two studies have shown a slight increase in gram-negative aerobic rods in the vagina of postmenopausal females. However, monilia, and Trichomonas are still the leading infectious organisms. The age of the patient should not negate the responsibility to do an adequate evaluation for infectious agents. Each year we see a number

of older patients who have had hysterectomies who have had long-standing Trichomonas infections. Their physicians could not believe that this was possible.

NONINFECTIOUS CAUSES

ATROPHIC VAGINITIS. Withdrawal of endogenous estrogen from ovarian failure results in regression of the secondary sex characteristics and atrophy of the genitalia. The degree of atrophy varies from patient to patient. The vaginal skin assumes a pale gray, smooth appearance with easy bruisability. Bacterial infection of this atrophic skin is common. Response to estrogen therapy is dramatic and results in spontaneous resolution of inflammation without specific antibiotic therapy.

EPITHELIAL DYSTROPHIES. These are numerous in type and may simulate infectious vulvitis. The disease varies from localized lesions to a more generalized involvement of the external genitalia. The salient features in diagnosis of the condition include severe pruritus, failure in demonstration of an offending organism and lack of response to antibiotic substances.

An important part of diagnosis of these dystrophies is biopsy of the lesion. The hypertrophic variety may be associated with or be a precursor to premalignant and malignant disease of the vulva.

ALLERGIC REACTIONS. The same diligent historical questioning is necessary here as in any age group to seek possible causes. Many times vulvar allergic reaction is indistinguishable from the vulvar dystrophies.

NEOPLASMS. Not uncommonly genital neoplasms present with symptoms and signs of vaginitis. If careful examination is not carried out, these lesions may be missed.

Lastly, a group of patients will be found in whom symptomatology is severe and recurrent, examination reveals little and treatment with a wide variety of agents fails. The diagnosis of psychosomatic vaginitis is made after exclusion of all other causes. Failure to recognize the psychosomatic nature of a patient's problem and repeated attempts at therapy for infectious agents serve to reinforce the patient's symptomatology without getting to the basic psychologic cause. This problem is perhaps more common in women of the reproductive age group.

Treatment of Refractory and Recurrent Vaginitis

Certain general rules can be established for the treatment of vulvovaginitis. An attempt to establish a diagnosis as accurately as possible requires a complete history, physical examination and laboratory tests. It is important to determine whether or not the cause is infectious and whether or not the agent is venereally transmitted. One must always consider multiple infecting organisms, which are present in 25 per cent of patients.

The male consort(s) should be treated in most situations involving infectious agents. It is important to emphasize this to the patient, since reinfection frequently arises from this source.

Topical treatment for the infectious causes of vulvovaginitis may not be successful as the only treatment modality. Some reasons for this are less patient compliance owing to a "messy" method of treatment, improper use, failure of the agent to eradicate deep-seated infections and failure to treat the urethral and rectal reservoir. Additional systemic treatment may help with some of these problems.

Some general measures include improving personal hygiene. The use of sitz baths as often as possible results in significant relief. Analgesic agents given orally or topically are often helpful. The use of tight-fitting underclothes should be discouraged. Wearing loose cotton underclothes during the day and sleeping "bare" at night is beneficial. Douching is useful for patients who have a profuse discharge in the initial phase of therapy; it provides a diluent effect leading to some symptomatic relief. By itself, it provides no specific long-term benefit.

Not uncommonly the treatment of recurrent and refractory vulvovaginitis may require cauterization of large cervical ectropions and nabothian follicles. We have found that cryocautery is substantially better than hot cautery.

Use of condoms by sexual partners is recommended until the treatment schedule is completed to prevent reinfection. Often one of the partners harbors infection that is not eradicated by conventional drug regimes. This may follow a prostatitis in the male or cervicitis in the female requiring more prolonged therapy. Continuation of condom use for such a patient is usually found to reduce the recurrence rate. It is not surprising on examining females who have used diaphragms for several years to find the cervix looking "clean," probably from protection by the occlusive device or the spermicidal agent, which is known to have bacteriostatic properties. Use should be made of this principle in patients with chronic cervicitis in order to suppress reinfection and allow healing to occur.

The various agents used in the treatment of the common infectious causes of vulvovaginitis are listed in Table 5.

As can be seen from Table 5, there is no specific therapy for recurrent genital herpes infection. It will spontaneously cure itself regardless of therapy. The physician can provide only symptomatic relief. Any therapy must shorten the course of the infection compared with a spontaneous cure. Therefore, the best therapy for the acute genital infection is keeping the infected area dry and using good hygiene, and using topical anesthetics (such as viscous lidocaine) as needed. The same is true for the recurrent infection. Many topical agents have been used, but either the studies are not controlled well or there are too few patients from which to draw a conclusion. The study problem for recurrent herpetic infection

TABLE 5. VARIOUS THERAPIES FOR COMMON CAUSES OF VULVOVAGINITIS

ORGANISM	CHOICE	OTHERS
Candida albicans	Clotrimazole Miconazole Nystatin Ketoconazole (systemic)	Gentian violet Boric acid Natural yogurt Potassium sorbate
Gardnerella vaginalis	Metronidazole ? Ampicillin	Sulfa creams Tetracycline
Trichomonas vaginalis	Metronidazole	Sulfa creams
Herpesvirus genitalis	—	—

is compounded by the facts that the infection is short-lived (usually less than 2 weeks); it is variable in degree and duration from patient to patient; and patients present for therapy over a variable time period so that the lesions are treated without taking into account the time for an expected spontaneous cure. Acyclovir has been shown to be somewhat effective as topical therapy only for the acute primary genital infection by herpesvirus.

Therapy to *prevent* recurrences of genital herpesvirus infection is another matter. The list goes from psychotherapy to vaccination with a variety of infectious agents such as vaccinia virus (smallpox), poliovirus, herpesvirus vaccines, *Corynebacterium parvum* and BCG. Needless to say, none has proven beneficial enough to recommend specific therapy.

An attempt was made in this chapter to provide the clinician with a general approach to the difficult problem of recurrent and refractory vulvovaginitis. We have emphasized accurate diagnosis and adequate therapy for the condition. Since infection of the vulva and vagina may affect significantly other biologic functions, the clinician is urged to renew his enthusiasm for the management of patients with seemingly simple problems that over a short time period can become psychologically and physically debilitating when they recur or become chronic.

REFERENCES

1. Amstey, M. S.: Genital herpesvirus infection. Clin. Obstet. Gynecol. 18:89, 1975.
2. Dunkelberg, W. E.: *Corynebacterium vaginale.* Sex. Transm. Dis. 4:69, 1977.
3. Galask, R. P., Larson, B., and Ohm, M. J.: Vaginal flora and its role in disease entities. Clin. Obst. Gynecol. 19:61, 1976.
4. Josey, W. E., McKenzie, W. J., and Lambe, D. W., Jr.: *Corynebacterium vaginale (H. vaginalis)* in women with leukorrhoea. Am. J. Obstet. Gynecol. 126:574, 1976.
5. Josey, W. E. and Lambe, D. W., Jr.: Epidemiologic characteristics of women infected with *Corynebacterium vaginale (Hemophilus vaginalis).* J. Am. Vener. Dis. Assoc. 3:9, 1976.
6. Josey, W. E.: Vaginitis: reducing the number of refractory cases. Postgrad. Med. 62:171, 1977.
7. Lang, W. R.: Pediatric vaginitis. N. Engl. J. Med. 253:1153, 1955.
8. Lewison, M. E., Lourdes, C. C., Carrington, E. R., and Kaye, D.: Quantitative microflora of the vagina. Am. J. Obstet. Gynecol. 127:80, 1977.
9. Miles, M. R., Ryan, M., Olsen, L., and Rogers, A.: Recurrent vaginal candidiasis importance of an intestinal reservoir. J.A.M.A. 238:1836, 1977.
10. Meisels, A., and Gagne, O.: Microbiology of the female reproductive tract v. changing patterns within one decade in a French Canadian population. J. Reprod. Med. 18:66, 1977.
11. Pathak, U. N., Sur, S. K., and Farrand, R. J.: Comparison of metronidazole/nystatin and nitrofuratel in the treatment of vaginitis. Br. J. Clin. Practice 29:270, 1975.
12. Zuspan, F. P.: Management of patients with vaginal infections. An invitational symposium. J. Reprod. Med. 9:1, 1972.

Editorial Comment

Of all the complications and problems that persist in gynecology the one that is most perplexing and difficult to handle is current and refractory vulvovaginitis. It is a common finding in the history of such a patient that she has been treated with almost every medication listed in the PDR for vaginitis. Additionally, many home remedies and suggestions from friends have also entered into therapy. This chapter attempts to focus on an approach to the problem. The controversy is what should be done and the approach to the problem.

It would appear, in my experience from referred patients I have seen, that most gynecologists have an aversion to the problem of chronic or recurrent vulvovaginitis and do not accept it as a serious condition in the patient. However, it is a major problem for the patient and requires a special concern. The basis of all therapy for vulvovaginitis is an attempt to return normal flora to the vagina and vulva. It must be remembered that unctions, ointments, solutions and medications all alter the vaginal flora. The patient and her physician should know that in addition to exogenous medications, anxiety can alter (increase) the pH of the vagina and promote recurrent vaginitis. There are two important issues when you examine a patient with this particular problem. First, take the complaint seriously, because this is indeed a problem for the patient. Second, make sure that you have an adequate evaluation of the patient, which means no vaginal medications, douching and so forth for at least five days before the examination.

The pH of the vagina is a reflection of its microbiology. Each examining area should have limited-scale pH paper available to help in evaluating the vagina on each examination. The pH paper is not a substitute for the microscope, but most situations of vaginitis can be diagnosed in the office. Cultures are used only to confirm your diagnosis and seldom are needed. (The exception are Chlamydia cultures.)

The authors of these articles point out that the normal pH of the vagina is 3.5 to 4.2. We have not observed any vaginal infection at this pH range. The pH will be higher following menstruation or if blood is present and, understandably, patients with increased bleeding will not have a normal pH, which may trigger their problem. A higher yield will be obtained if a drop of saline is put on the slide at the examining table and the swab immersed into the drop of saline for evaluation for Trichomonas, yeast or Hemophilus. The examination for yeast, especially Candida, can be done with a 10 per cent potassium hydroxide solution, which acts as a lytic agent on cells other than spores and filaments of the yeast. Hemophilus gives a musty sulfide odor. *Torulopsis glabrata* is a fungus seen mostly with spore formations that grows in a pH that approaches the normal pH of the vagina, i.e., near 4.5. It is not uncommon for a patient to have more than one vaginal infection, such as the association of Hemophilus in 25 per cent of cases with Trichomonas. It is not unusual that when one organism is treated another organism emerges as the problem. It is best to inform the patient before therapy that this may occur, so that expectations are appropriate.

Physicians argue about whether or not the sexual partner should be treated. It is known that Trichomonas, Hemophilus, herpes and usually yeast infections are forms that may afflict both partners. There are a number of ways to treat Hemophilus. The authors outline their form of therapy and point out that reinfection is higher if both partners are not treated. This is also true in Trichomonas, when a reinfection rate of greater than two times is seen if both are not treated. It is appropriate to instruct your female patients to use an antifungal vaginal suppository on a daily basis during broad-spectrum antibiotic therapy so they do not have a later complication of yeast vaginitis.

The promotion of normal vaginal hygiene assures that the lactobacillus will grow in an exuberant fashion, causing a pH (3.5 to 4.2) that is unacceptable for other organisms. We have found that a jelly (Aci-jel) or powder (micronized alumina) is an appropriate buffer to help stabilize and promote the growth of normal bacteria. When all else fails and our frustration titer is high we suggest that yogurt (must have active bacteria) eaten at least twice a week may be helpful. Some individuals have also been helped by taking a yogurt douche (cup yogurt with active cultures to douche bag water) several times a week for several weeks. It is an inexpensive method to promote the growth of "lacto-type" bacillus in the vagina.

Most women who have persistent and chronic vaginal infection tend to be tense individuals and we have been impressed that tension and anxiety can increase the vaginal pH, which does not promote the growth of normal bacteria.

What we all look for in women who have intractable vaginitis is a consultant, as we are often as frustrated and confused as the patient, but persistence and a systematic approach as outlined by these experts will yield beneficial results.

15
Galactorrhea Syndromes

Alternative Points of View

by R. Jeffrey Chang and Howard L. Judd
by David W. Keller and James C. Warren

Editorial Comment

Clinical Management of Galactorrhea

R. Jeffrey Chang, M.D.
Howard L. Judd, M.D.
UCLA Center for the Health Sciences

The advent of a precise and reliable radioimmunoassay for the measurement of serum prolactin has allowed the clinician to differentiate more readily functional galactorrhea from that arising as a result of disordered prolactin metabolism. The clinical significance of hyperprolactinemic galactorrhea is emphasized by recent reports of prolactin-secreting pituitary adenomas occurring in these patients.[1-3] The pathogenesis of abnormal prolactin metabolism and the natural history of associated disease—in particular, prolactin-secreting pituitary adenomas—are not clearly understood. These limitations have led to alternative and occasionally controversial approaches to the management of galactorrhea. An example of this is the management of infertility in patients with prolactin-secreting pituitary adenomas. The purpose of the following discussion is to address the problem of galactorrhea and to review its current clinical management.

Definition

Galactorrhea is defined as the secretion of milky fluid from the breast unassociated with pregnancy or the postpartum period. In contrast, milk production during and following pregnancy is a normal physiological event. Galactorrhea may appear spontaneously or occur following manipulation of the breast. Occasionally, breast secretion may not appear white, but rather discolored or almost clear. Desquamation of the ductal epithelium occurs regularly and may account for the discoloration. Breast secretion that appears thin and watery may reflect a lowered concentration of protein and carbohydrate. Normally, human milk is composed of nearly 90 per cent water. For these reasons, nearly all breast discharges may be considered as evidence of galactorrhea. The appearance of fat droplets on microscopic examination of the breast secretion or a positive fat stain usually confirms that the secretion is milk. Obviously, any breast secretion that contains blood must be fully evaluated for the possibility of breast carcinoma.

Lactogenesis

The capacity of the breast to produce milk involves several hormonal influences. The de-

436

velopment and maintenance of breast tissue is dependent on estrogen and progesterone. During puberty, coincident with ovulatory activity, the prepubertal breast undergoes a series of maturational changes that result in the formation of the adult female breast. The rising levels of circulating estrogen, which accompany the onset of ovulatory function, stimulate the ductal elements of the breast to grow and develop, while increased progesterone secretion serves to promote the alveolar development of the lobular tissue. The production of milk also involves prolactin, which gradually increases in the circulation during puberty as a result of stimulation of pituitary lactotrophs by estrogen. To date the only function attributed to prolactin in humans is the promotion of lactogenesis. In this regard, prolactin appears to replenish and increase the volume and fat content of breast milk.[4] Cortisol and insulin also contribute to lactogenesis; however, it is not clear whether thyroxine is involved in the process. Growth hormone, while lactogenic in animals, probably is not essential for milk production in humans, since growth hormone-deficient dwarfs lactate normally following delivery.

During pregnancy growth of the alveolar and ductal elements and milk production are stimulated by the increasing levels of circulating estrogen, progesterone and prolactin.[5] Human placental lactogen derived from the placenta also serves to further enhance milk production. In late pregnancy, the high concentrations of estrogen and progesterone, while contributing to the production of milk, exert a local cellular effect on the breast to inhibit milk release through an as yet undefined mechanism. Following delivery, sex steroid levels decline rapidly and milk release (milk let-down) mediated by oxytocin is allowed to proceed. This process involves mechanical stimulation of the nipple, which triggers a nerve impulse to release oxytocin. Oxytocin stimulates the myoepithelial cells of the ductal system to contract and express milk. Replenishment of milk is maintained by prolactin.

Prolactin levels usually return to normal prepregnant levels about seven days after delivery in nonnursing mothers, although higher levels may persist for several weeks.[6] During this time, the increased prolactin continues to exert its stimulating effect on milk production, and in the absence of lactation-suppressant drugs, some milk secretion occurs. In women who breast feed, a marked increase in serum prolactin occurs with suckling, which probably serves to replenish breast milk. Baseline prolactin levels may remain elevated before returning to normal nonpregnant levels after 80 to 100 days. Increases in serum prolactin in response to suckling also gradually diminish over time.[5]

Control of Prolactin Secretion

Prolactin secretion is controlled by an inhibitory factor originating in the hypothalamus, prolactin inhibitory factor (PIF), which as yet has not been identified. This inhibitory factor is transported along the pituitary stalk via portal venous blood vessels to the anterior pituitary, where it acts on the lactotrophic cells to regulate prolactin secretion. Current evidence indicates that PIF may be stimulated by dopamine or dopamine agonists acting at the level of the hypothalamus. The administration of L-dopa, which is converted to dopamine in the brain, decreases prolactin level. Dopamine agonists, such as the ergot alkaloid bromocriptine, also reduce the circulating level of prolactin.[7] The demonstration of dopamine receptors in the pituitary has led some investigators to hypothesize that dopamine is, in fact, PIF. Disorders that interfere with the hypothalamic production of dopamine or interrupt portal venous blood flow by compression of the pituitary stalk can result in decreased PIF activity, increased prolactin release and hyperprolactinemia. While evidence for a prolactin-releasing factor is lacking in humans, thyrotropin-releasing hormone (TRH) in pharmacologic amounts has been shown to stimulate prolactin secretion. Whether TRH has a significant role in the physiological regulation of normal prolactin release is unclear.

Incidence of Hyperprolactinemia

The presence of galactorrhea with or without amenorrhea suggests the possibility of hyperprolactinemia. In patients with normal ovulatory function, galactorrhea has been poorly correlated with hyperprolactinemia.[8] In these individuals, a prior history of lactotroph stimulation may be elicited, such as pregnancy, use of estrogen-dominant oral contraceptives, use of psychotropic drugs, stress, or breast or chest wall stimulation. This suggests that hyperprolactinemia was once present and resulted in galactorrhea, but the stimulus for prolactin secretion has ceased while the established galactorrhea has persisted. If the galactorrhea is accompanied by amenorrhea, the incidence of hyperprolactinemia is more frequent in comparison to that observed in patients with either galactorrhea or amenorrhea only. Most series have reported a 50 per cent or greater association.[3, 9] Some patients with amenorrhea but no demonstrable galactorrhea also may be suffering hyperprolactinemia. Approximately 20 per cent of amenorrheic patients have been found to have hyperprolactinemia.[10] The clinical significance of hyperprolactinemic amenorrhea is accentuated by the recent reports of prolactin-secreting pituitary adenomas occurring in these patients.

In the presence of hyperprolactinemia, the incidence of galactorrhea is approximately 30 to 40 per cent, although an incidence of 80 per cent was reported in one study.[11] This disparity was attributed to the select nature of the patient population and very careful breast examination in the latter study. In individual patients with hyperprolactinemia unaccompanied by galactorrhea, either the circulating concentration of prolactin may be insufficient for adequate breast milk production or factors that prime the breast for the action of prolactin may not be adequate.

Hyperprolactinemic States

Hyperprolactinemia may develop as a result of various physiological, pharmacologic or pathologic conditions. The physiological factors that result in hyperprolactinemia are the most common. As previously mentioned, increased prolactin levels accompany the pregnant state and occur postpartum during suckling by mothers who are nursing. In addition, it is well established that prolactin levels rise in association with sleep. Hyperprolactinemia may be induced by stress resulting from surgical manipulation (endoscopy) or nonsurgical stimuli, such as insulin-induced hypoglycemia and exercise.[12] Nipple stimulation may lead to mild elevation of serum prolactin, and, in some instances, galactorrhea.

Pharmacologically, hyperprolactinemia may be associated with the administration of antidepressants, sex steroids and antihypertensive medications.[13] Commonly, the use of psychotropic drugs such as the phenothiazines (chlorpromazine), tricyclic amines (Elavil or Triavil),

or butyrophenones (haloperidol) can be associated with hyperprolactinemia. Estrogen administration frequently leads to an elevation of circulating prolactin. Oral contraceptives may cause an increase in the mean level of prolactin, but values exceeding those of the normal range for prolactin are uncommon. Occasionally, hyperprolactinemia may be associated with the administration of antihypertensive drugs. Aldomet, acting as a false neurotransmitter, may stimulate an increase in prolactin levels. Reserpine and guanethidine also may increase prolactin concentration by preventing the uptake and storage of dopamine in the hypothalamus.

Among the pathologic disorders associated with hyperprolactinemia, pituitary tumors, hypothalamic disease and hypothyroidism appear to be the most common, although other endocrine and nonendocrine disturbances may be implicated.[14] With pituitary tumors, excessive prolactin production may result either from direct hormonal secretion by the neoplasm or from interruption of inhibitory hypothalamic control following compression of the pituitary stalk and portal blood flow by tumor mass. Prolactin-secreting pituitary adenomas probably comprise the majority of pituitary tumors. While it appears that pituitary neoplasms tend to grow slowly, the natural course of prolactin-secreting pituitary tumors is not clearly defined. In certain instances, marked tumor growth has been observed within a short period of time. Considering the vital structures that are in direct proximity to the pituitary, it is critical that the presence of a pituitary neoplasm be determined.

Hyperprolactinemia may result from disease or destruction of the hypothalamus or pituitary stalk. These conditions include primary (craniopharyngioma) or metastatic tumors, infiltrative disease, infarction and surgical or radiation ablation. The lesions probably disrupt catecholamine metabolism in the hypothalamus, which results in a loss of inhibitory control of prolactin. If the insult to the hypothalamus is severe, the gradual deprivation of tropic substances to the pituitary may eventually lead to panhypopituitarism without hyperprolactinemia. It is not known if the magnitude of hyperprolactinemia correlates with the extent of hypothalamic disease, although sleep-induced increases in prolactin are usually absent in these patients.

Patients with primary hypothyroidism may often demonstrate mild hyperprolactinemia associated with galactorrhea and amenorrhea.[15] Since serum TSH levels are usually elevated, it is presumed that the increase in prolactin results from enhanced thyrotropin-releasing hormone activity, although direct evidence is lacking. While lactotroph hyperplasia may accompany hyperprolactinemia in these hypothyroid patients, the development of a pituitary adenoma also has been observed.

Other endocrine-related disorders that may manifest hyperprolactinemia are acromegaly, Nelson's syndrome and Parkinson's disease. Nonendocrine diseases associated with abnormal prolactin metabolism include renal disease and ectopic prolactin production by malignant tumors.

Evaluation of Galactorrhea

Several tests have been utilized in the evaluation of galactorrhea, of which measurement of serum prolactin and evaluation of the sella turcica appear to be most useful. Additional studies may be necessary in order to complete the diagnosis in some cases. It is important for the physician to be cognizant of these tests and understand their clinical significance.

Serum prolactin levels are measured by radioimmunoassay and range between 3 to 30 ng/ml in normal cycling women. Variation in the upper normal limit may be encountered among individual laboratories performing the test. In prepubertal girls, prolactin levels are low (2 to 12 ng/ml) and gradually attain adult levels during puberty as a result of ovarian estrogen production. This incremental change in prolactin should be considered in the management of a young patient with galactorrhea, primary amenorrhea and a mildly elevated prolactin.

Accurate assessment of the sella turcica is accomplished by performing sella polytomography in the anteroposterior and lateral projections. It has been clearly demonstrated that sellar polytomography is a highly sensitive method for detecting subtle changes in the bony configuration of the sella turcica, which often are not demonstrated by plain cone-down views.[16] The utility of sellar polytomography is reflected in the diagnosis of small pituitary neoplasms.[2, 3] Pituitary adenomas tend to expand initially in an anterior-inferior direction against that portion of the sellar floor overlying the sphenoid sinus. For this reason, an early sign of an intrasellar mass is cortical bone thinning, resulting in a "blistered" appearance of the floor of the sella. Continued tumor growth may, in fact, lead to actual penetration of the sellar floor and expansion of tumor into the sphenoid sinus. Frequently, these changes are subtle and may be detected only by polytomographic technique. Consequently, this technique, in combination with a reliable method for the measurement of serum prolactin by radioimmunoassay, probably has led to the diagnosis of prolactin-secreting pituitary adenomas being made more frequently than previously occurred.

While the advantages of sellar polytomography over those of plain cone-down views are obvious, other clinical and practical considerations should be pointed out. Animal studies indicate that cataractal changes may result from massive doses of x-ray radiation to the lens.[17] In humans, no conclusive reports have appeared to confirm these findings, although a relationship has been suggested by one uncontrolled study.[18] Nevertheless, much of the potential problem may be avoided by shielding the lens with lead glasses, since lens exposure to radiation is greatest during anteroposterior polytomography. Another consideration is procedural costs incurred in diagnosis. In some instances, there is a large difference in expense between sellar polytomography and cone-down views.

While sellar polytomography may serve to detect infrasellar extension, suprasellar lesions must be evaluated by other techniques such as visual field examination, pneumoencephalography and computerized axial tomography. Unfortunately, each procedure has inherent limitations that detract from its applicability or acceptability. Visual field examination may suggest suprasellar extension by virtue of tumor impinging on the optic chiasm. However, by the time a field defect is discovered irreparable damage and significant tumor growth already may have occurred. Compared to visual field examination, pneumoencephalography affords a more sensitive estimation of suprasellar extension, but the procedure is associated with risk and marked discomfort. Acceptability of repeated pneumoencephalography is problematic. In an effort to overcome the disadvantages of pneumoencephalography and visual field examination, computerized axial tomography has been applied to the evaluation of extension of pituitary tumors. Reports have not been consistent regarding the ability of this technique to identify moderate suprasellar extension. We can hope that refinement of the technique will offer an acceptable method of assessing tumor extension. Thus, the most reasonable procedure that can be performed repeatedly for the detection of suprasellar extension appears to be examination of the visual fields.

Attempts to utilize anterior pituitary function tests for the diagnosis of a prolactin-secreting pituitary adenoma have been disappointing, with the possible exception of the administration of TRH.[19] The prolactin response to TRH stimulation is significantly blunted in patients with prolactin-secreting pituitary adenomas and probably reflects autonomous prolactin secretion by the tumor or a state of maximal lactotroph stimulation or both. Hyperprolactinemic patients without radiologic evidence of an intrasellar mass can also demonstrate similar blunted responses to TRH administration. Whether these patients harbor small but radiologically undetectable pituitary neoplasms has not been determined. Long-term follow-up studies are needed to determine if hyperprolactinemic patients are at risk for development of a pituitary adenoma.

The initial screening procedure for a patient with galactorrhea involves consideration of menstrual function, measurement of serum prolactin and assessment of thyroid function. Screening tests of thyroid function include measurement of free thyroxine concentration or free thyroxine index, and serum triiodothyronine, although the latter is less useful in the diagnosis of hypothyroidism. In the presence of thyroid dysfunction, subsequent evaluation and treatment would be determined by the nature of the disorder. Normal cycling women with galactorrhea may be adequately screened by a serum prolactin. If the prolactin level is normal, the patient may be followed yearly with a serum prolactin measurement. If the prolactin levels are elevated, the patient warrants evaluation of the sella despite the occurrence of regular menstrual cycles. Galactorrhea in the presence of amenorrhea or oligomenorrhea requires evaluation of both the serum prolactin level and the sella turcica. Thus, the initial evaluation serves to identify patients on the basis of prolactin level and the appearance of the sella turcica.

Management of Galactorrhea

Following completion of the initial evaluation, patients may be separated into various groups according to a normal or abnormal serum prolactin and sella turcica. Clinical management will vary among individual groups.

NORMAL PROLACTIN, NORMAL SELLA. In this group of patients the likelihood of a pituitary neoplasm is small. However, persistence of galactorrhea and amenorrhea requires that evaluation of the serum prolactin and sella turcica be performed yearly. In those patients with galactorrhea and regular menstrual cycles, a prolactin measurement obtained once a year serves as adequate management. Resolution of galactorrhea and resumption of normal menstrual function may be achieved by the administration of bromocriptine. Pregnancy is not contraindicated in this situation.

NORMAL PROLACTIN, ABNORMAL SELLA. Abnormalities in the configuration of the sella suggest the presence of an intrasellar mass. If the changes are subtle, it is very likely that a pituitary neoplasm is confined within the sellar space, but these findings do not preclude the existence of a dumbbell-shaped lesion. Assessment of suprasellar extension should be performed. Although pneumoencephalography provides the most sensitive measure, visual field examination may be more practical. In the presence of any extrasellar tumor extension, definitive ablative therapy is indicated. If there is no evidence of extrasellar extension, then the patient's case may be managed conservatively.

A normal serum prolactin concentration suggests that the neoplasm is not a prolactin-secreting pituitary adenoma but rather a non-hormone-secreting tumor. It also suggests that growth of the tumor probably has not been sufficient to cause an interruption of portal blood flow by compression of the pituitary stalk. It should be remembered that the growth pattern of a suspected intrasellar mass cannot be determined from an initial evaluation. There is evidence to suggest that non-hormone-secreting pituitary neoplasms are slow growing. With minor changes in the sella turcica, normal anatomic variation always should be considered. For these reasons, follow-up management consists of assessment of the sella and serum prolactin at yearly intervals. Any change indicative of tumor growth warrants sellar exploration. While pregnancy probably is not contraindicated in these patients, it may be advisable to wait one year, thereby providing some measure of possible tumor growth. In the absence of increased sellar size or elevation of serum prolactin, it is unlikely that a nonhormone-secreting pituitary adenoma would give rise to any major complication during pregnancy. However, some caution should be exercised in these patients because a normal pituitary gland may enlarge up to twice its original size in response to the changing hormonal milieu of pregnancy. If pregnancy should occur, frequent examination of the visual field is indicated.

ABNORMAL PROLACTIN, NORMAL SELLA. Patients with hyperprolactinemia and no x-ray evidence of an intrasellar mass may be suffering from a small but as yet radiologically undetectable pituitary adenoma, lactotroph hyperplasia or a hypothalamic lesion. A visual field examination or pneumoencephalography should be performed to rule out a suprasellar lesion. The management of these patients is complicated by the fact that small pituitary adenomas have been found in patients with extremely high prolactin levels and a normal sella turcica. The prolactin level obtained on the initial evaluation provides little information as to the progressive nature of a prolactin-secreting pituitary adenoma but does correlate significantly with the size of the neoplasm as determined at surgery.[2]

Clinical management should be based on subsequent determinations of serum prolactin at six-month intervals and evaluation of the sella at yearly intervals. If there is no further increase in prolactin levels and the sella remains normal, then progressive growth of a prolactin-secreting pituitary adenoma is not evident and no treatment is necessary. If progressive increases in serum prolactin occur without changes in the sella, then consideration must be given to the possible existence of a hypothalamic lesion or development of suprasellar extension of a small pituitary tumor.[20] In this situation, a repeat visual field examination or pneumoencephalogram is indicated. While the hyperprolactinemia may result from a focus of lactrotrophic hyperplasia or a small pituitary adenoma, the normal configuration of the sella turcica argues against any pituitary enlargement. If marked hyperprolactinemia (greater than 200 ng/ml) is present, it may prompt consideration of sellar exploration because the likelihood of a prolactin-secreting pituitary adenoma is increased.

Pregnancy is probably permissible in patients with hyperprolactinemia, a normal sella turcica and no evidence of a suprasellar lesion. In the absence of suprasellar disease hyperprolactinemic patients without evidence of an intrasellar mass have been reported to tolerate pregnancy without complications or sequelae.[21]

ABNORMAL PROLACTIN, ABNORMAL SELLA. In these patients, the probable diagnosis is a prolactin-secreting pituitary adenoma. Subsequent procedures should be performed to ascertain whether suprasellar extension has occurred. If the tumor is small and confined to the sella, surgical or medical management may be proposed. In this group of patients there is controversy over which therapy is better. This arises largely because of the unpredictability of progressive tumor growth. In many instances, treatment will be individualized according to the needs of the patient. These tumors can be removed selectively by transsphenoidal microdissection. It has been shown that this form of therapy is highly effective and affords the patients the benefit of cessation of galactorrhea and resumption of ovulatory function in most cases.[2] In addition, anterior pituitary function usually is not impaired postoperatively. Complications of the procedure are much less common and severe than those associated with craniotomy. The most common complication is transient diabetes insipidus. Postoperative follow-up of these patients is not extensive and little information has been accumulated concerning the rate of tumor recurrence.

In contrast to surgery, medical management has been directed toward alleviation of symptoms while maintaining close observation of prolactin levels and sellar size. Clinical trials have shown that the administration of bromocriptine effectively reduces or eliminates galactorrhea and restores regular menstrual function in about 75 per cent of cases. In vitro studies have suggested that bromocriptine inhibits lactotroph proliferation, and a recent case report indicated that regression of tumor was achieved during bromocriptine therapy.[22] Whether the focus of lactotroph neoplasia may be eradicated by long-term treatment is not known. Discontinuation of bromocriptine usually is followed by a recurrence of symptoms and hyperprolactinemia. Management of these patients with bromocriptine requires strict monitoring of prolactin levels at six-month intervals and evaluation of the sella at least yearly if not more frequently. Given the likelihood that the patient already has a pituitary adenoma, any evidence of increased tumor growth requires consideration of ablative therapy.

In the presence of marked suprasellar extension of the tumor, the management is less controversial, with surgery being the treatment of choice. The transsphenoidal approach is not appropriate and instead craniotomy may be preferred. The operative removal of a large pituitary neoplasm is associated with greater morbidity and an increased risk of permanent sequelae. Clinically, there usually is resolution of galactorrhea, but ovulatory function is frequently absent secondary to gonadotroph destruction by the tumor mass or surgery.

Unless surgery is contraindicated, radiation is not advised as a primary therapeutic modality. Irradiation of a large pituitary adenoma may be instituted primarily, or secondarily, following incomplete surgical resection. Radiation therapy may be administered by supravoltage irradiation, proton beam or heavy particle irradiation, or implantation of radioactive yttrium or gold within the sella. The abatement of galactorrhea is highly successful, although restoration of ovulatory function often does not occur. Complications associated with radiation therapy include hypopituitarism, damage to cranial nerves and adjacent neural structures, rhinorrhea and meningitis.

Medical management of large tumors is limited to symptomatic relief by the administration of bromocriptine, although inhibition of tumor growth also may occur. Since this drug effectively induces ovulation, an alternative method of contraception other than that of birth control pills should be offered.

With regard to pregnancy, it is becoming increasingly controversial whether or not to attempt removal of a prolactin-secreting pituitary adenoma confined to the sella prior to pregnancy. In the past, several isolated case reports have appeared describing sudden visual field loss in patients with prolactin-secreting pituitary tumors during pregnancy resulting from rapid growth of the tumor or generalized enlargement of the pituitary gland.[23, 24] In these cases, either total or partial removal of the pituitary was performed, which restored normal vision to patients for the remainder of pregnancy. Therefore, in an effort to avoid potential permanent visual field compromise or compressive erosion into surrounding vital structures, surgical resection of prolactin-secreting pituitary adenomas prior to pregnancy has been recommended.

Recently a possible alternative to surgical management has emerged. Several groups have discussed small series of patients with prolactin-secreting pituitary adenomas who were allowed to become pregnant without prior surgical intervention. Since clomiphene citrate therapy has not been very successful in these patients, induction of ovulation was achieved by the administration of bromocriptine.[25] Once pregnancy was suspected, bromocriptine therapy was discontinued. The majority of patients did not experience signs of tumor extension during pregnancy. In some patients, visual field defects were encountered, which proved to be temporary and resolved completely following delivery. There was no evidence of suprasellar extension in these patients prior to becoming pregnant and no maternal deaths were reported. Use of bromocriptine during pregnancy to treat progressive visual field loss has not been extensively studied, although in the few reported cases improvement was noted.[25]

Bromocriptine does not appear to be teratogenic in human pregnancy. These recent data are both encouraging and discouraging. Whereas pregnancy may be well tolerated in some patients with prolactin-secreting pituitary adenomas confined to the sella, the potential for marked pituitary or tumor enlargement and subsequent blindness during pregnancy remains. While evidence is not available, permanent visual field loss may be related to the severity and duration of chiasmatic compression during pregnancy.

The demonstration of a totally or partially empty sella by pneumoencephalography in a hyperprolactinemic patient with an enlarged sella poses additional considerations in clinical management. While pituitary adenomas have been found in these patients, sella enlargement more likely occurs as a result of arachnoid herniation through the sellar diaphragm rather than by tumor expansion. Consequently, the interpretation of follow-up sellar polytomography becomes problematical and emphasis should be placed on the measurement of serum prolactin and examination of visual fields. Surgical management of these patients also may be influenced by the presence of cerebrospinal fluid in the sella space and a compressed pituitary gland in which the normal anatomy has been distorted. These factors present a significant risk of postoperative cerebrospinal fluid rhinorrhea or hypopituitarism following surgery. There is little available information regarding pregnancy in hyperprolactinemic patients with an empty sella. However, symptomatic enlargement of the pituitary arising from extrasellar extension of tumor may be obviated by the relatively increased sellar space. In these patients, pregnancy is probably permissible.

REFERENCES

1. Jacobs, H. S.: Prolactin and amenorrhea. N. Engl. J. Med. 295:954, 1976.
2. Chang, R. J., Keye, W. R., Jr., Young, J., Wilson, C. B. and Jaffe, R. B.: Detection, evaluation, and treatment of pituitary microadenomas in patients with galactorrhea. Am. J. Obstet. Gynecol. 128:356, 1977.
3. Davajan, V., Kletzky, O., March, C. M., Roy, S. and Mishell, D. R., Jr.: The significance of galactorrhea in patients with normal menses, oligomenorrhea, and secondary amenorrhea. Am. J. Obstet. Gynecol. 130:894, 1978.
4. Tyson, J. E., Friesen, H. G. and Anderson, M. S.: Human milk secretion after TRH induced prolactin release. In Gual, C. (ed.): Hypothalamic Hypophysiotropic Hormones. New York, Excerpta Medica Foundation, 1973.
5. Tyson, J. E., Hwang, P., Guyda, H. and Friesen, H. G.: Studies of prolactin secretion in human pregnancy. Am. J. Obstet. Gynecol. 113:14, 1972.
6. Jaffe, R. B., Yuen, B. H., Keye, W. R. Jr. and Midgely, A. R., Jr.: Physiologic and pathologic profiles of circulating human prolactin. Am. J. Obstet. Gynecol. 117:757, 1973.
7. Leblanc, H., Lachelin, G. C. L., Abu-Fadil, S. and Yen, S. S. C.: Effects of dopamine infusion on pituitary hormone secretion in humans. J. Clin. Endocrinol. Metab. 43:668, 1976.
8. L'Hermite, M. and Robyn, C.: Pathological secretion of human prolactin. In Crosignani, P. G., James, V. H. T. (eds.): Recent Progress in Reproductive Endocrinology. London, Academic Press, 1975.
9. Archer, D. F., Nankin, H. R., Gabos, P. F., Maroon, J., Nosetz, S., Wadhwa, S. R. and Josimovich, J. B.: Serum prolactin in patients in inappropriate lactation. Am. J. Obstet. Gynecol. 119:446, 1974.
10. Franks, S., Murray, M. A. F., Jequier, A. M., Steel, S. K., Nabarro, J. D. N. and Jacobs, H. S.: Incidence and significance of hyperprolactinemia in women with amenorrhea. Clin. Endocrinol. 4:597, 1975.
11. Thorner, M. D. and Besser, G. M.: Hyperprolactinemia and gonadal function: results of bromocriptine treatment. In Crosignani, P. G., Robyn, C. (eds.): Prolactin and Human Reproduction. London, Academic Press, 1977.
12. Noel, G., Suh, K. J., Stone, G. and Frantz, A. G.: Human prolactin and growth hormone release during surgery and other conditions of stress. J. Clin. Endocrinol. Metab. 35:840, 1972.
13. Archer, D. F.: Current concepts of prolactin physiology in normal and abnormal conditions. Fertil. Steril. 28:125, 1977.
14. Chang, R. J.: Normal and abnormal prolactin metabolism. In Judd, H. L. (ed.): Clinical Obstetrics and Gynecology. Vol. 21, No. 1, March 1978.
15. Keye, W. R., Jr., Yuen, B. H., Knopf, R. F. and Jaffe, R. B.: Amenorrhea, hyperprolactinemia and pituitary enlargement secondary to primary hypothyroidism. Obstet. Gynecol. 45:497, 1976.
16. Vezina, J. L. and Sutton, T. J.: Prolactin-secreting pituitary microadenomas. Am. J. Roentgenol. 120:46, 1974.
17. Hanna, C.: Cataract of toxic etiology. A. Radiation cataract. In Bellows, J. G. (ed.): Cataract and Abnormalities of the Lens, New York, Grune and Stratton, 1974.
18. Merriam, G. R., Jr. and Focht, E. F.: A clinical study of radiation cataracts and the relationship to dose. Am. J. Roentgenol. 77:759, 1957.
19. Chang, R. J., Keye, W. R., Jr., Monroe, S. E. and Jaffe, R. B.: Pituitary function in amenorrhea associated with normal or abnormal serum prolactin concentration and sellar polytomography. J. Clin. Endocrinol. Metab. 4:830, 1980.
20. Burry, K. A., Schiller, H. S., Mills, R., Harris, B. and Heinrichs, L.: Actual visual loss during pregnancy after bromocriptine-induced ovulation. Obstet. Gynecol. 52:195, 1978.
21. Thorner, M. O., Besser, G. M., Jones, A., Dacie, J. and Jones, A. E.: Bromocriptine treatment of female infertility: report of 13 pregnancies. Br. Med. J. 4:694, 1975.
22. McGregor, A. M., Scanlon, M. F., Hall, K., Cook, D. B. and Hall, R.: Reduction in size of a pituitary tumor by bromocriptine therapy. N. Engl. J. Med. 300:291, 1979.
23. Swyer, G. I. M., Little, V. and Harries, B. J.: Visual disturbance of pregnancy after induction of ovulation. Br. Med. J. 4:90, 1971.
24. Kajtar, T. and Tomkin, G. H.: Emergency hypophysectomy in pregnancy after induction of ovulation. Br. Med. J. 4:88, 1971.
25. Bergh, T., Nillius, S. J. and Wide, L.: Clinical course and outcome of pregnancies in amenorrheic women with hyperprolactinemia and pituitary tumors. Br. Med. J. 1:875, 1978.

Management of Galactorrhea Syndromes

David W. Keller, M.D.
James C. Warren, M.D., Ph.D.
Washington University School of Medicine

The association of galactorrhea with amenorrhea has been recognized for many years.[1, 2] Inappropriate lactation has been reported to occur in 1 per cent of women with normal menstrual cycles compared with a 3 per cent incidence in anovulatory or amenorrheic women.[3] In patients with amenorrhea for 12 or more months, the rate of associated galactorrhea is 21 per cent.[4-6]

Galactorrhea has been associated with the

use of tranquilizers, antihypertensive agents and sex steroids, and with pituitary tumors, primary hypothyroidism and the empty sella syndrome.[7, 8] Inappropriate lactation has also been reported following surgical procedures including hysterectomy, thoracotomy and breast biopsy.[9] Hyperprolactinemia and even prolactin-secreting adenomas, however, have been found in amenorrheic women without galactorrhea.[10-12] Therefore, we operationally evaluate all patients with hyperprolactinemia.

Patient Identification

The obstetrician-gynecologist should evaluate serum prolactin levels in all patients who have galactorrhea. Even in the absence of galactorrhea, serum prolactin levels should be evaluated in all patients who present with a corpus luteum inadequacy, hypoestrogenic hypogonadatropic amenorrhea (whether primary or secondary) or ovulation failure. The only exception to this requirement would occur when patients with ovulation failure clinically have polycystic ovary syndrome of the Stein-Leventhal type: a distinct elevation of free serum testosterone and ratios of luteinizing hormone and follicle-stimulating hormone in serum that (when both expressed in mIU/ml) are in excess of 3. Thus, some patients will be identified as having the hyperprolactinemia syndrome by the presence of lactation and others will be identified by elevation of serum prolactin. If the patient with obvious galactorrhea has a normal serum prolactin, we routinely repeat that test. Ordinarily, we draw the first serum level without the use of the intravenous catheter (described later), but if the level is slightly elevated we are inclined to consider the possibility that stress may have induced the elevation and we do repeat with the indwelling catheter. We see an occasional patient who complains of slight, but significant discharge from the breast whose prolactin and menstrual periods are normal. We consider that this is probably a physiologic breast discharge, although we do routinely get yearly serum prolactin levels on such patients for three years. Should we find that the patient has an elevation of serum prolactin, with or without galactorrhea, we turn our attention to diagnosis.

Diagnosis

As we will see later, hyperprolactinemia is an ominous sign. The most serious cause, of course, is the prolactin-secreting pituitary adenoma. Unfortunately, many patients with elevated serum prolactin levels will be followed for several years before such a tumor becomes evident. Many patients originally assigned to the "idiopathic group" ultimately have diagnosis of adenoma. It is obvious that the obstetrician-gynecologist will do his patient a great service by a rigorous evaluation of her history and thyroid function and a search for the empty sella syndrome. Nothing is more satisfying to the physician than to define primary hypothyroidism as a cause of prolactin elevation and correct it with the administration of thyroid hormone, removing this patient from a high-risk group that otherwise must be followed with continuing uncertainty.

Detailed clinical history and careful physical examination will rule out the majority of etiologies for hyperprolactinemia, leaving basically two categories: that of idiopathic inappropriate lactation and that associated with pituitary tumor. Pituitary tumors 1 cm or less in diameter are referred to as microadenomas, while tumors greater than 1 cm in diameter, because they often cause sellar enlargement, are referred to as macroadenomas.[13] The single most valuable screening test in the diagnosis of pituitary tumor is the measurement of basal level of prolactin. Prolactin levels above 200 ng/ml are associated with prolactin-secreting adenomas in more than 80 per cent of cases.[14] Patients with an abnormal basal prolactin level should consequently be evaluated to rule out the presence of pituitary tumor. Basal prolactin levels, however, may be affected by stress.[15] Samples should ideally be drawn through an indwelling intravenous needle placed in a relaxed supine patient for an hour.[16] An alternative method of initial screening consists of determinations on several pooled serum prolactin specimens obtained from the ambulatory patient. Routine skull films and biplanar tomograms are useful in the early diagnosis of these tumors.[17] A common finding with tomography is tilting of the sellar floor with erosion of the anterior wall.[18] Frequent x-ray findings of "compatible with a microadenoma" changes of the sella turcica may represent a normal variant or extremely subtle changes secondary to the presence of a microadenoma. The presence of bony erosion or asymmetry of the sella exceeding 2 mm is most probably abnormal.[19]

Numerous provocative and suppressive procedures have been utilized to attempt to differentiate between idiopathic galactorrhea and pituitary tumor. Unfortunately, none reliably differentiates patients with tumor from those with idiopathic galactorrhea.[16, 20] Women with galactorrhea or hyperprolactinemia or both should also be screened for primary hypothyroidism with a thyroid-stimulating hormone determination even if they have an abnormal tomogram. When hypothyroidism is the cause, signs and symptoms may be reversed by thyroid replacement.[21] Finally, before the adenoma is removed surgically, computerized axial tomography or a pneumoencephalogram should be obtained to determine the presence of the "empty sella syndrome"[22] or suprasellar extension of the tumor.

Treatment

The treatment may be directed toward several aspects, depending upon the patient's needs. These aspects include elimination of lactation, resumption of ovulation in the anovulatory or amenorrheic patient, or prevention of progressive enlargement of an existing pituitary tumor. The modalities of treatment are pharmacologic, radiologic and surgical.

DRUG THERAPY. If no evidence for the existence of a pituitary tumor exists, pharmacologic therapeutic modalities are preferable. Pharmacologic therapy has included primary L-dopa and 2α-bromergocryptine. L-dopa therapy has generally been unsatisfactory.[23, 24] Bromergocryptine, a dopamine receptor agonist, is effective in decreasing serum prolactin, restoring menses, and inhibiting galactorrhea. It has been shown to be effective in women with prolactin-secreting adenomas.[25-27] The effect of bromergocryptine on the growth of pituitary tumors in vivo is debatable, but there is considerable evidence that it may reduce their size.[14, 28, 29] While bromergocryptine is quite successful in inducing ovulation in hyperprolactinemic women with pituitary tumors, there is evidence that pregnancy must be allowed with some caution and only after extensive discussion of possible complications and alternatives. Reports of rapid enlargement of microadenoma during pregnancy resulting in temporary or permanent loss of vision and necessitating emergency neurosurgical procedures are present in the literature.[30-32] We do not use bromergocryptine to attempt pregnancy with patients who have macroadenomas, believing the risk to be too high. Prevention of this complication has been achieved with pretreatment of the tumor with irradiation. However, there are two reports of visual loss occurring during

pregnancy following bromergocryptine treatment despite pre-pregnancy radiation.[31, 33] While the FDA proscribes use of bromergocryptine in patients with microademonas, successful pregnancy outcome has been achieved in over 90 per cent of patients treated with the drug. Nevertheless, the occurrence of pregnancy in a woman with a known or suspected pituitary tumor necessitates close observation of the patient during the pregnancy. Surgical removal of the tumor or radiation therapy should be considered when measurable visual field defects develop during pregnancy. Both forms of treatment have been successful in restoring vision with no adverse effect upon the outcome of the pregnancy.[34]

RADIATION THERAPY. Radiation therapy, cobalt beam, proton beam, and implantation of radioactive yttrium or gold within the sella have been employed in the treatment of pituitary tumors. Therapy may be followed by various degrees of hypopituitarism, visual field defects, occulomotor palsies, rhinorrhea and meningitis. These forms of therapy may arrest the growth of the tumor and may be followed by cessation of lactation, but return of normal menstrual function is unusual.[35] Radiation therapy is usually reserved for tumors that are not completely resectable and are associated with marked hyperprolactinemia following surgery.[36] The failure rate for radiation therapy appears to be approximately 20 per cent.[37]

SURGICAL THERAPY. Cure rates as high as 90 per cent have previously been reported in patients with adenomas of less than 10 mm in diameter and prolactin values of less than 200 ng/ml treated with transsphenoidal surgery. Patients with larger tumors and higher elevation of plasma prolactin have much lower cure rates.[38] This approach is suitable for the removal of intrasellar adenomas and tumors with minimal suprasellar extension. Complications include transient diabetes insipidus, hemorrhage, meningitis, rhinorrhea and panhypopituitarism.[36]

Conclusion

Patients with hyperprolactinemia syndromes may have lactation, ovulation failure, hypogonadatropic hypoestrogenic amenorrhea or corpus luteum inadequacy. Any of these findings necessitates quantitation of serum prolactin. During the first or second visit every effort should be made to elicit signs of pituitary tumor, history of drug intake (particularly tranquilizers, antihypertensive agents and sex steroids), and symptoms suggestive of primary hypothyroidism. If the first prolactin determination is elevated, a TSH determination and repeat of the serum prolactin are next carried out. While primary hypothyroidism is a cause of hyperprolactinemia only 2 to 3 per cent of the time, the patient is greatly benefited by this diagnosis. Should history and thyroid elevation be negative with prolactin levels remaining persistently elevated, skull x-rays (and if negative, tomograms of the sella) are ordered. If x-rays show abnormalities, CAT scan or pneumoencephalogram or both are indicated. Ultimately, this series of careful interrogations and laboratory testing will (once drugs and primary hypothyroidism are ruled out) place the patient in one of six categories. They are as follows:

1. Lactation, normal prolactin

2. Elevated prolactin with normal tomogram

3. Elevated prolactin with suspicious tomogram

4. Elevated prolactin with microadenoma

5. Elevated prolactin with macroadenoma

6. Elevated prolactin with empty sella

Management of a patient in any of these categories can be carried out only after discussion of her goals and explanation of risks and alternatives. The patient in category 1 can be followed with yearly prolactin determinations and instructed to avoid breast stimulation during sexual relations. If the problem persists, a trial of bromergocryptine is not unreasonable. In these instances, we often employ half a tablet twice daily for 30 days, increasing the dose to the full tablet twice daily only when improvement is not originally seen.

In patients who have elevated prolactin levels with normal or suspicious tomograms but no definite diagnosis of pituitary adenoma, management will depend upon desire for pregnancy, estrogen status and the duration of any hypoestrogenic state. In the United States, bromergocryptine is presently recommended by FDA for induction of ovulation in the absence of demonstrable pituitary tumor. We explain to the patient that the outcomes of some 1276 pregnancies have been reported, with no increase in congenital malformation or spontaneous abortion rate. If after this discussion she still desires pregnancy, we treat her with bromergocryptine (starting with one half tablet twice daily and going up to full tablet twice daily if normalization of prolactin

and resumption of normal menses do not occur on the lower dose). If the patient does not desire pregnancy, employment of bromergocryptine may be indicated if lactation is symptomatic or if she is severely hypoestrogenic.

Finally, there is evidence, particularly from Zarate and co-workers in Mexico,[12] that employment of bromergocryptine may slow the development of microadenomas. If the patient is not desirous of pregnancy and is not concerned about lactation or her estrogenic status, we have utilized careful follow-up with serum prolactin measurements at six-month intervals and repeat tomography at approximately two- to three-year intervals, or sooner if the prolactin level rises sharply. It should be pointed out that repeat tomograms may ultimately lead to cataract formation, and before doing them the practitioner should check with a radiologist to see how many will be safe for a given patient. Finally, in the young individual with amenorrhea and estrogen deficiency who already shows evidence of osteoporosis, we are inclined to originally give six months of treatment with bromergocryptine, realizing that the day may come when we must decide to give her estrogen. There is a strong sentiment and some evidence that estrogen administration may promote the growth of microadenomas, but we have used this therapy on occasion in carefully selected patients.

The optimal management of the patient in category 4 (elevated prolactin with microadenoma) is not completely clear at the moment. Until the natural history of pituitary microadenoma is known, and long-term follow-up of patients undergoing surgery as compared with those undergoing pharmacologic treatment is available, a conservative approach may well be indicated. Prolonged bromergocryptine therapy may possibly inhibit further growth of pituitary microadenoma with potential reversal of radiologic abnormalities. Thus, in the patient who does not desire pregnancy, we suggest that she utilize barrier contraception and take the bromergocryptine. If the patient does desire pregnancy, we discuss with her and her husband whether she would prefer to undergo a transsphenoidal surgical procedure or take the bromergocryptine and attempt pregnancy. It seems that some patients prefer to deal with their problems definitively and they immediately elect the surgery. Others select the medical therapy. Those who elect surgery are referred to the neurosurgeon, while those who elect medical therapy receive bromergocryptine. We advise the patient selecting medical therapy that there is a 5 per cent chance that she will have trouble during her pregnancy from tumor expansion, which may force surgical intervention.

For patients in category 5 who have a clear macroadenoma with or without suprasellar extension, it seems that operative or radiation therapy is indicated, and these patients are sent for neurosurgical consult. Finally, the patient with empty sella syndrome is usually in no danger (unless there is also a lurking adenoma). Thus, we treat her with bromergocryptine if pregnancy is her desire and she is anovulatory, or with estrogen and progesterone combinations if pregnancy is of no concern to her.

It is hard to define a management protocol for this syndrome because all the answers are not in. There is still considerable debate as to the basic etiology of these syndromes and the mechanism by which they are initiated. It is clear from basic physiological studies that the role of the hypothalamus is to inhibit the secretion of prolactin. Over 10 per cent of a general population coming to routine autopsy have pituitary adenomas and the majority of these are prolactin secreters. It is unknown whether birth control pills and other estrogens accelerate the growth of pituitary microadenomas. Nevertheless, it is not unreasonable to postulate a general physiologic mechanism whereby prolactin-inhibiting factor, if diminished by any one of a number of causes (probably including birth control pills and estrogens), leads first to a hyperplasia of lactotropes in the pituitary and utimately to the formation of the benign adenoma. Once that adenoma occurs, the correct choice of treatment is extremely difficult. It is possible that patients who come to surgery will (if the basic elevation of prolactin-inhibitory factor is not corrected) be coming back for second operations. It is attractive to give such patients bromergocryptine, but it is unknown what the ultimate complications of long-term therapy with bromergocryptine will be. Fortunately, several studies are now underway to answer these questions.

REFERENCES

1. Jones, J. R. and Gentile, G. P.: Incidence of galactorrhea in ovulatory and anovulatory females. Obstet. Gynecol. 45:13, 1975.
2. Shearman, R. P. and Turtle, J. R.: Secondary amenorrhea with inappropriate lactation. Am. J. Obstet. Gynecol. 106:818, 1970.
3. Shearman, R. P.: Prolonged secondary amenorrhea after oral contraceptive therapy. Lancet 2:64, 1971.
4. Shearman, R. P. and Smith, I. D.: Statistical analysis of relationship between oral contraceptives, secondary amenorrhea, and galactorrhea. J. Obstet. Gynaecol. Br. Commonwealth 79:654, 1972.
5. Kleinberg, D. L., Noel, G. L. and Frantz, A. G.: Galactorrhea: a study of 235 cases, including 48 with pituitary tumors. N. Engl. J. Med. 296:589, 1977.
6. Edwards, C. R. W., Forsyth, I. A. and Besser, G. M.: Amenorrhea, galactorrhea and primary hypothyroidism with high circulating levels of prolactin. Br. Med. J. 3:462, 1971.
7. Frantz, A. G.: Prolactin secretion and physiologic and pathologic human conditions measured by bioassay and radioimmunoassay. In Josimovich, J. B., Reynolds, M. and Cobo, E. (eds.): Lactogenic Hormones, Fetal Nutrition, and Lactation. New York, John Wiley & Sons, 1974, p. 379.
8. Argonz, J. and del Castillo, E. B.: A syndrome characterized by estrogenic insufficiency, galactorrhea and decreased urinary gonadotropin. J. Clin. Endocrinol. Metab. 13:79, 1953.
9. Forbes, A. P., Henneman, P. H., Griswold, G. L. and Albright, F.: Syndrome characterized by galactorrhea, amenorrhea and low urinary FSH: comparison with acromegaly and normal lactation. J. Clin. Endocrinol. Metab. 14:265, 1954.
10. Lewis, P. D. and Van Noorden, S.: "Nonfunctioning" pituitary tumors: a light and electron microscopical study. Arch. Pathol. 97:178, 1974.
11. Nader, S., Mashiter, K., Doyle, F. H. and Joplin, G. F.: Galactorrhea, hyperprolactinemia and pituitary tumors in the female. Clin. Endocrinol. (Oxf) 5:245, 1976.
12. Zarate, A., Canales, E. S., Villalobos, H. et al.: Pituitary hormonal reserve in patients presenting hyperprolactinemia, intrasellar masses, and amenorrhea with galactorrhea. J. Clin. Endocrinol. Metab. 40:1034, 1975.
13. Keye, W. R., Chang, R. J. and Jaffe, R. B.: Prolactin secreting pituitary adenomas in women with amenorrhea or galactorrhea. Obstet. Gynecol. Surv. 32:727, 1977.
14. Friesen, H. G. and Tolis, G.: The use of bromocriptine in the galactorrhoea-amenorrhoea syndromes: the Canadian Cooperative Study. Clin. Endocrinol. (Oxf) 6:Suppl:915, 1977.
15. Frantz, A. G., Habif, D. V., Hyman, G. A. et al.: Physiological and pharmacological factors affecting prolactin secretion including its suppression by L-dopa in the treatment of breast cancer. In Pasteels, J. L., and Robyn, C. (eds.): Human Prolactin. Amsterdam, Excerpta Medica Foundation, 1973, p. 273.
16. Adler, R. A., Noel, G. L., Wartofsky, L. and Frantz, A. G.: Failure of oral water loading and intravenous hypotonic saline to suppress plasma prolactin in man. J. Clin. Endocrinol. Metab. 41:383, 1975.
17. Vezina, J. L. and Sutton, T. J.: Prolactin-secreting microadenomas, roentgenologic diagnosis. Am. J. Roentgenol. 120:46, 1974.
18. Guiot, G. and Thibaut, B.: L'extirpation des adenomes hypophysaires par voie trans-sphenoidale. Neurochirugia (Stuttg) 1:133, 1959.
19. Davajan, V., Kletzky, O., March, C. M. et al.: The significance of galactorrhea in patients with normal menses, oligomenorrhea, and secondary amenorrhea. Am. J. Obstet. Gynecol. 130:894, 1978.

20. Tolis, G., Somma, N., Van Campenhout, J. and Friesen, H.: Prolactin secretion in sixty-five patients with galactorrhea. Am. J. Obstet. Gynecol. 118:91, 1974.

21. Keye, W. R., Jr., Yuen, B. H., Knopf, R. F. and Jaffe, R. B.: Amenorrhea, hyperprolactinemia and pituitary enlargement secondary to primary hypothyroidism, successful treatment with thyroid replacement. Obstet. Gynecol. 48:697, 1976.

22. Kaufman, B., Pearson, D. H. and Chamberlin, W. B.: Radiologic features of intrasellar masses and progressive asymmetric nontumorous enlargement of the sella turcica, the "empty" sella. *In* Kohler, P. O. and Ross, G. T. (eds.): Diagnosis and Treatment of Pituitary Tumors. Amsterdam, Excerpta Medica (International Congress Series No. 303), 1973, p. 100.

23. Turkington, R. W.: Inhibition of prolactin secretion and successful therapy of the Forbes-Albright syndrome with L-dopa. J. Clin. Endocrinol. Metab. 34:306, 1972.

24. Malarkey, W. B., Jacobs, L. S. and Daughaday, W. H.: Levadopa suppression of prolactin in nonpuerperal galactorrhea. N. Engl. J. Med. 285:1160, 1971.

25. Copinschi, G., L'Hermite, M., Pasteels, J. L. and Robyn, C.: 2-Br-α Ergocryptine (CB-154) inhibition of prolactin secretion and galactorrhea in a case of pituitary tumor. *In* Hubinot, P. O., Hendeles, S. M., and Premont, P., (eds.): (Hormones and Antagonists. Basel, Karger, 1972, p. 128.

26. Dickey, R. P. and Stones, S. C.: Effect of bromergocryptine on serum hPRrl, hLH, hFSH, and estradiol 17-β in women with galactorrhea-amenorrhea. Obstet. Gynecol. 48:84, 1976.

27. Jacobs, H. S.: Prolactin and amenorrhea. N. Engl. J. Med. 295:954, 1976.

28. L'Hermite, M., Caufriez, A. and Robyn, C.: Amenorrhea, hyperprolactinemia, and infertility in relation to prolactin producing pituitary adenomas. Fertil. Steril. 28:346, 1977.

29. Corenblum, B., Webster, R., Mortimer, C. B. and Ezrin, C.: Possible antitumor effect of 2 bromergo-criptine (CB-154, Sandoz) in two patients with large prolactin secreting adenomas. Clin. Res. 23:614A, 1975.

30. Child, D. F., Gordon, H. and Joplin, G. F.: Pregnancy, prolactin and pituitary tumors. Br. Med. J. 4:87, 1975.

31. Lamberts, S. W. J., Seldenrath, H. J., Kwa, H. G. and Birkenhager, J. C.: Transient bitemporal hemianopsia during pregnancy after treatment of galactorrhea-amenorrhea syndrome with bromergocriptine. J. Clin. Endocrinol. Metab. 44:180, 1977.

32. Jewelewicz, R., Zimmerman, E. A., and Carmel, P. W.: Conservative management of a pituitary tumor during pregnancy following induction of ovulation with gonadotropins. Fertil. Steril. 28:35, 1977.

33. Thorner, N. O., Besser, G. M., Jones, A. et al.: Bromocriptine treatment of female infertility: report of 13 pregnancies. Br. Med. J. 4:694, 1975.

34. Falconer, M. A. and Stafford-Bell, M. A.: Visual failure from pituitary and parasellar tumors occurring with favorable outcome in pregnant women. J. Neurol. Neurosurg. Psychiatr. 38:919, 1975.

35. Kramer, S.: Indications for and results of treatment of pituitary tumors by external radiation. *In* Kohler, P. O. and Ross, G. T., (eds.): Diagnosis and Treatment of Pituitary Tumors. Amsterdam, Excerpta Medica (International Congress Series No. 303), 1973, p. 217.

36. Chang, R. J., Keye, W. R., Jr., Young, J. R. et al.: Detection, evaluation and treatment of pituitary microadenomas in patients with galactorrhea and amenorrhea. Am. J. Obstet. Gynecol. 128:356, 1977.

37. Ontjes, D. A. and Ney, R. L.: Pituitary tumors. Cancer 26:330, 1976.

38. Hardy, J., Beauregard, H. and Robert, F.: Prolactin-secreting pituitary microadenomas: transsphenoidal microsurgical treatment. *In* Robyn, C. and Harter, M. (eds.): Progress in Prolactin Physiology and Pathology. North Holland, Elsevier, 1978, p. 361.

Editorial Comment

It should be recalled that not all breast discharges are galactorrhea and that the gynecologist will do more breast examinations and evaluate more breast discharges than any other medical practitioner. The surgeons, after all, do not believe in routine or in screening examinations and do breast examinations only on patients who are self-referred or physician-referred. The breast examination is, of course, an integral part of the routine gynecologic survey and breast discharges should be evaluated thoroughly. There are four types of breast discharges: (1) the clear or greenish-clear myoepithelial discharge that is a common, normal finding and therefore not of significance; (2) the serosanguineous discharge (usually clear amber in character) that must be evaluated for an intraductal papilloma; (3) the frankly bloody discharge that must be evaluated for malignancy; and (4) the milky discharge of true galactorrhea. Evaluation of the serum prolactin levels should not be restricted to patients with galactorrhea and should be done in evaluating any unphysiologic amenorrhea or menstrual aberration.

Differences of opinion regarding management of the patient with a microadenoma exist because the natural history of such adenomas is not yet known in a large population. While such information is being gathered the management will be evolving. It is now becoming more clear that small nonexpanding adenomas need not be routinely surgically removed. This is in contrast to our information of five years ago. Patients with small adenomas (microadenoma, less than 1 cm) usually do quite well with medical treatment. Once detected, of course, these adenomas do need to be followed as described by the authors of this chapter.

It does appear that all microadenomas do not continue to enlarge, that some regress spontaneously and that some may regress with bromergocryptine. It has only been within the last half dozen years that longitudinal studies utilizing accurate prolactin levels, polytomography and CT scans have been possible so that all impressions at this time are tentative and continued surveillance of all such patients is mandatory. However, it does appear that over a period of 10 years as few as 5 per cent of microadenomas may progress to the point of requiring surgery. The incidence of microadenomas is emerging to be greater than anyone suspected. It appears that some 10 per cent of patients with secondary amenorrhea may have such a lesion and some 25 per cent of patients with secondary amenorrhea and galactorrhea likewise may have such a lesion.

The proscription of pregnancy in the patient with microadenoma seems to be unnecessary. There have now been over 1000 pregnancies following bromergocryptine treatment, with good results. Only 5 per cent of such patients have symptoms referable to the microadenoma and a percentage less than that require surgery during the pregnancy. Certainly, surgical removal of the otherwise quiescent microadenoma is not indicated prior to pregnancy.

16
Prophylactic Antibiotics in Obstetrics and Gynecology

Alternative Points of View

by Susan R. Johnson, Marilyn Ohm-Smith,
and Rudolph P. Galask
by Richard H. Schwarz and William R.
Crombleholme

Editorial Comment

Prophylactic Antibiotics in Obstetrics and Gynecology

Susan R. Johnson, M. D.
Marilyn Ohm-Smith, M.S., M.T. (ASCP)
Rudolph P. Galask, M.D.
University of Iowa College of Medicine

Infection remains a major complication of any surgical procedure performed through a contaminated field, and efforts to reduce this type of morbidity continue to be a valid preoccupation of many physicians. Since antibiotics first became available in clinical practice, they have been used for prevention as well as treatment of infections. Early in the antibiotic era, studies of the use of prophylactic antibiotics were reported in several areas of medicine, including obstetrics and gynecology. These studies, in which penicillin and sulfonamides were used, were often poorly designed and yielded conflicting results. The emergence of antibiotic-resistant organisms necessitated limiting the indiscriminate use of antibiotics, and by the early 1950s antibiotic prophylaxis was restricted to only a few special situations.

The successful use of prophylactic antibiotics in effecting a reduction in infection following gastrointestinal surgery sparked renewed interest among gynecologists, especially in view of the increase in the number of vaginal hysterectomies with their high rate of postoperative infection. While the studies carried out during this period were primarily restricted to those precedures that had a high risk of postoperative infection, the protocols and the kinds of antibiotics used varied substantially, and comparisons and conclusions were difficult. In addition, most studies did not provide adequate information by which the overall (and potentially adverse) effects of prophylaxis could be judged.

Finally in 1975 Ledger et al.[1] proposed guidelines for the use of antibiotic prophylaxis in gynecologic surgery. They apply as well to obstetrics and remain pertinent today. First, the operation should carry significant risk of postoperative infection. Generally, this includes procedures at which intraoperative contamination of the operative field occurs. It also implies that the type of patient (malnourished, aged, immunosuppressed or seriously ill) and the skill of the physician be considered.[2] Second, the antibiotics used should show both in vitro and clinical evidence of effectiveness against possible contaminating microorganisms. Antibiotics needed against highly resistant organisms should not be used. Third, the antibiotic should be present in therapeutic concentration at the wound site during the operative procedure and should be used only for a short time thereafter. Finally, the benefits of antibiotic prophylaxis must be weighed against the adverse effects and only if the benefits clearly outweigh the dangers should prophylaxis be used.

Using these guidelines and the information provided by the many studies that have been done, we will in this chapter discuss the current role of prophylactic antibiotics in gynecology and obstetrics and indicate areas in which further research may be necessary.

Gynecology

VAGINAL HYSTERECTOMY

Vaginal hysterectomy carries a postoperative infection rate higher than any gynecologic procedure, with the possible exception of radical surgery for pelvic malignancies. At many hospitals over 50 per cent of women undergoing vaginal hysterectomy develop infections postoperatively; a rate of less than 30 per cent without the use of prophylactic antibiotics is rare. Therefore, the use of antibiotic prophylaxis in this procedure has been studied extensively. The results of selected prospective studies are summarized in Table 1.[3-21] Because the overall rate of febrile morbidity includes complications unaffected by antibiotic administration, only those studies that report postoperative infections separately have been included. The studies vary widely in composition of the study population, prophylactic antibiotic used, administration protocol and definition of morbidity. We have included and indicated studies that were not double-blind even though there exists a greater possibility of biased results.

Many studies have included an undefined mixture of premenopausal and postmenopausal women undergoing vaginal hysterectomy with or without attendant procedures such as colporrhaphy. Some investigators have tried to define subgroups that have either a higher or lower risk of morbidity. Postmenopausal women, for example, have been excluded from some studies because it is thought that they have a lesser risk of infection.[4, 7, 22] However, most recent studies in which the postmenopausal and premenopausal populations were considered separately suggest that the rates of postoperative morbidity are similar.[23, 24] The decision to use prophylactic antibiotics in postmenopausal women undergoing vaginal hysterectomy should be made by each gynecologic service.

Two studies have included women undergoing vaginal hysterectomy only, without attendant procedures.[6, 13] In both studies the group of patients that received prophylaxis had lower morbidity. It is of interest that the control groups, however, had lower rates of infection than control groups in most other studies in which patients underwent more involved procedures. This suggests that women undergoing vaginal hysterectomy alone are at less risk of postoperative infection than those undergoing vaginal hysterectomy with attendant colporrhaphy.

Two investigative teams have reported on the use of prophylactic antibiotics for women undergoing sequential conization and vaginal hysterectomy.[3, 9] In both studies the populations were small; however, the groups that received prophylactic antibiotics had a considerably lower rate of infection than the groups receiving placebo.

Many antibiotics have been used for prophylaxis. As outlined previously, an ideal agent should be effective against the contaminating organisms, should achieve high tissue levels, should have low toxicity and should not be needed for infections caused by resistant organisms.

Cephalosporins have been approved by the Food and Drug Administration for prophylactic use and have been the most common class of antibiotics used in gynecologic trials.[3-5, 7-9, 12, 14, 15, 18, 20, 21, 25] They are broad spectrum and bactericidal, and have an established record of safe clinical use. All routes of administration are available, increasing clinical usefulness. Equilibration between blood and tissue occurs rapidly, and sufficient tissue levels in the highly vascular pelvic region occur.[14] The most serious deficiency is the lack of activity against *Streptococcus faecalis* and *Bacteroides*

TABLE 1. STUDIES OF THE USE OF PROPHYLACTIC ANTIBIOTICS IN VAGINAL HYSTERECTOMY*

INVESTIGATORS	TYPE OF STUDY	PROPHYLACTIC ANTIBIOTICS	ADMINISTRATION SCHEDULE	NO. PATIENTS	TOTAL INFECTIOUS MORBIDITY	PELVIC INFECTIONS	AVE. NO. HOSPITAL DAYS
Allen et al.[3]	Prospective Double-blind	Cephalosporins	Preop. thru 5 POD	50 (C) 48 (A)	50% (C) 4% (A)	38% (C) 4% (A)	(A) 4 days less than (C)
Ledger et al.[4]	Prospective Double-blind	Cephalosporins	Preop. plus 2 doses	50 (C) 50 (A)	60% (C) 36% (A)	34% (C) 8% (A)	9.9 (C) 8.6 (A)
Ohm & Galask[5]	Prospective Double-blind	Cephalosporins	Preop. thru 4 POD	23 (C) 25 (A)	48% (C) 0% (A)	22% (C) 0% (A)	9.0 (C) 7.9 (A)
Harralson et al.[6]	Prospective Not double-blind	Penicillin/ streptomycin	Preop. thru 2 POD	100 (C) 100 (A)	25% (C) 3% (A)	19% (C) 1% (A)	6.3 (C) 5.0 (A)
Breeden & Mayo[7]	Prospective Double-blind	Cephalosporins	Preop. plus 2 doses	56 (C) 64 (A)	27% (C) 6% (A)	20% (C) 5% (A)	7.7 (C) 7.3 (A)
Bivens et al.[8]	Prospective Double-blind	Cephalosporins	Preop. thru 6 POD	30 (C) 30 (A)	43% (C) 13% (A)	20% (C) 13% (A)	8.1 (C) 7.5 (A)
Forney et al.[9]	Prospective Double-blind	Cephalosporins	Preop. thru 5 POD	14 (C) 18 (A)	43% (C) 0% (A)	29% (C) 0% (A)	6.7 (C) 4.7 (A)
Mayer et al.[10]	Prospective Not double-blind	Cephalothin/ kanamycin	Preop. thru 2 POD	21 (C) 23 (A)	43% (C) 4% (A)	24% (C) 4% (A)	Not given
Sengupta et al.[11]	Prospective Not double-blind	Penicillin/ streptomycin or kanamycin	Preop. thru 4 POD	20 (C) 10 (P/S) 10 (Kan.)	75% (C) 10% (A)	Not given	Not given
Lett et al.[12]	Prospective Double-blind	Cephaloridine or cefazolin	Preop. only (cefaz.) or preop. plus 2 doses (cephal.)	51 (C) 50 (Cephal.) 52 (Cefaz.)	49% (C) 12% (Cephal.) 8% (Cefaz.)	37% (C) 12% (Cephal.) 8% (Cefaz.)	7.2 (C) 5.3 (Cephal.) 4.9 (Cefaz.)

Roberts & Homesley[13]	Prospective Double-blind	Carbenicillin	Preop. thru 1 POD	26 (C) 26 (A)	35% (C) 8% (A)	12% (C) 0% (A)	7.8 (C) 6.2 (A)
Mendelson et al.[14]	Prospective Double-blind	Cephradine	Preop. only or preop. plus 4 doses	22 (C) 23 (A-single) 21 (A-multi)	82% (C) 9% (A-single) 0% (A-multi)	64% (C) 1% (A-single) 0% (A-multi)	10.7 (C) 7.5 (A-single) 6.7 (A-multi)
Grossman et al.[15]	Prospective Double-blind	Penicillin or cefazolin	Preop. thru 2 POD	24 (C) 26 (Pen.) 28 (Cef.)	67% (C) 39% (Pen.) 39% (Cef.)	25% (C) 8% (Pen.) 4% (Cef.)	7.6 (C) 6.8 (Pen.) 6.6 (Cef.)
Hemsell et al.[16]	Prospective Double-blind	Cefoxitin	Preop. plus 2 doses	49 (C) 50 (A)	61% (C) 16% (A)	57% (C) 8% (A)	7.6 (C) 4.8 (A)
Mickal et al.[17]	Prospective Double-blind	Cefoxitin	Preop. plus 2 doses	57 (C) 68 (A)	Not given	32% (C) 10% (A)	5.9 (C) 5.2 (A)
Peterson et al.[18]	Prospective Not double-blind Not random	Cephalothin	Preop. thru 3 POD	597 (C) 333 (A)	32% (C) 10% (A)	<2% in both groups	9.5/8.8 (C) 8.4 (A)
Wheeless et al.[19]	Prospective Double-blind	Doxycycline	Preop. thru 2 POD	31 (C) 59 (A)	35% (C) 7% (A)	Not given	Not given
Jennings[20]	Prospective Double-blind	Cefazolin/cephalexin	Preop. thru 2 POD	43 (C) 48 (A)	65% (C) 10% (A)	33% (C) 2% (A)	10.6 (C) 9.5 (A)
Holman et al.[21]	Prospective Double-blind	Cefazolin	Preop. plus 2 doses	44 (C) 40 (A)	36% (C) 10% (A)	23% (C) 0% (A)	6.5 (C) 5.6 (A)

*Study population includes patients with either vaginal hysterectomy alone or with colporrhaphy in addition to hysterectomy.
(C) Those who received placebo or no prophylactic antibiotic.
(A) Those who received prophylactic antibiotic.
POD, Postoperative day.

fragilis, both having been associated with postoperative infection.

Cefoxitin, a cephamycin derivative, has a broad spectrum similar to the cephalosporins but in addition has activity against *Bacteroides fragilis*. It has been used effectively in recent trials.[16, 17] Because this agent has potential usefulness in the treatment of serious pelvic infections,[26] its use as a prophylactic agent should perhaps be limited.

A few investigators have used two drugs to achieve broader coverage. Most commonly, a cephalosporin or penicillin has been used in combination with an aminoglycoside.[6, 10, 11] While these regimens have also achieved a significant reduction in morbidity, the potential toxicity of aminoglycosides makes their use unwarranted in most situations.

Bacteriostatic antibiotics have been used infrequently in studies of prophylactic antibiotics in vaginal hysterectomy.[19, 22, 27] Chloramphenicol prophylaxis was relatively ineffective in lowering postoperative morbidity,[22] whereas tetracycline appeared to be as effective as bactericidal antibiotics, including ampicillin used in one study.[19, 27] Recommendations regarding the use of bacteriostatic antibiotics cannot be made, however, since sufficient data with respect to their effectiveness are lacking.

Antibiotics needed to treat infections caused by organisms susceptible to a very limited number of drugs should *not* be used for prophylaxis because the danger is too great of emergence of resistant strains that are even more difficult to treat.

A major difference among reported studies is the length of time prophylactic antibiotics were administered. In the earliest of the modern studies and in the majority of studies that followed, the antibiotic was begun preoperatively and continued for several days postoperatively.[3, 5, 6, 8-11, 15, 18-20] All of these regimens resulted in a significant reduction in postoperative morbidity in the antibiotic group as compared with the placebo control group. The average postoperative hospitalization time was usually reduced by one to two days in the treated groups. In studies in which colonization or superinfection by resistant organisms was evaluated, no problems occurred. However, because the long-term use of prophylactic antibiotics has resulted in colonization and infection by resistant organisms in other specialties, the threat of similar occurrences exists in obstetrics and gynecology.

As a result of this concern, in 1973 Ledger

et al. presented a study in which three doses of prophylactic antibiotic were given on the day of surgery only.[4] With this regimen postoperative infections in patients who received prophylactic antibiotics were significantly fewer than in those who received the placebo. Both urinary tract and pelvic infections were decreased in the group that received antibiotic. Subsequently seven other studies in which short antibiotic administration schedules were used have shown similar results.[7, 12-14, 16, 17, 21] In six of these eight studies the average hospitalization time was also less in the group that received antibiotics. In two studies, hospitalization times were similar.[7, 17] Hamod et al.[25] compared a single 3-g dose of cephalothin given preoperatively with a regimen of 9 doses given over 2 days, and no significant difference was seen in the incidence of postoperative infection between the groups studied. These results suggest that it is both unnecessary and unwise to give prophylactic antibiotics for more than 24 hours postoperatively.

A major fear regarding the use of antibiotic prophylaxis is that early symptoms of infection will be masked, and what could have been treated as a minor problem may not be apparent until serious pelvic infection occurs. However, this problem has not been reported in any of the studies of prophylactic antibiotics in vaginal hysterectomy, including those in which patients were followed for several weeks after their hospital discharge.[4, 5, 9, 13, 21] In addition, this problem is theoretically less likely to occur if a short course of prophylaxis is used.

Although the development of colonization or superinfection by resistant organisms is a worrisome side effect of antibiotics, few investigators of prophylactic antibiotics have done careful aerobic and anaerobic microbiology studies either to determine the effect of prophylactic antibiotics on lower genital tract flora or to distinguish the effects of the prophylactic antibiotic from the effects of the vaginal surgery. Most of the data that have been included in published reports relate to organisms isolated from infection sites (usually urinary tract or operative bed). Ledger et al.[4] noted the occurrence of organisms resistant to the prophylactic antibiotics and other less commonly isolated organisms from infection sites of patients with morbidity who received prophylactic antibiotics. These organisms included Pseudomonas, *Enterobacter cloacae*, and *Candida albicans*. Others have not found this to occur.[6, 10, 13] *Escherichia coli* and Group D streptococci, common vaginal inhabitants, appeared to be the most common organisms isolated from infection sites of all patients with morbidity.[4, 5, 6, 10, 13, 15] Grossman et al. found no correlation between organisms found in intraoperative vaginal cuff cultures and those cultured at subsequent infections.[28]

When vaginal cuff cultures were obtained immediately postoperatively from all patients in studies of short-term prophylaxis,[4, 7] the flora of the women who received prophylactic antibiotics was similar to the flora of patients who received placebo. The most commonly isolated organisms were *E. coli*, enterococci, diphtheroids and coagulase-negative staphylococci. However, if cultures were taken four to five days postoperatively in studies of long-term prophylaxis, differences in flora between the antibiotic and placebo groups were apparent and included a greater incidence of organisms resistant to the antibiotic in the group of women who received prophylaxis.[8, 29] The resistant organisms included Enterobacter species and Pseudomonas. Also, the incidence of organisms common in indigenous endocervical flora (e.g., lactobacilli, diphtheroids, staphylococci) was less in women who received the antibiotic than in those who received placebo. It would be interesting to know if flora differences exist three to five days postoperatively between women who received short-term prophylaxis and those who received placebo, but this has not been studied.

In three studies data were presented such that comparison between preoperative and postoperative flora could be made.[8, 29, 30] *E. coli* was found in the postoperative cultures of both the antibiotic and the placebo groups more often than in the preoperative cultures in all three studies. Bivens et al. also reported a postoperative increase of streptococci (not further identified) in both the antibiotic and placebo groups.[8] Ohm and Galask showed a higher postoperative incidence of both Group D streptococci and *Bacteroides fragilis* in both the antibiotic and the placebo groups after a five-day course of antibiotics.[29] This was confirmed by Grossman et al. in a study in which a two-day course of prophylaxis was given.[30] Since these changes occurred in both the antibiotic and the placebo group, they were probably effects of surgery rather than of the prophylactic antibiotic. The most apparent effects of prophylactic antibiotics were two. First, the organisms comprising the preoperative indigenous flora occurred less fre-

quently in postoperative cultures of patients who received prophylactic antibiotic. Second, gram-negative rods other than *E. coli* (often resistant to the prophylactic antibiotic) were isolated more frequently from postoperative than from preoperative cultures of women who received antibiotic. The organisms included Enterobacter species,[8, 29, 30] *Pseudomonas aeruginosa*,[29] and Proteus species.[30]

The question of development of resistant organisms with the use of routine prophylaxis remains a critical one. Grossman et al. have presented hospital-wide epidemiologic data that suggest an increase in cephalosporin-resistant *E. coli* in their hospital after the introduction of cephalosporin prophylaxis.[31] This underscores the fact that continued microbiologic surveillance is critical when prophylaxis is used.

In general the use of prophylactic antibiotics decreased the overall incidence of febrile morbidity following vaginal hysterectomy but, more importantly, decreased febrile morbidity from pelvic infections in particular. This decrease in the incidence of pelvic infections occurred in all studies, despite differences in patient populations, prophylactic antibiotics, antibiotic administration schedules and criteria for determining morbidity. Hospitalization time was also decreased in the patient group receiving antibiotic prophylaxis in most studies. Adverse effects of antibiotic prophylaxis such as delayed recognition of infections or infections by highly resistant organisms have not been reported thus far, even though it has been shown that organisms resistant to the prophylactic antibiotic are more commonly isolated from those patients who receive prophylaxis.

In summary, with careful surveillance of specific organisms and antibiotic susceptibility patterns, antibiotic prophylaxis can be used safely as an adjunct to lower the rate of infection following vaginal hysterectomy in a patient population at risk.

ABDOMINAL HYSTERECTOMY

Fewer studies have been done to evaluate the use of prophylactic antibiotics in cases of total abdominal hysterectomy than in cases of vaginal hysterectomy. Those in which results could be tabulated in terms of postoperative infection rates[3, 10, 13, 15, 20, 21, 32, 33] are summarized in Table 2. The study populations included both women undergoing abdominal

TABLE 2. STUDIES OF USE OF PROPHYLACTIC ANTIBIOTICS IN TOTAL ABDOMINAL HYSTERECTOMY*

Investigators	Type of Study	Prophylactic Antibiotics	Administration Schedule	No. Patients	Total Morbidity†	Major Morbidity‡	Ave. No. Hospital Days
Allen et al.[3]	Prospective Double-blind	Cephalosporins	Preop. thru 5 POD	83 (C) 85 (A)	37% (C) 12% (A)	22% (C) 8% (A)	(A) 6 days less than (C)
Rosenheim[32]	Retrospective	Ampicillin or tetracycline	Day of surgery thru 5 POD	100 (C) 100 (A)	9% (C) 3% (A)	3% (C) 2% (A)	(A) greater than (C)
Ohm & Galask[33]	Prospective Double-blind	Cephalosporins	Preop. thru 4 POD	46 (C) 47 (A)	39% (C) 15% (A)	17% (C) 13% (A)	7.4 (C) 7.2 (A)
Mayer et al.[10]	Prospective Not double-blind	Cephalothin/ kanamycin	Preop. thru 2 POD	28 (C) 28 (A)	50% (C) 29% (A)	32% (C) 29% (A)	Not given
Roberts & Homesley[13]	Prospective Double-blind	Carbenicillin	Preop. thru 1 POD	22 (C) 25 (A)	54% (C) 4% (A)	14% (C) 4% (A)	10.5 (C) 7.7 (A)
Grossman et al.[15]	Prospective Double-blind	Penicillin or cefazolin	Preop. thru 2 POD	84 (C) 76 (Pen.) 79 (Cef.)	26% (C) 32% (Pen.) 35% (Cef.)	11% (C) 5% (Pen.) 11% (Cef.)	6.9 (C) 7.2 (Pen.) 7.1 (Cef.)
Jennings[20]	Prospective Double-blind	Cefazolin/ cephalexin	Preop. thru 2 POD	52 (C) 50 (A)	33% (C) 8% (A)	11.5% (C) 0.0% (A)	9.1 (C) 8.0 (A)
Holman et al.[21]	Prospective Double-blind	Cefazolin	Preop. plus 2 doses	38 (C) 42 (A)	71% (C) 19% (A)	34% (A) 5% (A)	8.5 (C) 6.9 (A)

*Study population may or may not include those who also underwent procedures related to abdominal hysterectomy, e.g., salpingo-oophorectomy.
†Total morbidity, infectious and/or febrile morbidity.
‡Major morbidity, pelvic and wound infections.
(C) Those who received placebo or no prophylactic antibiotic.
(A) Those who received prophylactic antibiotic.
POD, Postoperative day.

hysterectomy alone and those undergoing abdominal hysterectomy with salpingo-oophorectomy. The antibiotics for prophylaxis and the administration schedules were similar to those reported in studies of prophylactic antibiotics in vaginal hysterectomy. In all but one study[15] the incidence of postoperative morbidity was less in the group that received prophylactic antibiotics than in the group receiving placebo or no antibiotics. In four of eight studies the patients who received prophylaxis had less major morbidity and also had shorter hospital stays than those who received placebo.[3, 13, 20, 21] However, in the other four studies the incidence of pelvic infections or wound infections or both as well as the length of hospitalization was similar in the patients who received prophylaxis and in those who did not. A lower incidence of urinary tract infections was responsible for the decrease in overall morbidity of patients receiving prophylaxis in most studies.

Culture results from infection sites, which were reported in most of the studies, indicated that similar organisms were isolated both from patients receiving prophylaxis and from those receiving placebo. The most frequently occurring of these organisms were *E. coli*, *Streptococcus faecalis* and *Proteus mirabilis*. Anaerobic bacteria were isolated from patients in only three studies.[3, 15, 33] While no problems with resistant organisms or delayed infections were reported, Ohm and Galask[33] observed that the infections in the patients who received prophylactic antibiotics in their study were not as well defined as infections that occurred in patients who received placebo. The reason for this is not clear, although it may be related to the number of potential infection sites in patients who have undergone abdominal hysterectomy as opposed to vaginal surgery. Since this problem occurred only in the prophylaxis group, however, it may suggest that because prophylaxis decreases or alters symptoms, proper treatment may be delayed.

Complete microbiologic evaluation—cervical and vaginal apex cultures both preoperatively and postoperatively on all patients— was reported in only two studies.[30, 34] In the study by Ohm and Galask,[34] more antibiotic-resistant organisms were found postoperatively in women who received antibiotic prophylaxis than in those who did not. These organisms included Enterobacter species, *Pseudomonas aeruginosa* and Candida species. The incidences of *E. coli, Klebsiella*

pneumoniae and *Bacteroides fragilis* were greater postoperatively than preoperatively in both the antibiotic and the placebo groups. In the placebo group, Group D streptococci, *Proteus mirabilis*, *Peptostreptococcus anaerobius* and Bacteroides species other than *B. fragilis* were also isolated with greater frequency from postoperative than from preoperative specimens. The study of Grossman and Adams[30] included both abdominal and vaginal hysterectomies, and the microbiologic data were not presented separately, so specific conclusions are not possible. They did, however, isolate more anaerobes overall than did Ohm and Galask. Both of these studies confirm the fact previously discussed that an effect on the cervical and vaginal flora occurs from surgery alone.

Although some studies of the effect of prophylactic antibiotics on morbidity following total abdominal hysterectomy have shown that the use of prophylaxis can reduce postoperative febrile morbidity, we would not advocate routine prophylaxis for all patients undergoing this procedure. The decrease in the incidence of reported morbidity in the majority of published studies was due to a lower incidence of urinary tract infections. Since urinary tract infections can be treated symptomatically with little inconvenience or extra hospitalization time, the use of prophylactic antibiotics is not justified. Although four studies showed a greater incidence of wound or pelvic infection in patients who did not receive prophylactic antibiotics, the infections did not appear more serious than those that occurred in patients who did receive prophylaxis. The use of prophylactic antibiotics resulted in an increased incidence of antibiotic-resistant organisms in specimens obtained from the vaginal apex. Although this has not yet been demonstrated to be of clinical significance, it suggests that serious infection with resistant organisms is possible. Finally, it appears that the signs and symptoms of infections in patients receiving prophylactic antibiotics may be confusing, and prompt, correct treatment may be delayed. The benefits of antibiotic prophylaxis for total abdominal hysterectomy patients do not in our opinion appear to outweigh these risks.

OTHER GYNECOLOGIC PROCEDURES

Few reported studies of the use of prophylactic antibiotics in other gynecologic procedures appear in the literature. Prophylactic antibiotics are probably used routinely in cases of radical hysterectomy because the extent of the surgery and debilitation of the patient increase the risk of postoperative infection. Ledger et al.[35] reported that infectious morbidity following radical hysterectomy, radical vulvectomy or pelvic exenteration ranged from 80 to 100 per cent. Infectious morbidity following pelvic exenteration (100 per cent) occurred despite the routine use of antibiotic prophylaxis. Although it may be unethical to withhold prophylaxis from patients undergoing extensive pelvic surgery for gynecologic malignancies, studies could be done that would provide valuable information.

Cases of laparotomy and vaginal procedures other than hysterectomy have been included in studies of prophylactic antibiotics,[3, 11] but either the numbers of study patients were small or insufficient data were presented so results are difficult to evaluate. A single study of a prophylactic antibiotic for women undergoing first trimester abortion[36] and a single study of morbidity following cone biopsy of the cervix alone[37] suggest that routine use of prophylactic antibiotics is unnecessary for these procedures because the incidence of major complications was low. In most hospitals, gynecologic procedures other than hysterectomies do not appear to have an incidence of major postoperative infection high enough to warrant routine use of antibiotic prophylaxis.

Several alternatives to the use of prophylactic antibiotics to lower infectious morbidity following gynecologic surgery have been reported. Although Goosenberg et al.[22] and Grossman et al.[15] stated that postoperative morbidity was not related to the phase of the patient's menstrual cycle at the time of surgery, Prigg reported that an increased incidence of febrile morbidity occurred in women who underwent hysterectomy in the late secretory phase of their cycle.[24] In contrast, Neary et al. found more bacterial colonization of the vagina and a higher incidence of infection following abdominal hysterectomy in women who were operated on during the follicular phase of their cycle.[38] Although these studies offer conflicting results, they suggest that studies of bacterial colonization of the lower genital tract in relation to the menstrual cycle are needed to determine whether or not timing of surgery in relation to the cycle may be a way of reducing morbidity.

Several mechanical techniques for reduction of posthysterectomy morbidity have been studied. These methods have theoretical appeal because they eliminate the potential adverse reactions associated with antibiotics. Diefenbach investigated the use of carbazochrome salicylate, a systemic hemostatic agent in reducing perioperative blood loss, and serendipitously found that the treated group had no febrile morbidity.[39] This agent has not been studied further.

More recently Osborne et al. reported on the use of preoperative hot conization of the cervix in a retrospective analysis of 402 premenopausal women undergoing vaginal hysterectomy.[40] The comparative febrile morbidity was 49.1 per cent in 108 patients with no prophylaxis, 9.7 per cent in 134 patients who received perioperative antibiotics, and only 4.3 per cent in 160 women who had hot conization. Of particular interest, the conization group had a 1.9 per cent incidence of pelvic cellulitis, and no pelvic abscesses occurred. Although these groups were not randomized, the results would seem to warrant further prospective evaluation.

Swartz and Tanaree have extensively studied the use of suction drainage in both abdominal and vaginal hysterectomy.[41-43] The rationale for this technique is removal of the culture medium (serum) rather than the bacteria. Prospectively, these investigators showed a reduction in both overall febrile morbidity and pelvic infection equivalent to that in patients receiving antibiotics. The wound infection rate in abdominal hysterectomy was not affected. Their results suggest that postoperative drainage may be a reasonable adjunctive measure in certain patients undergoing either vaginal or abdominal hysterectomy.

Obstetrics

The use of antibiotic prophylaxis in obstetrics has been studied, as it has in gynecology, almost as long as antibiotics have been available. Numerous reports of the efficacy of antibiotic prophylaxis in obstetrics have been published; however, the controversy remains of when antibiotic prophylaxis should be used or if there is a place for routine use of prophylactic antibiotics in obstetric cases.

In the earliest studies, both patients undergoing vaginal delivery and those undergoing cesarean section were included. Keettel and Plass concluded that prophylactic antibiotics were unnecessary for women undergoing normal delivery.[44] However, the idea that women undergoing cesarean section were at "high risk" for postoperative infectious complications appears to have persisted, since most of the modern studies of prophylactic antibiotics have included only women undergoing cesarean section. Until recently, little or no differentiation regarding patient populations such as cases of primary cesarean section or repeat cesarean section, presence or absence of labor, or presence, absence or duration of ruptured membranes has been made. Therefore, in most studies, the population is a collection of unknown subpopulations that differ in various ways from the populations of other studies. Also the choice of prophylactic antibiotics and the administration schedules vary from study to study.

Table 3 presents summaries of studies of the use of prophylactic antibiotics in cesarean section.[45-60] Despite the differences in protocols and populations, in all the studies total morbidity following cesarean section was less in women who received prophylactic antibiotics.than in those who did not. In most studies the difference in the rates of morbidity between the two groups was statistically significant. The most common infectious complications occurring after cesarean section included urinary tract infection, wound infection and endometritis. It is important to note that in the studies the incidence of endometritis, the most frequent type of infection reported in women undergoing cesarean section, was reduced considerably when women received prophylaxis. The incidence of wound infection was also less in women who received prophylaxis, but it was not high in any of the study populations who did not receive prophylaxis. The postoperative occurrence of urinary tract infections was reduced by the use of prophylactic antibiotics in some studies[45-47, 50, 52, 55] but not in others.[49, 53, 54, 56-59]

Because it has become clear that there are many dangers inherent in the use of prophylactic antibiotics and because it is also clear that the value of prophylaxis may outweigh the risks in certain cases, investigators of antibiotic prophylaxis in obstetrics have begun to define more carefully the populations involved in studies and to try to determine which populations have a high risk of postoperative infection.

Gibbs et al.[47] were the earliest to present separate data for patients undergoing primary cesarean section and those undergoing repeat section. Their data showed that both groups had a high rate of infection when prophylactic antibiotics were not used. In contrast, Ohm-Smith and Galask found that serious pelvic infectious morbidity occurred at a low rate following elective cesarean section, and further that the use of prophylactic antibiotics did not significantly affect the rate.[55] The report of Phelan and Pruyn[57] agreed with the findings of Ohm-Smith and Galask. Most recent reports have excluded patients undergoing repeat cesarean section from study protocols.

Rothbard et al.[50] differentiated patients according to the presence or absence of labor, and showed that the infectious morbidity in patients who were not in labor and did not receive antibiotics was less than half the morbidity of the patients in labor who did not receive prophylaxis. More important, the group not in labor had no cases of endometritis whether or not prophylactic antibiotics were used. This historically was the first evidence that some patients had lesser risk of postoperative infection, and also provided a rationale for the difference between morbidity in repeat and primary cesarean section. Other investigators have since confirmed the increased risk of patients in labor.[48, 58, 59, 61]

Other factors have been studied in an attempt to further define the high-risk group. Green and Sarubbi subjected 15 variables to statistical analysis to determine which, if any, were associated with infection after cesarean section.[62] General anesthesia, a hematocrit less than or equal to 30, obesity, or labor prior to cesarean section was found to have a significant association with infection, while socioeconomic status, duration of interval after membrane rupture or fetal monitoring did not. In contrast, Kreutner et al. analyzed similar factors and found that only the presence of ruptured membranes (but not duration) had a significant association with a high risk of postoperative infection.[54] Wong et al., using the incidence of infection following various procedures, determined the high-risk population on their obstetric service to be women in labor who had internal fetal monitoring before cesarean section.[53] Gordon et al. demonstrated a significant increase in morbidity associated with the presence of labor, ruptured membranes or internal monitoring.[59]

From these studies it may be inferred that

TABLE 3. STUDIES OF USE OF PROPHYLACTIC ANTIBIOTICS IN CESAREAN SECTION*

INVESTIGATORS	TYPE OF STUDY	PROPHYLACTIC ANTIBIOTIC	ADMINISTRATION SCHEDULE	NO. PATIENTS	TOTAL MORBIDITY†	ENDOMETRITIS	AVE. NO. HOSPITAL DAYS
Miller & Crichton[45]	Prospective Not double-blind	Ampicillin	Preop. thru 6 POD	150 (C) 150 (A)	64% (C) 36% (A)	5% (C) 1% (A)	Not given
Weissberg et al.[46]	Prospective Not double-blind	Penicillin/ kanamycin	Preop. thru 3–5 POD	40 (C) 40 (A)	Not given	35% (C) 10% (A)	8.7 (C) 5.8 (A)
Gibbs et al.[47]	Prospective Double-blind	Ampicillin/ kanamycin	Preop. plus 2 doses	62 (C) 67 (A)	63% (C) 25% (A)	45% (C) 19% (A)	7.8 (C) 6.4 (A)
Morrison et al.[48]	Prospective Double-blind	Penicillin/ kanamycin	Preop. thru 3 POD	115 (C) 115 (A)	51% (C) 22% (A)	27% (C) 7% (A)	8.8 (C) 5.4 (A)
Moro & Andrews[49]	Prospective Double-blind	Cephalosporins	Preop. thru 4 POD	74 (C) 74 (A)	29% (C) 9% (A)	16% (C) 3% (A)	7.5 (C) 6.2 (A)
Rothbard et al.[50]	Prospective Not double-blind	Cephalothin/ kanamycin	Preop. thru 2 POD	53 (C) 47 (A)	43% (C) 13% (A)	15% (C) 2% (A)	No difference between (C) & (A)
Gibbs & Weinstein[51]	Prospective	Clindamycin/ gentamicin	Preop. plus 2 doses	0 (C)‡ 54 (A)	20% (A)	15% (A)	6.6 (A)
Green et al.[52]	Retrospective	Ampicillin	Preop. plus 2 doses	30 (C) 54 (A)	63% (C) 15% (A)	40% (C) 9% (A)	6.2 (C) 5.9 (A)
Wong et al.[53]	Prospective Double-blind	Cefazolin	Immed. post delivery plus 2 doses	45 (C) 48 (A)	67% (C) 46% (A)	51% (C) 29% (A)	Not given

Kreutner et al.[54]	Prospective Double-blind	Cefazolin	Preop. plus 2 doses	49 (C) 48 (A)	35% (C) 27% (A)	20% (C) 12% (A)	No difference. between (C) & (A)
Ohm-Smith & Galask[55]	Prospective Double-blind	Cephalosporins	Preop. thru 4 POD	19 (C) 22 (A)	42% (C) 14% (A)	16% (C) 9% (A)	5.9 (C) 6.1 (A)
Gall[56]	Prospective Double-blind	Cefazolin/ cephalothin	Preop. plus 3 doses	49 (C) 46 (A)	41% (C) 17% (A)	33% (C) 11% (A)	8.3 (C) 7.9 (A)
Phelan & Pruyn[57]	Prospective Double-blind	Cefazolin	Preop. plus 2 doses	39 (C) 37 (A)	38% (C) 16% (A)	15% (C) 11% (A)	Not given
Kreutner et al.[58]	Prospective Triple-blind	Cephalothin or cefamandole	Preop. plus 2 doses	29 (C) 48 (Ceph.) 43 (Cef.)	66% (C) 38% (Ceph.) 28% (Cef.)	59% (C) 31% (Ceph.) 23% (Cef.)	Not given
Gordon et al.[59]	Prospective Not double-blind	Ampicillin	3 doses: Preop. or after cord clamped	36 (C) 38 (Preop) 40 (Post)	39% (C) 11% (Preop) 7% (Post)	33% (C) 11% (Preop) 5% (Post)	6.0 (C) 5.1 (Preop) 4.7 (Post)
D'Angelo & Sokol[60]	Prospective Not double-blind	Cefazolin/ cephalexin	3 doses or 5 days	31 (C) 24 (3 dose) 25 (5 day)	Not given	65% (C) 29% (3 dose) 20% (5 day)	Not given

*Studies vary in regard to subgroups of cesarean section patients included in study population.
†Total morbidity = Total infectious and febrile morbidity.
‡Investigators use a control population those patients used as a control in a previous study (Ref. 47)
(C) Those who received placebo or no prophylactic antibiotic
(A) Those who received prophylactic antibiotic.
POD. Postoperative day.

women who are in labor prior to undergoing cesarean section have a higher risk of serious postoperative infection than those who are not. The independent significance of additional variables such as internal fetal monitoring, rupture of membranes or number of vaginal examinations has not been conclusively demonstrated. However, several recent reports in which limited and clearly defined high-risk groups have been studied have demonstrated a decreased morbidity and a decreased incidence of endometritis with the use of prophylactic antibiotics.[52, 53, 58, 60]

Because risk factors may vary from hospital to hospital, each obstetric service should define its own high-risk factors to determine the need for prophylaxis.

Most investigators have studied a cephalosporin or ampicillin and have reported equivalent results. More important, the use of a single antibiotic has been shown to be as effective as the use of a combination of antibiotics in lowering the incidence of infection. Even though early studies included antibiotic combinations such as the addition of an aminoglycoside, the potential for toxicity with little, if any, increase in efficacy does not justify the risk. The use of an antibiotic for prophylaxis such as clindamycin, which may be needed against an organism difficult to treat with other antibiotics, was not recommended.[1, 51]

Two studies have reported maternal serum levels of cephalosporins given as preoperative prophylaxis. Kreutner et al. studied maternal serum levels of cefamandole and cephalothin and found them to be in the therapeutic range.[58] Gall, who studied cefazolin, found maternal serum concentrations at 60 minutes following injection to be 30 to 60 mcg per ml, also within the therapeutic range.[56]

Although the duration of antibiotic administration has varied among reported studies, it is clear that a short course of prophylactic antibiotic administration was as effective as a long course in reducing morbidity. In a study comparing a 3-dose administration schedule with a 5-day schedule, it was shown that the effect on postoperative morbidity for the two antibiotic regimens was similar.[60]

There is limited evidence whether preoperative antibiotics have an effect on the newborn. Gordon et al. reported that birth weights and Apgar scores were similar in neonates delivered from mothers who received antibiotics prior to cesarean section

when compared with those in neonates whose mothers received the drug following interruption of umbilical cord blood flow.[59]

Concern about the effects prophylactic antibiotics have on the fetus and newborn prompted Wong et al. to study the effect that delaying prophylactic antibiotic administration until after the umbilical cord was clamped would have on morbidity.[53] Their study suggested that this regimen was effective in reducing postoperative morbidity. Further, in a placebo-controlled prospective randomized study, Gordon et al. compared the effect on morbidity of 3-dose antibiotic administration schedule beginning before cesarean section with antibiotic administration following umbilical cord flow restriction and found no difference between the antibiotic groups.[59] The data suggest that antibiotic administration following severance of the umbilical cord is equally as effective as preoperative administration in lowering postoperative morbidity. This is important because concern about the effect of drug remaining in the neonate is eliminated.

Microbiology studies have not been included in many reports of prophylactic antibiotics in cesarean section. In those studies in which the microorganisms associated with morbidity are discussed,[49-51, 54-59] similar microorganisms (E. coli, enterococci, anaerobic cocci and Bacteroides) were isolated both from patients with morbidity who received prophylaxis and from those who did not. The recovery of organisms resistant to the prophylactic antibiotics used has been reported in three studies, but any clinical significance was not reported in detail.[57-59]

In two studies results were reported of cultures taken from all study patients preoperatively and postoperatively. Kreutner et al. compared results of postoperative endometrial cultures with those of preoperative endocervical cultures.[54] Since the organisms were placed into broad classes, it is difficult to determine the significance of the postoperative variation in flora between the prophylactic antibiotic group and the placebo group. Enterobacteriaceae occurred more often in the postoperative cultures of women who received antibiotics than in those of women who received placebo; however, information regarding bacterial resistance to the prophylactic antibiotic was not reported.

In a study of preoperative and postoperative endocervical flora of women who underwent elective cesarean section and received prophylactic cephalosporins, Ohm-Smith and Galask found that over one third of the postoperative gram-negative rod isolates from women who received prophylactic cephalosporins were resistant to cephalosporins in vitro.[55] These resistant organisms occurred only postoperatively in women who received prophylaxis. Group D streptococci (usually resistant to cephalosporins) were also isolated more frequently from postoperative cultures of the antibiotic group. Almost all other organisms were isolated considerably more frequently from postoperative cultures of the placebo group. These results suggest that prophylactic antibiotics do reduce the indigenous endocervical flora and allow resistant organisms to colonize. Although this occurrence did not cause problems in this study, it emphasizes again the need for microbiologic surveillance when prophylactic antibiotics are used.

The problems with the design of many of the studies of prophylactic antibiotics in obstetrics have been summarized and discussed by Mead.[63] These include studies that are not double-blind, are poorly controlled, have inadequate criteria for defining infection and do not analyze data separately for subgroups of the patient population. Mead stated that antibiotic prophylaxis in cesarean section should be considered experimental and outlined an experimental protocol that would avoid the shortcomings of previous studies. We concur that further studies must follow a rigid protocol similar to that described. Before meaningful results can be obtained, the data must be analyzed in subgroups of the obstetric patient population such as length of interval after membrane rupture, use of fetal monitoring and length of labor. It is also necessary to do complete and careful preoperative and postoperative microbiologic studies on all patients to determine the effects of the prophylactic antibiotic. The usefulness of any regimen of prophylactic antibiotic cannot be completely evaluated without this information. If the prophylactic antibiotic is given preoperatively, follow-up of the newborn must also be done and reported.

Summary

The routine use of prophylactic antibiotics in gynecology at present appears to be indicated only for patients undergoing vaginal hysterectomy. Although prophylaxis is used routinely for radical hysterectomy, no data have been presented to indicate whether or not prophylaxis is beneficial.

At present the use of prophylactic antibiotics in patients who are in labor and undergoing primary cesarean section appears beneficial. Additional risk factors such as ruptured amniotic membranes would further support the use of a perioperative antibiotic for prophylaxis.

Combining conclusions drawn from the literature reviewed with the guidelines suggested by Ledger et al.,[1] we propose the following guidelines for the use of antibiotic prophylaxis in obstetrics and gynecology:

1. The procedure must have a significant postoperative infectious morbidity or the patient must be thought to have an altered host response to infection.

2. The operative procedure must be associated with a high probability of microbial contamination.

3. The drug must be of low toxicity, have an established record of patient safety and not be routinely utilized for serious infections.

4. The drug utilized must have a spectrum of activity that includes those microorganisms from the site of contamination that are most likely to cause infection.

5. The drug must achieve a reasonable tissue concentration during the procedure and be administered for a short duration.

6. The hospital must have a functioning infection surveillance program with established guidelines and maintain records of current antibiotic susceptibility patterns prior to initiating elective antibiotic prophylaxis for general use.

Because antibiotic prophylaxis remains a controversial subject to many students of infectious disease, each institution should establish a need and develop protocols for the use of antibiotic prophylaxis.

REFERENCES

1. Ledger, W. J., Gee, C. and Lewis, W. P.: Guidelines for antibiotic prophylaxis in gynecology. Am. J. Obstet. Gynecol. 121:1038, 1975.
2. Cutler, R., Westcott, D. and Ringrose, D.: Antibiotic prophylaxis and hysterectomy. Dimens. Health Serv. 53:34, 1976.
3. Allen, J. L., Rampone, J. F. and Wheeless, C. R.:

Use of a prophylactic antibiotic in elective major gynologic operations. Obstet. Gynecol. 39:218, 1972.

4. Ledger, W. J., Sweet, R. L. and Headington, J. T.: Prophylactic cephaloridine in the prevention of postoperative pelvic infections in premenopausal women undergoing vaginal hysterectomy. Am. J. Obstet. Gynecol. 115:766, 1973.

5. Ohm, M. J. and Galask, R. P.: The effect of antibiotic prophylaxis on patients undergoing vaginal operations. I. The effect on morbidity. Am. J. Obstet. Gynecol. 123:590, 1975.

6. Harralson, J. D., vanNagell, J. R., Roddick, J. W. and Sprague, A. D.: The effect of prophylactic antibiotics on pelvic infection following vaginal hysterectomy. Am. J. Obstet. Gynecol. 120:1046, 1974.

7. Breeden, J. T. and Mayo, J. E.: Low-dose prophylactic antibiotics in vaginal hysterectomy. Obstet. Gynecol. 43:379, 1974.

8. Bivens, M. D., Neufeld, J. and McCarty, W. D.: The prophylactic use of Keflex and Keflin in vaginal hysterectomy. Am. J. Obstet. Gynecol. 122:169, 1975.

9. Forney, J. P., Morrow, C. P., Townsend, D. E. and Disaia, P. J.: Impact of cephalosporin prophylaxis on conization-vaginal hysterectomy morbidity. Am. J. Obstet. Gynecol. 125:100, 1976.

10. Mayer, W., Gordon, M. and Rothbard, M. J.: Prophylactic antibiotics. N. Y. State J. Med. 76:2144, 1976.

11. Sengupta, B. S., Wynter, H. H., Hall, J. S., Ramchander, R., Alexis, A., Zamah, N. and Gajraj, K.: Prophylactic antibiotic in elective gynaecological and obstetrical major surgery. Int. J. Gynaecol. Obstet. 14:417, 1976.

12. Lett, W. J., Ansbacher, R., Davison, B. L. and Otterson, W. N.: Prophylactic antibiotics for women undergoing vaginal hysterectomy. J. Reprod. Med. 19:51, 1977.

13. Roberts, J. M. and Homesley, H. D.: Low-dose carbenicillin prophylaxis for vaginal and abdominal hysterectomy. Obstet. Gynecol. 52:83, 1978.

14. Mendelson, J., Portnoy, J., deSaint Victor, J. R. and Gelfand, M. M.: Effect of single and multidose cephradine prophylaxis on infectious morbidity of vaginal hysterectomy. Obstet. Gynecol. 53:31, 1979.

15. Grossman, J. H., Greco, T. P., Minkin, M. J., Adams, R. L., Hierholzer, W. J. and Andriole, V. T.: Prophylactic antibiotics in gynecologic surgery. Obstet. Gynecol. 53:537, 1979.

16. Hemsell, D. L., Cunningham, F. G., Kappus, S. and Nobles, B.: Cefoxitin for prophylaxis in premenopausal women undergoing vaginal hysterectomy. Obstet. Gynecol. 56:629, 1980.

17. Mickal, A., Curole, D. and Lewis, C.: Cefoxitin sodium: double-blind vaginal hysterectomy prophylaxis in premenopausal patients. Obstet. Gynecol. 56:222, 1980.

18. Peterson, L. F., Justema, E. J., Wiersma, A. F. et al.: Comparative efficacy of preoperative and postoperative cephalothin therapy in vaginal hysterectomy. Curr. Ther. Res. 22:792, 1977.

19. Wheeless, C. R., Dorsey, J. H. and Wharton, L. R.: An evaluation of prophylactic doxycycline in hysterectomy patients. J. Reprod. Med. 21:146, 1978.

20. Jennings, R. H.: Prophylactic antibiotics in vaginal and abdominal hysterectomy. South. Med. J. 71:251, 1978.

21. Holman, J. F., McGowan, J. E. and Thompson, J. D.: Perioperative antibiotics in major elective gynecologic surgery. South. Med. J. 71:417, 1978.

22. Goosenberg, J., Emich, J. P. and Schwarz, R. H.: Prophylactic antibiotics in vaginal hysterectomy. Am. J. Obstet. Gynecol. 105:503, 1969.

23. Boyd, M. E. and Garceau, R.: The value of prophylactic antibiotics after vaginal hysterectomy. Am. J. Obstet. Gynecol. 125:581, 1976.

24. Prigg, D. H.: Vaginal hysterectomy: effect of prophylactic use of antibiotics on morbidity. J. Am. Osteopath. Assoc. 76:664, 1977.

25. Hamod, K. A., Spence, M. R., Rosenshein, N. B. and Dillon, M. B.: Single dose and multidose prophylaxis in vaginal hysterectomy: a comparison of sodium cephalothin and metronidazole. Am. J. Obstet. Gynecol. 136:976, 1980.

26. Sweet, R. L. and Ledger, W. J.: Cefoxitin: single-agent treatment of mixed aerobic-anaerobic pelvic infections. Obstet. Gynecol. 54:193, 1979.

27. Bolling, D. R. and Plunkett, G. D.: Prophylactic antibiotics for vaginal hysterectomies. Obstet. Gynecol. 41:689, 1973.

28. Grossman, J. H., Adams, R. L., Hierholzer, W. J. and Andriole, V. T.: Endometrial and vaginal cuff bacteria recovered at elective hysterectomy during a trial of antibiotic prophylaxis. Am. J. Obstet. Gynecol. 130:312, 1978.

29. Ohm, M. J. and Galask, R. P.: The effect of antibiotic prophylaxis on patients undergoing vaginal operations. II. Alterations of microbial flora. Am. J. Gynecol. 123:597, 1975.

30. Grossman, J. H. and Adams, R. L: Vaginal flora in women undergoing hysterectomy with antibiotic prophylaxis. Obstet. Gynecol. 53:23, 1979.

31. Grossman, J. H., Adams, R. L. and Hierholzer, W. J.: Epidemiologic surveillance during a clinical trial of antibiotic prophylaxis in pelvic surgery. Am. J. Obstet. Gynecol. 128:690, 1977.

32. Rosenheim, G. E.: Prophylactic antibiotics in elective abdominal hysterectomy. Am. J. Obstet. Gynecol. 119:335, 1974.

33. Ohm, M. J. and Galask, R. P.: The effect of antibiotic prophylaxis on patients undergoing total abdominal hysterectomy. I. Effect on morbidity. Am. J. Obstet. Gynecol. 125:442, 1976.

34. Ohm, M. J. and Galask, R. P.: The effect of antibiotic prophylaxis on patients undergoing total abdominal hysterectomy. II. Alterations of microbial flora. Am. J. Obstet. Gynecol. 125:448, 1976.

35. Ledger, W. J., Reite, A. and Headington, J. T.: The surveillance of infection of an inpatient gynecology service. Am. J. Obstet. Gynecol. 113:662, 1972.

36. Hodgson, J. E., Major, B., Portmann, K. and Quattlebaum, F. W.: Prophylactic use of tetracycline for first trimester abortions. Obstet. Gynecol. 45:574, 1975.

37. DeCenzo, J. A., Malo, T. and Cavanagh, D.: Factors affecting cone-hysterectomy morbidity. Am. J. Obstet. Gynecol. 110:380, 1971.

38. Neary, M. P., Allen, J., Okubadejo, O. A. and Payne, D. J. H.: Preoperative vaginal bacteria and postoperative infections in gynaecological patients. Lancet 2:1291, 1973.

39. Diefenbach, E. J.: Comparative blood loss in hysterectomies. Obstet. Gynecol. 39:357, 1972.

40. Osborne, N. G., Wright, R. C. and Dubay, M.: Preoperative hot conization of the cervix: a possible method to reduce postoperative febrile morbidity following vaginal hysterectomy. Am. J. Obstet. Gynecol. 133:374, 1979.

41. Swartz, W. H. and Tanaree, P.: Suction drainage as an alternative to prophylactic antibiotics in hysterectomy. Obstet. Gynecol. 45:305, 1975.

42. Swartz, W. H. and Tanaree, P.: T-tube suction drainage and/or prophylactic antibiotics: a randomized study of 451 hysterectomies. Obstet. Gynecol. 47:665, 1976.

43. Swartz, W. H.: Prophylaxis of minor febrile and major infectious morbidity following hysterectomy. Obstet. Gynecol. 54:284, 1979.

44. Keettel, W. C. and Plass, E. D.: Prophylactic administration of penicillin to obstetric patients. J.A.M.A. 142:324, 1950.

45. Miller, R. D. and Crichton, D.: Ampicillin prophylaxis in cesarean section. So. Afr. J. Obstet. Gynaecol. 6:69, 1968.

46. Weissberg, S. M., Edwards, N. L. and O'Leary, J. A.: Prophylactic antibiotics in cesarean section. Obstet. Gynecol. 38:290, 1971.

47. Gibbs, R. S., Hunt, J. E. and Schwarz, R. H.: A follow-up study on prophylactic antibiotics in cesarean section. Am. J. Obstet. Gynecol. 117:419, 1973.

48. Morrison, J. C., Coxwell, W. L., Kennedy, B. S., Schreier, P. C., Wiser, W. L. and Fish, S. A.: The use of prophylactic antibiotics in patients undergoing cesarean section. Surg. Gynecol. Obstet. 136:425, 1973.

49. Moro, M. and Andrews, M: Prophylactic antibiotics in cesarean section. Obstet. Gynecol. 44:688, 1974.

50. Rothbard, M. J., Mayer, W., Wystepek, A. and Gordon, M.: Prophylactic antibiotics in cesarean section. Obstet. Gynecol. 45:421, 1975.

51. Gibbs, R. S. and Weinstein, A. J.: Bacteriologic effects of prophylactic antibiotics in cesarean section. Am. J. Obstet. Gynecol. 126:226, 1976.

52. Green, S. L., Sarubbi, F. A. and Bishop, E. H.: Prophylactic antibiotics in high-risk cesarean section. Obstet. Gynecol. 51:569, 1978.

53. Wong, R., Gee, C. L. and Ledger, W. J.: Prophylactic use of cefazolin in monitored obstetric patients undergoing cesarean section. Obstet. Gynecol. 51:407, 1978.

54. Kreutner, A. K., DelBene, V. E., Delamar, D., Huguley, V., Harmon, P. M. and Mitchell, K. S.: Perioperative antibiotic prophylaxis in cesarean section. Obstet. Gynecol. 52:279, 1978.

55. Ohm-Smith, M. J. and Galask, R. P.: Antibiotic prophylaxis in elective cesarean section. Unpublished data.

56. Gall, S. A.: The efficacy of prophylactic antibiotics in cesarean section. Am. J. Obstet. Gynecol. 134:506, 1979.

57. Phelan, J. P. and Pruyn, S. C.: Prophylactic antibiotics in cesarean section: a double-blind study of cefazolin. Am. J. Obstet. Gynecol. 133:474, 1979.

58. Kreutner, A. K., DelBene, V. E., Delamar, D., Bodden, J. L. and Loadholt, C. B.: Perioperative cephalosporin prophylaxis in cesarean section: effect on endometritis in the high-risk patient. Am. J. Obstet. Gynecol. 134:925, 1979.

59. Gordon, H. R., Phelps, D. and Blanchard, K.: Prophylactic cesarean section antibiotics: maternal and neonatal morbidity before or after cord clamping. Obstet. Gynecol. 53:151, 1979.

60. D'Angelo, L. J. and Sokol, R. J.: Short versus long-course prophylactic antibiotic treatment in cesarean section patients. Obstet. Gynecol. 55:583, 1980.

61. Rehu, M. and Nilsson, C. G.: Risk factors for febrile morbidity associated with cesarean section. Obstet. Gynecol. 56:269, 1980.

62. Green, S. L. and Sarubbi, F. A.: Risk factors associated with post-cesarean section febrile morbidity. Obstet. Gynecol. 49:686, 1977.

63. Mead, P. B.: Prophylactic antibiotics and antibiotic resistance. Sem. Perinatol. 1:101, 1977.

Contemporary Use of Prophylactic Antibiotics in Obstetrics and Gynecology

Richard H. Schwarz, M.D.

William R. Crombleholme, M.D.

State University of New York—Downstate Medical Center

It was probably inevitable that not long after the first availability of therapeutic antibiotics the concept of prevention would be introduced. Unfortunately, the initial venture in this area was somewhat ill-conceived. In it were utilized sulfonamides for prophylaxis against urinary tract infection following operative procedures, although it has since been shown that such infections are not amenable to prophylaxis. Falk[12] in 1946 reported on 193 patients given sulfonamides as prophylaxis against urinary tract infection. Of these, 23 per cent had morbidity compared with 18 per cent of 307 patients not on sulfonamides or to 21 per cent overall morbidity in the series. Not only was there little effect on the incidence of postoperative urinary tract infection, but as can be seen from the morbidity data, sulfonamides had little effect on overall morbidity as well.

More promisingly, Turner[58] in 1950 reported on the use of penicillin vaginal suppositories preoperatively in an effort to decrease febrile morbidity following vaginal hysterectomy. He noted a decrease in morbidity from 34.8 per cent in a comparable though not controlled series of patients to 7 per cent in 100 patients in whom penicillin suppositories were used. Similarly, Cron et al.[9] reported a diminution in postoperative febrile morbidity with use of penicillin suppositories. Reporting on one thousand consecutive hysterectomies, they noted a decrease in morbidity from 38 to 21 per cent for total abdominal hysterectomies, from 42 to 23 per cent for vaginal hysterectomies and from 51 to 28 per cent for subtotal abdominal hysterectomies. However, at the same time, the generally indiscriminate use of penicillin led to the emergence of resistant infections caused by beta-lactamase–producing staphylococci. Despite the fact that prophylaxis in clean surgery was not the only ill-advised use of penicillin and sulfa, the concept fell into disfavor for several years. It was not until the classic studies of Burke[6] utilizing experimental staphylococcal wound infection in guinea pigs in 1961 that interest was revived. He demonstrated unequivocally in that model that antibiotics administered within three hours of inoculation had a beneficial effect but that the optimal result was seen when the antibiotic level was achieved prior to the incision and inoculation of organisms. This became the basis for the now-accepted principle of preoperative initiation of antibiotics for surgical prophylaxis.

The classical clinical report came from Polk and Lopez-Mayor[50] in 1969 with the use of a cephalosporin in the prevention of postoperative intra-abdominal and wound infections in a group of patients undergoing gastrointestinal or pancreaticobiliary surgery. It is clear from this study that the use of prophylaxis in a short perioperative course was quite effective. Their work became a model for the subsequent use of antibiotic prophylaxis.

There is a strong analogy between the use of this approach in gastrointestinal and pancreaticobiliary surgery and its use in certain obstetric and gynecologic procedures, because the indigenous bacterial flora of the cervix and vagina is qualitatively if not quantitatively similar to that found in those areas. As one views modern microbiologic studies of the flora, one finds multiple opportunistic pathogens isolated from the cervix or vagina of all patients. (Modern studies generally have better technique and therefore better recovery of larger numbers of species, especially anaerobes.) Gorbach et al.[23] examined the cervical flora in 30 healthy women having routine gynecologic care. Only one patient had negative cultures, 27 per cent had aerobes alone and 70 per cent had both aerobes and anaerobes. The median number of isolates was four per specimen and one specimen had nine different species of microorganisms.

Developmentally one can trace the changing flora along with pH and glycogen content as a function of the endocrine milieu in the woman. The fetal cervix and vagina are presumably sterile but acidic, with a high glycogen content reflecting the maternal hormonal levels. Because this milieu persists in the early neonatal period the cervix and vagina are rapidly colonized after birth with organisms similar to those seen in the adult. As the maternal steroid levels wane, however, the infant and young girl will have a reduced vaginal bacterial population, a more alkaline pH and reduced glycogen content, a situation that persists until puberty.

During the reproductive period, the pH again becomes more acidic, glycogen increases and there is an increase in total organisms as well as numbers of species and especially an increase in the number of anaerobes present. With the advent of the menopause there occurs a dramatic change not only in the pH and glycogen content of the cervix and vagina but also in the number of organisms and species present in the flora. There is an especially notable decrease in the number of anaerobes. Although most authors have suggested that the difference in the morbidity between premenopausal and postmenopausal women having vaginal hysterectomy results from the increased vascularity and blood loss in the premenopausal group, the difference may in fact be related to the difference in flora, especially the frequency of anaerobes in the younger patients.

It has been suggested that morbidity with vaginal hysterectomy may be increased when it is performed in the secretory phase of the cycle and that this is due to the susceptability to infection of a recent ruptured follicle. This in fact must account for a comparatively small number of postoperative infections, however, since ovarian abscesses and oophoritis are quite rare. The impact of the menstrual phase in clinical practice appears to be relatively minor, but it is conceivable that this difference might be caused by differences in the cervicovaginal flora. Such changes have been demonstrated in relation to the estrous cycle in experimental animals.

The mechanism of action of prophylactic antibiotics is not clearly defined but several possibilities seem apparent. First, if the administration of preoperative antibiotics decreases the population of bacteria present at the operative site before the surgical procedure is begun, then the size of the inoculation will be reduced. Ohm and Galask[47, 49] have extensively examined the effects of prophylactic antibiotics on the vaginal flora of patients undergoing vaginal and abdominal hysterectomies. In comparisons of the preoperative and postoperative flora in patients undergoing such surgery, the patients on prophylaxis in both studies showed reductions postoperatively in aerobic gram-positive rods, aerobic gram-positive cocci, anaerobic gram-positive rods, anaerobic gram-positive cocci and anaerobic gram-negative cocci.

A factor of at least equivalent importance is the reduction of the number of bacterial species present. In their study of vaginal flora before and after vaginal hysterectomy, Ohm and Galask[47] demonstrated that in the placebo group 52 per cent of the patients had six or more species cultured preoperatively and 59 per cent had six or more species cultured postoperatively. In the patients on prophylaxis, however, 72 per cent had six or more species preoperatively but only 12.5 per cent had six or more species postoperatively. This is also evident by the observation that prophylaxis is effective despite the fact that all species are not covered by the drug selected. The effect is related to the principle of bacterial synergism, whereby two bacterial species acting symbiotically are more likely to produce an infection than either species acting alone. Another explanation for the efficacy of prophylactic antibiotics is the possibility that the drugs may actually be effective in treating established but not clinically apparent infection. This is especially likely when one deals with cesarean section in patients with ruptured membranes or established labor prior to the operation.

Indications For Use

As one considers the potential uses of this approach in obstetrics and gynecology, there

TABLE 1.   INDICATIONS FOR PROPHYLACTIC ANTIBIOTICS

SBE prophylaxis
Premenopausal vaginal hysterectomy
Cesarean section
Radical pelvic surgery
Postconceptional cerclage
Abdominal hysterectomy
Premature rupture of membranes
Infertility surgery

are a number of possible indications. We will discuss these individually, weighing the evidence pro and con from the most clear-cut to those indications for which there is little or no evidence. Despite the volumes that have been written supporting the use of prophylactic antibiotics in obstetrics and gynecology, the only absolute indication is in the prevention of subacute bacterial endocarditis. Progressively, as one scans this list, the evidence for the indications is less substantial (Table 1).

Patients with valvular heart disease and probably those with the less well-defined problems of mitral valve prolapse require prophylaxis when they undergo gynecologic surgery, delivery or perhaps more importantly the rather mundane procedures of routine dental care such as scaling of the teeth. Prophylaxis should be employed in any manipulation that might result in bacteremia. The selection of antibiotics must include penicillin as well as an aminoglycoside, since the risks are for infection with both streptococci and gram-negative enteric bacilli.

Questions are often raised concerning intrauterine contraceptive devices and the risk of subacute bacterial endocarditis. There is very little evidence upon which to base a judgment. Everett and colleagues[11] in 1976 studied 100 patients and found no evidence of bacteremia at intervals of 1, 3, 15, 30 and 90 minutes following insertion or removal; however, there is a case report in 1975 by De Swiet et al.[10] of endocarditis following insertion. Because endocarditis is so devastating when it occurs, it is advisable to utilize prophylaxis when inserting or removing an IUD, despite the scant evidence available.

VAGINAL HYSTERECTOMY

The best documentation for the use of prophylaxis in gynecologic and obstetric surgery is in vaginal hysterectomy in the premenopausal patient. There are several studies,[1, 3-5,]

[21, 22, 40] the first in 1969, of varying size and quality, in which several regimens were used. The investigators all seem to have reached a similar conclusion; there is a significant reduction in febrile morbidity and, when reported, in serious pelvic infections as well (Table 2).

If the average reduction in febrile morbidity is calculated in these 8 studies of 1307 patients, the controls showed a 51.7 per cent morbidity as opposed to 9.8 per cent in the study patients. Using the same liberty with hospital stay there was a reduction of 9.1 to 7.7 days. In addition to establishing the efficacy of the approach, these studies also underscore some of the important basic principles in prophylaxis. Vaginal hysterectomy in the premenopausal patient is a procedure that is accompanied by a significant febrile morbidity, ranging from 32 to 77 per cent in these studies, and therefore the use can be justified. One could not support the approach in a surgical procedure with as low a percentage of morbidity as 5 to 10 per cent.

In addition to the known high morbidity, vaginal hysterectomy fits the criteria in that there is an inevitable contamination of the operative site by the cervical and vaginal flora as opposed to, for example, the situation in a transabdominal ovarian cystectomy. Thus, based upon the data available it seems clear that prophylactic antibiotics are useful in premenopausal vaginal hysterectomy in that they do reduce febrile morbidity, perhaps decrease serious infections and shorten the hospital stay. The ominous threat of superinfections and emergence of resistant strains does not appear to have materialized in the reported material;[27] however, especially as concerns the latter, long-term surveillance is necessary. Indeed any increase in antibiotic use, be it therapeutic or prophylactic, creates pressures on the flora, which must be constantly monitored.

Two studies lend support to this concern. In 1975 Ohm and Galask[47] examined the effects on vaginal flora in patients receiving prophylaxis for vaginal hysterectomy. In comparing preoperative and postoperative cultures, the number of cultures positive for aerobic gram-negative rods was increased in both the placebo and the drug group. However, recovery of *Pseudomonas aeruginosa* was seen only in the postoperative cultures of the drug group, even though this organism was not associated with postoperative infection. In 1976 the same authors[49] examined the alterations in vaginal flora in patients on prophylaxis for abdominal hysterectomy. In this study, while there was no difference between the placebo and drug groups in the number of cultures positive for anaerobic gram-negative rods preoperatively compared to postoperatively, the postoperative cultures of the drug group showed a decrease in the number

TABLE 2. PROPHYLACTIC ANTIBIOTICS FOR VAGINAL HYSTERECTOMY

STUDY	YEAR	NO. PATIENTS	ANTIBIOTICS	COURSE	PERCENTAGE FEBRILE MORBIDITY	HOSPITAL STAY (DAYS)
Goosenberg	1969	202	Penicillin and streptomycin; chloromycetin	Preop + 5 days	Controls–77.5 Chloromycetin–52.5 Pen + Strep–7.5	Controls1–0 Study–7.5
Thomsen	1970	169	Cephaloridine ± penicillin	Preop + hospital stay	Controls–58 Study "virtually none"	"Decreased"
Allen	1972	98	Cephalothin	Preop + 72 hours	Controls–50 Study–4.1	Decreased by 4 days
Bolling	1973	296	Ampicillin, tetracycline	Preop + 7 days	Controls–32 Study–7	Not reported
Ledger	1973	100	Cephaloridine	Short perioperative (8 hrs)	Controls–46 Study–24	Controls–9.9 Study–8.6
Breeden	1974	120	Cephaloridine	Short perioperative (12 hrs)	Controls–52 Study–9	Controls–7.7 Study–7.3
Goodlin	1974	58	Cephaloridine	Preop + 4 days	Controls–66 Study–14	No change
Boyd	1976	264	Ampicillin	Postop for 5 days	Control–32.1 Study–2.7	Controls–8.7 Study–7.5

of Bacteroides species isolated compared to the placebo group, but a specific increased isolation of *Bacteroides fragilis*.

FIRST TRIMESTER ABORTION

In the category of procedures with low morbidity, one might consider the reported use of prophylactic tetracycline in first trimester abortions. In 1975 Hodgson et al.[31] examined the complications in a very large series of patients undergoing first trimester abortions. In two control groups of 1000 patients each the incidence of total complications was 9.1 and 8.8 per cent, respectively, encompassing all complications whether classified as minimal, minor or major. In the two groups treated prophylactically, again with 1000 patients each, the incidence of total complications was 3.4 and 2.9 per cent, respectively. Similarly, London et al.[42] reported on the use of doxycycline for prophylaxis in first trimester abortions. Here again a reported decrease incidence of complications was noted, from 10.5 for controls to 4.5 per cent for the drug-treated group. However, despite claims of statistical significance in these reductions in morbidity, it must be remembered that the bulk of these complications are not infectious in nature and that therefore the benefits to be expected from prophylaxis fall far short of exceeding the attendant risks of antibiotic usage.

CESAREAN SECTION

The second most frequently studied use of prophylaxis is in cesarean section. As with vaginal hysterectomy, there have been a large number of studies utilizing a variety of antibiotics for differing periods of time.[1, 17, 19, 34, 44, 45, 53, 61] Although their results look at least superficially as good as those on vaginal hysterectomy, they are considerably more difficult to interpret (Table 3). If one reviews the data on febrile morbidity, the averaged figures for 8 studies involving 850 patients indicate a reduction from 48 to 15 per cent overall, but there is extreme variation in the frequency of morbidity in the controls (25 to 85 per cent) as well as in the study patients (0 to 27.1 per cent). Only one study (Kreutner et al.[34]) shows an insignificant difference between control and study patients. There are not sufficient data to evaluate the frequency of serious infections and the information concerning the duration of hospitalization is inconclusive.

TABLE 3. PROPHYLACTIC ANTIBIOTICS FOR CESAREAN SECTION

STUDY	YEAR	No. PATIENTS	ANTIBIOTICS	COURSE	PERCENTAGE FEBRILE MORBIDITY	HOSPITAL STAY (DAYS)
Weisberg	1971	80	Penicillin Kanamycin	Preop + 3–5 days	Controls–85 Study–15	Shortened
Allen	1972	12	Cephalothin	Preop + 5 days	Control–42.9 Study–0	No change
Morrison	1973	230	Penicillin Kanamycin	Preop + 3 days	Control–51 Study–22	Shortened
Gibbs	1973	129	Ampicillin Kanamycin (Methicillin)	Short peri-operative	Control–65 Study–24	Shortened
Moro	1974	148	Cephalothin	Preop + 5 days	Control–29.2 Study–8.8	Shortened
Rothbard	1975	100	Cephalothin Kanamycin	Preop + 4 days	No Labor Control–25 Study–0 Labor Control–51.4 Study–19.4	No change
Gibbs	1976	54	Clindamycin Gentamicin	Short peri-operative	Study–20.4	–
Kreutner	1978	97	Cefazolin	Short peri-operative	Control–34.7 Study–27.1	No change

Two studies indicate that antibiotic pressures do bring about changes in flora after use, favoring organisms not covered by the drug selected. In 1976, Gibbs and Weinstein[19] examined the bacterial effects of a prophylactic regimen of clindamycin and gentamicin in cesarean section. In this study they noted an increased isolation in the drug group of enterococcus resistant to both clindamycin and gentamicin. Similarly, in 1978 Kreutner et al.[34] examined the effectiveness of cefazolin for prophylaxis in cesarean section. In the study group receiving cefazolin six patients developed endometritis; of these, five had positive cultures growing organisms resistant to cefazolin.

The major difficulty, however, that is faced in evaluating these reports is the extreme heterogeneity of the populations. There are so many variables, including labor, rupture of the membranes, presence or absence of meconium, examinations, monitoring techniques and the like that it would require a massive collaborative study to have sufficiently large subsets to make valid comparisons. A simple and rather gross example of this point can be seen in the Kreutner[34] study, in which the difference in the two groups is significant when one compares the frequency of endometritis and wound infections only (26.5 per cent in the control group compared with 12.5 per cent in the drug group) but not significant if total morbidity is assessed. This is an important point, since most authors have suggested that prophylaxis is not effective in preventing pulmonary or urinary tract infections.

In addition to the wide variation in efficacy depending upon the particular subset of patients, there is a considerable difference in the control incidence of morbidity in these groups. The febrile morbidity accompanying elective repeat cesarean section is in many instances far too low to justify the approach, while in other cases, such as the patient with prolonged labor and rupture of the membranes undergoing emergency cesarean section, the morbidity is exceedingly high and prophylactic antibiotics may not be effective. In this latter case the failure may be the result of an already established but not clinically apparent infection that might require more than the short perioperative approach.

Yet another concern with prophylaxis in cesarean section relates to exposure of the fetus to the antibiotic when it is administered preoperatively. This may interfere with the pediatricians' ability to obtain meaningful cultures, and in the eyes of some, necessitates treating the newborn regardless of its status. However, if the administration is delayed until after delivery or cord clamping, the full prophylactic effect may not be achieved. Most neonatologists would happily accept this problem in the case of treatment of active infection in the mother and fetus (overt chorioamnionitis) but question the exposure when the antibiotic is to be administered prophylactically.

To summarize the situation with regard to cesarean section, the evidence is not as clear as it would seem at first from the overall data. In some subsets of patients prophylaxis cannot be justified on the basis of known low morbidity rates. Although it may well be justified in other subsets of patients definably at risk, there is the suggestion that it may be less effective under those conditions in which subclinical infection may be present. Selective use and perhaps a full therapeutic course in the group at highest risk may be the answer.

GYNECOLOGIC ONCOLOGY

Still farther down the scale, largely because of lack of data, is prophylaxis in gynecologic oncology procedures. In a recent survey we conducted of directors of gynecologic oncology services (51 of 62 responded) information on patterns of use was acquired (Table 4). Only 5 (9.8 per cent) did not use prophylaxis routinely in any of the procedures listed. Forty-three (84.3 per cent) used the approach in pelvic exenteration, 30 (58.8 per cent) in radical hysterectomy and 28 (54.9 per cent) in radical vulvectomy. The oncologists responding utilized prophylaxis in vaginal hysterectomy in 37.3 per cent of cases, 19.6 per cent for vulvectomy and 13.7 per cent for abdominal hysterectomy. Single antibiotics were used by 53.7 per cent and multiple by 46.3 per cent, and the most common antibiotics em-

TABLE 4. USE OF ANTIBIOTIC PROPHYLAXIS BY GYNECOLOGIC ONCOLOGISTS[51]

Do not use routinely	9.8% (5)
Radical hysterectomy	58.8% (30)
Pelvic exenterations	84.3% (43)
Radical vulvectomy	54.9% (28)
Hysterectomy	
vaginal	37.3% (19)
abdominal	13.7% (7)
Vulvectomy	19.6% (10)

TABLE 5. ANTIBIOTICS SELECTED FOR
PROPHYLAXIS

Cephalosporins	30
Aminoglycosides	15
Ampicillin	11
Clindamycin	6
Penicillin	6
Tetracycline	2
Chloromycetin	1
Septra	1

ployed were cephalosporins, aminoglycosides and ampicillin in that order (Table 5). Therapy was instituted preoperatively in 91.3 per cent and the duration varied widely from a short perioperative course to 14 days.

Although there are no data specifically to support all these uses in gynecologic oncology, the application in total and posterior exenteration is justified by the information available from the general surgical literature, since bowel resection and colostomy are involved. The patterns of antibiotic selection and duration of treatment by the oncologists do not vary from the general ones, except perhaps for a greater use of aminoglycosides presumably in the exenteration patients. In the case of radical hysterectomy no studies are available, but in reading between the lines of the responses one feels the major concerns are for preventing urinary tract infections, despite the fact that many authors concede these are not likely to develop.

More critically, however, Forney et al.[13] studied the influence of prophylactic antibiotics on febrile morbidity following sequential cervical conization and vaginal hysterectomy. Previous authors[8, 59] had pointed out the significant morbidity associated with this sequence, but such risks have been thought to be justified because of the patients' diagnoses. Forney et al. noted that in 18 patients on prophylaxis there was no instance of postoperative febrile morbidity. However, of 14 women given placebos, six (43 per cent) developed febrile morbidity. While the number of patients in their study was small, the morbidity in the control group is comparable to that of vaginal hysterectomy alone without prophylaxis; further investigation with larger groups would certainly be warranted.

Postconceptional cerclage procedures for cervical incompetence are mentioned, also without any supporting data. It is suggested that when a degree of silent dilatation of the cervix has already occurred, exposing the dependent membranes to the cervicovaginal bacteria, focal chorioamnionitis may result, leading to rupture of the membranes as a mechanism of failure. There is no evidence to suggest that prophylactic antibiotics can in fact prevent this from occurring. Indeed it is possible that one may again in this case be dealing with established subclinical infection. Since the situation is relatively uncommon and the pregnancy risk high, it is unlikely that controlled clinical studies will be done.

Finally, in the case of abdominal hysterectomy, premature rupture of the membranes and infertility surgery, evidence to support the use of chemoprophylaxis does not seem to exist. In abdominal hysterectomy uncomplicated by pre-existent infection the rate of febrile postoperative morbidity is generally too low[52] to warrant prophylaxis, and when acute or subacute infection exists at the time of surgery it is therapeutic antibiotics, not prophylactic antibiotics, that are in order. As well, Ohm and Galask,[48] in evaluating the effect of prophylaxis on morbidity following total abdominal hysterectomy, found the data on febrile morbidity in the drug group in their study to be conflicting. This led them to suggest that the prophylactic drug may have altered the symptoms of infection or led to diagnostic confusion.

In the case of premature rupture of the membranes prophylactic antibiotics have been shown to be ineffectual in protecting the fetus, despite some reduction in postpartum endometritis.[32, 36] The reasons for the failure of fetal protection include the fact that the primary route of infecton for the fetus is via the amniotic fluid and the tracheobronchial tree and that amniotic fluid levels of antibiotics lag far behind fetal serum levels. Many investigators believe that, at least in late pregnancy, the amniotic fluid concentrations of antibiotics are achieved by fetal urination, accounting for this 4- to 5-hour lag. In addition, the distribution of the fetal circulation is such that blood flow is diverted away from the lung, the site of potential infections.

Many infertility surgeons employ prophylactic antibiotics at the time of tuboplasty or lysis of adhesions on the grounds that if an operative site infection does occur it would be disastrous and also because anti-inflammatory agents have sometimes been used concurrently. Until recently there have been no studies to support or refute this practice. However, a study at the Downstate Medical Center by Siegler and Kontopoulos, unpublished as of this writing, has shown no significant difference between control and study patients with a total of 85 patients. The study patients received a four-day course of cephalothin starting preoperatively. One might criticize this longer course as not being prophylactic but perhaps therapeutic. However, if anything, this longer course should make an even greater improvement in the results in the treated group. In viewing this preliminary data one might also suggest that the morbidity is so low to begin with that prophylaxis is difficult to justify.

Summary

To summarize, despite all the studies available, the only absolute indication for antibiotic prophylaxis in obstetrics and gynecology is prevention of subacute bacterial endocarditis. Good supportive data exist for use in premenopausal vaginal hysterectomy and perhaps in selective cases of cesarean section. In oncologic surgery, the application to total and posterior exenteration can be supported by the surgical literature, but there are no studies justifying the use in radical hysterectomy or vulvectomy, despite the fact that this is common practice. Finally, with regard to abdominal hysterectomy, premature rupture of the membranes and infertility surgery, the evidence available is to the contrary.

In arriving at a decision to utilize antibiotic prophylaxis in association with a surgical procedure, there are certain guidelines to be followed and these have been well stated by Ledger et al.[37] The following are the slightly modified guidelines proposed:

1. The procedure in question must be accompanied by a significant postoperative morbidity due to infection. This is obviously a matter for individual interpretation, but it is difficult to justify postoperative administration of antibiotics to all patients when risk of infection is low. An exception is in the case of subacute bacterial endocarditis, in which the infection is uniformly life-threatening.

2. The nature of the operation should be such that there is significant bacterial contamination of the operative site as an unavoidable occurrence.

3. The antibiotic selected should be effective against some but not necessarily all the potential opportunistic pathogens. The evidence for this lies in the fact that single drug prophylaxis, e.g., with a cephalosporin, has proved as effective in many cases as multiple drug regimens.

4. Best results are achieved when a tissue level of antibiotic is achieved at the operative site before operation is begun.

5. For most applications the short perioperative course is sufficient to provide true prophylaxis. Longer courses may be providing therapy rather than prevention. This latter approach may be justified in circumstances wherein established but subclinical infection is suspected.

6. The antibiotic selected should not be a "first-line" drug that might be needed to treat patients who are severely ill or have resistant infections.

7. There must be an ongoing program of surveillance of the antibiotic sensitivity patterns within the institution. It must be kept clearly in mind that the use of prophylactic antibiotics may have detrimental effects not only upon the patients receiving them but upon all patients in the hospital.

Finally, are there any reasonable alternatives to chemoprophylaxis in the patient at high risk for morbidity? One approach suggested by Swartz and co-workers[56, 57] in San Diego is to utilize suction drainage to reduce the accumulation of blood and serum that acts as a culture medium at the operative site. Their data would suggest an equivalent role for either suction drainage or antibiotics alone in decreasing postoperative infectious morbidity. Their study has also raised the possibility that a combination of suction drainage and antibiotics may act to decrease such morbidity even further. Other possibilities include timing of surgery when feasible to coincide with periods of more favorable indigenous flora or perhaps in some way to attempt manipulation of the flora by nonantibiotic means—for example, by endocrine manipulation—to produce a milieu less conducive to the presence of bacteria, especially anaerobes.

As with so many innovations in medicine, there are advantages as well as disadvantages. Early enthusiasm often yields to negative over-reaction and ultimately to what is a considered well-formulated position. Having been involved early on and throughout all the phases, the senior author feels a special obligation to attempt to place this rather controversial subject in a proper perspective and we hope we have done so.

REFERENCES

1. Allen, J., Rampone, J. and Wheeless, C.: Use of a prophylactic antibiotic in elective major gynecologic operations. Obstet. Gynecol. 39:218, 1972.
2. Atkinson, S. and Chappell, S.: Vaginal hysterectomy for sterilization. Obstet. Gynecol. 39:759, 1972.
3. Bolling, D. and Plunkett, S.: Prophylactic antibiotics for vaginal hysterectomies. Obstet. Gynecol. 41:689, 1973.
4. Boyd, M. and Garceau, R.: The value of prophylactic antibiotics after vaginal hysterectomy. Am. J. Obstet. Gynecol. 125:581, 1976.
5. Breeden, J. and Mayo, J.: Low-dose prophylactic antibiotics in vaginal hysterectomy. Obstet. Gynecol. 43:379, 1974.
6. Burke, J.: The effective period of preventive antibiotic action in experimental incisions and dermal lesions. Surgery 50:161, 1961.
7. Cavanagh, D. and Dahm, C.: The use of prophylactic antibiotics in obstetrics and gynecology. *In* Cavanagh, D., Rao, P., Camas, M., (eds.), Major Problems in Obstetrics and Gynecology, Vol. II. Philadelphia, W. B. Saunders Co., 1977, p. 123.
8. Cavanagh, D. and Rutledge, F.: The cervical cone biopsy-hysterectomy sequence and factors affecting the febrile morbidity. Am. J. Obstet. Gynecol. 80:53, 1960.
9. Cron, R., Stauffer, J. and Paegel, A.: Morbidity studies in 1000 consecutive hysterectomies. Am. J Obstet. Gynecol. 63:344, 1952.
10. De Swiet, M., Ramsay, I. D. and Rees, G. M.: Bacterial endocarditis after insertion of intrauterine contraceptive device. Br. Med. J. 3:76, 1975.
11. Everett, E. D., Reller, B., Droegemueller, W. and Greer, B.: Absence of bacteremia after insertion or removal of intrauterine devices. Obstet. Gynecol. 47:207, 1976.
12. Falk, A. and Bunkin, I.: A study of 500 vaginal hysterectomies. Am. J. Obstet. Gynecol. 52:623, 1946.
13. Forney, J., Morrow, P., Townsend, D. and DiSaia, P.: Impact of cephalosporin prophylaxis on conization—vaginal hysterectomy morbidity. Am. J. Obstet. Gynecol. 125:100, 1976.
14. Gassner, C. and Ledger, W.: The relationship of hospital-acquired maternal infection to invasive intrapartum monitoring techniques. Am. J. Obstet. Gynecol. 126:33, 1976.
15. George, J., Ansbacher, R., Otterson, W. and Rabey, F.: Prospective bacteriologic study of women undergoing hysterectomy. Obstet. Gynecol. 45:60, 1975.
16. Gibbs, R., DeCherney, A. and Schwarz, R. H.: Prophylactic antibiotics in cesarean section: A double-blind study. Am. J. Obstet. Gynecol. 114:1048, 1972.
17. Gibbs, R., Hunt, J. and Schwarz, R.: A follow-up study on prophylactic antibiotics in cesarean section. Am. J. Obstet. Gynecol. 117:419, 1973.
18. Gibbs, R. and Weinstein, A.: Puerperal infection in the antibiotic era. Am. J. Obstet. Gynecol. 124:769, 1976.
19. Gibbs, R. and Weinstein, A.: Bacteriologic effects of prophylactic antibiotics in cesarean section. Am. J. Obstet. Gynecol. 126:226, 1976.
20. Glover, M.and vanNagell J.: The effect of prophylactic ampicillin on pelvic infection following vaginal hysterectomy. Am. J. Obstet. Gynecol. 126:385, 1976.
21. Goodlin, R. C.: Prophylactic antibiotics. Obstet. Gynecol. 44:310, 1974.
22. Goosenberg, J., Emich, J. and Schwarz, R.: Prophylactic antibiotics in vaginal hysterectomy. Am. J. Obstet. Gynecol. 105:503, 1969.
23. Gorbach, S., Menda, K., Thadepalli, H. and Keith, L.: Anaerobic microflora of the cervix in healthy women. Am. J. Obstet. Gynecol. 117:1053, 1973.
24. Green, S. and Sarubbi, F.: Risk factors associated with postcesarean section febrile morbidity. Obstet. Gynecol. 49:686, 1977.
25. Green S., Sarubbi, F. and Bishop, E.: Prophylactic antibiotics in high-risk cesarean section. Obstet. Gynecol. 51:569, 1978.
26. Grossman, J., Adams, R., Hierholzer, W. and Andriole, V.: Endometrial and vaginal cuff bacteria recovered at elective hysterectomy during a trial of antibiotic prophylaxis. Am. J. Obstet. Gynecol. 130:312, 1978.
27. Grossman, J., Adams, R. and Hierholzer, W.: Epidemiologic surveillance during a clinical trial of antibiotic prophylaxis in pelvic surgery. Am. J Obstet. Gynecol. 128:690, 1977.
28. Harralson, J., vanNagell, J., Roddick, J. and Sprague, A.: The effect of prophylactic antibiotics on pelvic infection following vaginal hysterectomy. Am. J. Obstet. Gynecol. 120:1046, 1974.
29. Hilliard, G. and Harris, R.: Utilization of antibiotics for prevention of symptomatic postpartum infections. Obstet. Gynecol. 50:285, 1977.
30. Hodari, A. and Hodgkinson, P.: Iatrogenic bacteriuria and gynecologic surgery. Am. J. Obstet. Gynecol. 95:153, 1966.
31. Hodgson, J., Major, B., Portman, K. and Quattlebaum, F.: Prophylactic use of tetracycline for first trimester abortions. Obstet. Gynecol. 45:574, 1975.
32. Huff, R.: Antibiotic prophylaxis for puerperal endometritis following premature rupture of the membranes. J. Reprod. Med. 19:79, 1977.
33. Jackson, C. and Amstey, M.: Prophylactic ampicillin therapy for vaginal hysterectomy. Surg. Gynecol. Obstet. 141:755, 1975.
34. Kreutner, A. K., Del Bene, V., Delamar, D., Huguley, V., Harmon, P. and Mitchell, K.: Perioperative antibiotic prophylaxis in cesarean section. Obstet. Gynecol. 52:279, 1978.
35. Larsen, J., Weiss, K., Lenihan, J., Crumrine, M. and Heggers, J.: Significance of neutrophils and bacterial in the amniotic fluid of patients in labor. Obstet. Gynecol. 47:143, 1976.
36. Lebherz, T., Hellman, L., Madding, R., Anctil, A. and Arje, S.: Double-blind study of premature rupture of the membranes. Am. J. Obstet. Gynecol. 87:218, 1963.
37. Ledger, W., Gee, C. and Lewis, W.: Guidelines for antibiotic prophylaxis in gynecology. Am. J. Obstet. Gynecol. 121:1038, 1975.
38. Ledger, W., Kriewall, T. and Gee, C.: The fever index. A technic for evaluating the clinical response to bacteremia. Obstet. Gynecol. 45:603, 1975.
39. Ledger, W. and Puttler, O.: Death from pseudomembranous enterocolitis. Obstet. Gynecol. 45:609, 1975.
40. Ledger, W., Sweet, R. and Headington, J.: Prophylactic cephaloridine in the prevention of postoperative pelvic infections in premenopausal women undergoing vaginal hysterectomy. Am. J. Obstet. Gynecol. 115:766, 1973.
41. Lett, W., Ansbacher, R., Davison, B. and Otterson, W : Prophylactic antibiotics for women undergoing

vaginal hysterectomy. J. Reprod. Med. 19:51, 1977.

42. London, R., London, E., Siegelbaum, M. and Goldstein, P.: Use of doxycycline in elective first trimester abortion. South. Med. J. 71:672, 1978.

43. Miller, R. D. and Crichton, D.: Ampicillin prophylaxis in cesarean section. S. African J. Obstet. Gynaecol. 6:69, 1968.

44. Moro, M. and Andrews, M.: Prophylactic antibiotics in cesarean section. Obstet. Gynecol. 44:688, 1974.

45. Morrison, J., Coxwell, W., Kennedy, B., Schreier, P., Wiser, W. and Fish, S.: The use of prophylactic antibiotics in patients undergoing cesarean section. Surg. Gynecol. Obstet. 136:425, 1973.

46. Ohm, M. and Galask, R.: The effect of antibiotic prophylaxis on patients undergoing vaginal operations. I. The effect on morbidity. Am. J. Obstet. Gynecol. 123:590, 1975.

47. Ohm, M. and Galask, R.: The effect of antibiotic prophylaxis on patients undergoing vaginal operations. II. Alterations of microbial flora. Am. J. Obstet. Gynecol. 123:597, 1975.

48. Ohm, M. and Galask, R.: The effect of antibiotic prophylaxis on patients undergoing total abdominal hysterectomy. I. Effect on morbidity. Am. J. Obstet. Gynecol. 125:442, 1976.

49. Ohm, M. and Galask, R.: The effect of antibiotic prophylaxis on patients undergoing total abdominal hysterectomy. II. Alterations of microbial flora. Am. J. Obstet. Gynecol. 125:448, 1976.

50. Polk, H. and Lopez-Mayor, J.: Postoperative wound infection: A prospective study of determinant factors and prevention. Surgery 66:97, 1969.

51. Robert, J. and Homesley, H.: Low-dose carbenicillin prophylaxis for vaginal and abdominal hysterectomy. Obstet. Gynecol. 52:83, 1978.

52. Rosenheim, G.: Prophylactic antibiotics in elective abdominal hysterectomy. Am. J. Obstet. Gynecol. 119:335, 1974.

53. Rothbard, M., Mayer, W., Wystepek, A. and Gordon, M.: Prophylactic antibiotics in cesarean section. Obstet. Gynecol. 45:421 1975.

54. Sengupta, B. S., Wyner, H. H., Hall, S. J. et al.: Prophylactic antibiotic in elective gynaecological and obstetrical major surgery. Int. J. Gynaecol. Obstet. 14:417, 1976.

55. Sprague, A. and vanNagell, J.: The relationship of age and endometrial histology to blood loss and morbidity following vaginal hysterectomy. Am. J. Obstet. Gynecol. 118:805, 1974.

56. Swartz, W. and Tanaree, P.: Suction drainage as an alternative to prophylactic antibiotics for hysterectomy. Obstet. Gynecol. 45:305, 1975.

57. Swartz, W. and Tanaree, P.: T-tube suction drainage and/or prophylactic antibiotics. A randomized study of 451 hysterectomies. Obstet. Gynecol. 47:665, 1976.

58. Turner, S.: The effect of penicillin vaginal suppositories on morbidity in vaginal hysterectomy and on the vaginal flora. Am. J. Obstet. Gynecol. 60:806, 1950.

59. vanNagell, J., Roddick, J. Cooper, R. and Triplett, H.: Vaginal hysterectomy following conization in treatment of carcinoma in situ of the cervix. Am. J. Obstet. Gynecol. 113:948, 1972.

60. Wang, R., Gee, C. and Ledger, W.: Prophylactic use of cefazolin in monitored obstetric patients undergoing cesarean section. Obstet. Gynecol. 51(4):407, April 1978.

61. Weissberg, S., Edwards, L. and O'Leary, J.: Prophylactic antibiotics in cesarean section. Obstet. Gynecol. 38:290, 1971.

Editorial Comment

Most of us were taught that the use of antibiotics in a prophylactic manner was not only practicing medicine with no scientific basis but also that such practice would do harm by causing superinfections and resistant strains of organisms. Although there is a continued need to do longitudinal studies in regard to resistant strains developing after prophylactic antibiotic therapy there has been no great evidence to that effect and certainly superinfections are not a problem caused by prophylactic use.

It does appear that prophylactic antibiotics do not sufficiently reduce infection in routine vaginal hysterectomy, in premature rupture of the membranes or in infertility surgery. There does appear to be slightly less endometritis following antibiotic use in premature rupture of the membranes but no protection seems to be afforded the infant.

The problem we are discussing may well be a problem of semantics, because prophylaxis may be an ill-chosen word. Is this issue of use of prophylactic antibiotics still a controversy? Recent studies have indicated that staff patients with ruptured membranes and protracted labor who eventually came to cesarean childbirth have more than a 50 per cent chance of developing sepsis in the postoperative period. Is this then really prophylaxis or therapy to use antibiotics, since we now have data based upon known predicted statistics? A new investigative effort is now under study in the use of copious lavage of either saline or antibiotics in the uterine cavity at cesarean section. These preliminary results look promising and if the data hold up the method will provide a topical, mechanical method of diminishing sepsis that may eliminate the need for parenteral therapy.

It is no longer recommended that antibiotics be "hung" once general anesthesia begins. There have been at least four cases of death due to this practice—the reason is unknown. The patient should either receive therapy before or after the general anesthesia. The cause for this anaphylactic-like reaction is still unknown.

It is now our practice that if we are going to use "prophylactic antibiotics" that these be given "on call" to the operating room along with the preoperative medication. The antibiotic regimen is continued for no longer than 48 hours, since this is all the time needed for therapy. This difference of opinion of the time needed to treat or prevent sepsis is certainly new thinking. If we had only observed the lesson of our patients who had urinary tract infections, they would have taught us the same thing because most are asymptomatic by 48 hours, and the additional eight days of therapy will only improve the statistics by 10 per cent. The current concept of therapy should be large doses of antibiotics for no longer than 48 hours. It will take time and good clinical observations to see whether all of this new thinking is correct.

No matter how good the antibiotics seem to be, the surgical dictums of the past still take precedence, i.e., impeccable hemostasis and good drainage.

17
Endoscopy in Obstetrics and Gynecology

Alternative Points of View

by Luis A. Cibils
by Moon H. Kim
by David Pent

Editorial Comment

Endoscopy in Obstetrics and Gynecology

Luis A. Cibils, M.D.
The University of Chicago

The direct visualization of the female pelvic organs by means of optic instruments (besides laparotomy) may be accomplished at almost any stage of the vital cycle of a woman, with the exception of advanced pregnancy. On the other hand, the uterus may be viewed from the inside by insertion of appropriate optic instruments. These maneuvers constitute the areas of endoscopy applied to obstetrics and gynecology.

The visualization of the pelvic organs may be approached from either the abdominal or the vaginal route, thereby distinguishing the two techniques of laparoscopy and culdoscopy. Both give relatively easy access to the pelvic organs but they are technically rather different, and their clinical indications are not the same. For this reason they are discussed separately and their advantages and inconveniences pointed out.

Laparoscopy

When the optic instrument is introduced through the anterior abdominal wall the procedure is called laparoscopy, celioscopy or peritoneoscopy. First attempted in the early part of this century, it did not become an accepted technique in gynecology until the last decade. Either local or general anesthesia may be used, depending upon the indication and patient's cooperation. With the patient in supine position the orientation of the surgeon during the procedure is easy because it is exactly as during laparotomy.

INDICATIONS

Laparoscopy may be used for diagnostic as well as therapeutic purposes, and the benefits derived from it depend upon the skill and restraint of the surgeon. Properly applied it is relatively simple and may clarify diagnostic problems in a short time with minimal inconvenience to the patient. However, faulty technique or incorrect patient selection may create serious complications that should be completely preventable.

Its first indication in gynecology was in evaluation of the infertile patient. Currently it is a mandatory step in the adequate assessment of these patients, particularly as preoperatory evaluation prior to tubal surgery. It helps to avoid unnecessary laparotomy in a high percentage of patients in whom the pathology is so extensive that the chances of success are minimal.

In cases of amenorrhea, primary or secondary, it may be used to define etiology when malformations of internal genitalia are observed. In addition, biopsies may be taken for histologic studies of the gonads.

The most frequent indication of this procedure as a diagnostic tool in general gynecology is in cases of suspected ectopic pregnancy. With it prolonged periods of observation and uncertainty of the past are avoided, as is unnecessary laparotomy.

The presence of relatively small adnexal masses at pelvic examination often requires visual inspection for accurate diagnosis.

In many circumstances, acute salpingitis has been observed when the procedure has been done for clarification of sudden, obscure lower abdominal pain. Numbers of the group of patients with unexplained pelvic pain have been greatly reduced with the advent of laparoscopy, because it often has helped to diagnose cases of unsuspected endometriosis, pelvic congestion, chronic salpingo-oophoritis of various etiologies and so forth. It has also been applied in cases of uterine perforation during curettage when either intra-abdominal hemorrhage or bowel damage is suspected. It can help in making a rapid diagnosis and often prevent unwarranted laparotomy. In gynecologic oncology it has been used to evaluate the results of treatment in ovarian carcinomas as a substitute for "second-look" operations.

Many relatively minor surgical procedures may be carried out in conjunction with laparoscopy, such as ovarian biopsy, division of adhesions, electrocoagulation of small endometriotic foci or cauterization of bleeding follicles or corpora lutea.

Aspiration of ascitic fluid to collect a specimen for cytologic study has been done by some, as well as aspiration of fluid from small ovarian cysts.

The removal of intra-abdominal foreign bodies (intrauterine contraceptive devices) is a relatively frequent therapeutic manipulation done by laparoscopy instead of laparotomy, when a "lost IUD" is documented to be in the peritoneal cavity.

The most frequent indication of laparoscopy for therapeutic purposes is to produce permanent sterilization. Currently there are several techniques to accomplish this, among them electrocauterization of the fallopian tubes and application of clips or bands of synthetic material. A few operators have carried out successfully more complicated surgical procedures such as suspension of the uterus, catheterization of tubes, collection of ova and even appendectomy.

CONTRAINDICATIONS

In only a few circumstances is there a contraindication to laparoscopy. Furthermore, the contraindications may be relative but on occasion they may be absolute.

Absolute contraindications may be encountered when pathologic states hinder the mechanical manipulations necessary for a technically good procedure. The production of a good pneumoperitoneum is hindered by heart failure, conditions that diminish the pulmonary capacity and the presence of a diaphragmatic hernia. The introduction of the sharp trocar may be dangerous when there is generalized peritonitis, bowel distension from other diseases, advanced gestation, and a history of intra-abdominal pathology that produces extensive adhesions. The most important contraindication, however, is lack of experience in the operator.

Relative contraindications are more common and may not necessarily be observed by experienced and careful operators. Among these one may cite the presence of abdominal scars from previous operations, excessive obesity, and a history of extensive pelvic infection or a previous failure, particularly in the hand of an experienced endoscopist.

FAILURES

From the survey of the published reports it seems that the incidence of failure to visualize the pelvic cavity is in the range of 1 in 40 to 1 in 2000, the overall average being approximately 1 in 250. In our own hospital this has been 2 in 5000. The causes are varied, but the most common one is the subperitoneal injection of gas with subsequent improper insertion of the trocar. Most often this is the result of inexperience on the part of the operator, but on occasion it could be due to poor selection of patients (ignoring certain contraindications). Unrecognized malfunctioning of the equipment could also be the cause of failed procedures.

INSTRUMENTATION

The extraordinary variety of instruments available may be confusing for the uninitiated, but it is possible to perform diagnostic laparoscopy with only a few of them. The essential ones include a light source to which the fiber glass cable should be connected. The caliber of this depends upon the number of fibers encased (in the cable and the optic). These fibers control the amount of light transmitted; for viewing, only a small 2.5 to 4.5 mm diameter may be sufficient but for photography the larger ones need to be used.

The gas insufflator has to be provided with safety devices to prevent too-rapid injection and excessive pressure in order to avoid some of the most dangerous complications.

The optic should be adequate for the purpose of either viewing or obtaining photographs, the ones with 10 mm diameter being necessary for the latter. The angle of vision could be "direct" (180°), right angle (90°), or intermediate (oblique 135°), the direct one being the most common and easy to use because no special training is needed for appropriate orientation of the images. The models with angulated vision distort somewhat the anatomic view of the pelvic organs, and some training is required before the operator feels at ease with them. The so-called operating laparoscopes carry an accessory tube through which the operating instrument is introduced and manipulated.

The needle to produce pneumoperitoneum should preferably be the Verres type, provided with a blunt inner "cannula-lead;" however, some operators feel satisfied with using a simple spinal needle with a Touhey tip. The extra safety provided by the blunt spring-controlled lead of special needles is worth the difference in cost.

The trocar and cannula (or sleeve) should be the exact caliber to house the optic. The tip of the trocar could be conical or pyramidal with sharp edges, the latter being preferable. An accessory trocar, for the second puncture, allows the introduction of instruments to either manipulate the pelvic organs or execute surgical procedures.

The accessory instruments are innumerable and have been designed for every specialized purpose imaginable. Most often used and versatile are Palmer or Eder biopsy tongs, cautery guns, punch biopsy forceps, a great variety of electrodes and needles as well as scissors and grasping forceps and band applicators. When electrosurgery is to be performed, an electrosurgical unit is necessary to provide current for either unipolar or bipolar instruments.

TECHNIQUES

ANESTHESIA. Laparoscopy may be performed under either local or general anesthesia, depending upon the indication for the procedure, the patient's cooperation and condition and the availability of equipment. Some operators prefer to do it under local anesthesia, particularly when operating on patients in semiambulatory clinics. Others prefer general anesthesia with endotracheal intubation and hyperventilation in order to obtain a better pelvic view and avoid some of the problems of intra-abdominal injection of carbon dioxide under pressure. This technical requirement facilitates the production of hypercarbia because of rapid absorption of carbon dioxide from the peritoneal cavity. On the other hand, its great solubility in plasma is the reason for choosing carbon dioxide as a safe gas for insufflation. Attempts at using nitrous oxide have not been satisfactory, and currently carbon dioxide is practically the gas of choice for pneumoperitoneum.

General Anesthesia. With endotracheal intubation, this produces much better relaxation and control of respiratory and circulatory parameters, all of which facilitate performing ancillary operatory maneuvers under laparoscopy. It also prevents excessive hypercarbia, often observed under general anesthesia and spontaneous respiration, a situation further facilitated by using the Trendelenburg position required for adequate visualization of pelvic organs.

Local Anesthesia. A number of experienced laparoscopists prefer to use local anesthesia with good premedication, thus avoiding the possible complications of general anesthesia. This type of anesthesia is particularly suited for procedures done under semiambulatory conditions in which the surgeon deals with healthy young individuals with a minimal likelihood of complications. The only disadvantage is that it requires full patient cooperation, even when she develops the nagging feeling of "fullness" produced by the intra-abdominal injection of gas under pressure. The dull pain produced by cauterization or tubal clipping is not prevented unless local anesthetic is injected over the area to be manipulated.

Other anesthetic techniques such as conduction anesthesia (spinal, caudal, epidural) or so-called neuroleptanalgesia are used by some, but they constitute a small proportion of all techniques used in laparoscopy.

PNEUMOPERITONEUM. An extremely important step is aimed at facilitating the safe insertion of the trocar through the abdominal wall. To adequately accomplish this, the gas-injecting needle must be introduced into the peritoneal cavity where the unhindered gas flow should distend it symmetrically. There are at least three spots where the needle may be safely inserted to avoid abdominal wall vessels and intra-abdominal organs. Two of them located on the abdominal wall are shown in Figure 1, the subumbilical one being the most commonly used, in spite of the fact that it is less convenient and leads to more difficulties and complications than the other two. The left subcostal point is very safe; with it the penetration of each wall layer is perfectly controlled, the peritoneum being firmly attached to the fascia and therefore penetrated with ease (Fig. 2). The preferred point should be the posterior vaginal fornix, with which every house staff member is familiar from doing culdocentesis. In order to facilitate a successful insertion, the uterus must be moved against the anterior abdominal wall to unfold the pouch of Douglas; this is accomplished by using the intrauterine cannula and lifting it until the uterus is seen pushing above the pubis. The insertion of the needle is then simple (Fig. 3). Once the tip of the needle is in the peritoneum the carbon dioxide line is connected and the insufflation continued until a satisfactory distension has been obtained. This may require anywhere between 2.5 to 6 liters, variable with each individual, but not a fixed volume as so often suggested in many writings or teaching movies. An intra-abdominal pressure between 15 and 20 mg Hg is safe for the patient and satisfactory in obtaining good abdominal wall resistance.

When there are abdominal scars, and the likelihood of bowel adhesions exists, it is important to ascertain that adhesions are not present at the spot where the trocar is to be introduced. For this purpose, a well-lubricated glass syringe with a no. 18 or 20 needle

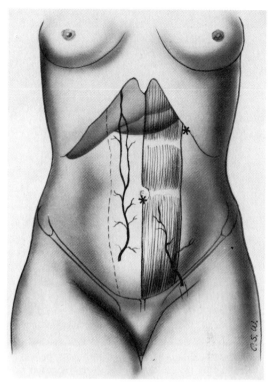

Figure 1. Schematic drawing showing the principal vessels supplying the anterior abdominal wall. On the left side of the patient is shown the superficial epigastric artery running superficial to the rectus abdominis. The right side, the rectus removed, shows running within its fascia but behind the muscle, the epigastric anastomosing with the internal mammary and their branches. The upper part projects the edges of the liver and greater curvature of the stomach. The points of choice for insertion of pneumoperitoneum needle are shown on the left subcostal margin and lower rim of umbilicus. (From Cibils, L.A.: Gynecologoic Laparoscopy. Diagnostic and Operatory. Philadelphia, Lea & Febiger, 1975.)

is inserted where the tip of the trocar is expected to penetrate the peritoneum (Fig. 4), usually about 3 to 4 cm below the entrance in the skin because of the slanted direction of the wound. When the needle enters the abdominal cavity, with carbon dioxide under pressure, the plunger will be quickly pushed up, whereas if it enters the lumen of an adherent bowel it will not be pushed up because of the lack of pressure in it. In that case, another site should be tested until a free space is found and only then the trocar inserted.

THE TROCAR. After the skin incision has been made, the trocar is fully held with the stronger hand, with the tip directed toward the center of the pelvis. The other hand *does*

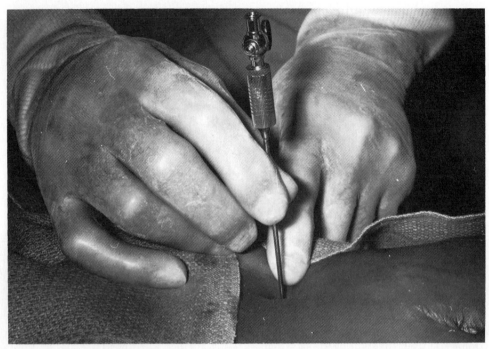

Figure 2. Technique of inserting the Veress needle on the left upper quadrant: perpendicular needle held from the middle by the hand "resting" over the costal margin. Only the fingers push the needle while the index of the other hand identifies the edge of the rib cage. (From Cibils, L.A.: Gynecologic Laparoscopy. Diagnostic and Operatory. Philadelphia, Lea & Febiger, 1975.)

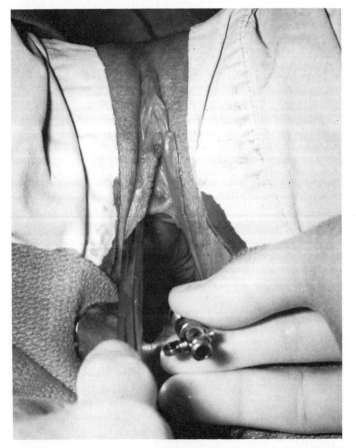

Figure 3. Inserting the pneumoperitoneum needle through the cul-de-sac. The operator "lifts" the uterus, with the intrauterine instrument, against the anterior abdominal wall opening the pouch of Douglas. The needle, held from below the hub for free movement of the stylet, is directed horizontally about 1 cm from the vaginal insertion and penetrates only 2 cm before the stylet springs free into the peritoneal cavity. (From Cibils, L.A.: Gynecologic Laparoscopy. Diagnostic and Operatory. Philadelphia, Lea & Febiger, 1975.)

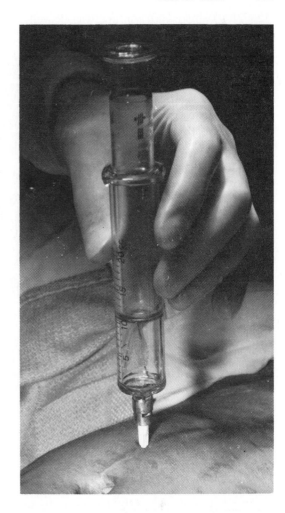

Figure 4. To test for possible bowel adhesions after good, symmetric distension, a well-lubricated syringe with a No. 20 needle, 50 cm long, is inserted perpendicular to the skin where the tip of the trocar is expected to enter the peritoneum (usually 3 to 4 cm below the skin incision). The plunger will be pushed up by the increased intraperitoneal gas under pressure. If the tip of the needle falls within bowel lumen or omental adhesion the plunger will not move, indicating the need to look for another point free from adhesions. (From Cibils, L.A.: Gynecologic Laparoscopy. Diagnostic and Operatory. Philadelphia, Lea & Febiger, 1975.)

not grab the abdominal wall but controls the movement of the sleeve (Fig. 5) to prevent any sudden penetration into the abdomen. Penetration should be obtained by a steady pressure of the pushing hand. (At no time in laparoscopy is a thrust with the instruments required; on the contrary, all gestures must be gentle, smooth and steady.) When the tip has penetrated the abdomen, the sleeve is pushed in while the trocar is held with the other hand, and then the optic, connected to the light source, is substituted. Recently Dingfelder has suggested the insertion of the trocar without prior pneumoperitoneum, an "innovation" taking us back to Jacobaeus. This may be successful in many cases but is definitely less safe than previous distension of the abdominal wall, which separates the wall from its contents and gives good resistance against the pushing instrument. Changes in technique should be introduced for a useful reason, not for the sake of doing it differently.

The second trocar, used routinely for operative laparoscopy, should always be introduced under direct visual control of the operator. The preferred site is the midline, which gives equally good access to both adnexa and is minimally vascularized, in contrast to the paramedian site, supplied by important vessels (see Fig. 1) and their branches. After the skin incision has been made, the instrument is pushed straight down, with either the little or the middle finger extended as "stopper" to avoid sudden penetration; this usually separates the peritoneum from the wall because here it is very loosely attached. This fact requires that patience be exercised for a smooth and complete penetration of the sleeve, which tends to "hook" in the peritoneum and pull it away. After complete penetration the operating instrument is substituted while the assistant manipulates the intrauterine instrument under the direction of the surgeon.

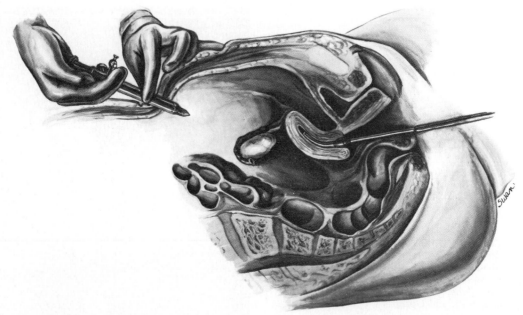

Figure 5. Schematic sagittal section of the female lower abdomen illustrating the safety precaution when the main trocar is inserted at the subumbilical point. Over one third of the instrument penetrates, slanted, before the tip perforates the peritoneum and the sleeve enters a bit. Note that two fingers of the free hand hold the trocar sleeve at all times to make for a controlled smooth penetration and prevent any sudden passage. Any further penetration of the trocar beyond this point only endangers the intraperitoneal organs. What should be done is to push in the sleeve, holding the trocar firm in its place. (From Cibils, L.A.: Gynecologic Laparoscopy. Diagnostic and Operatory. Philadelphia, Lea & Febiger, 1975.)

DIAGNOSTIC

Perhaps the most frequent indication for diagnostic laparoscopy is the complaint by the patient of lower abdominal pain. This may be either chronic or acute. In order to adequately diagnose the abnormal condition, the operator must be thoroughly familiar with the images of normal anatomic formations and their changes throughout the ovarian cycle.

CHRONIC PELVIC PAIN. This may be produced by a variety of pathologic conditions, the precise diagnosis being established only after visual inspection of the pelvis. Pelvic inflammatory disease is the most commonly given diagnosis in outpatient clinics of large university hospitals. It is true that often there is good history of previous pelvic infection and perhaps objective findings; however, often there is nothing to justify that diagnosis.

Chronic salpingitis may be experienced only as peritubo-ovarian adhesions, or it may be manifested as a bilateral hydrosalpinx (Fig. 6), usually with peritubal adhesions. When the tension within the tube is not high, these cases may be completely unsuspected. Less frequently observed are cases of tuberculous

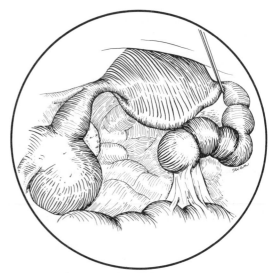

Figure 6. Panoramic view of uterus and tubes of a 27-year-old patient who never practiced contraception and had lower abdominal pain, and overdue menstrual period. To rule out ectopic pregnancy a laparoscopy was done; it revealed these dilated tubes of pale color, with peritubal adhesions to small bowel and uterus. The right side, pulled with the probe, is club-like and hides the ovary. The left, more distended, allows partial view of the ovary. Bilateral hydrosalpinx. (From Cibils, L.A.: Gynecologic Laparoscopy. Diagnostic and Operatory. Philadelphia, Lea & Febiger, 1975.)

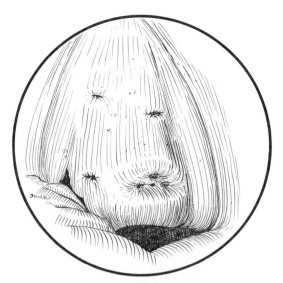 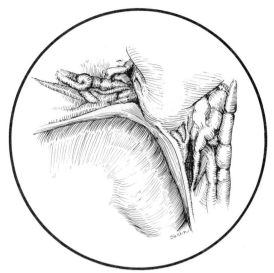

Figure 7. A 23-year-old woman, gravida 1, para 1, with persistent abdominal pain without dysmenorrhea. Close-up view of the pouch of Douglas outlined by sharp, normal uterosacral ligaments. Several dots of scar-like tissue break what should be a smooth peritoneal surface. At the bottom there is a small pool of blood collected after freeing the adherent ovary to endometriotic foci. Endometriosis of ovary and Douglas. (From Cibils, L.A.: Gynecologic Laparoscopy. Diagnostic and Operatory. Philadelphia, Lea & Febiger, 1975.)

Figure 8. A 22-year-old woman, gravida 3, para 2, with chronic pelvic pain suspected of having pelvic inflammatory disease. At laparoscopy the tubes and ovaries were free but the vessels of the broad ligament were markedly dilated as seen here, above sharp uterosacral ligaments and clean Douglas. Note the tortuous course of the vessels. Severe pelvic congestion. (From Cibils, L.A.: Gynecologic Laparoscopy. Diagnostic and Operatory. Philadelphia, Lea & Febiger, 1975.)

salpingitis, the confirmation of which requires a biopsy and identification of the acid-fast bacillus.

Among the noninfectious causes of chronic pelvic pain, endometriosis must be the most common pathologic condition (Fig. 7). The incidence of endometriosis has risen dramatically since the advent of widespread use of laparoscopy, because all the cases in early stages previously unsuspected or unconfirmed are now easily observed and are amenable to specific treatment.

Another condition, only vaguely mentioned in the past, is now a clinical reality when observed directly: pelvic congestion (Fig. 8) may mimic almost any syndrome and carries with it a number of distressing secondary effects such as dyspareunia, anorgasmia, chronic discharge and dysuria.

When none of these conditions is observed, attention should be turned to the appendix, which may show signs of chronic infection (adhesions, increased consistency, localized congestion).

If all accessible organs look normal the patient at least benefits from the certainty of excluding the possible diagnoses, and only

then the tentative diagnosis of idiopathic pelvic pain may be justified. (In older patients inspection of the sigmoid may disclose the presence of asymptomatic chronically inflamed diverticuli.)

ACUTE PELVIC PAIN. Laparoscopy has been such an important new aid in diagnosis that it is almost inconceivable now to observe a patient for more than 24 hours without making a firm diagnosis. Acute salpingitis is often suspected, but when the clinical picture is not very clear a laparoscopy may either confirm it or find another condition.

This has often been the acutely inflamed appendix, hidden behind bowels. When the adnexa appear normal it is mandatory to expose the whole length of the appendix because severe acute appendicitis can often be limited to the distal half of the organ.

In cases of suspected ectopic pregnancy, with or without positive culdocentesis, laparoscopy confirms the diagnosis (Fig. 9) or clarifies the source of pain or bleeding or both. The problem could be a bleeding corpus luteum, a ruptured follicle or passage of endometrial blood into the pelvic cavity (Fig. 10). Other conditions of acute pelvic pain have

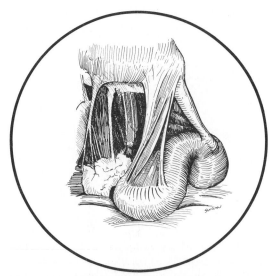

Figure 9. A 31-year-old woman, gravida 1, para 0, admitted for laparoscopy because she had passed "decidua" histologically, and was 8 weeks past her last menstrual period. Pregnancy test was negative and continuous spotting was present. This view of the uterine fundus and right tube shows this to be dilated, sausage shaped and with loose adhesions. It was burgundy color but there was no blood in the peritoneum. Unruptured ectopic pregnancy. (From Cibils, L.A.: Gynecologic Laparoscopy. Diagnostic and Operatory. Philadelphia, Lea & Febiger, 1975.)

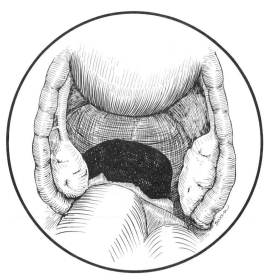

Figure 10. A 28-year-old woman, gravida 2, para 2, admitted for laparoscopy because of menometrorrhagia and diffuse pelvic pain at examination. Perfectly normal-appearing uterus, ovaries and tubes with non-clotted blood were seen in the pelvis. This was slowly dripping from the left tube, which, at "palpation" with the forceps, was normal in consistency, shape and size. At D&C "multiple endometrial polyps" was reported. Thus this was a case of menstrual blood in the peritoneal cavity. (From Cibils, L.A.: Gynecologic Laparoscopy. Diagnostic and Operatory. Philadelphia, Lea & Febiger, 1975.)

been clarified at laparoscopy, such as twisted adnexa, unsuspected uterine perforations and ruptured "chocolate" cysts. In acute pelvic pain, unless the diagnosis is clear, there is no justification in procrastinating for hours when a carefully executed laparoscopy can facilitate a precise diagnosis and a rapid, specific treatment.

MALFORMATIONS. The frustrating group of syndromes characterized by primary amenorrhea due to congenital anomalies of the genitalia became easier to diagnose with the advent of laparoscopy. In the past, after cumbersome and expensive work-ups, only laparotomy would really produce the diagnosis. Now it is possible to make a diagnosis in the early stages of a work-up with minimal inconvenience to the patient, when biopsies may be taken and further tests decided upon. Not infrequently the pelvic examination may be quite unrevealing because of the presence of a large uterus, but visual inspection and eventual biopsy may be definitive (Fig. 11). The whole gamut of incomplete development of genitalia may be observed, up to total agenesis of the uterus. When the diagnosis of testicular feminization syndrome is suspected (Fig. 12) it may be confirmed with a biopsy.

INFERTILITY WORK-UP. Laparoscopy is a necessary step for a complete work-up of the infertile patient and may be performed at different stages of the cycle, depending upon the history. As mentioned earlier, in cases of primary amenorrhea laparoscopy may be done as the first and definite step, whereas in cases of secondary amenorrhea or proven tubal factors it may be done before a surgical procedure to more precisely ascertain the extent of the problem and establish a prognosis. Often, when all tests are negative, a laparoscopy may reveal unsuspected endometriosis. It is a good practice at the same session to test tubal potency by injecting dye through the intrauterine cannula; this will confirm the patency previously found by hysterosalpingogram (HSG) or will demonstrate the exact point of obstruction when occlusion has been diagnosed by HSG. If the extension of peritubo-ovarian adhesions is minimal the prognosis may be excellent, while if they are extensive any attempt at corrective surgery may be futile and can thus be avoided.

ONCOLOGY WORK-UP. When intraperitoneal cancer, particularly early stages of ovarian cancer, is suspected, a laparoscopy gives the opportunity to survey the extent of the process and obtain biopsies for completing the work-

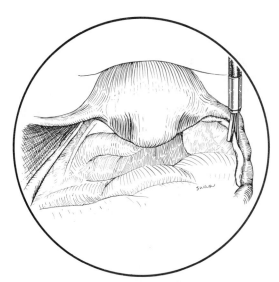

Figure 11. A 30-year-old patient with primary amenorrhea, normal external genitalia and palpable uterus. This is borderline small in size, with normal-appearing tubes. In place of the ovaries a pair of white streaks were seen, the one on the right held by the forceps; biopsied they were reported: "fibrous streaks, primary atrophy of ovary." Karyotyping was 46, XX, normal female, thus indicating that this was a case of primary ovarian failure. (From Cibils, L.A.: Gynecologic Laparoscopy. Diagnostic and Operatory. Philadelphia, Lea & Febiger, 1975.)

up and prognosis. However, laparoscopy is more useful in therapeutic oncology as a means to assess the success of a treatment, either radiation or chemotherapy (primary or complementary to surgery), instead of so-called second-look laparotomies. Under these conditions, extreme care must be exercised because of the possibility of adhesions against abdominal wall or between bowels and omentum.

BIOPSIES. Relatively often obtaining biopsy specimens is necessary in diagnostic laparoscopy; all endoscopists should be adequately trained in obtaining these. The most frequently biopsied organ is the ovary, which is also the most difficult to obtain a specimen from, unless the surgeon resorts to technical manipulations to expose and fix it properly. This should be attempted only through the "two-puncture" technique—that is, with accessory entrance for the forceps. With a grasping forceps the ovary must be taken and pulled out toward the center of the pelvis from its position under the tube. Then the uterus should be pushed back and against the corresponding lateral pelvic wall to serve as support for the ovary, which must "rest" on top of it. At this point the biopsy forceps is substituted for the grasping tool and the bites taken (Fig. 13). (During these steps the uterus must re-

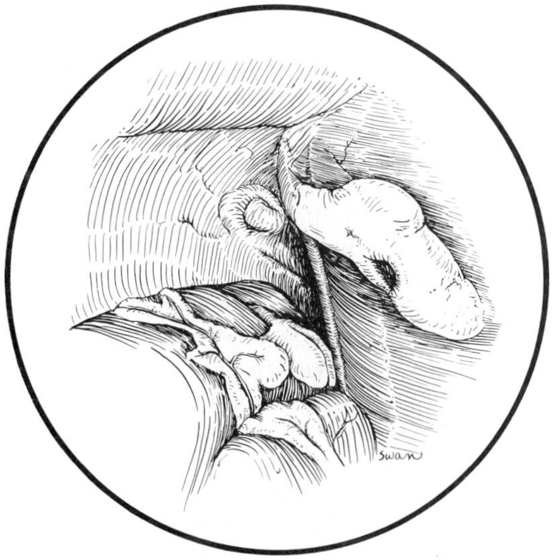

Figure 12. A 17-year-old patient with primary amenorrhea and absence of vagina, suspected of testicular feminization syndrome (46, XY karotype). The uterus and tubes were absent. Two gonads were present at the normal sites, the right one seen here with biopsy spot close to sigmoid. The frozen section, reported "primitive testicular tubules showing only Sertolli cells," confirmed the diagnosis. (From Cibils, L.A.: Gynecologic Laparoscopy. Diagnostic and Operatory. Philadelphia, Lea & Febiger, 1975.)

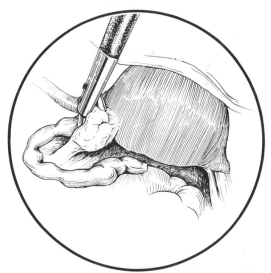

Figure 13. Technique of ovarian biopsy. The uterus is pushed against the hollow of the sacrum and the left side of the pelvis after the ovary had been "pulled-out" with the Palmer forceps and released, well exposed. In this view the Siegler forceps is biting on the anti-hilus side of the ovary to cut a specimen. If needed, after removing the specimen, the same forceps may be used to cauterize the crater. (From Cibils, L.A.: Gynecologic Laparoscopy. Diagnostic and Operatory. Philadelphia, Lea & Febiger, 1975.)

main fixed.) Occasionally there will be some oozing from the biopsy site and this needs to be cauterized with the tip of the forceps placed into the crater of the wound. When hemostasis is good the procedure is terminated. The specimen then is processed: either fixed for histologic study or seeded in tissue culture media if chromosomal studies are to be done or in bacteria culture media if bacteriologic tests are necessary.

When suspicious lesions are found in the peritoneal cavity or pelvic organs, they may be biopsied as well for appropriate studies, always taking into consideration that electro-coagulation may be necessary to obtain good hemostasis. Therefore, bowel lesions or those close to large vessels are not amenable to laparoscopic biopsy.

THERAPEUTIC

A number of definitive therapeutic procedures that in the past were possible only after laparotomy may now be safely performed under laparoscopy, with less physical discomfort and cost to the patient.

PERMANENT STERILIZATION. The extraordinary popularity of laparoscopy was mainly due to its application as a technique for sterilization. This may be performed with several techniques, the differences being established according to how the tubes are treated.

Cauterization. Using coagulation current the tubes are cauterized in either one or several spots. For some physicians this is sufficient to obtain occlusion of the tubes, while for the majority sectioning of the cauterized area (with or without removal of a piece of tube) is necessary in order to complete the operation. From experience in my institution and from reviewing the published reports, I believe that section and recauterization of the stumps (Fig. 14) gives additional chances of success in preventing pregnancy.

This procedure is usually performed between menstrual periods (so-called interval period), as a complement of voluntary abortion or in the early puerperal stage. (In the latter circumstance it seems to be a technical "acrobatic" procedure because a minilaparotomy is technically simpler, and not more physically taxing to the patient. Furthermore, the complications seem to be higher when operation is done in the puerperium.) The results are very satisfactory, the pregnancy rate (intrauterine or ectopic) being in the range of 0.5

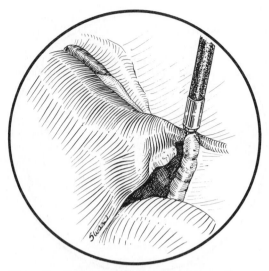

Figure 14. Technique of tubal cauterization. The tube is taken close to the uterus, held up isolated, and current passed. After blanching it may be cut, as shown in this view where the uterine side of the specimen has already been sectioned. To obtain a specimen, the other side must also be divided. It is a good practice to recauterize the uterine stump. Note the round ligament behind the forceps. (From Cibils, L.A.: Gynecologic Laparoscopy. Diagnostic and Operatory. Philadelphia, Lea & Febiger, 1975.)

to 1 per thousand. The majority of failures are due to the technical error of cauterizing the round ligaments instead of the tube, which thus remains patent.

The still more common way of applying current involves use of the unipolar electrode, with the inactive one applied on the patient's thigh or back. However, it is safer to use the now-available bipolar electrodes in which both electrodes are applied against the held tube, which is the only part of the patient through which current passes. This is a very important improvement to prevent accidental burning.

Clips. With the aim of avoiding the inherent danger of accidental burns, Hulka developed a gold-covered plastic clip to be applied at laparoscopy. After successful testing in animals it was applied to humans and the experience seems to be satisfactory. It may be applied with the two-puncture technique or with the operating laparoscope, requiring a larger trocar and sleeve than the standard. It seems to have an advantage over the other methods in that it has almost no chance of complications: a recent publication by Hulka reported no bleeding or other complications, which were still present in operations done with the other methods.

Bands. With the same purpose of preventing intra-abdominal burns, Yoon designed and tested a small vinyl ring to be applied to a loop of the tube with a special applicator, which may be used with either the two-puncture technique or the operating scope. As for all operatory procedures, it is preferable to use two separate sleeves for optic and operating instruments because this gives the operator a much better view and control of what is done. Application of the band is easy, safe and effective, provided all technical details are followed carefully. The special applicator has blunted prongs with which the tube only must be taken, and after adequate identification, this is slowly and gently pulled into the hollow of the applicator. There must not be resistance to this maneuver because the instrument has been designed to take in normal tubes. If there is tubal pathology, either thickening or adhesions, this will interfere with the "taking-in" effect of pulling and the tube may be lacerated, causing bleeding. (If there is evidence of this type of pathology, an alternative technique of treating the tubes should be used.) When the loop of tube is fully taken in, the band should be delivered by further pull on the prongs against the spring. The release of the ring can be seen clearly when separate sleeves are used for the operation, but this is impossible when the operating scope is used.

A final step to ascertain the successful application of the band is to slowly release the loop out of the hollow and inspect both parts of the tube before it is completely dropped (Fig. 15). When the operator does not take precautions to be sure of what was taken and "ligated," an incomplete taking of the tube or incorrect ligation may be overlooked. In Figure 16 is shown one such case in which the infundibulopelvic ligament on one side was mistaken for the tube and the band applied, leaving the tube on that side intact. The patient became pregnant two cycles later. Reapplication was performed along with voluntary abortion; the tube of the other side had been properly ligated.

Aranda et al.[A] have reported a series done in early puerperium with excellent results and very low complication rate. This experience proves that when there is a problem related to tubal size it may be an inflamed tube rather than one related to pregnancy because in this state the tubes do not seem to undergo marked hypertrophy.

The failure rate with this method seems to be slightly higher than with cauterization. From personal experience I believe it should be a good method, provided that the tube is well ligated, because there is little likelihood for the band to slip off the knuckle and allow the tube to regain its patency. All three lapa-

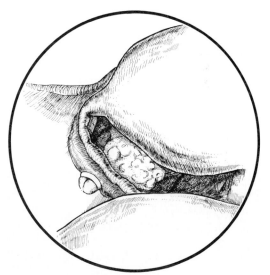

Figure 16. Laparoscopy on a 30-year-old woman, gravida 4, para 3, 16 weeks after tubal ligation and 8 weeks after her last menstrual period. Note the roundish profile of the uterine fundus, which was very soft, as it should be in pregnancy. The tube is intact in its whole length. The Silastic band had been applied on the infundibulopelvic ligament and was only minimally peritonized. The ovary had a corpus luteum over the inferior pole. Failure due to improper technique.

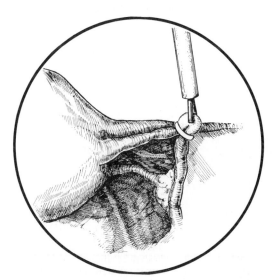

Figure 15. Technique of tubal ligation with Silastic band. The tube is being held from the "knuckle," which looks very pale after the band has been applied, to ascertain proper application. Note that the ampulla falls down covering the ovary, and that the round ligament runs behind the tube and applicator.

roscopic variations of technique have a much lower failure rate than the classical cold knife techniques, with the exception of the Uchida method. With a much shorter hospitalization period it seems highly justifiable to recommend laparoscopy as a good choice for the patient.

SEVERING OF ADHESIONS AND CAUTERIZATION OF TISSUES. Many limited procedures may be carried out under laparoscopy provided that the surgeon is prudent enough not to attempt the impossible and that he has available the appropriate special instruments. It was already mentioned that a variety of biopsies can be obtained if the proper forceps are available. Likewise, adhesions may be divided with either cutting scissors or hot cautery equipped with special electrodes. These may be adhesions of bowel to uterus, tubes, omentum, abdominal wall scars or between these various organs. Peritubal adhesions and veil adhesions covering the ovaries are particularly amenable to this type of management.

Endometriotic foci, which are limited in size and not close to vessels or bowel, can be successfully therapeutically cauterized and a laparotomy avoided.

REMOVAL OF FOREIGN BODIES. The unrecognized perforation of the uterus with passage of intrauterine contraceptive devices into the abdominal cavity provided a new possible application of laparoscopy to avoid laparotomy. Depending on the time elapsed since the passage of the IUD into the cavity, its type and location, the operation may be easy or one requiring a great deal of patience and skill and the use of accessory instruments to complete dissection of the imbedded foreign body.

It is critical to know the exact location of the IUD, particularly of those located outside the pelvic cavity. Anteroposterior and lateral x-ray films (Fig. 17) should orient the operator and help to limit the search to a relatively small area. Then if necessary, the operator can "feel" with the instruments to locate the IUD. Often it is either imbedded within the broad ligament or wrapped by omentum (Fig. 18) and not easily visualized. The need to dissect the IUD from surrounding tissues is determined by the fibrous reaction, usually related to the site of perforation and the type of device. Dalkon shields produce the toughest adhesions no matter where they are located. After completion of the removal it is mandatory to ascertain that there are no bleeding points; if these are present, they should be cauterized. The postoperative course is usually as benign as for diagnostic laparoscopy. In our experience of about 20 cases, we have seen Copper 7 attached to the appendix, Lippes loops imbedded between rectum and uterus, Dalkon shields buried between ovary and pelvic wall, as well as coils or loops "floating" free in the peritoneal cavity. When attempting this procedure we have not *yet* failed to complete it successfully.

COMPLICATIONS

As in any other surgical procedure, immediate or delayed complications may occur with a laparoscopy. The types of complications are related to the various steps involved in the procedure and are briefly discussed in that sequence.

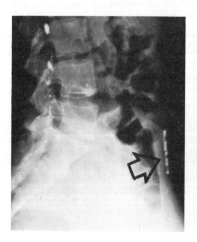 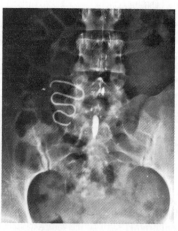

Figure 17. A 30-year-old gravida 3, para 2 patient had a Lippes loop inserted, followed by a full-term delivery 10 months later. Three years later these films were taken. The anteroposterior view, on the right, shows the loop projecting against the promontory and slightly to the right. The lateral view on the left shows, indicated by the arrow, the loop very close to the anterior abdominal wall, suggesting imbedding by the omentum. (From Cibils, L.A.: Gynecologic Laparoscopy. Diagnostic and Operatory. Philadelphia, Lea & Febiger, 1975.)

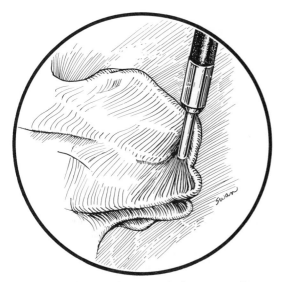

Figure 18. The same patient as in the previous figure. At laparoscopy nothing was seen, but with the Palmer forceps the omentum overlying the bowels was "palpated," in the area suggested by the films, and in the edge it was felt to be harder. Grasping and pulling showed the profile of the loop to be completely wrapped. It was possible to free it and remove safely. Slight oozing from omentum was cauterized. (From Cibils, L.A.: Gynecologic Laparoscopy, Diagnostic and Operatory. Philadelphia, Lea & Febiger, 1975.)

Anesthesia. Gastric regurgitation is a possibility always present, as is laryngospasm; less frequent but still worrisome is the occurrence of hypertension and collapse, often labeled "vasovagal reflex." More commonly observed are cardiac arrhythmias and extrasystoles generally due to excessive hypercapnia, particularly in cases in which no endotracheal intubation was performed. The extreme development of unrecognized untreated extrasystoles is ventricular fibrillation and cardiac arrest. Successful resuscitation has been reported in a few cases. The most dramatic, usually fatal and completely preventable complication is intubation of the esophagus instead of the trachea. This danger, inherent in anesthesia with intubation, has been reported to occur when laparoscopy is attempted, and it is especially unfortunate in these healthy young women.

Gas Needle. Subperitoneal injection is so common that it is almost taken for granted that it will occur in a given percentage of cases. In fact, it should not occur if the puncture site is properly chosen and the puncture executed with good technique and care. If unrecognized, it may extend into the mediastinum and be fatal. Puncture of intraperitoneal

small bowel, stomach and colon, as well as arteries and veins, has also been reported. All should be preventable with proper technique.

Trocars. As with the small needle, all intraperitoneal organs have been perforated with the large trocar: stomach, colon, small bowels. Most dangerous are lacerations of arteries (mesenteric, aorta, iliac) or veins (vena cava, iliac) because of the massive bleeding they cause. Delayed complications are hematomas of the abdominal wall, protrusion of omentum, bowel obstruction, infection. With the small trocar the bladder may be entered when it has not been catheterized.

Surgical Procedures. Bleeding from the site of a biopsy is a possibility if it is not cauterized with due care. Wounding of adjacent organs has occurred: ureters, infundibulopelvic ligament, appendix, tube. At the time of sectioning the tubes for permanent sterilization, bleeding occurs too predictably; adequate catheterization should prevent this. When tube bands are used, lacerations and subsequent bleeding have occurred; these also should be preventable with good technique, but when they occur cauterization is the procedure of choice to treat them.

Burns. Bowel burns have been recognized at the time of cauterizing the tube or endometriotic foci and therefore treated immediately. However, more often they have not been recognized and delayed peritonitis is manifested with dramatic suddenness after the burn site sloughs off. Of course this requires urgent laparotomy and partial bowel resection. Burns of the abdominal wall have also been observed, with extensive necrosis around the puncture site. These are all preventable complications if the instrumentation is in good order and sufficient attention is paid to detail in technique. In the majority of cases it has occurred because of inexperience or overconfidence of the operator. Less preventable is salpingo-oophoritis seen after tubal cauterization. Not preventable are thromboembolic accidents following laparoscopy; they may follow this as they may any other surgical procedure.

Culdoscopy

Visualization of pelvic organs, with the optic inserted through the posterior vaginal fornix, was introduced and popularized by Decker, who called it culdoscopy (or view through the cul-de-sac). Almost the only endoscopic procedure taught to gynecologists until the late 1960s, it is now a distant second choice to view the pelvic organs. This is because of several factors: the position the awake patient must assume (extreme genupectoral) is quite uncomfortable. (This particular problem was obviated by Palmer, who used lithotomy and Trendelenburg positions and gas injection through the fornix, with an intrauterine cannula for manipulation as in laparoscopy.) The view of the pelvic organs from "under" with a right angle optic mandates a thorough reorientation and relearning of the anatomy and the relationship among organs. This requires much more training than with the laparoscope. The two most important drawbacks of culdoscopy when compared with laparoscopy are the limited view obtained in which only the outer two thirds of the tubes and ovaries are well visualized, and inability to perform surgical procedures with the exception of a few (such as tubal ligation). More elaborate procedures may be carried out when the incision is extended to make a classical colpotomy. Among the advantages culdoscopy has over laparoscopy is the fact that it does not require general anesthesia (a "relative" advantage for some), and particularly that it does not require the injection of gas into the abdomen. With it air enters by negative, "sucking," pressure as soon as the lead is removed from the puncturing needle. Thereby all the complications inherent in gas injection are avoided. The only possible important complications that may occur at culdoscopy are perforation of the rectum with the trocar and bleeding of the wound. Both are relatively minor problems because appropriate suturing will correct then.

When the physician must choose between these ways to look into the pelvis, probably laparoscopy has to be chosen. However, a university hospital should be prepared to teach culdoscopy, for a fully trained gynecologist should have seen a few of them and be able to do one if laparoscopy is not possible.

Hysteroscopy

Direct viewing of the uterine cavity had been attempted for a long time but because of poor illumination and distension it had always met with failure. Both problems were solved almost simultaneously, and hysteroscopy has become an established endoscopic procedure in gynecology. When indicated and properly executed it may be a useful diagnostic or therapeutic tool. There still is some controversy with regard to its indications and advantages over other techniques in gynecology.

INSTRUMENTATION

The optic is similar to the child cystoscope with the sheath round or slightly ovoid depending upon the type of operating instruments used, and a caliber no. 7 or 8. The standard instruments are all rigid, although there is an experimental model with movable tip for better view and manipulation around the cornual areas and tubal ostia called "a steering hysteroscope." Illumination is provided by fiberoptic cable as for standard laparoscopes.

Distension of the uterine cavity may be accomplished by injecting carbon dioxide at a moderately high rate (80 to 150 ml per minute) as suggested by Lindeman, who uses an automatic injector. Quinones et al. use saline or dextrose solution rapidly dripping from an IV pole. These two excellent techniques have the inconvenience of requiring continuous high inflow of the distending substance because they escape quickly through the tubes into the peritoneal cavity. Therefore, to maintain a moderately high pressure in the uterus (80 to 150 mm Hg), a continuous injection is necessary. In order to obviate this problem, heavy dextran (70 per cent) is now more frequently used. This substance, having a high viscosity, escapes slowly through the tubes and allows for an excellent distension of the cavity. Furthermore, it mixes poorly with blood. Good viewing results, even when small amounts of bleeding are produced by manipulations. (With saline or dextrose solutions this creates an almost insurmountable problem.)

Accessory instruments have been devised to enable the operator to do a variety of procedures: scissors, biopsy forceps, grasping forceps, coagulating electrodes, plug applicators. All have been used with good results by experienced endoscopists.

TECHNIQUE

Hysteroscopy has to be carried out when there is no bleeding and endometrium is thin and without secretions that could cloud the view. Thus, the ideal time in the cycle is shortly after the menstrual period has ended, at about the eighth or ninth day during the proliferative phase.

The preparation is the same as for a dilatation and curettage. It may be easily done under paracervical anesthesia, although a few operators prefer general, especially in teaching institutions in which more than one viewer is usually participating. A good bilateral infiltration with a standard local anesthetic gives excellent tolerance (with complementary premedication) to the majority of procedures usually performed.

The uterus should be very gently sounded in order to ascertain the position and depth of the cavity. Following this, gentle dilatation up to one number less than the size of the instrument is performed, and then this is introduced slowly. As soon as the tip enters the cervical canal the assistant must start the injection of the distending substance (saline or dextran), or the carbon dioxide flow must be opened. Under direct view the optic is slowly advanced until the cavity is entered, then a short wait helps to obtain satisfactory distension and thus better perspective of the anatomy. Depending upon the objective of the procedure, the cavity is either carefully inspected or the planned manipulation executed.

INDICATIONS

The proponents of hysteroscopy have indicated its use for a variety of situations. However, the same, or better, information may be obtained by other less cumbersome procedures in a number of those situations, diagnostic or therapeutic.

Diagnostic. It has been proposed to use hysteroscopy in cases of suspicion of endometrial polyps, submucous fibroids, intrauterine adhesions (Asherman's syndrome), lost intrauterine contraceptive devices or adenomyosis. In all these conditions a hysterosalpingogram, done with water-soluble contrast medium, should help make an accurate diagnosis, with a procedure that is less elaborate and easier on the patient. The place of hysteroscopy as a diagnostic method is indeed limited, and one may dispense with it without inconvenience.

Therapeutic. Here again, hysteroscopy has been proposed to undertake therapeutic steps in many situations. Removal of polyps and sectioning and removal of pedunculated

fibroids have been accomplished by several authors. However, probably a good dilatation and curettage should obtain the same result with a much less serious operation. Where hysteroscopy is probably a better procedure is in cases of intrauterine adhesions, which may be lysed or resected under direct visual control; great skill and patience is required in these cases because the optic must be advanced extremely slowly, step by step only after the lower adhesions are lysed.

To remove intrauterine contraceptive devices, hysteroscopy has been used by a number of authors almost routinely. However, the majority of these devices may be removed without difficulty at routine curettage. Rarely, this is impossible; in these cases hysteroscopy is the only alternative to hysterotomy. These circumstances occur particularly when the IUD is imbedded in the mucosa and myometrium (Figs. 19 and 20), in which case even "feeling" it with the curette may be difficult. Good exposure of the free part of the device facilitates grasping, with a stronger instrument than the very delicate ones fitting into the operating sheath of the scope; often strong pull is needed to dislodge these devices.

The area in which more experience has been gathered with hysteroscopy is permanent sterilization. Significant experience was obtained

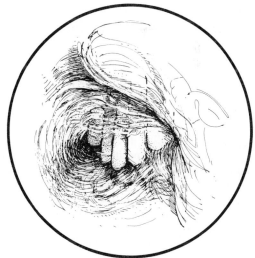

Figure 19. A 22-year-old woman, gravida 1, para 1, who wanted her IUD removed because she wanted to attempt another pregnancy. The string had broken and because of inability to remove the IUD in the office she had a D&C, at which it could not be recovered. Hysteroscopy done the following day showed the "fingers" of a Dalkon shield emerging from under the mucosa of the anterior uterine wall and against the left cornu.

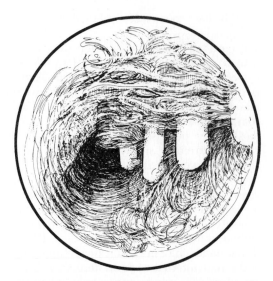

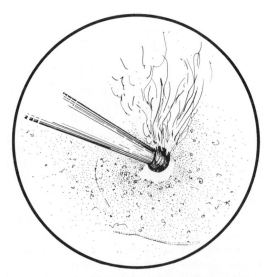

Figure 20. Close-up view of the same patient as in previous figure to better illustrate that the shield is partially "buried." With a strong forceps it was possible to grab the IUD and dislodge it intact.

Figure 21. Technique to electrocoagulate the tubal ostium under hysteroscopic control. The electrode is inserted, gently, making sure that part of the uninsulated area is visible as shown (to prevent excessive penetration); then the current is passed and the tissue blanches as bubbles form. The periphery of the ostium must be well blanched to ensure success, before the electrode is withdrawn.

outside this country by Lindeman in Europe, Sugimoto in Asia, and Quinones and Alvarado in Latin America before it was first tried in this country. Technically relatively easy, the high hopes of widespread application of hysteroscopy were dampened by a significant incidence of failures. Thus a hysterosalpingogram is needed before patients can be allowed unprotected intercourse. Technically the procedure requires the insertion of a small electrode into the tubal ostium and passage of coagulation current, which should produce necrosis, sloughing, scarring and retraction with closure of the ostium.

There are a few apparently minor but important technical details to be followed for a successful and safe coagulation. The electrode must have sufficient active surface, about 5 to 6 mm, with insulated tip to avoid heat dissipation toward the peritoneal surface of the uterus. In order to be sure that the electrode is inserted far enough but not too far, it is important to be able to see part of the uninsulated area at the opening of the ostium (Fig. 21) before the current is activated. This should pass until the mucosa blanches uniformly around. There are two types of current proposed for this step: high frequency for a short time (5 to 10 seconds), and low voltage for longer time (30 to 150 seconds). It is claimed that the latter is safer to prevent burn complications. The success of bilateral occlusion after a first operation ranges from 85 to 95 per cent, depending upon the series; both of these

figures are much lower than after any of the laparoscopic methods. However, after a second attempt the failure rate (for patency) is low to an acceptable less than 5 per cent. It seems clear that hysteroscopy should have a place in sterilization by cauterization, although it should be limited to a few selected patients not eligible for laparoscopy (obesity, scars, patients' desire).

Another technique to obtain a reversible sterilization by hysteroscopy has been proposed by Hosseinian[7a] and tested successfully in animals. It consists of inserting a "plug" in the ostium by means of an applicator, which delivers it after careful insertion. It has a set of hooks to anchor it in place and may be eventually removed when pregnancy is desired. So far it is experimental for humans.

Complications. A few problems have been reported with the use of carbon dioxide as distension substance; even fatal embolisms have occurred in patients when the gas was used without controlled insufflation apparatus. Uterine perforations have been observed by some and these are especially common when visualization is made difficult by blood or excessive secretions, as well as in uterine hyperflexions. When using cauterizing electrodes it is easy to create a "false way" even when not passing current; this probably is one of the causes of the failure to obtain occlusion. A much more serious complication is the possible perforation of the myometrium with burn of overlying bowels, an accident previously reported by us. The safeguard against this is the controlled insertion of the electrode and its "capping" with nonconductive material.

In conclusion, in our view, the clinical application of hysteroscopy is very limited, its main applicability being in a selected group of patients for permanent sterilization (may be reversible in the future), removal of intrauterine foreign bodies and lysis of adhesions. It probably does not have a place in diagnosis.

REFERENCES

A. Aranda, C., Prada, C., Broutin, A., Mangel, T., Edelman, D. A. and Goldsmith, A.: Laparoscopic sterilization immediately after term delivery: a preliminary report. J. Reprod. Med. 14:171, 1975.

1. Cibils, L. A.: Technique of cold ovarian biopsy at laparoscopy. J. Reprod. Med. 9:164, 1972.
2. Cibils, L. A.: Anesthesia for coelioscopy. Acta Europ. Fertil. 6:271, 1975.
3. Cibils, L. A.: Gynecologic Laparoscopy. Diagnostic and Operatory. Philadelphia, Lea & Febiger, 1975.
4. Cibils, L. A.: Permanent sterilization by hysteroscopic cauterization. Am. J. Obstet. Gynecol. 121:513, 1975.
5. Decker, A. and Cherry, T.: Culdoscopy: a new method in diagnosis of pelvic disease. Am. J. Surg. 64:40, 1944.
6. Dingfelder, J. R.: Direct laparoscope trocar insertion without prior pneumoperitoneum. J. Reprod. Med. 21:45, 1978.
7. Fourestier, N., Gladu, A. and Vulmiere, J.: Perfectionnements a l'endoscopie Realisation bronchoscopique. Presse Med. 60:1292, 1952.
7a. Hosseinian, A. H., Lucero, S. and Zaneveld, L. G. D.: Hysteroscopically delivered tubal plugs. In Sciarra, J. J., Zatuchni, G. and Speidel, J. (Eds.): Reversal sterilization. Hagerstown, Harper & Row, 1978, pp. 241–48.

8. Hulka, J. F.: Controlling tenaculum: Instrument for uterine mobilization during tubal sterilization. Am. J. Obstet. Gynecol. 112:865, 1972.
9. Hulka, J. F.: Relative risks and benefits of electric and nonelectric sterilization techniques. J. Reprod. Med. 21:111, 1978.
10. Hulka, J. F. and Omran, K. F.: Comparative tubal occlusion: rigid and spring-loaded clips. Fertil. Steril. 23:633, 1972.
11. Hulka, J. F., Thweatt, D. and Ulberg, L. C.: Contained cautery: studies toward safer laparoscopic sterilization techniques. Fertil. Steril. 24:912, 1973.
12. Jacobaeus, H. D.: Ueber die Moeglichkeit die Zystoskopie bei Undersachung seroeser. Hoehlungen anzuwenden. Muench. Med. Wochenschr. 57:2090, 1910.
13. Lindeman, H. J.: Transuterine Tubensterilisation per Hysteroskopie. Geburtsh. u. Frauenheilk. 33:709, 1973.
14. Neuwirth, R. S.: Hysteroscopy. Philadelphia, W. B. Saunders, 1975.
15. Palmer, R.: Technique et instrumentation de la coelioscopie gynecologique. Gynec. Obstet. (Paris) 46:420, 1947.
16. Phillips, J., Hulka, J., Hulka, B., Keith, D. and Keith, L.: American Association of Gynecologic Laparoscopists' 1976 Membership. J. Reprod. Med. 21:3, 1978.
17. Phillips, J., Keith, D., Keith, L., Hulka, J. and Hulka, B.: Survey of gynecologic laparoscopy for 1974. J. Reprod. Med. 15:45, 1975.
18. Quinones, R., Aznar, R. and Alvarado, A.: Tubal electrocauterization under hysteroscopic control. Contraception 7:195, 1973.
19. Rioux, J. E. and Cloutier, D.: Bipolar cautery for sterilization by laparoscopy. J. Reprod. Med. 13:6, 1974.
20. Sciarra, J. J., Butler, J. C. and Speidel, J. J.: Hysteroscopic sterilization, Miami Symposia Specialists, 1974.
21. Sugimoto, O.: Hysteroscopic control by electrocoagulation. In Sciarra, J. J., Butler, J. C., and Speidel, J. J. (eds.): Hysteroscopic sterilization, Miami, 1974, Symposia Specialists, pp. 107–20.
22. Yoon, I. B. and King, T. M.: A preliminary and intermediate report on a new laparoscopic tubal ring procedure. J. Reprod. Med. 15:54, 1975.

Endoscopy in Obstetrics and Gynecology

Moon H. Kim, M.D.

Ohio State University College of Medicine

With the advent of the fiberoptic cold light system the diagnostic and therapeutic uses of various endoscopes have become one of the most important advances in operative obstetrics and gynecology. Although endoscopy had been a known technique of investigation of pelvic pathology, it was revolutionized by the use of fiberoptic light and the newer instruments. Endoscopy has added an extra dimension not only to gynecology but also to obstetrics. This chapter reviews the current status of laparoscopy, culdoscopy, hysteroscopy and fetoscopy.

Laparoscopy (Peritoneoscopy, Celioscopy)

Endoscopic examination of the abdominal cavity in the human was first described by Jacobaeus,[1] and it was called laparoscopy. The technique was popularized as a diagnostic and surgical procedure in Europe. However, laparoscopy was not well accepted in the United States until late in the 1960s. Prior to this the conventional light system for laparoscopy was not satisfactory, and culdoscopy had been the method of inspecting the pelvic organs. Palmer[2] in France was responsible for the modernization of laparoscopy. Interest in laparoscopy in the United States was revived by the need to seek a safe and effective technique for tubal sterilization as a method of population control. Its impact on gynecology has become so substantial that it is essential in diagnostic and therapeutic gynecology. All trained gynecologists are expected to be familiar with the technique. The scope of operative laparoscopy depends upon the operator's imagination and experience.

INSTRUMENTS

Although there is a wide variety of laparoscopic instruments available, they consist essentially of endoscopes with variously angled view-fields, gas insufflator, fiberoptic light sources and other accessory instruments for diagnostic and surgical manipulation. With technologic improvement in the optical system, some laparoscopes are equipped with a magnifying lens. The gas insufflator regulates the flow of carbon dioxide or nitrous oxide to create an adequate level of pneumoperitoneum for safe entry into the peritoneal cavity and better visualization. Numerous accessory instruments are designed to allow such surgical manipulations as biopsy, cauterization, dissection and displacing and immobilizing organs. With the increasing interest in laparoscopic applications, new instruments have been developed constantly.

INDICATIONS AND CONTRAINDICATIONS

Before the indications for the procedure are discussed, the reader should remember that laparoscopy is a closed procedure with limitations. Although numerous reports of some rare applications of laparoscopy have appeared in the literature, its primary indications are for the diagnosis of pelvic pathology and therapeutic use in tubal sterilization.

The common diagnostic indications are the following:

1. Pelvic pain of unknown etiology
2. Infertility of unknown etiology, and of tubal pathology
3. Evaluation for possible tubal reconstructive surgery
4. Suspected pelvic endometriosis
5. Suspected ectopic pregnancy
6. Evaluation of gonads in certain endocrinologic and genetic disorders
7. Evaluation of gynecologic cancer.

It is obvious that laparoscopy reduces the need for exploratory laparotomy in many instances. Any organic cause of pelvic pain can be readily diagnosed by laparoscopy—that is, chronic pelvic inflammatory disease, endometriosis, uterine anomalies or an ovarian cyst. After an exhaustive medical investigation of the infertile patient, laparoscopy is indicated to evaluate other causes such as peritubal adhesions or endometriosis. Preoperative laparoscopy allows better selection of the patient for tuboplasty. With wide use of this procedure unruptured ectopic pregnancy is more frequently diagnosed. Although they are not common, unclear cases of polycystic ovaries or other endocrinologic conditions are better evaluated by laparoscopy. Recently many centers have begun utilizing laparoscopy in the evaluation of gynecologic cancer.

The major surgical indication of laparoscopy is for female tubal sterilization. With the use of various techniques the fallopian tubes can be partially excised after coagulation or occluded with Silastic rings (Yoon's) or Hulka clips. Other indications include lysis of pelvic adhesions, removal of foreign bodies (intrauterine contraceptive devices) in the abdominal cavity, fulguration and biopsies of endometriotic implants and aspiration of simple ovarian cysts. Usually secondary or tertiary punctures are needed to perform more extensive operative manipulation by introducing accessory instruments. The physician should remember that such manipulation will not provide the same degree of exposure as in laparotomy.

Contraindications to laparoscopy remain controversial, as some of them so regarded in the past are no longer considered contraindications. For example, previous laparotomy or salpingitis should not be considered as an absolute contraindication.

The following conditions are absolute or relative contraindications to laparoscopy:

Absolute contraindications:

1. Conditions contraindicating anesthesia
2. Diaphragmatic hernia, hiatal hernia
3. Intestinal obstruction or generalized peritonitis
4. Extensive bowel adhesions
5. Inability to establish pneumoperitoneum.

Relative contraindications:

1. Obesity
2. Acute pelvic inflammatory disease with peritonitis suspected
3. Advanced pregnancy
4. Hemoperitoneum.

TECHNIQUE

It is not intended here to describe various laparoscopic techniques in detail. The reader is referred to textbooks.[3, 4] However, it is important to point out the essentials of the technique.

The site of entry incision is selected with cosmetic consideration; usually a transverse incision in the lower margin of the umbilicus is made. For the diagnostic and surgical laparoscopy, the second or the third puncture can be made suprapubically in the midline or paramedian line. When a paramedian puncture is made, care should be taken not to injure the inferior epigastric vessels.

Achieving a pneumoperitoneum is the most important step to successful laparoscopy. It can be attained by placing a Verres needle subumbilically, or subcostally in the left upper abdomen. Although it is not preferred, an approach through the cul-de-sac can be made. When the patient requires excessive hyperventilation before endotracheal intubation, it is wise to use a nasogastric tube to ensure a deflated stomach. Among the gaseous substances, carbon dioxide is most widely used. In many institutes nitrous oxide is used, and it has the advantage of less irritation to the diaphragm when the procedure is performed under local anesthesia. In the obese patient, a long Verres needle may be used, but a classic Palmer approach through the left subcostal margin is often preferred. In most cases approximately 2 to 3 liters of gas will be sufficient to create an intra-abdominal pressure of about 10 mm Hg.

Anesthesia for laparoscopy varies, depending on the procedures involved. General anesthesia with endotracheal intubation allows for controlled ventilation to counteract the hypercarbia and respiratory acidosis associated with the readily absorbed carbon dioxide, decreasing the incidence of cardiac arrhythmias. In recent years there has been increasing use of local anesthesia for laparoscopy.[5] Its obvious advantage is that it can be performed in an outpatient facility. However, it should be used only for a short, uncomplicated procedure requiring only minimal manipulation, such as tubal sterilization. Under local or regional anesthesia, less pneumoperitoneum must be used. Thus it may restrict the effectiveness of the procedure. Despite some advantages of local anesthesia I believe that general anesthesia is superior for laparoscopy, particularly when an ambulatory surgical facility with anesthesia coverage is available.

The selection of trocar and laparoscope depends on the procedure and the operator's preference. Usually a smaller laparoscope (5 to 8 mm) is sufficient for diagnostic purposes. Manipulation of the tissues can be readily done through an extrapuncture site. For better visualization of the pelvic organs the patient should be placed in the Trendelenburg position. At the conclusion of the procedure the gas within the abdomen is allowed to escape completely following removal of the laparoscope and operative instruments. Then, skin incisions are closed with simple subcuticular sutures.

Complications from laparoscopy are relatively uncommon in the hands of trained operators. According to a recent survey,[6] the major complications (requiring laparotomy for bowel injuries, hemorrhages and so forth) occur at the approximate rate of 1 in 300 cases. The mortality from the procedure is approximately 1 per 20,000 cases. This survey indicated that the rate of complications was higher in the patients treated by presumably less qualified operators. It seems only logical that thorough understanding by the surgeon of the technique, the indications, the contraindications and the limitations of the procedure and adequate experience are essential to prevent complications.

Complications associated with pneumoperitoneum:

1. Retroperitoneal or subcutaneous infusion of gas
2. Perforation of blood vessels
3. Perforation of stomach, bowels, pelvic organs
4. Aggravation of subclinical hernia.

Complications associated with trocar insertion:

1. Perforation of blood vessels in the abdominal wall and within the abdominal cavity
2. Injuries to abdominal viscera.

Complications from surgical manipulation:

1. Hemorrhage from dissection or lysis
2. Injuries to the bowels and urinary tract (thermal or surgical)
3. Electric current injuries to the viscera and abdominal wall
4. Peritonitis (from chemicals or infections).

As a summary, laparoscopy has become an essential procedure in gynecologic practice. It often replaces laparotomy for diagnostic and therapeutic purposes. Although it is relatively safe, those performing it should have a thorough understanding of the procedure and adequate training.

Culdoscopy

While laparoscopy was popular in Europe, culdoscopy became the mainstay of pelvic endoscopy in the United States until the 1960s. Decker[7] popularized culdoscopy primarily as a diagnostic procedure. Although it has certain specific advantages over laparoscopy, the latter largely replaced it during the 1970s. However, because of the simplicity and other advantages of culdoscopy, it is wise to become familiar with the procedure.

INSTRUMENTS AND POSITIONING OF PATIENT

Unlike laparoscopy, generally culdoscopy needs only a trocar, a culdoscope and light source. Because of the limitation in mobility of the culdoscope, few accessory instruments for surgical manipulation have been made available. The patient is placed in knee-chest position. Thus, a natural pneumoperitoneum and displacement of bowel are created when the cul-de-sac is entered. Proper positioning is important; therefore, some supporting pads for shoulders, knees, chest and abdomen are often helpful. Because of this difficult positioning we have tried culdoscopy successfully by placing the patient in the dorsolithotomy position with the body in Trendelenburg position and establishing pelvic pneumoperitoneum by carbon dioxide. This allows displacement of the bowels into the upper abdomen, and good visualization of the ovaries and tubes can be obtained by pushing the uterus anteriorly with an intrauterine cannula.

INDICATIONS AND CONTRAINDICATIONS

The indications for culdoscopy are similar to those for diagnostic laparoscopy. These include infertility, pelvic pain, suspected ectopic pregnancy and evaluation of the ovaries. I personally believe that the laparoscopy gives better visualization in these conditions. However, for patients with obesity or suspected anterior abdominal adhesions from previous surgery, culdoscopy can serve well.

The contraindications to culdoscopy are inability to maintain the knee-chest position, obliteration of the cul-de-sac (endometriosis, fixed mass), acute or subacute pelvic inflammatory disease and hemoperitoneum (ruptured ectopic pregnancy). Other relative contraindications include severe vaginitis and cervicitis.

TECHNIQUE AND ANESTHESIA

The major advantage of culdoscopy over laparoscopy is its simplicity. The procedure can be easily performed under local anesthesia with some sedation. Intravenous administration of valium 10 mg and local infiltration of 1 per cent lidocaine into the posterior fornix of the vagina provide adequate anesthesia. The vagina should be thoroughly cleansed; the posterior lip of the cervix is grasped and displaced anteriorly, tenting the vaginal vault. After a small incision is made, the trocar is inserted at the apex of the vault in the midline. The surgeon should remember that the cul-de-sac is separated from the vaginal fornix only by thin tissues of vaginal mucosa and peritoneum. Care should be taken not to penetrate too deeply. Then the surgeon should insert the culdoscope while looking through it to avoid any tissue damage. Unlike the laparoscope, the culdoscope should be rotated for viewing of all angles. At the conclusion of the procedure the incision is closed with absorbable suture. With experience, it can be performed easily.

Minor operative manipulations can be done through the culdoscopy. However, colpotomy is usually required for more extensive manipulation. Some surgeons remain enthusiastic about the use of culdoscopy for such operative purposes as tubal sterilization.[8, 9] Despite this enthusiasm and the apparent simplicity of culdoscopy, it has been for the most part replaced by laparoscopy in recent years. Our recent experience with culdoscopy at The Ohio State University Hospital is presently quite limited. I think that culdoscopy remains primarily a diagnostic procedure to be used only in selected cases. Because of the inability to examine the anterior pelvic cavity with its use, laparoscopy is preferred in most situations.

Complications from culdoscopy are mostly minor and rare, if the cases are selected carefully. Inability to enter the cul-de-sac, rectal perforation (usually occurring in the patients with unrecognized cul-de-sac pathology), uterine puncture and bleeding from the vaginal incision are the more common complications seen. Rarely, peritonitis, embolism and subcutaneous emphysema can occur. A complication rate is approximately 2 to 3 per cent, excluding the inability to enter the peritoneal cavity (3 to 5 per cent).

Culdoscopy can be a valuable diagnostic procedure in gynecology. However, the scope of its use has diminished greatly because of the many advantages of laparoscopy over this procedure. It is relatively safe and simple in selected patients, and often requires only a minimal anesthesia.

Hysteroscopy

This endoscopic procedure for visualization of the uterine cavity is a relatively new addition to gynecologic endoscopy. Although it had been described in the literature almost a century ago, like laparoscopy it did not become popular until the introduction of the fiberoptic light system and the availability of substances capable of maintaining uterine distension. During the past decade many inves-

tigators have tried various materials to distend the uterine cavity—water, dextrose and water, carbon dioxide, dextran 70 and so forth. Since 1970, the hysteroscopic techniques have been more accepted by many gynecologists for diagnostic and surgical management of pathology of the uterine cavity.

The reintroduction of hysteroscopy in gynecology has been stimulated by the continuous search for a simpler method of tubal sterilization. The advantage in the characteristic of hysteroscopy of not requiring entrance into the peritoneal cavity has been compromised by its high failure rate as a sterilization technique. Although many hysteroscopic sterilization techniques using cauterization of the tubal ostia or uterotubal blocking devices (plug or hydrogel) have been under investigation, the major indications for hysteroscopy are diagnosis of intrauterine pathology and limited operative procedures.

INSTRUMENTS

Two kinds of hysteroscopes are available, rigid and steerable. The rigid one is derived from the principle of cystoscope. It consists of an endoscope, fiberoptic light source, cervical adaptors, a set of cervical dilators (Hegar's), and ancillary instruments such as scissors, probes, biopsy forceps, cutting loops and cautery. Media for distending the uterine cavity are dextran, 5 per cent dextrose in water and carbon dioxide. We have used dextran 70 (Hyskon) and found it superior. One of the advantages of using dextran is that it does not mix with blood or mucus and so provides excellent visibility. However, proper cleansing of instruments is necessary after its use. For gaseous media, one should have a flow-control apparatus (insufflator). Instillation of dextrose in water or carbon dioxide requires continuous flow pressure.[10]

TECHNIQUE

Hysteroscopy should be performed in a well-equipped operating room, whether it is in an ambulatory setting or in a hospital. The patient should be prepared as for any other surgical procedure. In most cases, paracervical block with 1 per cent lidocaine or 2 per cent chloroprocaine supplemented by moderate sedation is satisfactory. Because of cyclic changes of the endometrium, it is best to perform hysteroscopy in the early or mid follicular phase following cessation of menstrual flow.

After the cervix is exposed, the uterine cavity is sounded. The cervical canal is dilated to one size larger than the hysteroscope. The cervical adaptor may be placed. Then the hysteroscope is introduced through the endocervix under careful inspection. As one advances the scope into the uterine cavity, the entire cavity is inspected, as well as the uterotubal ostia. During the procedure, the cavity must be distended with dextran or other media. Operative manipulation can be done easily. The procedure is completed by removing the instruments.

INDICATIONS AND CONTRAINDICATIONS

Although there have been some reports of rather unusual operative procedures performed through hysteroscopy, such as excision of submucous fibroids, the common indications in clinical practice are somewhat limited. Intrauterine synechiae (Asherman's syndrome) is best diagnosed and managed by hysteroscopy. Lysis of synechiae under direct visualization offers the best therapeutic result. The procedure is used for locating retained intrauterine contraceptive devices or other foreign bodies for diagnosis and removal. Other indications are location of suspected submucous fibroids or polyps and intrauterine anomalies for diagnosis and possible removal. Diagnosis and treatment of persistent abnormal uterine bleeding is another indication.

Besides these indications hysteroscopy has been used to investigate postmenopausal bleeding, endometrial cancer, infertility and habitual abortions. Its use as a sterilization technique has also been under investigation.

The contraindications to the use of hysteroscopy are infection in pelvic organs, intrauterine pregnancy and heavy uterine bleeding. Because of the potential for dissemination of infection, hysteroscopy should not be done in patients with active pelvic inflammatory disease, endometritis, severe cervicitis and vaginitis. In the presence of heavy bleeding it is obvious that visualization will be unsatisfactory; therefore, the procedure should not be performed.

COMPLICATIONS

Complications of hysteroscopy are not common. The most serious complication is inadvertent perforation of the uterus. It occurs usually as a result of uterine sounding or cervical dilatation, not of the procedure itself. Infection of the pelvic organs and uterine bleeding are other uncommon complications. When electric coagulation is used, burning of adherent bowel can be a serious complication. Rarely, embolism of dextran or carbon dioxide may occur.

Hysteroscopy is now a proved practical method of gynecologic endoscopy. Although the technique is relatively simple, interpretation of the findings is far more difficult. Through personal experience I believe that interpretation is more difficult during the luteal phase. Therefore, the procedure is best done during the proliferative phase for diagnostic purposes. Hysteroscopy in managing intrauterine synechiae and removing retained intrauterine foreign bodies such as intrauterine contraceptive devices is unquestionably superior to the traditional blind method of dilatation and curettage.[11] In various indications it only complements other diagnostic and therapeutic techniques. Its simplicity and requirement for local anesthesia should make hysteroscopy more useful in gynecologic practice.

Fetoscopy

Fetoscopy is an endoscopic procedure to visualize the fetus in utero. As interest in prenatal evaluation of the intrauterine fetus has increased, this application of the fiberoptic endoscope was developed. Approximately 2.5 per cent of all human births are associated with a congenital defect. Since amniotic fluid analysis can diagnose only a minority of defects prenatally, direct visualization of the fetus could add one more dimension to the diagnosis of congenital defects.

Since the first description[12] in 1957, other investigators' experiences have been published.[13, 14] Modification of the endoscope to a needle "needlescope" and better localization of the placenta and fetal position with the use of ultrasonographic echogram have made this procedure realistically applicable to clinical obstetrics. Various terms have been used—hysteroscopy, endoamnioscopy, laparoamnioscopy and embryoscopy—but fetoscopy seems most descriptive and logical.

INSTRUMENTS AND TECHNIQUE

Most fetoscopes today consist of a 1.7 mm endoscope (needlescope) with 2 mm cannula and trocar, and fiberoptic light source. A pediatric cystoscope (3.5 mm in diameter) can be substituted. Auxiliary instruments include a 27-gauge needle for fetal blood sampling and a biopsy instrument. The cannula with a sharp trocar is inserted into the amniotic cavity transabdominally under local anesthesia, and the trocar is replaced by the fetoscope for visualization. Although the needlescope has made the visualization of the fetus considerably safer than earlier experiences with a pediatric cystoscope (5 to 6 mm scope), it has the disadvantages of a smaller visual field. The magnification used in fetoscopy makes it difficult to examine the entire fetus without a great deal of manipulation. A successful visualization of various fetal parts depends on the operator's experience and can be achieved in about 70 per cent of cases.[13, 14] The optimal time to perform fetoscopy for visualization is at 16 to 18 weeks' gestation, and for fetal blood sampling after 18 weeks. Since it is primarily for the diagnosis of congenital anomalies, it should only be done at institutions equipped with a complete genetic counseling team.

The potential indications are (1) for direct visualization of the fetus in utero to diagnose physical defects such as limb anomalies, anencephaly, meningocele, (2) for blood sampling from the placental and cord vessels for hemoglobin analysis, enzyme studies and chromosomal studies, (3) for tissue biopsy of amnion, skin and placenta, and (4) to aid intrauterine fetal transfusion, and in obtaining amniotic fluid. While the placenta and cord can be readily visualized, location of other fetal parts and particularly genitalia has been more difficult in most investigators' experience. In addition to the limitation of needlescope, fetal movements cause difficulties in visualizing certain fetal parts. Blood sampling is done with a 27-gauge needle with a success rate ranging from 57 to 100 per cent of the cases. Occasionally contamination with the maternal blood is encountered.

Fetal complications from fetoscopy seem to be related to the size of instrument and the technique (experience) of the operator. With the needlescope, the incidence of fetal death or abortion has declined markedly. Possible fetal complications are hemorrhage and fetal-maternal transfusion with maternal sensitization. Potential maternal risks are infection, leakage of amniotic fluid, uterine bleeding and injury to other organs. Although these risks have not been obvious, perhaps because of limited use, further close evaluation is needed.

It can be concluded from the available data that fetoscopy offers the potential for direct observation of the fetus in utero and for obtaining blood samples and tissue biopsies for prenatal diagnosis of congenital defects. In spite of enthusiasm and encouraging results, it is important to recognize that the safety and accuracy of fetoscopy have been evaluated in a limited number of pregnancies. At present it should be considered only for diagnosing serious fetal conditions at centers where expertise in fetoscopy and genetic counseling is available.

REFERENCES

1. Jacobaeus, H.: Ueber die Moglichkeit die Zystoscopie bei Untersuchung Seroser Hohlungen Anzuwenden. Muench. Med. Wochenschr. 57:2090, 1910.
2. Palmer, R.: Instrumentation et technique de la coelioscopie gynecologique. Gynecol. Obstet. (Paris). 46:422, 1947.
3. Cohen, M. R.: Laparoscopy, Culdoscopy and Gynecography; Technique and Atlas. Philadelphia, W. B. Saunders Co., 1970.
4. Cibils, L. A.: Gynecologic Laparoscopy. Philadelphia, Lea & Febiger, 1975.
5. Wheeless, C. R.: Outpatient laparoscopic sterilization under local anesthesia. Obstet. Gynecol. 39:767, 1972.
6. Proceedings of the Fifth Annual Clinical Symposium on Gynecologic Endoscopy, AAGL. J. Reprod. Med. 18:227, 1977.
7. Decker, A.: Culdoscopy. Am. J. Obstet. Gynecol. 63:654, 1952.
8. Chang, G. C. E., Khew, K. S., Chen, C. et al.: Culdoscopic ligation as an outpatient procedure. Am J. Obstet. Gynecol. 122:109, 1975.
9. Paldi, E., Timor-Tritsch, I., Abramovici, H. and Perez, B. A.: Operative culdoscopy. Br. J. Obstet. Gynecol. 82:318, 1975.
10. Neuwirth, R. S.: Hysteroscopy. Philadelphia, W. B. Saunders Co., 1975.
11. March, C. M., Israel, R. and March, A. D.: Hysteroscopic management of intrauterine adhesions. Am. J. Obstet. Gynecol. 130:653, 1978.
12. Westin, B.: Technique and estimation of oxygenation of the human fetus in utero by means of hysterophotography. Acta Pediatr. Scand. 46:117, 1957.
13. Benzie, R. J. and Doran, T. A. The "fetoscope"—A new clinical tool for prenatal genetic diagnosis. Am. J. Obstet. Gynecol. 121:460, 1975.
14. Hobbins, J. C. and Mahoney, M. J.: Fetoscopy and fetal blood sampling: the present state of the method. Clin. Obstet. Gynecol. 19:341, 1976.

Endoscopy in Obstetrics and Gynecology

David Pent, M.D.

University of Arizona College of Medicine

Only fifteen years ago an article on endoscopy in obstetrics and gynecology would have been limited to a discussion of culdoscopy. It would have been read with enthusiasm by the advocates of that technique, but the vast majority of gynecologists would have read the article with continued skepticism—if they read it at all—firm in the belief that no significant role existed for an endoscopic procedure in gynecologic practice. Laparoscopy has changed all that. As with any new procedure, however, it has been associated with a good deal of controversy.

In the beginning this dealt mainly with variations in techniques and the comparative roles of laparoscopy and culdoscopy in diagnosis and patient management, the latter being discussed in the last volume of *Controversies in Obstetrics and Gynecology*. At the present time disagreement involves the various laparoscopic techniques of tubal sterilization. Each technique has its enthusiastic supporters; at one end of the spectrum the advocates of minilaparotomy are in favor of doing away with laparoscopy altogether as a tool for sterilization.

No matter what the future role of laparoscopy in our discipline becomes, there can be no doubt that it has made many gynecologists into endoscopists. As a result of this, and the same technologic improvements that made laparoscopy feasible, gynecologists have begun looking inside the uterus via hysteroscopy, the lower female urinary tract via urethroscopy, and at the unborn baby via fetoscopy.

Laparoscopic Sterilization

All of the laparoscopic equipment produced during the early 1970s utilizes the familiar unipolar, or monopolar, current. When the active electrode is applied to the tissue, the current density at the point of application is high and the desired tissue destruction is achieved. The current is then dispersed through the patient's body and exits via a return electrode. This is a conductive plate with a large enough area so that the current density remains low and there is no burning of the patient's skin at the exit point. As all surgeons know, however, improper application of the return electrode plate can result in areas of high current density and subsequent burns. Similarly, breakdown in the insulation and errors in technique can result in unwanted areas of tissue destruction, and burns of the anterior abdominal wall were one of the early complications noted with laparoscopy.

Shortly thereafter a more serious problem arose, specifically burns involving the small bowel with subsequent necrosis, peritonitis and even death. Most of these burns were unrecognized at the time of surgery, and resulted in an acutely ill patient requiring major surgery and experiencing a stormy convalescence. Although the incidence of bowel burns is relatively small (the reported incidence is 1 in 2000 but the actual incidence is probably somewhat higher), the seriousness of the complication as well as the medicolegal problems associated with it has been the primary factor behind the effort to seek safer ways of performing tubal sterilizations.

The other major factor in seeking alternative methods of laparoscopic sterilization has been an effort to curtail the extent of tubal injury, so as to improve the chances for tubal reconstruction at some later date should that be desired. Large numbers of women are turning to surgical sterilization as a form of contraception. In older age groups laparoscopic sterilization is the most frequently used form of contraception, and some of these women will, for various reasons, return at a later date requesting reversal of the sterilization procedure. Although the percentage of women in this category is small, their total numbers will become more significant as the number of sterilizations performed continues to increase. If other forms of laparoscopic sterilization can offer the same advantages and effectiveness, then indeed it would be worthwhile to utilize those techniques that result in a more limited destruction of the tube.

THE BIPOLAR INSTRUMENT

One of the first efforts to reduce the risks associated with monopolar electrical procedures was the development of the bipolar forceps, which incorporates both the active and return electrodes within the instrument. The current travels down the active electrode and across the tissue to be coagulated, which is held within the prongs of the instrument, and then back up the return electrode. The burn is discrete and limited to the tissue grasped by the instrument. Except for that tissue, the patient is not a part of the electrical circuit. There were technical problems associated with the initial bipolar instruments, resulting in incomplete coagulation of the tissue, but these problems have been overcome in the current instruments.[1]

It is necessary to use special generators with the bipolar instruments, since their insulation may not be able to withstand the high voltages produced by standard generators. The use of these special low-power generators means a longer application of the current in order to ensure full occlusion of the tube. Since the burn to the tube is limited, it is necessary to coagulate the tube in two, three, or four places, or up to a total distance of approximately 1.5 cm. This is a disadvantage of the technique, but the limited nature of tissue destruction is an advantage when considering the possibility of future reanastomoses.

With only the tube being grasped, and not the mesosalpinx, there is no interference with tubo-ovarian blood supply. Intra-abdominal adhesions, especially those that involve the bowel, can be managed with the use of bipolar current. Monopolar current can be dangerous in such a situation, but discrete coagulation of the adhesion, followed by cutting with scissors, can be performed utilizing the bipolar technique.

Because of the risk of bleeding during the procedure, it has been generally recommended that monopolar back-up be available, to coagulate any bleeding vessels. However, Rioux points out that sterilization using the bipolar technique requires only coagulation, with no need for the subsequent division of the tube. He believes that there is therefore really no reason to cause any bleeding, and that the occasional bleeder can be taken care of by a bipolar unit. As would be expected by the very nature of the instrument, there have been no bona fide bowel burns resulting from intelligent use of bipolar diathermy.[2]

THERMOCOAGULATION

More recently, electricity has been used to heat a resistant wire with subsequent heating of the tissue, resulting in a thermal burn as opposed to an electrical burn. These units use a step-down transformer or a rechargeable battery, so that voltages are safely reduced to the range of 4 to 6 volts. In the instrument developed by Semm, the resistant wire is incorporated into one jaw of the instrument and the instrument is designed so that the temperature can be preselected.[3] The patient is totally separated from the electrical current. Only that portion of the tube which is grasped by the instrument, plus approximately 1 mm on each side, is affected by the coagulation process. In the unit marketed by the Waters Company the cauterization is provided by a spring-loaded hook, which retracts the fallopian tube into a Teflon shield where it is coagulated and transected. The coagulated area is approximately 10 mm in length.[4]

Both techniques are relatively new so there has not been adequate opportunity to collect meaningful statistics. They do provide a discrete burn of the fallopian tube with minimal disturbance of the ovarian blood supply, but some concern has been expressed over a possible slight increase in pregnancy rates. This is based on the extent of the coagulation and whether enough damage to the tubes has occurred to occlude them permanently. It is believed that since the ends of the tube remain in close proximity, recannulization may occur more easily than with some of the other techniques.

THE BAND

In order to totally circumvent the use of electricity in laparoscopic sterilizations attention has been directed to the development of nonelectrical occlusive devices. The first of these was the Silastic band, developed by Yoon, and marketed as the Falope ring. The fallopian tube is grasped by the tongs of the instrument, approximately 5 cm from the cornual area, and a loop of the tube is drawn up into the central cylinder of the ring applicator forceps. The band is then placed down onto the loop of tube by the outer cylinder of the forceps.

Complications have been reported in slightly more than 5 per cent of the cases, but fortunately most are not life-threatening. The major ones are mesosalpingeal tears and transection of the fallopian tube. The latter occurs in 2.5 to 3.5 per cent of cases.[5, 6] It can often be avoided by retracting and expelling the tube several times prior to drawing up the loop of tube into the instrument. Although experienced operators can manage the tubal transsection by applying an extra ring to each divided segment, the band technique really should not be used without monopolar back-up for hemostasis. Transsections of the tube occur almost always with inflamed, enlarged or fixed fallopian tubes, so if the tube is enlarged or if there are pelvic adhesions or even a history of pre-existing pelvic infection, it would be wise to consider a technique other than the band. Similarly, the ring probably should not be used routinely in the immediate postpartum period because of the increased diameter and vascularity of the tubes at that time.[7] Long-term follow-up has shown that the bands do not become displaced, and are usually covered over with fibrous tissue or peritoneum with no adhesions developing to the area of banding. There has been no peritoneal reaction to those bands inadvertently discharged into the peritoneal cavity.

A significant problem associated with the use of the band, however, is intraoperative and postoperative pain. Patients operated on under local anesthesia can even develop a shock-like state when the band is applied. Topical lidocaine applied to the tube will relieve the pain during the procedure, but these patients will still experience the same degree of postoperative pain. Microscopic examination of the tube, both proximal and distal to the loop, shows a perfectly normal fallopian tube. This has been cited as an advantage should an attempt be made at a later date to reanastomose the tubes. On the other hand, it has raised the question of the similarity of this procedure to the old Madlener technique of tubal ligation, in which the ends of the tube were held in close approximation by a nonabsorbable suture. This procedure was associated with a significantly higher pregnancy rate than the other commonly performed techniques and has been largely abandoned. At the present time pregnancy rates reported with the band technique appear to be in an acceptable range, Poliakoff reporting 11 pregnancies (excluding luteal phase pregnancies) in slightly more than 2000 cases.[6]

THE CLIP

The other nonelectrical occlusive technique is the spring clip, pioneered by Hulka. It consists of two Lexan plastic jaws that have teeth on their opposing surfaces, which penetrate the tube at the time of closure and prevent it from rolling out. The jaws are in an open position until the clip is loaded onto the special applying instrument. An upper ram then comes forward, closing the jaws of the clip and allowing its introduction into the peritoneal cavity. The clip is opened again just prior to its application onto the tube, and then when the tube is in the jaws of the clip it is closed again. At this time a lower ram is pushed forward, advancing a gold-plated stainless steel spring over the clip and firmly applying it to the fallopian tube. Only 3 to 4 mm of the tube is occluded, and this allows an excellent opportunity for successful reanastomosis.

The clip technique has not been associated with any problems with tubal transsection, and bleeding has been less than with the band technique. In two series of over 1000 patients no hemorrhage from the mesosalpinx and no bowel injury have been encountered, and Hulka believes that the need for electrocoagulation as a back-up has yet to be demonstrated.[5] As with the band technique, less pneumoperitoneum is required because there is no fear of an electrical burn. In contrast to other forms of laparoscopic sterilizations, the tube does not need to be lifted up or put on a stretch. This means that the clip can be used in the presence of adhesions, thickened tubes, or bowel adhesions to the adnexal areas in which electrical techniques might injure the bowel. In fact, the operator needs only to visualize the uterotubal junction and the first centimeter or two of the tube in order to be able to apply the clip. The use of the clip is associated with only about half of the postoperative pain seen with the band technique, but it is still about twice the discomfort noted with electrocoagulation. Manipulation of the tube is somewhat difficult with the clip technique and correct application of the clip to the tube requires more skill than is required with the other laparoscopic techniques.

OPEN LAPAROSCOPY

The blind introduction of the needle and trocar has resulted in penetration injuries to stomach, large and small bowel, bladder, and more importantly, to major intraabdominal blood vessels. It is also associated with a certain number of failed laparoscopies, often due to preperitoneal placement of the gas.

These problems can be largely eliminated with the use of the open laparoscopy technique developed by Hasson. A small subumbilical incision is made and carried down through the fascia, and a hemostat is thrust through the peritoneum so that the peritoneal cavity is entered under direct vision. The special Hasson cannula is then inserted and the cone-shaped flange is pulled up against the anterior abdominal wall to provide a gas-tight seal. The peritoneal cavity is then insufflated and the laparoscopy performed in a routine manner. At the conclusion of the procedure, the abdominal wall is closed in layers. There have been no significant complications associated with the insertion of the Hasson cannula, and the technique avoids blind punctures, assures creation of the pneumoperitoneum and permits correct anatomic repair of the abdominal wall.[8]

Minilaparotomy

Laparoscopy requires a certain degree of sophistication, both with regard to physician training and the instrumentation employed. Just as techniques to avoid the use of electricity with laparoscopy have been developed, techniques that avoid entirely the use of laparoscopy are receiving increasing attention. Foremost among these is minilaparotomy, the "mini-lap." The technique itself is rather simple. An incision is made 2.0 to 2.5 cm above the symphysis. It is approximately 1 inch long, but some operators extend it to 2 or 3 inches in length. The incision is carried down in layers until the peritoneal cavity is entered. The wound edges can be retracted with special retractors, or frequently an instrument such as a proctoscope is utilized for access to the tubes. The fundus is manipulated so that the cornual portion of the uterus presents itself and then any type of tubal occlusion can be performed. At the conclusion of the procedure, the abdominal wall is closed in layers.

By avoiding laparoscopy, the complications of laparoscopy are also avoided: penetration injuries, electrical burns and gas embolism. Many authorities also believe that the pregnancy rate following a standard Pomeroy ligation, as is done with the mini-lap, is less than that reported following laparoscopic sterilization. The technique is easily learned and utilizes relatively inexpensive standard surgical instruments that are less subject to breakdown than the laparoscopic equipment.

On the other hand, the field of view is limited, so that even with the abdomen "open" and the patient under a general anesthetic the ovaries are not visualized in one third of the patients and there is no view of the abdominal contents. Not all patients are candidates for minilaparotomy. Any obstacle to uterine movement such as adhesions from endometriosis or pelvic inflammatory disease, and uterine fibroids are relative contraindications, and at times one may be forced to widen the incision and essentially complete the procedure by performing a laparotomy. Obesity is another contraindication, but it becomes less of a problem with increasing operator experience.

There is no doubt that minilaparotomy is a safe, simple and highly effective method of surgical sterilization and that it is admirably suited for mass sterilization programs in underdeveloped countries (where, incidentally, most of the women are thin). On the other hand, laparoscopy has captured the imagination of gynecologists and has assumed a major role in the specialty, with widespread application outside the field of fertility control. As long as laparoscopic sterilization can be performed with an acceptable degree of safety and success, it is reasonable to expect that it will be performed by those physicians familiar with the endoscopic technique. For those doctors who do not know laparoscopy, minilaparotomy is unquestionably the procedure of choice for fertility control.

Failures

The failure rates associated with the various tubal sterilization procedures are difficult to determine. Not only do many of the pregnancies occur years after the operation, but the statistics reported in the literature are often the results achieved by experienced surgeons and do not accurately reflect the overall results of large numbers of physicians with varying degrees of training. The experience to date seems to indicate that all of the laparoscopic techniques for sterilization are highly effective and that their failure rates are in the same general range.

A serious problem, however, is the high incidence of ectopic pregnancy among those patients who do become pregnant following tubal sterilizations. The seriousness of this situation can be appreciated when one realizes that even today ectopic pregnancy accounts for up to 10 per cent of maternal mortality. There is some preliminary data to indicate that the proportion of ectopic pregnancies is higher with the coagulation only and band techniques and lowest with the spring clip.[9] What the statistics finally show will have an important bearing on which technique of tubal sterilization will be most frequently employed in the years ahead. All other things being equal, the technique with the lowest incidence of ectopic pregnancies would be the procedure of choice.

Reversibility

Tubal sterilization should be looked upon as an irreversible procedure, and this point needs to be emphasized to the patient. Still, no matter how thorough the preoperative counseling, there will be patients who will return seeking a reversal of the sterilization. Interestingly, this patient is not the young nulligravida who has decided that she never wants to have children but is usually a patient with several children who, since the operation, has been divorced, is now remarried and desires to have children with her new husband. In Gomel's series of 100 patients requesting reversal of their sterilization, almost two thirds had had a change in their marital status.[10] It appears that approximately 1 per cent of the patients will seriously request reversal. As the number of operations performed rapidly increases each year, so will the actual number of patients seeking to have the operation "undone." There is only limited data on the success rates following the various methods of tubal sterilization, and it will still be some time before enough reversals have been attempted on patients with the band and clip to provide meaningful statistics. The overall results reported so far look quite encouraging. Gomel, using microsurgery, has reported an intrauterine pregnancy rate of 64 per cent.[11] Peterson and Behrman have implanted the ampulla of the tube into the back of the uterus, a technique, they think, that is ideal for the patient whose tubes have been extensively burned by the electrocoagulation technique. They reported 6 pregnancies in their 10 patients.[12]

Postligation Syndrome

One of the perpetual controversies in gynecology has been concerned with the "postligation syndrome." Nobody knows for sure if it exists, and, if it does, nobody can adequately explain the etiology. In some uncontrolled studies up to 50 per cent of patients have exhibited dysfunctional uterine bleeding and dysmenorrhea subsequent to the sterilization procedure, although in most studies the incidence given for dysfunctional bleeding has been in the range of 13 to 39 per cent. The difficulty lies in obtaining a well-controlled study, with patients matched for race, age, social class, parity, blood loss and pain. Added to this is the unreliability of subjective determinations of menorrhagia and the difficulties in measuring pain.

A frequently quoted study is that of Neil and colleagues,[13] in which laparoscopic and abdominal tubal ligations were compared, using women whose husbands had had vasectomies as the controls. Dysfunctional uterine bleeding was found in 39 per cent of the laparoscopic patients, compared with 22 per cent of those with abdominal tubal ligations and 13 per cent in women whose husbands had a vasectomy. However, this study was based on a questionnaire sent out postoperatively, and only three fourths of these were returned. Furthermore, Stock points out that Neil's study did not take into account the prior use of oral contraceptives and made no use of preoperative questionnaires or operative findings.

With this in mind, Stock studied the problem and found the incidence of both subsequent menorrhagia and pelvic pain to be 6 per cent.[14] Edgerton compared two groups of approximately 500 patients each, in which one group had approximately twice the volume of tube and four times the area of mesosalpinx destroyed by the electrocoagulation (two different surgical techniques having been used). He found no significant difference in the incidence of abnormal uterine bleeding, subsequent pain, dysmenorrhea or the need for subsequent hysterectomy.[15] The International Fertility Research Program conducted a prospective study of menstrual pattern changes—duration, flow and dysmenorrhea—questioning women at the time of sterilization, 6 months postoperatively and 12 months postoperatively. Only women with no prior contraceptive method, or only barrier methods, were accepted into the study and patients who had used intrauterine devices or steroid contraceptives were excluded. Their results did not indicate a pattern of increased menstrual disturbances after electrosurgical tubal sterilization.[16]

What causes the increased postligation

problems seen by some observers? It may well be that the sterilization request is a manifestation of a stressful life situation: a woman with an unstable marriage is more motivated to seek out the most effective method of contraception. It might be that the sterilization procedure itself turns out to be more stressful to the patient than was thought, or that the husband's response is disturbing. Some recent work by Berger et al. shows decreased luteal function in patients with previous tubal sterilization, but the data are still preliminary.[17] The pain sometimes reported may be due to torsion of the distal portion of the tube, since cases of infarction of that segment of the tube have been reported. Finally, one of the major factors is the attitude of both patient and surgeon. Patients, especially those who have been taking birth control pills, often have a decreased tolerance toward menstrual irregularity and pelvic pain. Following surgery the patient seems to forget her previous irregular and painful menstrual periods and seems only to remember the more recent years of regular, pain-free "menses" while taking the oral contraceptives. The surgeon thinks that since the uterus is now "useless," there is very little sense in medical management (he certainly does not want to put the patient back on the pill) and so a hysterectomy is advised.

Obviously, some of these problems can be avoided by a more thorough and complete preoperative history and discussion with the patient. Some physicians find it helpful to have the patient discontinue birth control pills several months prior to surgery. This permits the patient an opportunity to assess her menstrual function off the pill and eliminates the tendency to associate the menstrual complaints with the surgical procedure.

Hysteroscopy

Improvements in technology have also spurred a reawakening of interest in hysteroscopy. Although the information that can be obtained from direct inspection of the uterine cavity may be invaluable, there is still debate concerning the indications for hysteroscopy and the clinical significance of the findings. To many gynecologists, hysteroscopy is largely "a procedure in search of an indication."

The technique itself is relatively simple. The cervical canal is dilated, as would be done for a dilatation and curettage, to allow the introduction of a No. 7 Hegar dilator. The cannula, which contains a channel for the hysteroscope and accessory channels for the introduction of solutions and operative instruments, is introduced into the uterus via the cervical canal. The uterine cavity can then be distended with either carbon dioxide gas or a liquid medium. Dextrose in water is a readily available and economic solution, but it is miscible with blood, so that any bleeding from the endometrium will tend to obscure the view. This problem can be overcome with the use of Hyskon (32 per cent dextran 70 in 10 per cent dextrose in water solution). Hyskon does not mix with blood, so a good view is afforded even with the performance of intrauterine surgical procedures.

Unlike laparoscopy, with its familiar view of the abdomen and pelvis, the view through the hysteroscope is an entirely new one to the gynecologist. The endometrium in its different phases presents different pictures, and errors occur both ways in comparing hysteroscopic findings and subsequent clinical results.

Attention was initially focused on hysteroscopy as a means of surgical sterilization, with the hope that such a procedure could be performed in the office without general anesthesia. Most of the experience has been with electrocoagulation, and the failure rates have been unacceptably high, between 15 and 30 per cent. Complications have included perforation of the fundus by both the hysteroscope and the wire electrode, and even bowel burns.[18]

Hysteroscopy can be of value in the patient with abnormal uterine bleeding who has had a previous dilatation and curettage or has failed to respond to hormonal therapy. In a D&C small focal lesions such as fibroids or polyps can often be missed, and hysteroscopy can help to "guide" the curette for a subsequent curettage. At the present time routine hysteroscopic examination in infertility patients yields little information, and should not be part of the initial evaluation. If the history and examination point to possible intrauterine pathology, if the hysterosalpingogram is abnormal or if there is a history of habitual abortion, then hysteroscopy can be of value. However, abnormal images on the x-rays can be due to clots, mucus or debris, so that a patient with an apparently abnormal HSG will often turn out to have a perfectly normal hysteroscopic examination. Similarly, abnormal findings have been reported in association with normal hysterosalpingograms.

The problem concerns the clinical significance of lesions, such as polyps, septa and synechiae, found on the endoscopic examination. Interestingly, in one series the hysteroscopic findings in infertile patients were compared with findings in a group of fertile women scheduled for laparoscopic sterilization. The investigators found the incidence of these lesions to be quite similar in both groups—38.9 and 32.2 per cent, respectively.[19]

Hysteroscopy is invaluable in the diagnosis of intrauterine adhesions and offers a less traumatic and more refined approach to lysis of the adhesions under direct vision. Similarly, it can be used to avoid a blind approach to the removal of a lost intrauterine device and may be used to avoid unnecessary surgery. Patients whose menstrual history raises the suspicion of submucous fibroids, or whose examination suggests the presence of uterine fibroids, may benefit from a hysteroscopic examination. Resection of fibroids, especially if they are pedunculated, has been accomplished hysteroscopically using a modified urologic resectoscope, but this is a procedure that should be done only by gynecologists with advanced endoscopic skills.[20]

Because of the increased possibility of uterine perforation, all difficult surgical procedures performed hysteroscopically need to have concomitant laparoscopic control. Postmenopausal bleeding is considered by some to be an indication for hysteroscopy, permitting an accurate evaluation of the source of the bleeding and, if it is due to a malignancy, more precise location of the lesion. Others, however, consider carcinoma of the endometrium as a possible contraindication to hysteroscopy because of concern about retrograde dissemination of cancer cells. Such dissemination probably does occur, but the unanswered question is whether or not the cells form a nidus of metastases.

Contraindications to hysteroscopy include pelvic infection, which may flare up secondary to the procedure, and known intrauterine pregnancy, because of the risk of infection, abortion or perforation of the soft, enlarged uterus. Other contraindications include cervical stenosis and profuse uterine bleeding.

Fetoscopy

One of the most interesting developments in obstetric and gynecologic endoscopy has been fetoscopy. The technique involves the use of a small telescope that incorporates the lens system and fiberoptic bundle within a diameter of only 1.7 mm. The cannula has an outside diameter of 2.2 mm, approximately the size of a 14-gauge needle. Preliminary evaluation by ultrasonography is absolutely essential for localization of the placenta and fetal parts and for selection of the insertion site. The trocar and cannula are then introduced through the central hole of an ultrasonic transducer, which permits precise determination of the location of the tip of the instrument throughout the procedure.[21] The amniotic cavity can be entered in more than 90 per cent of the cases. The procedure has been carried out with very low maternal and fetal morbidity, the overwhelming majority of patients continuing on with their pregnancy following the examination. Still, the procedure is not as simple as it sounds. The visual field is extremely limited and the membranes tend to sag down into that limited field of view. Furthermore, the amniotic fluid tends to become more opaque after 19 weeks' gestation, and significant amounts of meconium or pigments can make the examination impossible.[22]

One of the first uses for the technique was to inspect the fetus for anatomic defects. Recognition of fetal structures is difficult because only a very small portion of the fetus can be visualized at any one time. As expected, the ability to totally visualize the fetus improves with experience. Clinically, fetoscopy for visualization of the fetus has been limited to those patients with a child born previously with a recognizable and otherwise undiagnosable severe phenotypic abnormality. It is also indicated for the phenotypical defects that may be indicators of a more serious internal anomaly. The fetal scalp and the vessels on the fetal side of the placenta can be fairly consistently visualized, so that fetal skin sampling by scalp biopsy and fetal blood sampling can be performed. Cells from the fetal skin biopsy can be grown for cytogenetic examination in only seven to ten days, and, since healthy living cells are obtained, the samples are more suitable for biochemical analysis.[21] Fetal blood sampling is indicated for fetuses at risk for sickle cell disease or beta thalassemia, and an adequate sample for study has been obtained in more than 90 per cent of the cases in which blood sampling was attempted. It is possible to perform fetal blood transfusions under direct vision and to administer drugs directly to the fetus. Other future indications may include the detection of fetal infections, intrauterine malnutrition and the monitoring of the adequacy of fetal treatment in utero. On the other hand, its use may remain rather limited if other techniques are able to provide much the same information: ultrasound, for instance, has taken over in the prediction of fetal deformities. Performance of the technique dramatically improves with the experience of the operator, so that for the time being the procedure, still in its experimental stage, should be limited to a relatively few centers.

Urethroscopy

The large number of operative procedures for the correction of stress incontinence suggests that the cause of the problem is not operative failure but diagnostic failure. Although cystoscopy has been in use for a centruy, it has only been in recent years that urethroscopy has been utilized as a part of the urodynamic evaluation of the patient with urinary incontinence.[23]

Robertson has developed a gas urethroscope, 8 inches long and 24 French in diameter, with a straight head-on (180-degree) view. The gas used is carbon dioxide, which acts as an obturator and urethral dilator for the introduction of the telescope. The distal urethra is anesthetized with a topical agent and the urethroscope inserted. The urethral mucosa is inspected for evidence of pus, inflammation, diverticula and atrophy. The procedure can be easily performed in the office with minimal discomfort to the patient.

REFERENCES

1. Engel, T.: Laparoscopic sterilization: electrosurgery or clip application? J. Reprod. Med. 21:107, 1978.
2. Rioux, J. E.: The relative risks of unipolar versus bipolar electrocoagulation. *In* Phillips, J. M., (ed.): Endoscopy in Gynecology. Downey, Ca., American Association Gynecologic Laparoscopists, 1978.
3. Semm, K.: Endocoagulation: a new field of endoscopic surgery. J. Reprod. Med. 16:195, 1976.
4. Valle, R. F. and Battifora, H. A.: A new approach to tubal sterilization by laparoscopy. Fertil. Steril. 30:415, 1978.
5. Hulka, J. F.: Relative risks and benefits of electric and nonelectric sterilization techniques. J. Reprod. Med. 21:111, 1978.
6. Poliakoff, S. R., Yoon, I. B. and King, T. M.: A four-year experience with the Yoon ring. *In* Phillips, J. M., (ed.): Endoscopy in Gynecology. Downey, Ca., American Association Gynecologic Laparoscopists, 1978.
7. Ziegler, J. S., Schneider, G. T. and Caire, A. A.: A comparison of the Falope ring and laparoscopic tubal cauterization. J. Reprod. Med. 20:237, 1978.
8. Hasson, H. M.: Open laparoscopy: a report of 150 cases. J. Reprod. Med. 12:234, 1974.
9. Tatum, H. J. and Schmidt, F. H.: Contraceptive and sterilization practices and extrauterine pregnancy: a realistic perspective. Fertil. Steril. 28:407, 1977.
10. Gomel, V.: Profile of women requesting reversal of sterilization. Fertil. Steril. 30:39, 1978.
11. Gomel, V.: Tubal reanastomosis by microsurgery. Fertil. Steril. 28:59, 1977.
12. Peterson, E. P., Musich, J. R. and Behrman, S. J.: Uterotubal implantation and obstetric outcome after previous sterilization. Am. J. Obstet. Gynecol. 128:662, 1977.
13. Neil, J. R., Hammond, G. T., Nobel, A. D., Rushton, L. and Letchworth, A. T.: Late complications of sterilization by laparoscopy and tubal ligation. Lancet 2:699, 1975.
14. Stock, R. J.: Evaluation of sequelae of tubal ligation. Fertil. Steril. 29:169, 1978.
15. Edgerton, W. D.: Late complications of laparoscopic sterilization, II. J. Reprod. Med. 21:41, 1978.
16. Sciarra, J. J., Zatuchni, G. I. and Speidel, J. J.: Risks, benefits and controversies in fertility control. Hagerstown, Harper and Row, 1978.
17. Berger, G. S., Radwanska, E. and Hammond, J. E.: Possible ovulatory deficiency after tubal ligation. Am. J. Obstet. Gynec. 132:699, 1978.
18. Cibils, L. A.: Permanent sterilization by hysteroscopic cauterization. Am. J. Obstet. Gynecol. 121:513, 1976.
19. Siegler, A. M., Kemmann, E. and Gentile, O. P.: Hysteroscopic procedures in 257 patients. Fertil. Steril. 27:1267, 1976.
20. Neuwirth, R. S.: A new way to manage submucous fibroids. Contemp. Ob. Gyn. 12:101, 1978.
21. Hobbins, J. C. and Mahoney, M. J.: Fetoscopy and fetal blood sampling: the present state of the method. Clin. Obstet. Gynecol. 19:341, 1976.
22. Hobbins, J. C. and Mahoney, M. J.: Fetoscopy in continuing pregnancies. Am. J. Obstet. Gynecol. 129:440, 1977.
23. Robertson, J. R.: Who is the genitourinary surgeon for women? Trans. Pac. Coast Obstet. Gynec. Soc. 45:31, 1977.
24. Kassar, N. S., Huse, W. J. and Jonas, H. S.: The value of a urethroscopic evaluation in the treatment of stress incontinence. *In* Phillips, J. M. (ed.): Endoscopy in Gynecology. Downey, Ca., American Association Gynecologic Laparoscopists, 1978.
25. Younglove, R. H., Wall, L. A. and Newman, R. L.: Diagnosis and treatment of female urinary incontinence with the Robertson urethroscope. *In* Phillips, J. M. (ed.): Endoscopy in Gynecology. Downey, Ca., American Association Gynecologic Laparoscopists, 1978.

Editorial Comment

One of the most exciting advances in obstetrics and gynecology in the United States has occurred during the past 15 years and relates specifically to endoscopy, or the direct visualization of organs by means of optic instruments. Since the advent of fiberoptics, obstetrics and gynecology has advanced from a science of palpation and deductive reasoning to one of direct visualization of the pathology within or outside of specific organs. Many years ago the culdoscope was the only visual instrument used by the obstetrician-gynecologist to diagnose pelvic pathology. (A disagreement still exists as to whether endoscopy is appropriate and needed for diagnosis and therapy in our specialty.)

Each of the authors, Cibils, Kim and Pent, has covered the topic very well. Basically, obstetrics and gynecology has become a specialty of the seven "oscopies;" culd-, lapar-, fet-, hyster-, amni-, cyst- and colp-. Everybody agrees that the development of laparoscopy has been aided by the advent of superior optics and fiberoptics that have revolutionized diagnostics for us.

Early indications for the use of laparoscopy dealt with the infertile patient, since it has always been difficult to determine the anatomic and pathologic condition of the tubes and ovaries. The laparoscope, along with other endoscopes, has made possible a new realm of outpatient procedures.

It is now possible to evaluate patients by endoscopy who have problems of infertility in a critical manner by directly visualizing the injection of dye that is emitted from the fallopian tubes. An area that has been most life-saving in endoscopy has been in ruling out ectopic pregnancy. Now if an ectopic pregnancy is suspected it should be ruled out by laparoscopy. Ectopic pregnancy accounts for 1 out of every 12 maternal deaths, and such no longer need be the case.

Chronic pelvic pain is an enigma for the gynecologist and is best diagnosed by laparoscopy because there is now little reason to do a laparotomy for such a condition. The diagnosis of pelvic inflammatory disease is often difficult unless laparoscopy is done. Swedish gynecologists have shown that 65 per cent of women with a clinical diagnosis of pelvic inflammatory disease have the disease; however, 35 per cent do not. This precision in diagnosis is important for the long-term management of such individuals and appropriate to eliminate the stigma of this disease.

Other methods of endoscopy have found favor in our field and include hysteroscopy, with an ability now to diagnose uterine synechiae. Therapeutically the physician can alter this condition by cutting the adhesions as well as removing imbedded or "lost" intrauterine contraceptive devices. Tubal cautery by hysteroscopy has not found much favor in this country, even though it has been used extensively in Europe and Mexico.

More recent advances in endoscopy deal with female urology and urethroscopy, principally with the instillation of carbon dioxide into the bladder. In the diagnostic work-up of individuals who have stress incontinence, this has helped to identify those who would not benefit from operation. We have found that doing endoscopy of the urethra and bladder at the time of either anterior colporrhaphy with urethral suspension or retropubic urethropexy enables us to identify funneling at the bladder neck, to alter the angle and to achieve better results than ever before.

Obstetrics has a new area for endoscopy called fetoscopy. (The case of the second trimester abortion patient lends itself well to learning how this is done prior to the instillation of the abortificant medication.) Fetoscopy has a limited indication

508

and at this point is used principally for biochemical or tissue cytogenetic or enzyme studies to rule out potential congenital anomalies. Its major indication in Europe has been the diagnosis of thalassemia by fetal blood sampling. The problem in the United States is to find an appropriate indication and if this is done to then find someone competent to do the procedure.

If we look at methods of sterilization, this involves the decision of whether the individual patient should have closed laparoscopy, open laparoscopy, minilaparotomy or hysteroscopy, Many competent gynecologists prefer minilaparotomy as a means of sterilization because it carries with it morbidity similar to that for laparoscopy. It would seem that method choice would depend more upon patient preference and the skills of the operator since all the methods are effective.

There is a controversy among the laparoscopists as to whether the tube should be transsected and a portion removed, or whether neither should be done when coagulation of the fallopian tube is performed.

Most gynecologists have abandoned unipolar cautery and now use only bipolar cautery, which basically eliminates the entire patient from part of the current because the only current involved is at the tip of the instrument that is in contact with the tube. Additionally, it is almost impossible to create thermal burns of the bowel using bipolar cautery. The complications of unipolar cautery are mainly those of thermal bowel burns, which occur in approximately 1 in 2000 cauteries. However, when these do occur, they may cause generalized peritonitis and death. I have been called in consultation on the cases of three patients who have died as a result of cautery due to bowel burns, peritonitis and septic shock. One additional reason for its decline in use is that unipolar cautery destroys more of the tube and if a patient requests microsurgery reanastomosis, the results are better with bipolar cautery, the clip or the occluding ring than with unipolar cautery. There is a controversy at the present time as to whether or not the fallopian tube should be divided if bipolar cautery is used. It's obvious that if the cautery is done correctly the tube is completely occluded; however, I know of no way to tell externally whether or not this has been achieved. We still recommend cutting the tube after bipolar cautery, and this information is carefully recorded on the operative note.

The band and the clip are emerging as methods of sterilization that are especially adaptable to younger women in case the necessity arises in the future for tubal reanastomosis. The clip has the advantage of being able to fit on tubes that are larger and more edematous, and there is no problem with transsecting the tube. This situation occasionally occurs when the Silastic band is used. Use of the band carries with it postoperative bilateral lower abdominal discomfort that lasts for a short period of time, whereas use of the clip involves about half the amount of discomfort. What all of this gets down to is individual selection of patients as pointed out by Cibils, Kim and Pent. It is essential to know the absolute contraindications for laparoscopy with general intubation anesthesia. These include diaphragmatic hernia, intestinal obstruction, extensive bowel adhesions, inability to establish a pneumoperitoneum, as well as any specific contraindication to general anesthesia. Pent points out one of the problems encountered following laparoscopy sterilization: the so-called post-tubal ligation syndrome. Whether it really exists is a matter of controversy. We believe that most gynecologists think it does and in at least one study in which laparoscopy was compared to "mini-lap" and to vasectomy, there was a significant incidence. At the present time there are no good randomized prospective studies with excellent follow-up that can settle the dispute. There are many reasons, Pent says, why these situations occur, but the answers are not always easy to come by.

All of the authors have utilized culdoscopy in the past, and everyone thinks that there is little controversy here, since it is a useful tool. However, culdoscopy does not replace laparoscopy because there are few therapeutic maneuvers that can be done through the culdoscope. It is designed mainly for markedly obese patients in whom laparoscopy is contraindicated or for women who have abdominal wall adhesions, in which the pelvic contents need to be viewed.

The hysteroscope has been a useful instrument and is suited principally for diagnosis and therapy of intrauterine adhesions. The so-called "lost intrauterine contraceptive device" frequently in the uterus can be easily extracted with the hysteroscope. Therapy using thermal cautery of the fallopian tubes through the hysteroscope has never really caught on well in this country, and all agree that there are better ways to occlude the fallopian tubes. There was an era in which the hope was that the hysteroscope could be utilized in underdeveloped countries with local anesthesia used for tubal occlusions, but this has never really gone well.

During the past 15 years, the specialty of obstetrics and gynecology has certainly changed, and one of the reasons for its change has been the introduction of endoscopy. Our specialty now emerges as the most sophisticated one for endoscopy in medicine, since we now use it to peer into the abdomen, the pelvis, the urethra, the bladder, the uterus and the amniotic sac. There are few areas left that we have not been able to view, and all of this has led to superior diagnostic techniques and the privilege of preventing major surgery through use of procedures that create good reproductive organ rehabilitation with less morbidity for the patient.

18

Candidates for Reparative Uterine and Fallopian Tubal Surgery

Alternative Points of View

by I. Brosens
by Marvin A. Yussman

Editorial Comment

Diagnosis and Management of Urinary Incontinence

Jack R. Robertson, M.D.
University of Southern California, Santa Maria, California

Selection of candidates for reparative uterine and fallopian tube surgery remains a crucial problem in the treatment of female infertility. In this chapter I will attempt a critical review of investigative procedures, contraindications and reasons for failure.

Preoperative Investigations

Before reparative surgery of the uterus or fallopian tube is attempted, it is mandatory to investigate the couple and to ascertain that there is no other cause of infertility. This investigation includes history, postcoital test, sperm analysis, assessment of ovarian function by basal body temperature, and properly timed endometrial biopsy or plasma progesterone assay or both.

Hysterosalpingography and laparoscopy are complementary procedures for the preoperative assessment of the internal genital organs.[1-3] Although hysterosalpingography is a relatively simple procedure it can cause, even under antibiotic cover, a flare-up of a latent inflammatory condition. If it is carried out during the early or mid follicular phase of the cycle there is no interference with a potential pregnancy, but the risk of false occlusion due to spasm at the uterotubal junction appears to be higher during this period than during the immediate postovulatory period. Uterine anomalies, endometrial polyps, submucous fibroids and synechiae can be detected or suspected and must be differentiated from artefacts.

In cornual occlusion of the tubes it is important to find out if the intramural segment is patent, in which case tubocornual anastomosis can be performed. In mid tubal occlusion or after sterilization the length and the patency of the proximal tubal segment can be assessed and in terminal occlusion the structure and fold pattern of the ampullary segment are important factors in the prognosis.[4-6] Cornual polyps in otherwise patent tubes are not uncommon but are rarely diagnosed on the hysterosalpingogram. Such polyps can measure 1 to 4 mm in size and if they are bilateral they can cause infertility.[7] Protruding from the intramural portion into the isthmic segment, the polyps are seen as an umbrella-like picture on the hysterosalpingogram. They contain endometrial glandular stroma but are largely covered by ciliated tubal epithelium with no or few glandular openings (Fig. 1).

A normal hysterosalpingogram does not exclude significant tubal pathology such as periadnexal adhesions, infundibular phimosis or even a mild hydrosalpinx with a small opening.[3] Obviously, it is important to know the limitations of this investigative procedure.

It is now accepted not to proceed with reparative tubal surgery without preoperative laparoscopy. The procedure must be carried out with great care and by preference by the surgeon who will perform the reparative surgery. It may reveal unsuspected pelvic disease and permit a more accurate assessment of tubal damage prior to surgery. In general it is recommendable to perform laparoscopy in the early luteal phase. There are less false tubocornual blocks in this period, possibly because the isthmic mucus is thin at that time and the ovarian function can be evaluated. The use of a probe is very helpful to properly inspect the pelvic organs and to estimate the density of adhesions. Methylene blue or indigo carmine dye solution is injected transcervically to test tubal patency, but it should be remembered that even anesthesia does not prevent spasm of the uterotubal junction. It is estimated that by preoperative laparoscopy unnecessary laparotomies or those in patients who will not be helped by them can be avoided in one out of five cases.[3]

Hysteroscopy is an additional tool to explore the uterine cavity and to treat minor uterine abnormalities such as synechiae or endometrial polyps.

There is undoubtedly a great need for improved evaluation of the functional state of the fallopian tube. I have proposed a fimbrial microbiopsy technique,[8] but this has been criticized on the basis that microbiopsies are not representative. Pauerstein and his group recently proposed in vivo testing of the fallopian tube by electromyography.[9]

Indications and Contraindications

AGE. It seems reasonable to put a patient age limit on tubal plastic surgery, but it may be difficult to determine the age, particularly in the distressed patient anxious to obtain every possible help. The age limit is usually set arbitrarily at 37 years. The life table analysis shows that the fertility index starts to drop rather precipitously at age 35. However, it is reasonable to take into account three factors in addition to age. First is the type of tubal surgery; that is, the chances for conception are much better after tubal anastomosis for reversal of sterilization than after salpingostomy. Second is the family history of the patient. If you have a patient whose mother had three or four children after the age of 40 it is reasonable to offer her surgery. Third are psychological and social reasons. In some cultural groups even the slightest chance of conception may be a crucial factor in saving a marriage or a family.

Should patients be excluded on grounds of youth? Is it better to wait until a patient is more capable of understanding the importance of her operation or wants to conceive? (This may be a legitimate question if hydrosalpinx is discovered incidentally.) There are data suggesting that in tubal occlusion the lesions tend to get worse with time. In some patients it may therefore be advisable to try to restore patency even before they are considering a pregnancy. However, one should be careful and not become too enthusiastic with the knife.

ADDITIONAL FACTORS OF SUBFERTILITY. In many patients one or more additional factors of subfertility may be present, such as previous tubal (pelvic) surgery, anovulation, male subfertility or sterility or uterine malformation. Patients with one or more additional factors are not excluded if the additional factor can be corrected. However, such combined treatment is reasonable only if the tubal surgery has a good chance of restoring tubal function.

TYPE AND DEGREE OF TUBAL LESION. It is often difficult to assess accurately the etiology and extent of tubal lesion, as in tubal block.

Tubal Block. In several patients tubal occlusion diagnosed at HSG and laparoscopy is

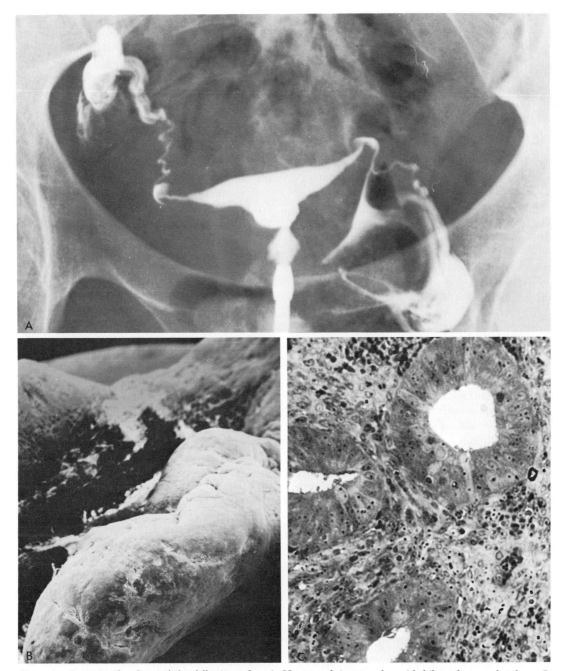

Figure 1. Intramural polyps of the fallopian tube. *A*, Hysterosalpingography with bilateral cornual polyps. *B*, Intramural polyp from right uterine horn measuring 4 mm in length (S.E.M. × 22). *C*, Postscanning histological section of polyp seen in *B:* the polyp has an endometrial glandular structure with small cell infiltration.

not confirmed at surgery. We all know of patients with "bilateral (cornual) block" who have conceived without surgery. Hysteroscopy and cannulation of the tube may improve the diagnosis. In tubal lesions without block, the lesions may include tubocornual polyps, salpingitis isthmica nodosa, tubal diverticula, tubal endometriosis, tubal tuberculosis.

Tubocornual polyps, even when they are large and bilateral, should not be treated primarily by microsurgery. The results are poor and it is not proved that they are a real cause of infertility. Frequently they are associated with other pathology such as endometriosis or endometrial polyps.

Salpingitis isthmica nodosa, if bilateral, may be an indication for surgery. The disease may progressively destroy the tube. Bilateral resection of the localized lesion in the isthmic segment followed by anastomosis may be successful.

Tubal diverticula are not an indication for operation, although they may be associated with an increased risk of ectopic pregnancy.

Hydrosalpinx. Bilateral hydrosalpinx is one of the major indications for tubal surgery; however, the results are still poor. Preoperative evaluation is difficult, but some criteria are important such as the presence or absence of folds on the hysterosalpingogram and the appearance of large distended or thick-walled hydrosalpinx at hysterosalpingogram or laparoscopy.

Unilateral Tubal Disease. Unilateral tubal lesions may be of different origin (congenital, infectious or systemic) and in general are not an indication for surgery. However, mild or moderate lesions such as phimosis or tuboovarian adhesions may be present in the contralateral apparently normal tube. If such lesions are present or suspected, operation may be justified.

"Frozen Pelvis"–Tubo-ovarian Mass. When the pelvic organs are immobilized by dense adhesions microsurgery is no more effective than conventional surgery. Such cases should be excluded, particularly if the condition is secondary to pelvic inflammatory disease or to previous surgery. A frozen pelvis secondary to pelvic endometriosis is a less unfavorable condition.

Combined proximal block and hydrosalpinx in both sides is no contraindication for surgery.

GENITAL TUBERCULOSIS. This is a major contraindication for reparative surgery, because the chances of an intrauterine pregnancy are extremely low. Any suspicion of genital tuberculosis should be explored by repeated examination of menstrual tissue to exclude the disease before reparative surgery is attempted. The disease has become rare in some countries but modern travel and migration is still a source of spread. Genital tuberculosis is suspected[10] on the hysterosalpingogram in several situations: (1) calcified lymph nodes or smaller, irregular calcifications in the adnexal areas; (2) obstruction of the fallopian tube in the zone of transition between the isthmus and the ampulla, often with sacculation of the terminal end; (3) multiple constrictions along the course of the fallopian tube (beaded appearance); (4) endometrial adhesions, and deformity or obliteration or both of the endometrial cavity in the absence of a history of curettage or abortion.

During laparoscopy miliary lesions in the pelvis can be observed and biopsied.

OTHER CONTRAINDICATIONS. Active pelvic inflammatory disease must be excluded by history, pelvic examination and blood analysis (erythrocyte sedimentation rate, WBC count).

Additional to the risk of surgery are the risks of subsequent pregnancy. Every patient should therefore be in good health and obviously there should be no contraindications for pregnancy. It is also unwise to attempt reparative surgery during acute illness such as ectopic pregnancy, ruptured ovarian cyst or appendicitis.

Reasons for Failure in Reparative Fallopian Tubal Surgery

The most careful preoperative investigation will not prevent a large number of patients from failing to conceive after surgical correction. It is obvious that surgery in the presence of progressive inflammatory disease leads to complete failure. Recurrent genital infection such as gonorrhea may also be a cause of subsequent failure.

Clearly, surgical repair of tubal patency is often not sufficient to restore tubal function. The functions of the fallopian tube are complex and still not exactly understood with regard to ovum pick-up and transport, sperm migration, fertilization and early embryo transport.

Salpingolysis and fimbrioplasty are relatively successful operations. Failures may result from adhesion or scar formation and alteration in the fimbrial-ovarian relationship. This relationship and the presence of the fimbria ovarica are probably important factors in the mechanism of ovum pick-up. Combined surgery of the equilateral fallopian tube and ovary is more likely to result in adhesion formation and subsequent defective ovum pick-up than extensive surgery of one of these organs only. From this point of view the Kistner classification[11] is a more logical approach to operative prognosis of endometriosis than the Acosta classification,[12] as it is based primarily on the number of organs involved. (It would, however, be more justifiable to have subdivisions for the extent of tubal involvement rather than for the actual size of ovarian endometriomas.)

The major unknown factor in prognosis is, however, the endosalpinx. A study of fimbrial microbiopsies in patients with periadnexal adhesions has shown that the endosalpinx is normal in most patients with endometriosis but that the percentage of ciliated cells is often reduced in patients with sequelae of pelvic inflammatory disease,[13] which is in keeping with the difference in pregnancy rates between both conditions following reparative surgery.

Salpingoneostomy is reportedly successful in one out of four patients. The fold pattern

on the hysterosalpingogram has some prognostic value. The large, thin-walled hydrosalpinx may indicate a better prognosis than the thick-walled hydrosalpinx, particularly if on the hysterosalpingogram a fold pattern persists at the isthmoampullary junction.[6]

A recent extensive study[14] of hydrosalpinx by scanning and transmission electron microscopy has revealed a variety of lesions of the endosalpinx such as attenuation and loss of the normal mucosal fold pattern, epithelial flattening, deciliation, pleomorphic aspect of the secretory cells and in severe cases defects in epithelium by necrosis or desquamation of the surface cells (Fig. 2). The reversibility of these

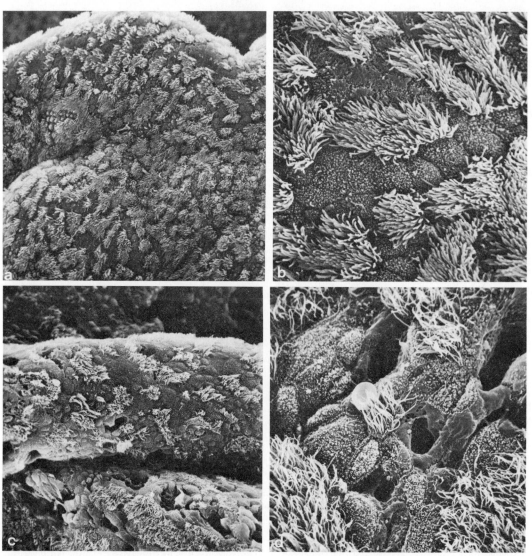

Figure 2. Changes of the endosalpinx in hydrosalpinx. *A,* Normal endosalpingeal fold of the ampulla (S.E.M. × 550). *B,* Normal pattern of ciliated and secretory cells in the ampulla (S.E.M. × 2200). *C,* Hydrosalpinx with deciliation (S.E.M. × 500). *D,* Hydrosalpinx with pleomorphic aspect of the secretory cells, deciliation and defects in the epithelium (S.E.M. × 2000).

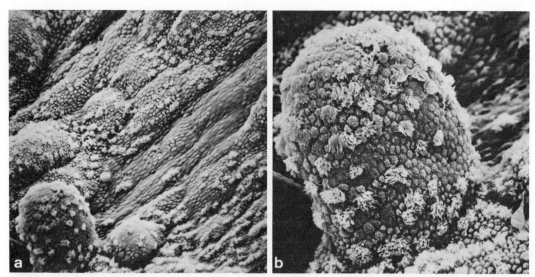

Figure 3. Tubal lesions following sterilization. *A,* The endosalpinx of the occluded segment on the uterine side (isthmus) contains small polyps and areas of deciliation (S.E.M. × 255). *B,* Small polyp arising on top of flattened fold in the isthmus (S.E.M. × 640).

lesions is probably the key to the ultimate outcome of the salpingoneostomy, and may also explain the observation that the majority of pregnancies follow after the first postoperative year.[20]

Tubotubal anastomosis for reversal of sterilization is becoming in some centers one of the most commonly performed reparative tubal operations. The prognosis depends largely on the extent of tubal damage and the technique of sterilization.[15] Sterilization by electrocoagulation and fimbriectomy are most unfavorable for reversal. Experimental and preliminary clinical data indicate that success of reversal is largely determined by the length of the remaining tube (more than 6 cm) and by the site of anastomosis (isthmoisthmic).

However, even after microsurgical anastomosis the pregnancy rate is not as high as the patency rate. A scanning electron microscopic study of tubal biopsies taken in previously sterilized women[16] showed that nearly half the patients had abnormalities of the tubal mucosa. The majority of the lesions occurred in the occluded isthmic segment on the uterine side with enlargement of the luminal diameter, formation of small polyps (varying between 50 and 600 μ in diameter) and loss of mucosal folds and deciliation (Fig. 3). Vasquez and colleagues also found a correlation between the occurrence of lesions and the duration of sterilization (Table 1).[16] Such lesions may play a role in the outcome of sterilization reversals, but their clinical significance needs further assessment (Table 2).

Cornual anastomosis by microsurgical techniques[17] is now replacing in many instances the classical technique of tubouterine implantation. Ehrler[18] demonstrated in 1965 that in cornual block the intramural or interstitial portion of the tube is usually patent. However, in a recent study of patients with cornual blocks, Vasquez and collaborators[14] observed the presence of small polyps in the intramural portion. These polyps are too small to be identified on the hysterosalpingogram.

TABLE 1. ISTHMIC TUBAL LESIONS FOLLOWING STERILIZATION

YEARS AFTER STERILIZATION	NO. PATIENTS	AGE (M ± S.D.)	FLATTENING OF FOLDS (N)	DECILIATION (N)	POLYPS (N)
Less than 5	16	32.4 ± 4.4	4[a]	3[b]	4[c]
More than 5	15	33.4 ± 3.4	14	8	11
Controls	8	36.6 ± 6.5	0[a]	0[b]	0[c]

P versus more than 4 years: [a]<0.001; [b]<0.05; [c]<0.01.

(From Vasquez, G., Boeckx, W., Winston, R. and Brosens, I.: Human Tubal Mucosa and Reproductive Microsurgery. IX: Microsurgery in Female Infertility. *In* Crosignani, P. G. and Rubin, B. L. (eds.): Proceedings of the Serono Clinical Colloquia on Reproduction I. New York, Academic Press, 1980.)

TABLE 2. PREGNANCY AFTER REVERSAL OF STERILIZATION

Sterilization-reversal interval	<5 years	>5 years
Number of patients	11	15
Age at reversal (m ± s.d.)	31 ± 1 years	33 ± 3 years
Pregnancy		
Successful	7 (63%)	3 (20%)
Miscarriage	0	2
Tubal	1	0

(From Vasquez, G., Boeckx, W., Winston, R. and Brosens, I.: Human Tubal Mucosa and Reproductive Microsurgery. IX: Microsurgery in Female Infertility. *In* Crosignani, P. G. and Rubin, B. L. (eds.): Proceedings of the Serono Clinical Colloquia on Reproduction I. New York, Academic Press, 1980.)

They do not always block the tube but can probably interfere with transport if they are not removed. The polyps associated with cornual blocks have a fibrous structure and are probably different from endometrial cornual polyps.

The possibility of ectopic implantation following fallopian tubal surgery is well known (Table 3). The basic question is whether this implantation is a consequence of restoring tubal patency in women at risk or is a surgical sequela arising from the formation of fibrosis, adhesions, stenosis or displacement. Clinical data seem to indicate that microsurgery does not reduce the risk of ectopic pregnancy following salpingostomy,[19] but the risk seems to be lower after microsurgical tubotubal and tubocornual anastomosis than after macrosurgical anastomosis or tubouterine implantation.[20] This may be a benefit of less surgical trauma and improved tissue handling during microsurgical operation. It would seem from reading the literature that the ectopic pregnancy rate following salpingostomy is particularly high during the first postoperative year. An ectopic pregnancy is probably more likely to occur in a fallopian tube with largely normal fold structure but with deciliation. The degree and extent of regeneration of the endosalpingeal folds and ciliogenesis may be important factors in determining the risk of ectopic pregnancy during the first postoperative year.

Congenital Malformations

Most uterine congenital malformations are discovered only by chance or as a result of abortion, usually rather late than early, premature labor or malpresentation of the fetus. Many pregnancies occur in the presence of uterine anomalies. Therefore, when some uterine anomaly is found in infertility patients it is not easy to decide whether this should be an indication for reparative surgery. Apparently such a condition either can be coincidental or can induce subfertility rather than infertility. It is therefore essential to investigate other possible factors in subfertility. In the young woman with no other factor of subfertility surgery is less indicated than in the older woman or in the presence of other factors of subfertility.

Rudimentary uterine horns, especially those not communicating with the main cavity, can be difficult to diagnose and require excision if they contain functional endometrium.

Pregnancy and Labor After Reparative Uterine Surgery

The management of pregnancy and labor following reparative surgery is still controversial. Strassman[21] believed that scars left after reshaping of a malformed uterus or after resection of a rudimentary horn are sufficiently strong to allow normal pregnancy and labor. This view, however, is not shared by all, and elective cesarean section before term is often advised. It is also often advised to delay pregnancy for six months or longer after surgery to allow complete healing of the scar. This practice, however, is not logical on the basis of principles of tissue healing and pregnancy changes. The healing process in the uterus may be enhanced by pregnancy changes; hyperplasia of muscular elements and increase in collagen result in improved strength of the scar. No matter how long the incision is, it is more logical to advise patients to conceive early after repair of the uterus. In my opinion the risk of uterine rupture in late pregnancy or labor is presently overestimated.

Fibromyoma

Many women with fibromyomas succeed in becoming pregnant and often the tumors are

TABLE 3. RISK OF TUBAL PREGNANCY AFTER TUBAL MICROSURGERY

	NO. PATIENTS	INTRAUTERINE PREGNANCIES	ECTOPIC PREGNANCIES
Reversal of sterilization	360	210 (58%)	18 (5%)
Tubocornual anastomosis	111	37 (33%)	14 (13%)
Salpingostomy	586	137 (23%)	52 (31%)

Leuven Colloquium on Microsurgery, July 4, 1980

only discovered during routine antenatal examination. Moreover, it is important to remember that in older infertile women the fibroids can be the result rather than the cause of sterility and that not infrequently fibromyomas are associated with pathology such as endometriosis. If the other causes of infertility are excluded it may be justified to operate on intramural or submucous myomas of even moderate size.

Cases of uterine rupture following myomectomy have been recorded, but in contrast to the scar of plastic uterine surgery, many gynecologists believe that the scar of a myomectomy can sustain a normal pregnancy and labor. It would, however, be wise to perform elective cesarean section after myomectomy.

Uterine Synechiae

Uterine synechiae that are sequelae of pelvic inflammatory disease are frequently associated with tubo-ovarian pathology. The indication for surgery should therefore be based on both laparoscopic and hysterographic findings. Even in the presence of patency the prognosis may be poor due to extensive mucosal lesions.

Conclusion

The selection of candidates for reparative fallopian tubal and uterine surgery requires detailed and complete investigation of the fertility of both partners. Such a procedure should always be carried out after discussion of the indication, prognosis and risk with the patient. If surgery is decided on, the basic principles of gentle tissue handling and conservative surgery should be applied. Exact knowledge of tubo-ovarian physiology is the basis in deciding on the extent to which function can be improved by a surgical procedure.

REFERENCES

1. Maathuis, J. B., Horbach, J. G. M. and Van Hall, E. V.: A comparison of results of hysterosalpingography and laparoscopy in the diagnosis of fallopian tube dysfunction. Fertil. Steril. 23:428, 1972.
2. Swolin, K. and Rosencrantz, M.: Laparoscopy vs. hysterosalpingography in sterility investigations. A comparative study. Fertil. Steril. 23:270, 1972.
3. Gomel, V.: Laparoscopy prior to reconstructive tubal surgery for infertility. J. Reprod. Med. 18:251, 1977.
4. Ozaras, H.: The value of plastic operations on the fallopian tube in the treatment of female infertility. A clinical and radiologic study. Acta Obstet. Gynecol. Scand. 47:489, 1968.
5. Young, P. E., Egan, J. E., Barlow, J. J. and Mulligan, W. J.: Reconstructive surgery for infertility at the Boston Hospital for Women. Am. J. Obstet. Gynecol. 108:1093, 1970.
6. Madelenat, P. and Palmer, R.: L'avenir des gros hydrosalpinx. J. Gynecol. Obstet. Biol. Repr. 6:557, 1977.
7. Bret, A. J. and Grepinet: Polypes endométriaux de la portion intramurale de la trompe. Leur rapport avec la stérilité et l'endométriose. Sem. Hôp. 43:183, 1967.
8. Brosens, I. A. and De Graef, R.: Microbiopsy of the fallopian tube as a method for clinical investigation of tubal function in infertility. Int. J. Fertil. 20:55, 1975.
9. Eddy, C., Azaher, D. and Pauerstein, C.: Electrophysiologic function of the rabbit oviduct following tubal microsurgery. Fertil. Steril. 28:23, 1978.
10. Klein, T. A., Richmond, J. A. and Mishell, D. R., Jr.: Pelvic tuberculosis. Obstet. Gynecol., 48:99, 1976.
11. Kistner, R. W., Siegler, A. M. and Behrman, S. J.: Suggested classification for endometriosis: relationship to infertility. Fertil. Steril. 28:1008, 1977.
12. Acosta, A., Buttram, V., Bresch, P., Malinak, R., Franklin, R., and Vanderheyden, J.: A proposed classification of pelvic endometriosis. Obstet. Gynecol. 42:19, 1973.
13. Brosens, I. and Vasquez, G.: Fimbrial microbiopsy. J. Reprod. Med. 16:171, 1976.
14. Vasquez, G., Boeckx, W., Winston, R. and Brosens, I.: Human Tubal Mucosa and Reconstructive Microsurgery IX: Microsurgery in Female Infertility. In Crosignani, P. G. and B. L. Rubin (eds): Proceedings of the Serono Clinical Colloquia on Reproduction 1. New York, Academic Press, 1980.
15. Brosens, I. and Winston, R. M. L.: Reversibility of Female Sterilization. New York, Academic Press, 1978.

16. Vasquez, G., Winston, R. M. L., Boeckx, W. and Brosens, I.: Tubal lesions subsequent to sterilization and their relation to fertility after attempts at reversal. Am. J. Obstet. Gynecol. 138:86, 1980.
17. Winston, R. M. L. : Microsurgical tubocornual anastomosis for reversal of sterilization. Lancet I:184, 1977.
18. Ehrler, P.: Anastomose intramurale de la trompe. Bull. Féd. Soc. Gynécol. Obstét. 17:866, 1965.
19. Gomel, V.: Salpingostomy by microsurgery. Fertil. Steril. 29:380, 1978.
20. Brosens, I., Boeckx, W., Vasquez, G. and Winston, R.: Implantation intra et extra-utèrine après microchirurgie tubaire. In F. Du Mensil du Buisson, A. Psychoyos, K. Thomas, L'Implantation de l'Oeuf. Paris, Masson, 1977.
21. Strassmann, E. O.: Plastic unification of double uterus. Am. J. Obstet. Gynecol. 64:25, 1952.

Candidates for Reparative Uterine and Fallopian Tube Surgery

Marvin A. Yussman, M.D.

University of Louisville School of Medicine

The long-stable incidence of venereal disease started its dramatic rise in the mid 1960s and finally plateaued in 1977. Approximately 13 per cent of individuals who contracted one case of gonorrhea during this period were subsequently infertile. The infertility rate rose to 75 per cent in individuals contracting their third case of gonorrhea.[1] During this same period, physicians succumbed to consumer pressures to abandon criteria for tubal sterilization. Such pressure, combined with the technical ease of laparoscopic sterilization, resulted in an increasing number of sterilized women of low parity. It has been estimated that 10 per cent of sterilized women have had sufficient regret to investigate the possibility of reversing their sterilization.[2] These two sources have created an increasing pool of patients who are candidates for reconstructive surgery. This pool is in addition to the 0.34 per cent of women with anomalies of the genital tract[3] and the 20 per cent of women with acquired noninfectious abnormalities such as uterine leiomyomas[4] and endometriosis.

This burgeoning infertile population has been the primary stimulus to a resurgence of interest in reconstructive surgery of the genital tract. The second important stimulus has been the adaption of microsurgical principles, attitudes and, to a lesser extent, techniques to gynecologic surgery. The use of the operating microscope has not yet been demonstrated to be a major advance in the overall reversal of anatomic causes for infertility.

However, the attitudes and principles of the microsurgeon are being increasingly applied by all reconstructive surgeons. These principles include: (1) using delicate handling of tissue by the finest instruments that will perform the task, (2) avoiding tissue trauma by packs and sponges, (3) obtaining a clear operating field by use of tourniquets and constant irrigation, (4) obtaining meticulous hemostasis by needlepoint unipolar cautery or by microbipolar cautery, (5) using nonreactive, delicate suture material and needles appropriate to the procedure, (6) avoiding unnecessary handling of tissue and (7) striving for meticulous reapproximation of tissue layers.

Experienced surgeons will recognize this list not as a list of recent discoveries but as a reaffirmation of fundamental principles that too long have gone unappreciated. The stimulus of the microsurgeon, then, has been to excite the gynecologist by the promise, yet to be realized, that improved fertility rates can be achieved by combining these principles with the increasing array of sophisticated materials and intriguing, intricate procedures.

Although these technical considerations are important and certainly titillating, the most important consideration in the success of any surgical procedure to reverse infertility is the differentiation of the patient who can be helped by a procedure from the one who cannot.

The reader must know that much material offered on the subject of patient selection is opinion. While overselection of patients will likely result in improved *rates* of fertility, it will decrease the total *number* of pregnancies by dooming to childlessness some individuals with borderline indications for repair. On the other hand, abandoning all guidelines will unnecessarily subject many patients to the expense and morbidity of surgery and the emotional upheaval of unrealized hope. It is to the proper balance between these that pelvic surgeons must address themselves and to which the remainder of this chapter is devoted.

Congenital Abnormalities of the Uterus

DIDELPHIC UTERUS

History, pelvic examination, hysterosalpingogram, intravenous pyelogram and laparoscopy remain the keystones on which patients are selected for repair of the didelphic uterus or the septate uterus. The addition of hysteroscopy to the evaluation has added an interesting, but not particularly useful, dimension to the evaluation.

Didelphic uterus occurs in .33 per cent of women. Approximately 50 per cent of women with this abnormality fail to have successful pregnancies.[3] The didelphic uterus offers little diagnostic challenge. It is usually accompanied by a vaginal septum. The dual cervices are missed only if the examination is done too casually. Inasmuch as the septum is frequently deviated against one vaginal wall, exposing only one cervix, embarrassing oversights occur. In the evident didelphic uterus, a hysterosalpingogram is usually obtained for confirmation, though I have never observed a case in which it failed to confirm the expected finding. Complete duplication of the uterus is the least likely of the müllerian fusion defects to cause primary reproductive failure.

I have had occasion to consider several patients with primary infertility to be candidates for unification. The criteria were: (1) presence of a potentially fertile mate as determined by a normal semen analysis, (2) exposure to pregnancy for at least one year, and (3) no other evident cause for the infertility after evaluation of ovulatory, luteal phase and cervical mucus factors. Hysterosalpingograms were obtained. Laparoscopy was performed to rule out other evident cause for the infertility such as endometriosis. Laparoscopy was also

considered necessary to assess whether the uterine horns were sufficiently mobile to allow unification. Unification procedures were performed as classic Strassman procedures. No effort was made to unify the two cervices in order to decrease the theoretic possibility of cervical imcompetence. The reported rate of pregnancy following unification is 75 to 80 per cent.[5] It should be pointed out that an intravenous pyelogram is the most essential diagnostic procedure associated with this condition, since approximately 30 per cent of patients with a didelphic uterus have accompanying renal abnormalities. The most common of these are agenesis or duplication.[6]

At my institution we have diagnosed a rare variant of the didelphic uterus in four patients during the past four years. In this condition, one of the uteruses discharges into a blind vaginal pouch while the other discharges into a patent vaginal canal. Each of these cases had similar characteristics. Each patient had a normal menarche; dysmenorrhea was severe. Each soon became amenorrheic; a mass was discovered high in the lateral vaginal wall extending into the pelvis. The mass was ultimately determined to be a hematocolpos, though this was not immediately evident. Confusion existed because one good vaginal passage could be demonstrated and a cervix was visible at its apex. The first patient underwent abdominal operation, to everyone's ultimate consternation. The condition in the three subsequent patients was easily diagnosed once it was suspected. Surgery consisted of vaginally removing the septum separating the closed pouch from the open vaginal canal. Three of these cases were associated with left renal agenesis. The fourth patient had a normal intravenous pyelogram.

More common than primary infertility is fetal wastage secondary to spontaneous abortion or prematurity. Approximately 43 per cent of women with didelphic uteruses exhibit this difficulty.[7] The question exists of how many abortions should be allowed to occur before operative repair is undertaken. Classically, three are suggested. The physical dangers of abortion are not great. The mortality associated with early spontaneous abortion followed by dilatation and curettage is negligible. However, infection, blood group sensitization and incompetent cervix are all potential complications that should be considered before it is suggested that the patient undergo "test" abortions. Physical complications aside, the emotional drain of an abortion in an infertility patient is so great that the suggestion to "try" an additional pregnancy when abortion is likely will usually meet with resistance from the patient. In my experience, when the full details are disclosed to the patient, she rarely elects to undertake additional pregnancies, and prefers early operative repair. In this circumstance, the second abortion is considered the indication to proceed with repair. Although I have not performed unification following a single pregnancy wastage, I would not consider it to be unreasonable if other causes for the reproductive failure have been ruled out.

A variant of the didelphic uterus has been described recently. The "T-shaped uterus" has been demonstrated by hysterosalpingography to exist in some patients exposed in utero to diethylstilbestrol.[11] Approximately 90 per cent of patients with demonstrable cervical or vaginal lesions have been demonstrated to have some variant of the T-shaped uterus. Variants include constricting bands in the uterine horns or in the fundus, irregular cavities and enlarged or "box-like" uterine cavities. The significance of these abnormalities has yet to be defined. Initial reports imply an increase in primary infertility and abortion when this condition exists. Since insufficient data on this condition are available, no recommendation concerning an approach can be made. It is strongly suggested that no attempt be made to repair the abnormality until the reproductive history of individuals with this condition is reasonably complete.

SEPTATE UTERUS

The septate or subseptate uterus is not so immediately apparent, inasmuch as there may be no palpable division in the fundus. These are usually suspected at D&C following abortion or discovered by hysterosalpingography that is being performed as part of the evaluation of repeated abortion or primary infertility. If it has not yet been performed, initial evaluation consists of a hysterosalpingogram to confirm the diagnosis and to determine the amount of uterine cavity available for unification. Laparoscopy is usually indicated in order to plan the appropriate procedure. I prefer to approach a divided myometrium by a Strassman[8] procedure. I approach a unified myometrium with a Jones[9] or a Tompkins[10] procedure. The choice of the latter procedures is based on the width of the septum and the adequacy of the uterine cavity. With a wide septum, a Jones excision is used. With a narrow septum, particularly if associated with a marked compromise of the available cavities, a Tompkins procedure is used. In fact, each of these procedures results in similar pregnancy rates.

The prerequisite for surgical repair is a history of repeated abortion with no other demonstrable cause. Our approach to the number of abortions "required" is similar to that for the didelphic uterus described previously. We routinely obtain repeat endometrial biopsies or serum progesterones to rule out luteal phase deficiencies, and endocervical cultures, including mycoplasma. Laparoscopy is performed. Hysteroscopy is performed, although it has proved to be of no clinically applicable value in our hands. Successful pregnancy rates should approach 80 per cent following repair.

Primary infertility with this condition is handled much the way as with the didelphic uterus. If there is a potentially fertile mate as demonstrated by semen analysis and no other evident cause after at least one year's infertility, a unification procedure is considered indicated.

Acquired Uterine Abnormalities

UTERINE LEIOMYOMA

Uterine leiomyoma is estimated to occur in 10 to 20 per cent of all women, with a higher percentage occurring in blacks. While 3 per cent of women who deliver term infants have demonstrable uterine leiomyomas, there is little doubt that the presence of such tumors interferes with reproductive capacity. These patients usually experience repeated abortion, though primary infertility may occur. There are various opinions concerning the relationship of leiomyomas to reproductive failure. While a few authors continue to deny any relationship at all, most sterologists estimate that 25 to 40 per cent[17] of patients with uterine leiomyomas experience some form of reproductive failure. Even in those patients who complete a pregnancy, fetal mortality is reported as high as 11 per cent.[12]

The causal relationship between leiomyoma and reproductive failure is conjectural. The vascularity overlying myomas is poor. The hormonal response of the endometrium is frequently out of phase, interfering with nidation. Interference with expansion of the enlarging uterus and distortion of the endometrial cavity caused by the hormonally stimulated, rapidly expanding myoma have all been suggested as causes for reproductive difficulty.

As in correcting other anatomic defects for infertility, myomectomy should be considered after other causes have been excluded as far as possible. These include establishing the potential fertility of the male and establishing adequate luteal function, adequate cervical mucus and absence of tubal disease. Other factors helpful in selecting patients for myomectomy include number, size and location of the tumors. Submucous and intramural leiomyomas that obviously distort the cavity are more likely candidates for excision. Those obstructing the cornu or deforming the cervical canal are also likely candidates.

Even in parous women, myomectomy should be considered as an alternative to hysterectomy in patients who desire further childbearing. Successful pregnancy rates following myomectomy differ. However, a figure between 25 and 50 per cent is reported by most authors.[12-15]

In recommending myomectomy, physicians should be clear that it is frequently a stopgap measure. While a recurrence rate as low as 3 per cent has been reported, my experience is that this figure is optimistically low. A more realistic figure would be that of Marlowe,[16] who reported that 11 per cent of patients who had removal of solitary tumors ultimately underwent total abdominal hysterectomy for recurrent symptomatic myomas. Somewhat over 20 per cent of patients who had excision of multiple growths ultimately underwent hysterectomy for symptomatic recurrent tumors.

Another note of caution should be offered to those performing myomectomy for infertility. Approximately one fourth of all reconstructive surgery in the pelvis for infertility is undertaken to correct defects that are the result of previous pelvic surgery.[2] This knowledge should serve as a reminder to undertake surgery only in those in whom it is truly indicated. It further serves to caution the surgeon that even a procedure as gross as a myomectomy should be undertaken with the same meticulous attention to hemostasis and tissue approximation as more obviously delicate procedures on the fallopian tubes.

ASHERMAN'S SYNDROME

Although the condition has been known since the late 1890s, Asherman in 1948[18] elaborated on the syndrome of postabortal intrauterine synechiae as a cause of secondary amenorrhea. As originally described, this syndrome consisted of postabortal adhesions in the uterine cervix with subsequent infertility. This was gradually classified into a rigidly defined syndrome of amenorrhea secondary to apposition of the anterior and posterior uterine walls resulting from endometrial destruction. This destruction was due to a combination of the mechanical trauma of curettage combined with infection following incomplete abortion. This highly restrictive definition eliminated many instances in which varying degrees of intrauterine adhesions resulted in equally varying symptoms. Among these are hypomenorrhea, dysmenorrhea, unexplained infertility, early repeated abortion, premature labor and abnormal placentation.[19]

The presence of some degree of intrauterine adhesions should be suspected in any infertility patient with a history of D&C having been performed between the second and the fifth weeks after spontaneous abortion. It is even more suggestive when infection was present, although this may not have been clinically evident. The classic symptoms of hypomenorrhea and dysmenorrhea occur in approximately 20 per cent of patients. Erikson and Kaestel[20] reported a 20 to 25 per cent incidence of intrauterine adhesions of some degree in all patients undergoing D&C within two months following delivery.

The diagnosis can be further suggested by failure to obtain adequate withdrawal flow following estrogen-progesterone cycling. Hysterosalpingograms will likely demonstrate subtle defects if a small amount of contrast medium is used but will show only gross defects if performed casually with a large amount of contrast medium. Our own experience confirms that of Dmowski and Greenblatt,[21] who reported that 1.5 per cent of hysterosalpingograms will demonstrate intrauterine adhesions. This is the only condition in which I have found the hysteroscope to be an aid in diagnosis. Fine adhesions not demonstrated by hysterosalpingogram can be readily observed through the hysteroscope. Because of this, it would seem reasonable that hysteroscopy should accompany the infertility laparoscopy in patients who have previously aborted. Experience with the hysteroscope demonstrates that intrauterine adhesions is more common than previously suspected.

Indications for repair in this condition are perhaps less rigid than for the conditions of the uterus previously discussed. This is because the repair in most cases is quite innocuous, usually done at the time of hysteroscopic discovery. In more extensive cases the physician should consider the poor prognosis, even though surgical repair remains relatively simple. Live birth rates following therapy have been reported to occur in only 10 per cent of cases.[19]

Our therapy used to be a simple curettage, followed by corticosteroids, estrogens and broad-spectrum antibiotics. In the markedly adherent uterus, this was accompanied by laparoscopy to discover occult perforations and to guide complete curettage. This has most recently been replaced by direct lysis under hysteroscopic visualization.

Adnexal Abnormalities

PATHOLOGIC

We classify adhesive adnexal disease according to a modification of the classification suggested by Hulka:[22]

Stage I—Peritubal adhesions with spill of dye from the tubal ostium.

Stage II—Hydrosalpinx. No spill of dye; more than 50 per cent of the ovary visible.

Stage III—Hydrosalpinx. No spill of dye; less than 50 per cent of the ovary visible.

Stage IV—Tubo-ovarian complex.

These stages are further subdivided into A or B, depending on whether the adhesions are filmy or vascular. Findings are those observed by laparoscopy.

It is generally conceded that a normal semen analysis in the patient's mate is a prerequisite for tubal repair. The logic for this requirement is simple. The purpose of tubal surgery is to achieve pregnancy. The absence of a fertile mate obviates pregnancy. This principle, however, fails to recognize that a legitimate goal of tubal surgery is restoration of fertility potential—when the *option* for pregnancy is the goal rather than the pregnancy itself. Such a situation may occur in the patient considering remarriage or in one in

whom artificial insemination may be required. Needless to say, much counseling is required in these circumstances. It is my point, however, that such patients should not be dismissed without due consideration to *their* goal, as opposed to the goal the physician sets for them. In some situations I have been willing to accept a good postcoital test as a substitute for a semen analysis. While purists may find this unacceptable, I find it is occasionally practical when the mate cannot otherwise produce a semen specimen. Again, one should be willing to individualize rather than follow an irrevocable set of criteria. Other causes for infertility such as anovulation, luteal phase deficiency and cervical mucus factors should be ruled out or corrected.

Hysterosalpingography and laparoscopy are the keystones on which the decision to repair adhesive adnexal disease is based. The hysterosalpingogram demonstrates the size of the hydrosalpinx. Those 3 cm or larger are unlikely to be successfully repaired. The absence of mucosal folds portends a poor result. The hysterosalpingogram is vital in determining the site of obstruction, a point not necessarily recognized at laparoscopy. The demonstration of a consistent proximal block by hysterosalpingography associated with a distal occlusion demonstrated by laparoscopy is considered by most surgeons to be an inoperable situation. My rare decision to ignore this rule has only confirmed its truth. No patient with a dual occlusion on whom I have operated has achieved a pregnancy.

After a candidate has been selected for repair by general work-up and hysterosalpingography, laparoscopy should be performed. It has been suggested that this be performed in the immediate postovulatory period if possible. Such timing allows anatomic assessment of the corpus luteum in addition to assessment of the fallopian tube. The extent of the adnexal adhesive disease is classified as previously described. We generally eliminate patients with dual occlusions and those with tuberculous salpingitis. Patients with adhesive disease on one side and completely normal adnexa on the other side are not considered candidates for repair. After laparoscopy, the patient is counseled on the advisability of repair using the previously described criteria. Without other complicating factors, we generally counsel that the postrepair live birth rate is 35 to 40 per cent with stage I, approximately 20 to

25 per cent with stage II, less than 10 per cent with stage III and 0 with stage IV.

The age of the patient should be considered. The normal fertility potential decreases after age 24, and declines rapidly after age 30.[23] We do not generally consider a patient over age 35 to be a candidate for surgical repair. Diseases that would adversely affect pregnancy or that would be adversely affected by pregnancy should be meticulously sought before final advice is given on the advisability of tubal repair.

From a practical point, I consider obesity to be a relative contraindication to tubal repair. Since the operating microscope has become an increasingly popular adjunct in the repair of adnexal adhesive disease, the obese patient presents a mechanical barrier to effective repair.

While one can assess anatomic abnormality, there is no clinically applicable means of assessing the functional capacity of the fallopian tube. While experimental techniques of hydrosalpinx fluid analysis, microbiopsy and ovum surrogates are interesting and even promising, they cannot be applied currently.[24]

Repair is not performed at the time of laparoscopy but scheduled for some future time. This is to allow full discussion prior to undertaking the procedure. From a practical point, it allows scheduling of sufficient operating room time for an unhurried repair. It has also been suggested that the infection rate is higher if the repair immediately follows laparoscopy.

IATROGENIC

PREVIOUS TUBAL STERILIZATION. Patients who desire reversal of tubal sterilization undergo the same evaluation as those with adnexal adhesive disease. It is preferable to have a fertile mate, although I no longer consider this an absolute prerequisite. Evidence of ovulation and adequate luteal function is particularly important in this generally older age group. A careful obstetric history is important. There have been requests for reversal from individuals who have had disastrous obstetric histories. Such individuals frequently need to be reminded of the original reason for their sterilization. By far, the most common reason for reversal requests is remarriage. Loss of a child is the second most common cause. Women planning remarriage

often request reversal to establish their fertility potential rather than to plan an immediate pregnancy. While this certainly should be permitted, it should be strongly discouraged. The failure rate following microsurgical tubal reanastomosis *in ideal candidates* varies from 30 to 40 per cent.[25, 26] A couple planning marriage following tubal reanastomosis must be willing to accept childlessness in their marriage. It has been my experience that individuals requesting reversal are, in large number, quite mercurial in personality. In my practice at least 50 per cent of them change their mind after laparoscopy. This is yet another reason not to combine the diagnostic procedure of laparoscopy with the repair.

Candidates for reversal should have a hysterosalpingogram to determine the length of remaining patent proximal tube. The sterilization operative note should be obtained if possible. However, the nature of the procedure must always be confirmed by laparoscopy. There are a surprising number of discrepancies between the operative note and the laparoscopic findings. Patients who have had fimbriectomy should be totally discouraged. Though a rare pregnancy occurs following a cuff salpingostomy after fimbriectomy, it never should be undertaken with any expectation of success. Patients who have had occlusion of their tubes with mechanical devices such as Silastic rings or Hulka clips are best candidates for repair. This is particularly so if the ring or the clip has been placed in the mid isthmus. Patients who have had Pomeroy or Madlener types of procedures are also good candidates, depending on the amount of residual tube and the location of the defect. An isthmic-isthmic reanastomosis has the best chance of success. This is followed, in order, by isthmic-cornual, isthmic-ampullary and ampullary-cornual repairs.

Patients who have had laparoscopic fulguration of the fallopian tubes may be candidates for repair, depending on the length of residual tube and the degree of peritubal fibrosis. The surgeon frequently finds such extensive obliteration of the fallopian tubes following fulguration that repair is not feasible. In such candidates, the surgeon should assess laparoscopically that at least 4 cm of reanastomosed tube will remain after repair, though successful pregnancies have been reported with as little as 3 cm of residual tube.[2] In performing the preoperative laparoscopy, the surgeon should recall that the extent of luminal damage exceeds that observed on the serosa. Again, laparoscopy should be a separate procedure from the repair to allow proper counseling and to schedule adequate time for careful reanastomosis.

PREVIOUS PELVIC SURGERY. One of the most common causes of adnexal adhesive disease is previous pelvic surgery. Wedge resection of the ovaries and ovarian cystectomy have been reported to account for as many as 25 per cent of cases of adnexal adhesions. Our experience confirms this observation. The immediate lesson from this figure is to re-alert the pelvic surgeon to the need for meticulous layered closure in doing "small" pelvic surgery in the menarchal woman. The second lesson is that the surgeon should be highly suspicious of adnexal adhesions in patients who have had previous wedge resections or ovarian cystectomies. Such patients are excellent candidates for repair inasmuch as intrinsic tubal disease rarely coexists.

Reoperating on previously repaired fallopian tubes is notoriously unsuccessful. This is particularly true in the case of hydrosalpinx. It is less so in the poststerilization reanastomosis. In those instances in which the initial repair was adequate but a few adhesion bands appear to alter tubal motility, lysis can be undertaken successfully. Reoperating on a tube that has re-formed a hydrosalpinx is usually futile and should be undertaken only as a "token tuboplasty." This makes it imperative that the surgeon undertaking the initial repair be highly selective in whom he treats surgically, selective in which procedure is applied and meticulous in applying the procedure properly.

REFERENCES

1. Westrom, L.: Effect of acute pelvic inflammatory disease in fertility. Am. J. Obstet. Gynecol. 121:707, 1975.
2. Winston, R. L.: Personal communication, 1978.
3. Editorial comment: Obstet. Gynecol. Surv. 31:660, 1976.
4. Kistner, R. W. and Patton, G. W.: *In* Atlas of Infertility Surgery. Boston, Little, Brown & Company, 1975, p. 88.
5. Chapler, F. K.: Year Book of Obstetrics and Gynecology. Chicago, Year Book Medical Publishers, 1971, p. 20.
6. Chapler, F. K.: Concomitant congenital reproductive tract and urinary tract anomalies. *In* Bushbaum, H. and Schmidt, J. (eds.): Gynecologic and Obstetric Urology. Philadelphia, W. B. Saunders Co., 1978.
7. Jones, H. W. and Wheeless, C. R.: Salvage of the reproductive potential of women with anomalous developmnt of the müllerian ducts. Am. J. Obstet. Gynecol. 104:348, 1969.
8. Kaufman, R. H., Binder, G. L., Gray, P. M. and Adam, E.: Upper genital tract changes associated with exposure in utero to diethylstilbestrol. Am. J. Obstet. Gynecol. 128:51, 1977.
9. Strassman, E. O.: Plastic unification of double uterus. Am. J. Obstet. Gynecol. 64:25, 1952.
10. Jones, H. W. and Jones, G. E. S.: Double uterus as an etiological factor in repeated abortion: indications for surgical repair. Am. J. Obstet. Gynecol. 65:325, 1953.
11. Kistner, R. W. and Patton, J. W.: *In* Atlas of Infertility Surgery. Boston, Little, Brown & Company, 1975, p. 81.
12. Davids, A. M.: The management of fibromyomas in infertility and abortion. Clin. Obstet. Gynecol. 2:837, 1959.
13. Bonney, V.: Fruits of conservatism. J. Obst. Gynaec. Br. Commonwealth 41:1, 1937.
14. Fenn, W. F. and Miller, P. F.: Abdominal myomectomy. Am. J. Obstet. Gynecol. 60:109, 1950.
15. Brown, A. B., Chamberlain, R. and TeLinde, R. W.: Myomectomy. Am. J. Obstet. Gynecol. 71:759, 1956.
16. Malone, L. J.: Myomectomy: recurrence after removal of solitary and multiple myomas. Obstet. Gynecol. 34:200, 1969.
17. Rubin, I. C.: Uterine fibromyomas and sterility. Clin. Obstet. Gynecol. 1:501, 1958.
18. Asherman, J: Amenorrhea tramatica (atretica). J. Obstet. Gynaecol. Br. Commonwealth 55:23, 1948.
19. Klein, S. M. and Garcia, Celso-Ramon: Asherman's syndrome: a critique and current review. Fertil. Steril. 24:722, 1973.
20. Erikson, J. and Kaestel, C.: The incidence of uterine atresia after postpartum curettage. Danish Med. Bull. 7:50, 1960.
21. Dmowski, W. P. and Greenblatt, R.: Asherman's syndrome and the risk of placenta accreta. Obstet. Gynecol. 34:288, 1969.
22. Hulka, J. F., Omran, K. and Burger, G. S.: Classification of adnexal adhesions: evaluation of its prognostic value. Fertil. Steril. 30:6, 1978.
23. Kistner, R. W. and Patton, J. W.: *In* Atlas of Infertility Surgery, Boston, Little, Brown & Company, 1975, p. 1.
24. Pauerstein, C. and Hodgson, B.: Rate of transport of radioactive ovum models in the oviducts of individual rabbits. Am. J. Obstet. Gynecol. 124:840, 1976.
25. Gomel, V.: Tubal reanastomosis by microsurgery. Fertil. Steril. 28:59, 1977.
26. Siegler, A. M.: Surgical treatment for tuboperitoneal causes of infertility since 1967. Fertil Steril. 28:1019, 1977.

Editorial Comment

The area of reparative fallopian tube surgery has mushroomed into an entire discipline in our specialty during the past five years. It is becoming an integral part of training in residency programs. Importantly, it is the approach to those problems not heretofore solvable that extends our expertise in clinical medicine. Future generations of trained gynecologists will be able to offer help to patients with specific problems of tubal occlusion. This approach of microsurgery also adds a different perspective in tissue handling and cannot help but result in better surgery, especially for patients with ectopic pregnancy. This is a very positive change from "destroying" tubes to repairing tubes.

There never was a major demand in past years for tubal reanastomosis until the numbers of individuals wishing sterilization performed on them increased to more than 600,000 per year and from this at least 1 per cent requested reanastomosis, which amounts of a minimum of 6000 to 7000 patients per year. Once these figures emerged and the necessity became clear, the obstetrician-gynecologist responded with training to become a microsurgeon and to increase success for pregnancy by a twofold factor over conventional methods with this method.

We have real problems in the area of training microsurgeons at the present time. There are many three-day courses that claim to demonstrate how to do it. Individuals take these, go home, purchase a very expensive operating microscope and essentially consider themselves trained. This is an inappropriate way for those in our specialty to behave. It is only after considerable experience and time on animals, most preferably the rabbit, or practice with the use of the umbilical cord by anastomosing the umbilical artery and vein, that an individual can become skilled. It is a whole different ball game to learn how to function under the microscope. Indeed it is not easy, because procedures take a minimum of three hours and often may take five hours if there is complication with many adhesions. Unless you have a personality of great patience we would advise you not to try to become a microsurgeon because this skill is not suited for everyone.

Once the gynecologist is trained, the next hurdle is the exquisite selection of patients and it is here that your success will emerge. The authors of this chapter identify in a very detailed fashion the work-up that is necessary prior to reparative surgery. It is underscored that the laparoscopy should be done by the gynecologist who will do the microsurgery. If this is the case, it will diminish by 20 per cent the need for a laparotomy, as many individuals are just not appropriate candidates.

Careful selection and work-up by a skilled microsurgeon who has prepared well on animals before working on humans will assure results considerably better than those produced by the individual who casually does microsurgery. We are not sure why all obstetrician-gynecologists seem to feel the need or compulsion to say they can do microsurgery. The demand for microsurgery is so slight that the regular obstetrician-gynecologist may not do more than one to three cases per year. Unless surgeons do more than one case per week they probably lose some of their initial skills. This type of patient is probably best handled by referral to a surgeon who does these on a regular basis; then everyone benefits.

The new controversy of the microsurgeons is whether to use optic loops or the microscope. The magnifying loops of three to four power attached to the glasses make it possible to use 8-0 suture without difficulty and are more available when there is an unexpected problem with the tube. It is more convenient and easier to

526

be able to move your head with the magnifying loops than to always have to move the operating microscope. The one main advantage of the operating microscope is an attachment for televising what takes place; it also provides an excellent teaching device.

Whether to use the operating microscope or magnifying loops is only one issue. Both authors identify that the most significant issue is patient selection. You must choose the patients who you know will have a good chance of success for tubal patency and pregnancy. Philosophically, then, the question arises as to whether you have the right to make decisions such as this, since the patient is requesting that something be done. Can you really be sure there is no hope? Other unsettled issues in this arena of microsurgery include randomized investigation dealing with the size of the suture, and use of corticoids and antibiotics after surgery. Most authors believe that antibiotics are a must and there is still some discussion as to whether corticoids are beneficial in decreasing the tissue reaction following surgery.

Another area of controversy is how to prevent adhesions both inside and outside the tube. The use of dextran 70 was an observation of serendipity a number of years ago when hysteroscopy with tubal cautery was done. A very high failure rate was encountered in patients who had dextran used as a medium to expand the uterine cavity, as contrasted to a higher tubal closure rate when carbon dioxide or saline was used. Since then at least one report on animals shows preventive value in adhesion formation with dextran 70. We have used this for a number of years to prevent adhesions after both abdominal surgery and microsurgery. It is not a good substitute for impeccable homeostasis. There is still no good randomized study to state whether or not this is beneficial in the human.

Microsurgery is an emerging field and good clinical investigation is necessary to answer some of the questions posed. Since it is an expensive investment in terms of both time and resources, there is even more need for immediate answers.

19
Surgical Contraception

Alternative Points of View

by Subir Roy and Daniel R. Mishell, Jr.
by William Droegemueller,
Louis Weinstein and Patrick Morell

Editorial Comment

The Optimal Method of Female Sterilization

Subir Roy, M.D.
Daniel R. Mishell, Jr., M.D.
University of Southern California School of Medicine

Overview

In the United States the incidence of female sterilization has increased from 9.7 per cent of all couples practicing contraception in 1970 to 22.6 per cent in 1975.[1] Male sterilizations have followed the same trend with an increase from 10.3 per cent in 1970 to 24.1 per cent in 1975.[1] Currently in the United States, sterilization is the most popular form of fertility regulation for couples married ten or more years.[1] One member of 43.5 per cent of these couples is sterilized.[1] It was estimated that during 1975, 674,000 female and 639,000 male sterilization procedures were performed in the United States.[2]

Since there are a variety of procedures used for female sterilization, it is necessary to review the efficacy, complications and side effects of these methods before a selection is made. Before this review, we will discuss the procedures that have proved useful in the selection of candidates for sterilization.

Selection of Candidates for Sterilization

Since sterilization is, and should be, considered a permanent method of fertility regulation, it is imperative that sound counseling be provided the patient regarding the risks, benefits and alternatives. Counseling should include testing of the patient after visual aid and didactic* instruction. Information pertaining to all types of sterilization procedures and their complications as well as anesthetic risks should be covered in this presentation.

In addition, since the guidelines on sterilization of the American College of Obstetricians and Gynecologists (the rule of 120[3] that age times parity should exceed 120 before a woman is sterilized) has been superseded,[4] it has been useful to have more than one phy-

---

*These materials may be obtained from Association for Voluntary Sterilization (AVS), Planned Parenthood Federation of America and the Department of HEW.

sician decide whether sterilization should be performed if the woman is less than 25 years of age with fewer than three living children. At least two physicians should concur with these patients' request for sterilization before it is performed.

Reversibility Considerations

The rationale for so careful a scrutiny of these younger candidates is that they tend to change their minds more often than older women, as they have a longer period of reproductive life in which divorce, remarriage or death among their children can take place. It has been estimated that 1 per cent of sterilized women will subsequently request reversal.[5] On the basis of the 1975 AVS survey, this means that approximately 7000 women per year will request reversal.

The most effective, least destructive method of tubal occlusion is the most desirable in these younger individuals because with it ovarian function and adhesion formation are diminished while the incidence of successful reversal procedures is increased.[5]

For this reason, until reversibility of the clip and band techniques has been more thoroughly evaluated, we recommend that the modified Pomeroy technique be used in patients who are less than 25 years of age. Reversal of this method of sterilization is associated with approximately a 40 to 60 per cent successful pregnancy rate,[6-10] which is higher than that reported following laparoscopic fulguration. Many patients in the latter group are not candidates for any reversal procedure when very little tube remains.[9, 11]

In order to determine the optimal method of sterilization for an individual, it is necessary to evaluate the patient's complete medical and physical condition. It is imperative to determine whether any pathology, either structural or functional, of the genital (vagina or uterus) or contiguous structures (bladder and rectum) exists. In this manner, the least amount of surgery should be performed consistent with the patient's needs. Patients may be categorized into four groups according to whether or not they have pathology or are pregnant.

The first group consists of patients who have no pathology and are not pregnant. In these, a tubal occlusion procedure is the treatment of choice. Controversy exists regarding the decision to perform a hysterectomy for sterilization in the absence of pathology.

There have been numerous reports of the "post-tubal ligation syndrome"[12] (see Chapter 17) in which patients who have had a previous tubal ligation develop abnormal uterine bleeding associated in some instances with ovarian cyst formation. It has been hypothesized that the tubal occlusion procedure interferes with the ovarian blood supply resulting in abnormal ovarian function (e.g., lower estradiol production), which results in abnormal or dysfunctional uterine bleeding. There have been no published prospective controlled studies using actuarial methods of analysis to determine whether abnormal bleeding is greater in women who have had a tubal ligation than in a control group of the same age and parity. However, as this syndrome may exist and because removal of the uterus would eliminate the chance of cervical or uterine cancer, elective hysterectomy has been advocated as an acceptable method to sterilize women in this group.[13]

Reducing the chance of developing cervical or uterine cancer by hysterectomy has not been demonstrated to be cost-effective.[14] The cost of elective hysterectomy exceeds the cost of treating the few cervical or uterine cancers that would be expected to occur in these patients. In some patients, however, the peace of mind that they seek by having this organ removed is more important to them than cost considerations. In any event, the ultimate decision for hysterectomy is dependent upon patient desires after thorough counseling with the physician. A mutual decision should be reached regarding the best procedure for the individual woman.

The second group consists of patients without pathology who are pregnant. These individuals need to have been counseled either before pregnancy or early enough in pregnancy that a valid decision for sterilization may be made without the added emotional influences of an unwanted pregnancy. A consent for sterilization should not be obtained during labor unless it is a formality for a patient who has already had the appropriate counseling. These patients are ideally suited for a postpartum or postabortion tubal occlusion procedure.[15]

The third group consists of patients with pathology who are pregnant. If the pathology is limited to the uterus, an abortion-hysterectomy or a hysterectomy after cesarean section is indicated. If the pregnancy is less than 12 weeks and the pelvic arch is adequate, a vaginal hysterectomy has been shown to be a safe and effective method of sterilization.[12, 16] It is best not to evacuate the uterus first as it has been reported that there is less blood loss if the uterus is not evacuated before the hysterectomy.[16] In pregnancies greater than 12 weeks an abdominal abortion-hysterectomy may be safely performed without evacuation of the uterus.[13] A hysterectomy after cesarean section is indicated in the patient who has completed her family and has uterine pathology.[17]

If the pathology exists in the contiguous structures such as the bladder or rectum, the appropriate procedures should be performed on an interval basis. There are experienced surgeons, however, who have stated that vaginal colporrhaphies performed at the time of vaginal abortion-hysterectomy are not associated with an increased morbidity.[18] These anecdotal verbal reports would indicate that the increased vascularity of the pregnant state is offset by the easier dissection of the tissue planes. A definitive answer to the question of whether corrective surgery should or should not be performed at the time of pregnancy termination must await the reports of well-designed prospective studies.

The final group of patients includes those who have pathology and are not pregnant. In these, interval corrective surgery should be performed.

Tubal Occlusive Procedures

CLASSICAL METHODS

The classical tubal occlusive techniques may be performed via laparotomy, minilaparotomy or colpotomy approaches. With the Madlener technique,[19] first reported in 1919, the midportion of the oviduct is formed into a loop, the base of which is crushed with a clamp and ligated with a nonabsorbable suture. The failure rates have been reported to range from 0.3 to 2.0 per cent.[20] Some have modified this technique by cutting off the loop. Whether this modification reduces the failure rate is not known.

Irving,[21] in 1924, reported a technique of dividing the oviduct between two absorbable suture ligatures and burying the proximal stump in the posterior myometrium. The failure rate is nil.[20] It does take more time and a larger incision than most tubal occlusion methods, but is more effective.

Colleagues of Pomeroy[22] published his method in 1930 after his death. It is the most popular method of tubal occlusion because of its simplicity. The oviduct is picked up near its midportion to form a loop. A ligature of absorbable suture is placed around the base of the loop and the portion of the oviduct above the ligature is then cut off. This procedure can be performed at any time through any incision. The usual failure rate for this procedure has been reported to range from 0.0 to 0.4 per cent.[20] Some investigators have reported an unexplained high failure rate of 2.5 to 5.0 per cent when this procedure is performed at the time of cesarean section.[23-25] Husbands,[26] however, reported no increase in the failure rate, 0.2 per cent, whether the procedure was performed at the time of cesarean section or as an interval procedure. Some modified the Pomeroy technique and coagulated[27] or applied phenol and alcohol[28] to the cut ends of the oviduct. In both these personal series no failures have been reported.

Aldridge[29] reported a technique in 1934 that is interesting for its lack of tissue destruction and its potential for reversibility. The fimbriae are inserted into a neo-bursa through an incision of the parietal peritoneum. Sutures between the tubal serosa and the peritoneum secure and separate the fimbrial ends of the tubes from the ovaries. Reversal is, theoretically, accomplished by opening the peritoneum over the neo-bursa and removing the fimbrial ends of the tubes. There have been only a few reports of this procedure being performed and none of the reversal.[29]

Fimbriectomy, or the Kroener procedure,[30] has been employed since 1935, although it was only reported in 1969. A double silk ligature is placed around the distal one third of the tube with excision of the fimbrial end. This method is particularly suited to the vaginal approach. The failure rate with this method has been reported as zero.[20] Hydrosalpinx formation has been reported after this procedure, which may necessitate further surgery.[31, 32]

The Uchida technique[33] reported in 1961 requires injection of a solution, either saline or epinephrine-saline (1:1000), beneath the serosa of the ampulla. The serosa is incised and the muscular portion of the tube dissected so that a 5 cm segment may be ligated with nonabsorbable suture at each end and then excised. The proximal stump is buried within the serosa while the distal end is left protruding into the peritoneal cavity; this end is encircled with a purse-string ligature of the serosa. The failure rate is nil.[20] This technique is performed by the abdominal approach only.

Tubal sterilization by colpotomy[12] is associated with greater morbidity than by laparotomy or minilaparotomy: Following colpotomy sterilization it has been reported that there is a greater incidence of secondary dysmenorrhea, dyspareunia, hydrosalpinx formation and tubo-ovarian abscesses than occurs when the same tubal occlusive procedures are performed by the abdominal route. However, no randomized comparative studies have been performed to date.

ENDOSCOPIC METHODS

The recently developed methods of tubal occlusion are all endoscopic. These include the laparoscopic, culdoscopic and hysteroscopic techniques.

The laparoscopic approach may be employed either as an interval or as a postabortal procedure.[16] Occlusion is most commonly performed by the use of electrocoagulation (or diathermy), which utilizes high frequency current. Laparoscopy may be performed either with the single- or double-puncture technique. The single-puncture technique requires greater experience than the double-puncture technique because of reduced visibility.[34, 35] In one series there was no difference in bowel burns between the one- and two-puncture techniques,[36] but the incidence of bowel burns is reported to be 0.5 per 1000 cases.[37]

In an attempt to eliminate the problem of bowel injury, bipolar forceps were developed[38] to supplant the unipolar apparatus. The latter method has a grounding plate attached to the patient through which the current passes, while in the bipolar system the current passes in one prong of the forceps through the tissue and out of the other prong, producing a controlled coagulation with destruction of a small segment of the oviduct. After coagulation, if division is to be performed, scissors or the Kleppinger forceps are introduced to cut or to transsect the oviduct. If division is not to be performed with the bipolar instrument, some operators perform a two- or three-contiguous-burn coagulation on each oviduct to ensure adequate obliteration of the lumen. In contrast, only a single burn on each oviduct is necessary with the unipolar apparatus. In the

bipolar method, therefore, the danger of electrical burns is, theoretically, restricted to those instances when because of anomalous structures or inadequate visualization the wrong tissue is grasped and electrocoagulated. There has been only one anecdotal report, without any details, of a bowel injury with the bipolar instrument.[39]

Regardless of whether the single- or double-puncture technique with unipolar or bipolar equipment is employed, the tube may be occluded by coagulation only, coagulation and division or coagulation, division and excision of an intervening segment of tube.[20] Failure rates reported with these techniques, respectively, have ranged from 1.0 to 2.0 per cent, 0.2 to 2.0 per cent and 0.0 to 0.6 per cent for intrauterine pregnancy rates.[20] The percentage of ectopic to total pregnancies following sterilization is higher (59 per cent) for coagulation with division and removal of a segment than for coagulation with division (19 per cent) or coagulation alone with unipolar (22 per cent) or bipolar (26 per cent) instruments.[40] During the 1970s the standard interval sterilization procedure used at our institution was coagulation with unipolar forceps followed by division with the same instrument employing a cutting current. The procedure was performed with a double-puncture laparoscopy under general anesthesia. Of the approximately 3500 such procedures performed since 1970, there have been only a few known failures and no known bowel injuries. Failures have all been the result of coagulation and division of structures other than the oviduct, such as the round ligament or a fold of peritoneum over the mesosalpinx. Factors to keep in mind when doing laparoscopic fulguration include the extent of tubal and mesosalpingeal damage. Much more tissue is damaged than that which turns white at the time of unipolar coagulation.[41] Two deaths have been reported following unrecognized bowel burns after unipolar sterilization procedures.[42] For this reason unipolar coagulation with or without division is no longer a recommended sterilization procedure.

At the time of diagnostic laparoscopy prior to attempting tubal reconstruction after previous sterilization by unipolar fulguration, we have usually observed very little oviduct remaining, usually just the fimbrial portion and therefore have not attempted a reversal procedure. Peterson et al. have, nonetheless, successfully implanted these short tubes in the posterior aspects of the uterus in 4 patients who had undergone laparoscopic cauterization and have had 3 intrauterine pregnancies within 12 or more months following surgery. They did not attempt implantation in 3 patients who were observed to have less than 3 cm of distal tube at the time of diagnostic laparoscopy.[11] They also recommended that patients having reversal of laparoscopic fulguration be delivered by cesarean section because they observed large myometrial defects at the implantation site. Therefore, these patients may require two operations in order to have a reversal of the sterilization.

Because of the problems of electrocoagulation with the unipolar instrument just discussed (bowel burns and extent of tissue destruction), efforts have been made to develop safer methods that produce less tissue destruction. One of the methods is low thermal coagulation.[43] With this method the grasping forceps brings a loop of the tube into a protective sheath where it is fulgurated through heating a wire in the forceps to about 120° to 140° C. Only low voltage such as that obtained from a car battery is needed. The heat and time of fulguration may be preselected. Only 1 millimeter on either side of the forceps is fulgurated prior to division; therefore, the extent of tubal and mesosalpingeal tissue destruction is diminished.

The nonelectrical tubal occlusion techniques that may be performed through the laparoscope are the tantalum,[44] plastic[45] and spring-loaded clips[46] and the Silastic band or Falope ring[47] (see Chapter 17). Each of these techniques requires a modification of the conventional laparoscope as well as specialized training in its use.

Insufficient data are available to evaluate completely the effectiveness of all these methods. It is possible to state, however, that failures occur with each. Clips made of tantalum, a nontissue–reactive metal, have been employed, but the failure rate has exceeded 10 per cent.[44] The lack of a spring to ensure closure of the tube has been one explanation offered for the high failure rate with this method. The plastic clip of Bleier is too new to evaluate. With the spring-loaded clip the explanation for method failure includes application of the clip to the round ligament, mesosalpinx or incomplete application to the ampullary portion of the tube.[46, 48] In one instance at subsequent hysterectomy the excised tissue around the clip revealed that only 3 mm of

each tube had been destroyed by the clip. There was no evidence of an intrinsic inflammatory reaction or adhesions to adjacent structures, and a transparent epithelium covered the clip.[48]

Technical difficulties with the spring-loaded clip method were originally greater than with the Silastic band or with electrocoagulation.[34] This reflected problems with a prototype instrument in the hands of individuals learning its use. Furthermore, when a single-puncture instrument is used, there is a greater obstruction of view with this method than with the Silastic band or electrocoagulation methods, which may explain the greater instances of misapplication of the clip.[34] This problem may be obviated if a double-puncture technique is employed. Local anesthesia to both sites could be used to decrease the anesthetic risk further. The advantages of the double-puncture technique include unobstructed vision, need to purchase only the appropriate trocar and clip applicator instead of an operating single-puncture laparoscope and easier maneuverability than that obtained with a single-puncture method. In one British study[49] there have been no failures in 533 cases of the spring-loaded clip in which a double-puncture technique was employed. With this method it is possible to reposition the clip on the fallopian tube if necessary before setting the spring. The intrauterine pregnancy failure rate of the new spring-loaded clip has been reported to be 0.2 per cent to 0.6 per cent,[20] while the rate of extrauterine to intrauterine pregnancies was 13 per cent.[40] Microsurgical reversal of clip sterilization has been followed by intrauterine pregnancy in 21 of 26 cases, with one ectopic pregnancy.[46, 51]

The Silastic* band method,[47] which employs bands 2 mm thick with 1 mm inner diameter, requires the use of a combination applicator and laparoscope. The developer of the method recommends that the tube be grasped 3 cm from the cornu,[52] while various published reports state that the tube may be grasped from 2 to 2.5 cm from the cornu.[53, 54] It is important to have a sufficient length of tube to manipulate, since the forceps and tube must be drawn into the inner cylinder of the applicator before the Silastic band is pushed off the outer cylinder enclosing the loop of tube in a Madlener type of tubal occlusion.

---

*Dimethylpolysiloxane with 5 per cent barium sulfate.

If the tube is grasped too close to the cornu, avulsion from the uterus may occur, or if the tube is thickened as a consequence of pregnancy (midtrimester) or previous or current salpingitis, the tube may be transsected when the band is applied.[34, 53-54] Cautery or laparotomy may be required if avulsion occurs. There are published reports of postoperative febrile morbidity thought to be related to pelvic inflammatory disease or to the development of tubo-ovarian abscesses in patients who had transected tubes following placement of the Silastic band.[58] Another problem with the bands is that they may fall off or be dropped.[54] In most instances they can be recovered with grasping forceps, and even if not recoverable, they do not cause tissue reaction. There have been several pregnancies reported after band application.[52, 55] Even if incorrect applications to the round ligament, utero-ovarian ligament, the serosa overlying the infundibular ligament as well as to the colon are eliminated, failures still have occurred, although the rate is less than 1 per 100 women-years at the end of 1 year following surgery.[56] Microsurgical reversal of band sterilization has been followed by intrauterine pregnancy in six of eight cases with no reported ectopic pregnancies to date.[51, 52]

One complication encountered with the band is postoperative pain: 32 per cent of patients in one study complained of pain that lasted for longer than one week and required analgesics stronger than aspirin to control.[53] Electrocoagulation is associated with only minimal pain. Electrocoagulation with only local anesthesia to the skin trocar sites causes pain during the procedure, but by destruction of nerve fibers in the tube, there is only minimal pain after the procedure. Local anesthesia to the trocar site and to the tubes before band application is associated with only minimal pain during the procedure, but subsequent tissue necrosis of the tube is conveyed by the patent nerve fibers and accounts for the pain after the procedure.

Culdoscopy provides another avenue for endoscopic tubal occlusion and, theoretically, all the methods used by laparoscopy could also be utilized by culdoscopy. Most gynecologists are not trained in this method and considerable retraining would be necessary before they would feel comfortable observing the pelvic structures from this orientation. The knee-chest position is also quite uncomfortable for the patient, especially if only local anesthetics

and analeptic drugs are employed. There does not seem to be any major advantage to employ this avenue for the tubal occlusion.

With the technique of hysteroscopy electrocoagulation, thermocoagulation and nonelectrical chemical or physical agents have been used to achieve tubal occlusion. With the advent of nitrous oxide and dextran to distend the uterus and the newer hysteroscopic equipment, electrocoagulation of the cornu has been attempted with high-frequency current following passage of an electrode into the ostia.[57] In some instances uterine anomalies, polyps or long uterine horns may preclude correct placement of the electrode, and in only 75 per cent of attempts could the ostia be localized.[58] Various currents for variable durations have been employed with uniformly poor results, both in terms of tubal patency and in terms of pregnancy.[59] The pregnancies have been interstitial and cornual in location. The small spermatozoa may traverse the partially occluded tube, while the larger, fertilized zygote may not. Electrocoagulation of the ostia transcervically is inadvisable at present.

Thermocoagulation was employed in an attempt to improve the poor results obtained with high-frequency electrocoagulation of the ostia.[60, 61] This low-voltage device, which has a controllable temperature and therefore reduces the risk of burns to adjacent structures, was not able to reduce the patency rate below 12 per cent. Because of the lack of success in achieving tubal occlusion, this method has been abandoned.

Several chemical agents have been formulated for intrauterine delivery indirectly via a blind catheter. These agents, such as quinacrine[62] and 10 per cent silver nitrate,[63] are sclerosing in nature, while methylcyanoacrylate (MCA) monomer[64] is additionally a tissue adhesive. They destroy tubal epithelium and promote fibrous tissue formation. If tubal spillage occurs, injury to the intestines or adhesion formation or both may occur. At best these methods require several administrations and many weeks to achieve tubal occlusion rates that are less than 90 per cent. They are not reversible and are often associated with abdominal pain and recanalization. None is recommended at present.

Of the nonsclerosing substances, Silastic, especially with the addition of a catalyst that results in the formation of a plug in approximately 4 minutes, may be a promising new method of hysteroscopic or intrauterine administration for tubal occlusion.[65] Whether this method may be reversible is not known at present.

NEW TECHNIQUES

A tubal plug made of Silastic that may be introduced via laparoscopy, laparotomy or minilaparotomy through the fimbriae into the ampullary region of the tube and kept in place with tantalum clips has been developed by Steptoe.[66] This method has been employed in 40 women with one intrauterine pregnancy when the plug fell out. This failure suggests that no permanent tubal damage is produced by the placement of the plug and indicates that reversal is possible by removal of the plug. This could be done via laparoscopy, although this has not been attempted to date.

Fimbriopexy, which is the placement of a cap or hood over the fimbrial end of the tube, was proposed as a potentially reversible tubal occlusive technique.[67] It would, theoretically, not require a laparotomy for reversal as with the Aldridge method after which it was modeled. The need in some instances of attaching the device to the broad ligaments to secure them and the dense adhesion formation in some individuals indicates that this method will not be easy to perform or to reverse. Newer techniques with different materials may simplify this approach.

Conclusion

With our operating thesis that the least amount of surgery should be performed consistent with the patient's needs, this review has described a wide variety of procedures. The central issues are patient selection and the choice of the appropriate means of sterilization for that patient. No method should be proposed as being potentially reversible.

If a tubal occlusion technique of sterilization is chosen, the surgeon should tailor the method of sterilization to the patient's age and parity. The failure rates, both in terms of intrauterine and ectopic pregnancies, are similar for bipolar coagulation with or without division, spring-loaded clip and Silastic band. Even if the nonelectrical methods are preferred, it is necessary to have electrocoagulation available as a backup procedure because mesosalpingeal injury with hemorrhage that

may be amenable to cautery may occur, especially with the Silastic band technique. For this reason one experienced laparoscopist has recommended that bipolar sterilization on one site of the isthmic portion of the tube with division of the coagulated tissue is the best method of sterilization at the present time in his hands.[68]

Of the newer techniques, the bipuncture application of the spring-loaded clip and the Silastic band have been successfully used, but both these methods as well as any new technique require careful retraining. For this reason it is probably best that the practitioner employ the technique with which he is most familiar until he can be retrained in the other techniques.

REFERENCES

1. Westoff, C. F. and Jones, E.F.: Contraception and sterility in the United States, 1965–1975. Fam. Plann. Perspect. 9:153, 1977.
2. Female sterilizations now surpass vasectomies. Association of voluntary sterilization (AVS) News, September 1976.
3. American College of Obstetricians and Gynecologists: Manual of Standards, 1968.
4. American College of Obstetricians and Gynecologists: Manual of Standards, 1970.
5. Hulka, J. F.: Current status of elective sterilization in the United States. Fertil. Steril. 28:515, 1977.
6. Williams, G. F. J.: Fallopian tube surgery for reversal of sterilization. Br. Med. J. 1: 599, 1973.
7. Umezaki, C., Katayama, K. P., and Jones, H. W.: Pregnancy rates after reconstructive surgery on the falllopian tubes. Obstet. Gynecol. 43:428, 1974.
8. Siegler, A. M. and Perez, R. J.: Reconstruction of fallopian tubes in previously sterilized patients. Fertil. Steril. 26:388, 1975.
9. Winston, R. M. L.: Microsurgical tubocornual anastomosis for reversal of sterilisation. Lancet 1:284, 1977.
10. Gomel, V.: Tubal reanastomosis by microsurgery. Fertil. Steril. 28:59, 1977.
11. Peterson, E. P., Musich, J. R. and Behrman, S. J.: Uterotubal implantation and obstetric outcome after previous sterilization. Am. J. Obstet. Gynecol. 128:662, 1977.
12. Rioux, J. E.: Late complications of female sterilization: a review of the literature and a proposal for further research. J. Reprod. Med. 19:329, 1977.
13. Hibbard, L. T.: Sexual sterilization by elective hysterectomy. Am. J. Obstet. Gynecol. 112:1076, 1972.
14. Cole, P. and Berlin, J.: Elective hysterectomy. Am. J. Obstet. Gynecol. 129:117, 1977.
15. Whitson, L. G., Ballard, C. A. and Israel, R.: Laparoscopic tubal sterilization coincident with therapeutic abortion by suction curettage. Obstet. Gynecol. 41:677, 1973.
16. Ballard, C. A.: Therapeutic abortion and sterilization by vaginal hysterectomy. Am. J. Obstet. Gynecol. 118:891, 1974.

17. Hofmeister, F. J.: Tubal ligation versus cesarean hysterectomy. Clin. Obstet. Gynecol. 12:676, 1969.
18. Ballard, C. A.: Personal communications.
19. Madlener, M.: Uber sterilisierende Operationen an den Tuben (About sterilization operations on the tubes). [GE] Zentralbl. Gynaekol. 43(20):380, 1919.
20. Wortman, J.: Tubal sterilization review of methods. Population Reports C: 73, 1977.
21. Irving, F. C.: A new method of insuring sterility following cesarean section. Am. J. Obstet. Gynecol. 8:335, 1924.
22. Bishop, E. and Nelms, W. F.: A simple method of tubal sterilization. N. Y. State J. Med. 39:214, 1930.
23. Garb, A. E.: A review of tubal sterilization failures. Obstet. Gynecol. Surv. 12:291, 1957.
24. Poulson, A. M.: Analysis of female sterilization techniques. Obstet. Gynecol. 42:131, 1973.
25. Overstreet, E. W.: Techniques of sterilization. Obstet. Gynecol. 7:109, 1964.
26. Husbands, M. E., Jr., Pritchard, J. A. and Pritchard, S. A.: Failure of tubal sterilization accompanying cesarean section. Am. J. Obstet. Gynecol. 107:966, 1970.
27. Shipp, J. F.: Sterilization procedures. Letters to the Editor. Am. J. Obstet. Gynecol. 114:1109, 1972.
28. Barr, S. J.: A method of tubal ligation. Am. J. Obstet. Gynecol. 107:324, 1970.
29. Rioux, J. E. and Yuzpe, A. A.: A guide to sterilization procedures. Contemp. Ob/Gyn 12:33, 1978.
30. Kroener, W. F., Jr.: Surgical sterilization by fimbriectomy. Am. J. Obstet. Gynecol. 104:247, 1969.
31. Roe, R. E., Laros, R. K. and Work, B. A.: Female sterilization: the vaginal approach. Am. J. Obstet. Gynecol. 112:1031, 1972.
32. Akhter, M. S.: Vaginal versus abdominal tubal ligation. Study at Victoria General Hospital. Am. J. Obstet. Gynecol. 115:491, 1973.
33. Uchida, H.: Uchida tubal sterilization. Am. J. Obstet. Gynecol. 121:153, 1975.
34. Brenner, W. E. and Edelman, D. A.: Laparoscopic sterilization with electrocautery, spring-loaded clips, and Silastic bands: technical problems and early complications. Fertil. Steril. 27:256, 1976.
35. Lieberman, B. A.: A clip applicator for laparoscopic sterilization. Fertil. Steril. 27:1036, 1976.
36. Thompson, B. H. and Wheeles, C. R.: Gastrointestinal complications of laparoscopy sterilization. Obstet. Gynecol. 41:669, 1973.
37. Phillips, J. M., Keith, D., Hulka, J. F., Hulka, B. and Keith, L.: Gynecologic laparoscopy in 1975. J. Reprod. Med. 16:105, 1976.
38. Rioux, J. E. and Cloutier, D.: A new bipolar instrument for laparoscopic tubal sterilization. Am. J. Obstet. Gynecol. 119:737, 1974.
39. Hulka, J. F.: Relative risks and benefits of electrical and non-electrical sterilization techniques. J. Reprod. Med. 21: 111, 1978.
40. Phillips, J. M., Hulka, J., Hulka, B., Keith, D. and Keith, L.: American Association of Gynecologic Laparoscopists, 1976 Membership Survey. J. Reprod. Med. 21:3, 1978.
41. Fishburne, J. I. and Hulka, J. G.: Tubal healing following laparoscopic electrocoagulation. J. Reprod. Med. 16:129, 1976.
42. Peterson, H. B., Ory, H. W., Greenspan, J. R. and Tyler, C. W., Jr.: Deaths associated with laparoscopic sterilization by unipolar electrocoagulatory

43. Semm, K.: Tubal sterilization finally with cauterization or temporary with ligation via pelviscopy. *In* Phillips, J. M. and Keith, L. (eds.): Gynecological Laparoscopy Principles and Techniques. New York, Stratton Intercontinental, 1974, pp. 337-359.
44. Haskins, A. L.: Oviductal sterilization with tantalum clips. Am. J. Obstet. Gynecol. 114:370, 1972.
45. Bleier, W.: Indications and statistics of tubal sterilization using a synthetic clip. Arch. Gynaekol. 244: 41, 1982.
46. Hulka, J. F.: Spring clip sterilization: one-year follow-up of 1000 cases. *In* Sciarra, J. J., Droegemueller, W. and Speidel, J. J. (eds.): Advances in Female Sterilization Technology. Hagerstown, Harper and Row, 1976, pp. 51-58.
47. Yoon, I.B. and King, T. M.: The laparoscopic Falope ring procedure. *In* Sciarra, J. J., Droegemueller, W. and Speidel, J. J. (eds.): Advances in Female Sterilization Technology. Hagerstown, Harper and Row, 1976, pp. 59-68.
48. Kumarasamy, T., Hulka, J. F., Mercer, J. P. et al.: Laparoscopic sterilization with a spring loaded clip. *In* Philips, J. M. and Keith, L. (eds.): Gynecologic Laparoscopy Principles and Techniques. New York, Stratton Intercontinental, 1974, p. 361-370.
49. Lieberman, B. A., Gordon, A. G. and Bostock, J. F: Laparoscopic sterilization with spring-loaded clips: double puncture technique. J. Reprod. Med. 18: 241, 1977.
50. Letchworth, A. T. and Lieberman, B. A.: Successful reversal of clip sterilization. Lancet 2:902, 1976.
51. Female Sterilization. Population Reports. C:97-123, 1980.
52. Yoon, I. B., King, T. M. and Parmley, T. H.: A two-year experience with the Falope ring sterilization procedure. Am. J. Obstet. Gynecol. 127:109, 1977.
53. Kumarasamy, T., and Hurt, W. G.: Laparoscopic sterilization with silicone rubber bands. Obstet. Gynecol. 50:351, 358, 1977.
54. Levinson, C. J. and Daily, H. I.: Nonelectric laparoscopic sterilization—Experience with a Silastic band. Obstet. Gynecol. 48:494, 1976.
55. Ziegler, J. S., Schneider, G. T. and Caire, A. A.: A comparison of the Falope ring and laparoscopic tubal cauterization. J. Reprod. Med. 20:237, 1978.
56. Mumford, S. D. and Bhiwandiwaca, P. P.: Tubal ring sterilization: Experience with 10,086 cases. Obstet. Gynecol. 57:150, 1981.
57. March, C. M. and Israel, R.: A critical appraisal of hysteroscopic tubal fulguration for sterilization. Contraception 12:261, 1975.
58. Quinones, R., Alvarado, A. and Ley, E.: Tubal electrocoagulation under hysteroscopic control (350 cases). Am. J. Obstet. Gynecol. 121:1111, 1975.
59. Israngkun, C. and Phaosavasdi, S.: Hysteroscopic sterilization: Complications in 296 cases. *In* Sciarra, J. J., Droegemueller, W., and Speidel, J. J. (eds): Advances in Female Sterilization Technology. Hagerstown, Harper and Row, 1976, pp. 148-152.
60. Semm, K.: Tubal sterilization finally with cauterization or temporary with ligation via pelviscopy. *In* Phillips, J. M. and Keith, L. (eds.): Gynecological Laparoscopy: Principles and Techniques. New York, Stratton Intercontinental, 1974, pp. 337-359.
61. Lindemann, H. J. and Mohr, J.: Review of clinical experience with hysteroscopic sterilization. *In* Sciarra, J. J., Droegemueller, W. and Speidel, J.

J. (eds.): Advances in Female Sterilization Technology. Hagerstown, Harper and Row, 1976, p. 153-161.

62. Zipper, J., Stracchetti, E. and Medel, M.: Transvaginal chemical sterilization: clinical use of quinacrine plus potentiating adjuvants. Contraception 12:11, 1975.

63. Richart, R. M., Gutierrez-Najar, A. J. and Neuwirth, R. S.: Transvaginal human sterilization: a preliminary report. Am. J. Obstet. Gynecol. 111:108, 1971.

64. Stevenson, T. C.: Methyl cyanoacrylate (MCA) for tubal occlusion. *In* Sciarra, J. J., Droegemueller, W. and Speidel, J. J. (eds.): Advances in Female Sterilization Technology. Hagerstown, Harper and Row, 1976, pp. 216-224.

65. Erb, R. A., Davis, R. H., Balin, H. and Kyriazis, G. A.: Device and technique for blocking the fallopian tubes: A method for reversible contraceptive sterilization. *In* Schima, M. E., Lubell, I., Davis, J.

E. and Connell, E.: Advances in Voluntary Sterilization. Amsterdam, Excerpta Medica, 1974, pp. 336-337.

66. Steptoe, P. C.: Intratubal devices for reversible sterilization. *In* Philips, J. M. and Keith, L. (eds.): Gynecological Laparoscopy Principles and Techniques. New York, Stratton Intercontinental, 1974, pp. 309-314.

67. Laufe, L. E., Hassler, C. and Lower, B. R.: A laboratory prototype for reversible female sterilization. *In* Duncan, G. W., Falb, R. D. and Speidel, J. J. (eds.): Female Sterilization. Proceedings of a workshop on Female Sterilization, Airlie, Virginia, Dec. 2-3, 1971, New York, Academic Press, 1972, p. 65-69.

68. Frangenheim, H.: The effectiveness of different methods of laparoscopic tubal sterilization (author's translation). Geburtshilfe Frauenheilkd, 1980, pp. 896-900.

Surgical Contraception: The Optimal Method

William Droegemueller, M.D.

Louis Weinstein, M.D.

Patrick Morell, M.D.

University of Arizona Medical Center

"There are very few operations and surgery which offer more relief from anxiety. . . . and hardly any for which the surgeon can give as high a chance of success."[1]

The first reported tubal sterilization was performed in Toledo, Ohio, in 1880. One hundred years later our society is experiencing a sexual revolution. Dramatic advances in medicine have accomplished in vitro fertilization and therefore the prerequisites of tubal patency and sexual intercourse may not be essential for conception in the future.

In recent years sterilization has become the most common means of birth control. The dramatic and almost geometric rise in numbers of sterilization procedures is related to a complex interplay of changes in our cultural attitudes, especially recognition of equal rights for women. Relaxation of barriers, recent emphasis on complications associated with the pill and intrauterine device and advances in surgical techniques have altered the thinking of patients and physicians alike.

Developments in technology, women's liberation and the "sexual revolution" have all made an impact on the choice of the most appropriate sterilization operation. Presently, the topic promotes dynamic and rapidly changing debate. Of the many unresolved issues, we have selected five for discussion:

1. What should the physician do about informed consent?
2. Which partner should have the sterilization operation?
3. When is the most appropriate time to perform surgery?
4. Which operative technique should be used for female sterilization?
5. Does the post-tubal ligation syndrome actually exist?

We have partial answers for these questions. Obviously, our statements are intended for the majority of couples. Certainly, we appreciate that there are overriding individual arguments and situations that would lead any prudent physician to differing conclusions.

Informed Consent

Informed consent is a lawyer's dream and a physician's nightmare. In litigations surrounding "wrongful birth," damages in excess of a half million dollars have been awarded.

Physicians have an inherent reluctance to completely fulfill the requirements of informed consent that are presently being proposed by the federal government and activist groups. The intent of third parties is well justified, although in reality for the patient, it may produce an increase in anxiety and apprehension. Providing adequate informed consent invariably requires more time than the indicated sterilization procedure. Because of the present medical, legal and social climate, a physician must overlook the impact on the physician-patient relationship and strive to comply with the requirements of informed consent.[2-3]

Therefore, it is important that the physician discuss with the patient and her mate the risks, alternatives and short-term and long-term complications of the procedure. Obviously, the discussion should emphasize the failure rates and the fact that sterilization operations are not easily or readily reversible. For the physician's own protection, he must document in writing the occurrence of this conversation. If litigation occurs, the physician will have to prove to a lay jury that the discussion was adequate, thorough and understood by the couple.

An educator would believe that this should be accomplished by both a pretest and posttest. Pragmatically, standard consent forms are often ridiculed by the plaintiff's attorney during the trial process. A handwritten letter from the couple to the physician will help to impress the lay jury that there was a discussion concerning the surgical procedure. The use of audiovisual aids such as movies, tapes or pamphlets is useful, but does not replace the confirmation of understanding implied by the personal letter written by the patient.

In a healthy adult, there should be only one contraindication to a sterilization operation: that is, the request must be entirely voluntary. If there is suspicion of coercion from any source, this procedure should be postponed and re-evaluated. In 1976, the United States Supreme Court ruled that a husband's signature is not required for a woman to have a tubal ligation.

In summary, the hallmarks of "informed consent" are that a mature adult has made a voluntary decision after considering the risks and alternatives. It is important that there has been an opportunity to ask and answer all questions and a reasonable period of time between the initial decision and surgical procedure.

Which Partner?

Scientifically and practically, vasectomy is simpler and more easily reversible than tubal ligation, with less immediate morbidity and expense. Most importantly, the success of vasectomy can be measured by a laboratory test. Recently, there have been preliminary reports in subhuman primates of the association of accelerated atherosclerotic cardiovascular changes following vasectomy.[4] Because of the longer reproductive life span and anxiety of sexual performance in males, there is probably a higher incidence of psychological sequelae following vasectomy than tubal ligation.

In discussing the sterilization procedure, the physician should involve both partners in making the decision of which to use. Important facets of the discussion are age, current health and individual emotional maturity. Coercion by mate or peer pressure may lead to emotional conflicts.

Several studies have looked at the "profile" of women requesting reversal of sterilization. Presently, it is estimated that approximately 1 to 2 per cent of women regret their initial decision to have a tubal ligation and request an operation to restore their fertility. In a study by Gomel of 100 consecutive patients, the major reasons for requesting sterilization reversal were changes in marital status (65 per cent), crib death (17 per cent), and the desire for more children in the same marriage (10 per cent). Ironically, all 17 patients who experienced the tragedy of a crib death in their family had received postpartum sterilizations.[5-6] Many patients retrospectively stated that there were significant marital problems prior to and at the time of the sterilization operation. Hindsight is rarely cloudy; however, women should be cautioned that a sterilization procedure rarely saves a marriage.

In 1970, approximately 80 per cent of sterilization operations were vasectomies. However, the surgical pendulum has recently swung toward the female. Presently, more than 60 per cent of operations that result in sterility are performed on the female. We anticipate that this trend will continue for the next few years.

When is the Most Appropriate Time?

The foundations of effective population programs have stressed postpartum tubal ligation. However, many times this is not optimal for the individual couple. Permanent sterilization is a major decision that may affect the person's future emotional and physical well-being. Therefore, the decision should be made at a time of psychological tranquility.[7]

Many tubal ligations are performed in the early postpartum period because of convenience, financial savings and ease of technique. We believe this is acceptable if a proper amount of thought and discussion regarding this decision occurred during the pregnancy. However, a commitment made late in pregnancy or the puerperium is like "adopting religion on the battlefield." It is a commitment that may not last throughout the reproductive life of the individual. Another rare but catastrophic event that must be considered in the scheduling of a postpartum tubal ligation is the occurrence of sudden infant death syndrome. Because of the complexity of ambivalent feelings that surround either a spontaneous or a therapeutic abortion, the postabortal period is less optimal for sterilization surgery than the time following a live birth.

Unique factors that must be considered in female sterilization include the possibility of luteal phase pregnancy and current contraceptive usage. To prevent the former, the surgery should be scheduled prior to ovulation or curettage should be performed at the same time as the tubal ligation procedure. Removal of an intrauterine contraceptive device coincidental with a sterilization operation may result in an increase in infectious morbidity.[8] Therefore, we advocate removal of the device one month prior to surgery. If the IUD is removed or left in place at the time of surgery, the patient should receive prophylactic broad-spectrum antibiotics. Lastly, one should consider the hypercoagulable state produced by oral contraceptives in scheduling any elective surgery.[9] Ideally, oral contraceptives should be discontinued three weeks prior to surgery and barrier contraceptives utilized.

In summary, ideal timing is an *interval* sterilization procedure, when the couple has mutually agreed that they have completed their family. The longer the interval from the last term pregnancy or abortion, the less likely the chance that the decision will be regretted. Once again, the necessity to counsel both partners cannot be overemphasized.

Which Operative Technique?

The ideal safe, simple, inexpensive method of female sterilization has yet to be discovered. It is important for the surgeon to individualize the choice of sterilization technique with consideration of both the present and potential future wishes of the patient. At the present time, the most prominent issue is the choice between laparoscopy or minilaparotomy.[10-12]

The glamour of elaborate equipment, Band-Aid incision and reported speed of surgery and recovery with laparoscopy have captured the popular press, lay public and most American gynecologists. Recently, we have regressed from our initial enthusiasm for the "silver tube" and presently select minilaparotomy for the majority of sterilization procedures. Laparoscopy is an excellent technique and is extensively used in our practice for the differential diagnosis of pelvic pain and the work-up of infertility patients. We believe that it is the optimal method for sterilization of the moderately obese female. In performing a laparoscopic sterilization, the Silastic band or spring-loaded clip is preferred over electrocoagulation.[13, 14]

In making the transition from electrocoagulation to Silastic bands or clips, many surgeons have encountered technical difficulties, especially when the tubes are large or thickened by previous pelvic infections. The patients usually experience more immediate postoperative pelvic and abdominal pain with the nonelectrical techniques. However, the major advantage is avoiding the rare but catastrophic burn to structures other than the fallopian tube. With less tissue damage, it is anticipated that there will be a higher potential for reversibility.

Initially, major complications related to electrical injury and pneumoperitoneum with the use of the laparoscope stimulated interest in minilaparotomy.[16] Unless one is an accomplished laparoscopist, by definition a surgeon performing a minimum of 500 procedures, a minilaparotomy is the preferable procedure. The surgical technique is easier to learn. Another advantage of minilaparotomy is less variability in the time of the surgical procedure. The minor difficulties such as exposure or bleeding are everyday problems with common solutions. With the minilaparotomy procedure, we perform the Pomeroy or Uchida method of tubal ligation.[17] The isolated fimbriectomy procedure is never selected because long-term follow-up studies have documented an unacceptable pregnancy rate. Regardless of surgical technique with the fimbriectomy operation, tubal fistulas do develop.[18] Pregnancies following the fimbriectomy operation do not occur as rapidly as other tubal ligation failures, but in time they do appear at an alarming rate.

Irrespective of the operative technique selected, the isthmic portion of the fallopian tube is where the ligation should be performed. Some consideration should be given to preservation of tubal length and blood supply. The highest pregnancy rates following tubal microsurgery occur in end-to-end anastomosis of the isthmic portion.

In summary, because of individualizing the procedure it is difficult to make didactic statements. Usually, we would select a Pomeroy tubal ligation of the isthmic portion of the tube for younger women and a Uchida procedure for older patients.

"Post-Tubal Ligation Syndrome:" A Definite Entity?

Standard textbooks discuss only two long-term sequelae of tubal ligation, the occasional patient who regrets her decision and a woman who has a pregnancy related to failure of the original operation. Recent literature from England and Canada has established a specific syndrome that develops subsequent to tubal ligation.[19-21] Major components of the post-tubal ligation syndrome are dysfunctional uterine bleeding and pelvic pain. Most often the abnormal bleeding is menorrhagia and the pelvic pain includes dysmenorrhea and dyspareunia.

The incidence of this condition is difficult to establish and many American authors have yet to recognize the association of the previous tubal surgery and the subsequent pelvic symptoms. Definite statistics will not be available until prospective studies are completed. However, it is our opinion that a definite syndrome does exist. A small percentage of previously asymptomatic women develop pelvic complaints following tubal ligation. Often, these chronic symptoms are severe enough for the patient to request a hysterectomy.

Although it is difficult to separate this syndrome from a psychosomatic complaint, we have been impressed by the specificity with which patients describe their symptoms. The pelvic pain that these women experience is usually related to movement or activity. On pelvic examination, the uterus is freely mobile and normal in size. Pelvic tenderness is usually noted in the parametrial areas. The menorrhagia is not invariably related to anovulatory bleeding and the pelvic pain is not relieved by oral contraceptives or other medical management. Hysterectomy is successful in alleviating the symptoms.

Colleagues who remain skeptical of this association believe that these women become symptomatic from endometriosis, adenomyosis or a small myoma. They postulate that the syndrome is overdiagnosed or that it is merely a phenomenon of aging. The debate continues that recent oral contraceptive therapy or an intervening pregnancy has caused the woman to forget her previous similar symptoms. Nevertheless, we have identified women with the triad of symptoms, who were not postpartum and were not taking oral contraceptives prior to their sterilization procedure.

The etiology of this syndrome remains as obscure as scientific data substantiating the incidence. One theory is that the pain may be related to intermittent torsion of the fimbria or ovary or both. Other investigators believe that the symptoms result from compromise of the delicate vascular network between the uterus and the ovary. We believe that the pain is secondary to retrograde menstruation into the closed segment of the fallopian tubes. Observations made during peritoneal dialysis and laparoscopy performed at the time of the menstrual period demonstrate that approximately 50 per cent of normal women experience retrograde menstruation. It is possible that this normal variant is the precipitating factor in the development of the pelvic pain.

One must put in perspective that if 15 per

cent of women develop this syndrome, 85 per cent do not. Therefore, it would seem illogical to use the post-tubal ligation syndrome as an over-riding argument to propose hysterectomy with sterilization as the primary indication. We select vaginal hysterectomy as the primary operation if there are pelvic symptoms such as uterine prolapse or dysfunctional uterine bleeding accompanying the request for sterilization.

In summary, we believe that a small percentage of patients will develop the post-tubal ligation syndrome. Therefore, patients are counseled about this possibility prior to sterilization. However, anticipation of the syndrome should not lead either the patient or the physician to choose hysterectomy as the operation of choice for sterilization.

The Future

The most significant developments in sterilization technology in the past five years have been the Silastic band and modifications of the spring-loaded clip.

Two novel techniques of transcervical sterilization may result in a method with ease of reversal. Hosseinian has developed a uterotubal plug that is inserted via the hysteroscope.[22] Pregnancies were obtained in baboons following removal of the device. Similarly, the Silastic plug developed by Erb had encouraging results in animal experiments.[23] The plug is presently in preliminary clinical trials.

Other investigators have focused their interest on transcervical outpatient sterilization. These include uterine injections of sclerosing agents such as methylcyanoacrylate or quinacrine and thermal damage to the uterotubal junction by cryosurgery, electrocautery or laser beam.[24-26] Research continues on these methods but none have achieved acceptable failure rates. Reversibility is obviously a low priority in programs attempting to develop a new method for outpatient sterilization.

REFERENCES

1. Staff of the Margaret Pyke Center. One Thousand Vasectomies. Br. Med. J. 4:216, 1973.
2. Laforet, E. G.: The fiction of informed consent. J.A.M.A. 235:1579, 1976.
3. Schneider, J.: Ideas and actions. Obstet. Gynecol. 42:778, 784, 1973.
4. Alexander, N. J. and Clarkson, T. B.: Vasectomy increases the severity of diet-induced atherosclerosis in Macaca Fascicularis. Science 201:538, 1978.

5. Gomel, V.: Profile of women requesting reversal of sterilization. Fertil. Steril. 30:39, 1978.
6. Thomson, P. and Templeton, A.: Characteristics of patients requesting reversal of sterilization. Br. J. Obstet. Gynaecol. 85:161, 1978.
7. Emens, J. M. and Olive, J. E.: Timing of female sterilization. Br. Med. J. 2:1126, 1978.
8. Taylor, E. S., McMillan, J. H., Greer, B. E., Droegemueller, W. and Thompson, H. E.: The intrauterine device and tubo-ovarian abscess. Am. J. Obstet. Gynecol. 123:338, 1975.
9. von Kaulla, E., Droegemueller, W., Aoki, N. and von Kaulla, K. N.: Antithrombin III depression and thrombin generation acceleration in women taking oral contraceptives. Am. J. Obstet. Gynecol. 109:868, 1971.
10. Pelland, P. C.: Instruments and methods. Obstet. Gynecol. 50:106, 1977.
11. Hefnawai, F., Badraoui, M. H. H. and Serour, G. I.: Minilaparotomy for female sterilization: a feasibility study of a new technique. Int. J. Gynecol. Obstet. 14:390, 1976.
12. Dassenaike, A., Saha, A. and McCann, M. F.: Female sterilization via minilaparotomy. J. Reprod. Med. 17:119, 1976.
13. Engel, T.: Laparoscopic sterilization: electrosurgery or clip application? J. Reprod. Med. 21:107, 1978.
14. Yoon, I. B., King, T. M. and Parmley, T. H.: A two-year experience with the Falope ring sterilization procedure. Am. J. Obstet. Gynecol. 127:109, 1977.
15. Hulka, J. F., Mercer, J. P., Fishburne, J. I. et al.: Spring clip sterilization: one-year follow-up of 1079 cases. Am. J. Obstet. Gynecol. 125:1039, 1976.
16. Engel, T. and Harris, F. W.: The electrical dynamics of laparoscopic sterilization. J. Reprod. Med. 15:33, 1975.
17. Uchida, H.: Uchida tubal sterilization. Am. J. Obstet. Gynecol. 121:153, 1975.
18. Metz, K. G. P.: Failures following fimbriectomy. Fertil. Steril. 28:66, 1977.
19. Chamberlain, G. and Foulkes, J.: Long-term effects of laparoscopic sterilization on menstruation. South. Med. J. 69:1474, 1976.
20. Neil, J. R., Hammond, G. T. et al.: Late complications of sterilization by laparoscopy and tubal ligation. Lancet 1:699, 1975.
21. Ringrose, C. A.: Post-tubal ligation menorrhagia and pelvic pain. Int. J. Fertil. 19:168, 1974.
22. Hosseinian, A. H., Lucero, S. and Kim, M. H.: Hysteroscopic implantation of uterotubal junction blocking devices. *In* Sciarra, J. J., Droegemueller, W. and Speidel, J. J. (eds.): Advances in Female Sterilization Techniques. Hagerstown, Harper & Row, 1976.
23. Erb, R. A.: Silastic: a retrievable custom-molded oviductal plug. *In* Sciarra, J. J., Droegemueller, W. and Speidel, J. J. (eds.): Advances in Female Sterilization Techniques. Hagerstown, Harper & Row, 1976.
24. Richart, R. M., Neuwirth, R. S., Bolduc, L. R.: Single-application fertility-regulating device: Description of a new instrument. Am. J. Obstet. Gynecol. 127:86, 1977.
25. Zipper, J., Stacchetti, E. and Medel, M.: Transvaginal chemical sterilization: clinical use of quinacrine plus potentiating adjuvants. Contraception 12:11, 1975.
26. Droegemueller, W., Greer, B. E., Davis, J. R. et al.: Cryosurgery of the endometrium. Am. J. Obstet. Gynecol. 131:1, 1978.

Editorial Comment

It is difficult to appreciate the changes in attitude about surgical contraception during the past 15 years. The changes toward a more liberal policy of sterilization in this country have been directed to benefit the married, divorced and single woman. It is fortunate that our former sterilization rules, such as the "120 rule," no longer apply, as when we were residents and junior faculty. The "120 rule" holds that the woman had to be 30 years of age and have four children; i.e., the product of the pregnancies and age should equal 120 or more. It was also necessary that she and her husband sign papers that were then signed by two physicians who presented the case to a departmental or hospital committee that voted upon whether or not it was permissible to perform the surgical sterilization. Most of these sterilizations were performed in the immediate postpartum period. There were very few if any surgical sterilizations performed as interim procedures. If the patient was not sterilized within the first 48 hours after the delivery, she would then have to wait until after her next baby.

The women's liberation movement has done much to alter the perception that males control female surgical sterilization; we no longer require a husband to sign permission for his wife to be sterilized. This does not mean that we do not advocate counseling the male, but it does mean that in present-day society the woman has control over her own fertility.

Litigation following tubal ligation is now commonplace, but few if any lawsuits have been settled in favor of the plaintiff if the procedure has been done correctly. The most single important event in informed consent, as pointed out by Droegemueller and others, is that it must be *entirely voluntary*. There should be no coercion or suspicion of coercion for this procedure. Yes, there will be regrets after tubal ligation, but with proper education of individuals and well-informed patients this should be kept to a minimum.

Many years ago we did a follow-up study of tubal ligation patients and found that if patients voluntarily wanted the tubal ligation, 95 per cent were pleased and would have it done again, whereas 5 per cent were very unhappy. Most of the unhappy individuals were those who had a true medical indication for the tubal ligation; even though they understood that they should not become pregnant, their emotions affected their view of the situation.

I don't believe that there is any question that vasectomy is a simpler operation. Vasectomy has always been known as the physicians' sterilization operation. There has been recent controversy about the development of antibodies to sperm following vasectomy. These reports were in subhuman primates and showed accelerated arteriosclerotic cardiovascular changes following vasectomy. What this all means we do not know, except that it has become only a mild deterrent to male sterilization.

More women are now sterilized as an interim procedure than postpartum. The reason for this great upsurge in interim sterilization procedures has been the development of fiberoptics and the ability to visualize the pelvic contents by the laparoscope. Tubal cautery, which was first done by unipolar current and is now done by bipolar current, should be reserved for the patient over 30 years of age. The emergence in the past five years of the fallopian clip and Silastic ring have added a greater impetus to interim procedures, especially in younger women who may later wish tubal reanastomosis. It now appears that one surgical procedure begets another. An example would be the young woman who is sterilized by a fallopian ring or clip. She then gets divorced and remarried, and wishes more children; hence, the development of a new specialty of microsurgery with results that assure tubal patency in 80 per cent of carefully selected patients and pregnancy in 60 per cent.

Female sterilization increased from 1970 to 1975 from 10 to 23 per cent and male sterilization from 10 to 24 per cent. Interestingly, an equal number of males and females are now currently being sterilized. The most dramatic of all statistics involves the 1 to 2 per cent of individuals who request reversal; this is a very important issue in choosing the proper method of sterilization. This does not sound like many individuals, but it amounts to somewhere between 7000 to 14,000 women per year who will request reversal for various reasons. A true reversible form of tubal sterilization is needed. Cautery has little place any more in sterilization, except in those individuals who have medical problems that preclude a safe pregnancy. The majority of hazards from laparoscopy sterilization have come from unipolar cautery with adjacent burns of the viscera. It is not appropriate to argue whether minilaparotomy is better than laparoscopy, except to state that every obstetrician-gynecologist should know how to perform both in an equally expertise fashion. The Kroener procedure, which is removal of the fimbriae, should be done only in those patients who have medical problems that preclude pregnancy. The Pomeroy procedure, which is probably the simplest of all tubal ligation procedures, is an easy procedure for the minilaparotomy, as is the Uchida method of sterilization.

None of the authors mentioned other forms of surgical sterilization: vaginal hysterectomy, total abdominal hysterectomy and cesarean section hysterectomy. Cesarean section hysterectomy has been a common operation in the past in populations that are principally Catholic or that have a high incidence of cervical or uterine pathology. The patient of the physician who does only an occasional cesarean section hysterectomy may have complications; hence, this is not a procedure that is designed as a casual operation. Total abdominal hysterectomy is seldom done as a primary means of sterilization unless there is some form of adnexal and myometrial pathology. Vaginal hysterectomy is a common operation done principally in the South as a form of surgical sterilization and not infrequently is done in conjunction with either an anterior or posterior colporrhaphy. It is an excellent operation and the operation of the gynecologist; however, unless there is some specific pathology present such as consistent abnormal bleeding, adenomyosis, enlarged uterus, fibroids, dysplasia of the cervix or carcinoma in situ, it is a major operation to achieve the benefit of no more children. It has been the favorite operation in institutions in which tubal ligation is not an acceptable operative procedure.

The point we are trying to make is that all these operations have merit and it is important to determine with each patient which is best for her at this time in her life. Once this decision has been made, it is important that a very positive attitude be taken by the physician and the patient toward the procedure to be done. Fortunately, complications are rare and individuals seldom die from this surgical procedure, but death can occur.

New methodology for tubal occlusion includes hysteroscopy plugs, injecting sclerosing chemical substances through the hysteroscope, hysteroscopy cautery and fimbriotexy. All these have been designed principally to be used in less developed countries and are probably not appropriate for the sophisticated level of health care available in the United States.

20
Appropriate Uses of Medical and Surgical Therapy in Endometriosis

Alternative Points of View

by W. P. Dmowski and A. Scommegna
by Brooks Ranney

Editorial Comment

The Appropriate Uses of Medical and Surgical Therapy in Endometriosis

W. P. Dmowski, M.D., Ph.D.

A. Scommegna, M.D.

University of Chicago Pritzker School of Medicine

More than a century after its original histologic description by Rokitansky[1] and over half a century after Sampson[2] coined its name, endometriosis remains one of the enigmatic diseases with unknown etiology and poorly understood histogenesis. It affects women in their reproductive years, limits their fertility and seriously impairs their health, although it is not life-threatening. It is not known why some women acquire this disease, but it is widely accepted that its persistence and spread are stimulated by cyclic secretion of ovarian hormones. The unknown etiology of endometriosis precludes a cure of this disease. All of the currently employed therapeutic methods offer at best a temporary remission and are in essence only palliative. The only definitive method of treatment that ensures permanent cure of the disease is associated with castration.

The disease interferes with the reproductive function of the patient and, on the other hand, it is the function of the gonads that stimulates the spread of the disease. Pregnancy is generally beneficial but difficult to achieve in the presence of endometriosis. Hormonal treatment is indicated in infertile patients, but the therapy itself prevents conception during several months of its use.

The choice of treatment in endometriosis is frequently influenced by the bias of the physician; this bias is generally based on his expertise with the specific therapeutic method. Thus the results of treatment, especially when the operative approach is involved, vary significantly. Positive results often cannot be duplicated by physicians less experienced.

The symptoms and findings of endometriosis are variable, and the disease in no two patients is alike. Severe, incapacitating dysmenorrhea and pelvic pain are often observed with minimal endometriosis, while extensive disease is at times symptom free and found on a routine examination. Extensive, bilateral ovarian endometriosis may be occasionally observed in teenagers, while only a minimal cul-de-sac disease may be found coincidentally in perimenopausal women.

Unknown etiology of endometriosis, poor understanding of its natural course and until recently, inadequate diagnostic techniques, produced multiple myths, half-truths and misconceptions.[3] The most common of these, in which the incidence of endometriosis was related to the race and social stratum of the patient, has been a frequent reason for misdiagnosing endometriosis as pelvic inflammatory disease among poor black populations treated in hospital clinics.

Endometriosis, as probably few other conditions in our specialty, still remains surrounded by a great deal of controversy.

Principles of Diagnosis and Therapy

The clinical or presumptive diagnosis of endometriosis is based on presenting symptoms and findings of the pelvic examination. These, however, may at times be misleading and the diagnosis must be confirmed through direct visualization of the lesions. This is especially important if prolonged hormonal treatment is contemplated. In questionable cases, a tissue specimen should be obtained for histologic examination at the time of visualization of the lesions.

Traditionally, and until recently almost exclusively, exploratory laparotomy had been the procedure during which suspected diagnosis of endometriosis was confirmed. It was usually performed to identify the origin of an adnexal mass; therefore, it took place relatively late in the course of the disease. The surgeon usually felt committed to more or less complete resection of the organs affected, and medical treatment, if any, was supplementary and reserved only for those patients with residual lesions.

During the past decade laparoscopy has become the most common method for visualization of the pelvic organs and for diagnosis of pelvic endometriosis. Consequently, the disease is being diagnosed with increasing frequency in symptomatic women without pelvic findings and at much earlier stages of the disease. The laparoscopic appearance of endometriosis and especially that of mild and moderate disease is characteristic.

Bluish-brown elevated peritoneal implants are commonly located in the cul-de-sac, on uterosacral ligaments, on the posterior wall of the uterus and on ovaries. "Powderburn" ecchymotic areas, "puckered nodules," "mulberry spots" or "peritoneal pockets" are commonly noted telltale signs of the disease. Small endometriomas and surface lesions release thick, brownish "chocolate" contents when touched with the probe or biopsied. Characteristically, pelvic adhesions are observed in the absence of tubal disease. Advanced endometriosis with massive adhesions between the reproductive system and neighboring organs may be, however, difficult to evaluate and diagnose through the laparoscope. In questionable cases biopsies of endometriotic implants or suspected lesions are generally feasible with laparoscopic instruments.

"Second-look" laparoscopy, to evaluate the results of treatment, identify the need for additional therapy and detect pelvic adhesions, a potential sequelae of healing, is becoming an acceptable procedure in patients with endometriosis. Minor surgical procedures, such as lysis of pelvic adhesions and cautery of minor endometriotic implants, has been recommended and performed by experienced laparoscopists at the time of the second-look laparoscopy.

There is no cause-directed therapy for endometriosis, since the etiology of the disease is unknown. Considering, however, that the focus of endometriosis begins with a few endometrial cells proliferating and functioning under endocrine stimulation, not visible to the naked eye and not amenable to surgical excision, the most desirable therapy for this disease should be the one effective at the level of the endometrial cell. Recent data seem to suggest that endometriosis develops in females with deficient cellular immunity.[4] If further studies confirm that immune deficiency is causally related to the development of endometriosis, specific immunotherapy may become available for the treatment of this condition.

Conservative surgery for endometriosis is the time-sanctioned approach favored by many gynecologists as the primary treatment.[5] Postsurgical results, in terms of recurrence and conception rates, which are used most frequently to evaluate the effectiveness of the endometriosis therapy, have been variable—in some hands higher than those achieved with the medical approach. There is no doubt that a skillful operator experienced in the surgical excision of this "benign cancer" may achieve excellent results in a small, selected group of patients. There is, however, no doubt also that even such an operator will not be able to remove all ectopic endometrial implants unless each lesion is large enough, isolated and well-circumscribed. Although it can be argued that not all endometriotic cells have to be removed, since endometriosis is not a neoplastic disease, it is widely known that even minimal endometriotic implants may be associated with infertility or severe symptoms and may give origin to the earlier postsurgical recurrence. Thus, it is the medical treatment of endometriosis as the primary approach that should be recommended for the average gynecologist with average surgical expertise. Conservative surgery, if required, should follow the hormonal treatment. This combined approach limits the extent of the surgical procedure and allows lysis of pelvic adhesions that might have formed during healing of the disease.

The most effective medical treatment of endometriosis at the present time is induction of pseudomenopause with danazol. The results in terms of clinical improvement and post-treatment pregnancy rates have been comparable to or better than those reported in selected series after conservative operations.[3, 5-9] Therapy with danazol is more effec-

tive, better tolerated and has fewer and less serious side effects than pseudopregnancy induced with estrogen-progestogen preparations. Treatment of endometriosis with testosterone or estrogens offers limited advantages and many disadvantages and it is not generally accepted.

Observation and symptomatic treatment may be the best choice of therapy in a woman with mild endometriosis and without immediate plans for conception. If such a patient desires contraception, strongly progestational oral contraceptives may be prescribed on a cyclic basis. They limit the degree of endometrial proliferation, may have ameliorating effect on dysmenorrhea and should control proliferation and spread of endometriosis. Preparations most likely to induce "salient periods" are the best choice for this purpose.

Pregnancy as a form of therapy for endometriosis should be considered in all patients with unproved fertility who are willing to conceive. They should be advised accordingly. Those with other causes of infertility should receive appropriate treatment to facilitate conception.

The choice of therapy for endometriosis is dictated by the age of the patient, family status, desire for conception, severity of symptoms and extent of the disease. Schematic outlines of the management of endometriosis in common clinical situations are demonstrated in Figures 1 to 4.

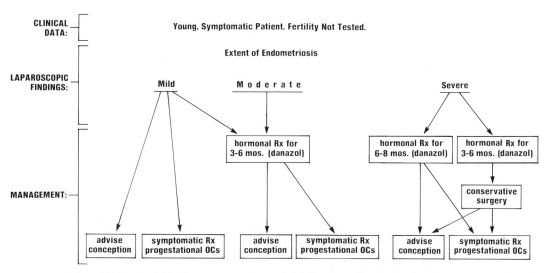

Figure 1. Management of endometriosis in a young, symptomatic patient with fertility not tested. (From Dmowski, W. P.: Current concepts in the management of endometriosis. *In* Wynn, R. M. (ed.): Obstetrics and Gynecology Annual, vol. 10. New York, Appleton-Century-Crofts, 1981, p. 304.)

MANAGEMENT OF ENDOMETRIOSIS

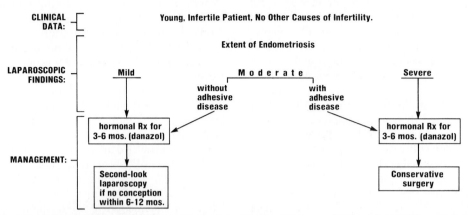

Figure 2. Management of endometriosis in a young, infertile patient without other causes of infertility. (From Dmowski, W. P.: Current concepts in the management of endometriosis. *In* Wynn, R. M. (ed.): Obstetrics and Gynecology Annual, vol. 10. New York, Appleton-Century-Crofts, 1981, p. 305.)

Medical Treatment

Hormonal treatment of endometriosis is based upon clinical observations that improvement in symptoms and findings of the disease occurs during amenorrhea of pregnancy and menopause. The hormonal suppressive treatment stops cyclic endometrial stimulation by endogenous estrogens and progesterone and inhibits cyclic proliferative, secretory and desquamative changes and induces amenorrhea. Proliferation of endometriotic lesions is arrested and repeated peritoneal bleeding does not occur. Atrophy of both uterine and ectopic endometrium results, and healing of endometriosis begins. The effect of treatment is essentially the same on uterine as on ectopic endometrium, thus the histologic pattern of the former reflects well the changes of the latter.

There are two currently acceptable and reasonably effective methods of medical treatment: induction of pseudopregnancy and induction of pseudomenopause. Just as pregnancy is less consistent in inducing atrophic changes in the ectopic endometrium[10] in comparison with surgical or physiologic menopause, pseudopregnancy has less consistent effect on endometriosis than pseudomenopause. Pseudomenopause is more effective, has fewer and better tolerated side effects and requires less time to achieve a desirable improvement.

PSEUDOMENOPAUSE

Endometriosis undergoes regression with menopause. An assumption can be made that the hypoestrogenic state of the menopause

MANAGEMENT OF ENDOMETRIOSIS

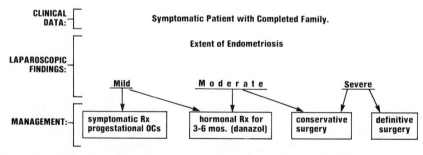

Figure 3. Management of endometriosis in a symptomatic patient with completed family. (From Dmowski, W. P.: Current concepts in the management of endometriosis. *In* Wynn, R. M. (ed.): Obstetrics and Gynecology Annual, vol. 10. New York, Appleton-Century-Crofts, 1981, p. 305.)

MANAGEMENT OF ENDOMETRIOSIS

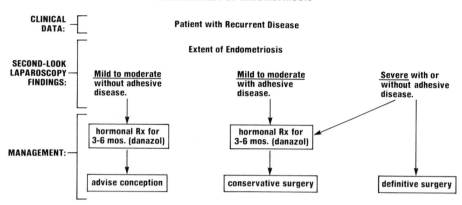

Figure 4. Management of endometriosis in a patient with recurrent disease. (From Dmowski, W. P.: Current concepts in the management of endometriosis. *In* Wynn, R. M. (ed.): Obstetrics and Gynecology Annual, vol. 10. New York, Appleton-Century-Crofts, 1981, p. 306.)

results not only in atrophy of the uterine endometrium and in amenorrhea but also in atrophy of the ectopic endometrium and thus in improvement in the findings and symptoms of endometriosis. A similar situation is observed after oophorectomy—that is, during surgical menopause.

During pseudomenopause induced with danazol, plasma estradiol levels are significantly suppressed.[11] They remain either undetectable or fluctuate in the early follicular range, while the preovulatory surge and post-ovulatory rise characteristic of normal cycles are not observed. Suppressed plasma estradiol and plasma progesterone in the follicular range are the result of suppressed FSH and LH secretion and suppressed ovarian function by the antigonadotropin.

Danazol inhibits pituitary secretion of both FSH and LH, and the effect is dose dependent.[12] Results of LHRH testing to determine the mechanism of danazol action at the hypothalamopituitary level have been inconsistent. It is unclear at this point whether danazol inhibits the response of the pituitary to LHRH or whether it acts through suppression of hypothalamic LHRH secretion. Furthermore, an inhibitory effect of danazol on ovarian steroidogenesis has been demonstrated[13] and a direct action at the endometrial level has been postulated.[14]

Clinically, in patients treated with the drug, amenorrhea develops along with symptoms and findings of lowered estrogen effect. In about 8 per cent of patients, hypoestrogenic state is associated with development of clinical symptoms of menopause such as hot flashes, night sweats and other signs of vasomotor instability.[15] For this reason, the temporary state of ovarian suppression induced with danazol and resembling in many respects menopause has been named pseudomenopause.[11]

To induce pseudomenopause, danazol is administered continuously in a daily dose of 800 mg for three to nine months, depending on the initial extent of the disease and on the patient's response. The drug has more consistent effect if administered in four divided doses and not BID as recommended in the package insert. It is quickly metabolized and excreted, with half-life in the plasma of about 4.5 hours.[16, 17] Eight hours after administration, plasma levels of danazol become undetectable. In many patients, daily dose lower than 800 mg may be adequate to induce pseudomenopause.[18]

The therapy should begin with the first day of the menstrual cycle. Starting danazol later on in the cycle may delay the onset of amenorrhea and may be associated with irregular bleeding during the first few weeks of therapy. Furthermore, unless treatment coincides with the beginning of the cycle, early conception cannot be excluded and although the drug does not appear to have teratogenic effects, it should not be used in pregnancy.

The primary evidence of adequate clinical response is prompt development of amenorrhea. It indicates that intraperitoneal bleeding is not occurring and that ectopic endometrium is undergoing atrophy. Atrophy of the ectopic endometrium is followed by its resorption and healing of endometriosis. In symptomatic patients, there is usually prompt relief of symptoms. Ovarian endometriomas and other palpable lesions gradually decrease in size, and the time of their complete disappearance may be used to determine the length of treatment required. Nodularities of the uterosacral ligaments and rectovaginal septum frequently persist and may never disappear completely.

Pseudomenopause induced with danazol has been found beneficial to patients with pelvic endometriosis in several studies.[6-8, 19] Symptomatic improvement was noted in 70 to 93 per cent of patients and improvement in pelvic findings in about 80 per cent. Laparoscopy before and after the course of treatment revealed marked decrease in the extent of endometriosis in all patients treated.[7]

However, in spite of marked improvement, a three-year follow-up on 99 patients treated demonstrated a recurrence rate of 39 per cent.[8] The interval between the end of the treatment and the time of recurrence was less than a year in 23 per cent of patients and increased annually thereafter by about 5 per cent. It should be emphasized, however, that at an average of 37 months after the end of treatment, 61 per cent of patients were symptom-free and had no pelvic findings suggestive of recurrence.

The return of menstrual function and fertility after discontinuation of the pseudomenopause has been prompt in the experience of all investigators. The first menstrual period usually occurs within four to six weeks after discontinuation of the treatment. The first cycle is frequently ovulatory, as indicated by conceptions that have taken place without a menstrual period between iatrogenic amenorrhea and the amenorrhea of pregnancy.[8]

The post-treatment pregnancy rate has been comparable to that observed after conservative surgery and generally higher than that after pseudopregnancy. In two separate studies, the corrected pregnancy rates after danazol treatment were 72 per cent and 76 per cent.[6, 8] The majority of conceptions occurred within the first year after discontinuation of the drug. It appears that post-treatment conception offers further protection from recurrence, since the recurrence rate was 50 per cent lower and the time of recurrence was twice as long among patients who conceived as compared with all patients treated.[8]

Endometriosis tends to recur at an annual rate between 10 to 15 per cent, regardless of the method of treatment. This probably reflects the natural course of the disease and indicates that unknown etiologic or predisposing factors are present in some women and

are not altered by the therapy.[12] The interval between the end of the treatment and the time of recurrence is variable, as is the natural course of the disease. There are no contraindications to repeated danazol treatment in patients with recurring endometriosis. However, if the recurrence is early and if palpable lesions are present, alternative methods such as conservative or definitive surgery should be considered.

Danazol is relatively well-tolerated, has few and rather minor side effects and few contraindications. Most side effects are related to the anabolic and mildly androgenic properties of the drug. Weight gain, skin oiliness, acne and occasional increase in hair growth or deepening of the voice have been reported.[15] Clitoral enlargement or frank virilization were not observed. About 8 to 15 per cent of patients complain of hot flashes, sweats and other vasomotor disturbances characteristic of the hypoestrogenic state. The drug is excreted through the biliary system; therefore, it should not be administered to patients with markedly impaired liver function. Other contraindications listed include undiagnosed abnormal uterine bleeding, pregnancy, breast feeding and impaired renal or cardiac function.

PSEUDOPREGNANCY

The beneficial effect of pregnancy in some patients with endometriosis has been repeatedly observed by clinicians. Unfortunately, pregnancy as a treatment for endometriosis may be applied only seldom, since a significant proportion of patients affected by this disease is infertile. A hormonal status similar to that of pregnancy may be achieved with continuous administration of estrogens and progestogens in high doses. Such treatment of endometriosis, introduced by Kistner[20] in 1958, has been aptly called pseudopregnancy.

Exogenous estrogen-progestogen preparations suppress pituitary secretion of FSH and LH and as a consequence inhibit ovarian function. There is little or no ovarian estrogen synthesis and plasma progesterone is in the follicular range because of suppressed ovulation. Cyclic endometrial stimulation by endogenous steroids is replaced by the continuous effect of exogenously supplied hormones. Exogenous estrogen-progestogen preparations in contrast to endogenous steroids suppress ectopic and uterine endometrium for two reasons: (1) their effect is continuous and not cyclic, and (2) progestogen is administered simultaneously with estrogen with a strongly progestational overall effect.

During treatment with pseudopregnancy, both uterine and ectopic endometrium undergo characteristic histologic changes. The initial stimulation phase is characterized by increased endometrial proliferation and hypertrophy, increased vascularity and stromal edema and deciduation of the stromal cells. With continued treatment, the endometrial glands become small, with little mitotic activity, and "out of phase" with deciduously changed stroma. Necrobiosis and atrophy of the endometrium then follow, and tissue resorption and healing begin to take place in the ectopic locations.

Symptomatically, some patients feel worse during the initial three to four months of treatment, which correspond to the period of endometrial hypertrophy, increased vascularity and edema. Pelvic pain may also become more severe and, in addition, multiple side effects related to pseudopregnancy may appear, such as nausea, vomiting, fluid retention and hypertension. Hypertrophic uterine endometrium may be expelled in the form of a uterine cast and in association with uterine bleeding and cramps. If treatment is continued, gradual improvement coincides with regressive and atrophic changes that take place in the endometriotic foci.

A variety of preparations have been recommended to induce pseudopregnancy. Those found most effective have been oral contraceptives with strong progestational properties, such as norethynodrel 10 mg plus mestranol 100 μg, norethindrone 10 mg plus mestranol 60 μg, and norgestrel 0.5 mg plus ethinyl estradiol 50 μg. The usual therapeutic regimen consists of one tablet daily continuously for six to nine months, with an increase by one tablet for each episode of breakthrough bleeding. In this way, the lowest effective dose is determined individually for each patient. The use of progestational preparations alone has been associated with much higher incidence of breakthrough bleeding, and generally addition of an estrogenic component is recommended.

The results achieved by pseudopregnancy, if continued, have been found satisfactory by many investigators. Improvement in symptoms was reported as high as 94 per cent.[21] The post-treatment pregnancy rates have been variable but, in general, lower than those after conservative surgery.[5] Kistner, who has reported the largest series, noted a post-treatment pregnancy rate of 55 per cent,[22-24] while Andrews and Larsen observed a post-treatment conception rate of 43 per cent.[25]

The recurrence rate of endometriosis after treatment is higher during the first year and then varies between 5 per cent and 10 per cent annually. Riva et al.[26] reported 18 per cent recurrence after an average of 11 months and Kistner[22] reported a 17 per cent rate after a similar period of time. The recurrence rate appears to be similar regardless of the method of treatment.

Side effects of pseudopregnancy, as mentioned earlier, are frequent and many patients tolerate them poorly. Contraindications to its use are the same as to oral contraceptives: thromboembolic and vascular disorders, markedly impaired liver function, estrogen-dependent neoplasms, pregnancy and undiagnosed uterine bleeding.

TREATMENT WITH ANDROGENS

Androgens such as testosterone and methyltestosterone have been employed for many years in the treatment of endometriosis. Several reports are on record indicating their beneficial effect on endometriosis and specifically on amelioration of symptoms such as pelvic pain, dyspareunia and dysmenorrhea.[27-31] There is no exact explanation as to the mechanism of this effect. The dose of androgen is not high enough to suppress ovarian function, at least not consistently. Ovulations and conceptions have been reported to occur during therapy. A direct effect of androgens on the endometrium has been suggested, but histologic studies of the endometriotic tissue in monkeys on androgen treatment did not reveal microscopic changes that could be attributable to the therapy.[32]

The most common therapeutic regimen consists of methyltestosterone linguets administered continuously for a period of about six months in a daily dose of 5 to 10 mg. The therapy should be discontinued immediately if conception occurs; therefore, use of contraception or early diagnosis of pregnancy are necessary. Symptomatic improvement in the severity of dysmenorrhea, dyspareunia and pelvic pain has been observed in about 75 per cent of patients treated.[31] However, in most patients, the relief is only partial and temporary, and the symptoms tend to recur within a few cycles after discontinuation of treatment.

The pregnancy rate within a year after discontinuation of treatment is variable and has been reported in the range of 11 to 19 per cent.[30, 31] The major advantage of the use of androgens as opposed to other therapeutic regimens is their apparent lack of the inhibitory effect on ovulation. The clinical results and post-treatment pregnancy rate are not as good with androgens as those achieved with other modes of treatment.

Side effects of androgen therapy may be significant and are related to their inherent endocrine properties. Hirsutism, acne, deepening of the voice and clitoral enlargement have been observed. If conception occurs during treatment, virilization of the female fetuses may occur. Large doses of androgens may occasionally inhibit or delay ovulation.

TREATMENT WITH ESTROGENS

Continous administration of large doses of estrogens to induce "hyperhormonal amenorrhea" has been advocated for treatment of endometriosis by a few investigators.[33, 34] Although symptomatic improvement has been observed in some patients on this regimen, atrophic changes in the ectopic endometrium could not be demonstrated histologically.[35] On the contrary, endometrium, as expected, responds with the development of cystic and adenomatous hyperplasia.[36] The risks of such therapy—especially those related to the development of hyperplastic endometrial changes and thromboembolic disease, along with multiple side effects such as peripheral edema, nausea, mastodynia and heavy vaginal bleeding—make this regimen currently not acceptable.

Combination of Medical and Surgical Treatments

The extent and location of endometriotic lesions or the type of a therapeutic response may at times dictate a combined medical and surgical treatment. The choice of which approach should be used first and which should follow usually depends on individual indications and on the personal preference of the physician. If the diagnosis is made at the time of laparotomy, the surgeon usually makes an attempt to resect the endometriotic tissues, but unless the disease is circumscribed it cannot be removed completely. In such cases hormonal treatment may follow surgery.

A combination of conservative surgery and hormonal treatment has been evaluated by several investigators for pseudopregnancy and androgen therapy and generally found without a particular advantage.[9, 25, 31] If used prior to conservative surgery, pseudopregnancy increases pelvic vascularity and edema and usually makes dissection and hemostasis more difficult. Androgens, having little effect on the endometrium, probably do not influence surgical dissection one way or the other. Used after conservative surgery, the treatment with pseudopregnancy or androgens appears not to change significantly the course of the disease or influence the post-treatment conception rates.[5]

Danazol, on the other hand, appears to be better suited as the adjuvant treatment preceding or following the conservative surgery. If a course of danazol precedes the surgical approach, atrophic endometrial changes induced by the drug limit the extent of required dissection. Decreased edema and pelvic vasocongestion observed after pseudomenopause facilitate surgical dissection and decrease blood loss during the procedure.[7] Furthermore, adhesions that potentially could have formed as a result of healing of the disease during medical treatment can be lysed and pelvic anatomy can be restored to normal, facilitating or increasing chances for conception. For these reasons, induction of pseudomenopause prior to conservative surgery offers additional advantages in the treatment of more extensive endometriosis. If conservative surgery as the primary treatment is incomplete and endometriotic implants remain, a course of postoperative danazol can facilitate further regression of the disease.

Surgical Treatment

Surgical procedures utilized in the treatment of endometriosis may be divided in two broad categories: conservative and definitive. Conservative surgery aims at resection of endometriosis and preservation of the fertility potential, while definitive surgery involves castration hysterectomy with excision or destruction of all visible areas of endometriosis.

CONSERVATIVE SURGERY: OPERATIVE ENDOSCOPY

Laparoscopy is the most common technique utilized for visualization of the pelvic organs and hence is of special importance in the diagnosis of endometriosis. Although primarily of diagnostic value, the laparoscopic approach may be supplemented by minor surgical procedures performed with accessory instruments inserted through one or more puncture wounds in the abdominal wall. Some authors consider operative laparoscopy as an accepted and, at times, preferred surgical technique for the treatment of mild endometriosis.

Endoscopic surgery requires clear visualization of the pelvic structures, good quality instruments and an experienced laparoscopist. Biopsies, lysis of adhesions, cautery of endometriotic implants, transection of uterosacral ligaments and even uterine suspension have been performed with this technique.

As already mentioned, operative laparoscopy is indicated only in patients with mild endometriosis. In patients with a more extensive disease, second-look laparoscopy (after a course of hormonal therapy) may also be combined with minor endoscopic procedures such as cautery of isolated endometriotic foci or lysis of peritoneal adhesions. It cannot be overemphasized, however, that such procedures may be technically difficult and should be attempted only by experienced endoscopists. The risk of serious injury to vital organs such as bowel, bladder, ureters and blood vessels is high. Prompt recognition of such injury and ability to initiate the appropriate corrective measures are necessary. Furthermore, because the exposure is never as good as with laparotomy, there is always the possibility of overlooking some endometriotic lesions too close to vital structures.

Meticulous hemostasis at the conclusion of the procedure is essential, since any blood left in the pelvis may well be the cause of further pelvic adhesions. Therefore, irrigation and aspiration of the irrigating solution are used routinely at the conclusion of the operative laparoscopy.

CONSERVATIVE SURGERY: LAPAROTOMY

Conservative surgery for endometriosis consists of resection of endometriotic lesions and reconstruction of the pelvic anatomy. In a young infertile woman with a mild or moderate disease and few symptoms, it is performed with the primary purpose of improving fertility. On the other hand, the primary purpose of conservative surgery may be relief of symptoms and resection of diseased organs in a patient who wants to retain her reproductive capacity but is not concerned with immediate conception.

In either case, since the procedure is performed to enhance or preserve the patient's reproductive potential, techniques similar to those used for tuboplasty are utilized. These include the use of optical loupes or operative microscope for better visualization, scrupulous hemostasis, avoidance of intraperitoneal pads or sponges to prevent future adhesions, constant irrigation and suction to maintain a clear field, dissection with the aid of an electrocautery needle to minimize bleeding and peritonealization of the raw areas at the conclusion of the procedure. Endometriotic implants are excised or cauterized. Large endometriomas are resected with preservation of healthy ovarian tissue whenever possible. At times, excision of severely affected adnexal structures on one side and preservation of the contralateral ovary and fallopian tube may be indicated.

A variety of ancillary surgical procedures have also been recommended. These include anterior uterine suspension, appendectomy, presacral neurectomy and free omental or peritoneal grafts to cover any raw surface. Among these, uterine suspension has been more widely accepted. Its purpose is to suspend the uterus and adnexa away from the cul-de-sac and help prevent their subsequent fixation in the pelvis. It should be performed when moderate or severe disease affects the pouch of Douglas or in the presence of a retroverted or retroflexed uterus. Corticosteroids in pharmacologic doses and antihistamines administered systemically before and for three days after surgery as well as instilled intraperitoneally during surgery have been advocated for the prevention of postoperative adhesions. Low molecular weight dextran, instilled intraperitoneally before abdominal closure, has also been used for this purpose. The value, if any, of such treatment modalities has not been conclusively demonstrated.

Many gynecologists pointing to the results of Acosta et al.[37] who reported pregnancy rates of 75 per cent and 50 per cent within two years after conservative surgery in patients suffering mild and moderate endometriosis, respectively, consider surgery a preferred method of treatment in these patients.[5] However, it is difficult to compare the results obtained with conservative surgery to those obtained by hormonal therapy because most often the characteristics of patients in each group are different. In general, patients with mild endometriosis tend to be treated with conservative surgery, while those with more extensive disease are treated either by definitive surgery or with hormonal medications. A pregnancy rate of 72 to 76 per cent after danazol treatment,[6, 8] comparable or better than that obtained after conservative surgery and higher than that after pseudopregnancy, makes pseudomenopause preferable to surgery as the first therapeutic approach in the treatment of this disease.

In our opinion, conservative surgery for endometriosis in a young infertile woman should be performed as a primary therapeutic approach only if a well-circumscribed unilateral endometrioma is present. Such isolated lesions can be excised completely and pregnancy may be attempted shortly after surgery. In the majority of patients, pseudomenopause either alone or followed by conservative surgery should be the treatment of choice. In some patients when the disease recurs after hormonal treatment or in those who cannot tolerate the medication, conservative surgery is the preferable treatment.

DEFINITIVE SURGERY

This therapeutic approach is usually reserved for the management of extensive endometriosis in older patients who are past the childbearing period or who have completed their families. However, patients in whom an unacceptable degree of symptoms have recurred after medical or surgical treatment are also candidates for definitive surgery.

The operation involves abdominal hysterectomy, bilateral salpingo-oophorectomy and resection of the endometriosis. Although preservation of the ovaries has been advocated in younger women, the possibility that the preserved ovarian function would stimulate undetected endometriotic foci makes hysterectomy without castration undesirable. It should be emphasized that if the extent of the endometriosis and severity of symptoms justify removal of the uterus, this procedure in effect terminates reproductive function of the patient. Preservation of the ovaries in such patients, exclusively for their hormonal function, does not justify the risks of the recurrence of endometriosis. Controlled amounts of estrogen or estrogen and androgen combination can be used for the relief or prevention of symptoms and changes resulting from estrogen deficiency. If, by chance, small foci of endometriosis left behind are stimulated by the exogenous estrogen, the medication can be stopped and a low-dose estrogen-progestogen combination substituted.

REFERENCES

1. Von Rokitansky, C.: 1860, as quoted in Ridley, J. H.: The histogenesis of endometriosis: a review of facts and fancies. Obstet. Gynecol. Surv. 23:1, 1968.
2. Sampson, J. A.: Perforating hemorrhagic (chocolate) cysts of the ovary, their importance and especially their relation to pelvic adenomas of the endometrial type. Arch. Surg. 3:245, 1921.
3. Sotrel, G. and Dmowski, W. P.: Endometriosis and its management. Obstet. Gynecol. Digest 15:26, 1976.
4. Dmowski, W. P., Steele, R. W. and Baker, G. F.: Deficient cellular immunity in endometriosis. Am. J. Obstet. Gynecol. 141:377, 1981.
5. Hammond, C. B. and Haney, A. F.: Conservative treatment of endometriosis: 1978. Fertil. Steril. 30:497, 1978.
6. Friedlander, R. L.: The treatment of endometriosis with danazol. J. Reprod. Med. 10:197, 1973.
7. Dmowski, W. P. and Cohen, M. R.: Treatment of endometriosis with an antigonadotropin, danazol: a laparoscopic and histologic evaluation. Obstet. Gynecol. 46:147, 1975.
8. Dmowski, W. P. and Cohen, M. R.: Antigonadotropin (danazol) in the treatment of endometriosis: evaluation of post-treatment fertility and three-year follow-up data. Am. J. Obstet. Gynecol 130:41, 1978.
9. Hammond, C. B., Rock, J. A. and Parker, R. T.: Conservative treatment of endometriosis: the effects of limited surgery and hormonal pseudopregnancy. Fertil. Steril. 27:756, 1976.
10. McArthur, J. W. and Ulfelder, H.: The effect of pregnancy upon endometriosis. Obstet. Gynecol. Surv. 20:709, 1965.
11. Dmowski, W. P. and Scommegna, A.: The rationale for treatment of endometriosis with danazol. *In* Greenblatt, R. B. (ed.): Recent Advances in Endometriosis. Amsterdam, Excerpta Medica, 1976, p. 87.
12. Dmowski, W. P.: Endocrine properties and clinical applications of danazol. Fertil. Steril. 31:237, 1979.
13. Barbieri, R. L., Canick, J. A., Makris, A. et al.: Danazol inhibits steroidogenesis. Fertil. Steril. 28:809, 1977.
14. Worley, R. J. and Podratz, K. C.: Estrogenic and antiestrogenic effects of danazol administration in estradiol receptor binding studies. Abstract 8, Pro-

gram of the 48th Annual Meeting of the Central Association of Obstetricians and Gynecologists, Minneapolis, 1980.

15. Rakoff, A. E.: Side effects of danazol therapy. *In* Greenblatt, R. B. (ed.): Recent Advances in Endometriosis. Amsterdam, Excerpta Medica, 1976, p. 108.

16. Davison, C., Banks, W. and Fritz, A.: The absorption, distribution and metabolic fate of danazol in rats, monkeys, and human volunteers. Arch. Int. Pharm. Ther. 221:294, 1976.

17. Williams, T. A., Edelson, J. and Ross, R., Jr.: A radioimmunoassay for danazol (17α-Pregna-2,4-dien-20-yno [2,3-d] isoxazole-17-ol). Steroids 31:205, 1978.

18. Ward, G. D.: Dosage aspects of danazol therapy in endometriosis. J. Int. Med. Res. 5:75, 1977.

19. Greenblatt, R. B., Dmowski, W. P., Mahesh, V. B. and Scholer, H. F. L.: Clinical studies with an antigonadotropin—danazol. Fertil. Steril. 22:111, 1971.

20. Kistner, R. W.: The use of newer progestins in the treatment of endometriosis. Am. J. Obstet. Gynecol. 75:264, 1958.

21. Andrews, M. C., Andrews, W. C. and Strauss, A. F.: Effects of progestin-induced pseudopregnancy on endometriosis: clinical and microscopic studies. Am. J. Obstet. Gynecol. 78:776, 1959.

22. Kistner, R. W.: Infertility with endometriosis. A plan of therapy. Fertil. Steril. 13:237, 1962.

23. Kistner, R. W.: The effects of new synthetic progestogens on endometriosis in the human female. Fertil. Steril. 16:61, 1965.

24. Kourides, I. A. and Kistner, R. W.: Three new synthetic progestins in the treatment of endometriosis. Obstet. Gynecol. 31:821, 1968.

25. Andrews, W. C. and Larsen, G. D.: Endometriosis: treatment with hormonal pseudopregnancy and/or operation. Am. J. Obstet. Gynecol. 118:643, 1974.

26. Riva, H. L., Wilson, J. H. and Kawaski, D. M.: Effect of norethynodrel on endometriosis. Am. J. Obstet. Gynecol. 82:109, 1961.

27. Hirst, J. C.: Conservative treatment and therapeutic test for endometriosis by androgens. Am. J. Obstet. Gynecol. 53:483, 1947.

28. Creadick, R. N.: The non-surgical treatment of endometriosis. NC Med. J. 11:576, 1950.

29. Preston, S. N. and Campbell, H. B.: Pelvic endometriosis: treatment with methyltestosterone. Obstet. Gynecol. 2:152, 1953.

30. Katayama, K. P., Manuel, M., Jones, H. W. and Jones, G. S.: Methyltestosterone treatment of infertility associated with pelvic endometriosis. Fertil. Steril. 27:83, 1976.

31. Hammond, M. G., Hammond, C. B. and Parker, R. T.: Conservative treatment of endometriosis externa: the effects of methyltestosterone therapy. Fertil. Steril. 29:651, 1978.

32. Scott, R. B. and Wharton, L. R., Jr.: The effect of testosterone on experimental endometriosis in rhesus monkeys. Am. J. Obstet. Gynecol. 78:1020, 1959.

33. Karnaky, K. J.: The use of stilbestrol for endometriosis. South. Med. J. 41:1109, 1948.

34. Hoskins, A. L. and Woolf, R. B.: Stilbestrol-induced hyperhormonal amenorrhea for the treatment of pelvic endometriosis. Obstet. Gynecol. 5:113, 1955.

35. Kistner, R. W.: Management of endometriosis in the infertile patient. Fertil. Steril. 26:1151, 1975.

36. Douglas, C. F. and Weed, J. C.: Endometriosis treated with prolonged administration of diethylstilbestrol: report of a case. Obstet. Gynecol. 13:744, 1959.

37. Acosta, A. A., Buttram, V. C., Jr., Besch, P. K., Malinak, R. L., Franklin, R. R. and Vanderheyden, J. D.: A proposed classification of endometriosis. Obstet. Gynecol. 42:19, 1973.

Operative Treatment of Endometriosis

Brooks Ranney, M.D.

University of South Dakota School of Medicine

In general, patients who have significant endometriosis that causes infertility, pelvic pain, dysmenorrhea, deep dyspareunia or palpably abnormal pelvic findings are best treated by operative therapy. Observations of individual patients have convinced me that hormonal therapy of endometriosis is essentially palliative, temporarily decreasing the cyclic responses of glands and stromas in the ectopic endometrium, but seldom, if ever, truly eliminating these ectopic endometrial glands. Assuming adequate peripheral blood supply, these ectopic glands will retain the potential ability to respond to cyclic female hormonal stimulation. The interval of quiescence varies with the stage of the disease, type and duration of hormonal "suppression," and each patient's individual inherited characteristics, but is seldom long-lasting or permanent. To obtain long-lasting results, significant endometriosis needs to be completely excised.

Operative management of significant endometriosis depends upon many individually variable factors, such as age and desire for pregnancy of the patient, duration of infertility, stage or extent of the disease, severity of symptoms, associated pelvic pathologic lesions and the possibility of preserving ovarian tissue with a good blood supply and the possibility that a subsequent pelvic operation may be needed.

Palliative hormonal therapy of endometriosis, using progestogens to produce "pseudopregnancy," or using danazol to cause "pseudomenopause," has been described elsewhere. Both types of therapy can be associated with significant complications and therefore should not be utilized prior to an exact diagnosis of endometriosis. Such a diagnosis may be made by laparoscopic observation and biopsy or may be made during other abdominal or pelvic operations that permit observation and excision of biopsy specimens. In general, we do not favor coagulation or other attempts at limited operative treatment of significant endometriosis through the laparoscope for reasons that will be described later.

If symptoms and findings warrant abdominal section for treatment of potential endometriosis, a preceding laparoscopy seems to be a waste of operating room time and an extension of anesthesia time for the patient. However, if the presumptive diagnosis is unclear, the laparoscope is an excellent diagnostic tool.

All experienced gynecologic surgeons carefully evaluate the extent of endometriosis and utilize this information while determining how best to treat each patient. Several recent attempts to standardize the preoperative extent of endometriosis into a formal staging of the disease have been summarized by Malinak.[12]

Types of Operative Treatment

In general, there are three types of operative treatment that may be indicated for patients with endometriosis. The first of these is conservative operative treatment with preservation of reproductive function. The second is conservative operative treatment with removal of the uterus and preservation of ovarian hormonal function. The third method of operative treatment includes removal of the uterus, tubes, ovaries and resection of all available endometriosis. For lack of a better term, this final therapy may be called a complete operation.

CONSERVATIVE OPERATIVE TREATMENT WITH PRESERVATION OF REPRODUCTIVE FUNCTION

If the patient is young, if the reproductive potential is to be saved, if the extent of the endometriosis is not too great, if the symptoms have not been too severe and if there is not an indication to remove the pelvic organs because of other abnormalities, an attempt may be made to resect all endometriosis, preserving the cervix, uterus, tubes and at least part of one ovary. Although there is a wide range of individual variability, if it is necessary to remove all of one ovary and *more* than two thirds of the other ovary, the chance of the remaining fragment of normal ovarian tissue functioning physiologically is relatively small. Therefore, at least a sixth of the normal ovarian tissue with a good blood supply should be retained in order to achieve reasonable reproductive success postoperatively.

When a patient with endometriosis needs a conservative operation, this should be performed by a well-trained, experienced gynecologist who understands reproductive physiology. A second operation can seldom undo unsatisfactory changes caused by an injudicious first operation.

Preoperatively, using a model of the female pelvis to illustrate respective anatomy and physiology, the physician can discuss with the patient the purposes and extent of the operation and can inform her of the possible outcome. However, final decisions concerning extent of operation should be based upon observations that can only be made when the abdomen is open. Therefore, patients should understand the necessity for this latitude in judgment during the operation.

During operative procedures of this type, it is important to evaluate the amount of endometriosis that may have affected the ovarian hilum. If endometriosis severely involves the blood supply of both ovaries, complete resection of the endometriosis will interfere with the blood supply to both ovaries and will result in poor ovarian function or none postoperatively. Incomplete resection of the endometriosis will result in continuation of symptoms and infertility. Conversely, if it is possible to conserve as much as one third of one ovary with a good blood supply, subsequent ovarian function should be satisfactory.

Deep involvement of the wall of bowel, bladder or ureter usually should be a contraindication to attempts at conservative operation with retention of reproductive function, because if such endometriosis is retained, in many such instances the patient will have debilitating symptoms or will not be fertile or both.

When all of these factors have been taken

into consideration, there is often good reason to resect endometriosis and retain reproductive function when feasible in young women who wish to conceive and whose mates are fertile, because approximately 60 to 85 per cent of these patients will conceive within one month to two years postoperatively. About 15 per cent of these patients may need subsequent pelvic operations within the next 20 years after resection of endometriosis. Most of these subsequent operations are not needed for recurring endometriosis but are usually needed for removal of other pelvic tumors that develop during intervening years, such as leiomyofibromas, adenomyosis, recurring endometrial polyps and ovarian cysts.

I prefer not to use preoperative progestogens because they soften the plaques of endometriosis, interfering with palpation of otherwise sharp borders and because the more friable tissues bleed more during resection. I also prefer not to use postoperative progestogens because many infertile patients may conceive within the first several months after resection of endometriosis, and this tendency should not be inhibited.

CONSERVATIVE OPERATIVE TREATMENT WITH PRESERVATION OF OVARIAN FUNCTION

Among about a third of patients who have significant pelvic endometriosis with symptoms, the husband or the wife has other serious causes of infertility, no children are wanted, or the patient has other significant pelvic abnormalities requiring hysterectomy. Usually these patients tend to be in the age group of 30 to 35 years, or older. Likewise, they usually have been infertile for long periods of time.

If it is possible to resect all or most of the endometriosis and to remove the uterus and if good ovarian tissue with a good blood supply can be retained, these patients will continue to have relatively normal ovarian function for their allotted number of years postoperatively. If the resection of endometriosis has been done in a thorough manner, a few of these patients (less than 1 per cent) will need a subsequent pelvic operation, either because of recurring endometriosis or because of development of other pelvic abnormalities.

Technically, it would be easier to castrate such women and not to resect the endometriosis. This would eliminate the source of fluctuating female hormones (which are the "generators" and stimulators of endometriosis). Residual endometriosis would be expected to resolve gradually into quiescent glands and stromas, surrounded by scar. However, such castration would also produce menopausal symptoms in many patients. Any subsequent attempts to treat the patient's menopausal symptoms with hormones would tend to restimulate the quiescent endometriosis, producing more pain or tumor. Therefore, resection of all endometriosis and hysterectomy is the best physiologic way to treat these patients who are still some years from climacteric.

COMPLETE OPERATION

Patients who are mostly older, who have no desire for preservation of reproductive potential and who have either severe endometriosis or any endometriosis found in association with other significant pelvic tumors are better served by removal of the uterus, tubes, and ovaries and resection of the endometriosis. Again, the key location of endometriosis is in the hilar region of the ovaries. Deep involvement of the hilar regions of both ovaries makes it impossible to resect endometriosis and to retain any ovarian tissue with a good blood supply.

Removal of the ovaries also removes the female hormones. However, if these patients have menopausal symptoms and if significant endometriosis has been retained in the pelvic tissues, treatment of the menopausal symptoms with estrogen therapy will result in resurgence of endometriosis. Therefore, even in these patients who have their ovaries removed, it is important to try to resect all possible endometriosis so that postoperative postmenopausal symptoms may be treated by estrogen therapy for preservation of the patient's future health.

One group of patients merits special discussion. These are somewhat younger women whose moderate or severe endometriosis has been softened by either endogenous or exogenous progestogens, producing a secretory or decidual response not only in the endometrium but also in endometriotic tissues. Sometimes, without warning, these softened, adherent, endometriotic surfaces may be avulsed from each other. These highly vascular tissues bleed into the abdomen, producing hemoperitoneum, severe pain and sometimes acute shock-like symptoms. Emergency operation may be needed. In these patients, one can rarely preserve either reproductive or ovarian function. Meticulous resection of hemorrhagic, softened endometriosis is difficult. Results of conservative operations are poor. Rarely after such operations will these patients conceive, and about one fourth may require operations within the next ten years to remove symptomatic endometriosis. Therefore, it is usually best to remove the uterus, adnexa and as much endometriosis as possible during the initial emergency operation in these unfortunate young women.

I have seen a series of ten postmenopausal patients whose pelvic pain or tumors or both were caused by symptomatic endometriosis, which was restimulated by resurging endogenous hormones or by exogenous hormones. These patients required complete operation with removal of the uterus, adnexa and resection of endometriosis. These women were from 1 to 20 years postmenopausal and ranged in age from 50 to 74 years.

Rarely, one may find carcinoma or sarcoma in endometriosis. It is worthwhile to resect these tissues as completely as possible. Four such patients of mine are alive and well years after resection of endometriosis and extirpation of the uterus, tubes and ovaries.

POSTOPERATIVE TREATMENT. Unless there are specific contraindications to estrogen therapy, patients who have had "complete operation" (hysterectomy, bilateral salpingo-oophorectomy and resection of endometriosis) may be treated for significant menopausal symptoms postoperatively in the following manner: (1) If the operator was able to remove all endometriosis, patients may receive supportive estrogen therapy (0.02 mg Estinyl [ethinyl estradiol]) daily, starting on the second or third postoperative day. (2) If most significant endometriosis has been resected, similar estrogen therapy for menopausal symptoms may be started on the fourth or fifth postoperative day and in most instances may be continued because there will be no adverse postoperative effect. However, in rare instances it will be necessary to discontinue hormonal estrogen therapy for the menopausal symptoms, because of bleeding from bowel or bladder or pelvic pain, and to utilize other palliative methods of treatment. (3) If large amounts of significant endometriosis are retained postoperatively, it is not wise to attempt to treat postoperative menopausal symptoms with estrogen therapy because the residual endometriosis will almost certainly respond to hormonal therapy and will become symptomatic postoperatively. In these patients other palliative methods of treatment of menopausal symptoms will be needed.

Methods of Resection of Endometriosis

There is one very practical reason for excising small endometriomas or tiny areas of endometriosis rather than treating them with electrocautery, cryotherapy or carbon dioxide laser. Usually the observed portion of endometriosis is merely the tip of the iceberg; palpation often reveals a much larger area surrounding and deep to the smaller point the surgeon may see. Electrocautery, cryotherapy or carbon dioxide laser may treat only a part of the true lesion. Also, such treatments may inadvertently be extended too deeply, near bowel, bladder or ureter.

A combination of observation and palpation used alternately, interspersed with careful dissection and snipping with fine scissors while upward traction is applied with tissue forceps, may be used to excise an area of endometriosis meticulously and completely. If the surgeon plans to remove the uterus, endometriosis around the uterosacral ligaments may be dissected medially, away from the ureter or the uterine artery, and may be turned in toward the cervix before the hysterectomy is completed. After resection of an endometrioma, arteries in the base of the crater are clamped and ligated. Then peritoneum is approximated and "dead space" is obliterated with fine sutures.

There is one theoretical advantage to cutting out endometriosis and sewing up the peritoneal defect rather than coagulating, freezing or desiccating the region. The latter three methods usually will involve healing with more tissue reaction—leading to more potential adhesions—than will meticulous cutting and sewing.

The major disadvantage of dissection and excision of endometriosis is that the procedure requires a considerable amount of time and exact attention to detail. Microscopic magnification is rarely useful, but occasionally low-power operating loupes may be helpful.

In general, those areas of endometriosis that are on the side wall of the pelvis, often just lateral to and sometimes adherent to the ovary, first must be dissected and separated from the adjacent ovary, using finger dissection, and scissor dissection alternately. Usually, dense scar ruptures and "chocolate cysts" drain; their contents must be aspirated from the pelvis and the pelvis should be irrigated with saline. Endometriotic cysts and smaller lesions usually can be cut from normal ovarian cortex with a plastic-bladed scalpel. Then traction is applied to the lesion with Allis forceps while it is dissected from deeper ovarian tissues with the handle of the scalpel.

One must identify the location of the ureter by palpation and observation, accurately enough to make certain that dissection of the endometriosis will not jeopardize it. In most instances this is possible without elaborate dissection of the ureter. When the ureter is severely involved with endometriosis and surrounding inflammation and scar, one must identify normal ureter above the lesion and make a small peritoneal incision just lateral to this. Then the ureter and endometriosis may be dissected carefully away from the pelvic side wall and adjacent vessels. The endometriosis usually can be dissected off the ureter. In rare, severe cases, to save kidney function, it may be necessary to remove a badly involved segment of ureter and to implant the free ureter into the bladder.

If endometriosis involves the surface of bowel (large or small), it is almost always isolated to the serosa and subserosa. Usually, it may be snipped carefully off the bowel surface, and the peritoneum may be approximated with fine silk sutures and sewn in a transverse manner to avoid narrowing the bowel lumen.

Even during careful dissections of endometriosis in the cul-de-sac, we have inadvertently entered the lumen of densely adherent sigmoid bowel in four patients. However, if the submucosa is closed with continuous fine catgut, if the serosa is sutured with interrupted fine silk, if the patient receives appropriate antibiotics, if she receives nothing orally until rectal gas passes and then only liquids for three more days, then these small lumenal defects should heal without incident.

In five patients, finger palpation revealed that the large or small bowel lumen was seriously narrowed by the scar of an endometrioma or there was acute angulation of bowel caused by unresectable endometriosis. In these rare cases we have performed either wedge-shaped excision of the involved antimesenteric bowel or bowel resection, removing only the involved loop of bowel, followed by end-to-end anastomosis. With appropriate postoperative care, all have had good healing.

If the uterus is markedly retrodisplaced, so that healing ovarian surfaces will be closely adjacent to healing cul-de-sac suture lines, the surgeon may decrease the tendency for postoperative adhesion formation by performing a uterine suspension. We have not done this routinely but rather occasionally, as needed. Since ventrosuspensions of the uterus, in which round ligaments are attached to the abdominal wall, frequently result in a tacky, dragging-down sensation for the patient thereafter, we have avoided this operative procedure. A satisfactory and fairly permanent anteversion of the uterus can be produced by the modified Baldy-Webster suspension procedure, in which (1) the bladder is advanced higher toward the fundus of the uterus, (2) the round ligaments are brought through the broad ligaments and are tacked to the back of the uterus with the fundus anteverted, and (3) the uterosacral ligaments are shortened and plicated to the back of the cervix. If a lesser (and only temporary) procedure is needed, the surgeon can accomplish anteversion of the uterus by simply "reefing" the round ligaments with a nonabsorbable suture. The suture is started anterior to the attachment of the round ligament into the uterus, is continued through the round ligament for a reasonable distance, is plicated back through the round ligament and reattached to the anterior wall of the uterus. When this suture is drawn up and tied, the round ligament is shortened.

If there is likely to be central pelvic pain after healing is completed caused by retention of nonresectable endometriosis in the pelvis, and if this patient has had dysmenorrhea, a presacral neurectomy may be performed before the abdomen is closed. It is important that the operator remember that an adequate presacral neurectomy removes all autonomic nervous fibers, medial to the ureters, posterior to the peritoneum and anterior to the promontory of the sacrum, for a distance of approximately 7 cm. While making such a dissection, it is quite easy to jeopardize pelvic veins, the anterior vertebral artery and veins and arteries posterior to the loops of the rectosigmoid bowel on the left side of the pelvis, so the dissection must be careful and meticulous. With such a careful, meticulous and thorough presacral neurectomy, the patient likely will have freedom from central pelvic pain. However, she may have interference with emptying of the bladder and lower bowel for some time postoperatively and may be chronically constipated. Likewise, if she becomes pregnant, she probably will have difficulty in recognizing the onset and progress of labor.

As it is seen at the operating table, endometriosis has a number of recognizable gross pathologic characteristics. A small blue-domed cyst, the size of a blueberry or smaller, may be surrounded by puckering, tough scar. Previous rupture and extrusion of blood pigments may have caused tan or brownish staining of adjacent peritoneum. Repeated rupture and sealing of endometriosis usually will cause dense adhesions between adjacent peritoneal surfaces. Portions of the cul-de-sac may be obliterated by this dense scar, and endometriomas of the ovary often are semifixed to the posterior aspects of the broad ligament or to adjacent bowel.

In contradistinction to carcinoma (which is usually initiated on an epithelial surface and which then grows into subjacent fibromuscular wall), endometriosis is usually initiated on or near a peritoneal surface and then tends to grow downward into subjacent fibromuscular structures. This often helps in differentiating grossly between more advanced lesions of endometriosis and cancer.

The age of endometriotic lesions in ovaries cannot be estimated, nor the severity judged exactly by the size or appearance of the ovaries. In general, however, observation will disclose the superficial lesions and palpation the deeper ones. Thick-walled cysts ranging up to 5 or 6 cm in size may have been caused by repeated extravasation of blood into ovarian endometriomas, and the contents usually are concentrated dark, old pigments of variable viscosity, ranging from watery to syrupy ("chocolate cysts"). Symptoms do not correlate well with the duration of the lesions. Probably this is because newer lesions are closer to nerve endings and cause irritation of those nerve endings during subsequent menses. On the other hand, older lesions have been sealed off and encased in an armor of scar, which tends to separate their activity from adjacent nerve endings.

Because of the dense adhesions that surround endometriosis and chocolate cysts of the ovaries, these can seldom be dissected without being ruptured. There is always some degree of distortion of tissues caused by the dissection of the dense adhesions, so it is almost impossible to send to the pathologic laboratory a specimen that resembles the pathologic appearance in vivo. For this reason, the gross appearance of endometriosis cannot be learned well in the pathologic laboratory but must be observed in the operating room. This marked distortion of tissues, resulting from dissection and excision of the tough scar around endometriosis, makes it extremely difficult for the pathologist to determine sites for microscopic section from the gross specimen. Therefore, if the gynecologic surgeon desires uniform microscopic confirmation of the gross operative findings, small individual specimens should be excised and sent to the pathologist in individually labeled containers of fixative. Alternately, pins should be placed in the larger gross specimen to identify areas from which microscopic sections may demonstrate endometriosis. If this is not done, microscopic confirmation of the gross findings will be quite incomplete. Even with these special efforts, microscopic verification is seldom 100 per cent.

Cervical endometriosis probably results from implantation of endometrial particles that descend during menses and lodge in defects in the cervical mucosa caused by tenaculum holes, biopsy punches, cervical cautery or cryotherapy. To avoid cervical endometriosis, it would seem logical to limit extensive operative treatment of the cervix to the early days after a menstrual cycle, so that healing will be complete prior to the next menstrual cycle. Small areas of endometriosis of the cervix may be treated with electrocoagulation or -cautery and often will heal well prior to the next menstrual period if the timing is early in the cycle.

Operative procedures such as salpingectomy or tubal ligation that leave a tubal stump very close to the cornual portion of the uterus may be followed by mild to severe endosalpingosis growing out of this ligated or coagulated tubal stump. During salpingectomy such postoperative endosalpingosis can usually be avoided by resecting a small wedge out of the corner of the uterus at the time of salpingectomy. During tubal coagulation or ligation, it seems likely that if the procedure is performed well away from the cornual portion of the uterus, there probably will be a decreased incidence of endosalpingosis thereafter. Such endosalpingosis can grow (as demonstrated by Sampson) for distances up to 12 cm from the corner of the uterus and can produce dense, painful scar. Ordinarily, resection of this endosalpingosis and adjacent scar and hysterectomy are needed to relieve the associated pelvic pain.

REFERENCES

1. Andrews, M. C., Andrews, W. C. and Strauss, A. F.: Effects of progestin-induced pseudopregnancy on endometriosus. Am. J. Obstet. Gynecol. 78:776, 1959.
2. Andrews, W. C.: Medical versus surgical treatment of endometriosis. Clin. Obstet. Gynecol. 23:917, 1980.
3. Ansbacher, R.: Treatment of endometriosis with danazol. Am. J. Obstet. Gynecol. 121:283, 1975.
4. Behrman, S. J.: The surgical management of endometriosis. *In* Greenblatt, R. B. (ed.): Recent Advances in Endometriosis. Amsterdam, Excerpta Medica, 1976, p. 62.
5. Cohen, J. R.: Laparoscopic diagnosis and pseudomenopause treatment of endometriosis with danazol. Clin. Obstet. Gynecol. 23:901, 1980.
6. Devereaus, R. P.: Endometriosis: long-term observations with particular reference to incidence of pregnancy. Obstet. Gynecol. 22:444, 1963.
7. Gardner, G. H.: Pelvic endometriosis. Northwest Med. 38:367, 1939.
8. Gray, L. A.: Endometriosis. Clin. Obstet. Gynecol. 3:472, 1960.
9. Gray, L. A.: The management of endometriosis involving the bowel. Clin. Obstet. Gynecol. 9:309, 1966.
10. Green, T. H.: Conservative surgical treatment of endometriosis. Clin. Obstet. Gynecol. 9:293, 1966.
11. Kistner, R. W.: The use of newer progestins in the treatment of endometriosis. Am. J. Obstet. Gynecol. 75:264, 1958.
12. Malinak, L. R.: Infertility and endometriosis: operative technique, clinical staging, and prognosis. Clin. Obstet. Gynecol. 23:925, 1980.
13. Meigs, J. W.: Endometriosis—a possible etiologic factor. Surg. Gynecol. Obstet. 67:253, 1938.
14. Moore, J. G., Hibbard, K. T., Growden, W. A. and Shifferan, B. S.: Urinary tract endometriosis, enigmas of diagnosis and management. Am. J. Obstet. Gynecol. 134:162, 1979.
15. Mostoufizadeh, G. H., Mahpareh and Scully, R. E.: Malignant tumors arising in endometriosis. Clin. Obstet. Gynecol. 23:951, 1980.
16. Pratt, J. H. and Williams, T. J.: Indications for complete pelvic operations and more radical procedures in the treatment of severe or extensive endometriosis. Clin. Obstet. Gynecol. 23:937, 1980.
17. Ranney, B.: Endometriosis I. Conservative operations. Am. J. Obstet. Gynecol. 107:743, 1970.
18. Ranney, B.: Endometriosis II. Emergency operations due to hemoparitoneum. Obstet. Gynecol. 36:437, 1970.
19. Ranney, B.: Endometriosis III, Complete operations. Am. J. Obstet. Gynecol. 109:1137, 1971.
20. Ranney, B.: Endometriosis: Pathogenesis, symptoms, and findings. Clin. Obstet. Gynecol. 23:865, 1980.
21. Ranney, B.: Etiology, prevention and inhibition of endometriosis. Clin. Obstet. Gynecol. 23:875, 1980.
22. Sampson, J. A.: Postsalpingectomy endosalpingosis. Am. J. Obstet. Gynecol. 23:443, 1930.
23. Scott, R. B., ReLinde, R. W. and Wharton, L. R., Jr.: Further studies on experimental endometriosis. Am. J. Obstet. Gynecol. 66:1082, 1953.
24. Weed, J. C. and Arquembourg, P. C.: Endometriosis: can it produce an autoimmune response resulting in infertility? Clin. Obstet. Gynecol. 23:885, 1980.
25. Weed, J. C.: Prostaglandins as related to endometriosis. Clin. Obstet. Gynecol. 23:895, 1980.

Editorial Comment

This chapter represents a true controversy in that a surgical proponent (Ranney) and medical endocrine proponents (Dmowski and Scommegna) voice their views. There is much agreement among these authors as to the basic understanding of endometriosis, but the disputed issue is how it should be managed once the diagnosis is made. Importantly, both agree that an exact diagnosis of endometriosis is necessary or therapy should not be instituted. It is now known that medical therapy, such as pseudomenopause (danazol) or pseudopregnancy (progesterone), costs considerable effort as well as money. (The average course of danazol for four to six months of therapy will cost approximately $700.) Ranney contends that all hormonal therapy is palliative and seldom long-lasting and that long-lasting results in significant endometriosis can be achieved only by excision. The diagnosis can be made by laparoscopy; however, there are all degrees of diagnosis. Ranney condemns laparoscopy coagulation because it will not eradicate the disease but only touch the tip of the iceberg of the problem. Additionally, he states that laparoscopy can produce only a presumptive diagnosis and to be certain a laparotomy and tissue diagnosis are necessary.

Ranney proposes different types of operative therapy: (1) conservative with preservation of reproductive function; (2) conservative with removal of the uterus and preservation of ovarian tissue and (3) complete clean-out.

It is important to understand reproductive physiology for the future well-being of the patient before a specific decision is made concerning therapy. Ranney states that endometriosis that affects the hilum of the ovary often will affect the blood supply and if one third of a good ovary with a good blood supply can be conserved, this is worth doing; otherwise, the ovary should be extirpated. If endometriosis involves the bowel, bladder or other foreign sites, conservative therapy in general is not good. The percentage of patients conceiving following surgical therapy is almost the same as those conceiving after hormonal therapy, 60 to 85 per cent from one month to two years. Ranney emphasizes that he does not use progestogens preoperatively or postoperatively as a form of therapy. It is important if a clean-out is done that much time is spent extirpating all the endometriosis lesions so that the menopausal symptoms that persist can be treated with appropriate estrogen therapy. If endometrial implants are not removed, there will be a recurrence with estrogen therapy. It is important in conservative therapy of endometriosis to excise the implants, suspend the uterus and do a presacral neurectomy; then the batting average for success is quite high.

Dmowski and Scommegna identify the persistence and spread of endometriosis that is stimulated by the cyclic secretion of ovarian hormones; they state that blocking the cyclic secretion will at least abate the spreading process. They agree that all current therapy at best is given only for temporary remission and state that the disease is now diagnosed much more frequently since laparoscopy has become a commonplace surgical procedure. The controversy exists as to whether second-look laparoscopy is helpful because it may only reveal whether or not surgery or more therapy is indicated. These authors propose cautery at the second look, whereas Ranney does not feel that cautery is appropriate.

Dmowski and Scommegna ask why it is that some women get endometriosis and others do not. Perhaps it develops in women who have a deficiency in cellular immunity.

Dmowski and Scommegna propose that if conservative surgical therapy is done it should be followed with hormonal therapy, that is, a course of danazol. They and Ranney agree that the choice of therapy should be dictated by the age of the patient, the family status, the desire for contraception and the patient's symptoms; hence, the treatment of endometriosis is individualized. Dmowski and Scommegna point out that 800 mg a day of danazol for three to nine months is probably appropriate therapy and that the medication should be taken four times a day rather than as two tablets twice a day, because the half-life is roughly 4.5 hours. Their statistics for relief of symptoms are 70 to 95 per cent, and 80 per cent of the patients have improvement on examination.

Endometriosis will emerge as a much more important diagnosis in the future. In the past it has been demonstrated that in a private hospital where major gynecologic surgical procedures are done, at least one third of all patients who are operated on for some specific reason have endometriosis. Since women are now delaying childbearing and are electing not to have children, the incidence of endometriosis should increase. Individualization of therapy is stressed in both articles, and the reader must choose the most appropriate means of therapy. Everyone agrees that endometriomas or large ovarian chocolate cysts cannot be treated with danazol because the disease is too overt. Surgery should be done first. The next question is whether or not pseudomenopausal therapy with danazol should be utilized following surgery, and here there is a difference of opinion.

21

Diagnosis and Management of Stress Urinary Incontinence

Alternative Points of View

by Jack R. Robertson
by Stuart A. Weprin and
Frederick P. Zuspan

Editorial Comment

Diagnosis and Management of Urinary Incontinence

Jack R. Robertson, M.D.

University of Southern California, Santa Maria, California

Historical Perspective

The genital and urinary tracts are as intimately related in women as in men. Kelly realized that gynecologists must be trained as genitourinary surgeons for women; he established the first residency program in gynecology at Johns Hopkins. Kelly developed a cystoscope, a hollow tube with a handle. He examined patients in the knee-chest position, with light for vision reflected from a head mirror.

A superior instrument, the indirect water cystoscope, became available. Urologists recognized endoscopy as a major advance in medicine, and the water cystoscope became the cornerstone for their exact scientific specialty. Urologists are genitourinary surgeons for men and urinary surgeons for women.

Cystoscopy disappeared from gynecology.

The gynecologist is a genital surgeon for women, but there are no genitourinary surgeons for women. This compartmentalization of medicine has isolated the lower urinary tract from the pelvis in the female patient.

The conventional male panendoscope is 35 cm long and has a 30-degree viewing angle. A 27-mm opening at the distal end of the sheath permits the use of a deflector for inserting ureteral catheters.

Urologists use the female urethra as a rest for the male endoscope while they look around in the bladder. Examination of the female urethra is unsatisfactory because the urethra collapses around the objective of the telescope (Fig. 1). Only 20 per cent of the female urethra can be seen. To correct these problems, I have developed new equipment.[1, 2]

The urethra is the most accessible portion of the urinary tract for investigation. It is

561

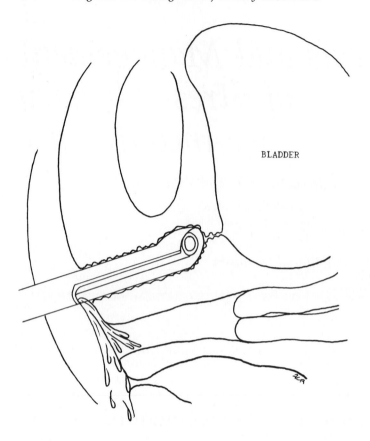

BLADDER

Figure 1. The McCarthy panendoscope has a 27-mm opening at the tip to allow passage of ureteral catheters. For this reason distention of the female urethra is poor, and at best only about 20 per cent of the female urethra can be visualized. It is difficult to inflate the female urethra with water. The patient gets a minidouche and an excellent perineal wash.

palpable in its entire length through the anterior vaginal wall. Its lumen can be delineated by contrast media and its angles measured by bead chains. Despite this, little is known of its function.

The development of a female urethroscope and a carbon dioxide cystometer makes the objective work-up of the female patient with genitourinary problems an office procedure.[3]

Definitions

The term stress incontinence is improperly used as a diagnosis, causing confusion. The International Continence Society defines stress incontinence as follows:[4]

1. The symptom "stress incontinence" describes the patient's statement of involuntary loss of urine when exercising.

2. The sign "stress incontinence" denotes the observation of involuntary loss of urine from the urethra immediately upon an increase of abdominal pressure.

3. The condition "genuine stress incontinence" is involuntary loss of urine at the time when the intravesical pressure exceeds the

maximum urethral pressure, occurring only in the absence of detrusor activity.

"Genuine stress incontinence," therefore, refers to deficiency of the urethral closure mechanism and does not involve the detrusor. The symptom and the sign of stress incontinence are unreliable in indicating whether the problem is sphincter weakness or detrusor activity or both.

Equipment

The Robertson™ gas urethroscope, which has a straight-ahead view, is eight inches long with a 24 French tapered sheath. The fiberoptic light cord and gas tubing attach to the handle (Fig. 2).

The Robertson™ endoscopy monitor records opening urethral pressures, uroflowmetry and cystometrograms under endoscopic control. A continuous simultaneous graph of the pressure and volume of gas delivered to the patient is recorded on a precison X-Y recorder. The flow rate is optional; I prefer to use a flow rate of 150 ml per min.

Analysis of voiding problems in male patients is easy — the urologist observes the male patient voiding. Force of stream, hesitancy and dribbling are noted. Psychological factors prevent this type of observation in females.

Uroflowmetry

Uroflowmetry is performed by connecting a uroflowmeter to the Robertson™ endoscopy monitor. Uroflowmetry makes the indirect measurement of flow rate possible (Fig. 3). The total time of micturition is divided into the volume or urine voided to get the urinary flow in millimeters per second.

The control switch is operated by the patient. The system is nonelectronic.

The following terms for uroflowmetry are generally accepted: *flow rate* is the volume of urine expelled through the urethra per unit of time, expressed in millimeters per second. *Flow time* is the time over which measurable flow occurs. *Time of maximum flow* is the time from onset of flow to maximum flow. *Maximum flow rate* (peak flow) is the maximum value of the flow rate. *Voided volume* is the volume expelled through the urethra. *Average flow rate* is the voided volume divided by the flow time.[5]

Uroflowmetry has limitations as an isolated measurement. A noninvasive procedure, it is valuable in screening and is useful in assessing results of treatment and the progression of disease.

An alternate method is *audible voiding*. Gas is left in the bladder at the end of examination. The patient voids the gas, which is clearly audible. The volume is known, and the pitch and voiding time are recorded on a tape recorder.

Technique

The patient is instructed to come to the office with a full bladder. She initiates the uroflow by touching the chair control switch.

After urination the patient is placed in the lithotomy position, and a pelvic examination is done. The saddle area of the perineum is checked by pinprick sensation. Innervation of this area is from dermatomes arising in sacral roots S2, S3 and S4, which is the portion of the spinal cord receiving sensory impulses from the bladder.

A Sims speculum is inserted into the vagina to spread the labia and make the urethral meatus easily available. As the patient contracts and relaxes the pelvic floor, the movement of the speculum is observed. Motor innervation to the pelvic floor is through the pudendal nerve from S2 to S4. The reflex micturitional arc is checked by stroking the clitoris and observing contraction of the anal sphincter.

The tapered end of the scope is placed at the meatus, and the carbon dioxide flow rate is set at 150 ml per min. The gas acts as the obturator and overcomes urethral resistance

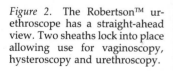

Figure 2. The Robertson™ urethroscope has a straight-ahead view. Two sheaths lock into place allowing use for vaginoscopy, hysteroscopy and urethroscopy.

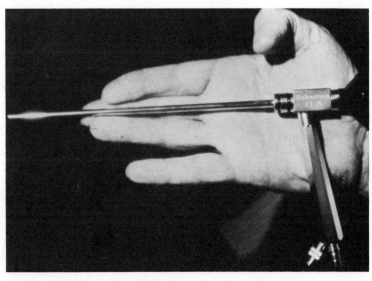

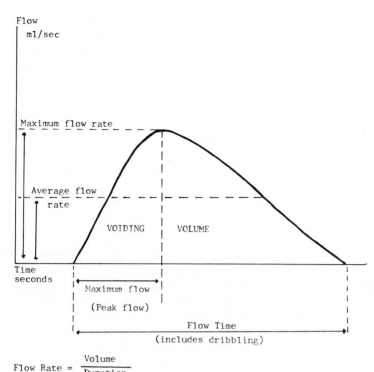

Figure 3. Uroflowmetry formula for indirect measurement of flow rate. The curve shown is normal.

as the urethroscope is threaded through the urethra, and the examiner views the urethra endoscopically.

The opening urethral pressure is recorded. The average opening urethral pressure is 80 cm of water pressure. Patients with true anatomic incontinence tend to have a low opening urethral pressure. Patients with bladder instability tend to have a normal or high opening urethral pressure.

When the urethroscope enters the bladder, the carbon dioxide is turned off. Urinary residual is collected, and the carbon dioxide is turned on again.

The scope is withdrawn from the bladder until the tip is approximately 0.5 cm distal to the vesical neck (Fig. 4A). The empty bladder has a horseshoe-shaped opening between 5 and 7 o'clock. The action of the vesical neck is observed as the bladder is insufflated with carbon dioxide (Fig. 4B–D).

Findings

NORMAL

The bladder and urethra function as a unit, with the urethra elongating as the bladder fills. As the bladder expands with carbon dioxide, the inferior rim of the urethra forms, replacing the horseshoe opening. At approximately 100 ml of insufflation the patient experiences the sensation of bladder filling. Bladder fullness is usually noted by the patient when the vesical neck closes.

Several maneuvers are performed to challenge the vesical neck. Two of these are:

1. The vesical neck is noted to be supported when the patient "bears down" (Valsalva maneuver). A squeeze is noted, and the vesical neck does not open (Fig. 5, Normal).

2. The vesical neck opens and closes, looking like a sphincter, when the scope is maneuvered back and forth through the vesical neck with the gas flowing at 150 cc per min. The "sphincter" is quick to form as the scope is withdrawn (Fig. 6, Normal).

ANATOMIC (GENUINE) STRESS INCONTINENCE

A low entering urethral pressure is recorded. The vesical neck may close sluggishly during bladder filling. Bladder capacity is normal. Manipulation of the scope reveals loss of support of the vesical neck (Fig. 5, Anatomic).

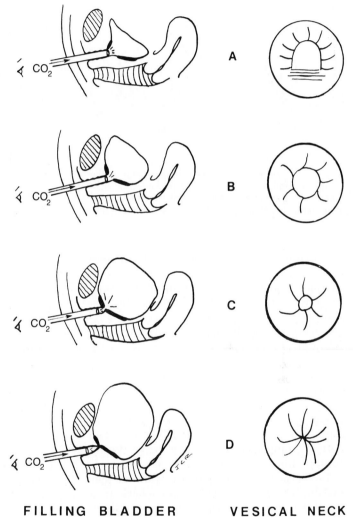

Figure 4. A, Horseshoe closure. Visualization of the vesical neck with the bladder empty reveals a horseshoe configuration with the open end of the horseshoe between 5 and 7 o'clock. *B,* As the bladder fills normally, the open end of the horseshoe disappears. It is at this time that the patient has the sensation that the bladder is filling. *C,* When the vesical neck has nearly closed, the patient experiences the sensation of having to void. *D,* When the bladder neck has closed, maximum capacity has been reached. *Note:* As the vesical neck closes, the urethroscope appears to recede down the urethra. At closure of the vesical neck, the tip of the urethroscope is located in what is now the proximal urethra.

FILLING BLADDER   **VESICAL NECK**

NORMAL

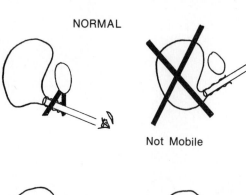

Not Mobile

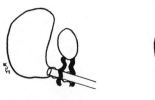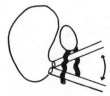

Mobile

ANATOMICAL

Figure 5. The vesical neck is normally behind the symphysis and is not mobile. The pubourethral ligaments have been stretched in the patient with genuine anatomical incontinence, and the vesical neck is mobile.

When these patients bear down, the vesical neck opens and a sharp rise in pressure is registered on the graph. The tip of the scope is withdrawn back and forth through the vesical neck, and the urethra is noted to funnel and close sluggishly (Fig. 6, Anatomic). The intravesical pressure is normal.

UNSTABLE BLADDER

The opening urethral pressure is average or high. Bladder capacity is usually small. The patient complains of urgency early during bladder filling. The vesical neck may not close.

In 50 per cent of patients with bladder instability urine may splash secondary to a small detrusor contraction (Fig. 7, Unstable). The spike may or may not be recorded on the graph. Intravesical pressure is high (greater than 15 cm of water pressure). Fine bladder trabeculations may be noted.

The patient is asked to suppress the contraction. Patients with normal bladder function can suppress a detrusor contraction, while patients with bladder instability cannot (Fig. 8). This is the most important test for determining bladder instability.

It is occasionally necessary to position the

patient standing to demonstrate bladder instability. To observe the urethra in the standing position, a teaching telescope is attached to the urethroscope.[6] A detrusor contraction is triggered, and the vesical neck can be observed to open by viewing it through the teaching attachment. Again, the patient with bladder instability cannot suppress the contraction.

Neurogenic Bladder

There are basically two types of neurogenic bladder, although various combinations or incomplete lesions occur. A *hypertonic* bladder is caused by an upper motor neuron lesion, and a *hypotonic* bladder is caused by a lower motor neuron lesion. Hypertonic bladders

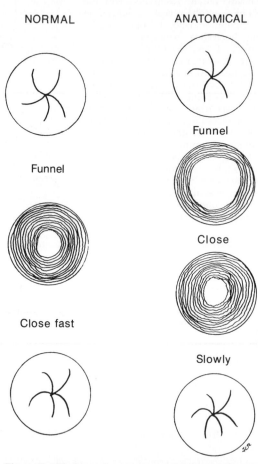

NORMAL   ANATOMICAL

Funnel

Funnel

Close

Close fast

Slowly

Figure 6. Pushing the urethroscope back and forth through the vesical neck is a detrusor-activating procedure. The normal vesical neck closes fast, looking like a sphincter. The patient with genuine anatomical incontinence has a sluggish vesical neck that is slow to close.

usually have a high entering urethral pressure and hypotonic bladders a low entering urethral pressure. Both types carry urinary residual and have bladder trabeculations. Hypotonic bladders have a large capacity and hypertonic bladders a small capacity.

Cystometry

Cystometrograms under endoscopic control give the following information:

1. Function of the vesical neck during bladder filling.

2. The patient's ability to contract and relax the sphincter on command with the bladder at rest and full.

3. Presence or absence of a detrusor reflex.

4. The patient's ability to suppress the detrusor reflex.

5. Bladder sensation during filling.

6. Pressure-to-volume relationship (least important).

Treatment of Urinary Incontinence

URETHRITIS

Generations of gynecologists have been taught that stress incontinence is due to sphincter weakness secondary to pelvic floor damage caused by the trauma of childbirth. It is not appreciated that urinary incontinence may be secondary to urethral obstruction.

The most common cause is chronic urethritis. Urinary incontinence from urethritis cannot be distinguished from sphincter incompetence by history. Uroflowmetry and urethroscopy are essential for proper diagnosis. Patients with urinary incontinence secondary to chronic urethritis have a high opening

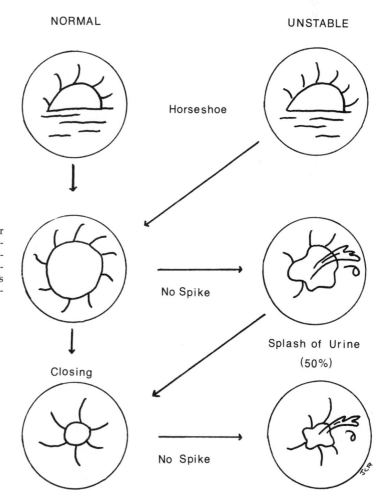

NORMAL   UNSTABLE

Horseshoe

No Spike

Splash of Urine
(50%)

Closing

No Spike

Figure 7. In patients with bladder instability observation of the vesical neck during bladder filling reveals that 50 per cent have detrusor contractions during filling. This may not register on the cystometer.

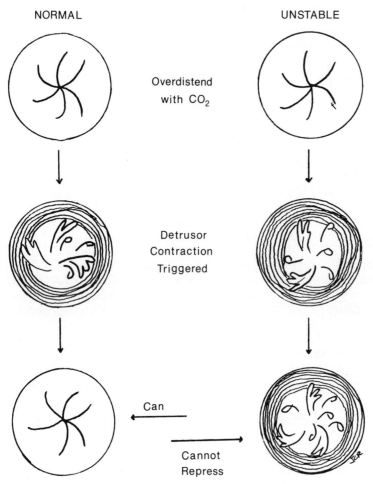

NORMAL

UNSTABLE

Overdistend
with CO_2

Detrusor
Contraction
Triggered

Can

Cannot
Repress

Figure 8. The detrusor-activating procedure (riding the urethroscope back and forth through the vesical neck with CO_2 flowing at 150 cc/min) may trigger a detrusor contraction in a normal patient. If so, she can suppress it. The patient with bladder instability cannot repress a detrusor contraction.

urethral pressure and endoscopic evidence of chronic granular urethritis.

Patients with genuine stress incontinence are usually "supervoiders," whereas patients with incontinence secondary to urethritis have a poor urinary stream as measured by uroflowmetry (Figs. 9 to 11).

Urethral obstruction is relieved by urethral dilation. This is an empiric procedure. The urethroscope is used as a dilator, and carbon dioxide distends the urethra aided by two fingers in the vagina to elevate the vesical neck against the symphysis.

The urethra is massaged with the fingers, similar to the manner in which the male prostate is massaged. Urethroscopy shows that epithelial debris, lymph and pus are milked from the periurethral glands. The urethral dilations drain infected periurethral glands, relieving obstruction. Urethral dilations are indicated if there is evidence of improvement

of urinary flow or endoscopic evidence of drainage of infected periurethral glands.

Urethral dilations should be covered by 24 hours of antibiotics. Antispasmodics are adjunctive therapy.

Unstable Bladder

Treatment for the unstable bladder is unsatisfactory. The bladder is activated by acetylcholine through the parasympathetic nervous system. Therefore, anticholinergic drugs are used, but results are disappointing. Side effects are common.

Oxybutynin chloride (Ditropan) exerts a direct antispasmodic effect on smooth muscle and inhibits the muscarinic action of acetylcholine on smooth muscle. It increases bladder capacity, diminishes the frequency of uninhibited bladder contractions and delays the

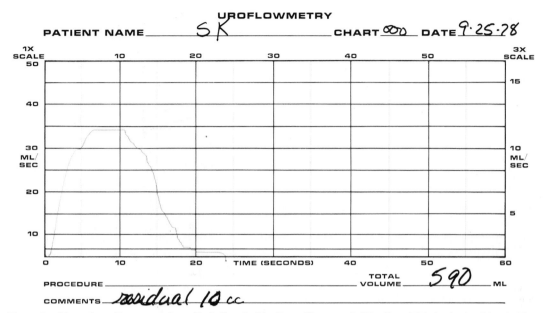

Figure 9. Normal reading on uroflow. Peak flow is 34 ml/sec. Flow rate is 25 ml/sec. This is obtained by dividing volume by time.

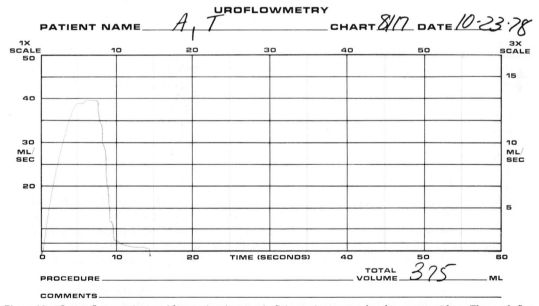

Figure 10. Super flow: patients with genuine (anatomical) incontinence tend to be super voiders. The peak flow is 39 ml/sec, and the flow rate is 27 ml/sec.

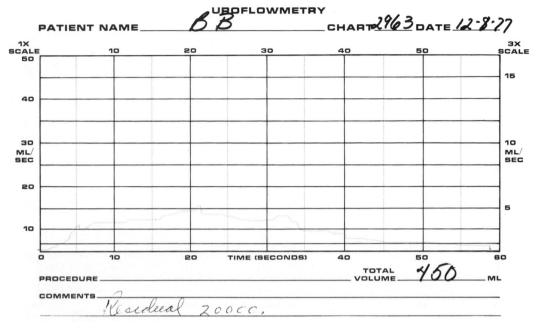

Figure 11. Peak flow is only 16 ml/sec. Flow rate is only 8 ml/sec. Residual is 200 cc. This patient's "stress incontinence" is on the basis of overflow incontinence.

initial desire to void. Unfortunately, side effects are common. They are dose related, and there is individual patient susceptibility.

Flavoxate hydrochloride (Urispas) acts on the muscle receptor to produce smooth muscle relaxation. It is comparable to propantheline (Pro-Banthine), with fewer side effects.

Imipramine (Tofranil), a tricyclic antidepressant, is excellent for some patients. It is an alpha-adrenergic stimulator, causing constriction at the vesical neck as well as having parasympathetic activity.

In my experience, patients operated on unsuccessfully two or more times develop a dysfunctional lower urinary tract. They may have the "battered bladder syndrome" with a frozen urethra. They become sexual and bladder cripples. In my opinion, no operative procedure will be successful unless it is preceded by medical therapy. This treatment includes anticholinergics, application of estrogen vaginal cream, urethral suppositories with cortisone and Kegel's isometric exercises. After six weeks of this therapy, the entering urethral pressure may increase from 0 to 20 cm of water pressure. Then and only then should surgery be attempted.

Surgery for Incontinence

Enhörning proposed that continence is achieved when the urethrovesical junction and proximal urethra are elevated into the abdominal zone of pressure.[7] Any sudden rise in abdominal pressure is equally transmitted to the bladder and proximal urethra. Incontinence occurs when intra-abdominal pressure is not transmitted equally to the proximal urethra and intravesical pressure exceeds intraurethral pressure.

The aim of surgery is to restore the vesical neck and proximal urethra to their normal intra-abdominal positions. In my opinion this is best accomplished by a urethropexy procedure.

TECHNIQUE

The patient is draped in a semilithotomy position. The surgeon operates in the space of Retzius, and the assistant works through the vagina. The assistant locates the vesical neck with the urethroscope, which helps in accurately restoring the vesical neck to its proper location. The tip of the scope is palpated at the vesical neck by the surgeon, and the second operator straddles it with two fingers (Fig. 12). The surgeon touches fingers with the second operator. The surgeon picks up the tissue over the assistant's fingers with two long Allis clamps.

A double bite with 0 polyglycolic acid suture is taken on each side of the vesical neck as the assistant monitors through the urethroscope.

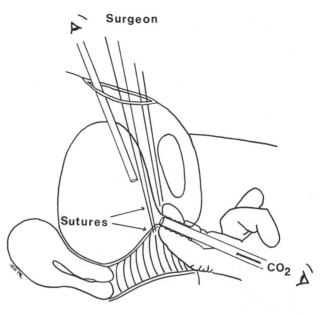

Surgeon

Sutures

CO_2

Assistant

Figure 12. The vesical neck is identified with certainty with the urethroscope. If the operator identifies the vesical neck with the balloon of a Foley catheter, he may pull the catheter into the upper part of the urethra, which gives a false identification. Also, he pulls the vesical neck beneath the symphysis, making the placing of sutures very difficult.

The vesical neck is supported behind the symphysis by placing the sutures through the periosteum or where the conjoined tendon inserts into the symphysis.

If it is possible to elevate the vagina to Cooper's ligaments, I prefer the Burch procedure. The vesical neck may be observed on the intravesical side by inserting the telescope into the bladder through an extraperitoneal opening into the bladder. The vesical neck is observed as the operator pulls on the sutures. It is important not to buckle the urethra or the trigone. Unilateral or even bilateral ureteral obstruction can occur if sutures are placed blindly.

After the telescope is removed, a suprapubic catheter is inserted through the opening for drainage.

Conclusion

The number of operative procedures for "stress incontinence" suggests that the problem is poorly understood. Poor results do not come about from operative failure but from diagnostic failure. The compartmentalization of medicine leads to the treatment of one problem (anatomic incontinence) while another is ignored (urethritis).

The diagnosis of urinary incontinence must be established by objective methods. Genuine stress (anatomic) incontinence is uncommon

as an isolated finding. A combination of problems of urethritis, bladder instability and anatomic incontinence is common. Other causes are neurogenic bladder, urethral diverticula, urinary retention with overflow, valvular vesicovaginal fistula and ectopic ureter opening below the sphincter.

Urinary incontinence is a complex problem and will not respond to simplistic answers such as the concept of the posterior urethral vesical angle. No patient should be operated upon for "stress incontinence" until that diagnosis has been established by objective methods.

REFERENCES

1. Robertson, J. R.: Gynecologic urethroscopy. Am. J. Obstet. Gynecol. 115:986, 1973.
2. Robertson, J. R.: Gas cystometrogram with urethral pressure profile. Obstet Gynecol. 44:72, 1974.
3. Robertson, J. R.: Ambulatory gynecologic urology. Clin. Obstet. Gynecol. 17:255, 1974.
4. International Continence Society: First report on standardization of terminology of lower urinary tract function. Br. J. Urol. 48:39, 1976.
5. Robertson, J. R.: CO_2 urethroscopy in gynecologic urologic problems. Clin. Obstet. Gynecol. 21:744, 1978.
6. Robertson, J. R.: Genitourinary Problems In Women. Springfield, Charles C Thomas, 1978.
7. Enhörning, G.: Simultaneous recording of intravesical and intraurethral pressure. Acta Chir. Scand. (Suppl.) 276:1, 1961.

Urinary Stress Incontinence: A Practical Approach

Stuart A. Weprin, M.D.

Frederick P. Zuspan, M.D.

Ohio State University School of Medicine

During the past 20 years a multitude of new and interesting diagnostic techniques have been introduced into the field of urodynamics. Concomitant with the interest in urodynamics, there has been a continued effort to improve the treatment of female urinary incontinence. Numerous medical and surgical approaches have been described. The purpose of this article is to present a practical yet complete approach toward diagnosis and management of the female with symptomatic urinary incontinence.

Diagnosis

The most important contribution that urodynamics has made to the field of female incontinence is its emphasis on determining the cause of the incontinence. Although most lists of causes of female incontinence are complex, the majority of patients coming to the gynecologist with incontinence will have either descent of the urethrovesical angle or uninhibited bladder contractions. Other causes of anatomic abnormalities are abnormally short urethra (less than 1.5 cm), extrinsic pelvic mass, fistulas and congenital anomalies. Neurogenic causes of incontinence include reflex neurogenic bladder, motor neurogenic bladder, sensory neurogenic bladder and autonomous neurogenic bladder.[1,2] There is also the rare patient whose incontinence is purely on a psychological basis (Table 1).

All patients with symptomatic incontinence require a complete history, physical examination, urine culture and cystometrics for accurate diagnosis (Fig. 1).

TABLE 1. CAUSES OF FEMALE URINARY INCONTINENCE

Uninhibited contractions
Descent of the urethrovesical angle
Other

HISTORY

The first step in evaluating female incontinence is obtaining a thorough history. The history is important in characterizing the extent of a patient's disease and in formulating proper treatment. The duration and extent of the problem should be documented. The classic history for pure stress incontinence is intermittent incontinence associated with the Valsalva maneuver in which urine is expelled instantaneously in spurts. Patients with resting incontinence, urgency incontinence or enuresis are suspect for uninhibited bladder contractions. Many patients have a mixed symptom complex. It is important to clarify the symptoms that are most distressing to the patient. All patients should have complete documentation of fluid intake and voiding frequency.

A thorough review of past medical history is helpful in both diagnosis and treatment. Patients who are obese, who smoke, who have chronic lung disease or failed previous operative repairs are at a high risk for surgical failures in the treatment of stress incontinence. A history of nulliparity, frequent urinary tract infections or known neurologic abnormalities is suggestive of uninhibited bladder contractions or neurogenic bladder.

PHYSICAL EXAMINATION

Physical examination should include a complete pelvic study with special emphasis on the status of the anterior vaginal wall. Removal of the anterior blade of the vaginal speculum and separation of the labia will aid in visualization. The demonstration of a cystocele or uterine prolapse will aid in deciding upon an operative approach. Descent of the urethrovesical angle with the Valsalva maneuver is suggestive of an anatomic basis for the incontinence. If urine loss is demonstrated, the

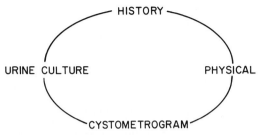

Figure 1. Evaluation of the patient with symptomatic incontinence.

Bonney test may be performed. Although a positive test suggests that an anatomic abnormality is the cause of the patient's incontinence, it does not exclude uninhibited bladder contractions.

After a thorough history and physical examination are obtained, all patients should have urinalysis and culture. Abnormal results are treated appropriately. Those patients with normal results should have cystometrics performed. Either carbon dioxide or water may be used.[3-5] No patient with incontinence should have an operative repair without a cystometrogram.

CYSTOMETRICS

The role of cystometry in the evaluation of female incontinence is to rule out causes of incontinence other than anatomic defects. The primary objective is the identification of the patient with uninhibited bladder contractions. Terms such as destrusor dyssynergia, bladder hyperreflexia, irritable bladder and unstable bladder all describe patients with uninhibited bladder contractions and normal neurologic examination. Uninhibited contractions are present in 6 to 66 per cent of females with urinary incontinence.[6-10] The importance in making a diagnosis of uninhibited contractions prior to surgery is apparent because their presence is associated with poor surgical outcome.[6-9] Preoperative recognition of the patient with uninhibited contractions may lead to medical cure and needless surgery can be avoided.

Most investigators have been unable to identify by history and physical those patients who do not need cystometry; therefore, all patients deserve this as part of a complete evaluation of urinary incontinence.[10, 11] Although some patients' history will seem to be clear, a mixed symptom complex is seen in many cases. This is especially true in those patients with more pronounced disease or recurrent disease. This problem exists because the uninhibited bladder will be stimulated to contract with the same Valsalva maneuvers that will produce incontinence in patients with weak sphincters.

At Ohio State University we perform cystometrograms with a Foley catheter connected to a plastic polyethylene tube to a carbon dioxide cystometer. Filling rates of 120 cc per min are used. Residual urine is noted and urinalysis and culture are obtained. Urethral length is recorded. All patients are first tested standing, then supine. Uninhibited bladder contractions of at least 30 mm Hg are considered clinically significant (Fig. 2). There is no problem in distinguishing true bladder activity at 30 mm Hg from increased intra-abdominal pressure secondary to patient movement or Valsalva maneuver. All patients are instructed to inhibit any urge to void; Valsalva maneuvers are not performed. The test is completed when the third segment of the cystometrogram is reached or the patient becomes uncomfortable. The uncomfortable sensation is often experienced between 300 and 400 cc volume.

Other authors have found that standard supine cystometry will reveal uninhibited bladder contractions in less than half of the patients.[10-13] In our experience, diagnosis in 67 per cent of those with uninhibited bladders is only made with the patient in the standing position. The standing cystometrogram produces significantly different results when compared with the supine cystometrogram (P less than .05) and is the study of choice. We have not seen a patient have a normal standing test in the presence of an abnormal supine test (Table 2). Provocative measures including changing the position from supine to upright, performing Valsalva maneuvers and walking in place have been used to elicit uninhibited bladder contractions. Such maneuvers require simultaneous rectal pressure measurements to determine true bladder activity. We have found that use of the erect filling cystometrogram eliminates the need to perform provocative maneuvers and simplifies the study of bladder dynamics.

The human is an erect mammal and has problems that relate to gravity. Since most patients experience their incontinence in the erect position, it seems logical to test them in that position.

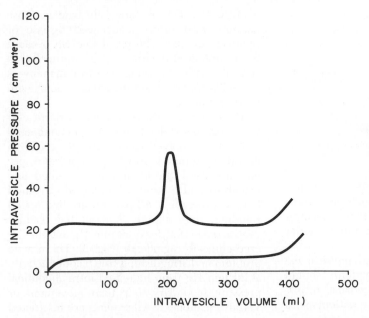

Figure 2. The top cystometrogram was obtained in the standing position from an incontinent female. Note the uninhibited bladder contraction. The bottom curve is a supine cystometrogram from the same patient. Treatment with anticholinergic medicine resulted in a cure of her incontinence. (From Weprin, S. A. and Zuspan, F. P.: The standing cystometrogram. Am. J. Obstet. Gynecol. 138:369, 1980.)

Following performance of the cystometrogram, 200 to 300 cc of normal saline are instilled into the bladder. Next, the Foley catheter is removed and the patient is instructed to cough in the supine and standing position. The demonstration of incontinence during the stress test helps confirm the diagnosis. Knowing the nature of the incontinence (urine expelled by spurt or continuous stream) is sometimes useful in difficult cases. The failure to demonstrate water loss during the stress test does not exclude stress incontinence or uninhibited contractions.

In most patients with symptomatic incontinence, the clinical demonstration of an anatomic defect along with normal cystometrics will make the diagnosis of urinary stress incontinence clear. However, in some patients the status of the urethrovesical angle is uncertain on the basis of the physical examination. This is especially true in patients with recurrent urinary stress incontinence. Numerous techniques have been devised to solve this problem. Simultaneous urethral and bladder pressure studies and various radiologic procedures including the voiding cystourethrogram, chain cystourethrography, and simultaneous cine–pressure flow cystography have been proposed. Although most of these procedures are of academic interest, they have not met with widespread clinical acceptance. During the past ten years carbon dioxide urethral pressure studies and urethroscopy have been introduced.

URETHRAL PRESSURE MEASUREMENTS

The urethral pressure profile is but one method to study urethral physiology. It is an artifactual assessment of urethral response to distention. The urethral pressure profile has been defined by the International Continence Society as the intraluminal pressure along the length of the urethra with the bladder at rest. The maximum urethral pressure is the maximum pressure of the measured length. The maximum urethral closure pressure is the maximum urethral pressure minus bladder pressure.[14] The functional profile length is the length of the urethra along which the urethral pressure exceeds the bladder pressure (Fig. 3). Water and gas measurements are statistically identical when low flow rate water infu-

TABLE 2. RESULTS OF STANDING AND SUPINE CYSTOMETROGRAMS IN 91 CASES OF INCONTINENCE

RESULTS OF CYSTOMETROGRAM	TYPE OF CYSTOMETROGRAM	
	Standing	*Supine*
Normal	76 (84%)	86 (95%)
Uninhibited contractions	15 (16%)	5 (5%)

From Weprin, S. A. and Zuspan, F. P.: The standing cystometrogram. Am. J. Obstet. Gynecol. 138:369, 1980.

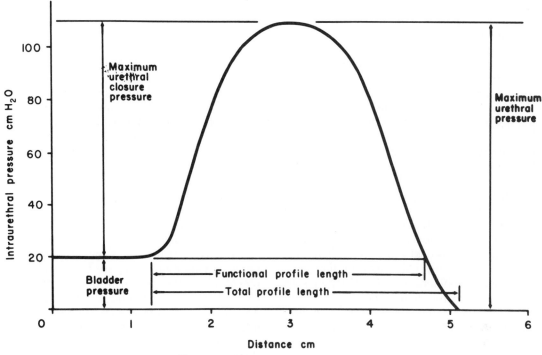

Figure 3. The urethral pressure profile.

sion (2 ml per min) is compared to carbon dioxide infusion performed with a ratio of flow rate to catheter withdrawal rate of at least 20 ml per cm.[15]

Over the past few years, numerous studies have been published in which altered urethral pressure profiles in females with stress incontinence are reported. The most consistent findings have been depressed maximum urethral closure pressures.[16-20] Although there is a difference between the profiles of normal and stress-incontinent females, the overlap between the two groups has limited the diagnostic value of the test. Numerous modifications have been proposed to overcome this problem.[18-22] Despite these investigations, the clinical value of urethral pressure profiles in the assessment of urinary stress incontinence is limited. However, in complicated cases, the test is often useful as an adjunct to the history and physical and cystometric examinations.

URETHROSCOPY

Carbon dioxide urethroscopy has been popularized by Robertson.[23-25] His technique of direct visualization of the vesical neck is illustrated in Figure 4. With the urethroscope at the vesical neck the patient is asked to bear down. In those patients with true stress incontinence, the vesical neck will funnel (open and

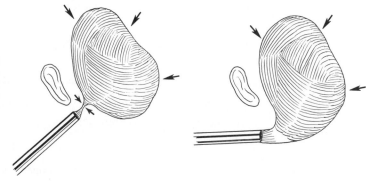

Figure 4. A, The normal patient will close her urethra during Valsalva maneuvers. B, The patient with stress incontinence will funnel her bladder neck during Valsalva maneuvers.

drop). Well-controlled studies using this technique for diagnosing stress incontinence are unavailable.

The additional benefit of evaluation of the urethra for intrinsic disease seems to add to the instrument's utility. Carbon dioxide urethroscopy affords much more satisfactory visualization of the urethral mucosa than does water urethroscopy. Although we do not believe that urethroscopy is necessary in all patients with stress incontinence, it is often helpful in those patients in whom the etiology of their symptoms is not clear on the basis of the history, physical examination and cystometrics.

Prior to an operative repair for stress incontinence, an intravenous pyelogram should be performed. Occasionally we find it helpful to perform cystoscopy. Although uroflowmetry and external sphincter electromyelograms are useful as research tools, they are of little practical value in the diagnosis and treatment of the female with stress incontinence.

Management

Once the diagnosis of urinary stress incontinence has been established, therapy may be instituted. Although the mainstay of treatment is surgical, much can be done with medical therapy. Most patients should undergo a trial of medical management prior to surgical intervention. Regardless of the form of management, attempts to correct obesity, cigarette smoking, infrequent voiding, excessively large fluid intake and urinary infection will often be helpful.

NONSURGICAL MANAGEMENT

Medical management of stress incontinence is based on urethral anatomy and physiology. The urethra is composed of smooth muscle that is a continuum of the detrusor muscle. Although the urethra is mostly smooth muscle, skeletal muscle is found at its mid portion. The proximal urethra functions as the internal urethral sphincter and the mid urethra as the external sphincter. Innervation of the urethra is via sacral roots S2 to S4. The smooth muscle innervation is parasympathetic (pelvic nerve) and the skeletal muscle is somatic (pudendal nerve). In addition, there are functional alpha receptors at the proximal urethra that are controlled by sympathetic nerves originating from T11 to L3. Stimulation of either type of urethral musculature will improve stress incontinence and is the basis of medical therapy (Fig. 5).

Perineal floor exercises are the most commonly accepted form of medical management. The goal of the exercises is to increase the tone of the skeletal muscle of the external sphincter and thereby decrease stress incontinence. As both the pelvic floor musculature and the levator ani muscle are intimately connected with the external sphincter, patients are taught the exercises by squeezing around the examiner's index finger during a pelvic or rectal examination. In addition, in-

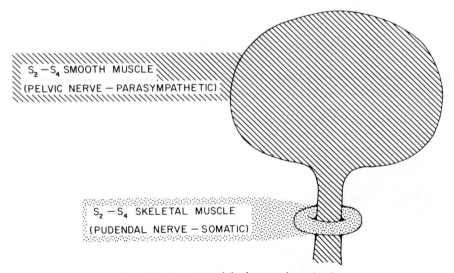

$S_2 - S_4$ SMOOTH MUSCLE
(PELVIC NERVE — PARASYMPATHETIC)

$S_2 - S_4$ SKELETAL MUSCLE
(PUDENDAL NERVE — SOMATIC)

Figure 5. Anatomy of the lower urinary tract.

TABLE 3. RESULTS OF EXERCISES INVOLVING
THE PERINEAL FLOOR

AUTHOR	EXERCISE ROUTINE	RESULTS	
Kegel (1955) 455 cases	5 times every half hour	Improved	90%
		Failed	10%
Wharton (1953) 63 cases	15 times 3 times a day	Improved	81%
		Failed	19%
Jones (1967) 117 cases	10 times every half hour	Improved	69%
		Failed	31%

terruption of the urinary stream during voiding will help in teaching the exercises. Kegel was the first to describe these exercises; his results, along with those of Wharton and Jones, are shown in Table 3.[26-28] The exercises are useful regardless of the severity of incontinence.[27, 28] One half of Kegel's patients had had previous surgery.

Electrical stimulating devices have been used in the treatment of urinary incontinence since the mid 1960s. A continuous pulsed current is applied through a vaginal pessary, an anal mold or a surgically implanted stimulator. The current works by improving the tone of the skeletal muscle of the external sphincter. Since the success rate with either internal or external stimulating devices is no better than with pelvic floor exercises, they are not commonly used.[29-31]

Medical therapy with alpha-stimulants has recently been advocated in the management of female stress incontinence. The goal of the therapy is to increase the tone of the smooth muscle of the proximal urethra and thereby decrease stress incontinence. Both ephedrine and Ornade have been used with some success. Overall the results are less successful than the use of perineal floor exercises.[32-35]

Whether the two used concomitantly offer any additional advantage remains to be shown.

Estrogens have been advocated in the medical management of stress incontinence. There are few good studies supporting this view. The mechanism of improvement is also unclear, although the medication may improve urethral pressure via an alpha-receptor–stimulating effect. Nevertheless, since estrogens are indicated in treating atrophic urethritis, they are often useful as adjunctive therapy in the postmenopausal patient with a mixed symptom complex.

If medical management is unsuccessful, an operation should be considered. In those patients who are poor operative risks, vaginal prostheses may be used.[29, 31]

SURGICAL MANAGEMENT

Surgical management of stress incontinence may be accomplished with either a vaginal or retropubic approach. Depending on patient selection, an anterior repair will be successful between 60 and 90 per cent of the time.[36-40]

Although gynecologists in England and the United States have attempted to select operative procedures by measuring urethrovesical angles, these techniques have been abandoned by most investigators and clinicians because of inaccuracies, cost of doing the procedure and patient inconvenience.[25, 41-44] Until a better method is described, selection should be based on the results of a thorough history and physical. Patients with severe incontinence or previous operative failures are at high risk for a failed anterior repair.[36, 38] Obesity, chronic smoking, chronic lung conditions and excessive degrees of activity are also factors to consider. Patients with mild degrees of stress incontinence and prolapse

Figure 6. A, In the patient with stress incontinence, the urethrovesical angle is not an abdominal organ and therefore does not close with increased abdominal pressure. *B,* After a retropubic suspension the urethrovesical angle becomes an abdominal organ and therefore closes with increased abdominal pressure.

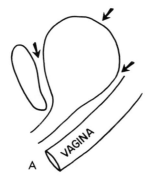
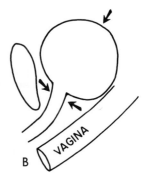

are excellent candidates for a vaginal approach.

The anterior repair most commonly used today is the basic Kelly stitch and plication along the length of the urethra.[45-47] Its probable mechanism of action is based on the creation of scar tissue along the bladder base and urethra to prevent funneling. This is an entirely different mechanism from retropubic procedures.

Many gynecologists have advocated the routine performance of a posterior colporrhaphy at the time of anterior repair. Since the urethral musculature, pelvic floor musculature and levator ani muscle are interrelated, tightening of the posterior vaginal wall should strengthen the pelvic diaphragm, decrease the mobility of the anterior wall and improve the operative results. Good studies are needed to verify this long-standing clinical impression.

Retropubic operations for stress incontinence date back to the early nineteen hundreds. The original procedures were fascial sling suspensions. In 1949, Marshall, Marchetti and Krantz introduced a retropubic procedure that was much simpler than the fascial sling procedures.[47, 48] Retropubic procedures will be effective 90 per cent of the time.[37, 49] All patients who do not qualify for an anterior repair should have a retropubic procedure.

Although there are many modifications of the original Marshall-Marchetti-Krantz procedure, they all have one thing in common: elevation of the urethrovesical angle into the abdominal cavity. Changing the urethrovesical angle from a vaginal to an abdominal organ will ensure proper pressure transmission during periods of increased abdominal pressure.[16, 49, 50] In this position, the urethra closes with stress and continence results (Fig. 6). The urethral lengthening that often occurs with retropubic suspensions is considered to be coincidental rather than responsible for the surgical results.

It is not important that the gynecologist learn all the modifications of the Marshall-Marchetti-Krantz procedure. All that is necessary is that he become familiar with a technique that establishes the desired urethrovesical elevation. We routinely place a hand in the vagina and a Foley catheter in the bladder for identification of the urethrovesical angle. Two to three sutures are placed on each side

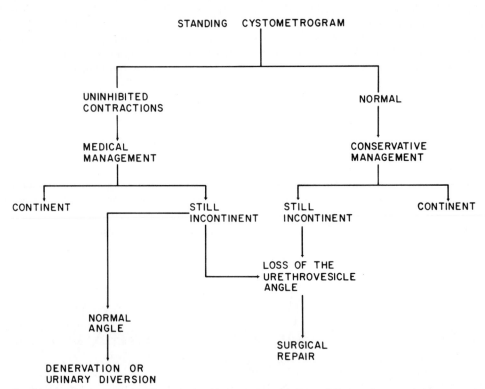

Figure 7. Management of the female patient with incontinence. (From Weprin, S. A. and Zuspan, F. P.: The standing cystometrogram. Am. J. Obstet. Gynecol. 138:369, 1980.)

of the urethra and sutured to the symphysis or to the ileopectineal ligament. The exact placement of the suture is individualized to each patient's anatomy. The critical sutures are at the urethrovesical angle; additional periurethral sutures are often unnecessary.

Most failures of the Marshall-Marchetti-Krantz procedure are a result of improper diagnosis, poor surgical technique and failure to achieve the clinical result because of a short anterior vaginal wall or because of weak fascia. Often a sling procedure can overcome these problems. Sling operations are more extensive than the Marshall-Marchetti-Krantz procedure and are not routinely used as primary procedures. A new surgical approach using a surgically implanted prosthetic urinary sphincter has been reported.[51-53] Although it will probably be more useful for male incontinence, it may be helpful in selected female patients.

In those patients with both uninhibited contractions and urinary stress incontinence, the uninhibited contractions should be treated first.[10, 25, 54] After the cystometrogram demonstrates suppression of uninhibited contractions, a reassessment of the patient's symptomatology is in order. If her incontinence is still a problem and an anatomic defect exists, a surgical repair is indicated. Occasionally, a surgical repair may be attempted in the face of unsuccessful medical management. This should only be done if an anatomic defect exists and the patient is willing to accept a higher failure rate.[8, 53] If an anatomic defect is not present, denervation procedures or urinary diversion may be necessary[55, 56] (Fig. 7).

REFERENCES

1. Wear, J. B.: The Diagnosis of Neurogenic Bladder. Presented at 6th Annual Meeting of American Urological Society, Inc., San Francisco, CA, May 1969.
2. Lapides, J. (ed.): Urological Clinics of North America, Vol. 1, No. 1, 1974.
3. Gleason, D. M. et al.: Comparison of cystometrograms and urethral profiles with gas and water media. Urology 9:155, 1977.
4. Wein, A. J. et al.: The reproducibility and interpretation of carbon dioxide cystometry. J. Urol. 120:205, 1978.
5. Lewis, S. D.: Carbon dioxide versus electronic urethrocystometry for the detection of detrusor dyssynergia. Am. J. Obstet. Gynecol. 133:371, 1979.
6. Hodgkinson, C. P. et al.: Dyssynergic detrusor dysfunction in the apparently normal female. Am. J. Obstet. Gynecol. 117:805, 1973.
7. Arnold, E. P. et al.: Urodynamics of female inconti-

nence: factors influencing the results of surgery. Am. J. Obstet. Gynecol. 117:805, 1973.
8. Beck, R. P. et al.: Results in treating 210 patients with detrusor dyssynergia overactivity incontinence of urine. Am. J. Obstet. Gynecol. 125:593, 1976.
9. Bates, C. P. et al.: The objective study of incontinence after repair operations. Surg. Gynecol. Obstet. 136:17, 1973.
10. Weprin, S. and Zuspan, F.: The standing cystometrogram. Am. J. Obstet. Gynecol. 138:369, 1980.
11. Turner-Warwick, R. T.: Some clinical aspects of detrusor dysfunction. J. Urol. 113:539, 1975.
12. Mayo, M. E.: Detrusor hyperreflexia: the effect of posture and pelvic floor activity. J. Urol. 119:635, 1978.
13. Arnold, E. P.: Cystometry — postural effects in incontinent women. Urol. Int. 29:185, 1974.
14. International Continence Society: First Report on the Standardization of Terminology of Lower Urinary Tract Function. Br. J. Urol. 48:39, 1976.
15. Tegue, C. F. and Merrill, D. C.: Laboratory comparison of urethral profilometry techniques. Urology 13:221, 1979.
16. Enhörning, G.: Simultaneous recording of intravesicular and intraurethral pressure. Acta Chir. Scand. 276:1 (Suppl.), 1961.
17. Hodgkinson, C. P.: Direct urethrocystometry. Am. J. Obstet. Gynecol. 79:648, 1960.
18. Awad, S. A. et al.: Urethral pressure profile in female stress incontinence. J. Urol. 120:475, 1978.
19. Gleason, D. M. et al.: The urethral continence zone and its relation to stress incontinence. J. Urol. 112:81, 1974.
20. Low, J. A. and Ming-Shian, K.: Intravesical and intraurethral pressure as a measure of urethral sphincter function. J. Obstet. Gynecol. 40:627, 1972.
21. Anderson, J. T. and Bradley, W. E.: Urethral pressure profilometry: assessment of urethral function by combined intraurethral pressure and electromyographic recording. J. Urol. 118:423, 1977.
22. Bright, T. C.: Urethral pressure profile: current concepts. J. Urol. 118:418, 1977.
23. Robertson, J. R.: Ambulatory gynecologic urology. Clin. Obstet. Gynecol. 17:255, 1974.
24. Robertson, J. R.: Urethroscopy — The neglected gynecologic procedure. Clin. Obstet. Gynecol. 19:315, 1976.
25. Robertson, J. R.: Genitourinary Problems in Women. Springfield, Charles C Thomas, 1978.
26. Kegel, A. H.: Stress incontinence of urine in women: physiologic treatment. J. Int. Coll. Sur. 25:487, 1956.
27. Jones, E. G.: Nonoperative treatment of stress incontinence. Clin. Obstet. Gynecol. 6:220, 1963.
28. Wharton, L. R.: The nonoperative treatment of stress incontinence in women. Am. J. Obstet. Gynecol. 66:1121, 1953.
29. Caldwell, K. P. S. (ed.): Urinary Incontinence. London, Sector Publishing, Ltd., 1975, Chapters 5 and 6.
30. Doyle, P. T.: Treatment of urinary incontinence by external stimulating devices. Urol. Int. 29:450, 1974.
31. Stanten, S. L.: Female Urinary Incontinence. London, Lloyd-Luke Ltd., 1977, pp. 70–84.
32. Stewart, B. H.: Stress incontinence: conservative therapy with sympathomimetic drugs. J. Urol. 115:558, 1976.

33. Awad, S. A. et al.: Alpha-adrenergic agents in urinary disorders of the proximal urethra, Part l. Sphincteric incontinence. Br. J. Urol. 50:332, 1978.

34. Raushbaum, M. and Mandelbaum, C. C.: Nonoperative treatment of urinary incontinence in women. Am. J. Obstet. Gynecol. 56:777, 1948.

35. Diokno, A. C. and Taub, M.: Ephedrine in treatment of urinary incontinence. Urology 5:624, 1975.

36. Low, J. A.: Management of anatomic urinary incontinence by vaginal repair. Am. J. Obstet. Gynecol. 97:308, 1967.

37. Green, T. H.: Urinary stress incontinence: differential diagnosis, pathophysiology and management. Am. J. Obstet. Gynecol. 122:368, 1975.

38. Beck, R. P. et al.: Surgical results in the treatment of pressure equalization stress incontinence. Am. J. Obstet. Gynecol. 100:483, 1968.

39. Cullen, P. K. and Welch, J. S.: Ten year results of the Kelly and Kennedy types of procedures in urinary stress incontinence. Surg. Gynecol. Obstet. 85, July 1961.

40. Jeffcoate, T. N. A.: The principles governing the treatment of stress incontinence of urine in the female. Br. J. Urol. 37:633, 1965.

41. Corlett, R. C.: Gynecologic urology. Curr. Probl. Obstet. Gynecol. 1:35, 1978.

42. Greenwald, S. W. et al.: Cystourethrography as a diagnostic aid in stress incontinence. Obstet. Gynecol. 29:324, 1967.

43. Kitzmiller, J. L. et al.: Chain cystourethrogram and stress incontinence. Obstet. Gynecol. 39:333, 1972.

44. Drutz, H. P. et al.: Do static cystourethrograms have a role in the investigation of female incontinence? Am. J. Obstet. Gynecol. 130:516, 1978.

45. Kelly, H. A.: Incontinence of urine in women. Urol. Cut. Rev. 17:291, 1913.

46. Kelly, H. A. and Drumm, W. M.: Urinary incontinence in women without manifest injury to the bladder. Surg. Gynecol. Obstet. 18:444, 1914.

47. Mattingly, R. F.: TeLinde's Operative Gynecology, 5th ed. Philadelphia, J. B. Lippincott Co., pp. 535–548, 1977.

48. Marshall, U. F. et al.: The correction of stress incontinence by simple vesicourethral suspension. Surg. Gynecol. Obstet. 88:509, 1949.

49. Hodgkinson, C. P.: Stress urinary incontinence — 1970. Am. J. Obstet. Gynecol. 1:1141, 1973.

50. Beck, R. P.: Urinary stress incontinence. Ob/Gyn Dig. 15:19, 1976.

51. Scott, F. B. et al.: Treatment of urinary incontinence by implantable prosthetic sphincter. Urology 1:252, 1973.

52. Scott, F. B. et al.: Treatment of urinary incontinence by an implantable prosthetic urinary sphincter. J. Urol. 112:75, 1974.

53. Diokno, A. C. and Taub, M. E.: Experience with the artificial urinary sphincter at Michigan. J. Urol. 116:496, 1976.

54. Ostergard, D. R.: The effect of drugs on the lower urinary tract. Obstet. Gynecol. Surv. 34:424, 1979.

55. Ingelman-Sundberg, A.: Partial denervation of the bladder. Acta Obstet. Gynecol. Scand. 38:487, 1959.

56. Diokno, A. C., Vinton, R. K. and McGillicuddy, J.: Treatment of the severe uninhibited neurogenic bladder by selective sacral rhizotomy. J. Urol. 118:299, 1977.

Editorial Comment

Dr. Jack Robertson, an author in this chapter, should be given credit for almost singlehandedly returning cystoscopy and urethroscopy to the gynecologist. He rightly points out that Kelly, a gynecologist, developed a cystoscope and used this with a light source and head mirror. The cystoscope then disappeared from the gynecologist's armamentarium except at Johns Hopkins University. During the past decade, Robertson introduced, with enthusiasm, the cystoscope for the female and pioneered the use of carbon dioxide urethroscopy and cystoscopy. His persistence as a scientific exhibitor at the American College of Obstetricians and Gynecologists meeting year after year finally paid off and the cystoscope has become an accepted tool of the gynecologist. I would like to think that the fiberoptic light source certainly helped bring this to the forefront, as well as Robertson's own personal enthusiasm and magnetism.

There is much common content in the articles in this chapter. The authors, Robertson and Weprin and Zuspan, agree that the patient's history is important and that there are many causes of incontinence. The physical examination in conjunction with the Valsalva maneuver and a complete urinalysis are essential. Weprin and Zuspan believe that no patient with incontinence of urine should have operative repair without a cystometrogram. The basis of the cystometrogram is to rule out causes other than anatomic defects that can account for incontinence, such as uninhibited bladder contractions. Both sets of authors agree that the physician cannot diagnose the precise cause of stress incontinence only by a history and physical examination. These provide a general idea of what problems exist, with the physical examination used to confirm or deny anatomic defects. Weprin and Zuspan state that the standing cystometrogram is significantly better than the supine, but I am not sure that this view is shared by others. The urethral pressure profile, which was first thought to be an exciting diagnostic tool, has been found to have limited value, since there is a great overlapping of results. Robertson speaks of the funneling at the bladder neck; however, Weprin and Zuspan point out that there have been no well-controlled studies utilizing carbon dioxide to identify such problems.

Robertson discusses urethral dilatations as an indication if infected periurethral glands are seen, and this would certainly fall under the category of "urethral syndrome," which is a large wastebasket diagnosis used for many conditions. Weprin and Zuspan question whether urethral dilatations are really of any long-term significant benefit. Robertson is a proponent of the retropubic approach for surgical repair, whereas Weprin and Zuspan think that this should be individualized and that the vaginal approach for stress urinary incontinence can be most appropriate if done correctly. Robertson has a very unique method in executing the retropubic approach in that there are two operators, one above and one below. The one below locates the vesical neck with the urethroscope and then inserts two fingers that straddle the scope. The abdominal operator palpates the second assistant's fingers and with an Allis clamp elevates the tissue; a stitch is then applied. This is monitored with the scope and is most commendable. Robertson also prefers to utilize elevation of the vagina, using the Burch procedure that Weprin and Zuspan do not use. We have seen patients who had several ureters ligated because of use of the Burch approach. The operators have gone out too far laterally and a suture is placed around the ureter. We know of at least three cases in which this has happened.

If the vaginal approach is used, it is important not to go out too far laterally, but basically to do almost the identical procedure that is done retropubically in that the urethra is attached securely beneath the periosteum of the pubic ramus.

The proper choice of the patient is essential if results are to be good. Chronic conditions should be ruled out before an attempt is made — especially obesity, smoking and chronic pulmonary disease cough.

22
Diagnosis and Management of Endometrial Disease

Alternative Points of View

by F. J. Hofmeister and
C. Robert Stanhope
by S. B. Gusberg and G. Deppe
by John H. Isaacs
by H. Jack Schmidt and John R. Davis

Editorial Comment

Diagnosis and Management of Endometrial Disease

F. J. Hofmeister, M.D.
Wauwatosa, Wisconsin

C. Robert Stanhope, M.D.
Rochester, Minnesota

Vaginal bleeding, except when associated with menstrual function, pregnancy or a known traumatic incident causing vulvovaginal injury, must be carefully investigated to rule out or to prove the presence of gynecologic malignancy. During the past decade many statements have appeared concerning the increased incidence of endometrial malignancy. The problem has been compounded because of the attempt to relate this increase to the use of exogenous estrogen.[1-10]

What logically is the necessary approach? One of us (FJH) has long had interest in the investigation of the endometrial cavity in an attempt to detect, diagnose and promptly initiate therapy for endometrial cancer in its earliest stages. The results of this investigation will be presented.

The purpose of this article is to stimulate thought and call attention to the following analogy: Patients have benefited from early investigation of the cervix by the Papanicolaou smear when malignancy was detected in its early stages. So then, by more aggressive investigation of the endometrial cavity, can women benefit if physicians make concerned efforts to gain baseline knowledge about the status of the endometrium before estrogen is given?

We recognize that ultimately cytologic evaluations may become more practical, less expensive and even more accurate. At this time, however, the best results have been achieved by the evaluation of histologic specimens. This has also been noted by others such as Schmidt and Davis elsewhere in this chapter, who indicate that none of the cytologic techniques compare in accuracy with endometrial biopsy in the diagnosis of early adenocarcinoma.[11, 12]

The recommendation of the American College of Obstetricians and Gynecologists relating to this controversial subject has been that cautious observation and the lowest possible dose of estrogen replacement therapy should be used. It was further stated that while a certain hazard with the use of estrogen does exist, this hazard is related to indiscriminate use without adequate monitoring and to those instances in which estrogen is used as a cure-all without specific indications.

A Method of Clinical Investigation and Patient Monitoring

One of us (FJH) has attempted to develop a screening method for the endometrium comparable to the Papanicolaou smear in success and value for detecting cervical carcinoma. Endometrial biopsy has been highly effective in determining the cause of uterine bleeding. Early use of endometrial biopsy was made by Jordan at Memorial Hospital in New York in 1946.[12] Wall published his first appeal to consider this approach in 1954.[13] Several methods of uterine washing and aspiration for cancer detection have been developed and some are presently still being investigated. These include Vakutage, Mi-Mark, Vabra Aspirator and Isaacs' Endometrial Sampler. Use of the Gravlee Jet Wash, once quite popular, has been discontinued at the present time. The thrust of these methods continues to be toward detection of endometrial carcinoma by cytology effectively and economically.

We have found in doing simultaneous studies using wash and aspiration performed on over 300 patients that when tissue is obtainable (1) the results are more accurate, (2) special preparation of the specimen is necessary for endometrial cytologic evaluation and (3) these procedures are not presently practical for general use by clinicians because not all laboratories, especially clinical laboratories, have personnel trained in the preparation and interpretation of endometrial cytologic specimens.[11]

Physicians rightly continue to fear patient loss and even inaccurate diagnosis due to the patient's pain and fear, and thus inadequate biopsies are obtained. In light of these factors, it is recommended that the following equipment be placed in the examining rooms so as to permit more effective use of endometrial biopsy: Novak and Randall curettes of sizes varying from $7/64$ to $3/16$ of an inch, a 20 cc syringe, a bottle containing 10 per cent formalin for the specimen and 5 cc of 4 per cent lidocaine.* To minimize the fear of pain and increase the efficiency of the endometrial evaluation, it is necessary to always carefully explain the procedure and the fact that there could be some discomfort. During the past three years, we have initiated the use of topical 4 per cent lidocaine into the uterine cavity. We determined that when lidocaine is cautiously instilled and permitted to remain for several minutes before the endometrial evaluation is done, discomfort is reduced and the procedure is made more tolerable. This has been studied in over 200 patients with no adverse effects noted. The author emphasizes that the use of 4 per cent lidocaine has greatly decreased the patients' discomfort.

Review of Experiences With Endometrial Biopsies

The women in this study were seen between March 1, 1949 and July 1, 1978. A total of 22,598 endometrial biopsies were performed and 252 endometrial carcinomas were detected. During this time, the detection of endometrial carcinoma rose from 0.81 per cent, as originally reported in a series from March 1, 1949 to January 1, 1958, to 0.9 per cent in the series ending July 26, 1973 and to 1.11 per cent in the total series being discussed here. Of the 252 patients in whom endometrial carcinomas were detected, 216 (85 per cent) presented with bleeding and 38 (15 per cent) were asymptomatic. Papanicolaou smears were not done or were negative in 186 (73.2 per cent) of the patients, and were atypical, suspicious or positive in 66 (26.8 per cent) (Table 1).[11] The first 4560 endometrial biopsies were performed whenever a Papanicolaou smear was taken or when indicated by bleeding. Thereafter, they were selectively performed on high-risk patients. Table 2 lists the criteria used in selection.

Additional studies were made of certain patients on whom endometrial biopsies were performed, and additional patients treated

---

*More recently Hofmeister has devised endometrial curettes of similar dimensions.

TABLE 1. RESULTS OF 22,598 ENDOMETRIAL BIOPSIES PERFORMED BETWEEN
MARCH 1, 1949 AND JULY 1, 1978

	NO. PATIENTS	PERCENTAGE
Endometrial carcinomas detected by biopsy	254	1.12
Patients with symptoms (bleeding)	216	85.00
Patients without symptoms	38	15.00
Pap smear negative or not done	186	73.00
Pap smear atypical, suspicious, positive	66	27.00

during the period since 1973 were questioned concerning their use of estrogen.

In an attempt to determine the relationship of exogenous estrogen use to hyperplasia, 146 consecutive endometrial biopsies were reviewed. Hyperplasia was diagnosed 17 times (11.6 per cent). Only 3 of these 17 patients with hyperplasia had been on estrogen (17.6 per cent). Two additional patients had taken birth control pills (11.7 per cent). Thus, of the 17 with hyperplasia, exogenous estrogen was a contributing factor in only five instances (29.4 per cent). One of the 17 instances of hyperplasia was atypical and hysterectomy revealed a well-differentiated adenocarcinoma in situ. In another case, atypical hyperplasia unrelated to estrogen was diagnosed adenomyosis at hysterectomy. Thus, when atypical indications are present, further investigation is essential and hysterectomy may be necessary.

In this study, exogenous estrogen was involved in a significantly small number of instances when endometrial hyperplasia and endometrial carcinoma were diagnosed. Table 3 indicates the incidence of exogenous estrogen use by 254 patients with endometrial carcinomas detected by endometrial biopsy. In 165

TABLE 2. CRITERIA FOR SELECTION OF PATIENTS
FOR ENDOMETRIAL BIOPSY

1. Over 40 years of age
2. Obesity
3. Diabetes
4. Hypertension
5. Infertility
6. Polycystic ovary syndrome
7. Endometrial hyperplasia
8. Erratic menstrual bleeding
9. Bleeding between periods
10. Bleeding on sexual contact
11. Postmenopausal bleeding with or without estrogen
12. Postmenopausal patient to be started on estrogens
13. Change of geographic environment

patients (64.9 per cent), no estrogen had been administered prior to diagnosis. Seventy (27.1 per cent) had used estrogen before diagnosis, and in 19 (8 per cent), estrogen use was unknown.

Table 4 indicates the results in a study of 100 of the most recently detected and diagnosed endometrial carcinomas. The following observations were made: In 50 of the patients who had been on estrogen, 32 (64 per cent) of the malignancies were noninvasive focal malignancies, and only the remaining 18 (36 per cent) were invasive. The other 50 patients had not been on estrogen and 22 (44 per cent) of these malignancies were noninvasive, while 28 (56 per cent) were invasive.

Similar experiences have been reported in other studies as indicated by Table 5.

Table 6 shows findings in an attempt to evaluate the relationship between the prevalence of cervical and endometrial carcinoma in 33,818 patients seen during a 27-month period. During this time, the prevalence of cervical and endometrial carcinoma almost parallel each other in the patient population. It is apparent that a more concerted effort will yield results of detecting those malignancies that could be missed without persistent effort.

We have been impressed with the necessity of a continuous process of evaluation of estrogen administration and diligent monitoring of patients. Three case histories are cited to illustrate this point.

CASE HISTORIES

Case 1. The patient, 54 years of age, with a history of no period in 8 years, requested estrogen because "hot flashes" awakened her every night. Before estrogen administration, Papanicolaou smear and endometrial biopsy were performed and proved positive for adenocarcinoma. The surgical specimen removed after irradiation confirmed these findings.

TABLE 3. EXOGENOUS ESTROGEN USE BY 254 PATIENTS WITH ENDOMETRIAL CARCINOMAS
DETECTED BY ENDOMETRIAL BIOPSY

HISTORY	NO. PATIENTS	PERCENTAGE
Estrogen administered before diagnosis	70	27.1
No estrogen administered before diagnosis	165	64.9
Estrogen use unknown	19	8.0
		100.0

Case 2. A 64-year-old woman, seen for bladder symptoms, had a negative Papanicolaou smear and negative pelvic findings. She had had no bleeding for 14 years and had not at any time taken estrogen. One week after the initial examination, the patient had bleeding. Endometrial biopsy performed the following day revealed adenocarcinoma. The surgical specimen confirmed the findings.

Case 3. The patient, 69 years of age, was first seen in 1971 for spotting. The Papanicolaou smear was negative for tumor cells but showed atrophic cells; the endometrial biopsy was negative. Because of the atrophic cells, Dienestrol Cream, one half applicator twice weekly, was prescribed. When seen in 1972, she reported no bleeding. The Papanicolaou smear was negative and the maturation index had become normal. In 1973, the tests were negative and there was no bleeding. In 1974, the same reports were obtained. She continued to use the Dienestrol Cream sporadically. In September, 1975, there was a pink discharge. She was seen in June, 1976, for spotting. The Papanicolaou smear was negative with atrophic cells present. No endometrial cells were obtained on endometrial aspiration. In November, 1976, the patient had an episode of bleeding. Dilatation and curettage revealed adenocarcinoma of the endometrium, moderately differentiated. A hysterectomy in January, 1977, revealed adenocarcinoma with minimal invasion. The radiologist advised no further therapy. The patient recovered but is being followed at three-month intervals. It should be noted that this patient did not take oral or injectable exogenous estrogen; the amount of the cream was minimal but sufficient to change the vaginal characteristics by topical application.

If estrogen had been given, even for several weeks, to any of these patients, it would doubtless have been implicated. It must be emphasized that estrogen should not be used when conditions exist that might be aggra-

vated by its use. The physician should be responsible for determining the presence of pathology by adequate screening detection methods.

Guidelines for Selecting and Monitoring Patients Taking Estrogen

The following guidelines are suggested as a practical procedure for evaluating the patient's need for estrogen and for monitoring patients using estrogen (Fig. 1).

THE HISTORY. Periodic examination, properly utilized, can be an accurate method of determining the need for estrogen and of monitoring dosage, duration of usage and estrogen effect. The patient is encouraged to have a total physical evaluation at her initial visit and annually or if symptoms occur. During the initial part of the examination, general health information is gathered and special attention is directed to age, weight and existence of hypertension, diabetes, malignancies or other conditions that necessitate re-evaluation more frequently than on an annual basis. Medications such as estrogen, used orally or vaginally, are noted. The menstrual history and all previous operations are listed. Examination of the reproductive and accessory organs should be tailored to conform to the information gained from the history.

THE PHYSICAL EXAMINATION. The following protocol for physical examination is useful in routine periodic examinations or in a patient, regardless of age, in whom abnormal vaginal bleeding has occurred. (Bleeding is

TABLE 4. REVIEW OF 100 PATIENTS WITH ENDOMETRIAL CARCINOMAS

HISTORY	NO. PATIENTS	PERCENTAGE
On estrogen (50 patients)		
Non-invasive carcinomas	32	64
Invasive carcinomas	18	36
Not on estrogen (50 patients)		
Non-invasive carcinomas	22	44
Invasive carcinomas	28	56

TABLE 5.　SURVEY OF EXPERIENCE WITH ESTROGEN AND ENDOMETRIAL CARCINOMA

GEOGRAPHICAL LOCATION OR GROUP	CARCINOMAS FOUND	PATIENT AGES	ESTROGEN USED	ESTROGEN USE NOT KNOWN	ESTROGEN NOT USED
Eau Claire (1971–1976)	16	34–71	3 (18.7%)	3 (18.7%)	10 (62.4%)
Medical College of Wisconsin Dept. of Radiotherapy	76		21 (27.6%)		55 (72.3%)
St. Joseph Hospital Denver, Colorado	73		46 (64.39%)*	1 (0.1%)	26 (35.6%)
Casper Clinic, Wyoming (1970–1975)	8	46–71	6 (75.0%)		2 (25.0%)
Skemp-Grandview Clinic La Crosse, Wisconsin (1971–1975)	12		4 (33.0%)†		8 (66.0%)
TOTAL	185		80 (43.2%) −7* 73 (39.4%)	4 (2.2%)	101 (54.5%)

*Seven of the patients (11.39%) were short-term users: 3 used estrogen for 1 week, 1 for 2 weeks, 2 for 1 month and 1 for 2 months. It is probable that a preadministration evaluation would have revealed these before the initial dose of estrogen was prescribed.
†Either estrogen or birth control pills (BCP) in excess of one year.

TABLE 6. Prevalence of Cervical and Endometrial Carcinoma Diagnosed in 33,818 Office Visits During the 27 Months Between July 1, 1973 and October 1, 1975

Procedure	No. Procedures	Percentage
Pap smear	26,445	
Cervical carcinoma (detected by Pap-colposcope-biopsy)	26	0,09
Incidence of cervical carcinoma in 33,818 procedures		0.08
Endometrial biopsy	823	
Endometrial carcinoma (detected by endometrial biopsy)	38	4.61
Incidence of endometrial carcinoma in 33,818 office visits		0.11

considered abnormal when the interval between periods is shorter or longer or when the flow is heavier than normal; scant episodes must also be considered abnormal.) The vagina is examined by speculum visualization. Clinically, the appearance of the vagina may offer a clue as to the estrogen level. For postmenopausal women and those on estrogen, a maturation index is advisable.

If a subtotal hysterectomy has been done and the cervix is present, a Papanicolaou smear of the cervix and vaginal vault is taken. The cervix is probed and a careful endocervical evaluation is done with the Novak or Randall curette or a cytology specimen is obtained by an aspiration technique.

The presence of a uterine corpus calls for careful evaluation of the endometrial cavity by complete circumferential endometrial biopsy as well as an examination of the endocervix. The endometrial biopsy is most valuable. The Papanicolaou smear has very limited value in detecting endometrial carcinoma, having proved helpful in only 26.5 per cent of patients in the study.

Rectovaginal abdominal examination completes the pelvic evaluation.

A careful breast evaluation is performed, during which the technique of breast self-examination is described and its value stressed.

Following the physical examination, the patient is given all information and, when possible, reassured about her physical status. Any questions should be answered. When indicated, further testing is planned to investigate abnormalities. The treatment course is determined. Estrogen therapy can be considered and discussed for the patient who no longer has periods or has erratic periods or vasomotor symptoms when not under stress (i.e., is awak-

ened by them during the night). If the evaluation and tests are negative, estrogen can be initiated beginning in small, preferably interrupted doses and increased when indicated by symptoms. Estrogen, 0.625 mg daily for several weeks, is the usual approach; thereafter, the estrogen is taken for five days of the week and omitted for two days. The dose may be increased to 1.25 mg or decreased to 0.3 mg. We prefer this approach to the 20 days on, 7 days off routine because with it hot flashes are better controlled and bleeding due to hyperplasia is less frequent.

Comment

Any bleeding in postmenopausal women should be thoroughly investigated and not be assumed to be due to estrogen; any abnormal bleeding in any age group should be investigated by endometrial biopsy. There is considerable evidence that exogenous estrogen, if administered for certain indications in appropriate dosage in a monitored patient, can be of value to postmenopausal women. It has been identified that unopposed estrogens in selected individuals can result in alterations of the endometrium. The youngest patient we have seen with endometrial carcinoma, who had not taken estrogen and had her full gynecologic organ system, was 33 years of age. She developed abnormal bleeding that proved to be endometrial cancer. Although the incidence of endometrial carcinoma in women younger than 40 is reported to be an incidence of 2.2 per cent of endometrial carcinoma and few deaths have been reported when low-grade lesions are detected, it is mandatory that every woman be completely investigated when abnormal bleeding occurs.

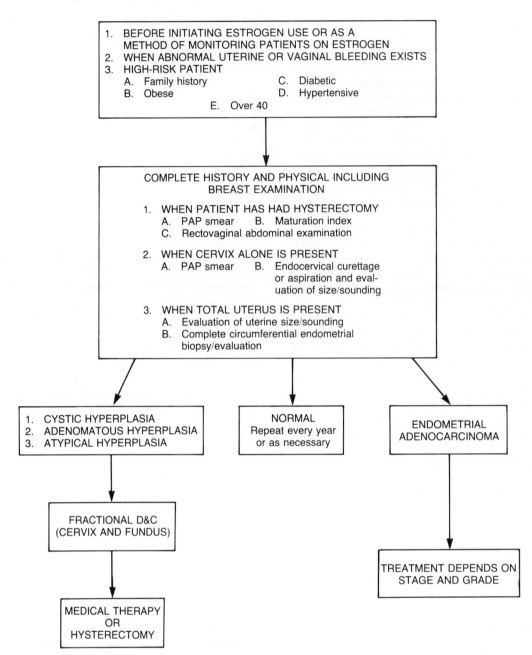

Figure 1. Guidelines for evaluating women before or during estrogen therapy.

Any patient taking estrogen, even when she is symptom free, must be carefully monitored annually or, when there are symptoms, more frequently. When uterine enlargement or irregularity exists and when hyperplasia of the endometrium is diagnosed, particular caution must be exercised, possibly including use of laparoscopy. If the endometrial biopsy is negative but symptoms continue, a more definitive approach such as dilatation and curettage in a hospital or hysterectomy may be advisable. Even when the endometrial biopsy is positive, it may be advisable to do a hospital dilatation and curettage to diagnose, stage and grade the lesion and thus more accurately initiate therapy. The advantage of early detection by endometrial biopsy in cases of malignancy cannot be overstressed.

The prevalence of cervical cancer detected in office practice by the authors has decreased since 1943 because of use of early detection methods—Papanicolaou smear, biopsy and colposcopy. The prevalence of endometrial carcinoma, however, has increased during this same period. An explanation for this phenomenon was offered by Hertig, who suggested that the increase in endometrial carcinoma is apparently due to more intelligent and aggressive investigation and does not constitute a real increase.[14] This has also been stated by Casey, who says, "Perhaps the increasing incidence of reported endometrial cancer is due to greater vigilance on the part of patients and their physicians."[15]

We believe that estrogen, as indicated by our experience, has stimulated early symptomatic bleeding and thus has instigated earlier investigation. The result has been detection of the superficial lesion in a great number of instances in which exogenous estrogen had been given. Early detection must include increased patient awareness of the importance of recognizing abnormal signs and symptoms such as increased discharge, spotting, bleeding or pressure and of having regular, complete examinations, including thorough breast examination.

It is the presence of endometrial abnormalities, with emphasis on the precursors of malignancy, to which all physicians must be especially alert. Precursors to invasive endometrial adenocarcinoma have been recognized for many years and include cystic hyperplasia, adenomatous hyperplasia, atypical hyperplasia and carcinoma in situ of the endometrium. Invasive endometrial cancer includes grade 1, grade 2 and grade 3 adenocarcinoma, adenoacanthoma, adenosquamous carcinoma, endometrial stromal sarcoma and mixed mesodermal sarcoma. The histologic appearance of each of these is easily recognizable following either endometrial biopsy or curettage.

Endometrial Adenocarcinoma Precursors

Cystic hyperplasia is associated with a voluminous endometrial specimen and must be differentiated, microscopically, from cystic atrophy of the endometrium, which is commonly associated with a scant endometrial specimen. In both conditions, large dilated glands, often filled with debris and histiocytes, coexist with small rounded glands. In cystic hyperplasia, the glandular epithelial cells are plump, appear proliferative and are often stratified in comparison to the flattened or cuboidal layer of epithelial cells seen in cystic atrophy. The stroma in cystic hyperplasia is increased so that the many dilated glands do not appear closely packed. In cystic hyperplasia, the nuclei of the stromal cells are larger and mitoses may be seen (Fig. 2A).

Adenomatous hyperplasia is characterized by distorted hyperplasic glands having increased angularity and abnormal shapes. Typically, small buds project from the larger glands into the supporting stroma. The projections may separate from the parent glands into the supporting stroma so that many small glands appear to be arranged close to the large glands (Fig. 2B).

Atypical hyperplasia represents a progression from adenomatous hyperplasia. Large glands are packed closely with little intervening stroma. The glandular cells are larger and have large nuclei; however, the nucleoli are indistinct or absent. Cytoplasmic eosinophilia of the glandular cells is frequently seen. Not uncommonly, adenomatous hyperplasia and atypical hyperplasia coexist (Fig. 2C).

Carcinoma in situ of the endometrium is characterized by large nuclei, stratified glandular cells and intraglandular bridging. Hyperchromatic nuclei with clumping of the chromatin and cytoplasmic eosinophilia are also seen (Fig. 2D).

Management of Endometrial Adenocarcinoma Precursors

Endometrial adenocarcinoma precursors are usually detected during evaluation of abnormal uterine bleeding in both premenopausal and postmenopausal patients. Reversals of these conditions with progestin therapy have been observed and this medication may be recommended for selected premenopausal patients who are desirous of childbearing and for certain postmenopausal patients who are unable to undergo surgery. It is necessary to evaluate and treat each patient individually; however, several guidelines can be set forth.

Following dilatation and curettage, when only cystic or adenomatous hyperplasia is found, patients may be followed with endometrial sampling every four to eight months. If abnormal bleeding recurs or adenomatous hyperplasia persists, hysterectomy should be considered.

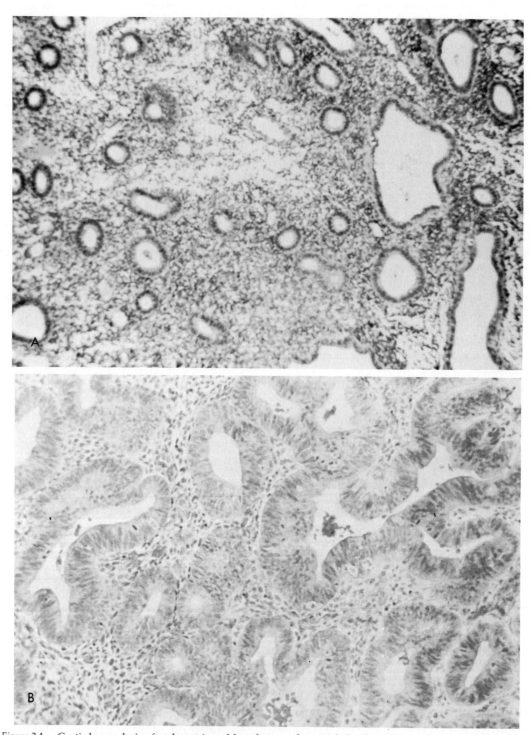

Figure 2A. Cystic hyperplasia of endometrium. Many large endometrial glands with low columnar epithelial cells mixed with small glands are seen. The amount of stroma appears increased.

Figure 2B. Adenomatous hyperplasia of endometrium. Endometrial glands have increased angularity and abnormal shape. Clusters of small glands have separated from the parent glands. Stroma separates the glands.

Illustration continued on opposite page

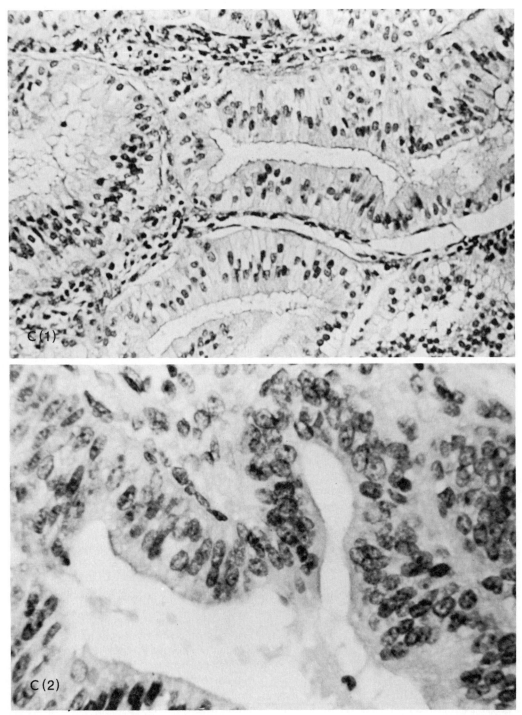

Figure 2C. Atypical hyperplasia of endometrium. Large glands are packed close together with little intervening stroma. (One, low power.) Atypical hyperplasia of endometrium. Glandular cells are stratified and have large nuclei with prominent hyperchromatin material. (Two, high power.)

Illustration continued on following page

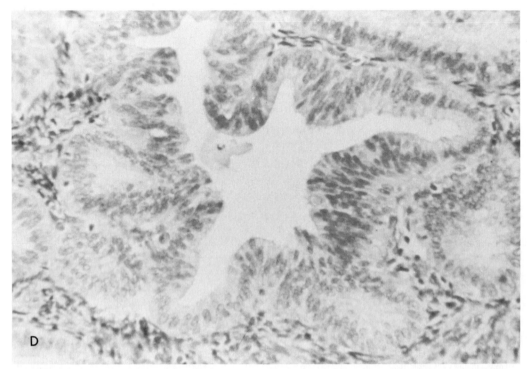

Figure 2D. Carcinoma in situ. Glandular cells are stratified and nuclei are larger with more clumping of chromatin. Eosinophilic cytoplasm and intraglandular bridging are frequently described.

In selected premenopausal patients with atypical hyperplasia or carcinoma in situ of the endometrium, cautious conservative management using clomiphene citrate, wedge resection or progestins may be appropriate. However, generally, hysterectomy is advised. In employing conservative management, clomiphene citrate or wedge resection of the ovaries is favored in patients with polycystic ovarian syndrome, while progestin therapy is used in patients without polycystic ovaries. Clearly, however, in postmenopausal patients with these abnormalities, definitive hysterectomy and bilateral salpingo-oophorectomy are indicated. If surgery is contraindicated in postmenopausal patients, reversal with progestins may be attempted.

Carcinomas of the Endometrium

Adenocarcinoma of the endometrium may be grade 1 (well-differentiated), grade 2 (well-differentiated carcinoma with partly solid areas) and grade 3 (poorly differentiated with predominantly solid areas).

Grade 1 lesions are recognized by back-to-back glands without intervening stroma. The epithelial cells appear piled up with intraglandular bridges (Fig. 3A). The chromatin is usually clumped and frequent abnormal mitoses may be seen. The stromal cells seem to be replaced by neutrophils or lipid-laden macrophages.

In grade 2 lesions areas of abnormal glands as just described are present along with areas of tumor cells showing no tendency to form glandular lumens and failing to show evidence of basement membranes (Fig. 3B).

Grade 3 lesions are composed predominantly of solid areas with occasional abortive attempts to form glands. In addition, necrosis and degeneration are usually quite prominent (Fig. 3C).

Foci of squamous metaplasia may be associated with some well-differentiated lesions. This squamous epithelium has a characteristic benign appearance. Patients with adenoacanthoma respond to treatment, grade for grade, in a similar way to patients with adenocarcinoma (Fig. 3D). The presence of benign squamous epithelium does not affect the response to treatment.

The mixed adenosquamous carcinomas differ significantly from adenoacanthoma in both histology and aggressiveness of tumor behav-

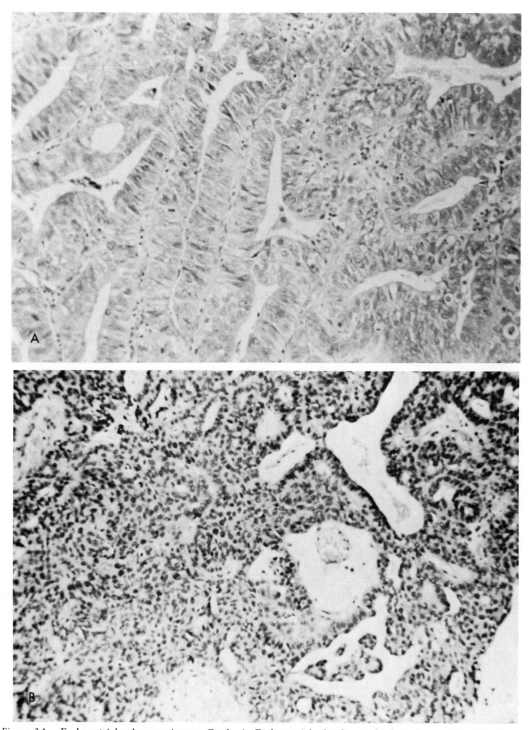

Figure 3A. Endometrial adenocarcinoma Grade 1. Endometrial glands are back to back with little, if any, intervening stroma. Nuclei are large with abnormal shapes, clumped chromatin and frequent mitotic figures.

Figure 3B. Endometrial adenocarcinoma Grade 2. Glandular areas show increasing abnormalities but in addition some areas are partly solid with no tendency to form glands.

Illustration continued on following page

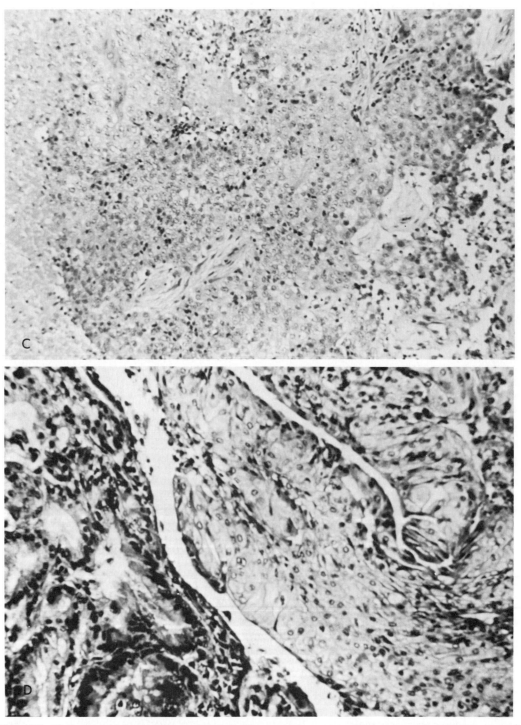

Figure 3C. Endometrial adenocarcinoma Grade 3. The tumor is composed predominently of solid areas with little or no attempt to form glands.

Figure 3D. Adenocanthoma of the endometrium. Foci of benign squamous metaplasia are associated with well-differentiated adenocarcinoma.

Illustration continued on opposite page

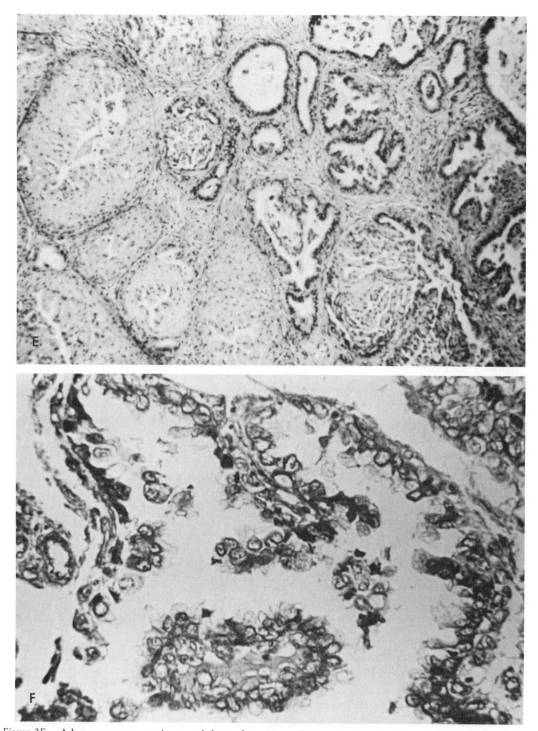

Figure 3E. Adenosquamous carcinoma of the endometrium. Foci or sheets of malignant squamous epithelium associated with adenocarcinoma of the endometrium.

Figure 3F. Clear cell adenocarcinoma of the endometrium. Papillary adenocarcinoma composed of cells having clear cytoplasm admixed with "hobnail" cells.

ior. In this mixed form, the squamous epithelium is histologically malignant and usually invades the surrounding stroma as extension from the malignant glandular elements (Fig. 3E).

Another rarer type of endometrial carcinoma is the mesonephroid or clear cell type. This tumor may grow in a papillary or solid pattern but characteristically the cells have voluminous clear cytoplasm. The clear cells are admixed with "hobnail" cells (Fig. 3F).

Management of Endometrial Carcinoma

Survival rate of patients with endometrial carcinoma decreases when cancer extends beyond the uterine corpus to involve either the cervix, pelvic or para-aortic lymph nodes, ovaries or other extrauterine sites. Pretreatment evaluation of a patient with endometrial cancer must be directed toward determining the extent or the stage of the cancer.

Measuring the length of the uterine canal in patients with early-stage lesions is important because it may correlate with the volume of tumor present. A larger uterine cavity may contain a greater volume of cancer. Correlations have been shown to exist between larger volumes of cancer and decreased survival. Similarly, extension of cancer through the uterine cervix is of major importance because of the greater potential for spread of cancer to pelvic and para-aortic lymph nodes. Cervical involvement can be identified by careful sampling of the cervix and endocervix. It is much more difficult to identify, on clinical examination, ovarian involvement or pelvic nodal involvement. It is possible, however, to estimate the likelihood of nodal involvement based on correlations that exist between the histologic grade of a tumor and the presence of metastatic nodal disease.

The current basis for determining the treatment of endometrial cancer rests with assessment of uterine size, careful clinical examination to detect possible endocervical or cervical involvement and careful histologic evaluation to determine histologic grade of tumor. In addition, efforts to identify metastatic spread must be made, including use of intravenous pyelogram and chest x-ray. Cystoscopy, proctoscopy and barium enema may be needed in specific instances when bladder or rectal involvement is suspected. The International Federation of Gynecology and Obstetrics (IFGO) staging system for endometrial carcinoma is shown in Table 7.

The treatment developed by the authors for endometrial carcinoma is based on the stage and grade of the lesion as shown in Table 8. Patients with adenoacanthoma or with clear cell carcinoma are treated according to the stage of disease and the grade of the adenomatous element. Adenosquamous carcinoma is considered poorly differentiated and treatment is approached in the same manner as in patients with other grade 3 lesions.

Both surgery and radiation are effective in the treatment of endometrial cancer. It has been suggested that, except for the patient with a small uterus and well-differentiated cancer, the combination of surgery and radiation increases survival over treatment with either surgery or radiation alone. Furthermore, it has been accepted that the incidence of vaginal recurrence is reduced following either preoperative or postoperative intracavitary radium. Jones, in a review of the literature, found a 10.3 per cent incidence of vaginal recurrence in 770 patients who were treated with surgery alone but only 4.6 per cent incidence in 1378 patients who were treated preoperatively with radium and 5.2 per cent incidence in 116 patients who were treated with postoperative radium.[16]

TABLE 7. INTERNATIONAL FEDERATION OF GYNECOLOGY AND OBSTETRICS STAGING SYSTEM ADOPTED FOR ENDOMETRIAL CARCINOMA (APRIL, 1970)

Stage 0	Carcinoma in situ. Histologic findings are suspicious of malignancy.
Stage I	Carcinoma is confined to the corpus.
IA	Uterine cavity length is 8 cm or less.
IB	Uterine cavity length is more than 8 cm.

Stage I cases should be subgrouped as follows:
- G-1 Highly differentiated adenomatous carcinomas.
- G-2 Differentiated adenomatous carcinomas with partly solid areas.
- G-3 Predominantly solid or entirely undifferentiated carcinomas.

Stage II	Carcinoma has involved the corpus and the cervix.
Stage III	Carcinoma has extended outside the uterus but not outside the true pelvis.
Stage IV	Carcinoma has extended outside the true pelvis or has obviously involved the mucosa of the bladder or rectum.

TABLE 8. TREATMENT PLAN FOR ENDOMETRIAL CANCER

STAGE	GRADE	TREATMENT
1A	1	Vaginal or abdominal hysterectomy and bilateral salpingo-oophorectomy (BSO)
1A	2	Intracavitary radium, total abdominal hysterectomy (TAH) and BSO*
1B small uterus	1–2	Intracavitary radium, TAH and BSO*
1B large uterus	1–2	External radiation plus intracavitary radium, TAH and BSO
1A–1B	3	External radiation plus intracavitary radium, TAH and BSO
11	1–2–3	External radiation plus intracavitary radium, TAH and BSO
111–IV		Individualize treatment; radiotherapy, surgery, hormonal and chemotherapy

*Postoperative external radiation is given in addition if, on pathologic examination of the uterus, the cervix is involved, or more than 50% of the uterine wall is involved or if grade 3 carcinoma predominates.

Patients who have medical contraindications to surgery or who have unresectable lesions are treated solely with radiation therapy, which consists of a combination of external and intracavitary radiation. The important role and efficacy of intracavitary radiation therapy recently has been demonstrated in a group of such patients who were treated with external radiation therapy alone at the M. D. Anderson Hospital. Landgren et al. evaluated 372 patients who were treated with intracavitary radiation alone and found fewer pelvic failures in this group than in a group of patients who were treated with external radiation plus a diminished amount of intracavitary radiation. In both groups of patients, however, the same incidence of failure due to distant metastases occurred.[17]

The routine use of radical hysterectomy for stage I or stage II endometrial carcinoma has not proved feasible because equally high or higher survival rates have been obtained using improved radiation methods and conservative hysterectomy.[18] In addition, the older-age patients most likely to develop endometrial cancer are often obese or have medical conditions that limit the applicability of radical surgery by increasing the complication rate.

Patients who have had previous radiotherapy and then develop endometrial cancer should not be retreated with radiation, if at all possible, but should be treated primarily with surgery.

Stromal sarcomas are divided into two groups of tumors: those that are locally aggressive with a good prognosis, such as endolymphatic stromal myosis, and those with the capacity to metastasize widely with a poor prognosis, such as endometrial stromal sarcoma. Endometrial stromal sarcoma lacks the prominent connective tissue support and circumscribed margins that its less aggressive counterpart, endolymphatic stromal myosis, has. Frequently, stromal sarcoma presents with polypoid intraluminal growths that infiltrate into the myometrium so that the tumor blends into the adjacent myometrium, separating the muscle fibers. Mitotic figures are common in endometrial stromal sarcoma (Fig. 4).

Treatment of endolymphatic stromal myosis with total abdominal hysterectomy and bilateral salpingo-oophorectomy is usually quite adequate. More aggressive stromal sarcoma is treated, however, with preoperative external and intracavitary radiation followed by hysterectomy and salpingo-oophorectomy. Recurrent or metastatic stromal sarcoma is ideally managed with a combination of radiation plus chemotherapy utilizing the combination vincristine, actinomycin D and cyclophosphamide (VAC) (Table 9). Metastases from the less aggressive stromal sarcomas may be hormone dependent and respond to progestin therapy.[19] If metastases from less aggressive stromal sarcomas do not respond to progestin therapy, they must also be treated with the VAC regimen.

Mixed mesodermal sarcoma is a composite of epithelial carcinoma plus stromal sarcoma. The epithelial element may resemble endometrial adenocarcinoma, cervical adenocarcinoma, serous papillary carcinoma or even squamous carcinoma. The sarcomatous element has a fibrosarcoma-like pattern with prominent spindle-shaped cells; however, foci

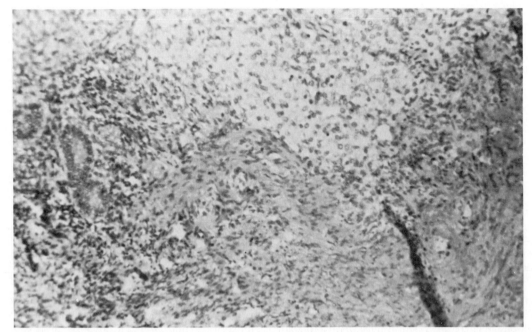

Figure 4. Endometrial stromal sarcoma of endometrium. In this field normal glandular elements and normal smooth muscle of the myometrium are seen; however, normal endometrial stroma is replaced by small plump oval cells with scant cytoplasm and larger than normal hyperchromatic nuclei.

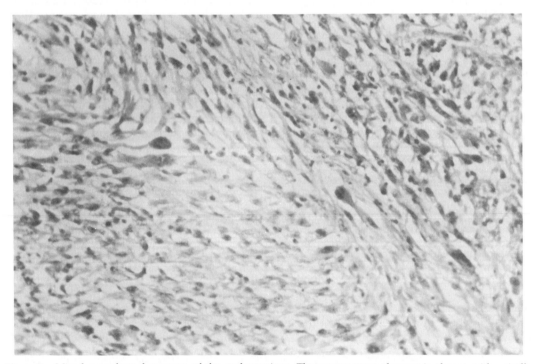

Figure 5. Mixed mesodermal sarcoma of the endometrium. The sarcomatous element is shown with spindle-shaped sarcoma cells resembling fibrosarcoma or rhabdomyosarcoma. The adenocarcinomatous element is not shown.

TABLE 9.   REGIMEN FOR TREATMENT OF UTERINE
SARCOMAS

Vincristine, actinomycin D, cyclophosphamide (VAC)

Vincristine
  1.5 mg/M² IV weekly for 12 weeks (2.5 mg maximum
  single dose)

Actinomycin D
  0.5 mg IV daily for 5 days

Cyclophosphamide
  6 mg/kg IV daily for 5 days

Cycles of actinomycin D and cyclophosphamide repeated every 4 weeks

---

of other homologous elements such as leio-
myosarcoma or heterologous elements such as
rhabdomyosarcoma, chondrosarcoma, liposar-
coma or osteosarcoma may be present (Fig.
5). The general treatment plan for mixed mesodermal sarcoma includes whole pelvis x-ray
therapy and intracavitary radium followed by
hysterectomy four to six weeks after irradiation. For patients with distant metastases,
persistent or recurrent disease, combination
VAC chemotherapy is used.

REFERENCES

1. Rosenberg, L., Armstrong, B. et al.: Myocardial infarction and estrogen therapy in post-menopausal women. N. Engl. J. Med. 294:1256, 1976.
2. Estrogen drugs; do they increase the risk of cancer? Science 191:838, 1976.
3. Weiss, N., Szekely, D. et al.: Increasing incidence of endometrial cancer in the United States. N. Engl. J. Med. 294:1259, 1976.
4. Mack, T. and Pike, M.: Estrogens and endometrial cancer in a retirement community. N. Engl. J. Med. 294:1262, 1976.
5. Ziel, H. and Finkle, W.: Increased risk of endometrial carcinoma among users of conjugated estrogens. N. Engl. J. Med. 293:1167, 1975.
6. Smith, D., Prentice, R. et al.: Association of exoge-nous estrogen and endometrial carcinoma. N. Engl. J. Med. 293:1164, 1975.
7. Burch, J. C., Byrd, B. F. and Vaughn, W. K.: The effects of long term estrogen on hysterectomized women. Am. J. Obstet. Gynecol. 118: March 15, 1974.
8. Kase, N.: Yes or no on estrogen replacement therapy? A formulation for clinicians. Clin. Obstet. Gynecol. 19:825, 1976.
9. Greenblatt, R.: Estrogens and endometrial cancer. In Beard, R. J. (ed.): The Menopause—A Guide to Current Research and Practice. London, MTP Press, Ltd., 1977.
10. Sommers, S. C.: The significance of endometrial hyperplasia and its early diagnosis. In Gynecologic Oncology. Baltimore, Williams and Wilkins, 1970.
11. Hofmeister, F. J., Savage, G. W. and Wolfe, C.: An analysis of office cancer detection in the private practice of gynecology. Am. J. Obstet. Gynecol. 77:June, 1959.
12. Anderson, D.: Cytologic diagnosis of endometrial adenocarcinoma. Am. J. Obstet. Gynecol. 125:376, 1976.
13. Wall, J. A., Fletcher, G. H. and MacDonald, E. J.: Endometrial biopsy as standard diagnostic tech-nique; review of 446 cases. Am. J. Roentgenol. 71:95, 1954.
14. Hertig, A.: Personal communication, 1976.
15. Casey, M. J.: Age-specific incidence rates of endo-metrial cancer. J.A.M.A. 238:213, 1977.
16. Jones, H. W.: Treatment of adenocarcinoma of the endometrium. Obstet. Gynecol. Surv. 30:147, 1975.
17. Landgren, R. D., Fletcher, G. H., Gallagher, H. S., Declos, L. and Wharton, J. T.: Treatment failure sites according to irradiation technique and histol-ogy in patients with endometrial cancer. Cancer 40:131, 1977.
18. Baggish, M. and Woodruff, D.: Uterine stromatosis: clinico-pathologic features and hormone depend-ency. Obstet. Gynecol. 40:487, 1972.
19. Rutledge, F.: The role of radical hysterectomy in adenocarcinoma of the endometrium. Gynecol. On-col. 2:331, 1974.

Diagnosis and Management of Preinvasive Endometrial Disease

S. B. Gusberg, M.D.

G. Deppe, M.D.

Mount Sinai School of Medicine of the City University of New York

Adenocarcinoma of the endometrium is the most common invasive gynecologic cancer in the United States today. If previous mortality rates continue, it is estimated that 37 per cent of females with cancer will die of recurrent or metastatic disease. It would appear, therefore, that carcinoma of the endometrium has become a critical problem. Diagnosis and treatment of preinvasive disease is the key to better control of this malignant tumor.

Advancement in control of endometrial carcinoma can be helped by:

1. Definition and acceptance of adenomatous hyperplasia as an endometrial cancer precursor.

2. Knowledge of high-risk factors for developing endometrial carcinoma such as obesity, infertility, failure of ovulation, dysfunctional uterine bleeding and long-term estrogen administration.

3. Introduction of aspiration curettage, an outpatient method for screening the high-risk patient and discovering the endometrial cancer precursor adenomatous hyperplasia. Histologic screening in the current era will be more efficient than cytologic screening; the latter is relatively inefficient for disclosing endometrial carcinoma when the cytologic smears are taken in the traditional manner, while the former enables the diagnosis of adenomatous hyperplasia to be made readily. This is not possible with cytologic screening.

Types of Precursors

Precursors of invasive endometrial carcinoma include adenomatous hyperplasia and carcinoma in situ.

Adenomatous hyperplasia is characterized by crowded glands, frequently back to back; there is pseudostratification of the glandular epithelium, a characteristic pallor or eosinophilic stain reaction of these glands with intense proliferation of the glandular epithelium, forming buds and islands within the gland lumen. Types I, II and III adenomatous hyperplasia are differentiated in an increasing order of severity. Each of these lesions has a distinctive histologic appearance but transitions between them are frequent.

We have repeatedly emphasized the relationship between adenomatous hyperplasia and carcinoma of the endometrium. Our own prospective studies of patients with adenomatous hyperplasia have indicated a cumulative risk of 30 per cent progression to endometrial cancer at 10 years.

However, the true incidence of progression of adenomatous hyperplasia to invasive endometrial cancer has not yet been and perhaps never will be unequivocally established. We prefer the term type III adenomatous hyperplasia rather than carcinoma in situ because of the impure criteria for invasion in the endometrium. We have reserved the diagnosis of carcinoma in situ for those lesions of undoubted invasion of the stroma, well differentiated with confinement to a local area of the endometrium, described in the past as adenoma malignum. This lesion is not reversible, though it may be removed at times by local excision—that is, by curettage.

Diagnosis

Accurate histologic samples of the endometrial cavity can be obtained with ease by suction curettage. This device consists of a cannula curette only 3 mm in its outside diameter connected to a negative-pressure source. It is an outpatient method, requires no anesthesia and has a high degree of patient acceptance. With aspiration curettage the physician can obtain an excellent general sample of endometrium. The onset of most invasive endometrial cancers can be prevented by diagnosis of these precursor lesions.

600

Treatment

Premenopausal adenomatous hyperplasia, occasionally discovered in young patients with anovulatory uterine bleeding or polycystic ovary syndrome, may be treated by induction of ovulation if infertility is a problem; in others a trial of the administration of progesterone or progestational agents may induce regression of the hyperplasia. Therapy of this kind should be monitored by repeat evaluation of the endometrial cavity after three to four months of therapy to rule out the presence of a missed endometrial cancer.

Patients with perimenopausal adenomatous hyperplasia type I or type II may be observed or be treated with progestational agents only. Repeat endometrial sampling at six-month intervals is necessary. In some patients hysterectomy will be preferred by patient and physician.

Patients with type III adenomatous hyperplasia and carcinoma in situ are best treated with hysterectomy because it is clear that they are at high risk for developing endometrial cancer.

Treatment of adenomatous hyperplasia in the postmenopausal age should be individualized so that each patient may be treated optimally. In lesions produced iatrogenically by the use of estrogen the physician may observe the condition after estrogen withdrawal without hormonal medication and await reversion to normal. In those patients in whom adenomatous hyperplasia occurs without medication, hysterectomy is indicated. One must weigh the patient's operability against the advantage of prophylaxis by considering the patient's age, general medical condition, psy-choemotional state and opportunity and willingness for repeated observation.

Conclusions

With the use of the aspiration curettage as a histologic screening measure, it is possible to evaluate all high-risk women with or without symptoms and all menopausal and postmenopausal women with uterine bleeding. In this manner we may be able to control cancer of the endometrium by detecting its precursor, adenomatous hyperplasia.

REFERENCES

1. Cohen, C. J. and Gusberg, S. B.: Screening for endometrial cancer. Clin. Obstet. Gynecol. 18:27, 1975.
2. Creasman, W. T. and Weed, J. C.: Screening techniques in endometrial cancer. Cancer 38:436, 1976.
3. Gray, L. A., Christopherson, W. M. and Hoover, R. N.: Estrogens and endometrial carcinoma. Obstet. Gynecol. 49:385, 1977.
4. Gusberg, S. B.: Precursors of corpus carcinoma, estrogens and adenomatous hyperplasia. Am. J. Obstet. Gynecol. 54:905, 1947.
5. Gusberg, S. B. and Kaplan, A. L.: Precursors of corpus cancer. IV. Adenomatous hyperplasia as stage O carcinoma of the endometrium. Am. J. Obstet. Gynecol. 87:662, 1963.
6. Gusberg, S. B., Chen, S. Y. and Cohen, C. J.: Endometrial cancer: factors influencing the choice of treatment. Gynecol. Oncol. 2:308, 1974.
7. Gusberg, S. B.: The individual at high risk for endometrial carcinoma. Am. J. Obstet. Gynecol. 126:535, 1976.
8. Inglis, R. M. and Weir, J. H.: Endometrial suction biopsy: appraisal of a new instrument. Am. J. Obstet. Gynecol. 125:1070, 1976.
9. MacMahon, B.: Risk factors for endometrial cancer. Gynecol. Oncol. 2:122, 1974.
10. Vellios, F.: Endometrial hyperplasia and carcinoma-in-situ. Gynecol. Oncol. 2:152, 1974.

Diagnosis and Management of Endometrial Disease

John H. Isaacs, M.D.

Stritch School of Medicine, Loyola University of Chicago

Normally uterine bleeding is a cyclic physiological event occurring during the reproductive years of the nonpregnant woman. Much of our current understanding of cyclic endometrial changes was developed by the work of investigators such as Bartelmez, Markee and Noyes.[1-3] Menstruation is a complex process involving functional interrelationships between the higher cerebral centers of the brain, hypothalamus, pituitary, ovaries and the endometrium. Interplay between these organs and the thyroid and adrenal glands complicates the process. The exact mechanism of the onset of menstruation is poorly understood. There are five theories as to the cause of menstruation and these include estrogen deprivation, progesterone deprivation, inadequate endometrial lymphatic drainage, menstrual toxin(s) and endometrial depolymerization. The interested reader is referred to the excellent review on the subject presented by Israel et al.[4]

The endometrium may be affected by disorders of pregnancy, inflammation, trauma, hormonal imbalance and benign or malignant tumors. These conditions usually manifest themselves by some deviation in the bleeding pattern; bleeding may be scant, heavy, prolonged, too frequent, too infrequent, intermenstrual or postmenopausal. Disease may make itself manifest by absence of bleeding. The disorders of pregnancy and the inflammatory and traumatic problems that affect the endometrium will not be covered in this article. The discussion will be confined to functional bleeding disorders and endometrial neoplasia.

Functional Bleeding Disorders

Nonorganic uterine bleeding is a poorly understood and often inappropriately managed menstrual disorder. It has been estimated that over 50 per cent of such patients are 45 years of age or older, about 20 per cent are adolescents and the remaining 30 per cent are of various reproductive ages.[5]

Many gynecologic endocrinologists would prefer the term dysfunctional uterine bleeding to be used only for anovulatory bleeding and would prefer to limit the discussion to those problems associated with such anovulatory bleeding. Such a limited definition does not seem practical, however, because most often the clinician is confronted with a patient whose menstrual cycle has deviated from her expected norm (not necessarily anovulatory), and she is seeking reassurance and help for her problem. Sutherland reviewed 1000 patients with dysfunctional uterine bleeding and found normal endometrium in over 50 per cent, with many endometria exhibiting secretory changes.[6] Taw reviewed 1520 patients who had uterine curettage for abnormal bleeding and found that 20 per cent had a secretory endometrium.[7] In reviewing my own series of

576 patients with abnormal uterine bleeding, secretory endometrium was found in 177 (30.8 per cent) patients. The clinician must bear in mind that this bleeding is probably an end organ phenomenon and that the exact mechanism whereby hormonal changes bring about such bleeding is as yet undetermined.

EVALUATION

The history is most important. A family history of bleeding problems may suggest an inherited blood dyscrasia. The history must include details as to medication the patient is taking, including salicylates, hormones, anticoagulants, vitamins and digitalis. Dietary changes causing either rapid weight loss or gain must be considered, because such fluctuations may markedly affect normal menstrual flow. Additionally, the history should elicit any chronic illnesses such as essential hypertension, diabetes, congestive heart failure or liver disease.

During the reproductive years, many factors can interrupt or delay normal pituitary-ovarian-uterine function. Psychogenic causes are frequently to blame. Some of the problems may include marital or sexual discord, broken family relationships, social pressures and alcohol or drug abuse.

A general physical examination is essential in any patient with abnormal uterine bleeding. The general appearance of the patient should be noted. Evidence of chronic disease or signs of blood dyscrasia such as ecchymoses or splenomegaly must be checked. The abdominal examination is important to diagnose either intra-abdominal or intrapelvic tumors. The pelvic examination should confirm that the blood is indeed uterine in origin. Particular attention should be paid to the vaginal hormonal status, whether hyperestrogenic or hypoestrogenic, and Papanicolaou smear will be helpful even in the face of bleeding. Local reasons for the abnormal bleeding may be discovered, including benign or malignant neoplasia or vaginal or cervical infection. A careful bimanual examination may detect leiomyomas, ovarian masses, ectopic pregnancy, complications of intrauterine pregnancy, foreign bodies, misplaced tampons or pessaries or a partially expelled intrauterine contraceptive device. The rectovaginal examination is important to exclude pelvic masses in the cul-de-sac, nodules suggestive of endometriosis on the uterosacral ligaments or rectal polyps, and hemorrhoids or carcinoma.

In addition to a complete blood count, other laboratory tests may be necessary. The literature is replete with reports citing excessive menstrual flow as the only symptom of idiopathic thrombocytopenic purpura in young women.[8, 9] Blood coagulation studies must be considered in any patient with abnormal bleeding. It is important to check for deficiencies in blood factor V, VII or X and for von Willebrand's disease. Iron deficiency has also been reported[10] in ovulatory dysfunctional bleeding, and testing of the serum iron level as well as the serum iron–binding capacity level may be indicated.

CLINICAL MANAGEMENT

In the adolescent, bleeding may present as an acute medical and emotional emergency with a hysterical mother and a terrified patient calling frantically about excessive vaginal bleeding. In such instances, the clinician can be reasonably certain that the bleeding is due to prolonged unopposed estrogen stimulation resulting in either a thick lush hyperplastic endometrial lining or a scanty denuded one, either of which can result from unopposed endogenous estrogen stimulation. If the bleeding is profuse and of relatively short duration, the endometrium is most likely hyperplastic. The heavy bleeding may be curtailed by high doses of exogenous estrogen followed by progesterone administered in a cyclic fashion. On the other hand, if the patient reports prolonged bleeding (3 to 5 weeks), it is more likely that the endometrial cavity is basically denuded. In such a situation, the use of a low-dose exogenous estrogen for two or three weeks will rebuild the endometrial lining. The estrogen therapy should be followed with progesterone for five days. After the estrogen and progesterone are discontinued, the resulting withdrawal bleeding will be more physiologic. Almost all of these adolescent bleeding problems correct themselves as the pituitary-ovarian axis matures.

The patient with abnormal bleeding that is most challenging to the clinician is the patient in her reproductive years, when normal pituitary-ovarian-uterine coordination is expected. When such patients experience vagaries in their menstrual flow, they became concerned and seek early gynecologic evaluation. In many such instances a careful history will elicit a tale of some psychogenic upset as the underlying cause of the menstrual irregularity. Obviously a careful history and physical examination is mandatory and further laboratory studies are indicated if any systemic disease, inappropriate use of medication or a suspicion of a hematologic disorder is suspected. Frequently a cervical cytologic smear and an intrauterine cytologic smear will assure the patient that any neoplastic changes have been excluded.

A sympathetic and attentive approach by the physician will reassure the patient. If all findings are within normal limits, all that is required initially is a suggestion that the patient keep a careful record of her bleeding disorder and return for re-evaluation in two to three months. In the majority of instances the bleeding irregularity will correct itself and no further therapy is necessary. In those instances in which the bleeding irregularity continues, specific investigation is necessary. Endometrial biopsy may be employed, but only a minimal amount of the surface area is sampled; therefore, this procedure may not be too reassuring to the patient. It has been my practice to suggest that if the condition has extended this long, an evaluation of the pelvis under anesthesia and a thorough uterine curettage is the procedure of choice. In many cases this procedure is not only diagnostic but in the majority of instances therapeutic. In order to validate this clinical impression, the records of 576 patients with abnormal uterine bleeding managed over a 20-year period and undergoing curettage were evaluated. In each instance the patient had a history of at least a three-month interval of abnormal bleeding before surgical intervention was suggested. Three hundred and seventy-three patients or 64.7 per cent required no further treatment; an additional 24 patients required a second D&C or hormonal therapy for a short duration. The findings in these cases are noted in Table 1. The remaining 179 patients ultimately (1 to 16 years later) required a hysterectomy. In 29 patients no specific pathology was found, but in the remaining 150 patients there was additional pathology that accounted for the abnormal bleeding.

Although we are beginning to have access to accurate assays for both the steroid and protein hormones that regulate uterine bleeding, it does not seem that we are on the brink of solving the aberration of bleeding by inge-

TABLE 1.   RESULTS OF D&C IN 397 PATIENTS WITH ABNORMAL UTERINE BLEEDING

NUMBER	HISTOLOGY	FOLLOW-UP
33	Endometrial hyperplasia	32 No further treatment 1 Hormonal therapy
180	Proliferative endometrium	168 No further treatment 8 Needed a second D&C 4 Hormonal therapy
141	Secretory endometrium	130 No further treatment 9 Needed a second D&C 2 Hormonal therapy
19	Endometrial polyp	19 No further treatment
12	Unspecified benign endometrium	12 No further treatment
5	Mixed endometrium	5 No further treatment
3	Endometritis	3 No further treatment
4	Leiomyoma	4 No further treatment
397 TOTAL		

nious manipulation of these substances. If one were to treat such patients with hormone therapy, what would be the rationale behind such therapy? As Zondek points out: "Since bleeding can take place at such widely varying phases in the development of the endometrium, with such different degrees of vascularization and with either decreasing or constant hormonal levels, the mechanism cannot be the same in every case."[11] It has been my custom therefore to perform curettage for those patients with prolonged abnormal bleeding as described rather than attempting any hormonal therapy. Most of the patients in the reproductive and perimenopausal age will be completely relieved of their bleeding problem following a thorough curettage. In few instances, however, some slight aberration will persist. What is the clinician to do with such patients? To offer them hormonal therapy that is not totally understood does not, to me, seem logical. It would seem wiser to assure the patient that there is no evidence of organic disease but that careful surveillance of the endometrium is mandatory. This can be done by periodic examination and endometrial cytology sampling.

Types of Endometrial Disease

ENDOMETRIAL HYPERPLASIA

Some retrospective studies[12, 13] have revealed that invasive endometrial carcinoma has often been preceded by a hyperplastic change in the endometrium. Vuopala has reviewed the literature on the subject and has estimated that the tendency of cystic glandular hyperplasia to progress to endometrial carcinoma is between 1 and 3 per cent, that of adenomatous hyperplasia is approximately 20 per cent and that of atypical adenomatous hyperplasia is approximately 25 per cent.[14]

Endometrial hyperplasia of any type may be found in patients of any age group. The management must differ depending on the age, desire for childbearing and as far as possible elimination of the risk of subsequent development of endometrial carcinoma.

Abnormal bleeding is not unusual in the adolescent and on occasions may be associated with some type of endometrial hyperplasia. In most instances, it is not practical to obtain histologic evidence of the exact state of the endometrium in this age group. It is reasonably safe to assume, however, that in most instances the bleeding is anovulatory in type. In the adolescent in whom curettage is necessary because of uncontrolled bleeding, a histologic diagnosis of endometrial hyperplasia may be found. In such cases, periodic addition of exogenous progesterone will allow for a more physiologic shedding of the endometrium. This regimen may be continued until such time as the pituitary-ovarian-uterine axis matures so that normal ovulatory cycles develop.

The second group of patients for consideration are those women in the childbearing

TABLE 2. ENDOMETRIAL HYPERPLASIA	
Cystic hyperplasia	46
Adenomatous hyperplasia	14
Unspecified hyperplasia	13
Total	73

age. Once the diagnosis is established by either endometrial biopsy or curettage, the patient's wants must be taken into consideration. If she desires more regular menses and additionally wants to maintain her childbearing function, careful follow-up is mandatory. Many of these patients are fearful of hormonal therapy and in my own experience hormones may not be helpful. In a review of personal records of patients in the childbearing age, 73 were diagnosed as having endometrial hyperplasia. The exact histologic report is shown on Table 2.

Hormonal therapy was minimal and in 33 cases a single curettage was adequate therapy except in one instance in which progestational therapy was employed cyclically for four months. The remaining 40 patients were followed several years and ultimately required hysterectomy. It is interesting that in eight of these patients an additional one or two D&Cs were performed prior to hysterectomy. Further evaluation of these 40 patients revealed that in 29, additional pathology was found in the excised specimen. These lesions included leiomyomas, adenomyosis and endometriosis. Obviously, these patients must be removed from the dysfunctional uterine bleeding group because organic pathology was discovered. In the other 11 patients the only apparent cause for the bleeding was hyperplasia.

It might be argued that hormonal therapy might have obviated the need for some of these hysterectomies, but it was noted that in only 14 of these cases was the patient 40 years of age or less and in only 5 cases was the hysterectomy necessary because of hyperplasia alone.

It is my belief that these patients may be safely managed with careful evaluation of the pelvic findings every three to six months combined with cervical-vaginal-endocervical cytologic smear and intrauterine endometrial cytology sampling.

ENDOMETRIAL POLYP

An endometrial polyp is a sessile or pedunculated mucosal projection that is composed of either hypertrophied, hyperplastic or neoplastic endometrial glands and stroma. Such tumors may occur at almost any age group. Their symptomatology is hard to define because they are often associated with uterine pathology such as leiomyomas and endometriosis. In our own series of 576 patients with abnormal bleeding, endometrial polyps were found in 33 instances, almost always in association with other uterine pathology.

ENDOMETRIAL CARCINOMA

There is mounting evidence that the incidence of endometrial carcinoma is rising.[15-17] This predominance of endometrial cancer may be the result of pure age-related rise in incidence; more people live longer, giving women an ever greater postmenopausal span. Additionally, the onset of menopause a generation ago was in the mid forties but now comes in the fifties, with a fair number of women still menstruating at age 54 or 55.

The overall strategy for the control of cancer is to find its cause and prevention, to achieve earlier diagnosis and to develop adequate therapeutic measures regardless of the stage at which the disease is found. The cause and prevention and the ideal therapy are still unclear, and so as clinicians we must turn our attention to early diagnosis. We must be aware of the patient at greatest risk and must be familiar with methods to help establish an earlier diagnosis. Obesity can increase the risk factor by as much as ninefold.[18] Those women who are tall are also at risk, even independent of obesity.[18] Nulliparity produces a risk that is two times greater than that in women with one child.[19] Additionally, diabetes and late menopause increase the risk by twofold to threefold.[19] Whether exogenous estrogen therapy is a factor in the development of endometrial carcinoma remains controversial.[20]

The physical examination may be helpful in determining which patient is more likely to be harboring endometrial carcinoma. If the pelvic examination reveals a cervix that is softer and more easily dilated and the uterus itself is softer and larger than normal, the clinician should be suspicious.

When the clinician selects those patients at greatest risk and those patients suffering from abnormal bleeding, which diagnostic procedures will be helpful? Cytologic screening is probably the most helpful and will be discussed under techniques for endometrial monitoring.

Usually the diagnosis of endometrial carcinoma is made by means of a fractional curettage. Once the diagnosis has been established a plan of therapy must be carried out. In this country, radiotherapy has generally been given preoperatively in keeping with the theory that this can prevent tumor spread at the time of surgery and to utilize the uterus as a radium carrier. There have been a number of reports,[21-23] however, that challenge the usefulness of preoperative radiation. Additionally, Jones surveyed the literature, comparing the five-year survival with surgery alone and the survival with radiation plus surgery in the treatment of endometrial carcinoma in over 6000 patients.[24] In only one series was he able to show a statistically significant improvement in the five-year survival rate for patients treated with a combination of radiation plus surgery.

Over the past few years a number of studies have suggested that treatment might better be tailored to the individual patient depending upon the type and extent of the tumor. In 1962 Barber et al. showed a positive relationship between stage of disease and the grade of the tumor.[25] It was later noted by Cheon that myometrial invasion is a significant prognostic factor.[26] Prognostic factors were clearly identified by Creasman et al., who concluded that myometrial invasion and the extent of lymph node metastases cannot be established preoperatively and that surgical staging to determine the extent of the disease may be useful in determining appropriate therapy for the individual patient.[27] This same basic philosophy is suggested by the Mayo Clinic group,[28] who believe that the treatment should be total abdominal hysterectomy and bilateral salpingo-oophorectomy with postoperative irradiation on an individual basis.

At present it would seem there are some compelling reasons for the initial therapy to be primary surgery. Such reasons include the following: (1) Unless external beam therapy is used in addition to intracavitary irradiation, there is little effect on the pelvic lymph nodes. (2) If preoperative radiation is employed, the physician is deprived of the information about the depth of myometrial invasion and possible occult spread to the cervix. (3) The radiation may interfere with the physician's ability to do progesterone receptor studies and thus valuable information may be lost in treating some patients. (4) Considerable morbidity is sometimes associated with radiation. (5) There does not seem to be any logical reason to irradiate and then to remove the organ shortly thereafter. This is not generally accepted in the management of other malignancies. (6) There is no convincing proof of the superiority of preoperative irradiation.

It would seem logical therefore in treating all patients suffering from endometrial carcinoma that the initial approach when medically feasible is to perform a total abdominal hysterectomy and bilateral salpingo-oophorectomy. This treatment should be supplemented with postoperative irradiation depending on the surgical and pathologic findings. Even the vaginal route may be acceptable in some instances, as has been demonstrated by Pratt et al.[29] More recently Candiani et al. have emphasized the use of vaginal surgery for the very obese and the poor surgical risk patient. Prem has also advocated this route in selected cases.[31]

Following surgery, radiation should be added if the histologic grade is 2 or 3 or if the cervix is involved or if there is deep myometrial invasion (greater than one half the thickness of the uterine wall) or if there is adnexal spread. A total of 5000 rads should be delivered to the pelvis. Postoperative intravaginal radiation may also be added on a selective basis.

ENDOMETRIAL SARCOMAS

Sarcomas comprise 1 to 2 per cent of all uterine cancers. The variety and uncertain behavior of endometrial stromal tumors have led to several designations, such as stromal adenomyosis, stromatosis, endolymphatic stromal myosis, stromal sarcoma, angioblastomatosis and hemangiopericytoma. Norris and Taylor reviewed the material available at the Armed Forces Institute of Pathology and have helped to eliminate some of the confusion. All mesenchymal tumors of the uterus involving the endometrium may be classified as shown in Table 3.

TABLE 3. ENDOMETRIAL SARCOMAS

1. Stromal tumors
   A. Tumors with pushing margins (stromal nodules)
   B. Tumors with infiltrating margins
      (1) Endolymphatic stromal myosis
      (2) Stromal sarcoma
2. Mixed mesodermal tumors
3. Carcinosarcomas

STROMAL TUMORS

Stromal nodules are composed of cells similar to those found in normal endometrial stroma and should be considered as benign. These patients' symptoms and physical findings were not different from those patients having other uterine tumors. Only three patients in Norris and Taylor's series were asymptomatic. Patients with these tumors have an excellent prognosis; none of the lesions recurred after definitive surgery.

Stromal tumors with infiltrating margins were separated on the basis of mitotic activity. These tumors were of the same cell type as tumors with pushing margins but at the margins the tumor extended irregularly between muscle bundles and along vascular spaces. Infiltrating tumors were divided into two groups on the basis of mitotic activity. Those tumors containing fewer than 10 mitotic figures in 10 high-power fields (HPF) were categorized as endolymphatic stromal myosis. Those tumors containing 10 or more mitotic figures in 10 HPF were considered to be stromal sarcoma. This classification seems appropriate based on the five-year survival rate of 100 per cent in the endolymphatic stromal myosis group and a 55 per cent survival at five years in the stromal sarcoma group.

In a retrospective view of therapy it would appear that hysterectomy and bilateral salpingo-oophorectomy was the treatment of choice and that external beam radiation appeared to be of benefit to those patients with symptomatic extrauterine tumor. This view has recently been emphasized by Yoonessi and Hart.[35]

MIXED MESODERMAL TUMORS

It was noted by Norris et al. that in most reported series of mixed mesodermal tumors these tumors are collections of several types of sarcoma.[33] Little specific information is given about mixed mesodermal tumors containing heterologous elements only. The study of Norris et al. consisted of patients with heterologous elements only. Of the 31 patients in their series most complained of abnormal uterine bleeding; only two were asymptomatic. The median age was 62. These tumors tend to spread by the lymphatics rather than being "blood-borne" as previously thought.

There were only 6 of 31 patients who survived five years. In none of these six patients had the tumor spread beyond the uterus. Additionally, the presence of cartilage and absence of striated muscle were favorable findings because the tumors of all survivors contained cartilage and none contained striated muscle cells.

The distribution of metastatic lesions was similar to that of adenocarcinoma of the endometrium, and for that reason hysterectomy with bilateral salpingo-oophorectomy, wide parametrial excision and pelvic lymph node dissection would appear to be the treatment of choice. This viewpoint has been substantiated by recent studies instituted under the auspices of the Gynecologic Oncology Group and the National Cancer Institute.[36]

CARCINOSARCOMAS

Carcinosarcoma tumors are those neoplasms having intermingled carcinomatous and sarcomatous elements. In histologic evaluations frequent invasion of the lymphatic spaces has been noted. The two elements should be so closely admixed to exclude the possibility that they represent collision tumors, which may on rare occasions be found in the uterus. In the study by Norris and Taylor, all the patients were postmenopausal and the median age was 62. The principal symptom was abnormal uterine bleeding.

The treatment should be total abdominal hysterectomy and bilateral salpingo-oophorectomy, wide parametrial excision and pelvic lymph node dissection. Radiation may not be helpful based on the fact that 5 out of 11 patients survived whose lesions were confined to the uterus and who were treated by surgery alone. Only 3 out of 10 patients survived whose lesions were confined to the uterus and who were treated with a combination of surgery and radiation.

In the study of Norris and Taylor, it was noted that the survival rate of those patients with carcinosarcoma is significantly better than that of patients with mixed mesodermal tumors.

Techniques for Endometrial Monitoring

If patients with abnormal bleeding are to be followed and if early endometrial neoplasms and their precursors are to be detected, the clinician must be able to evaluate the endometrium. Some of the techniques now employed include routine VCE smear, endometrial biopsy, hysterogram, hysteroscopy and intrauterine aspiration cytology.

The vaginal-cervical-endocervical (VCE) smear has been shown to be most effective in the detection of cervical carcinoma and its precursors. The diagnostic accuracy of the VCE smear in a study of over 1400 endometrial carcinomas, however, was only 42.2 per cent.[14] The finding of normal exfoliated cells on a routine VCE smear, however, may be of help to the clinician. Endometrial cells do not exfoliate continuously but exfoliate only during menstruation and for a few days thereafter. Postmenopausally, the endometrium gradually involutes and the exfoliation of cells ceases. Thus if exfoliated normal endometrial cells are noted on a VCE smear in the latter half of a menstrual cycle or after the menopause, it is significant. In those patients in whom endometrial cells were found in the latter half of the cycle, Ng reported that 21.6 per cent had adenomatous polyps of the endometrium, 4.9 per cent had endometrial hyperplasia and 2.0 per cent had endometrial carcinoma.[37] When normal endometrial cells were found in VCE smear after the menopause, 35.4 per cent had adenomatous polyps, 13.2 per cent had endometrial hyperplasia and 5.7 per cent had adenocarcinoma. The clinician must bear in mind, however, that there are other causes for endometrial cells to exfoliate abnormally, and these include hormonal therapy, submucosal leiomyomas, cervical or vaginal endometriosis, the presence of an intrauterine contraceptive device and endometritis.

Several authors[38, 39] have noted high estrogen values in the vaginal Papanicolaou smears of patients with endometrial neoplasias. Other investigators,[40] however, have made different observations, showing the hormonal composition as reflected in the vaginal smear to be similar to that of healthy subjects of the same age. In a series of patients with known endometrial carcinoma, Liu found the vaginal smears to be hyperestrogenic in 10 per cent of the cases, while 62 per cent showed no superficial cells and 38 per cent were clearly atrophic.[41]

The endometrium may also be monitored by means of outpatient tissue sampling; this is the most widely accepted method today. Various types of biopsy instruments have been utilized, but the one most popular today is the Vabra Aspirator. The instrument is 3 mm in diameter. After it is inserted into the uterine cavity, approximately 600 mm Hg of suction is applied to withdraw tissue samples from the uterine wall. Some of the disadvantages to this technique are that irregularities of the uterine cavity produced by either retroversion, myomas or large polyps may prevent the instrument from reaching the areas in which the abnormal cells are located. In the multiple series collection (4354 cases) by Vuopala, it was noted that because of the relatively large diameter of the instrument the procedure was unsuccessful in 10.1 per cent of the cases, and inadequate samples were noted in an additional 6.5 per cent.[14] Even Cohen and Gusberg, who have been strong supporters of Vabra aspiration, have suggested that this is probably impractical and may be unnecessary or undesirable except in those patients at high risk for the development of endometrial carcinoma.[42] A recent study[14] of 722 patients in whom the Vabra curettage was employed, it was noted that 60 of those patients were found to have endometrial hyperplasia by conventional curettage, but the Vabra curettage was able to detect only 27 of these cases and most importantly missed the only atypical hyperplasia in the group.

On the basis of these findings and the acknowledged difficulty and impracticality of routine tissue sampling, intrauterine endometrial cytology must be given more serious consideration by the practicing clinician. If endometrial cytopathologic methods are to be developed to a level of excellence comparable to cervical cytopathology, greater utilization of aspiration cytology is necessary. The technique is basically as follows: a metal or plastic cannula is introduced into the uterine cavity and the contents of the cavity are aspirated into a syringe connected to the cannula and then expelled onto a glass slide, fixed and stained according to Papanicolaou's method. This technique uses an instrument of only 1.8 mm in diameter that is capable of sealing off the cervix so that negative pressure of 600 mm Hg may be obtained.[43]

The cytologic characteristics of the different precursor lesions have been discussed particularly by Reagan and Ng.[44] Additionally, Vuopala has set down criteria for the cytologic diagnosis of cystic and adenomatous hyperplasia. Hutton et al. have recently reported on the use of intrauterine aspiration cytology in assessing the endometrial state.[45] In their series of 121 patients they were able to obtain

TABLE 4.   ENDOMETRIAL CYTOLOGY IN 205 PATIENTS WITH POSTMENOPAUSAL BLEEDING (ISAACS)

| | | CYTOLOGY | |
	HISTOLOGY	Positive Pos/Susp	Negative
Endometrial carcinoma	44	42	2
Atypical hyperplasia	3	2	1
Adenomatous hyperplasia	9	4	5
Benign	149	26	123

False negative 2/44 for carcinoma	(95.5%)	
False positive 26/149	(17.4%)	

satisfactory aspirates for cytological diagnosis in 91 per cent of cases and correctly diagnosed the condition of 16 out of 17 patients subsequently found to have endometrial hyperplasia on curettage or in a surgical specimen.

Segadal and Iversen in a recent study of 150 women with premenopausal and postmenopausal bleeding found that in diagnosis of postmenopausal endometrial disease cytologic specimens were more effective than histologic specimens obtained at the time of curettage. On the basis of this experience they plan to change their methods of evaluation of the patient with postmenopausal bleeding. Instead of routinely performing curettage, they plan to accept a normal clinical examination combined with normal endometrial cytologic findings and normal cervical cytology as sufficient examination. Only if abnormalities are detected will a curettage be performed.

In our own experience with a prospective study in patients with postmenopausal bleeding we have obtained endometrial cytological specimens in the last 205 patients admitted to the hospital for postmenopausal bleeding. There were 44 cases of endometrial carcinoma among this group and in only one instance was a suspicious or a positive diagnosis of carcinoma undetected, and in a second instance the slide was not properly prepared (Table 4).

Hysterography, although employed frequently in routine evaluation of the infertile patient, should be used more often in the patient with abnormal uterine bleeding. This technique may help to diagnose an unsuspected submucous myoma or an endometrial polyp. In some instances the extent of endometrial carcinomatous growth may be ascertained. Hysteroscopy seems to be gradually coming into its own.[47] Those physicians interested in infertility problems have been able to dissect uterine adhesions and have discovered unsuspected uterine polyps and myomas. Perhaps as interest in careful evaluation of the endometrium develops and perhaps to reduce the number of major surgical procedures now used for unexplained uterine bleeding, use of outpatient endometrial sampling and hysteroscopy will help the clinician monitor the endometrium more scientifically.

REFERENCES

1. Bartelmez, C. W.: Menstruation. Physiol. Rev. 17:28, 1937.
2. Markee, J. E.: Menstruation in intraocular transplants in the rhesus monkey. Contr. Embryol. Carneg. Inst. 28:219, 1940.
3. Noyes, R. W., Hertig, A. T. and Rock, J.: Dating the endometrial biopsy. Fertil. Steril. 1:3, 1950.
4. Israel, R., Mishell, D. R., Jr. and Labudovich, C. D. R.: Mechanism of normal and dysfunctional uterine bleeding. Clin. Obstet. Gynecol. 13:386, 1970.
5. Scommegna, A. and Dmowski, W. P.: Dysfunctional uterine bleeding. Clin. Obstet. Gynecol. 16:221, 1973.
6. Sutherland, A. M.: Histology of the endometrium in organic uterine hemorrhage. Lancet 2:742, 1950.
7. Taw, R. L.: Review of menstrual disorders in which a secretory endometrium was found. Am. J. Obstet. Gynecol. 122:490, 1975.
8. Quick, A. J.: Menstruation in bleeding disorders. Obstet. Gynecol. 28:37, 1966.
9. Snaith, L.: Menorrhagia due to essential thrombocytopenia. Lancet 2:684, 1940.
10. Taymor, M. L., Sturgis, S. H. and Yahia, C.: The etiological role of chronic iron deficiency in production of menorrhagia. J.A.M.A. 18:323, 1964.
11. Zondek, B.: On the mechanism of uterine bleeding. Am. J. Obstet. Gynecol. 68:310, 1954.
12. Vellios, F.: Endometrial hyperplasia, precursors of endometrial carcinoma. Pathol. Annu. 7:201, 1972.
13. Cramer, D. W. and Cutler, S. J.: Incidence and histopathology of malignancies of the female genital organs in the United States. Am. J. Obstet. Gynecol. 118:443, 1974.
14. Vuopala, S.: Diagnostic accuracy and clinical applicability of cytological and histological methods for investigating endometrial carcinoma. Acta Obstet. Gynecol. Scand. (Suppl.)10:1, 1977.
15. Smith, D. C., Prentice, R., Thompson, D. J. and Hermann, W. L.: Association of exogenous estrogen and endometrial carcinoma. N. Engl. J. Med. 293:1164, 1975.
16. Weiss, N. S., Szekely, D. R. and Austin, D. F.:

Increasing incidence of endometrial cancer in the United States. N. Engl. J. Med. 294:1259, 1976.

17. Salmi, T.: Risk factors in endometrial carcinoma with special reference to the use of estrogens. Acta Obstet. Gynecol. Scand. (Suppl.)86:1, 1979.

18. Wynder, E. L., Escher, G. C. and Mantel, N.: An epidemiologic investigation of cancer of the endometrium. Cancer 19:489, 1966.

19. MacMahon, B.: Risk factor for endometrial cancer. Gynecol. Oncol. 2:122, 1974.

20. Jelovsek et al.: Risk of exogenous estrogen therapy and endometrial cancer. Am. J. Obstet. Gynecol. 137:85, 1980.

21. Graham, J.: The value of preoperative or postoperative treatment by radium for carcinoma of the uterine body. Surg. Gynecol. Obstet. 132:855, 1971.

22. Shah, A. and Green, T. H., Jr.: Evaluation of current management of endometrial carcinoma. Obstet. Gynecol. 39:500, 1972.

23. Nilsen, P. A. and Loller, O.: Carcinoma of the endometrium in Norway 1957–1960 with special reference to treatment results. Am. J. Obstet. Gynecol. 105:1099, 1969.

24. Jones, H. W., III: Treatment of adenocarcinoma of the endometrium. Obstet. Gynecol. Surv. 30:147, 1975.

25. Barber, K. W., Jr., Dockerty, M. B., Pratt, J. H. and Hunt, A. B.: Prognosis in endometrial carcinoma by modified Dukes' typing. Surg. Gynecol. Obstet. 114:155, 1962.

26. Cheon, H. K.: Prognosis of endometrial carcinoma. Obstet. Gynecol. 34:680, 1969.

27. Creasman, W. T., Boronow, R. C., Morrow, C. P., DiSaia, P. J. and Blessing, J.: Adenocarcinoma of the endometrium: its metastatic lymph node potential. Gynecol. Oncol. 4:239, 1976.

28. Malkasian, G., Jr., McDonald, T. W. and Pratt, J. H.: Carcinoma of the endometrium: Mayo Clinic experience. Mayo Clin. Proc. 52:175, 1977.

29. Pratt, J. H., Symmonds, R. E. and Welch, J. S.: Vaginal hysterectomy for carcinoma of the fundus. Am. J. Obstet. Gynecol. 88:1063, 1964.

30. Candiani, G. B., Mangioni, C. and Marzi, M. M.: Surgery in endometrial cancer: age, route, and operability rate in 854 stage I and II fresh consecutive cases: 1915–1976. Gynecol. Oncol. 6:363, 1978.

31. Prem, K. A., Adcock, L. L., Okagaki, T. and Jones, T. K.: The evaluation of a treatment program for adenocarcinoma of the endometrium. Am. J. Obstet. Gynecol. 133:803, 1979.

32. Norris, H. J. and Taylor, H. B.: Mesenchymal tumors of the uterus. I. A clinical and pathological study of 53 endometrial stromal tumors. Cancer 19:755, 1966.

33. Norris, H. J., Roth, E. and Taylor, H. B.: Mesenchymal tumors of the uterus. II. A clinical and pathological study of 31 mixed mesodermal tumors. Obstet. Gynecol. 28:57, 1966.

34. Norris, H. J. and Taylor, H. B.: Mesenchymal tumors of the uterus. III. A clinical and pathological study of 31 carcinosarcomas. Cancer 19:1459, 1966.

35. Yoonessi, M. and Hart, W. R.: Endometrial stromal sarcomas. Cancer 40:898, 1977.

36. DiSaia, P. J., Morrow, G. P., Boronow, R., Creasman, W. and Mittelstaedt, L.: Endometrial sarcoma: lymphatic spread pattern. Am. J. Obstet. Gynecol. 130:104, 1978.

37. Ng, A. B. P., Reagan, J. W., Hawliczek, S. and Wentz, W. B.: Significance of endometrial cells in the detection of endometrial carcinoma and its precursors. Acta Cytol. 18:356, 1974.

38. Wachtel, E.: The diagnostic accuracy of vaginal smears for detection of endometrial carcinoma. Acta Cytol. 2:582, 1958.

39. Berg, J. W. and Durfee, G. R.: The cytological presentation of endometrial carcinoma. Cancer 11:158, 1958.

40. Weid, G. L.: Hormonal evaluation by means of vaginal cytology of patients with endometrial carcinoma. Acta Cytol. 2:629, 1958.

41. Liu, W.: Hypoestrogenism and endometrial carcinoma. Acta Cytol. 14:583, 1970.

42. Cohen, C. J. and Gusberg, S. B.: Screening for endometrial cancer. Clin. Obstet. Gynecol. 18:27, 1975.

43. Isaacs, J. H. and Wilhoite, R. W.: Aspiration cytology of the endometrium; office and hospital sampling procedures. Am. J. Obstet. Gynecol. 118:679, 1974.

44. Reagan, J. W. and Ng, A. B. P.: The cells of uterine adenocarcinoma, 2nd ed. Monographs in Clinical Cytology. Basel, S. Karger, 1973.

45. Hutton, J. D., Morse, A. R., Anderson, M. C. and Beard, R. W.: Endometrial assessment with Isaacs cell sampler. Br. Med. J. 1:947, 1978.

46. Segadal, E. and Iversen, O. E.: The Isaacs cell sampler: an alternative to curettage. Br. Med. J. 281:364, 1980.

47. Behrman, S. J.: Hysteroscopy: an overview. Clin. Obstet. Gynecol. 19:307, 1976.

Diagnosis and Treatment of Endometrial Neoplasia

H. Jack Schmidt, M.D.
John R. Davis, M.D.
University of Arizona Health Sciences Center

Despite advances in early detection and control of cervical cancer, no substantial progress has been attained in dealing with early endometrial neoplasia. Invasive cervical carcinoma has shown an absolute increase, reversing the ratio between the cancers of several decades ago. It has been established that carcinoma of the endometrium is the most common malignancy of the female reproductive tract. The projected number of new cases is 28,000 per year, which will result in 3300 deaths.[1] A renewed interest in management has therefore surfaced, and the review of previously established and often dogmatic treatment policies is being carried out in many institutions.

Etiology

Many etiologic factors have been implicated as influencing the endometrium to undergo malignant change. These include anatomic and physiologic factors such as obesity, low parity and late "bloody" menopause. Ovarian abnormalities resulting in the production of unopposed estrogen have been implicated.[2] Exogenous factors, including previous pelvic irradiation and the administration of systemic estrogens, have been demonstrated to have an association with endometrial neoplasia. Estrogen administration would appear to be related both to dosage and duration of use.[3] However, conclusive proof of the relationship of exogenous estrogen and endometrial cancer remains to be defined. Improved living standards with increased longevity as well as a decreasing incidence of invasive cervical cancer may also play a role in bringing endometrial malignancy to the forefront of gynecologic cancer.

Cytology

We have witnessed a definite improvement in cytodiagnostic approaches for detecting endometrial neoplasia. From the initially proposed vaginal pool to endocervical aspirates to direct fundal aspiration or brushing, a progressive enhancement in cytodiagnostic accuracy has occurred. Samples from the lower tract include cervical epithelia, and evaluation of endometrial cells may be compromised. Our experience with endocervical aspiration cytology reflects the sampling problem of this technique. Because of endocervical topography and dependency upon exfoliation of endometrial cells, in one third of our endocervical aspirates that contained abnormal glandular cells, the cells were derived from cervical lesions (reparative changes, dysplastic cervical glands and squamous dysplasias). This error can be avoided by direct sampling of the fundus by the brush technique described in succeeding paragraphs. We have adopted the technique at our institution with satisfying results. The Gravlee Jet Washer has also been shown to be highly effective in sampling the fundus cytologically and histologically.[4]

Direct fundic cytological sampling is an office procedure. Perhaps it should be directed as a screening test to all women beyond 50 years with closer monitoring of high-risk individuals (sustained anovulation, perimenopausal bleeding and so forth). The full potential of the cytologic method will not be realized if the postmenopausal woman is not tested periodically but seeks medical help only with the appearance of bleeding, as is usually the case. It would seem desirable to cultivate early detection if an impact upon the control of endometrial cancer is to be made.

Histopathology

GLANDULAR HYPERPLASIA

Instead of recreating an ambiguous and often subjective classification of potentially precancerous growth disturbances of the endometrium, attention will be directed to several problem areas.

EXTENT OF HYPERPLASIA. The usual concept of hyperplasia is that of excessive tissue readily recognized in either a hysterectomy specimen as thickened, lush endometrium or in curettings as voluminous samples. Hyperplasia may be focal and microscopic without satisfying the gross criteria for recognition, yet its biologic significance is not necessarily changed. Polypoid hyperplasia is an example of focal growth disturbance that retains features of excessive tissue. Since polyps are focal mucosal excrescences, they do not necessarily denote precancerous lesions. Polyps may consist of normal endometrium, hyperplasia (glands, stroma or both), or carcinoma. The clinical significance of polyps may be derived from the polyp itself (its bulk and threatened vasculature) independent of tissue composition.

INADEQUATE BIOPSY SPECIMEN. The occasional endometrial biopsy that a laboratory labels "insufficient for diagnosis" deserves comment. Certainly biopsy specimens obtained in an office procedure may be small and perplexing to the pathologist, but the information available may be significant to the gynecologist. Even a tiny specimen consisting of a few fragmented glands helps to exclude a profuse hyperplastic or malignant lesion. The character and mitotic activity of the epithelium may be quite helpful in assessing the growth activity and orderliness of the tissue. Careful scrutiny of tiny biopsy specimens may provide the surgeon with sufficient information to design management without forcing the significant procedure of dilatation and curettage. Pathologists should be urged to abandon reporting "no diagnosis" and to strive for descriptions of glandular epithelium regardless of the gland number. Due caution is appropriate in dealing with small specimens lest the gynecologist presume that they are fully representative of the endometrium.

TYPE OF HYPERPLASIA. The histopathologic recognition of endometrial hyerplasia requires an appreciation of normal cycling, noncycling and well-differentiated malignant endometria. Problems in diagnosis are found at either end of the structural spectrum. Physiologic growth of endometrium in the cycling tissue retains a pattern of orderly, uniform gland size, distribution and profile with regular cytologic characteristics. In hyperplasia some or all of these features are irregular. Following a series of anovulatory cycles, the appearance of sustained proliferative endometrium may approach a hyperplastic pattern with no reliable morphologic criteria available for distinguishing one from the other. A comparable problem occurs in attempting to separate morphologically an atypical or severe degree of hyperplasia from well-differentiated carcinoma. Pathologists should strive to communicate any lack of clear distinction. Decisions of management rest with the gynecologist, and should not be confounded by inappropriate classification when morphologic distinctions are not valid.

Characterization of the type of hyperplasia has suffered from overclassification and ambiguous terminology;[5] simplification would be helpful. That glandular hyperplasia possesses a precancerous potential is well accepted,[6] and the most useful indicator of biological behavior is the epithelial abnormality. Distinction between cystic and adenomatous hyperplasia may not be particularly useful, even though the former is acknowledged to be less a risk factor in cancer. Cystic change is usually an atrophic process and should not be confused with active cellular hyperplasia. Attention is appropriately directed to epithelial abnormality, not solely glandular conformation.

Hyperplastic epithelium has mitoses and usually takes the form of increased number of glandular units, so that their concentration per unit area is increased. It remains useful to grade the degree of abnormality in terms of mild (orderliness of epithelium remains), moderate (gland profiles irregular but cells fairly regular and orderly), and severe ("marked," "atypical": pleomorphic nuclei with orientation aberrations). Grading serves a role in management decisions, although it is not an infallible guide to risk of malignancy. In this context "carcinoma in situ" is not a particularly useful designation, since a comparable danger signal is registered by "severe (or atypical) adenomatous hyperplasia."

ADENOCARCINOMA

The type of adenocarcinoma influences design of therapy and prognosis. It has become well accepted that adenocarcinoma with mature squamous metaplasia (adenoacanthoma) has neither a better nor a worse prognosis than pure adenocarcinoma. However, a rise in the incidence of adenosquamous carcinoma has occurred and does affect prognosis.[7] In this malignancy both glandular and squamous components are morphologically malignant and invasive. Stage for stage, this neoplasm is comparable to adenocarcinoma but tends to present at a more advanced stage and is biologically more aggressive.

Grading remains a useful characterization by which to represent degree of differentiation. The Broders system uses grades 1 through 4; grade 1 is well differentiated. Although it is invasive into stroma, it otherwise resembles the gland pattern of hyperplastic endometrium; grade 4 is poorly differentiated or anaplastic. The International Federation of Gynecology and Obstetrics (IFGO) system of grading uses grades 1 through 3; grade 1 is composed of Broders' grade 1 and 2 (see p. 596).

Diagnosis

Peak incidence of endometrial cancer occurs in the postmenopausal age group, and accordingly postmenopausal bleeding is the prime presenting symptom. Formal fractional dilatation and curettage under anesthesia has remained the keystone for evaluating abnormal uterine bleeding. Unfortunately, standardized technique is not always adhered to, outpatient biopsy and cytologic techniques are often bypassed, and misdiagnosis (particularly of cervical extension of tumor) has been reported to be as high as 22 per cent.[8] Both surgical technique and histologic criteria are important in avoiding this discrepancy. Our suggested approach to evaluating the cancer suspect follows.

OUTPATIENT CYTOLOGY AND BIOPSY

Many patients can be effectively and economically evaluated for abnormal bleeding in the office setting. Patient acceptance is directly related to the time and effort used in explaining the procedure as well as using careful technique. Paracervical block can be effectively used as deemed necessary or routinely if desired. Our usual procedure is as follows:

1. A routine pelvic and rectovaginal examination is carried out, and cervical cytology (including a scraping and endocervical aspiration) is obtained.

2. Endocervical curettage with a standard endocervical curette is done *before sounding or dilating* of the endocervical canal.

3. The uterine cavity is sounded and the depth recorded in centimeters.

4. A sleeved endometrial brush (Cystayd) is inserted, the sleeve withdrawn and the endometrium sampled by rotating the brush within the cavity. The material is then spread on two glass slides, placed in 95 per cent alcohol fixative and submitted for staining and evaluation by the usual "Pap smear" technique.

5. Endometrial biopsy specimens (four quadrants or more) are taken with a small sharp curette or Novak aspiration curette and submitted for histologic evaluation.

Utilizing these techniques when applicable has been both accurate and rewarding in evaluating abnormal bleeding. The studies by Creasman and Weed, as well as others, support the accuracy of similar screening techniques in evaluating the endometrium.[9] Their findings indicate a greater than 90 per cent accuracy and approach 100 per cent when negative findings associated with a recent D&C are eliminated. It must be emphasized, however, that in order to rely on these techniques, adequate samples should be obtained. If adequate sampling is not achieved, formal dilatation and curettage is indicated.

FRACTIONAL DILATATION AND CURETTAGE UNDER ANESTHESIA

This technique should be implemented under the following circumstances, procedurally following the previously described techniques:

1. Persistent bleeding in spite of adequate but negative cytology and biopsy.

2. Inadequate sampling on outpatient basis.

3. Patient unsuitability for office cytology and biopsy.

Another point of emphasis is that a diagnosis of endocervical involvement with tumor should be made only when adequate endocervical tissue is obtained with either gross tumor or microscopic tumor in continuity with endocervical tissue. In this way "floaters" may be disregarded and the accuracy of staging maintained.

Pretreatment Evaluation

Pretreatment evaluation routinely includes CBC, renal and liver function studies, chest x-ray and intravenous pyelogram. Cystoscopy, radiologic evaluation of the bowel and proctoscopy are optional procedures employed on an individual basis only. Lymphangiography has been advocated by some to detect node metastasis and to direct adjuvant therapy. Our preference is to sample pelvic and para-aortic lymph nodes during surgical staging and implement adjuvant therapy on the basis of histologic findings. This will be further addressed. However, lymphangiography may be helpful in the nonsurgical candidate.

Treatment

Treatment of noninvasive endometrial neoplasia has been adequately discussed in the preceding edition.[10] The treatment of endometrial cancer over the years has fallen into a rather standardized regimen. Stage I disease has been treated surgically alone, in combination with irradiation or in some circumstances with irradiation alone.[11, 12] In fact, one can find a literature-supported series to justify a variety of treatment plans. Unfortunately, lack of standardization in comparing various studies has made interpretation difficult. Current standardized protocols through group study efforts will perhaps clarify optimal treatment programs in the future.

Our current treatment approach is based on the proven value of both surgery and irradiation but is individualized on the basis of the clinical, histologic and surgical staging. This includes the sampling of pelvic and para-aortic lymph nodes as outlined by Creasman et al.[13] In stage I disease, primary surgery or surgery immediately following irradiation (48 to 72 hours) is utilized in order to better define and preserve histologic indicators. The safety and low morbidity of this approach as reported by Underwood[12] and others reflects our experience. The treatment plan and options are as follows:

STAGE IAG1. Primary treatment in this lesion is surgical, consisting of laparotomy with peritoneal washings, total hysterectomy with bilateral salpingo-oophorectomy and selective pelvic and para-aortic node sampling. Careful histologic evaluation is carried out with adjunctive irradiation added as follows:

1. Superficial disease (inner one third myometrium) with negative nodes, no further treatment.

2. Disease beyond inner third but less than 50 per cent with negative nodes, postoperative vaginal cuff radium.

3. Fifty per cent invasion or greater, positive nodes, or occult cervical extension, whole pelvic irradiation with para-aortic additive when indicated.

STAGE IAG2–G3 OR IBG1–G3. In these stages preoperative tandem and Colpostat radium application is utilized followed by immediate surgery (48 to 72 hours) to include pelvic and para-aortic node sampling. Postoperative whole pelvic and split field irradiation is added based on the findings of greater than 50 per cent myometrial invasion, positive nodes or gross cervical extension.

STAGE II. Several options are utilized in managing cervical extension of endometrial cancer. If the disease is judged to be clinically superficial, our approach is the same as described in the preceding paragraph—namely preoperative radium followed by surgery with node sampling. Postoperative external irradiation may be added on the basis of histologic findings. With gross cervical involvement, however, preoperative whole pelvic irradiation, radium and hysterectomy with para-aortic node sampling is utilized, with para-aortic irradiation given later if nodes are positive.

STAGE III. Primary treatment of disease beyond the uterus is radiotherapeutic using combined external and internal irradiation with hysterectomy utilized on a selective basis.

STAGE IV. Disease extending beyond the pelvis is treated selectively with combined irradiation and chemotherapy. Progesterone is a first-line choice; with the availability of receptor site assays, individuals can be selected upon a rational basis for adjuvant therapy. Other chemotherapeutic agents (Adriamycin, Cytoxan, Melphalan and fluorouracil) have been utilized with some response.

Comment

With the ascendancy of endometrial cancer, an optimal and more specific therapeutic approach is bound to evolve. Current studies with estrogen-progesterone receptor assays reveal their potential importance in the management of endometrial cancer. They should be obtained when available at the time of surgery or by biopsy in cases of metastatic disease.[14, 15] Another prognostic indicator being defined is the presence of positive peritoneal cytology at the time of surgery for endometrial cancer. Positive cytology has been associated with a significant recurrence rate in spite of adequate therapy by current standards.[16]

REFERENCES

1. Cancer Facts and Figures: American Cancer Society, 1978.
2. Chamlian, D. L. and Taylor, H. B.: Endometrial hyperplasia in young women. Obstet. Gynecol. 36:659, 1970.
3. Gray, L. A., Christopherson, W. M. and Hoover, R. N.: Estrogens and endometrial carcinoma. Obstet. Gynecol. 49:385, 1977.
4. White, A. J., Buchsbaum, H. J. and Rodman, N. F.: Accuracy of the Gravlee Jet Washer in detecting endometrial adenocarcinoma. Am. J. Obstet. Gynecol. 116:1169, 1973.
5. Gore, H.: The Uterus, International Academy of Pathology Monograph. Baltimore, Williams and Wilkins, 1973.
6. Dallenbach-Hellweg, G.: Histopathology of the Endometrium. New York, Springer-Verlag, 1971.
7. Ng, A. B. P., Reagan, J. W., Storaasli, J. P. and Wentz, W. B.: Mixed adenosquamous carcinoma of the endometrium. Am. J. Clin. Pathol. 59:765, 1973.
8. Welander, C., Griem, M. L., Newton, M. and Marks, J. E.: Staging and treatment of endometrial carcinoma. J. Reprod. Med. 8:41, 1972.
9. Creasman, W. T. and Weed, J. C., Jr.: Screening techniques in endometrial cancer. Cancer 28:436, 1976.
10. Reid, D. E. and Christian, C. D.: Controversy in Obstetrics and Gynecology II. Philadelphia, W. B. Saunders Co., 1974.
11. Keller, D., Kempson, R., Levine, G. and McLennon, C.: Management of the patient with early endometrial carcinoma. Cancer 33:1108, 1974.
12. Underwood, P., Lutz, M., Kreutner, A., Miller, M. and Johnson, R., Jr.: Carcinoma of the endometrium. Radiation followed immediately by operation. Am. J. Obstet. Gynecol. 128:86, 1977.
13. Creasman, W. T., Boronow, R. C., Morrow, C. P., DiSaia, P. J. and Bleasing, J.: Adenocarcinoma of the endometrium: 2 + 2 metastatic lymph node potential. A preliminary report. Gynecol. Oncol. 4:239, 1976.
14. Kohom, E. I.: Gestagens and endometrial carcinoma. Gynecol. Oncol. 4:398, 1976.
15. Ehrlich, C. E.: Response of endometrial adenocarcinoma to progestin therapy related to concentration of receptors in cancer cells. Presented to Gynecologic Oncology Group, Beverly Hills, California, July, 1977.
16. Creasman, W. T.: Personal communication.

Editorial Comment

How to manage a patient with an abnormal endometrium may become a matter of controversy. Adenomatous hyperplasia of the endometrium may be a precursor to carcinoma of the endometrium. The statistics on this occurrence are rather solid in that some 30 per cent of these lesions progress over a 10-year period to carcinoma of the endometrium. Gusberg has been a pioneer in elucidating the fact that adenomatous hyperplasia is a precursor to carcinoma of the endometrium and in educating us about this. The clear and simple statements of the controversy and the solutions are vintage Gusberg, but careful reading is necessary. Mild and moderate adenomatous hyperplasia (types I and II) may lead to carcinoma of the endometrium but at much lower percentages than severe (type III) adenomatous hyperplasia. Patients with mild and moderate hyperplasia may be followed with appropriate sampling and treated with progestational agents.

Hysterectomy is not indicated every time the word hyperplasia appears on the pathology report from endometrial sampling. The gynecologist must be aware of what the pathologist means by his terminology; hence, the importance of also examining the biopsy material. It is disconcerting to see an automatic hysterectomy performed whenever "hyperplasia" appears on a report, since this may not be in the best interests of the patient.

There currently is much wringing of hands regarding the association between exogenous estrogen therapy and carcinoma of the endometrium. We welcome the solid data and believe that such incidence figures put us in a much better position to properly care for our patients. It is clear that with exogenous estrogen compounds in amounts of or equivalent to 1.25 mg of conjugated estrogen increase the incidence of carcinoma of the endometrium some fourfold if taken for as long as three to four years. But the common denominator is important—fourfold of what incidence? The de novo incidence of carcinoma of the endometrium is one per thousand women over 50 years of age per year (1/1000/year). Thus therapy as just mentioned means this increases the incidence to 4/1000/year, a risk many women may gladly accept when symptoms of the menopause and problems of osteoporosis are considered. This increased risk ratio of 4 moves back to 1 in a period of 2 years after the estrogen is stopped. It should be remembered that this is exactly the patient who is under surveillance and who should have the endometrium monitored periodically. We find no basis for handwringing but take great comfort from the fact that such incidence figures are known—would that such could be the case for all medications. No incidence figures are available to ascertain the effect of the way estrogen is administered and the effect of its use in conjunction with progesterone, but we believe these effects are much less severe than those produced by estrogen alone. Our method of administering estrogen to the postmenopausal woman results in less bleeding. We believe that estrogen should be administered orally, in the lowest dose necessary to prevent symptoms, Monday through Friday but not Saturday and Sunday. This permits endometrial blood vessel regression in 2 of 7 days and prevents overstimulation. Additionally, every three months oral progesterone in conjunction with the estrogen is administered for 7 days and stopped. If uterine bleeding follows, the regimen is continued until no more uterine bleeding takes place, at which time the progesterone medication is then given at cycles twice a year.

It is important to reassure the patient that the endometrium is normal or atrophic. This can be done only by using the endometrial sampling techniques outlined by the authors in this chapter. Hofmeister and Stanhope utilize the Novak endometrial curette or the Hofmeister curette while Isaacs uses the Isaacs endometrial sampler. They are both excellent techniques, and the procedure provides an exact method of reassurance that the patient's endometrium is normal and that estrogen therapy may be continued.

There is no disagreement about the remainder of the material contained in the chapter.

23
Carcinoma in Situ

Alternative Points of View

by Bengt Bjerre and Nils-Otto Sjöberg
by William T. Creasman and John C.
Weed, Jr.

Editorial Comment

Role of Conization in the Treatment of Dysplasia and Cervical Carcinoma in Situ

Bengt Bjerre, M.D.
Nils-Otto Sjöberg, M.D., Ph.D.
Allmänna Sjukhuset, University of Lund

Some 20 years ago, when many cases of carcinoma in situ of the uterine cervix began to be detected cytologically, most gynecologists believed that if left untreated, this lesion would soon become invasive. Therefore, hysterectomy or even more extensive measures were considered indicated. As far back as the 1950s several gynecologists started to use conization not only as a diagnostic procedure but also as a therapeutic measure in this disease.[3, 7, 21, 24, 29] In the 1960s this practice was adopted in most hospitals in Scandinavia[1, 4, 5, 22] as well as in some places in Canada[8] and the United States.[17, 18] But many gynecologists still believe that a diagnosis of cervical carcinoma in situ indicates hysterectomy without delay.

Since experience has taught that the frequency of complications attending conization is low, that the procedure means only a minor operation for the patient and a much smaller burden for the hospital than hysterectomy[5] and that it is still adequate for this disease,[6] we think that hysterectomy is not warranted in most cases of cervical carcinoma in situ.

When cytology is used over a considerable period, the newly diagnosed cases will be found mostly in young women,[11, 13, 14] who, at least in Sweden, often wish to preserve their fertility.[1, 6] This means a strong argument for conservative management of most cases of this disease detected nowadays.

The problem is, however, not only how to treat cervical carcinoma in situ but also how to treat dysplasia. The relationship between dysplasia, cervical carcinoma in situ and invasive cancer has puzzled many. Koss, who published a survey of the problem,[23] stressed that it is often impossible not only for the cytologist but also for the pathologist to differentiate between cervical carcinoma in situ and severe dysplasia. It therefore appears natural to choose the same kind of treatment for both types of lesions. Since even mild dysplasia might progress to cervical cancer,[30] these lesions should also be eradicated. The number of women who must be examined and treated because of cytologic changes is large. Therefore, therapeutic measures even less extensive than conization have been proposed. Wedge excision,[2, 15] cryosurgery[9, 10, 12, 13, 19, 31, 34] or

617

electrocoagulation[16] after colposcopic examination may be sufficient in selected cases. Since the alternative treatment in these cases seems to be knife conization, it might be of interest to compare the advantages and disadvantages of the various methods.

Since assessment of the reliability of conization in cervical cancer or dysplasia requires a long follow-up, we must use a series of patients in whom treatment was begun in past years. Between 1960 and 1970, 2099 women underwent conization at the Women's Clinic in Malmö, University of Lund, because of abnormal cytologic findings.[5, 6] During the period in question only 67 women were primarily treated in some way other than conization, and then because of coexisting findings.

Indications for Conization

It is practically always abnormal smears that lead to a diagnosis of cervical carcinoma in situ or dysplasia. In our opinion, an abnormal smear always warrants colposcopic examination. Such an examination will generally enable the gynecologist to decide whether further diagnostic procedures such as punch biopsy are warranted or if therapeutic measures such as conization should be performed without delay. In 1975 Nelson et al. wrote an excellent paper for the American Cancer Society, entitled "Dysplasia and Early Cervical Cancer." We agree with most of the points they made but would at the same time mention that in the 1960s—when our large series of patients who had conization were being treated—we did not take full advantage of colposcopy. At that time, when changes in smears were thought to be consistent with either carcinoma in situ or severe dysplasia, we usually performed conization without preceding punch biopsy.

Reliability of Cytology

Both the cytologic and histopathologic nomenclature may vary among different laboratories,[35] making comparisons between different series material difficult. The cytologist should not be expected to be able to make a firm diagnosis. His report should, however, be a guide for the gynecologist as to the histologic diagnosis to be expected at examination of an *adequate* biopsy specimen.

In 1960 to 1970 a cytologic report of a "positive" or "suspicious" smear at our hospital was regarded as indicating conization if clinical examination did not reveal invasive cancer. If a smear was "positive" we expected to find a histologic diagnosis of invasive cancer, carcinoma in situ or severe dysplasia. In 10 per cent of our patients having conization because of a "positive" smear, the histologic examination showed slight dysplasia, an inflammatory process or a totally benign condition. Serial sections of the cone might have shown more serious changes, but we believe that the 20 to 30 routinely examined blocks from the cone usually gave the desired information. We also think a cytologic "overdiagnosis" of 10 per cent is acceptable in order to keep down the false-negative rate.

In cases reported as "suspicious smear" our false-positive rate, by the same definition, was 18 per cent. We think this is acceptable. Thus, in our department, a cytologic report of a "positive" or "suspicious" smear in the 1960s was an indication for conization without preceding punch biopsy, provided that the clinical examination had not produced evidence of invasive cancer.

Large Cones and Small Cones

The technique used in conization varies widely,[32] which may explain the lack of agreement on the therapeutic value of the operation as well as differences in the frequency of complications. Some gynecologists remove only an extremely small portion of the cervix, an operation that would more appropriately be called ring biopsy. Such an operation is warranted only if colposcopic examination strongly suggests that all the atypical epithelial tissue can be removed with it. On the other hand, some gynecologists remove almost the entire cervix—virtually cervical amputation. In these cases the chances of removing all the epithelium affected are good, but such a radical operation markedly increases the risk of complications, especially in subsequent pregnancies. Owing to these differences in the amount of tissue removed it is impossible to get more than a vague idea of cure rates and frequency of complications of conization if the technique used for it is not specified.

Our Technique of Conization

Sutures are placed on both sides of the cervix and include the descending branches of the uterine artery. These sutures provide an excellent grip of the cervix, which is particularly valuable in the event of postoperative bleeding. Synthetic vasopressin solution is injected into the cervix to secure hemostasis. Lugol's solution is applied to the cervix (Schiller's test) to determine how wide the base of the cone should be. Hegar dilators are used to determine the position of the internal os and thus the height of the cone. Especially in younger women it is essential that the tip of the cone should not reach the internal os. Conization is performed with a special curved knife (Häljestrand). The wound is left unsutured and undressed. During the operation the patient is given 1 g of Cyklokapron (tranexamic acid) intravenously in 200 ml of 5.5 per cent glucose. This fibrinolytic antagonist reduces bleeding during operation. After operation it is given by mouth in a dose of 1 g 4 times a day for 10 days.[33]

Histologic Examination

The cones are fixed in 10 per cent neutral formalin. After fixation the cut surfaces are painted with 10 per cent lapis for marking and the cones are cut into sections 2 mm thick and embedded in paraffin. The top of the cone is cut transversely, the rest sagittally. As a rule, 20 to 30 paraffin blocks are obtained. The sections are stained with hematoxylin and eosin. When the cones are low or ragged, no transverse sections can be obtained and the entire cone is cut into sagittal sections. Such raggedness also sometimes makes it difficult to decide whether the operation is radical.

Radical and Not Radical Conization

The therapeutic effect of conization depends mainly on whether all the pathologic epithelium has been removed or not. The histologist must therefore carefully examine the resection margins. When these are free from changes we regard the operation as radical irrespective of the size of the cone. When the examination shows atypical epithelium at any of the resection margins, the operation is called "not radical." In some instances in this series the cone was low or ragged, which made the result of the histologic examination of the resection margins uncertain. In these cases the conization was said to be "doubtful."

Complications After Conization

For uncomplicated conization the average number of hospital days in our series was four. Postoperative bleeding was the most common complication and occurred in 11 per cent of patients. Since introduction of preoperative vasopressin infiltration of the cervix and prophylactic use of Cyklokapron, postoperative bleeding has been less severe. The bleeding can usually be controlled by further infiltration of vasopressin solution. Of the last 1060 women in our series undergoing conization, only 4 required blood transfusion or suture of the cervix. The only serious complication of conization was perforation of the cervix in the pouch of Douglas, which occurred in five cases in the beginning of our series and made laparotomy necessary. However, this complication has not occurred in any of the 2500 women undergoing conization since that time.

In 4 per cent conization was followed by dysmenorrhea. In two thirds of these cases there was clear stenosis of the cervix, which could usually be cured by dilatation of the cervix with Hegar dilators. Only rarely does cervical stenosis persist during pregnancy and require special measures such as manual dilatation of the cervix during delivery.

Pregnancies After Conization

Pregnancies before and after conization in 1285 women who had undergone conization and who were younger than 40 years of age at the time of the operation were counted. The numbers of deliveries and of spontaneous and legal abortions are given in Table 1. Of the 1112 children born before conization and whose birth weights were known, 122 (11 per cent) weighed 2500 g or less. The corresponding figure for the 311 children born after conization was 32 (10 per cent). The frequency of low birth weight was twice as high in this material as in the country as a whole, but the

TABLE 1. OUTCOME OF PREGNANCIES IN 1285 WOMEN BEFORE AND AFTER CONIZATION

	BEFORE CONIZATION		AFTER CONIZATION	
	No.	Percentage	No.	Percentage
Delivery	2029	83.7	331	70.0
Spontaneous abortion	280	11.6	81	17.1
Legal abortion	114	4.7	61	12.9
Pregnancies	2423		473	

frequency was equally high before as after conization. The parous women had a low birth weight rate of 8 per cent after conization, while women who had delivered their first child after conization had a low birth weight frequency of 16 per cent. The difference was not statistically significant, but similar figures have been reported in another Swedish investigation.[25] It is possible that there is a greater risk of removing too much tissue of the smaller cervix of nulliparous women than of parous women, who often have a larger cervix.[27]

The frequency of spontaneous abortion of 12 per cent before conization corresponded well to that in our total population. After conization it was slightly but significantly higher (17 per cent). Practically all the abortions occurred in early pregnancy, but since some of the patients had been treated outside our hospital, it is not possible to assess the ratio between early and late abortions with certainty. It is, of course, possible that other factors, such as advancing age, are responsible for part of the increase observed.[26] The rise in the frequency of legal abortion corresponded to a similar rise in the total population. In some instances, however, long-standing sterility was cured by conization. In none of our cases did conization *cause* sterility.

Follow-up After Conization

Regardless of the type of therapy used in cervical carcinoma in situ or dysplasia a close follow-up is imperative. In our material we obtained smears 3, 6, and 12 months after conization. If such checks reveal nothing remarkable, annual review should be sufficient.

Conization as Treatment of Carcinoma in Situ

In 1500 women who underwent conization at the Womens' Clinic in Malmö from 1960 to 1970, the histologic diagnosis was carcinoma in situ. During the follow-up the uterine cervix was removed from 81 patients because of uterine myoma or prolapse. One hundred thirty-two women were lost to follow-up. After the primary conization, the vaginal smears from 1099 showed no further abnormalities. Our patients were followed for 9 to 19 years (mean 10.6) with a total of 11,630 observation years.

Only 188 of the 1500 patients with carcinoma in situ in the primary cone needed further treatment indicated by a pathologic vaginal smear. Of the 188 women, 172 had pathologic smears at the first follow-up after the primary conization (Table 2). The other 16 also required further treatment, although the first smears after the primary conization had been of normal appearance (Table 2).

When histologic examination of the first cone showed normal epithelium at the resection margins, the smears at follow-up were normal in 94 per cent of these patients (Table 2). This could suggest that in 6 per cent the disease was multifocal. Therefore, even if a conization is considered "radical," the patient must be followed closely. In patients with abnormal epithelium at the resection margins of the cone, smears at follow-up were normal in a significantly lower frequency. On the other hand, "not radical" conization was followed by normal smears in as many as 62 per cent of patients (Table 2). Table 3 gives the histologic diagnosis after reconization in the 172 patients with persistent pathologic smears after primary conization.

Data on the 16 patients in whom the smears after the conization were initially normal are given in Table 4. In four of them the smears showed changes within one year after the primary conization. In these cases reconization and histologic examination showed cervical carcinoma in situ. The other 12 had normal smears for 3 to 13 years. Five of them underwent reconization and one hysterectomy, and the histologic diagnosis was carcinoma in situ in these cases. In three cases colposcopically directed biopsy showed slight dysplasia. Two of the remaining patients had normal smears for six years. They failed to report for their

TABLE 2. VAGINAL SMEARS AFTER PRIMARY CONIZATION

SMEARS	First Cone Considered			TOTAL
	Radical	Doubtful	Not Radical	
Normal	771	154	174	1099
Still pathological after primary conization	37	32	103	172
Initially normal after primary conization	10	2	4	16

TABLE 3. Histological Diagnosis at Further Treatment in 172 Patients with Persistent Pathologic Smears After Primary Conization for Carcinoma in Situ

Histological Diagnosis After Further Treatment	First Cone Considered			Total
	Radical	Doubtful	Not Radical	
Invasive cancer	3	2	6	11
Carcinoma in situ	24	25	88	137
Dysplasia	4	2	3	9
Benign	6	3	6	15
Total	37	32	103	172

cytologic examination and when seen again 3 and 13 years later, respectively, invasive cancer was suspected. The histologic diagnosis from biopsy specimens verified the clinical diagnosis. The last patient had normal smears for five years and thereafter a pathologic smear. Reconization was performed on her at the age of 54. The histologic diagnosis was microinvasive cancer.

Selective Local Excision

At the Womens' Clinic in Lund, University of Lund, all patients with cytologic abnormalities are examined with colposcopy. Patients with small areas of colposcopically abnormal epithelium in the transformation zone are treated with local excision.[2] This is performed by means of one or several punch biopsies with Schubert biopsy forceps. In the cytologic screening program in 1967 to 1974 cervical carcinoma in situ or severe dysplasia was diagnosed in 698 patients. Of these, 366 (52 per cent) were considered candidates for local excision. After the operation cervical cytology reverted to normal or showed slight atypical patterns in 61 per cent. One hundred fifty-three patients have been followed from one to seven years. Failure of removal of the entire lesion was discovered within the first year of follow-up in all but ten of the patients.

Residual Disease and Recurrence

Irrespective of the method used in the treatment of dysplasia or cervical carcinoma in situ, the risk of residual lesions and recurrence must be assessed. Residual lesions are more common after local excision than after conization. In our opinion local excision or ring biopsy is warranted only after colposcopic examination has revealed no signs of invasive cancer and also made it probable that at operation all the affected epithelium will be removed. Our series of local excision is not large enough to warrant assessment of the recurrence rate, but so far no invasive cancer has occurred in this series. All our patients have accepted the necessity of follow-up.

In our larger series of conization, the first vaginal smear after conization showed changes suggesting residual lesions in 13 per cent of the patients. At the following operation, the residual changes were most often found in the cervical canal and were detected by cytology. Since most of the women were young and wanted to preserve their fertility, we consider the figure of 13 per cent residual changes acceptable, provided that the patients can be examined regularly. If smears remain pathologic we usually perform reconization. However, what is not acceptable is that 11 of 172 women treated for residual disease at a subsequent operation showed invasive cancer. For different reasons, further treatment in

TABLE 4. Histological Diagnosis at Further Treatment in 16 Patients with Carcinoma in Situ in the First Cone and Initially Normal Smears After the Conization

Smears Initially Normal After Conization	First Cone Considered			Histological Diagnosis After Further Treatment	
	Radical	Doubtful	Not Radical		
Pathologic within one year	2	1	1	Carcinoma in situ	(4)
Pathologic within 3–13 years	8[°+]	1[+]	3*	°Dysplasia	(3)
				[+]Invasive cancer IB	(2)
				*Invasive cancer IA	(1)
				Carcinoma in situ	(6)

Number of patients within parenthesis.

these patients had been delayed for more than one year after the primary conization. These experiences stress the need of a thorough examination of the cone specimen, a close follow-up with colposcopy and adequate endocervical sampling for cytology. If any of the findings is abnormal, further diagnostic or therapeutic steps should not be delayed without very good reason. Kolstad found as many as 7 cases of invasive cancer in follow-up of 795 women treated with conization for cervical carcinoma in situ.[22] His experience also stresses the need for thorough follow-up after hysterectomy. In his material of 238 hysterectomies, 3 patients had a recurrence of carcinoma in situ and 5 developed invasive cancer.

True recurrence after conization seems to be rare. In only 16 of 1115 patients followed for more than 5 years were initially normal smears later followed by abnormal ones. Four of these ten patients showed pathologic smears within one year after conization. This finding may indicate residual lesions also in these patients. Few investigators differentiate between residual disease and recurrence, but Sheffield[20] stresses the necessity of doing so.

The frequency of a real recurrence increases with time after primary treatment. It is therefore better to relate the recurrence frequency to the number of observation years than to the number of patients. In our experience 1099 patients with normal smears after primary conization have been followed for a total of 11,630 observation years. Sixteen patients initially had normal smears but were later treated because of pathologic smears. If all these 16 represent real recurrences appearing within 11,630 observation years, they mean a recurrence frequency of 1.4 per 1000 observation years. This is roughly the same as the incidence of carcinoma in situ.[4, 11, 14, 20, 35]

The Role of Conization

The choice of therapy for cervical carcinoma in situ and dysplasia depends on several factors. In our opinion, all patients with cytologic changes should undergo colposcopic examination. In many cases the cytologic changes are caused by infection, which must be treated before a proper assessment of the patient's condition is possible.

The cytologic suggestion of a diagnosis of cervical carcinoma in situ or dysplasia must

always be confirmed by histology. Quadrant biopsy and cervical curettage without previous colposcopy involves the risk (4 per cent) of missing an early invasive cancer. In an earlier series without colposcopy,[4] when quadrant biopsies and curettage had shown cervical carcinoma in situ, 186 patients underwent conization within six weeks. In eight cases histologic examination of the cone showed early invasive cancer. Thus, without the aid of colposcopy, the cytologic suggestion of cervical cancer or dysplasia ought to warrant diagnostic conization, which in most instances will also be therapeutic.

Colposcopy gives the possibility of individualizing treatment. Early invasive cancer can be detected on the ectocervix and proper therapy can be given without delay. If invasiveness is ruled out by colposcopy and there is a small, wholly visible lesion, the histologic differentiation between dysplasia or cervical carcinoma in situ is not essential from a therapeutic point of view as long as the entire lesion is removed by local excision, wedge excision or ring biopsy. These patients must be followed with cytology and colposcopy, and if any of these studies show residual changes or recurrence, further steps must be taken.

Cryotherapy might perhaps be applied in cases of mild and moderate dysplasia in which the whole lesion is colposcopically visible. The main disadvantage of cryotherapy is that histologic confirmation of only part of the lesion can be obtained. Furthermore, we think that experience with cryotherapy is still too limited to warrant the use of the method in cervical carcinoma in situ and severe dysplasia.

If only a part of the lesion is visible, conization is indicated because the endocervical part of the lesion might be invasive and early invasive cancer cannot be ruled out by curettage. This also applies to cases in which no lesion is visible at colposcopy. Only in the event of coexisting indications for therapy, such as myoma, do we perform hysterectomy as primary treatment of cervical carcinoma in situ and dysplasia.

The practice just set forth means that some patients with mild or moderate dysplasia might be "overtreated" by conization in order not to miss any cases of early invasive cancer. This is in our opinion acceptable, since the frequency of complications of conization with our technique is low. From a therapeutic point of view, severe dysplasia and cervical cancer in situ are to be considered as the same disease. These lesions should be removed surgically.

In many cases the choice of therapy for cervical cancer in situ is between conization and hysterectomy. Most of these cases can be managed by conization provided that adequate follow-up is arranged. A cytologic sample must always be taken from the endocervix. This usually offers no difficulty in young women, but it might sometimes do so in older women because of cervical stenosis after conization. If colposcopic examination and adequate smears show nothing remarkable during the first year after conization, the risk of recurrence is of the same order as the incidence of cervical carcinoma in situ in the general population.

REFERENCES

1. Ahlgren, M., Ingemarsson, I., Lindberg, L. G. and Nordqvist, S. R. B.: Conization as treatment of carcinoma in situ. Obstet. Gynecol. 46:135, 1975.
2. Ahlgren, M., Lindberg, L. G. and Nordqvist, S. R. B.: Management of carcinoma in situ of the uterine cervix by selective local excision. Acta Obstet. Gynecol. Scand. 56:531, 1977.
3. Bickenbach, W. and Soost, H. J.: *In* Symposium on cervical lesions. Acta Cytol. 6:163, 1962.
4. Bjerre, B.: Studies on population screening for early carcinoma of the uterine cervix. Acta Obstet. Gynecol. Scand. 48:Suppl 6, 1969.
5. Bjerre, B., Eliasson, G., Linell, F., Söderberg, H. and Sjöberg, N-O.: Conization as only treatment of carcinoma in situ of the uterine cervix. Am. J. Obstet. Gynecol. 125:143, 1976.
6. Bjerre, B., Sjöberg, N-O. and Söderberg, H.: Further treatment after conization. J. Reprod. Med. 21:232, 1978.
7. Boyes, D. A. and Fidler, H. K.: *In* Symposium on cervical lesions. Acta Cytol. 6:163, 1962.
8. Boyes, D. A., Worth, A. J. and Fidler, H. K.: The result of treatment of 4389 cases of preclinical cervical squamous carcinoma. J. Obstet. Gynaecol. Br. Commonwealth 77:769, 1970.
9. Creasman, W. T., Weed, J. C., Curry, S. L., Johnston, W. W. and Parker, R. T.: Efficacy of cryosurgical treatment of severe cervical intraepithelial neoplasia. Obstet. Gynecol. 41:501, 1973.
10. Crisp, W. E.: Cryosurgical treatment of neoplasia of the uterine cervix. Obstet. Gynecol. 39:495, 1972.
11. Dunn, J. E. Jr. and Martin, P. L.: Morphogenesis of cervical cancer. Findings from San Diego County Cytologic Registry. Cancer 20:1899, 1967.
12. Einerth, Y.: Cryosurgical treatment of dysplasia and carcinoma in situ of the cervix uteri. Acta Obstet. Gynecol. Scand. 57:361, 1978.
13. Feldman, M. J., Kent, D. R. and Pennington, R. L.: Intraepithelial neoplasia of the uterine cervix in the teenager. Cancer 41:1405, 1978.
14. Fidler, H. K., Boyes, D. A. and Worth, A. J.: Cervical cancer detection in British Columbia. J. Obstet. Gynaecol. Br. Commonwealth 75:392, 1968.
15. Fish, C. R.: Cervical intraepithelial neoplasia: ration-ale of investigation and management. Med. Clin. North Am. 58:743, 1974.
16. Hollyock, V. E. and Chanen, W.: Electrocoagulation diathermy for the treatment of cervical dysplasia and carcinoma in situ. Obstet. Gynecol. 47:196, 1976.
17. International forum. Int. J. Gynecol. Obstet. 7:148, 1969.
18. International forum. Int. J. Gynecol. Obstet. 7:207, 1969.
19. Kaufman, R. H., Strama, T., Norton, P. K. and Conner, J. S.: Cryosurgical treatment of cervical intraepithelial neoplasia. Obstet. Gynecol. 42:881, 1973.
20. Kirkup, W., Singer, A. and Hill, A. S.: Follow-up of women treated for cervical precancer: an argument for a more rational approach. Lancet 2:22, 1979.
21. Kofler, E. and Kremer, H.: Zur Frage der Früherkennung und Behandlung des sog. präinvasiven Carcinom des Collum uteri. Arch. Gynäkol. 194:223, 1960.
22. Kolstad, P. and Klein, V.: Long-term follow-up of 1121 cases of carcinoma in situ. Obstet. Gynecol. 48:125, 1976.
23. Koss, L. G.: Dysplasia, a real concept or a misnomer? Obstet. Gynecol. 51:374, 1978.
24. Krieger, J. S. and McCormack, L. J.: The indications for conservative therapy for intraepithelial carcinoma of the uterine cervix. Am. J. Obstet. Gynecol. 76:312, 1958.
25. Larsson, G., Grundsell, H., Gullberg, B. and Svennerud, S.: Outcome of pregnancy after conization. Acta Obstet. Gynecol. Scand. Accepted for publication.
26. Lee, N. H.: The effect of cone biopsy on subsequent pregnancy outcome. Gynecol. Oncol. 6:1, 1978.
27. Leiman, G., Harrison, N. A. and Rubin, A.: Pregnancy following conization of the cervix: complications related to cone size. Am. J. Obstet. Gynecol. 136:14, 1980.
28. Nelson, J. H., Averette, H. E. and Richart, R. M.: Detection, diagnostic evaluation and treatment of dysplasia and early carcinoma of the cervix. American Cancer Society. Professional education publ. 1975.
29. Ober, K. G. and Bötzelen, H. P.: Technik, Vor- und Nachteile der Konisation der Cervix uteri. Geburthilfe Frauenheilkd 12:1051, 1959.
30. Richart, R. M. and Barron, B. A.: A follow-up study of patients with cervical dysplasia. Am. J. Obstet. Gynecol. 105:386, 1969.
31. Richart, R. M., Townsend, D. E., Crisp, W., et al.: An analysis of long-term follow-up results in patients with cervical intraepithelial neoplasia treated by cryotherapy. Am. J. Obstet. Gynecol. 137:823, 1980.
32. Rubio, C. A., Thomassen, P., Söderberg, G. and Kock, Y.: Big cones and little cones. Histopathology 2:133, 1978.
33. Rybo, G. and Westerberg, H.: The effect of tranexamic acid (AMCA) on postoperative bleeding after conization. Acta Obstet. Gynecol. Scand. 51:347, 1972.
34. Tredway, D. R., Townsend, D. E., Hovland, D. N. and Upton, R. T.: Colposcopy and cryosurgery in cervical intraepithelial neoplasia. Am. J. Obstet. Gynecol. 114:1020, 1972.
35. Walton Report: Can. Med. Assoc. J. 114:1003, 1976.

Diagnosis and Management of in Situ Carcinoma, Microinvasive Carcinoma and Stage I Invasive Carcinoma of the Cervix

William T. Creasman, M.D.

John C. Weed, Jr., M.D.

Duke University School of Medicine

Fifty years ago, more women died from uterine cancer (predominantly cervical) than any other malignancy.[1] Since 1930, the death rate from uterine cancer has dropped precipitously from 27.5 to 8 per 100,000 annually. Presently, carcinomas of the breast, colon, lung and ovary account for more deaths than does cancer of the cervix. The death rate had begun to drop before the publication of Papanicolaou and Traut's monograph on genital cytology in 1943;[2] however, this diagnostic technique has been the major factor leading to the earlier diagnosis, the more effective treatment and thereby the improved survival for cervical neoplasia.

Most investigators agree that cancer of the cervix begins at the cellular level and progresses through the various degrees of cervical intraepithelial neoplasia (CIN) to finally penetrate the basement membrane, becoming a microinvasive carcinoma. In time, clinical cancer of the cervix develops. All CIN lesions, particularly the early ones, do not necessarily progress to invasion; however, some obviously do.[3] Unfortunately, current techniques do not allow us to determine which lesions have truly invasive potential. The more advanced the CIN lesion is at the time of diagnosis, the greater the chance of a developing invasive lesion. Kottmeier noted that in a small number of patients, carcinoma in situ progressed to invasion in 71 per cent of the cases.[4] However, the time needed for progression from CIN is extremely variable. This interval may vary from 3 to 20 years, depending on the surveillance techniques, whether cytology alone or with biopsy confirmation.

Etiology

The cause of CIN and the subsequent development of invasive carcinoma of the cervix remains unknown. Epidemiologic studies have established the rarity of squamous carcinoma of the cervix in the virginal female and the importance of the age of first coitus in the subsequent development of cervical neoplasia.[5] The beginning of coitus during the mid-adolescent years is associated with an increased likelihood of developing cervical neoplasia as compared with first coitus in the late teens or twenties. Presently, it is recognized that cervical neoplasia is acquired venereally, and patients utilizing barrier contraception may have lower rates of neoplasia than those who do not.

Many substances have been investigated in an effort to identify the responsible agent. Bacteria, fungi, protozoa, viruses and chemicals have been studied. The most promising studies are those relating herpes simplex virus type 2 (HSV-2) to cervical neoplasia. The circumstantial evidence of elevated antibody titers to HSV-2 in patients with cervical cancer has prompted considerable investigation. Many variables such as age, race and onset of coitus must be studied. Studies regarding this virus are inconclusive or contradictory.[6] Recently, a viral coded antigen (AG-4), which is a structural component of the HSV-2 virion, has been identified and it has been adapted for use as an immunodiagnostic tool.[7] However, a cause-and-effect relationship has not been established.

Investigators from Australia and Europe have proposed that sperm may be the initiating factor in the development of cervical neoplasia. It would appear that the arginine-rich histone in the sperm has capabilities of transforming DNA into a malignant potential.[8] These same investigators have noted the existence of a so-called "high-risk" male; the risk is related to the amount of arginine-rich histone found in his sperm. This correlates with the incidence of carcinoma of the cervix in different social classes as determined by the male's occupation. This theory seems plausible

624

but considerably more investigation is needed before sperm can be established as the etiologic agent.

Other factors such as circumcision of the male, the number of pregnancies, hormonal factors and the type of contraception used have been investigated. Currently, it would appear that the two firmly established clinical associations concerning the etiology of cervical neoplasia are the following: early intercourse (in mid adolescent years), and multiple sexual partners.

Carcinoma In Situ

Carcinoma in situ is the most advanced of the spectrum of intraepithelial disease that has been termed cervical intraepithelial neoplasia (CIN). This includes the various degrees of dysplasia, as well as what is commonly known as carcinoma in situ. It must be recognized and remembered that this is a true spectrum and not four separate disease entities as may be connoted by the use of the terms mild dysplasia, moderate dysplasia, severe dysplasia and carcinoma in situ. Previous diagnoses of severe or marked dysplasia and carcinoma in situ have been included in the CIN III category. To state that these two diagnoses are definite and absolute is incorrect because the diagnosis rendered by one pathologist may be different from that of another pathologist and even from that of the same pathologist at different time intervals. It is in this context that "carcinoma in situ" will be discussed.

To comprehend the natural history of CIN, one must understand the transformation zone of the cervix. It is that portion of the uterine cervix that lies between the original squamocolumnar junction and the new or functional squamocolumnar junction. The area is covered by new squamous epithelium derived from columnar cells through the process of metaplasia. The columnar epithelium exists on the ectocervix in the majority of females during the premenarchal and adolescent years. At puberty, the metaplastic process probably is accelerated because of hormonal changes and acidification of the vagina. It has been proposed that CIN begins during the dynamic phases of metaplasia. Although metaplasia can occur at other times in a woman's life, the dynamic phase of metaplasia during adolescence is the first time in which an "environmental" factor (sexually transmitted agent) influences the metaplastic process. Sexual activity during the so-called dynamic phases of metaplasia appears to increase the chance of developing CIN.

Genital cytology has proved to be the best screening technique for identifying the patient with CIN. Twelve to fifteen cervical neoplasias per thousand patients screened may be identified in the unscreened population, and the detection rate is much lower in the screened population. A 10 to 20 per cent false-negative rate for the Papanicolaou smear is recognized; nevertheless this technique is still an excellent screening tool. Sampling errors probably account for the highest number of false-negative smears. It is extremely important to sample the endocervix cytologically as well as the ectocervix. The vaginal pool technique is considered inadequate in detecting cervical disease because of its failure to adequately and consistently sample the endocervix. Once an individual has an abnormal Pap smear, further diagnostic procedures are required.

Since cervical intraepithelial neoplasia begins within the transformation zone, usually at the squamocolumnar junction, the lesion may be identified with the colposcope. The colposcope allows a 10 to 20 times magnification of the cervix and the recognition of certain patterns indicative of intraepithelial disease. Colposcopy as a part of the routine pelvic examination adds only a few minutes to this examination. After the spectrum has been inserted into the vagina and the cervix visualized, a repeat Pap smear is obtained and a cleansing solution of 3 per cent acetic acid is placed on the cervix to help dissolve the mucus as well as to enhance the colposcopic patterns. Colposcopically, the original transformation zone can be identified easily by a fine thin line on the ectocervix with a metaplastic epithelium medial. It is not unusual to find gland ostia present throughout the transformation zone. The columnar epithelium is readily identified by its villus-like appearance, appearing red to the naked eye. Standard nomenclature for abnormal colposcopic findings is as noted:

1. Atypical transformation zone
   A. Keratosis
   B. White epithelium
   C. Mosaicism
   D. Punctation
   E. Atypical vascular pattern
2. Suspected invasive cancer
3. Unsatisfactory colposcopic examination

Colposcopic findings of white epithelium, mosaicism and punctation after the application of acetic acid are indicative of an intraepithelial neoplasia. The lesion should be visualized in its entirety and the most prominent area should be selected for biopsy. Using cytology, the colposcopic findings and the biopsy, the physician should be able to rule out invasive disease in essentially 100 per cent of examinations. There are, however, about 15 to 20 per cent of patients so evaluated in whom invasion cannot be ruled out. Therefore, a conization of the cervix is mandatory. The indications for conization after colposcopy and directed biopsies are as follows:

1. If the entire limits of the lesion are not seen,
2. A Pap smear or colposcopic examination suggestive of invasive disease but not verified on biopsy,
3. Either cytological or histologic evidence of "microinvasion,"
4. Significant CIN on the endocervical curettage.

In those patients in whom conization of the cervix is required, colposcopy can help determine the type of cone necessary. If there is very little or no intraepithelial disease on the portio, then only a narrow cone is required, removing the endocervical canal up to the internal os. As a result, a large amount of the cervical stroma is not removed and complications such as hemorrhage can be decreased considerably. When there is extensive disease on the portio and involvement of the canal, a larger amount of ectocervix needs to be removed in order to adequately evaluate the disease. The use of Lugol's solution by itself to determine the extent of the cone is inaccurate because there is a false-positive and false-negative correlation. After colposcopy the cervix can be stained with Lugol's solution and if the lesion and the staining match, Lugol's can be used in the operating room as a guide for the outer margins of the conization. If the two do not match, appropriate adjustments for the cone have to be made. It appears that the largest number of patients who require conization because the disease has not been adequately identified are postmenopausal women in whom the transformation zone does extend into the canal. In these patients, it is most helpful to have them use local estrogen cream in order to facilitate the colposcopic examination. Occasionally a mildly abnormal Pap smear may be overread owing to atrophic changes in the postmenopausal woman, and cytology returns to normal after the application of local estrogen.

Endocervical curettage is mandatory in those patients in whom a lesion is not seen on the portio, the lesion extends into the canal and the upper margin cannot be seen, and in individuals who have cytology indicative of invasive disease that cannot be identified on clinical examination. Endocervical curettage, however, is most useful in all patients examined as an objective procedure to rule out disease within the endocervical canal.

When cytology, colposcopic examination and directed biopsies indicate only intraepithelial neoplasia, several therapies are available for use depending upon the individual needs of the patient. Small lesions, usually less than one quadrant of the cervix, may be treated adequately by excisional biopsies. These may be done easily in the office with either a pair of sharp curved scissors or the biopsy forceps. Similar or larger lesions may be adequately treated with either electrocautery or cryosurgery. Electrocautery has proved efficacious, particularly in Australia and Europe; however, general anesthesia is usually required for the extensive destruction of the transformation zone required. Therefore, this technique loses its appeal as an outpatient modality. On the other hand, cryosurgery appears to be efficacious as an outpatient modality of therapy that causes very little discomfort to the patient. As a result, this is much more acceptable to physicians and patients in the United States.[9]

It appears that the size of the lesion is important in regard to the ability of cryosurgery to destroy it. With use of the so-called double-freeze technique, there is a greater rate of disease destruction, particularly with a large lesion. As a result, we favor the double-freeze technique in all patients with CIN. We prefer an endocervical probe with a base of 19 mm. This will usually encompass the lesion on the ectocervix but occasionally the flat probe must also be used to cover the portio lesion. A thin layer of KY Jelly is applied to the probe and a freeze using either nitrous oxide or carbon dioxide is used so that a 4 to 5 mm iceball around the probe is obtained. The cervix is then allowed to thaw and the freeze is repeated. Normally, only a minute and a half to two minutes is required to obtain an adequate iceball. It is extremely important to have adequate pressure in the refrigerant tank both before and after the freeze. Cryosurgery is equally efficacious using carbon dioxide or nitrous oxide.

Definitive surgical procedures have been advocated both in the United States and abroad. Conization of the cervix as the definitive surgical procedure has been advocated outside the United States for many years.[10] Long-term follow-up after this surgical procedure has noted good results.

For years hysterectomy, usually via the vaginal route, has been the treatment of choice for carcinoma in situ of the cervix in this country.[11] Since lesser procedures can be done with a high degree of destruction of the CIN lesion, one may question the primary use of surgery for treating these lesions. Hysterectomy should be restricted to the patient who desires sterilization or who has some other gynecologic problem such as uterine myoma, pelvic inflammatory disease, adenomyosis or pelvic relaxation. When hysterectomy is used, a simple surgical procedure is all that is required. Only when the intraepithelial disease extends onto the vagina as determined by colposcopy is it necessary to remove part of the upper vagina. This occurs probably less than 5 per cent of the time and to routinely remove the upper 2 cm of vagina as advocated by some investigators is without basis.

When invasive disease has not been ruled out by cytology, colposcopy and directed biopsies, conization of the cervix must be done for diagnosis. If only intraepithelial disease is noted, the conization can also be therapeutic. If in fact invasive disease is present, then the type of therapy required can be planned depending upon the extent of disease; conization may be adequate or simple hysterectomy may be all that is necessary. If on the other hand occult invasive disease is noted, either radical surgical or radiation therapy is required.

It would appear that cytology, colposcopy and colposcopically directed biopsies have several advantages over conization of the cervix in all patients with abnormal cytology and without clinical disease on the cervix. These diagnostic procedures all can be performed on an outpatient basis, saving patients time, expense and morbidity. Conization should be reserved for those individuals in whom invasion cannot be ruled out as just outlined. In the pregnant and the young patient, colposcopy and directed biopsies are certainly the diagnostic methods of choice. Conization of

the cervix does carry a higher morbidity in the pregnant patient. In the young patient, because of the size of the cervix, particularly the nulliparous cervix, a cone may remove a considerable amount of the cervix and thereby render the young patient more susceptible to infertility and possible cervical incompetence.

Microinvasion

Early invasion of the cervix is now recognized as a definite entity. The lesion can only be diagnosed microscopically in a conization specimen. Abnormal cytology can identify a patient with an early invasive lesion; however, the sophistication required to diagnose microinvasion on a cytologic basis is not as uniform as with intraepithelial neoplasia or invasive disease.

The suggestion of any early invasive lesion of the cervix by cytology or directed biopsy mandates a conization for adequate evaluation. Only with adequate histologic preparation can the lesion be delineated accurately and proper treatment applied. Unfortunately, opinions differ as to the exact diagnosis and the most appropriate therapy of early squamous cell carcinoma of the uterine cervix.

Ruch[12] called this lesion "a confusing dilemma." He was able to find 15 different names for the disease entity, as well as six histologic definitions from a review of the literature over only a four-year time interval. The International Federation of Obstetricians and Gynecologists (IFGO) has not defined this lesion histologically. In fact, IFGO has probably added somewhat to the confusion over this lesion, because the definition and staging of this entity has been changed four times since 1960.

In an attempt to better define this lesion, the Society of Gynecologic Oncologists in 1973 accepted the following statements on microinvasive carcinoma of the cervix uteri: (1) A case of intraepithelial carcinoma with questionable invasion should be regarded as intraepithelial carcinoma. (2) A cervix with microinvasion should be defined as one in which the neoplastic epithelium invades the stroma in one or more places to a depth of 3 mm or less below the basement membrane and in which lymphatic or vascular involvement is not demonstrated. Although this definition was not unanimously accepted, it does offer a definition for discussion purposes. Notwithstanding the considerable concern over the depth of invasion, vascular or lymphatic involvement and confluency, the virulence of the lesion probably is related to the volume of disease and volume, to a certain degree, is reflected by these histologic parameters. As more data have become available, it appears that more of these lesions can be treated in a conservative fashion. Presently, the consensus is that lesions with less than 1 mm of stromal invasion below the basement membrane may be treated with less than radical surgery—that is, with conization or simple hysterectomy.

Lohe et al.,[13] in a recent assessment of microinvasive carcinoma from their own material and a review of the world's literature, have added considerable information to our knowledge of this disease entity. They further broke down early invasive disease into two categories as follows: (1) early stromal invasion, projections of tumor penetrating the subepithelial connecting tissue, and (2) microinvasion, carcinoma involving the stroma to a maximum length and width of 10 mm and a maximum depth of 5 mm. The authors meticulously evaluated the histologic preparations from their patients, of whom 285 had early stromal invasion and 134 had microinvasion. In reviewing the 285 patients with early stromal invasion plus an additional 895 from the literature, they noted that radical surgery was performed in only about one fifth of the patients. Of these 285 patients, none died of their early stromal invasion, although 4 patients were considered to have recurrence. Of the 895 patients, 13 had tumor recurrence (1.5 per cent), but only 4 of these patients (0.4 per cent) died from their disease. In these authors' 134 patients with microinvasive carcinoma plus 435 identified from the literature, radical therapy was performed in about one half. Of the 435 patients from the literature, 24 (5.5 per cent) developed recurrence, of which 14 (3 per cent) died. Of these authors' 134 patients with microinvasive carcinoma, three had tumor recurrence and all died of their disease. It should be noted, however, that 10 of the 14 patients from the literature who died of their microcarcinoma probably had disease greater than 5 mm of stromal invasion. Lohe et al. concluded that the risk of dying of early stromal invasion, regardless of treatment modality, was rather small, as none of their 285 patients and only four of 895 from the literature (0.4 per cent) succumbed to their disease. The risk of dying of microinvasive carcinoma is higher, in that

3 per cent of those from the literature and 2 per cent of the authors' patients died from their disease. It is interesting to note that 75 percent of the authors' patients with early stromal invasion and over half of their microcarcinoma patients had restricted cancer therapy, and yet a five-year survival of 94.9 and 93.9 per cent, respectively, were obtained. Lohe and colleagues further make the point that the large number of patients cured of early cervical carcinoma after restricted treatment indicates that total extirpation of the tumor by whatever means seems to be sufficient therapy. They note, "The decisive criterion for successful treatment is the total elimination of the tumor from the cervix."

The incidence of lymph node metastasis in stage IA carcinoma of the cervix is low. Lohe, in his literature review and from his own material, concluded that less than 1 per cent of patients with early invasion of the cervix had lymph node metastasis.[14] Therefore, it would appear that with rare exception radical surgery is not indicated if the histologic lesion fulfills Lohe's requirement.

The incidence and significance of vascular and lymphatic involvement with tumor cells within the surgical specimen is unclear at the present time. Leman and associates in a thorough review of radical hysterectomy and lymphadenectomy specimens done for stage IA carcinoma of the cervix noted that over 24 per cent of the patients had capillary-like space invasion.[15] None of the patients had lymph node metastasis. Other investigators have found a lower incidence of lymphatic or vascular channel involvement, and yet there is the suggestion of correlation between intraluminal invasion and lymph node metastasis.[16] Lohe noted that in 134 patients with microcarcinomas, three patients died from their cancer and all three had invasion of lymphatic spaces.[14] Further evaluation of this histologic parameter must be made.

In view of these data, as well as our own, currently our institutional policy for therapy of stage IA (microinvasive carcinoma of the cervix) is as follows: (1) When the lesion is less than 3 mm in depth with only limited foci of stromal invasion, vaginal or abdominal hysterectomy with conservation of the ovaries if indicated is done. The removal of a wide vaginal cuff in some and not in others has not affected the prognosis. A conization may be adequate—obviously a highly individualized decision. (2) When the penetration of invasive foci of cells is 3 to 5 mm in depth, particularly if confluent, radical hysterectomy and pelvic lymphadenectomy are performed. (3) When lymphatic or vascular channels are invaded, regardless of the depth of invasion, radical therapy is utilized.[17] Further evaluation of the histologic definition of this disease entity as well as applicable therapy is on-going at our institution.

Stage I Carcinoma of the Cervix

Stage I carcinoma of the cervix is defined as invasive cancer confined to the cervix. Stage IA is microinvasive and has already been discussed. Stage IB disease is clinically invasive carcinoma that is confined to the cervix. Stage IB "OCC" is histologically invasive carcinoma of the cervix that could not be detected on routine clinical examination but that was diagnosed on a large biopsy, the cone or the amputated portio. Since most investigators feel that stage IB occult disease should be treated as a clinical stage IB lesion, these two substages will be considered together.

Stage I disease is being identified in a higher proportion of patients because of better detection techniques and the wider use of the Papanicolaou smear. Since the disease is now clinical, the chances of spread beyond the cervix is also increased. In stage IB carcinoma of the cervix, regional lymph node metastasis occurs in approximately 20 per cent of the patients. As a result, therapy for this disease entity must take this spread pattern into account. Unlike advanced disease in which radiation therapy is the only treatment applicable to all lesions, a patient with stage IB disease has a choice of treatment modalities. Radical hysterectomy and pelvic lymphadenectomy is the treatment of choice by the gynecologic oncologist in many women with this stage disease, while obviously radiation therapy with a combination of external and radium implantation is the treatment of choice of the radiotherapist. Surgical series, by definition, are somewhat selective. In many clinics, particularly in this country, the old, obese or medically ill patient is not considered for surgery. On the other hand, the radiotherapists will treat essentially all patients. There are, however, some clinics abroad as well as an occasional one in this country in which these lesions are treated with radical surgery in essentially all patients. Unfortunately, there is only one small study available to use for review in which, in a perspective randomized fashion, patients with stage I carcinoma of the cervix were treated with radiation therapy or surgery.[18] Survival rates in the two groups of patients were similar.

It would appear that in using either radical surgery or irradiation therapy survival in patients with stage I carcinoma of the cervix should be in the 85 to 90 per cent category because these figures have been reported by several investigators.[19, 20] The proponents of radical surgery state that with surgery the tumor can be removed in toto, along with a margin of normal tissue, and therefore cannot recur centrally. The true spread of the disease can be determined accurately with the exploratory laparotomy in identifying disease in the lymph nodes, both in the pelvic and para-aortic area. True disease spread in the parametrium can also be further evaluated. In the young patient, the ovaries can be conserved. The vaginal membrane also remains unaltered and sexual function is continued without difficulty. The complication rate from radical surgery in the past has mainly been related to a high rate (10 to 15 per cent) of genitourinary fistulas. With better surgical and drainage techniques, these complications should be no more than 1 to 2 per cent. With better medical care, anesthesia, and blood, fluid and electrolyte replacement, more patients with early cancer of the cervix are now candidates for radical surgery.

On the other hand, radiation therapists state that some of the prior objections to radiation therapy are no longer valid. Tumor radioresistance and therefore the lack of local tumor control is probably no longer applicable with high-voltage irradiation. Less than 3 per cent local recurrence rate in early carcinoma of the cervix has been seen with modern radiation therapy. Radiation therapy certainly can destroy metastasis in lymph nodes, but whether it is more effective in this regard compared with radical surgery is unknown. Possibly in early disease in those patients with positive lymph node metastasis the combination of surgery and radiation therapy is applicable. Morbidity from radiation injury varies with the skill of the therapist and the techniques and facilities used for radium application as is applicable to the morbidity resulting from surgery. However, significant morbidity should be no higher than 1 to 2 per cent in these patients. Radiation therapy does destroy ovarian function and alter the upper vaginal membrane. Postradiation therapy care to the vagina and hormone replacement allow these women to remain sexually active.

Since good radiation therapy and good surgery are available to the patient with stage IB carcinoma of the cervix, the cure rate and the morbidity from the two therapeutic modalities should essentially be equal. Radical surgery does offer the advantage of ovarian conservation and vaginal sparing to the young patient.

REFERENCES

1. Cancer Statistics, 1978. Cs 28:17–32, 1978.
2. Papanicolaou, G. N. and Traut, H. E.: Diagnosis of Uterine Cancer by the Vaginal Smear. New York, Commonwealth Fund, 1943.
3. Peterson, O.: Spontaneous course of cervical precancerous conditions. Am. J. Obstet. Gynecol. 72:1063, 1956.
4. Kottmeier, H. L.: Evolution et traitement des epitheliomas. Rev. Franc. Gynecol. 56:821, 1961.
5. Rotkin, I. D.: A comparison review of key epidemiological studies in cervical cancer for transmissible agents. Cancer Res. 33:1351, 1973.
6. Rawls, W. E., Adam, E. and Melnick, J. L.: An analysis of seroepidemiological studies of Herpesvirus type 2 and carcinoma of the cervix. Cancer Res. 33:1477, 1973.
7. Aurelian, L., Strand, B. C. and Smith, M. F.: Immunodiagnostic potential of a virus-coded, tumor-associated antigen (AG4) in cervical cancer. Cancer 39:1834, 1977.
8. Singer, A., Reid, B. L. and Coppleson, M.: A hypothesis: The role of a high-risk male in the etiology of cervical carcinoma. Am. J. Obstet. Gynecol. 126:110, 1976.
9. Creasman, W. T., Weed, J. C., Jr., Curry, S. L., Johnston, W. and Parker, R. T.: Efficacy of cryosurgical treatment of severe cervical intraepithelial neoplasia. Obstet. Gynecol. 41:501, 1973.
10. Coppleson, M.: Management of preclinical carcinoma of the cervix. In Jordan, J. A. and Singer, Q. (eds.): The Cervix. Philadelphia, W. B. Saunders Co., 1976.
11. Creasman, W. T. and Rutledge, F. N.: Carcinoma in situ of the cervix. Obstet. Gynecol. 39:373, 1972.
12. Ruch, R. M.: Microinvasive carcinoma of the cervix. A confusion dilemma. South. Med. J. 63:1123, 1970.
13. Lohe, K. J., Burghardt, E., Hillemanns, H. G., Kaufmann, C., Ober, K. G. and Zander, J.: Early squamous cell carcinoma of the uterine cervix. Gynecol. Oncol. 6:31,1978.
14. Lohe, K. J.: Early squamous cell carcinoma of the uterine cervix. III. Frequency of lymph node metastases. Gynecol. Oncol. 6:51, 1978.
15. Leman, M. H., Benson, W. L., Kurman, R. J. and Park, R. C.: Microinvasive carcinoma of the cervix. Obstet. Gynecol. 48:571, 1976.
16. Bohm, J. W., Krupp, P. J., Lee, F. Y. L. and Batson, H. W. K.: Lymph node metastasis in microinvasive epidermoid cancer of the cervix. Obstet. Gynecol. 48:65, 1976.
17. Creasman, W. T. and Parker, R. T.: Microinvasive carcinoma of the cervix. Clin. Obstet. Gynecol. 16:261, 1973.
18. Newton, M.: Radical hysterectomy or radiotherapy for stage I cervical cancer. Am. J. Obstet. Gynecol. 123:535, 1975.
19. Parker, R. T., Wilbanks, G. D., Yowell, R. K. and Carter, F. B.: Radical hysterectomy and pelvic lymphadenectomy with and without preoperative radiotherapy for cervical cancer. Am. J. Obstet. Gynecol. 99:933, 1967.
20. Fletcher, G. H. and Rutledge, F. N.: Overall results in radiotherapy for carcinoma of the cervix: modern treatment. Clin. Obstet. Gynecol. 5:958, 1968.

Editorial Comment

The Duke group, namely Drs. Creasman and Weed, have extended their part of the controversy to include microinvasive carcinoma and stage I invasive carcinoma of the cervix. The controversy rests with what to do with the patient who has severe dysplasia or carcinoma in situ or both. The controversy in the treatment of microinvasive carcinoma and stage I invasive carcinoma of the cervix is a debate between gynecologists and radiation therapists. They each wish to use their own techniques in an appropriate fashion.

As one might expect, the reproductive oncologists would prefer to do surgery on patients with microinvasive carcinoma and stage I invasive carcinoma of the cervix, whereas the gynecologic radiation therapists would prefer radiation therapy for stage I invasive carcinoma. The Duke group points out that the cure rate of stage IB carcinoma of the cervix, whether treated with radiation or adequate surgery, should basically be the same. Radical surgery, however, provides an advantage of ovarian conservation and vaginal sparing to the young patient. The surgeon, of course, always says that if there is central recurrence, the patient can either be reconsidered for additional surgery or a course of radiation therapy can be implemented.

Pelvic lymphadenectomy that is done in conjunction with radical hysterectomy is most likely the best indication of extent of disease and is predictive for long-term outcome. It is known that regional lymph node metastasis occurs in up to 20 per cent of patients with stage IB; however, that would be a pessimistic approach and if you are an optimist you would say that 80 per cent of the time there are no metastatic lymph nodes. Since the cure rate of the stage IB is 85 to 90 per cent, this correlates closely with the presence or absence of lymph node involvement, which is basically a predictor of outcome.

There is a controversy about microinvasion, and this is worldwide since there is no specific and identified histologic definition of this entity. The International Federation of Obstetricians and Gynecologists should come to grips with this problem. In the meantime, the Society of Gynecologic Oncologists has made specific statements about this particular problem: (1) Intraepithelial carcinoma with questionable invasion should be considered as an intraepithelial carcinoma. (2) Microinvasion as a specific entity should be defined as a lesion in which the neoplastic epithelium invades the stroma in one or more places to a depth of 3 mm or less below the basement membrane, and in which lymphatic or vascular involvement or both is *not* demonstrated.

This all sounds very good, but we know how imprecise the microscope and sectioning process becomes in specifically defining the depth of invasion. It is indeed difficult to have complete serial sections of the conization specimen to determine this. I believe that the society's first statement is probably correct in that if you do have a patient with microinvasion and if you are precise and certain about it, then it's a different entity, but if you are *in doubt,* it should be considered as a case of intraepithelial carcinoma. The next decision, which is controversial, is whether you should use x-ray therapy or surgery, and I believe that most departments of obstetrics and gynecology would opt for radical hysterectomy. The very least would be a simple hysterectomy. The current thinking is that in lesions that have less than 1 mm of stromal invasion below the basement membrane (if you can be positive about this), less than radical surgery can be utilized as cure, i.e., a therapeutic conization or simple hysterectomy. Since prognosis for the disease has to do with the virulence and the volume of the tumor, examination of the specimen is extraordinarily important.

Wouldn't it be helpful if we knew which cervical intraepithelial neoplasia (CIN) lesions would finally penetrate the basement membrane and become full carcinoma or which would regress to less troublesome types of lesions? Even at this time, clinicians cannot predict the malignant potential of premalignant lesions with sophisticated computer pattern recognition cellular studies. Most investigators would agree that severe dysplasia and carcinoma in situ can, in selected patients and over a variable number of years, progress to invasive cancer. The problem is which will and which won't. One major contribution the cytologists and gynecologists have made in medicine is that with a periodic Pap smear as screening tool in CIN disease, it has been possible to practically eliminate advanced carcinoma of the cervix. This is one cancer that over the past 25 years has shown a decline in late disease; hence, screening is important and should be done at periodic intervals. We don't wish to get into the debate of whether the American Cancer Society is correct in stating that if your patient is a young woman who has two normal Pap smears, it is not necessary to do this on an annual basis. We joined the protestors who wrote letters to the American Cancer Society stating that we believed this to be an inappropriate statement because more than a Pap smear is done on an annual examination. The female, because of the Pap smear, has been afforded better health care than the male because many other types of diseases are also identified during the time of the Pap smear, and the annual examination and Pap smear are also part of good psychotherapy since the cost is not extravagant. An annual examination we still believe is essential and part of good health care.

Approximately 15 cervical neoplasias per 1000 patients initially screened will be identified. It should be remembered that at least a 25 per cent false-negative rate for the Pap smear is recognized and accepted; hence, more than one smear is necessary to reassure the patient that disease is not present. The appropriate way· to obtain sampling from the cervix is important because the transitional zone is the important area.

The approach to a scientific understanding of CIN has been aided by the use of the colposcope; with it the transitional zone can be identified and abnormal colposcopic findings can be noted, such as atypical transformation zone with keratosis, white epithelium, mosaicism, punctation and atypical vascular pattern, as well as a suspected invasive cancer. We believe that colposcopy should be part of all residents' training and that they should be competent colposcopists when they finish the program. It does not mean that all women should have colposcopy done, but that the cytology as a screening tool could be followed by colposcopy and microbiopsy, as well as the crucial endocervical curettage. We still like the use of Lugol's solution to identify the areas of the cervix for nonstaining; however, this is used only after saline and acetic acid viewing of the area is completed by colposcopy. The Duke group and the Swedish group believe that cytology, colposcopy and colposcopy-directed biopsy have some advantages over conization of the cervix in all patients with abnormal cytology because they can be performed principally on an outpatient basis. These investigators prefer cryosurgery if the lesion is amenable to such therapy. This is especially important in the pregnant patient, in whom at the present time conization seldom should be done because it is extraordinarily bloody and may precipitate premature labor. Most would agree that it is unwise to do conizations during pregnancy if it is possible to adequately evaluate the patient with cytology and colposcopy, and then re-evaluate the patient at a later date after pregnancy is completed before specific decisions are made. The important issue here is to rule out invasive cancer that can occur in pregnancy.

The group from Sweden (article by Bjerre and Sjöberg) has the largest series of conizations of the cervix as treatment for dysplasia and carcinoma in situ of the cervix in the world today. Their study began 20 years ago. It is important to understand that the Swedish system of health care has an excellent computerized follow-up system because all citizens have a socialized health care number and excellent follow-up care is available. This means that statistics for the 7 million people in Sweden are most precise and a good index of health in a rather homogenous population group. It is also important to understand that hysterectomy in Europe is not as prevalent as in the United States; hence, the preservation of the uterus appears to be more important to European and Scandinavian women than to American women. Perhaps we should say it's more important for the United States physician to do hysterectomies than it is for the Scandinavian and European gynecologist. The opinion of the Scandinavian group is that conization is adequate for carcinoma in situ of the cervix and that hysterectomy is not warranted in most cases.

They are also fully aware that there are different types of conizations, including the superficial, which they call a ring biopsy. This is warranted only if colposcopic examination strongly suggests that such a conization or removal of the epithelial changes can be easily done. If there is more extensive involvement of the cervix, a more generous conization is done.

The Swedish method of conization is somewhat different from that done in this country. They use a hemostatic agent—synthetic vasopressin—that is injected into the cervix to help secure hemostasis. (We have used for many years either a dilute solution of epinephrine or Neo-Synephrine to achieve the same goal.) Lugol's solution is applied to the cervix to determine how wide the base of the cone should be, and a Hegar dilator is used to determine the position of the internal os and the height of the cone. This is especially important in younger women and it is essential that the tip of the cone not reach the internal os. This is identical to the procedure we have followed over the years and yields minimal complications. Conization is performed with a special curved knife and the wound is left unsutured and undressed. This is different from the method used in many areas of this country, in which sutures are placed to close the wound. The Swedes do use sutures on the descending branches of the cervical artery prior to doing the conization. They have given one gram of tranexamic acid intravenously during the surgery and then give this orally, 1 gram 4 times a day for 10 days, following surgery. They believe that this reduces the tendency for bleeding following a conization, but we would question whether this has ever been proved in a randomized study.

The most critical issue now is evaluating the conization specimen to determine whether the margins are free from any cellular changes. If there is any doubt about this, the specimen is called either "doubtful" or "margins not free." The method that they have used in their last 1060 patients in whom conization was done has required only four to receive blood transfusions or later suturing of the cervix.

They have had minimal complications in 2500 women who they have "coned" during this period of time. They have looked at the conception rate following this to see whether there were problems with prematurity, and of 1112 children born before the conization, 11 per cent weighed less than 2500 grams and following conization, 10 per cent; hence, there was no association with prematurity and conization. However, there was a higher incidence of spontaneous abortion after conization, 17 per cent, as compared with the figure of 12 per cent before conization. Their figures of 1500 patients who had carcinoma in situ showed that 175 of these needed further treatment because the conization specimen showed further pathology. Their mean follow-up time is 8.3 years, which should be ample time for any other cellular changes to develop.

One of the big items of controversy has been the multifocal origin of carcinoma in situ, and they have been able to demonstrate that when the first conization showed normal epithelial margins, 95 per cent of the patients were cured; hence, 5 per cent of the patients had multifocal origin of the disease. This is an important finding in that many United States physicians think that if the patient has carcinoma in situ and no further pregnancies are desired, the uterus should be taken out regardless of the histologic findings. It would appear that if the Swedish cervix and vagina are similar to the American cervix and vagina, this in all likelihood is a practice of the past that we should reconsider.

It would appear that there is a special way to handle and treat patients who have severe dysplasia or carcinoma in situ, and first and most important is individualization of therapy. Once the patient has been identified as having a problem, the next step is colposcopy with microbiopsy and endocervical curettage. Depending upon the finding at this particular time, the decision is made concerning the choice of cryosurgery, localized cautery, or, if the lesion is more extensive, conization of the cervix. If the woman is young and if she desires more children, conization indeed may be curative and is all that is necessary for her. This is all predicated upon the basis that the patient will come back for periodic follow-up and colposcopy as needed. If follow-up is not possible, then perhaps more heroic measures such as hysterectomy should be undertaken. Since the development of this modern approach to diagnosis and therapy, there have been few indications for doing conization of the cervix in pregnancy. Colposcopy with microbiopsy is essentially all that is necessary and then re-evaluation of the patient following termination of pregnancy. Interestingly, often vaginal delivery will denude the epithelium enough when carcinoma in situ or severe dysplasia was present, and Pap smear and colposcopy after pregnancy will be normal. This does not imply that the procedures are curative and that the changes will not return, but that statements made to patients about the need for urgent hysterectomy following delivery probably no longer should be made.

Index

Page numbers in *italic* type refer to illustrations and tables.